Recommended Dietary Allowances (RDA) and Adequate Intakes (AI) for Vitamins

Age (yr)	Thiamin RDA (mg/day)	Riboflavin RDA (mg/day)	Niacin RDA (mg/day)[a]	Biotin AI (µg/day)	Pantothenic acid AI (mg/day)	Vitamin B6 RDA (mg/day)	Folate RDA (µg/day)[b]	Vitamin B12 RDA (µg/day)	Choline AI (mg/day)	Vitamin C RDA (mg/day)	Vitamin A RDA (µg/day)[c]	Vitamin D RDA (µg/day)[d]	Vitamin E RDA (mg/day)[e]	Vitamin K AI (µg/day)
Infants														
0–0.5	0.2	0.3	2	5	1.7	0.1	65	0.4	125	40	400	10	4	2.0
0.5–1	0.3	0.4	4	6	1.8	0.3	80	0.5	150	50	500	10	5	2.5
Children														
1–3	0.5	0.5	6	8	2	0.5	150	0.9	200	15	300	15	6	30
4–8	0.6	0.6	8	12	3	0.6	200	1.2	250	25	400	15	7	55
Males														
9–13	0.9	0.9	12	20	4	1.0	300	1.8	375	45	600	15	11	60
14–18	1.2	1.3	16	25	5	1.3	400	2.4	550	75	900	15	15	75
19–30	1.2	1.3	16	30	5	1.3	400	2.4	550	90	900	15	15	120
31–50	1.2	1.3	16	30	5	1.3	400	2.4	550	90	900	15	15	120
51–70	1.2	1.3	16	30	5	1.7	400	2.4	550	90	900	15	15	120
>70	1.2	1.3	16	30	5	1.7	400	2.4	550	90	900	20	15	120
Females														
9–13	0.9	0.9	12	20	4	1.0	300	1.8	375	45	600	15	11	60
14–18	1.0	1.0	14	25	5	1.2	400	2.4	400	65	700	15	15	75
19–30	1.1	1.1	14	30	5	1.3	400	2.4	425	75	700	15	15	90
31–50	1.1	1.1	14	30	5	1.3	400	2.4	425	75	700	15	15	90
51–70	1.1	1.1	14	30	5	1.5	400	2.4	425	75	700	15	15	90
>70	1.1	1.1	14	30	5	1.5	400	2.4	425	75	700	20	15	90
Pregnancy														
≤18	1.4	1.4	18	30	6	1.9	600	2.6	450	80	750	15	15	75
19–30	1.4	1.4	18	30	6	1.9	600	2.6	450	85	770	15	15	90
31–50	1.4	1.4	18	30	6	1.9	600	2.6	450	85	770	15	15	90
Lactation														
≤18	1.4	1.6	17	35	7	2.0	500	2.8	550	115	1200	15	19	75
19–30	1.4	1.6	17	35	7	2.0	500	2.8	550	120	1300	15	19	90
31–50	1.4	1.6	17	35	7	2.0	500	2.8	550	120	1300	15	19	90

NOTE: For all nutrients, values for infants are AI. The glossary on the inside back cover defines units of nutrient measure.

[a]Niacin recommendations are expressed as niacin equivalents (NE), except for recommendations for infants younger than 6 months, which are expressed as preformed niacin.

[b]Folate recommendations are expressed as dietary folate equivalents (DFE).

[c]Vitamin A recommendations are expressed as retinol activity equivalents (RAE).

[d]Vitamin D recommendations are expressed as cholecalciferol and assume an absence of adequate exposure to sunlight.

[e]Vitamin E recommendations are expressed as α-tocopherol.

Recommended Dietary Allowances (RDA) and Adequate Intakes (AI) for Minerals

Age (yr)	Sodium AI (mg/day)	Chloride AI (mg/day)	Potassium AI (mg/day)	Calcium RDA (mg/day)	Phosphorus RDA (mg/day)	Magnesium RDA (mg/day)	Iron RDA (mg/day)	Zinc RDA (mg/day)	Iodine RDA (µg/day)	Selenium RDA (µg/day)	Copper RDA (µg/day)	Manganese AI (mg/day)	Fluoride AI (mg/day)	Chromium AI (µg/day)	Molybdenum RDA (µg/day)
Infants															
0–0.5	120	180	400	200	100	30	0.27	2	110	15	200	0.003	0.01	0.2	2
0.5–1	370	570	700	260	275	75	11	3	130	20	220	0.6	0.5	5.5	3
Children															
1–3	1000	1500	3000	700	460	80	7	3	90	20	340	1.2	0.7	11	17
4–8	1200	1900	3800	1000	500	130	10	5	90	30	440	1.5	1.0	15	22
Males															
9–13	1500	2300	4500	1300	1250	240	8	8	120	40	700	1.9	2	25	34
14–18	1500	2300	4700	1300	1250	410	11	11	150	55	890	2.2	3	35	43
19–30	1500	2300	4700	1000	700	400	8	11	150	55	900	2.3	4	35	45
31–50	1500	2300	4700	1000	700	420	8	11	150	55	900	2.3	4	35	45
51–70	1300	2000	4700	1000	700	420	8	11	150	55	900	2.3	4	30	45
>70	1200	1800	4700	1200	700	420	8	11	150	55	900	2.3	4	30	45
Females															
9–13	1500	2300	4500	1300	1250	240	8	8	120	40	700	1.6	2	21	34
14–18	1500	2300	4700	1300	1250	360	15	9	150	55	890	1.6	3	24	43
19–30	1500	2300	4700	1000	700	310	18	8	150	55	900	1.8	3	25	45
31–50	1500	2300	4700	1000	700	320	18	8	150	55	900	1.8	3	25	45
51–70	1300	2000	4700	1200	700	320	8	8	150	55	900	1.8	3	20	45
>70	1200	1800	4700	1200	700	320	8	8	150	55	900	1.8	3	20	45
Pregnancy															
≤18	1500	2300	4700	1300	1250	400	27	12	220	60	1000	2.0	3	29	50
19–30	1500	2300	4700	1000	700	350	27	11	220	60	1000	2.0	3	30	50
31–50	1500	2300	4700	1000	700	360	27	11	220	60	1000	2.0	3	30	50
Lactation															
≤18	1500	2300	5100	1300	1250	360	10	13	290	70	1300	2.6	3	44	50
19–30	1500	2300	5100	1000	700	310	9	12	290	70	1300	2.6	3	45	50
31–50	1500	2300	5100	1000	700	320	9	12	290	70	1300	2.6	3	45	50

NOTE: For all nutrients, values for infants are AI. The glossary on the inside back cover defines units of nutrient measure.

Tolerable Upper Intake Levels (UL) for Vitamins

Age (yr)	Niacin (mg/day)[a]	Vitamin B₆ (mg/day)	Folate (µg/day)[a]	Choline (mg/day)	Vitamin C (mg/day)	Vitamin A (µg/day)[b]	Vitamin D (µg/day)	Vitamin E (mg/day)[c]	
Infants									
0–0.5	—	—	—	—	—	600	25	—	
0.5–1	—	—	—	—	—	600	38	—	
Children									
1–3	10	30	300	1000	400	600	63	200	
4–8	15	40	400	1000	650	900	75	300	
9–13	20	60	600	2000	1200	1700	100	600	
Adolescents									
14–18	30	80	800	3000	1800	2800	100	800	
Adults									
19–70	35	100	1000	3500	2000	3000	100	1000	
>70	35	100	1000	3500	2000	3000	100	1000	
Pregnancy									
≤18	30	80	800	3000	1800	2800	100	800	
19–50	35	100	1000	3500	2000	3000	100	1000	
Lactation									
≤18	30	80	800	3000	1800	2800	100	800	
19–50	35	100	1000	3500	2000	3000	100	1000	

[a]The UL for niacin and folate apply to synthetic forms obtained from supplements, fortified foods, or a combination of the two.
[b]The UL for vitamin A applies to the preformed vitamin only.
[c]The UL for vitamin E applies to any form of supplemental α-tocopherol, fortified foods, or a combination of the two.

From Whitney/Rolfes, *Understanding Nutrition*, 13E. © 2013 Cengage Learning.

Tolerable Upper Intake Levels (UL) for Minerals

Age (yr)	Sodium (mg/day)	Chloride (mg/day)	Calcium (mg/day)	Phosphorus (mg/day)	Magnesium (mg/day)[d]	Iron (mg/day)	Zinc (mg/day)	Iodine (µg/day)	Selenium (µg/day)	Copper (µg/day)	Manganese (mg/day)	Fluoride (mg/day)	Molybdenum (µg/day)	Boron (mg/day)	Nickel (mg/day)	Vanadium (mg/day)
Infants																
0–0.5	—	—	1000	—	—	40	4	—	45	—	—	0.7	—	—	—	—
0.5–1	—	—	1500	—	—	40	5	—	60	—	—	0.9	—	—	—	—
Children																
1–3	1500	2300	2500	3000	65	40	7	200	90	1000	2	1.3	300	3	0.2	—
4–8	1900	2900	2500	3000	110	40	12	300	150	3000	3	2.2	600	6	0.3	—
9–13	2200	3400	3000	4000	350	40	23	600	280	5000	6	10	1100	11	0.6	—
Adolescents																
14–18	2300	3600	3000	4000	350	45	34	900	400	8000	9	10	1700	17	1.0	—
Adults																
19–50	2300	3600	2500	4000	350	45	40	1100	400	10,000	11	10	2000	20	1.0	1.8
51–70	2300	3600	2000	4000	350	45	40	1100	400	10,000	11	10	2000	20	1.0	1.8
>70	2300	3600	2000	3000	350	45	40	1100	400	10,000	11	10	2000	20	1.0	1.8
Pregnancy																
≤18	2300	3600	3000	3500	350	45	34	900	400	8000	9	10	1700	17	1.0	—
19–50	2300	3600	2500	3500	350	45	40	1100	400	10,000	11	10	2000	20	1.0	—
Lactation																
≤18	2300	3600	3000	4000	350	45	34	900	400	8000	9	10	1700	17	1.0	—
19–50	2300	3600	2500	4000	350	45	40	1100	400	10,000	11	10	2000	20	1.0	—

[d]The UL for magnesium applies to synthetic forms obtained from supplements or drugs only.

NOTE: An upper Limit was not established for vitamins and minerals not listed and for those age groups listed with a dash (—) because of a lack of data, not because these nutrients are safe to consume at any level of intake. All nutrients can have adverse effects when intakes are excessive.

SOURCE: Adapted with permission from the *Dietary Reference Intakes for Calcium and Vitamin D*, © 2011 by the National Academies of Sciences, Courtesy of the National Academies Press, Washington, D.C.

NUTRITION FOR HEALTH AND HEALTH CARE

seventh edition

Linda Kelly DeBruyne

Kathryn Pinna

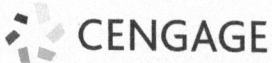

CENGAGE

Australia • Brazil • Mexico • Singapore • United Kingdom • United States

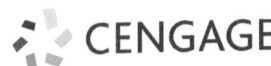

Nutrition for Health and Health Care,
Seventh Edition
Linda Kelly DeBruyne, Kathryn Pinna

Product Team Manager: Kelsey V. Churchman

Associate Product Manager: Courtney Heilman

Project Manager: Julie Dierig

Product Assistant: Lauren R. Monz

Content Manager: Carol Samet

Production Service: Charu Verma, MPS Limited

Intellectual Property Project Manager:
Erika A. Mugavin

Intellectual Property Analyst:
Christine M. Myaskovsky

Photo Researcher: Nishabhanu Beegan,
Neha Patil, Lumina Datamatics

Text Researcher: Sriranjani Ravi,
Lumina Datamatics

Copy Editor: Heather Dubnick

Art Director: Helen Bruno

Text Designer: Pam Verros

Cover Designer: Lisa Delgado

Cover Image: CatLane/E+/Getty Images

Compositor: MPS Limited

For product information and technology assistance, contact us at
**Cengage Customer & Sales Support, 1-800-354-9706
or support.cengage.com.**

For permission to use material from this text or
product, submit all requests online at
www.cengage.com/permissions.

Library of Congress Control Number: 2018946256
ISBN: 978-0-357-02246-7

Cengage
20 Channel Center Street
Boston, MA 02210
USA

Cengage is a leading provider of customized learning solutions with employees residing in nearly 40 different countries and sales in more than 125 countries around the world. Find your local representative at **www.cengage.com.**

Cengage products are represented in Canada by Nelson Education, Ltd.

To learn more about Cengage platforms and services, register or access your online learning solution, or purchase materials for your course, visit **www.cengage.com.**

Printed in the United States of America
Print Number: 01   Print Year: 2018

To my grandchildren, Ryder, Cruz, and Skyler, with love from the luckiest Nani in the world.

Linda Kelly DeBruyne

To my mom, Tina C. Pinna, who started me on the path to good nutritional practices in my earliest years.

Kathryn Pinna

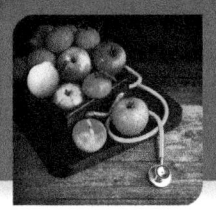

About the Authors

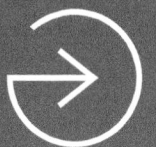

LINDA KELLY DEBRUYNE, M.S., R.D., received her B.S. and M.S. degrees in nutrition and food science at Florida State University. She is a founding member of Nutrition and Health Associates, an information resource center in Tallahassee, Florida, where her specialty areas are life cycle nutrition and fitness. Her other publications include the textbooks *Nutrition and Diet Therapy* and *Health: Making Life Choices.* She is a registered dietitian and maintains a professional membership in the Academy of Nutrition and Dietetics.

KATHRYN PINNA, PH.D., R.D., received her M.S. and Ph.D. degrees in nutrition from the University of California at Berkeley. She taught nutrition, food science, and human biology courses in the San Francisco Bay Area for over 25 years and also worked as an outpatient dietitian, Internet consultant, and freelance writer. Her other publications include the textbooks *Understanding Normal and Clinical Nutrition* and *Nutrition and Diet Therapy.* She is a registered dietitian and a member of the American Society for Nutrition and the Academy of Nutrition and Dietetics.

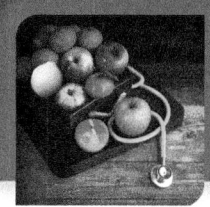

Brief Contents

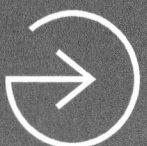

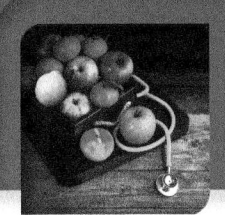

Contents

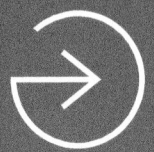

Contents

Preface

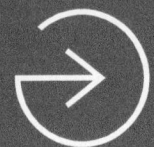

of *Nutrition for Health and Health Care*, which provides a solid foundation in nutrition science and the role of nutrition in clinical care. Health professionals and patients alike rank nutrition among their most serious concerns, as good nutrition status plays critical roles in both disease prevention and the appropriate treatment of illness. Moreover, medical personnel are frequently called upon to answer questions about foods and diets or provide nutrition care. Although much of the material has been written for nursing students and is relevant to nursing care, this textbook can be useful for students of other health-related professions, including nursing assistants, physician assistants, dietitians, dietary technicians, and health educators.

Each chapter of this textbook includes essential nutrition concepts along with practical information for addressing nutrition concerns and solving nutrition problems. The introductory chapters (Chapters 1 and 2) provide an overview of the nutrients and nutrition recommendations and describe the process of digestion and absorption. Chapters 3 through 5 introduce the attributes and functions of carbohydrates, lipids, and protein and explain how appropriate intakes of these nutrients support health. Chapters 6 and 7 introduce the concepts of energy balance and weight management and describe the health effects of overweight, underweight, and eating disorders. Chapters 8 and 9 introduce the vitamins and minerals, describing their roles in the body, appropriate intakes, and food sources. Chapters 10 through 12 explain how nutrient needs change throughout the life cycle. Chapters 13 and 14 explore how health professionals can use information from nutrition assessments to identify and address a patient's dietary needs. The remaining chapters (Chapters 15–23) examine nutrition therapy and its role in the prevention and treatment of common medical conditions.

CHANGES FOR THIS EDITION

Each chapter of this book is based on current nutrition knowledge and the latest clinical practice guidelines, and features new learning objectives for each major section.

Some major content changes in this edition include the following:

Chapter 1
Added a new section on marketing and food choices. Added a discussion of processed and ultra-processed foods versus whole foods and included definitions for each term. Expanded the discussion of Healthy People goals and progress made so far. Enhanced the Nutrient Intake Recommendation figure. Enhanced the Accurate/Inaccurate View of Nutrient Intakes figure. Added information about job duties of dietitians to the Nutrition In Practice.

Chapter 2
Reworked the Gastrointestinal Tract figure to indicate the digestive tract and accessory organs. Added a new section on GI tract health, regulation, and microbiota. Enhanced the table showing refrigerator home storage for fresh and processed foods.

Chapter 3
Added information about added sugars in ultra-processed foods. Included additional individual characteristics that influence a person's blood glucose response to food in the Nutrition in Practice.

Chapter 4
Added a new discussion and a table of the Mediterranean diet to the Nutrition in Practice.

Chapter 5
Added the definition of processed meat. Added a table of the Healthy Vegetarian Eating Pattern to the Nutrition in Practice.

Chapter 6
Added a brief discussion of intermittent fasting. Added and defined a new term, adiposity-based chronic disease. Added information about metabolically health obesity.

Chapter 7
Added a brief discussion about ghrelin, sleep duration, and obesity. Simplified the discussion of over-the-counter weight loss drugs and herbs. Enhanced the

discussion of energy density and weight loss. Reworked the section on behavior modification and deleted the food diary figure to emphasize mobile applications to track food and activity.

Chapter 8

Simplified the figure of the blood-clotting process. Reorganized the Niacin section. Deleted How to Estimate Dietary Folate Equivalents. Added a section about choline. Shortened and simplified some sections in the Nutrition in Practice. Added definitions of soy related terms: edamame, miso, and soy milk.

Chapter 9

Deleted the figure called what processing does to sodium and potassium contents of foods. Replaced drawings in figures showing good sources of certain nutrients with photos. Included a new figure of a supplement label in the Nutrition in Practice.

Chapter 10

Rewrote parts of the beginning of the chapter. Deleted the infant mortality figure. Shortened and enhanced the figure comparing nonpregnant, pregnant, and lactating women's nutrient needs. Added a new table of advice for pregnant and lactating women eating fish. Added a new table listing signs and symptoms of preeclampsia.

Chapter 11

Improved and simplified the table of supplement recommendations for infants. Added a new section called How to Feed Infants that includes and defines responsive feeding. Added information about hunger and satiety signals to the table of infant development and recommended foods. Included updated American Academy of Pediatrics juice recommendations for infants and children. Rewrote and shortened the section on nutrition at school.

Chapter 12

Deleted the table of Ineffective dietary strategies for arthritis. Shortened and simplified discussion of food insufficiency and obesity.

Chapter 13

Updated laboratory values in the table on routine laboratory tests.

Chapter 14

In the Nutrition in Practice about CAM, updated statistics, terminology, and tables related to herbal products.

Chapter 15

Refined the terms related to nutrition support: introduced the terms *specialized nutrition support* and *oral nutrition support*. Modified the table comparing tube feeding routes.

Reorganized the sections about administrating tube feedings. Modified sections on formula safety and initiating and advancing tube feedings. In the Nutrition in Practice about inborn errors, modified the dietary recommendations for phenylketonuria.

Chapter 16

Revised the section on micronutrient needs in acute stress. Added information about the types of oxygen equipment available for patients on oxygen therapy.

Chapter 17

Added a discussion about gastroparesis. Modified some material in the sections on gastroesophageal reflux disease, gastritis, and bariatric surgery; added glossary definitions for *acid regurgitation, heartburn, bloating,* and *pernicious anemia.*

Chapter 18

Added calcium channel activators to the table of laxatives and bulk-forming agents. Revised the table of foods that increase intestinal gas. Revised some information about nutrition therapies for acute and chronic pancreatitis and cystic fibrosis. Added some gluten sources to the table describing the gluten-free diet. In the Nutrition in Practice on probiotics, modified the sections about dietary sources of probiotics and safety concerns associated with the use of probiotics.

Chapter 19

Shortened the paragraph on the nutrition treatment for hepatitis. Updated the table of laboratory values for the evaluation of liver disease, and modified the table listing the clinical features of hepatic encephalopathy. Revised the section on the nutrition therapy for cirrhosis, including the table summarizing nutrition recommendations.

Chapter 20

Updated statistics throughout the chapter. Modified the sections on type 1 diabetes, prevention of type 2 diabetes, insulin use in type 2 diabetes, and physical activity in diabetes management. In the section on diabetic neuropathy, distinguished between peripheral and autonomic neuropathy. Revised various sections on nutrition therapy to reflect updated clinical guidelines. Modified the table on insulin preparations. Added a box showing the glycemic goals for pregnant women with diabetes. In the Nutrition in Practice on metabolic syndrome, modified the section about obesity's influence on hypertension.

Chapter 21

Updated statistics throughout the chapter. Revised various paragraphs in the sections on CVD lifestyle management and hypertension treatment. Updated the box showing how blood pressure measurements are classified. Updated the table of recommended lifestyle modifications for blood pressure reduction. Added a box describing the effects of drugs used in hypertension treatment. In the Nutrition in Practice on feeding disabilities, changed the photo showing an example of adaptive feeding equipment.

Chapter 22

Updated statistics throughout the chapter. Revised the section on malnutrition in chronic kidney disease and introduced the term *protein-energy wasting*. Revised the table on dietary guidelines for chronic kidney disease. In the section on kidney stones, introduced *hypocitraturia* as a risk factor for calcium kidney stones. Reformatted the table of foods high in oxalates. In the Nutrition in Practice on dialysis, revised the description of the different types of hemodialysis.

Chapter 23

Updated statistics throughout the chapter, and updated the tables on factors that influence cancer risk. Revised the section on cancer immunotherapy. Included information about prophylactic medications used in persons at risk of HIV exposure. Updated the definition of AIDS-wasting syndrome to reflect current guidelines. In the Nutrition in Practice on ethical issues, revised some glossary definitions and modified the discussion about the effectiveness of advance directives in medical care.

FEATURES OF THIS TEXT

Students of nutrition often begin a nutrition course with some practical knowledge of nutrition; after all, they may purchase food, read food labels, and be familiar with common nutrition problems such as obesity or lactose intolerance. After just a few weeks of class, however, the nutrition student realizes that nutrition is a biological and chemical science with a fair amount of new terminology and new concepts to learn. This book contains abundant pedagogy to help students master the subject matter. Within each chapter, definitions of important terms appear in the margins. How To skill boxes help readers work through calculations or give practical suggestions for applying nutrition advice. The Nursing Diagnosis feature enables nursing students to correlate nutrition care with nursing care. Review Notes summarize the information following each major heading; these summaries can be used to preview or review key chapter concepts. The Self Check at the end of each chapter provides questions to help review chapter information.

In the life cycle and clinical chapters, Case Studies guide readers in applying nutrition therapy to patient care. Diet-Drug Interaction boxes in the clinical chapters identify important nutrient-drug and food-drug

interactions. Clinical Applications throughout the text encourage readers to practice mathematical calculations, synthesize information from previous chapters, or understand how dietary adjustments affect patients. Nutrition Assessment Checklists remind readers of assessment parameters relevant to specific stages of the life cycle or medical problems.

The Nutrition in Practice sections that follow the chapters explore issues of current interest, advanced topics, or specialty areas such as dental health or dialysis. Examples of topics covered include foodborne illness, the glycemic index, vegetarian diets, alcohol in health and disease, nutritional genomics, metabolic syndrome, and childhood obesity and chronic disease. The appendixes support the book with a wealth of information on U.S. nutrient intake recommendations, food lists for diabetes, physical activity and energy requirements, nutrition assessments, enteral formulas, and aids to calculations.

MINDTAP: EMPOWER YOUR STUDENTS

MindTap is a platform that propels students from memorization to mastery. It gives you complete control of your course, so you can provide engaging content, challenge every learner, and build student confidence. Customize interactive syllabi to emphasize priority topics, then add your own material or notes to the eBook as desired. This outcomes-driven application gives you the tools needed to empower students and boost both understanding and performance.

ACCESS EVERYTHING YOU NEED IN ONE PLACE

Cut down on prep with the preloaded and organized MindTap course materials. Teach more efficiently with interactive multimedia, assignments, quizzes, and more. Give your students the power to read, listen, and study on their phones, so they can learn on their terms.

EMPOWER STUDENTS TO REACH THEIR POTENTIAL

Twelve distinct metrics give you actionable insights into student engagement. Identify topics troubling your entire class and instantly communicate with those struggling. Students can track their scores to stay motivated towards their goals. Together, you can be unstoppable.

CONTROL YOUR COURSE—AND YOUR CONTENT

Get the flexibility to reorder textbook chapters, add your own notes, and embed a variety of content including Open Educational Resources (OER). Personalize course content to your students' needs. They can even read your notes, add their own, and highlight key text to aid their learning.

GET A DEDICATED TEAM, WHENEVER YOU NEED THEM

MindTap isn't just a tool, it's backed by a personalized team eager to support you. We can help set up your course and tailor it to your specific objectives, so you'll be ready to make an impact from day one. Know we'll be standing by to help you and your students until the final day of the term.

ANCILLARIES

- A test bank is available through **Cengage Learning Testing Powered by Cognero**, a flexible online system that allows instructors to author, edit, and manage test bank content from multiple Cengage Learning solutions; create multiple test versions in an instant; and deliver tests from an LMS, a classroom, or wherever the instructor wants.

- The password-protected **Instructor Companion Site** offers everything an instructor needs for the course in one place! This collection of book-specific lecture and class tools is available online via www.cengage.com/login. Access and download PowerPoint presentations, images, an instructor's manual, videos, and more.

Acknowledgments

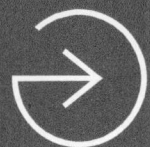

Among the most difficult words to write are those that express the depth of our gratitude to the many dedicated people whose efforts have made this book possible. A special note of appreciation to Sharon Rolfes for her numerous contributions to the chapters and Nutrition in Practice sections as well as to the Dietary Reference Intakes on the inside front cover and the appendices. Many thanks to Fran Webb for sharing her knowledge, ideas, and resources about the latest nutrition developments. Thanks also to David L. Stone for his assistance with multiple sections in the clinical chapters. We are indebted to our production team, especially Tara Slagle for seeing this project through. We would also like to acknowledge Jake Warde for his design recommendations. To the many others involved in designing, indexing, typesetting, dummying, and marketing, we offer our thanks. We are especially grateful to our associates, family, and friends for their continued encouragement and support and to our reviewers who consistently offer excellent suggestions for improving the text.

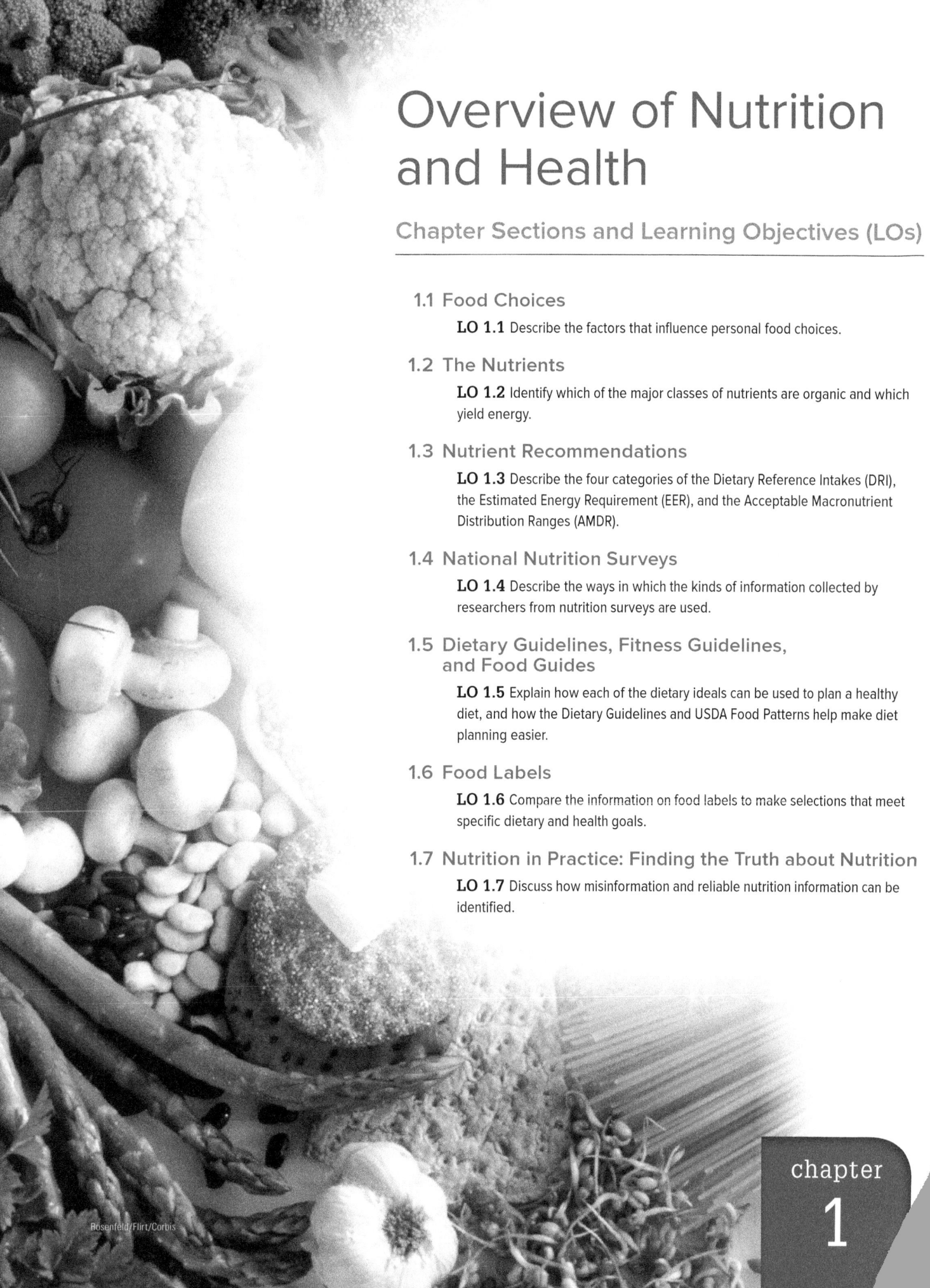

Overview of Nutrition and Health

Chapter Sections and Learning Objectives (LOs)

Rosenfeld/Flirt/Corbis

chapter

1

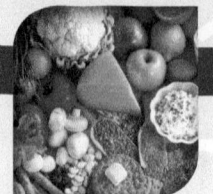

improve your **health** or harm it. Each choice may influence your health only a little, but when these choices are repeated over years and decades, their effects become significant.

The choices people make each day affect not only their physical health but also their **wellness**—all the characteristics that make a person strong, confident, and able to function well with family, friends, and others. People who consistently make poor lifestyle choices on a daily basis increase their risks of developing diseases. Figure 1-1 shows how a person's health can fall anywhere along a continuum, from maximum wellness on the one end to total failure to function (death) on the other.

As nurses or other health care professionals, when you take responsibility for your own health by making daily choices and practicing behaviors that enhance your well-being, you prepare yourself physically, mentally, and emotionally to meet the demands of your profession. As health care professionals, however, you have a responsibility to your clients as well as to yourselves.* You have unique opportunities to make your clients aware of the benefits of positive health choices and behaviors, to show them how to change their behaviors and make daily choices to enhance their own health, and to serve as role models for those behaviors.

This text focuses on how nutrition choices affect health and disease. The early chapters introduce the basics of nutrition to promote good health and reduce disease risks. The later chapters emphasize medical nutrition therapy and its role in supporting health and in treating diseases and symptoms.

1.1 Food Choices

Sound **nutrition** throughout life does not ensure good health and long life, but it can certainly help to tip the balance in their favor. Nevertheless, many people choose foods for reasons other than their nourishing value. Even people who claim to choose foods primarily for the sake of health or nutrition will admit that other factors also influence their food choices. Because food choices become an integral part of their lifestyles, people sometimes find it difficult to change their eating habits. Health care professionals who help clients make diet changes must understand the dynamics of food choices because people will alter their eating habits only if their preferences are honored. Developing **cultural competence** is an important aspect of honoring individual preferences, especially for health care professionals who help clients to achieve a nutritious diet.[1]

Preference Why do people like certain foods? One reason, of course, is their preference for certain tastes. Some tastes are widely liked, such as the sweetness of sugar and the savoriness of salt.[2] Research suggests that genetics influence people's taste preferences, a finding that may eventually have implications for clinical nutrition.[3] For example, sensitivity to bitter taste is an inheritable trait. People born with great sensitivity to bitter tastes tend to avoid foods with bitter flavors such as broccoli, cabbage, brussels sprouts, spinach, and grapefruit juice. These foods, as well as many other fruit and vegetables, contain **bioactive food components—phytochemicals** and nutrients—that may reduce the risk of cancer. Thus, the role that genetics may play in food selection is gaining importance in cancer research.[4] Nutrition in Practice 8 addresses phytochemicals and their role in disease prevention.

Habit Sometimes habit dictates people's food choices. People eat a sandwich for lunch or drink orange juice at breakfast simply because they have always done so. Eating a familiar food and not having to make any decisions can be comforting.

health: a range of states with physical, mental, emotional, spiritual, and social components. At a minimum, health means freedom from physical disease, mental disturbances, emotional distress, spiritual discontent, social maladjustment, and other negative states. At a maximum, health means *wellness.*

wellness: maximum well-being; the top range of health states; the goal of the person who strives toward realizing his or her full potential physically, mentally, emotionally, spiritually, and socially.

nutrition: the science of foods and the nutrients and other substances they contain, and of their ingestion, digestion, absorption, transport, metabolism, interaction, storage, and excretion. A broader definition includes the study of the environment and of human behavior as it relates to these processes.

cultural competence: an awareness and acceptance of one's own and others' cultures, combined with the skills needed to interact effectively with people of diverse cultures.

bioactive food components: compounds in foods (either nutrients or phytochemicals) that alter physiological processes in the body.

---

*Health care professionals generally use either *client* or *patient* when referring to an individual under their care. The first 12 chapters of this text emphasize the nutrition concerns of people in good health; therefore, the term *client* is used in these chapters.

FIGURE 1-1 The Health Line

No matter how well you maintain your health today, you may still be able to improve tomorrow. Likewise, a person who is well today can slip by failing to maintain health-promoting habits.

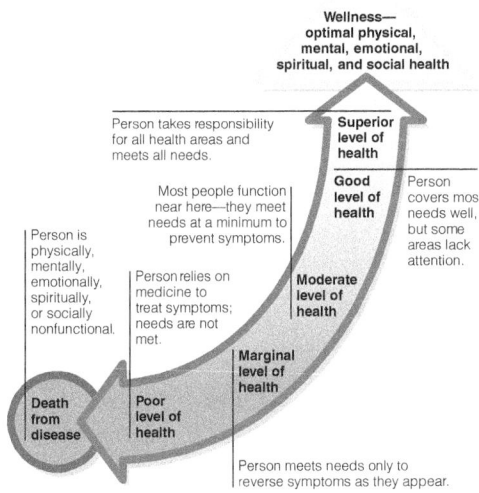

phytochemicals (FIGH-toe-CHEM-ih-cals): compounds in plants that confer color, taste, and other characteristics. Some phytochemicals are bioactive food components in functional foods. Nutrition in Practice 8 provides details.

foodways: the eating habits and culinary practices of a people, region, or historical period.

ethnic diets: foodways and cuisines typical of national origins, races, cultural heritages, or geographic locations.

Associations People also like foods with happy associations—foods eaten in the midst of warm family gatherings on traditional holidays or given to them as children by someone who loved them. By the same token, people can attach intense and unalterable dislikes to foods that they ate when they were sick or that were forced on them when they weren't hungry.

Ethnic Heritage and Regional Cuisines Every country, and every region of a country, has its own typical foods and ways of combining them into meals (see Photo 1-1). The **foodways** of North America reflect the many different cultural and ethnic backgrounds of its inhabitants. Many foods with foreign origins are familiar items on North American menus: tacos, egg rolls, lasagna, sushi, and gyros, to name a few. Still others, such as spaghetti and croissants, are almost staples in the "American diet." North American regional cuisines such as Cajun and TexMex blend the traditions of several cultures. Table 1-1 presents selected **ethnic diets** and food choices.

Values Food choices may reflect people's environmental ethics, religious beliefs, and political views. By choosing to eat some foods or to avoid others, people make statements that reflect their values. For example, people may select only foods that come in containers that can be reused or recycled. A concerned consumer may boycott fruit or vegetables picked by migrant workers who have been exploited. People may buy vegetables from local farmers to save the fuel and environmental costs of foods shipped from far away. Labels on some foods carry statements or symbols—known as *ecolabels*—that imply that the foods have been produced in ways that are considered environmentally favorable.

Religion also influences many people's food choices. Jewish law sets forth an extensive set of dietary rules. Many Christians forgo meat on Fridays during Lent, the period prior to Easter. In Islamic dietary laws, permitted or lawful foods are called *halal*. Other faiths prohibit some dietary practices and promote others. Diet planners can foster sound nutrition practices only if they respect and honor each person's values.

Photo 1-1

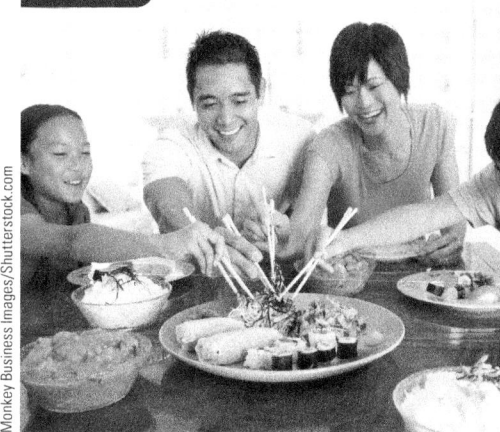

Monkey Business Images/Shutterstock.com

Ethnic meals and family gatherings nourish the spirit as well as the body.

TABLE 1-1   Selected Ethnic Cuisines and Food Choices

	GRAINS	VEGETABLES	FRUIT	PROTEIN FOODS	MILK
Asian	Millet, rice, rice or wheat noodles	Baby corn, bamboo shoots, bok choy, leafy greens (such as amaranth), cabbages, mung bean sprouts, scallions, seaweed, snow peas, straw mushrooms, water chestnuts, wild yam	Kumquats, loquats, lychee, mandarin oranges, melons, pears, persimmon, plums	Pork; duck and other poultry; fish, octopus, sea urchin, squid, and other seafood; soybeans, tofu; eggs; cashews, peanuts	Soy milk
Mediterranean	Bulgur, couscous, focaccia, Italian bread, pastas, pita pocket bread, polenta, rice	Artichokes, cucumbers, eggplant, fennel, grape leaves, leafy greens, leeks, onions, peppers, tomatoes	Berries, dates, figs, grapes, lemons, melons, olives, oranges, pomegranates, raisins	Fish and other seafood, gyros, lamb, pork, sausage, chicken, fava beans, lentils, almonds, walnuts	Feta, goat, mozzarella, parmesan, provolone, and ricotta cheeses; yogurt and yogurt beverages
Mexican	Hominy, masa (corn flour dough), tortillas (corn or flour), rice	Bell peppers, cactus, cassava, chayote, chili pepper, corn, jicama, onions, summer squash, tomatoes, winter squash, yams	Avocado, bananas, guava, lemons, limes, mango, oranges, papaya, plantain	Beans, refried beans, beef, goat, pork, chorizo, chicken, fish, eggs	Cheese, flan (baked caramel custard), milk in beverages

Becky Luigart-Stayner/ Encyclopedia/Corbis

Photodisc, Inc./ Getty Images

Mitch Hrdlicka/ Photodisc/Getty Images

Social Interaction Social interaction is another powerful influence on people's food choices. Meals are often social events, and the sharing of food is part of hospitality. Social customs invite people to accept food or drink offered by a host or shared by a group—regardless of hunger signals.[5] Food brings people together for many different reasons: to celebrate a holiday or special event, to renew an old friendship, to make new friends, to conduct business, and many more. Sometimes food is used to influence or impress someone. For example, a business executive invites a prospective new client out to dinner in hopes of edging out the competition. In each case, for whatever the purpose, food plays an integral part of the social interaction.

Emotional State Emotions guide food choices and eating behaviors.[6] Some people cannot eat when they are emotionally upset. Others may eat in response to a variety of emotional stimuli—for example, to relieve boredom or depression or to calm anxiety. A depressed person may choose to eat rather than to call a friend. A person who has returned home from an exciting evening out may unwind with a late-night snack. Eating in response to emotions can easily lead to overeating and obesity but may be appropriate at times. For example, sharing food at times of bereavement serves both the giver's need to provide comfort and the receiver's need to be cared for and to interact with others as well as to take nourishment.

Marketing Another major influence on food choices is marketing. The food industry competes for our food dollars, persuading consumers to eat more—more food, more often. These marketing efforts pay off well, generating more than $900 billion in sales each year. In addition to building brand loyalty, food companies attract busy consumers with their promises of convenience.

Availability, Convenience, and Economy The influence of these factors on people's food selections is clear. You cannot eat foods if they are not available, if you cannot get to the grocery store, if you do not have the time or skill to prepare them, or if you cannot afford them. Consumers who value convenience frequently eat out, bring home ready-to-eat meals, or have food delivered. Whether decisions based on convenience meet a person's nutrition needs depends on the choices made. Eating a banana or a candy bar may be equally convenient, but the fruit provides more vitamins and minerals and less sugar and fat.

Given the abundance of convenient food options, fewer adults are learning the cooking skills needed to prepare meals at home, which has its downside. People who are competent in their cooking skills and frequently eat their meals at home tend to make healthier food choices.[7] Not surprisingly, when eating out, consumers choose low-cost fast-food outlets over more expensive fine-dining restaurants. Foods eaten away from home, especially fast-food meals, tend to be high in nutrients that Americans overconsume (saturated fat and sodium) and low in nutrients that Americans underconsume (calcium, fiber, and iron)—all of which can contribute to a variety of health problems.[8]

Some people have jobs that keep them away from home for days at a time, require them to conduct business in restaurants or at conventions, or involve hectic schedules that allow little or no time for meals at home. For these people, the kinds of restaurants available to them and the cost of eating out so often may limit food choices.

Age Age influences people's food choices. Infants, for example, depend on others to choose foods for them. Older children also rely on others but become more active in selecting foods that taste sweet and are familiar to them and rejecting those whose taste or texture they dislike. In contrast, the links between taste preferences and food choices in adults are less direct than in children. Adults often choose foods based on health concerns such as body weight. Indeed, adults may avoid sweet or familiar foods because of such concerns.

Body Weight and Image Sometimes people select certain foods and supplements that they believe will improve their physical appearance and avoid those they believe might be detrimental. Such decisions can be beneficial when based on sound nutrition and fitness knowledge but may undermine good health when based on fads or carried to extremes. Eating disorders are the topic of Nutrition in Practice 6.

Medical Conditions Sometimes medical conditions and their treatments (including medications) limit the foods a person can select. For example, a person with heart disease might need to adopt a diet low in certain types of fats. The chemotherapy needed to treat cancer can interfere with a person's appetite or limit food choices by causing vomiting. Allergy to certain foods can also limit choices. The second half of this text discusses how diet can be modified to accommodate different medical conditions.

Health and Nutrition Finally, of course, many consumers make food choices they believe are nutritious and healthy (see Photo 1-2). Making healthy food choices 100 years ago was rather easy when the list of options was relatively short and markets sold mostly fresh, **whole foods**. Examples of whole foods include vegetables and legumes; fruit; seafood, meats, poultry, eggs, nuts, and seeds; milk; and whole grains. Today, tens of thousands of food items fill the shelves of super-grocery stores and most of those items are **processed foods**. Whether a processed food is a healthy choice depends, in part, on how extensively the food was processed. When changes are minimal, processing can provide an abundant, safe, convenient, affordable, and nutritious product.[9]

Examples of minimally processed foods include frozen vegetables, fruit juices, smoked salmon, cheeses, and breads. The nutritional value diminishes, however, when changes are extensive, creating **ultra-processed foods**. Ultra-processed foods no longer resemble whole foods; they are made from substances that are typically used in food preparation, but not consumed as foods themselves (such as oils, fats, flours, refined starches, and sugars). These substances undergo further processing by adding little, if any, processed foods, salt and other preservatives, and additives such as flavors and colors. Examples of ultra-processed foods include soft drinks, corn chips, fruit gummies, chicken nuggets, canned cheese spreads, and toaster pastries. Notably, these foods cannot be made in a home kitchen using common grocery ingredients. Dominating the

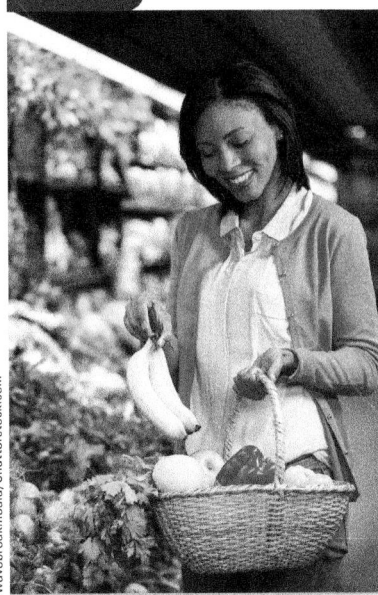

wavebreakmedia/Shutterstock.com

Nutrition is only one of the many factors that influence people's food choices.

whole foods: fresh foods such as vegetables, grains, legumes, meats, and milk that are unprocessed or minimally processed.

processed foods: foods that have been intentionally changed by the addition of substances, or a method of cooking, preserving, milling, or such.

ultra-processed foods: foods that have been made from substances that are typically used in food preparation, but not consumed as foods by themselves (such as oils, fats, flours, refined starches, and sugars) that undergo further processing by adding a little, if any, minimally processed foods, salt and other preservatives, and additives such as flavors and colors.

Review Notes

- A person selects foods for many different reasons.
- Food choices influence health—both positively and negatively. Individual food selections neither make nor break a diet's healthfulness, but the balance of foods selected over time can make an important difference to health.
- In the interest of health, people are wise to think "nutrition" when making their food choices.

global market, ultra-processed foods tend to be attractive, tasty, and cheap—as well as high in fat and sugar.[10] Consumers wanting to make healthy food choices will select fewer ultra-processed foods and more whole foods and minimally processed foods.[11]

1.2 The Nutrients

You are a collection of molecules that move. All these moving parts are arranged in patterns of extraordinary complexity and order—cells, tissues, and organs. Although the arrangement remains constant, the parts are continually changing, using **nutrients** and energy derived from nutrients.

Almost any food you eat is composed of dozens or even hundreds of different kinds of materials. Spinach, for example, is composed mostly of water (95 percent), and most of its solid materials are the compounds carbohydrates, fats (properly called lipids), and proteins. If you could remove these materials, you would find a tiny quantity of minerals, vitamins, and other compounds.

Six Classes of Nutrients

Water, carbohydrates, fats, proteins, vitamins, and minerals are the six classes of nutrients commonly found in spinach and other foods. Some of the other materials in foods, such as the pigments and other phytochemicals, are not nutrients but may still be important to health. The body can make some nutrients for itself, at least in limited quantities, but it cannot make them all, and it makes some in insufficient quantities to meet its needs. Therefore, the body must obtain many nutrients from foods. The nutrients that foods must supply are called **essential nutrients**.

Carbohydrates, Fats, and Proteins Four of the six classes of nutrients (carbohydrates, fats, proteins, and vitamins) contain carbon, which is found in all living things. They are therefore **organic** (meaning, literally, "alive").* During metabolism, three of these four (carbohydrates, fats, and proteins) provide energy the body can use.† These **energy-yielding nutrients** continually replenish the energy you expend daily.

Vitamins, Minerals, and Water Vitamins are organic but do not provide energy to the body. They facilitate the release of energy from the three energy-yielding nutrients. In contrast, minerals and water are **inorganic** nutrients. Minerals yield no energy in the human body, but, like vitamins, they help to regulate the release of energy, among their many other roles. As for water, it is the medium in which all of the body's processes take place.

kCalories: A Measure of Energy

The amount of energy that carbohydrates, fats, and proteins release can be measured in **calories**—tiny units of energy so small that a single apple provides tens of thousands of them. To ease calculations, energy is expressed in 1000-calorie metric units known

nutrients: substances obtained from food and used in the body to provide energy and structural materials and to serve as regulating agents to promote growth, maintenance, and repair. Nutrients may also reduce the risks of some diseases.

essential nutrients: nutrients a person must obtain from food because the body cannot make them for itself in sufficient quantities to meet physiological needs.

organic: in chemistry, substances or molecules containing carbon–carbon bonds or carbon–hydrogen bonds. The four organic nutrients are carbohydrate, fat, protein, and vitamins.

energy-yielding nutrients: the nutrients that break down to yield energy the body can use. The three energy-yielding nutrients are carbohydrate, protein, and fat.

inorganic: not containing carbon or pertaining to living organisms. The two classes of nutrients that are inorganic are minerals and water.

calories: a measure of *heat* energy. Food energy is measured in **kilocalories** (1000 calories equal 1 kilocalorie), abbreviated **kcalories** or kcal. One kcalorie is the amount of heat necessary to raise the temperature of 1 kilogram (kg) of water 1°C. The scientific use of the term *kcalorie* is the same as the popular use of the term *calorie*.

---

*Note that this definition of *organic* excludes coal, diamonds, and a few carbon-containing compounds that contain only a single carbon and no hydrogen, such as carbon dioxide (CO_2).

†*Metabolism* is the set of processes by which nutrients are rearranged into body structures or broken down to yield energy.

as **kilocalories** (shortened to **kcalories**, but commonly called "calories"). When you read in popular books or magazines that an apple provides "100 calories," understand that it means 100 kcalories. This book uses the term *kcalorie* and its abbreviation *kcal* throughout, as do other scientific books and journals.* kCalories are not constituents of foods; they are a measure of the energy foods provide. The energy a food provides depends on how much carbohydrate, fat, and protein the food contains.

Carbohydrate yields 4 kcalories of energy from each gram, and so does protein. Fat yields 9 kcalories per gram. Thus, fat has a greater **energy density** than either carbohydrate or protein. Chapter 7 revisits energy density with regard to weight management. If you know how many grams of carbohydrate, protein, and fat a food contains, you can derive the number of kcalories potentially available from the food. Simply multiply the carbohydrate grams times 4, the protein grams times 4, and the fat grams times 9, and add the results together (Box 1-1 describes how to calculate the energy a food provides).

Energy Nutrients in Foods Most foods contain mixtures of all three energy-yielding nutrients, although foods are sometimes classified by their predominant nutrient. To speak of meat as "a protein" or of bread as "a carbohydrate," however, is inaccurate. Each is rich in a particular nutrient, but a protein-rich food such as beef contains a lot of fat along with the protein, and a carbohydrate-rich food such as cornbread also contains fat (corn oil) and protein. Only a few foods are exceptions to this rule, the common ones being sugar (which is pure carbohydrate) and oil (which is pure fat).

Energy Storage in the Body The body first uses the energy-yielding nutrients to build new compounds and fuel metabolic and physical activities. Excesses are then rearranged into storage compounds, primarily body fat, and put away for later use. Thus, if you take in more energy than you expend, the result is an increase in energy stores and weight gain. Similarly, if you take in less energy than you expend, the result is a decrease in energy stores and weight loss.

Alcohol, Not a Nutrient One other substance contributes energy: alcohol. The body derives energy from alcohol at the rate of 7 kcalories per gram. Alcohol is not a nutrient, however, because it cannot support the body's growth, maintenance, or repair. Nutrition in Practice 19 discusses alcohol's effects on nutrition.

energy density: a measure of the energy a food provides relative to the amount of food (kcalories per gram).

| Box 1-1 | *HOW TO* Calculate the Energy a Food Provides |

To calculate the energy available from a food, multiply the number of grams of carbohydrate, protein, and fat by 4, 4, and 9, respectively. Then add the results together. For example, one slice of bread with 1 tablespoon of peanut butter on it contains 16 grams of carbohydrate, 7 grams of protein, and 9 grams of fat:

16 g carbohydrate × 4 kcal/g = 64 kcal

7 g protein × 4 kcal/g = 28 kcal

9 g fat × 9 kcal/g = 81 kcal

Total = 173 kcal

From this information, you can calculate the percentage of kcalories each of the energy nutrients contributes to the total.

To determine the percentage of kcalories from fat, for example, divide the 81 fat kcalories by the total 173 kcalories:

81 fat kcal ÷ 173 total kcal = 0.468 (rounded to 0.47)

Then multiply by 100 to get the percentage:

0.47 × 100 = 47%

Dietary recommendations that urge people to limit fat intake to 20 to 35 percent of kcalories refer to the day's total energy intake, not to individual foods. Still, if the proportion of fat in each food choice throughout a day exceeds 35 percent of kcalories, then the day's total surely will, too. Knowing that this snack provides 47 percent of its kcalories from fat alerts a person to the need to make lower-fat selections at other times that day.

---

*Food energy can also be measured in kilojoules (kJ). The kilojoule is the international unit of energy. One kcalorie equals 4.2 kJ.

Review Notes

- Foods provide nutrients—substances that support the growth, maintenance, and repair of the body's tissues.
- The six classes of nutrients are water, carbohydrates, fats, proteins, vitamins, and minerals.
- Vitamins, minerals, and water do not yield energy; instead, they facilitate a variety of activities in the body.
- Foods rich in the energy-yielding nutrients (carbohydrates, fats, and proteins) provide the major materials for building the body's tissues and yield energy the body can use or store.
- Energy is measured in kcalories.

Dietary Reference Intakes (DRI): a set of values for the dietary nutrient intakes of healthy people in the United States and Canada. These values are used for planning and assessing diets.

Recommended Dietary Allowances (RDA): a set of values reflecting the average daily amounts of nutrients considered adequate to meet the known nutrient needs of practically all healthy people in a particular life stage and gender group; a goal for dietary intake by individuals.

Adequate Intakes (AI): a set of values that are used as guides for nutrient intakes when scientific evidence is insufficient to determine an RDA.

requirement: the lowest continuing intake of a nutrient that will maintain a specified criterion of adequacy.

1.3 Nutrient Recommendations

Nutrient recommendations are used as standards to evaluate healthy people's energy and nutrient intakes. Nutrition experts use the recommendations to assess nutrient intakes and to guide people on amounts to consume. Individuals can use them to decide how much of a nutrient they need to consume.

Dietary Reference Intakes

Defining the amounts of energy, nutrients, and other dietary components that best support health is a huge task. Nutrition experts have produced a set of standards that define the amounts of energy, nutrients, other dietary components, and physical activity that best support health. These recommendations are called **Dietary Reference Intakes (DRI)** and reflect the collaborative efforts of scientists in both the United States and Canada.* The inside front covers of this book present the DRI values. (A set of nutrient recommendations developed by the World Health Organization for international use is presented in Appendix B.)

Setting Nutrient Recommendations: RDA and AI One advantage of the DRI is that they apply to the diets of individuals. The DRI committee offers two sets of values to be used as nutrient intake goals by individuals: a set called the **Recommended Dietary Allowances (RDA)** and a set called **Adequate Intakes (AI)**.

Based on solid experimental evidence and other reliable observations, the RDA are the foundation of the DRI. The AI values are based on less extensive scientific findings and rely more heavily on scientific judgment. The committee establishes an AI value whenever scientific evidence is insufficient to generate an RDA. To see which nutrients have an AI and which have an RDA, turn to the inside front cover.

In the last several decades, abundant new research has linked nutrients in the diet with the promotion of health and the prevention of chronic diseases. An advantage of the DRI is that, where appropriate, they take into account disease prevention as well as an adequate nutrient intake. For example, the RDA for calcium is based on intakes thought to reduce the likelihood of osteoporosis-related fractures later in life.

To ensure that the vitamin and mineral recommendations meet the needs of as many people as possible, the recommendations are set near the top end of the range of the population's estimated average requirements (see Figure 1-2). Small amounts above the daily **requirement** do no harm,

FIGURE 1-2 Nutrient Intake Recommendations

The nutrient intake recommendations are set high enough to cover nearly everyone's requirements (the boxes represent people). The Estimated Average Requirement (EAR) meets the needs of about half of the population (shown here by the red line). The Recommended Dietary Allowance (RDA) is set well about the EAR, meeting the needs of about 98 percent of the population (shown here by the purple line).

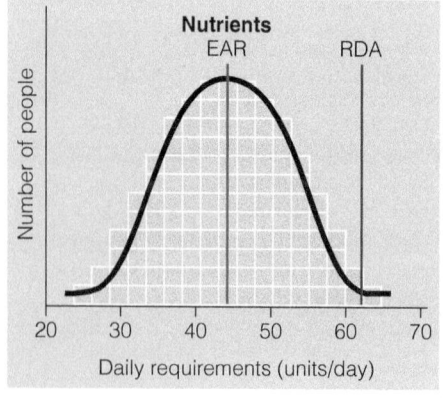

*The DRI reports are produced by the Food and Nutrition Board, Institute of Medicine of the National Academies, with active involvement of scientists from Canada.

whereas amounts below the requirement may lead to health problems. When people's intakes are consistently **deficient**, their nutrient stores decline, and over time this decline leads to deficiency symptoms and poor health.

Facilitating Nutrition Research and Policy: EAR In addition to the RDA and AI, the DRI committee has established another set of values: **Estimated Average Requirements (EAR)**. These values establish average requirements for given life stage and gender groups that researchers and nutrition policymakers use in their work. Nutrition scientists may use the EAR as standards in research. Public health officials may use them to assess nutrient intakes of populations and make recommendations. The EAR values form the scientific basis on which the RDA are set.

Establishing Safety Guidelines: UL The DRI committee also establishes upper limits of intake for nutrients posing a hazard when consumed in excess. These values, the **Tolerable Upper Intake Levels (UL)**, are indispensable to consumers who take supplements. Consumers need to know how much of a nutrient is too much. The UL are also of value to public health officials who set allowances for nutrients that are added to foods and water. The UL values are listed on the inside front cover.

Using Nutrient Recommendations Each of the four DRI categories serves a unique purpose. For example, the EAR are most appropriately used to develop and evaluate nutrition programs for *groups* such as schoolchildren or military personnel. The RDA (or AI, if an RDA is not available) can be used to set goals for *individuals*. The UL help to keep nutrient intakes below the amounts that increase the risk of toxicity. With these understandings, professionals can use the DRI for a variety of purposes.

In addition to understanding the unique purposes of the DRI, it is important to keep their uses in perspective. Consider the following:

- The values are recommendations for safe intakes, not minimum requirements; except for energy, they include a generous margin of safety. Figure 1-3 presents

deficient: in regard to nutrient intake, describes the amount below which almost all healthy people can be expected, over time, to experience deficiency symptoms.

Estimated Average Requirements (EAR): the average daily nutrient intake levels estimated to meet the requirements of half of the healthy individuals in a given age and gender group; used in nutrition research and policymaking and as the basis on which RDA values are set.

Tolerable Upper Intake Levels (UL): a set of values reflecting the highest average daily nutrient intake levels that are likely to pose no risk of toxicity to almost all healthy individuals in a particular life stage and gender group. As intake increases above the UL, the potential risk of adverse health effects increases.

FIGURE 1-3 Inaccurate versus Accurate View of Nutrient Intakes

The RDA (or AI) for a given nutrient represents a point that lies within a range of appropriate and reasonable intakes between toxicity and deficiency. Both of these recommendations are high enough to provide reserves in times of short-term dietary inadequacies, but not so high as to approach toxicity. Nutrient intakes above or below this range may be equally harmful.

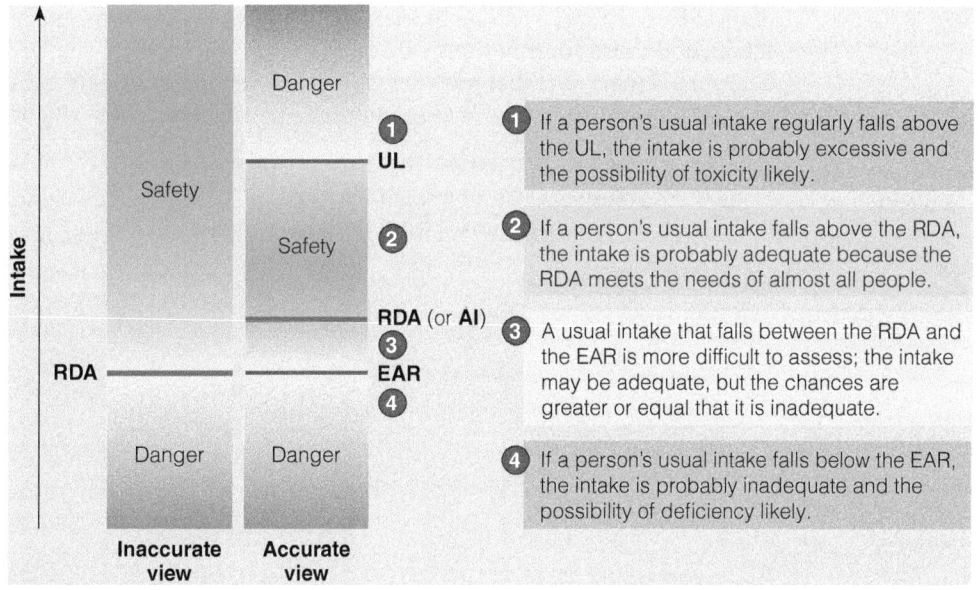

① If a person's usual intake regularly falls above the UL, the intake is probably excessive and the possibility of toxicity likely.

② If a person's usual intake falls above the RDA, the intake is probably adequate because the RDA meets the needs of almost all people.

③ A usual intake that falls between the RDA and the EAR is more difficult to assess; the intake may be adequate, but the chances are greater or equal that it is inadequate.

④ If a person's usual intake falls below the EAR, the intake is probably inadequate and the possibility of deficiency likely.

an accurate view of how a person's nutrient needs fall within a range, with danger zones both below and above the range.

- The values reflect daily intakes to be achieved on average, over time. They assume that intakes will vary from day to day, and they are set high enough to ensure that body nutrient stores will meet nutrient needs during periods of inadequate intakes lasting a day or two for some nutrients and up to a month or two for others.
- The values are chosen in reference to specific indicators of nutrient adequacy, such as blood nutrient concentrations, normal growth, and reduction of certain chronic diseases or other disorders when appropriate, rather than prevention of deficiency symptoms alone.
- The recommendations are designed to meet the needs of most healthy people. Medical problems alter nutrient needs, as later chapters describe.
- The recommendations are specific for people of both genders as well as various ages and stages of life: infants, children, adolescents, men, women, pregnant women, and lactating women.

Setting Energy Recommendations In contrast to the vitamin and mineral recommendations, the recommendation for energy, called the **Estimated Energy Requirement (EER)**, is not generous because excess energy cannot be excreted and is eventually stored as body fat. Rather, the key to the energy recommendation is balance. For a person who has a body weight, body composition, and physical activity level consistent with good health, energy intake from food should match energy expenditure, so the person achieves energy balance. Enough energy is needed to sustain a healthy, active life, but too much energy leads to obesity. The EER is therefore set at a level of energy intake predicted to maintain energy balance in a healthy adult of a defined age, gender, weight, height, and physical activity level.* Another difference between the requirements for other nutrients and those for energy is that each person has an obvious indicator of whether energy intake is inadequate, adequate, or excessive: body weight. Because *any* amount of energy in excess of need leads to weight gain, the DRI committee did not set a Tolerable Upper Intake Level.

Acceptable Macronutrient Distribution Ranges

As noted earlier, the DRI committee considers prevention of chronic disease as well as nutrient adequacy when establishing recommendations. To that end, the committee established healthy ranges of intakes for the energy-yielding nutrients—carbohydrate, fat, and protein—known as **Acceptable Macronutrient Distribution Ranges (AMDR)**. Each of these three energy-yielding nutrients contributes to a person's total energy (kcalorie) intake, and those contributions vary in relation to each other. The DRI committee has determined that a diet that provides the energy-yielding nutrients in the following proportions provides adequate energy and nutrients and reduces the risk of chronic disease:

- 45 to 65 percent of kcalories from carbohydrate
- 20 to 35 percent of kcalories from fat
- 10 to 35 percent of kcalories from protein

Estimated Energy Requirement (EER): the dietary energy intake level that is predicted to maintain energy balance in a healthy adult of a defined age, gender, weight, and physical activity level consistent with good health.

Acceptable Macronutrient Distribution Ranges (AMDR): ranges of intakes for the energy-yielding nutrients that provide adequate energy and nutrients and reduce the risk of chronic disease.

Review Notes

- The Dietary Reference Intakes (DRI) are a set of nutrient intake values that can be used to plan and evaluate dietary intakes for healthy people.
- The Estimated Average Requirement (EAR) defines the amount of a nutrient that supports a specific function in the body for half of the population.

(Continued)

---

*The EER for children, pregnant women, and lactating women includes energy needs associated with the deposition of tissue or the secretion of milk at rates consistent with good health.

1.4 National Nutrition Surveys

How do nutrition experts know whether people are meeting nutrient recommendations? The Dietary Reference Intakes and other major reports that examine the relationships between diet and health depend on information collected from nutrition surveys. One of the first nutrition surveys, taken before World War II, suggested that up to a third of the U.S. population might be eating poorly. Programs to correct **malnutrition** have been evolving ever since.

A national food and nutrient intake survey, called *What We Eat in America*, collects data on the kinds and amounts of foods people eat. Researchers then calculate the energy and nutrients in the foods and compare the amounts consumed with standards such as the DRI. *What We Eat in America* is conducted as part of a larger research effort, the National Health and Nutrition Examination Surveys (NHANES), which examine the people themselves using nutrition assessment methods. The data provide valuable information on several nutrition-related conditions such as growth retardation, heart disease, and nutrient deficiencies.

The resulting wealth of information can be used for a variety of purposes. For example, Congress uses this information to establish public policy on nutrition education, assess food assistance programs, and regulate the food supply. The food industry uses the information to guide decisions in public relations and product development. Scientists use the information to establish research priorities. These data also provide the basis for developing and monitoring national health goals.

National Health Goals

Healthy People is a program that identifies the nation's health priorities and guides policies that promote health and prevent disease. At the start of each decade, the program sets goals for improving the nation's health during the following 10 years. Nutrition is 1 of 42 topic areas of Healthy People 2020, each with numerous objectives (www.healthypeople.gov). Table 1-2 (p. 12) lists the nutrition and weight status objectives for 2020.

Progress in meeting the 2020 goals is mixed. The objective to meet physical activity and muscle-strengthening guidelines has been achieved, but the objective to eat more fruit and vegetables showed no improvement.[12] Trends in overweight and obesity actually worsened slightly. Clearly, to achieve the Healthy People goals, "what we eat in America" must change.

National Trends

What do we eat in America and how has it changed over the last 45 years? The short answer to both questions is "a lot." We eat more meals away from home, particularly at fast-food restaurants. We eat larger portions. We drink more sweetened beverages

malnutrition: any condition caused by deficient or excess energy or nutrient intake or by an imbalance of nutrients.

Healthy People: a national public health initiative under the jurisdiction of the U.S. Department of Health and Human Services (DHHS) that identifies the most significant preventable threats to health and focuses efforts toward eliminating them.

TABLE 1-2   Healthy People 2020 Nutrition and Weight Status Objectives

- Increase the proportion of adults who are at a healthy weight
- Reduce the proportion of adults who are obese
- Reduce iron deficiency among young children and females of childbearing age
- Reduce iron deficiency among pregnant females
- Reduce the proportion of children and adolescents who are overweight or obese
- Increase the contribution of fruit to the diets of the population aged 2 years and older
- Increase the variety and contribution of vegetables to the diets of the population aged 2 years and older
- Increase the contribution of whole grains to the diets of the population aged 2 years and older
- Reduce consumption of saturated fat in the population aged 2 years and older
- Reduce consumption of sodium in the population aged 2 years and older
- Increase consumption of calcium in the population aged 2 years and older
- Increase the proportion of worksites that offer nutrition or weight management classes or counseling
- Increase the proportion of physician office visits that include counseling or education related to nutrition or weight
- Eliminate very low food security among children in U.S. households
- Prevent inappropriate weight gain in youth and adults
- Increase the proportion of primary care physicians who regularly measure the body mass index of their patients
- Reduce consumption of kcalories from solid fats and added sugars in the population age 2 years and older
- Increase the number of states that have state-level policies that incentivize food retail outlets to provide foods that are encouraged by the Dietary Guidelines
- Increase the number of states with nutrition standards for foods and beverages provided to preschool-age children in childcare
- Increase the percentage of schools that offer nutritious foods and beverages outside of school meals

Source: www.healthypeople.gov.

and eat more energy-dense, nutrient-poor foods such as candy and chips. We snack frequently. As a result of these dietary habits, our energy intake has risen and, consequently, so has the incidence of overweight and obesity. Overweight and obesity, in turn, profoundly influence our health—as Chapter 6 explains.

Review Notes

- Nutrition surveys measure people's food consumption and evaluate the nutrition status of populations.
- Information gathered from nutrition surveys serves as the basis for many major diet and nutrition reports, including Healthy People.

1.5 Dietary Guidelines, Fitness Guidelines, and Food Guides

Today, government authorities are as concerned about **overnutrition** as they once were about **undernutrition**. Research confirms that dietary excesses, especially of energy, sodium, certain fats, and alcohol, contribute to many **chronic diseases**, including heart disease, cancer, stroke, diabetes, and liver disease.[13] Only one other lifestyle habit has more influence on health than a person's choice of diet: smoking and other tobacco use. Table 1-3 lists the leading causes of death in the United States; notice that three of the top four are nutrition related (and related to tobacco use). Note, however, that although diet is a powerful influence on these diseases, they cannot be prevented by a healthy diet alone; genetics, physical activity, age, gender, and other factors also play a role. Within the range set by genetic inheritance, however, disease development is strongly influenced by the foods a person chooses to eat.

Sound nutrition does not depend on the selection of any one food. Instead, it depends on the overall **eating pattern**—the combination of many different foods and beverages at numerous meals over days, months, and years.[14] So how can health care professionals help people select foods to create an eating pattern that supplies all the needed nutrients in amounts consistent with good health? The principle is simple enough: encourage clients to eat a variety of foods that supply all the nutrients the body needs. In practice, how do people do this? It helps to keep in mind that a nutritious diet achieves six basic ideals.

Dietary Ideals

A nutritious diet has the following six characteristics:

- Adequacy
- Balance
- kCalorie (energy) control
- Nutrient density
- Moderation
- Variety

The first, **adequacy**, was already addressed in the earlier discussion on the DRI. An adequate diet has enough energy and enough of every nutrient (as well as fiber) to meet the needs of healthy people. Second is **balance**: the food choices do not overemphasize one nutrient or food type at the expense of another. Balance in the diet helps to ensure adequacy.

The essential minerals calcium and iron illustrate the importance of dietary balance. Meat is rich in iron but poor in calcium. Conversely, milk is rich in calcium but poor in iron. Use some meat for iron; use some milk for calcium; and save some space for other foods, too, because a diet consisting of milk and meat alone would not be adequate. For other nutrients, people need to consume other protein foods, whole grains, vegetables, and fruit.

The third characteristic is **kcalorie (energy) control**: the foods provide the amount of energy needed to maintain a healthy body weight—not more, not less. The key to kcalorie control is to select foods that deliver the most nutrients for the least food energy. The fourth characteristic of a nutritious diet, **nutrient density**, promotes adequacy and kcalorie control. To eat well without overeating, select nutrient-dense foods—that is, foods that deliver the most nutrients for the least food energy.[15] Consider foods containing calcium, for example. You can get about 300 milligrams of calcium from either 1½ ounces of cheddar cheese or 1 cup of fat-free milk, but the cheese delivers about twice as much food energy (kcalories) as the milk. The fat-free milk, then, is twice as calcium dense as the cheddar cheese; it offers the same amount of calcium

TABLE 1-3 Leading Causes of Death in the United States

The diseases in bold italics are nutrition related.

1. ***Heart disease***
2. ***Cancers***
3. Chronic lung diseases
4. Accidents
5. ***Strokes***
6. Alzheimer's disease
7. ***Diabetes mellitus***
8. Pneumonia and influenza
9. Kidney disease
10. Suicide

Source: J. Xu and coauthors, Mortality in the United States, 2015, *NCHS Data Brief* 267, December 2016.

overnutrition: overconsumption of food energy or nutrients sufficient to cause disease or increased susceptibility to disease; a form of malnutrition.

undernutrition: underconsumption of food energy or nutrients severe enough to cause disease or increased susceptibility to disease; a form of malnutrition.

chronic diseases: diseases characterized by slow progression, long duration, and degeneration of body organs due in part to such personal lifestyle elements as poor food choices, smoking, alcohol use, and lack of physical activity.

eating pattern: customary intake of foods and beverages over time.

adequacy: the characteristic of a diet that provides all the essential nutrients, fiber, and energy necessary to maintain health and body weight.

balance: the dietary characteristic of providing foods in proportion to one another and in proportion to the body's needs.

kcalorie (energy) control: management of food energy intake.

nutrient density: a measure of the nutrients a food provides relative to the energy it provides. The more nutrients and the fewer kcalories, the higher the nutrient density.

empty kcalories: kcalories provided
by added sugars and solid fats with
few or no other nutrients.

nutrient profiling: ranking foods
based on their nutrient composition.

moderation: the provision of enough,
but not too much, of a substance.

solid fats: fats that are not usually liquid
at room temperature; commonly found
in most foods derived from animals
and vegetable oils that have been
hydrogenated. Solid fats typically contain
more saturated and *trans* fats than most
oils (Chapter 4 provides more details).

added sugars: sugars, syrups, and other
kcaloric sweeteners that are added to
foods during processing or preparation
or at the table. Added sugars do not
include the naturally occurring sugars
found in fruit and in milk products.

variety: consumption of a wide selection
of foods within and among the major
food groups (the opposite of monotony).

for half the kcalories. Both foods are excellent choices for adequacy's sake alone, but to achieve adequacy while controlling kcalories, the fat-free milk is the better choice. (Alternatively, a person could select a low-fat cheddar cheese providing kcalories comparable to fat-free milk.)

Just as a financially responsible person pays for rent, food, clothes, and tuition on a limited budget, healthy people obtain iron, calcium, and all the other essential nutrients on a limited energy (kcalorie) allowance. Success depends on getting many nutrients for each kcalorie "dollar." For example, a can of cola and a handful of grapes may both provide about the same number of kcalories, but grapes deliver many more nutrients. A person who makes nutrient-dense choices, such as fruit instead of cola, can meet daily nutrient needs on a lower energy budget. Such choices support good health.

Foods that are notably low in nutrient density—such as potato chips, cakes, pies, candy, and colas—deliver **empty kcalories**. The kcalories these foods provide are called "empty" because they deliver a lot of energy (from added sugars, solid fats, or both) but little or no protein, vitamins, or minerals.

The concept of nutrient density is relatively simple when examining the contributions of one nutrient to a food or diet. With respect to calcium, milk ranks high and meats rank low. With respect to iron, meats rank high and milk ranks low. But which food is more nutritious? Answering that question is a more complex task because we need to consider several nutrients—those that may harm health and those that may be beneficial.[16] Ranking foods based on their overall nutrient composition is known as **nutrient profiling**. Researchers have yet to agree on an ideal way to rate foods based on the nutrient profile, but when they do, nutrient profiling will be quite useful in helping consumers identify nutritious foods and plan healthy diets.[17]

The fifth characteristic of a nutritious diet is **moderation**. Moderation contributes to adequacy, balance, and kcalorie control. Foods rich in **solid fats** and **added sugars** often provide some enjoyment and lots of energy but relatively few nutrients. In addition, they promote weight gain when eaten in excess. A person who practices moderation eats such foods only on occasion and regularly selects foods low in solid fats and added sugars, a practice that automatically improves nutrient density. Returning to the example of cheddar cheese and fat-free milk, the milk not only offers more calcium for less energy, but it contains far less fat than the cheese.

Finally, the sixth characteristic of a nutritious diet, **variety**, improves nutrient adequacy. A diet may have all the virtues just described and still lack variety if a person eats the same foods day after day. People should select foods from each of the food groups daily and vary their choices within each food group from day to day, for a couple of reasons. First, different foods within the same group contain different arrays of nutrients. Consider fruit, for example, strawberries are especially rich in vitamin C while apricots are rich in vitamin A. Second, no food is guaranteed to be entirely free of substances that, in excess, could be harmful. The strawberries might contain trace amounts of one contaminant, the apricots another. By alternating fruit choices, a person will ingest very little of either contaminant.

Dietary Guidelines for Americans

Many countries set dietary guidelines to answer the question, "What should I eat to stay healthy?" In the United States, for example, the U.S. Department of Agriculture published its *Dietary Guidelines for Americans 2015–2020* as part of an overall nutrition guidance system. While the DRI set nutrient intake goals, the Dietary Guidelines for Americans offer food-based strategies for achieving them. If everyone followed their advice, people's energy intakes would match their requirements and most of their nutrient needs would be met.* Table 1-4 presents the *Dietary Guidelines for Americans 2015–2020* and key recommendations.

---

*USDA Food Patterns may not provide recommended intakes of vitamin D and potassium.

TABLE 1-4 2015–2020 Dietary Guidelines for Americans: The Guidelines and Key Recommendations

THE GUIDELINES

The following guidelines "encourage healthy eating patterns, recognize that individuals will need to make shifts in their food and beverage choices to achieve a healthy pattern, and acknowledge that all segments of our society have a role to play in supporting healthy choices."

1. **Follow a healthy eating pattern across the lifespan.** All food and beverage choices matter. Choose a healthy eating pattern at an appropriate kcalorie level to help achieve and maintain a healthy body weight, support nutrient adequacy, and reduce the risk of chronic disease.

2. **Focus on variety, nutrient density, and amount.** To meet nutrient needs within kcalorie limits, choose a variety of nutrient-dense foods across and within all food groups in recommended amounts.

3. **Limit kcalories from added sugars and saturated fats and reduce sodium intake.** Adopt an eating pattern low in added sugars, saturated fats, and sodium. Cut back on foods and beverages higher in these components to amounts that fit within healthy eating patterns.

4. **Shift to healthier food and beverage choices.** Choose nutrient-dense foods and beverages across and within all food groups in place of less healthy choices. Consider cultural and personal preferences to make these shifts easier to accomplish and maintain.

5. **Support healthy eating patterns for all.** Everyone has a role in helping to create and support healthy eating patterns in multiple settings nationwide, from home to school to work to communities.

KEY RECOMMENDATIONS

The following key recommendations provide more detailed tips on how individuals can establish healthy eating patterns to meet the guidelines.

Adopt a healthy eating pattern that accounts for all foods and beverages within an appropriate kcalorie level.

A healthy eating pattern includes:

- A variety of vegetables from all of the subgroups—dark green, red and orange, legumes (beans and peas), starchy, and other.
- Fruit, especially whole fruit.
- Grains, at least half of which are whole grains.
- Fat-free or low-fat dairy, including milk, yogurt, cheese, and/or fortified soy beverages.
- A variety of protein foods, including seafood, lean meats and poultry, eggs, legumes (beans and peas), and nuts, seeds, and soy products.
- Oils.

A healthy eating pattern limits:

- Saturated fats and *trans* fats to less than 10 percent of kcalories per day.
- Added sugars to less than 10 percent of kcalories per day.
- Sodium to less than 2300 milligrams per day.
- If alcohol is consumed, it should be consumed in moderation—up to one drink per day for women and up to two drinks per day for men—and only by adults of legal drinking age.

Meet the *Physical Activity Guidelines for Americans* (health.gov/paguidelines).

Note: These guidelines and key recommendations are designed for individuals 2 years of age or older and should be applied in their entirety; they are interconnected, and each dietary component can affect the others.

Source: U.S. Department of Health and Human Services and U.S. Department of Agriculture, *2015–2020 Dietary Guidelines for Americans,* 8th ed. (2015): health.gov /dietaryguidelines/2015/guidelines/.

People who follow the Dietary Guidelines—that is, those who do not overconsume kcalories, who take in enough of a variety of nutrient-dense foods and beverages, and who make physical activity a habit—often enjoy the best possible health. Only a few people in this country meet this description, however. Instead, about half of American adults suffer from one or more *preventable* chronic diseases related to poor diets and sedentary lifestyles.

Note that the Dietary Guidelines do not require that you give up your favorite foods or eat strange, unappealing foods. They advocate achieving a healthy dietary pattern through wise food and beverage choices and not by way of nutrient or other dietary supplements except when medically necessary. With a little planning and a few adjustments, almost anyone's diet can contribute to health instead of disease. The Dietary

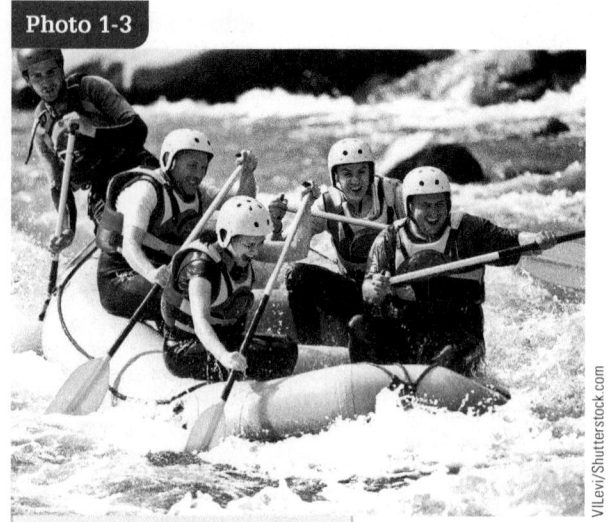

Photo 1-3

Physical activity helps you look good, feel good, and have fun, and it brings many long-term health benefits as well.

Guidelines also challenge the nation and local communities to change their policies in ways that make health and disease prevention high priorities. Part of the plan must be to increase individuals' physical activity to help achieve and sustain a healthy body weight, and the next section offers some guidelines.

Fitness Guidelines

Extensive evidence confirms that regular physical activity promotes health and reduces the risk of developing a number of diseases.[18] Yet, despite an increasing awareness of the health benefits physical activity confers, only about 20 percent of adults in the United States meet physical activity guidelines.[19] Like smoking and obesity, physical inactivity is linked to the degenerative diseases that are the primary killers of adults in developed countries: heart disease, cancer, stroke, diabetes, and hypertension.[20] Therefore, one of the most important challenges health care professionals face is to motivate more people to become physically active (see Photo 1-3). To motivate others, health care professionals must first become more physically active themselves, thereby enhancing their own health. Second, they can include regular physical activity as a component of therapy for their clients. As a person becomes physically fit, the health of the entire body improves. In general, physically fit people enjoy:

- *More restful sleep*. Rest and sleep occur naturally after periods of physical activity. During rest, the body repairs injuries, disposes of wastes generated during activity, and builds new physical structures.
- *Improved nutritional health*. Physical activity expends energy and thus allows people to eat more food. If they choose wisely, active people will consume more nutrients and be less likely to develop nutrient deficiencies.
- *Improved body composition*. A balanced program of physical activity limits body fat and increases or maintains lean tissue. Thus, physically active people may have relatively less body fat than sedentary people at the same body weight.[21]
- *Improved bone density*. Weight-bearing physical activity builds bone strength and protects against osteoporosis.[22]
- *Enhanced resistance to colds and other infectious diseases*. Fitness enhances immunity.*
- *Lower risks of some types of cancers*. Lifelong physical activity may help to protect against colon cancer, breast cancer, and some other cancers.[23]
- *Stronger circulation and lung function*. Physical activity that challenges the heart and lungs strengthens both the circulatory and respiratory systems.
- *Lower risks of cardiovascular disease*. Physical activity lowers blood pressure, slows resting pulse rate, lowers total blood cholesterol, and raises HDL cholesterol, thus reducing the risks of heart attacks and strokes.[24] Some research suggests that physical activity may reduce the risk of cardiovascular disease in another way as well—by reducing intra-abdominal fat stores.[25]
- *Lower risks of type 2 diabetes*. Physical activity normalizes glucose tolerance.[26] Regular physical activity reduces the risk of developing type 2 diabetes and benefits those who already have the condition.
- *Reduced risk of gallbladder disease*. Regular physical activity reduces the risk of gallbladder disease—perhaps by facilitating weight control and lowering blood lipid levels.[27]

aerobic physical activity: activity in which the body's large muscles move in a rhythmic manner for a sustained period of time. Aerobic activity, also called *endurance activity*, improves cardiorespiratory fitness. Brisk walking, running, swimming, and bicycling are examples.

---

*Moderate physical activity can stimulate immune function. Intense, vigorous, prolonged activity such as marathon running, however, may compromise immune function.

- *Lower incidence and severity of anxiety and depression.* Physical activity may improve mood and enhance the quality of life by reducing depression and anxiety.[28]
- *Stronger self-image.* The sense of achievement that comes from meeting physical challenges promotes self-confidence.
- *Long life and high quality of life in the later years.* Active people live longer, healthier lives than sedentary people do.[29] Even as little as 15 minutes a day of moderate-intensity activity can add years to a person's life.[30] In addition to extending longevity, physical activity supports independence and mobility in later life by reducing the risk of falls and minimizing the risk of injury should a fall occur.[31]

What does a person have to do to reap the health rewards of physical activity? To gain substantial *health* benefits, most guidelines recommend a minimum amount of time performing **aerobic physical activity**. The minimum amount of time depends on whether the activity is **moderate-intensity physical activity** or **vigorous-intensity physical activity**. Whether moderate- or vigorous-intensity, a minimum length of 10 minutes for short bouts of aerobic physical activity is recommended.[32] Of course, more time and greater intensity bring even greater health benefits: maintaining a healthy body weight and further reducing the risk of chronic diseases.

In addition to providing health benefits, physical activity helps to develop and maintain **fitness**. Table 1-5 presents the American College of Sports Medicine (ACSM) guidelines for physical activity.[33] Fitness and health both depend on maintaining an active lifestyle every day.

moderate-intensity physical activity: physical activity that requires some increase in breathing and/or heart rate and expends 3.5 to 7 kcalories per minute. Walking at a speed of 3 to 4.5 miles per hour (about 15 to 20 minutes to walk one mile) is an example.

vigorous-intensity physical activity: physical activity that requires a large increase in breathing and/or heart rate and expends more than 7 kcalories per minute. Walking at a very brisk pace (>4.5 miles per hour) or running at a pace of at least 5 miles per hour are examples.

fitness: the characteristics that enable the body to perform physical activity; more broadly, the ability to meet routine physical demands with enough reserve energy to rise to a physical challenge; the body's ability to withstand stress of all kinds.

TABLE 1-5 American College of Sports Medicine's Guidelines for Physical Activity

	CARDIORESPIRATORY	STRENGTH	FLEXIBILITY
Type of activity	Aerobic activity that uses large-muscle groups and can be maintained continuously	Resistance activity that is performed at a controlled speed and through a full range of motion	Stretching activity that uses the major muscle groups
Frequency	5 to 7 days per week	2 or more nonconsecutive days per week	2 to 7 days per week
Intensity	Moderate (equivalent to walking at a pace of 3 to 4 miles per hour)[a]	Enough to enhance muscle strength and improve body composition	Enough to feel tightness or slight discomfort
Duration	At least 30 minutes per day	8 to 12 repetitions of 8 to 10 different exercises (minimum)	2 to 4 repetitions of 15 to 30 seconds per muscle group
Examples	Running, cycling, swimming, inline skating, rowing, power walking, cross-country skiing, kickboxing, jumping rope; sports activities such as basketball, soccer, racquetball, tennis, volleyball	Pull-ups, push-ups, weight-lifting, pilates	Yoga

[a]For those who prefer vigorous-intensity aerobic activity such as walking at a very brisk pace (>4.5 mph) or running (5 mph), a minimum of 20 minutes per day, 3 days per week is recommended.

Sources: American College of Sports Medicine position stand, Quantity and quality of exercise for developing and maintaining cardiorespiratory, musculoskeletal, and neuromotor fitness in apparently healthy adults: Guidance for prescribing exercise, *Medicine and Science in Sports and Exercise* 43 (2011): 1334–1359; W. L. Haskell and coauthors, Physical activity and public health: Updated recommendation for adults from the American College of Sports Medicine and the American Heart Association, *Medicine and Science in Sports and Exercise* 39 (2007): 1423–1434.

The USDA Food Patterns

To help people achieve the goals set forth by the Dietary Guidelines for Americans, the USDA provides a **food group plan**—the **USDA Food Patterns**—that builds a diet from categories of foods that are similar in vitamin and mineral content. Thus, each group provides a set of nutrients that differs somewhat from the nutrients supplied by the other groups. Selecting foods from each of the groups eases the task of creating an adequate and balanced diet. The DASH Eating Plan, presented in Chapter 21, is another dietary pattern that meets the goals of the Dietary Guidelines for Americans.

Figure 1-4 (pp. 20–21) presents the major food groups and their subgroups. The plan assigns foods to five major food groups—fruit, vegetables, grains, protein foods, and milk and milk products. The USDA specifies portions (ounce or cup equivalents) of various foods within each group that are nutritional equivalents and thus can be treated interchangeably in diet planning. Figure 1-4 lists the key nutrients of each group, information worth noting and remembering, and also sorts foods within each group by nutrient density.

Recommended Amounts All food groups offer valuable nutrients, and people should make selections from each group daily. Table 1-6 presents the recommended daily amounts from each food group for one of the USDA Food Patterns—the Healthy U.S.-Style Eating Pattern. (Nutrition in Practice 4 introduces the Healthy Mediterranean-Style Eating Pattern, and Nutrition in Practice 5 includes the Healthy Vegetarian Eating Pattern.) As Table 1-6 shows, an adult needing 2000 kcalories a day, for example, would select 2 cups of fruit; 2½ cups of vegetables; 6 ounces of grain foods; 5½ ounces of protein foods; and 3 cups of milk or milk products.* Additionally, a small amount of unsaturated oil, such as vegetable oil or the oils of nuts, olives, or fatty fish, is required to supply needed nutrients. Estimated daily kcalorie needs for sedentary and active men and women are shown in Table 1-7. Chapter 6 explains how to determine energy needs.

All vegetables provide an array of vitamins, fiber, and the mineral potassium, but some vegetables are especially good sources of certain nutrients and beneficial phytochemicals. For this reason, the vegetable group is sorted into five subgroups. The dark green vegetables deliver the B vitamin folate; the red and orange vegetables provide vitamin A; legumes supply iron and protein; the starchy vegetables contribute carbohydrate energy; and the other vegetables fill in the gaps and add more of these same nutrients.

In a 2000-kcalorie diet, then, the recommended 2½ cups of daily vegetables should be varied among the subgroups over a week's time. In other words, eating 2½ cups of potatoes or even nutrient-rich spinach every day for seven days does *not* meet the recommended vegetable intakes. Potatoes and spinach make excellent choices when consumed in balance with vegetables from the other subgroups. One way to help ensure selections for all of the subgroups is to eat vegetables of various colors—for example, green broccoli, orange sweet potatoes, black beans, yellow corn, and white cauliflower. Intakes of vegetables are appropriately averaged over a week's time—it isn't necessary to include every subgroup every day.

For similar reasons, the protein foods group is sorted into three subgroups. Perhaps most notably, each of these subgroups contributes a different assortment of fats. Table 1-8 (p. 22) presents the recommended *weekly* amounts for each of the subgroups for vegetables and protein foods.

Notable Nutrients As Figure 1-4 notes, each food group contributes key nutrients. This feature provides flexibility in diet planning because a person can select any food from a food group (or its subgroup) and receive similar nutrients. For example, a person can choose milk, cheese, or yogurt and receive the same key nutrients. Importantly, foods provide not only these key nutrients, but small amounts of other nutrients and phytochemicals as well.

Legumes contribute the same key nutrients—notably protein, iron, and zinc—as meats, poultry, and seafood. They are also excellent sources of fiber, folate, and potassium, which

---

*Milk and milk products also can be referred to as dairy products.

TABLE 1-6	USDA Food Patterns: Healthy U.S.-Style Eating Pattern							
FOOD GROUP	1600 kcal	1800 kcal	2000 kcal	2200 kcal	2400 kcal	2600 kcal	2800 kcal	3000 kcal
Fruit	1 ½ c	1 ½ c	2 c	2 c	2 c	2 c	2 ½ c	2 ½ c
Vegetables	2 c	2 ½ c	2 ½ c	3 c	3 c	3 ½ c	3 ½ c	4 c
Grains	5 oz	6 oz	6 oz	7 oz	8 oz	9 oz	10 oz	10 oz
Protein foods	5 oz	5 oz	5 ½ oz	6 oz	6 ½ oz	6 ½ oz	7 oz	7 oz
Milk	3 c	3 c	3 c	3 c	3 c	3 c	3 c	3 c
Oils	5 tsp	5 tsp	6 tsp	6 tsp	7 tsp	8 tsp	8 tsp	10 tsp
Limit on kcalories available for other uses*	130 kcal	170 kcal	270 kcal	280 kcal	350 kcal	380 kcal	400 kcal	470 kcal

*The limit on kcalories for other uses describes how many kcalories are available for foods that are not in nutrient-dense forms.

Source: U.S. Department of Health and Human Services and U.S. Department of Agriculture, *2015–2020 Dietary Guidelines for Americans,* 8th ed. (2015): health.gov/dietaryguidelines/2015/guidelines/.

are commonly found in vegetables. To encourage frequent consumption of these nutrient-rich foods, legumes are included as a subgroup of both the vegetable group and the protein foods group, and thus can be counted as either.[34] In general, people who regularly eat meat, poultry, and seafood count legumes as a vegetable, and vegetarians and others who seldom eat meat, poultry, or seafood count legumes in the protein foods group.

The USDA Food Patterns encourage greater consumption from certain food groups to provide the nutrients most often lacking in the diets of Americans—dietary fiber, choline, vitamin A, vitamin C, Vitamin D, Vitamin E, calcium, magnesium, and potassium. In general, most people need to eat:

- *More* vegetables, fruit, whole grains, seafood, and fat-free or low-fat milk and milk products.
- *Less* sodium, saturated fat, and *trans* fat, and *fewer* refined grains and foods and beverages with solid fats and added sugars.

Nutrient-Dense Choices A healthy eating pattern emphasizes nutrient-dense options within each food group. By consistently selecting nutrient-dense foods, a person can obtain all the nutrients needed and still keep kcalories under control. In contrast, eating foods that are low in nutrient density makes it difficult to get enough nutrients without exceeding energy needs and gaining weight. For this reason, consumers should select nutrient-dense foods from each group and foods without solid fats or added sugars—for example, fat-free milk instead of whole milk, baked chicken without the skin instead of hot dogs, green beans instead of french fries, orange juice instead of fruit punch, and whole-wheat bread instead of biscuits. Notice that Figure 1-4 indicates which foods *within each group* contain solid fats and/or added sugars and therefore should be limited. Oil is a notable exception: even though oil is pure fat and therefore rich in kcalories, a small amount of oil from sources such as nuts, fish, or vegetable oils is necessary every day to provide nutrients lacking from other foods. Consequently, these high-fat foods are listed among the nutrient-dense foods (see Nutrition in Practice 4 to learn why).

TABLE 1-7	Estimated Daily kCalorie Needs for Adults	
	SEDENTARY[a]	ACTIVE[b]
Women		
19–25 yr	2000	2400
26–30 yr	1800	2400
31–50 yr	1800	2200
51–60 yr	1600	2200
61+ yr	1600	2000
Men		
19–20 yr	2600	3000
21–35 yr	2400	3000
36–40 yr	2400	2800
41–55 yr	2200	2800
56–60 yr	2200	2600
61–75 yr	2000	2600
76+ yr	2000	2400

[a]*Sedentary* describes a lifestyle that includes only the activities typical of day-to-day life.
[b]*Active* describes a lifestyle that includes physical activity equivalent to walking more than 3 miles per day at a rate of 3 to 4 miles per hour, in addition to the activities typical of day-to-day life. In addition to gender, age, and activity level, energy needs vary with height and weight (see Chapter 6).

FIGURE 1-4   USDA Food Patterns: Food Groups and Subgroups

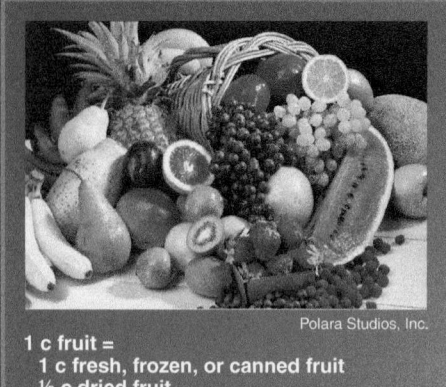

Fruit contributes folate, vitamin A, vitamin C, potassium, and fiber.

Consume a variety of fruit, and choose whole or cut-up fruit more often than fruit juice.

Apples, apricots, avocados, bananas, blueberries, cantaloupe, cherries, grapefruit, grapes, guava, honeydew, kiwi, mango, nectarines, oranges, papaya, peaches, pears, pineapples, plums, raspberries, strawberries, tangerines, watermelon; dried fruit (dates, figs, prunes, raisins); 100% fruit juices

Limit fruit that contains solid fats and/or added sugars:
Canned or frozen fruit in syrup; juices, punches, ades, and fruit drinks with added sugars; fried plantains

Polara Studios, Inc.

1 c fruit =
  1 c fresh, frozen, or canned fruit
  ½ c dried fruit
  1 c 100% fruit juice

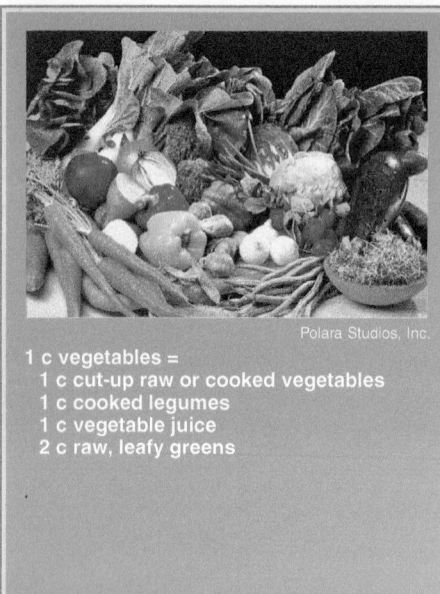

Vegetables contribute folate, vitamin A, vitamin C, vitamin K, vitamin E, magnesium, potassium, and fiber.

Consume a variety of vegetables each day, and choose from all five subgroups several times a week.

Dark-green vegetables: Broccoli and leafy greens such as arugula, beet greens, bok choy, collard greens, kale, mustard greens, romaine lettuce, spinach, turnip greens, watercress

Red and orange vegetables: Carrots, carrot juice, pumpkin, red bell peppers, sweet potatoes, tomatoes, tomato juice, vegetable juice, winter squash (acorn, butternut)

Legumes: Black beans, black-eyed peas, garbanzo beans (chickpeas), kidney beans, lentils, navy beans, pinto beans, soybeans and soy products such as tofu, split peas, white beans

Starchy vegetables: Cassava, corn, green peas, hominy, lima beans, potatoes

Other vegetables: Artichokes, asparagus, bamboo shoots, bean sprouts, beets, brussels sprouts, cabbages, cactus, cauliflower, celery, cucumbers, eggplant, green beans, green bell peppers, iceberg lettuce, mushrooms, okra, onions, seaweed, snow peas, zucchini

Limit these vegetables that contain solid fats and/or added sugars:
Baked beans, candied sweet potatoes, coleslaw, french fries, potato salad, refried beans, scalloped potatoes, tempura vegetables

Polara Studios, Inc.

1 c vegetables =
  1 c cut-up raw or cooked vegetables
  1 c cooked legumes
  1 c vegetable juice
  2 c raw, leafy greens

Grains contribute folate, niacin, riboflavin, thiamin, iron, magnesium, selenium, and fiber.

Make most (at least half) of the grain selections whole grains.

Whole grains: Amaranth, barley, brown rice, buckwheat, bulgur, cornmeal, millet, oats, quinoa, rye, wheat, wild rice and whole-grain products such as breads, cereals, crackers, and pastas; popcorn

Enriched refined products: Bagels, breads, cereals, pastas (couscous, macaroni, spaghetti), pretzels, white rice, rolls, tortillas

Limit these grains that contain solid fats and/or added sugars:
Biscuits, cakes, cookies, cornbread, crackers, croissants, doughnuts, fried rice, granola, muffins, pastries, pies, presweetened cereals, taco shells

Polara Studios, Inc.

1 oz grains =
  1 slice bread
  ½ c cooked rice, pasta, or cereal
  1 oz dry pasta or rice
  1 c ready-to-eat cereal
  3 c popped popcorn

(Continued)

FIGURE 1-4 USDA Food Patterns: Food Groups and Subgroups *(continued)*

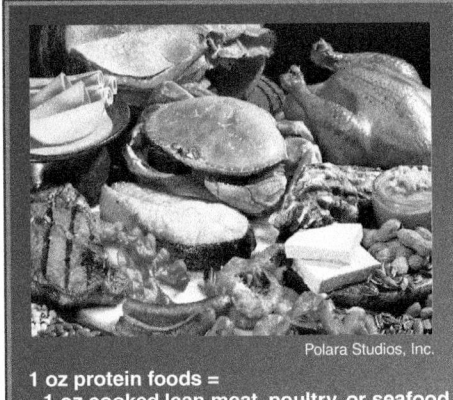

Polara Studios, Inc.

1 oz protein foods =
1 oz cooked lean meat, poultry, or seafood
1 egg
¼ c cooked legumes or tofu
1 tbs peanut butter
½ oz nuts or seeds

Protein foods contribute protein, essential fatty acids, niacin, thiamin, vitamin B_6, vitamin B_{12}, iron, magnesium, potassium, and zinc.

Choose a variety of protein foods from the three subgroups, including seafood in place of meat or poultry twice a week.

Seafood: Fish (catfish, cod, flounder, haddock, halibut, herring, mackerel, pollock, salmon, sardines, sea bass, snapper, trout, tuna), shellfish (clams, crab, lobster, mussels, oysters, scallops, shrimp)

Meats, poultry, eggs: Lean or low-fat meats (fat-trimmed beef, game, ham, lamb, pork, veal), poultry (no skin), eggs

Nuts, seeds, soy products: Unsalted nuts (almonds, cashews, filberts, pecans, pistachios, walnuts), seeds (flaxseeds, pumpkin seeds, sesame seeds, sunflower seeds), legumes, soy products (textured vegetable protein, tofu, tempeh), peanut butter, peanuts

Limit these protein foods that contain solid fats and/or added sugars:
Bacon; baked beans; fried meat, seafood, poultry, eggs, or tofu; refried beans; ground beef; hot dogs; luncheon meats; marbled steaks; poultry with skin; sausages; spare ribs

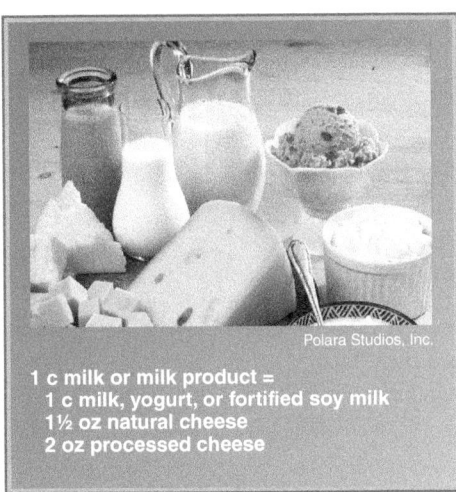

Polara Studios, Inc.

1 c milk or milk product =
1 c milk, yogurt, or fortified soy milk
1½ oz natural cheese
2 oz processed cheese

Milk and milk products contribute protein, riboflavin, vitamin B_{12}, calcium, potassium, and, when fortified, vitamin A and vitamin D.

Make fat-free or low-fat choices. Choose other calcium-rich foods if you don't consume milk.

Fat-free or 1% low-fat milk and fat-free or 1% low-fat milk products such as buttermilk, cheeses, cottage cheese, yogurt; fat-free fortified soy milk

Limit these milk products that contain solid fats and/or added sugars:
2% reduced-fat milk and whole milk; 2% reduced-fat and whole-milk products such as cheeses, cottage cheese, and yogurt; flavored milk with added sugars such as chocolate milk, custard, frozen yogurt, ice cream, milk shakes, pudding, sherbet; fortified soy milk

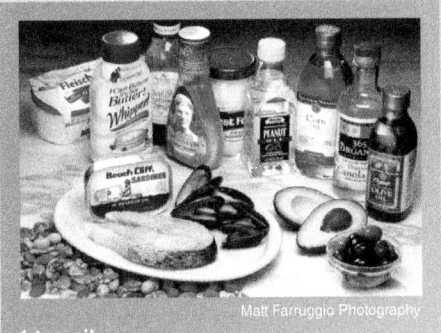

Matt Farruggio Photography

1 tsp oil =
1 tsp vegetable oil
1 tsp soft margarine
1 tbs low-fat mayonnaise
2 tbs light salad dressing

Oils are not a food group, but are featured here because they contribute vitamin E and essential fatty acids.

Use oils instead of solid fats, when possible.

Liquid vegetable oils such as canola, corn, flaxseed, nut, olive, peanut, safflower, sesame, soybean, sunflower oils; mayonnaise, oil-based salad dressing, soft *trans*-free margarine; unsaturated oils that occur naturally in foods such as avocados, fatty fish, nuts, olives, seeds (flaxseeds, sesame seeds), shellfish

Limit these solid fats:
Butter, animal fats, stick margarine, shortening

TABLE 1-8 **Recommended Weekly Amounts from the Vegetable and Protein Foods Subgroups**

VEGETABLES SUBGROUPS	1600 kcal	1800 kcal	2000 kcal	2200 kcal	2400 kcal	2600 kcal	2800 kcal	3000 kcal
Dark green	1 ½ c	1 ½ c	1 ½ c	2 c	2 c	2 ½ c	2 ½ c	2 ½ c
Red and orange	4 c	5 ½ c	5 ½ c	6 c	6 c	7 c	7 c	7 ½ c
Legumes	1 c	1 ½ c	1 ½ c	2 c	2 c	2 ½ c	2 ½ c	3 c
Starchy	4 c	5 c	5 c	6 c	6 c	7 c	7 c	8 c
Other	3 ½ c	4 c	4 c	5 c	5 c	5 ½ c	5 ½ c	7
PROTEIN FOODS SUBGROUPS								
Seafood	8 oz	8 oz	8 oz	9 oz	10 oz	10 oz	10 oz	10 oz
Meats, poultry, eggs	23 oz	23 oz	26 oz	28 oz	31 oz	31 oz	33 oz	33 oz
Nuts, seeds, soy products	4 oz	4 oz	5 oz	5 oz	5 oz	5 oz	6 oz	6 oz

Note: Table 1-6 specifies the recommended amounts of total vegetables and protein foods per day. This table shows those amounts dispersed among five vegetable and three protein foods subgroups per *week*.

Source: U.S. Department of Health and Human Services and U.S. Department of Agriculture, *2015–2020 Dietary Guidelines for Americans,* 8th ed. (2015): health .gov/dietaryguidelines/2015/guidelines/.

Solid Fats, Added Sugars, and Alcohol Reduce Nutrient Density As noted earlier, solid fats and added sugars add empty kcalories to foods, reducing their nutrient density. Solid fats include:

- Naturally occurring fats such as milk fat and meat fats.
- Added fats, such as butter, cream cheese, hard margarine, lard, sour cream, and shortening.

Added sugars include:

- All kcaloric sweeteners, such as brown sugar, honey, molasses, sugar, and syrups; and foods made from them, such as candy, jelly, and soft drinks.

Table 1-6 includes a limit on kcalories available for other uses. If all food choices are nutrient-dense, a small number of kcalories remain within the overall kcalorie limit of the eating pattern. These kcalories can be used for solid fats, added sugars, or to eat additional amounts of nutrient-dense foods. Alternatively, a person wanting to lose weight might choose to *not* use these kcalories.

Alcoholic beverages are a top contributor of kcalories to the diets of many U.S. adults, but they provide few nutrients. People who drink alcohol should monitor and moderate their intakes, not to exceed one drink per day for women and two for men. People in many circumstances should never drink alcohol (see Nutrition in Practice 19).

Cup and Ounce Equivalents Recommended daily amounts for fruit, vegetables, and milk are measured in cups, and those for grains and protein foods in ounces (see Photo 1-4). Figure 1-4 provides the equivalent measures for foods that are

Photo 1-4

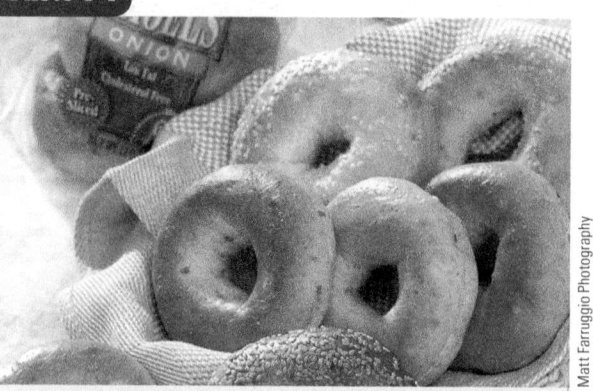

A portion of grains is 1 ounce, yet most bagels today weigh 4 ounces or more—meaning that a single bagel can easily supply four or more portions of grains, not one, as many people assume.

Matt Farruggio Photography

not readily measured in cups and ounces. For example, 1 ounce of grains is considered equivalent to 1 slice of bread or $^1/_2$ cup of cooked rice.

Consumers using the USDA Food Patterns can learn how to estimate the cups or ounces in their usual **portion sizes** by determining the answers to questions such as these: What fraction of a cup is a small handful of raisins? Is a "helping" of mashed potatoes more or less than a half cup? How many ounces of cereal do you typically pour into your bowl? How many ounces does the steak at your favorite restaurant weigh? How many cups of milk does your glass hold? For quick and easy estimates, visualize each portion as being about the size of a common object:

portion sizes: the quantity of food served or eaten at one meal or snack; *not* a standard amount.

- $^1/_4$ c dried fruit or nuts = a golf ball
- 1 c fruit or vegetables = a baseball
- 3 oz meat = a deck of cards
- 2 tbs peanut butter = a ping pong ball

Mixtures of Foods Some foods—such as casseroles, soups, and sandwiches—fall into two or more food groups. With a little practice, users can learn to divide these foods into food groups. From the USDA Food Patterns' point of view, a taco represents four different food groups: the taco shell from the grains group; the onions, lettuce, and tomatoes from the vegetable group; the ground beef from the protein foods group; and the cheese from the milk group.

Vegetarian Food Guide Vegetarian diets are plant-based eating patterns that rely mainly on grains, vegetables, legumes, fruit, seeds, and nuts. Some vegetarian diets include eggs, milk products, or both. People who do not eat meats or milk products can use the USDA Healthy Vegetarian Eating Pattern to create an adequate diet.[35] Nutrition in Practice 5 defines vegetarian terms and provides details on planning healthy vegetarian diets.

Ethnic Food Choices People can use the USDA Food Patterns and still enjoy a diverse array of culinary styles by sorting ethnic foods into their appropriate food groups. For example, a person eating Mexican foods would find tortillas in the grains group, jicama in the vegetable group, and guava in the fruit group. Table 1-1 (p. 4) features ethnic food choices.

MyPlate

The USDA created an educational tool called MyPlate to illustrate the five food groups and remind consumers to make healthy food choices. The MyPlate icon, shown in Figure 1-5, divides a plate into four sections, each representing a food group—fruit, vegetables, grains, and protein foods. The sections vary in size, indicating the relative proportion each food group contributes to a healthy diet. A circle next to the plate represents the milk group (dairy).

The MyPlate icon does not stand alone as an educational tool. A wealth of information can be found at the MyPlate website (www.choosemyplate.gov). The USDA's MyPlate online suite of information makes applying the USDA Food Patterns easier. Consumers can create a personal profile to estimate kcalorie needs and determine the kinds and amounts of foods they need to eat each day based on their height, weight, age, gender, and activity level. Information is also available for children, pregnant and lactating women, and vegetarians. In addition to creating a personal plan, consumers can find daily tips to help them improve their diet and increase physical activity. A key message of the website is to enjoy food, but eat less by avoiding oversized portions.

FIGURE 1-5 MyPlate

Note that vegetables and fruit occupy half the plate and that the grains portion is slightly larger than the portion of protein foods.

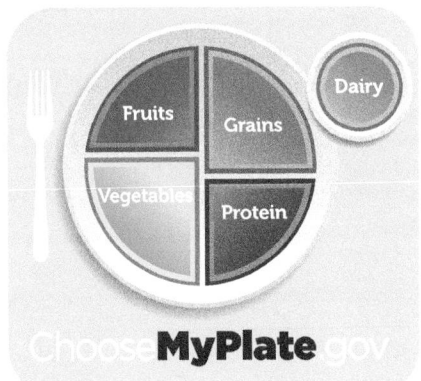

Source: USDA, www.choosemyplate.gov.

1.6 Food Labels

Today, consumers know more about the links between diet and disease than they did in the past, and they are demanding still more information on disease prevention. Many people rely on food labels to help them select foods with less saturated fat, *trans* fat, and sodium and more vitamins, minerals, and dietary fiber. Food labels appear on virtually all packaged foods, and posters or brochures provide similar nutrition information for fresh fruit, vegetables, and other foods. A few foods need not carry nutrition labels: those contributing few nutrients, such as plain coffee, tea, and spices; those produced by small businesses; and those prepared and sold in the same establishment. Markets selling nonpackaged items may voluntarily present nutrient information, either in brochures or on signs posted at the point of purchase.

Restaurants with 20 or more locations must provide menu listings of an item's kcalories, grams of saturated fat, and milligrams of sodium. In addition, kcalorie information must be provided for prepared foods and beverages sold in supermarkets, convenience stores, movie theaters, and vending machines. Other restaurants need not supply nutrition information for menu items unless claims such as "low-fat" or "heart healthy" have been made. When ordering from menus, keep in mind that restaurants tend to serve large portions—two to three times standard serving sizes. In general, most consumers support restaurant menu labeling and use the kcalorie information when making selections.[36]

The Ingredient List

All packaged foods must list *all* ingredients on the label in descending order of predominance by weight. Knowing that the first ingredient predominates by weight, consumers can glean much information. Compare these products, for example:

- A beverage powder that contains "sugar, citric acid, natural flavors . . ." versus a juice that contains "water, tomato concentrate, concentrated juices of carrots, celery . . . ."
- A cereal that contains "puffed milled corn, sugar, corn syrup, molasses, salt . . ." versus one that contains "100 percent rolled oats. . . ."

In each comparison, consumers can tell that the second product is the more nutrient dense.

CHAPTER 1 Overview of Nutrition and Health

Nutrition Facts Panel

The Food and Drug Administration (FDA) requires food labels to include key nutrition facts. The "Nutrition Facts" panel provides such information as serving sizes, Daily Values, and nutrient quantities. Updated revisions to the nutrition facts panel reflect current nutrition science, actual serving sizes, and an improved design (see Figure 1-6).[37]

Serving Sizes Food labels must identify the serving size (food quantity) for which nutrition information is presented. The FDA has established specific serving sizes for various foods and requires that all labels for a given product use the same serving size. By law, serving sizes must be based on the amounts of food or beverage people actually consume, not what they "should" consume. In general, people are eating and drinking more today than 20 years ago when the label was first designed, so the FDA is updating the reference values for serving sizes that manufacturers use, to better reflect what people really eat and drink. For example, the proposed standard serving size for all ice creams is ²/₃ cup. The use of specific serving sizes for various foods facilitates comparison shopping. Consumers can see at a glance which brand has more or fewer kcalories or grams of fat, for example. However, these serving sizes

FIGURE 1-6 Original and Proposed Nutrition Facts Panel

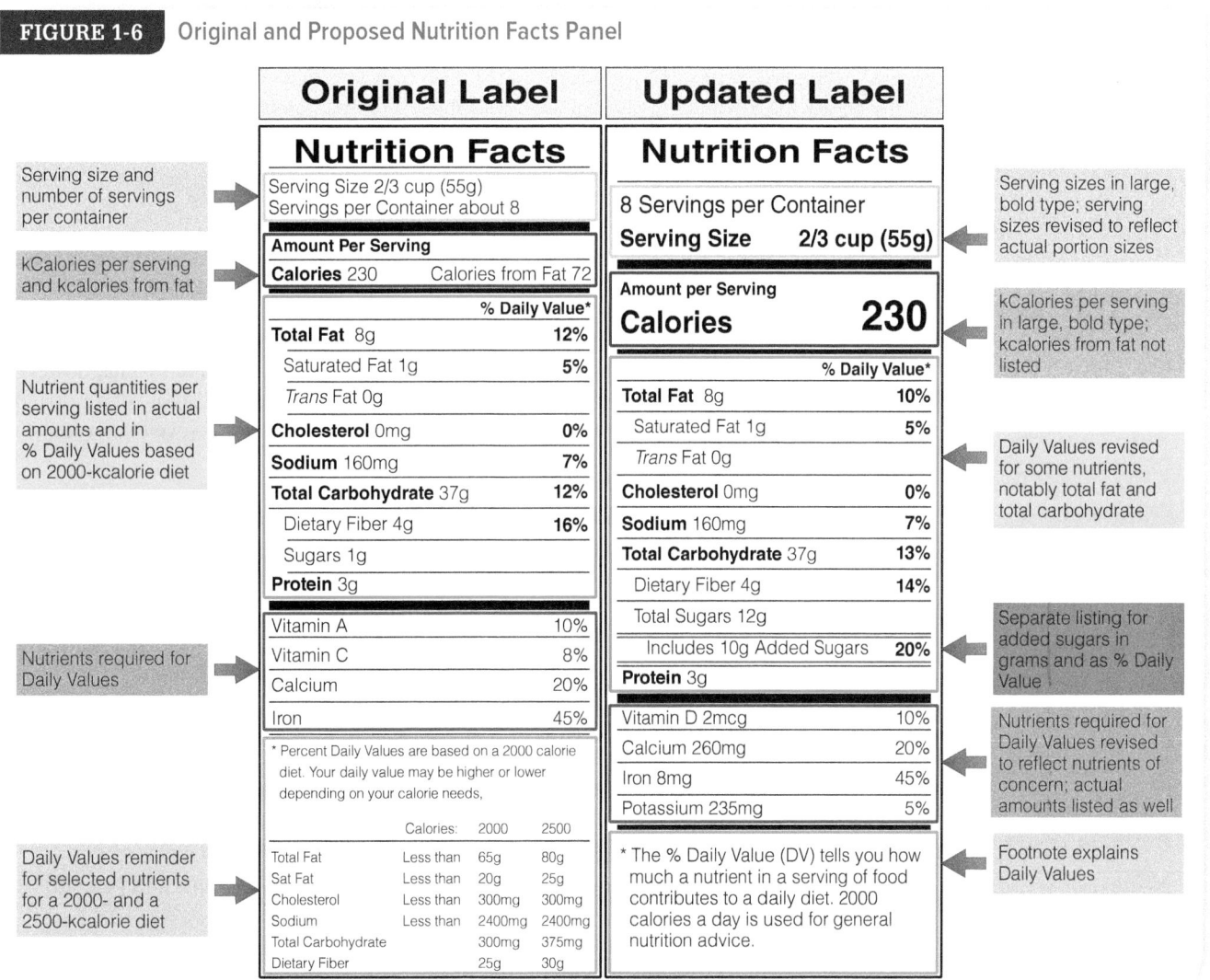

TABLE 1-9	Household and Metric Measures

- 1 teaspoon (tsp) = 5 milliliters (mL)
- 1 tablespoon (tbs) = 15 mL
- 1 cup (c) = 240 mL
- 1 fluid ounce (fl oz) = 30 mL
- 1 ounce (oz) = 28 grams (g)

Note: The Aids to Calculation section at the back of the book provides additional weights and measures.

do not provide a standard for desirable consumption. Standard serving sizes are expressed in both common household measures, such as cups, and metric measures, such as milliliters, to accommodate users of both types of measures (see Table 1-9).

In addition to updating serving sizes for certain products, the FDA is requiring some food and beverage containers previously labeled as more than one serving to be labeled as a single serving because people typically eat or drink the contents in one sitting. Examples are a 20-ounce soda and a 15-ounce can of soup. Certain larger packages may have a two-column label because some people may consume them in one sitting while others consume them in two or three sittings. For example, a 24-ounce bottle of soda or a pint of ice cream might be one serving for one person but not for another.

When examining the nutrition information on a food label, consumers need to compare the serving size on the label with how much they actually eat and adjust their calculations accordingly. For example, if the serving size is four cookies and you only eat two, then you need to cut the nutrient and kcalorie values in half; similarly, if you eat eight cookies, then you need to double the values. The number of servings per container is listed just above the serving size on the updated label.

The Daily Values To help consumers evaluate the information found on labels, the FDA created a set of nutrient standards called the **Daily Values** specifically for use on food labels. The Daily Values do two things: they set adequacy standards for nutrients that are desirable in the diet such as protein, vitamins, minerals, and fiber, and they set moderation standards for other nutrients that must be limited, such as fat, saturated fat, and sodium.

The "% Daily Value" column on a label provides a ballpark estimate of how individual foods contribute to the total diet. It compares key nutrients in a serving of food with the daily goals of a person consuming 2000 kcalories. Although the Daily Values are based on a 2000-kcalorie diet, people's actual energy intakes vary widely; some people need fewer kcalories, and some people need many more. This makes the Daily Values most useful for comparing one food with another and less useful as nutrient intake targets for individuals. By examining a food's general nutrient profile, however, a person can determine whether the food contributes "a little" or "a lot" of a nutrient, whether it contributes "more" or "less" than another food, and how well it fits into the consumer's overall diet.

Nutrient Quantities In addition to the serving size and the servings per container, the FDA requires that the Nutrition Facts panel on a label present nutrient information in two ways—in quantities (such as grams) and as percentages of the Daily Values. The updated Nutrition Facts panel must provide the nutrient amount, percent Daily Value, or both for the following:

- Total food energy (kcalories)
- Total fat (grams and percent Daily Value)—note that the updated label does not include kcalories from fat
- Saturated fat (grams and percent Daily Value)
- *Trans* fat (grams)
- Cholesterol (milligrams and percent Daily Value)
- Sodium (milligrams and percent Daily Value)
- Total carbohydrate, which includes starch, sugar, and fiber (grams and percent Daily Value)
- Dietary fiber (grams and percent Daily Value)
- Total sugars, which includes both those naturally present in and those added to the food (grams)

Daily Values: reference values developed by the FDA specifically for use on food labels.

- Added sugars, which includes only those added to the food (grams and percent Daily Value)—note that the original label does not include a separate line for added sugars.
- Protein (grams)
- The updated labels will no longer include information for vitamins A and C, but must present nutrient content information in actual amounts and as a percent Daily Value for the following nutrients: vitamin D, calcium, iron, and potassium.

The FDA developed the Daily Values for use on food labels because comparing nutrient amounts against a standard helps make them meaningful to consumers. A person might wonder, for example, whether 1 milligram of iron is a little or a lot. As Table 1-10 shows, the Daily Value for iron is 18 milligrams, so 1 milligram of iron is enough to take notice of: it is more than 5 percent.

Front-of-Package Labels Some consumers find the many numbers on Nutrition Facts panels overwhelming. They want an easier and quicker way to interpret information and select products. Some food manufacturers responded by creating front-of-package labels that incorporate text, color, and icons to present key nutrient facts.[38] Without any regulations or oversight, however, different companies used a variety of different symbols to describe how healthful their products were. To calm the chaos and maintain the voluntary status of front-of-package labels, major food industry associations created a standardized presentation of nutrient information called Facts Up Front (see Figure 1-7). In general, consumers find front-of-package labeling to be a quick and easy way to select products.[39]

Claims on Labels

In addition to the Nutrition Facts panel, consumers may find various claims on labels. These claims include nutrient claims, health claims, and structure–function claims.

Nutrient Claims Have you noticed phrases such as "good source of fiber" on a box of cereal or "rich in calcium" on a package of cheese? These and other **nutrient claims** may be used on labels only if the claims meet FDA definitions, which include the conditions under which each term can be used. For example, in addition to having less than 2 milligrams of cholesterol, a "cholesterol-free" product may not contain more than 2 grams of saturated fat and *trans* fat combined per serving. Table 1-11 defines nutrient terms on food labels, including criteria for foods described as "low," "reduced," and "free."

TABLE 1-10	Daily Values for Food Labels

FOOD LABELS MUST PRESENT THE "% DAILY VALUE" FOR THESE NUTRIENTS.	
FOOD COMPONENT	**DAILY VALUE**
Fat (total)	65 g
Saturated fat	20 g
Cholesterol	300 mg
Sodium	2300 mg
Carbohydrate (total)	275 g
Sugars	50 g
Fiber	28 g
Vitamin D	20 μg
Potassium	4700 mg
Calcium	1300 mg
Iron	18 mg

Note: Daily Values were established for adults and children over four years old. The values for energy-yielding nutrients are based on 2000 kcalories a day.

FIGURE 1-7	Facts Up Front

This example of front-of-package labeling (created by the Grocery Manufacturers Association and the Food Marketing Institute) presents key nutrient facts.

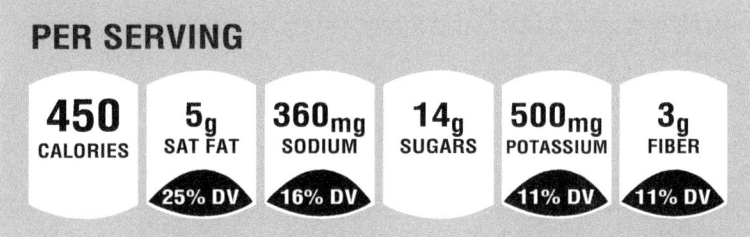

PER SERVING

450 CALORIES	5g SAT FAT	360mg SODIUM	14g SUGARS	500mg POTASSIUM	3g FIBER
	25% DV	16% DV		11% DV	11% DV

nutrient claims: statements that characterize the quantity of a nutrient in a food.

TABLE 1-11 Terms Used on Food Labels

GENERAL TERMS

free: "nutritionally trivial" and unlikely to have a physiological consequence; synonyms include *without, no,* and *zero.* A food that does not contain a nutrient naturally may make such a claim but only as it applies to all similar foods (for example, "applesauce, a fat-free food").

gluten-free: a food that contains less than 20 parts per million of gluten from any source: synonyms include *no gluten, free of gluten,* or *without gluten.*

good source of: the product provides between 10 and 19 percent of the Daily Value for a given nutrient per serving.

healthy: a food that is low in fat, saturated fat, cholesterol, and sodium and that contains at least 10 percent of the Daily Values for vitamin A, vitamin C, iron, calcium, protein, or fiber.

high: 20 percent or more of the Daily Value for a given nutrient per serving; synonyms include *rich in* or *excellent source.*

less: at least 25 percent less of a given nutrient or kcalories than the comparison food (see individual nutrients); synonyms include *fewer* and *reduced.*

light or lite: one-third fewer kcalories than the comparison food; 50 percent or less of the fat or sodium than the comparison food; any use of the term other than as defined must specify what it is referring to (for example, "light in color" or "light in texture").

low: an amount that would allow frequent consumption of a food without exceeding the Daily Value for the nutrient. A food that is naturally low in a nutrient may make such a claim but only as it applies to all similar foods (for example, "fresh cauliflower, a low-sodium food"); synonyms include *little, few,* and *low source of.*

more: at least 10 percent more of the Daily Value for a given nutrient than the comparison food; synonyms include *added* and *extra.*

organic (on food labels): at least 95 percent of the product's ingredients have been grown and processed according to USDA regulations defining the use of fertilizers, herbicides, insecticides, fungicides, preservatives, and other chemical ingredients.

ENERGY

kcalorie-free: fewer than 5 kcalories per serving.

low kcalorie: 40 kcalories or less per serving.

reduced kcalorie: at least 25 percent fewer kcalories per serving than the comparison food.

FAT AND CHOLESTEROL[a]

percent fat free: may be used only if the product meets the definition of *low fat* or *fat free* and must reflect the amount of fat in 100 grams (for example, a food that contains 2.5 grams of fat per 50 grams can claim to be "95 percent fat free").

fat free: less than 0.5 gram of fat per serving (and no added fat or oil); synonyms include *zero-fat, no-fat,* and *nonfat.*

low fat: 3 grams or less fat per serving.

less fat: at least 25 percent less fat than the comparison food.

saturated fat free: less than 0.5 gram of saturated fat and 0.5 gram of *trans* fat per serving.

low saturated fat: 1 gram or less saturated fat and less than 0.5 gram of *trans* fat per serving.

less saturated fat: at least 25 percent less saturated fat and *trans* fat combined than the comparison food.

***trans* fat free**: less than 0.5 gram of trans fat and less than 0.5 gram of saturated fat per serving.

cholesterol-free: less than 2 milligrams cholesterol per serving and 2 grams or less saturated fat and *trans* fat combined per serving.

low cholesterol: 20 milligrams or less cholesterol per serving and 2 grams or less saturated fat and *trans* fat combined per serving.

less cholesterol: at least 25 percent less cholesterol than the comparison food (reflecting a reduction of at least 20 milligrams per serving), and 2 grams or less saturated fat and *trans* fat combined per serving.

extra lean: less than 5 grams of fat, 2 grams of saturated fat and *trans* fat combined, and 95 milligrams of cholesterol per serving and per 100 grams of meat, poultry, and seafood.

lean: less than 10 grams of fat, 4.5 grams of saturated fat and *trans* fat combined, and 95 milligrams of cholesterol per serving and per 100 grams of meat, poultry, and seafood. For mixed dishes such as burritos and sandwiches, less than 8 grams of fat, 3.5 grams of saturated fat, and 80 milligrams of cholesterol per reference amount customarily consumed.

(Continued)

| **TABLE 1-11** | Terms Used on Food Labels *(continued)* |

CARBOHYDRATES: FIBER AND SUGAR

high fiber: 5 grams or more fiber per serving. A high-fiber claim made on a food that contains more than 3 grams fat per serving and per 100 grams of food must also declare total fat.

sugar-free: less than 0.5 gram of sugar per serving.

SODIUM

sodium-free and salt-free: less than 5 milligrams of sodium per serving.

low sodium: 140 milligrams or less per serving.

very low sodium: 35 milligrams or less per serving.

ᵃFoods containing more than 13 grams total fat per serving or per 50 grams of food must indicate those contents immediately after a cholesterol claim. As you can see, all cholesterol claims are prohibited when the food contains more than 2 grams saturated fat and *trans* fat combined per serving.

Some descriptions *imply* that a food contains, or does not contain, a nutrient. Implied claims are prohibited unless they meet specified criteria. For example, a claim that a product "contains no oil" implies that the food contains no fat. If the product is truly fat free, then it may make the no-oil claim, but if it contains another source of fat, such as butter, it may not.

Health Claims **Health claims** describe the relationship of a food or food component to a disease or health-related condition. In some cases, the FDA authorizes health claims based on an extensive review of the scientific literature. For example, the health claim that "diets low in sodium may reduce the risk of high blood pressure" is based on enough scientific evidence to establish a clear link between diet and health. Such reliable health claims have a high degree of scientific validity.

In cases where there is emerging—but not established—evidence for a relationship between a food or food component and disease, the FDA allows the use of *qualified* health claims that must use specific language indicating that the evidence supporting the claim is limited. A qualified health claim might state that "Very limited and preliminary research suggests that eating one-half to one cup of tomatoes and/or tomato sauce a week may reduce the risk of prostate cancer. The FDA concludes that there is little scientific evidence supporting the claim."

Structure–Function Claims **Structure–function claims** describe the effect that a substance has on the structure or function of the body but do not make reference to a disease—for example, "calcium builds strong bones." Unlike health claims, which require food manufacturers to collect scientific evidence and petition the FDA, structure–function claims can be made without any FDA approval. Product labels can claim to "slow aging," "improve memory," and "support immunity and digestive health" without any proof. The only criterion for a structure–function claim is that it must not mention a disease or symptom. Unfortunately, structure–function claims can be deceptively similar to health claims. Consider these statements:

- "May reduce the risk of heart disease."
- "Promotes a healthy heart."

Although most consumers do not distinguish between these two types of claims, the first is a health claim that requires FDA approval, whereas the second is an unproven, but legal, structure–function claim. Figure 1-8 compares the three types of label claims.

health claims: statements that characterize the relationship between a nutrient or other substance in food and a disease or health-related condition.

structure–function claims: statements that describe how a product may affect a structure or function of the body; for example, "calcium builds strong bones." Structure–function claims do not require FDA authorization.

FIGURE 1-8 Label Claims

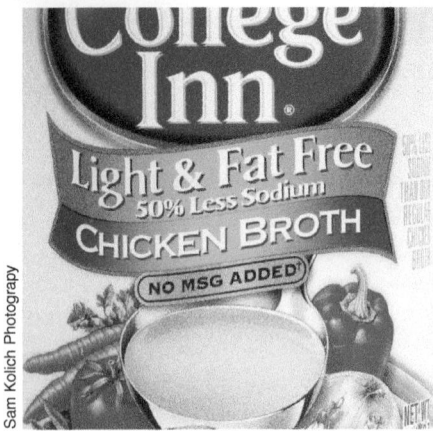

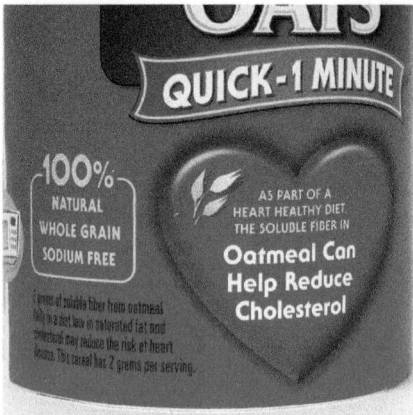

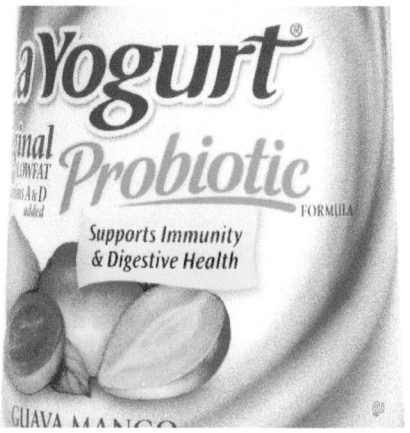

Sam Kolich Photograpy

Nutrient claims characterize the level of a nutrient in the food—for example, "fat free" or "less sodium."

Health claims characterize the relationship of a food or food component to a disease or health-related condition—for example, "soluble fiber from oatmeal daily in a diet low in saturated fat and cholesterol may reduce the risk of heart disease" or "a diet low in total fat may reduce the risk of some cancers."

Structure/function claims describe the effect that a substance has on the structure or function of the body and do not make reference to a disease—for example, "supports immunity and digestive health" or "calcium builds strong bones."

Review Notes

- Food labels list the ingredients, the serving size, the number of kcalories provided, and the key nutrient quantities in a food—information consumers need to select foods that will help them meet their nutrition and health goals.
- Daily Values are a set of nutrient standards created by the FDA for use on food labels.
- Reliable health claims are backed by the highest standards of scientific evidence.

Self Check

1. When people eat the foods typical of their families or geographic area, their choices are influenced by:
   a. occupation.
   b. nutrition.
   c. emotional state.
   d. ethnic heritage or regional cuisine.

2. The energy-yielding nutrients are:
   a. fats, minerals, and water.
   b. minerals, proteins, and vitamins.
   c. carbohydrates, fats, and vitamins.
   d. carbohydrates, fats, and proteins.

3. The inorganic nutrients are:
   a. proteins and fats.
   b. vitamins and minerals.
   c. minerals and water.
   d. vitamins and proteins.

4. Alcohol is not a nutrient because:
   a. the body derives no energy from it.
   b. it is organic.
   c. it is converted to body fat.
   d. it does not contribute to the body's growth or repair.

5. The nutrient standards in use today include all of the following except:
   a. Recommended Dietary Allowances (RDA).
   b. Adequate Intakes (AI).
   c. Daily Minimum Requirements (DMR).
   d. Tolerable Upper Intake Levels (UL).

6. Which of the following is consistent with the Dietary Guidelines for Americans?
   a. Limit intakes of fruit, vegetables, and whole grains.
   b. Shift to healthier food and beverage choices.
   c. Choose a diet with plenty of whole-milk products.
   d. Eat an abundance of foods to ensure nutrient adequacy.

7. In a food group plan such as the USDA Food Patterns, foods within a given food group provide similar amounts of:
   a. energy.
   b. proteins and fibers.
   c. vitamins and minerals.
   d. carbohydrates and fats.

8. A slice of apple pie supplies 350 kcalories with 3 grams of fiber; an apple provides 80 kcalories and the same 3 grams of fiber. This is an example of:
   a. kcalorie control.
   b. nutrient density.

c. variety.
d. essential nutrients.

9. According to the USDA Food Patterns: Food Groups and Subgroups, which of the following fruit/vegetables should be limited?
   a. Carrots
   b. Avocados
   c. Baked beans
   d. Potatoes

10. Food labels list ingredients in:
   a. alphabetical order.
   b. ascending order of predominance by weight.
   c. descending order of predominance by weight.
   d. the manufacturer's order of preference.

Answers: 1. d, 2. d, 3. c, 4. d, 5. c, 6. b, 7. c, 8. b, 9. c, 10. c

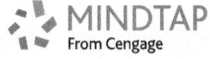 MINDTAP
From Cengage   For more chapter resources visit **www.cengage.com** to access MindTap, a complete digital course.

Clinical Applications

1. Make a list of the foods and beverages you've consumed in the past two days. Look at each item on your list and consider why you chose the particular food or beverage you did. Did you eat cereal for breakfast because that's what you always eat (habit), or because it was the easiest, quickest food to prepare (convenience)? Did you put fat-free milk on the cereal because you want to control your energy intake (nutrition)? In going down your list, you may be surprised to discover exactly why you chose certain foods.

2. As a health care professional, you can uncover clues about a client's food choices by paying close attention. You may be surprised to discover why a client chooses certain foods, but you can then use this knowledge to serve the best interests of the client. For example, an elderly, undernourished widower may eat the same sandwich for lunch every day. In talking with the client, you discover that this is what he and his wife fixed together each day. Consider ways you might be able to help the client learn to eat other foods and vary his choices.

3. Using the list of foods and beverages from exercise #1, compare your day's intake with the USDA Healthy U.S.-Style Food Pattern. Did you vary your choices within each food group? Did your intake match the daily recommended amounts from each group? If not, list some changes you could have made to meet the recommendations.

Notes

1. Think globally, practice locally: Culturally competent dietetics, *Journal of the Academy of Nutrition and Dietetics* 115 (2015): Entire supplement; M. Truong, Y. Paradies, and N. Priest, Interventions to improve cultural competency in healthcare: A systematic review of reviews, *BMC Health Services Research* 14 (2014): 99.

2. J. A. Mennella, Ontogeny of taste preferences: Basic biology and Implications for health, *American Journal of Clinical Nutrition* 99 (2014): 704S–711S; E. Stice, K. S. Burger, and S. Yokum, Relative ability of fat and sugar tastes to activate reward, gustatory, and somatosensory regions, *American Journal of Clinical Nutrition* 98 (2013): 1377–1384.

3. K. Keller and S. Adise, Variation in the ability to taste bitter thiourea compounds: Implications for food acceptance, dietary intake, and obesity risk in children, *Annual Review of Nutrition* 36 (2016): 157–182; H. B. Loper and coauthors, Taste perception, associated hormonal modulation, and nutrient intake, *Nutrition Reviews* 73 (2015): 83–91; Y. Shafaie and coauthors, Energy intake and diet selection during buffet consumption in women classified by the 6-n-propylthiouracil bitter taste phenotype, *American Journal of Clinical Nutrition* 98 (2013): 1583–1591; S.V. Lipchock and coauthors, Human bitter perception correlates with bitter receptor messenger RNA expression in taste cell, *American Journal of Clinical Nutrition* 98 (2013): 1136–1143.

4. Position of the Academy of Nutrition and Dietetics: Nutritional genomics, *Journal of the Academy of Nutrition and Dietetics* 114 (2014): 299–313.

5. T. Cruwys, K. E. Bevelander, and R. C. Hermans, Social modeling of eating: A review of when and why social influence affects food intake and choice, *Appetite* 86 (2015): 3–18; E. Robinson and coauthors, What everyone else is eating: A systematic review and meta-analysis of the effect of informational eating norms on eating behavior, *Journal of the Academy of Nutrition and Dietetics* 114 (2014): 414–429.

6. J. Reichenberger and coauthors, No haste, more taste: An EMA study of the effects of stress, negative and positive emotions on eating behavior, *Biological Psychology*, 2016, doi: 10.1016/biopsycho.2016.09.002.

7. J. A. Wolfson and S. N. Bleich, Is cooking at home associated with better diet quality or weight-loss intention? *Public Health Nutrition* 18 (2015): 1397–1406; C. Hartmann, S. Dohle, and M. Siegrist, Importance of cooking skills for balanced food choices, *Appetite* 65 (2013): 125–131.

8. T. L. Barnes and coauthors, Fast-food consumption, diet quality and body weight: Cross-sectional and prospective associations in a community sample of working adults, *Public Health Nutrition* 19 (2016): 885–892; A. Jaworowska and coauthors, Nutritional challenges and health implications of takeaway and fast food, *Nutrition Reviews* 71 (2013): 310–318.

9. C. M. Weaver and coauthors, Processed foods: Contributions to nutrition, *American Journal of Clinical Nutrition* 99 (2014): 1525–1542.

10. C. A. Monteiro and coauthors, Ultra-processed products are becoming dominant in the global food system, *Obesity Reviews* 14 (2013): 21–28.

11. E. M. Steele and coauthors, Ultra-processed foods and added sugars in the US diet: Evidence from a nationally representative cross-sectional study, *BMJ Open* 6 (2016): e009892.

12. National Center for Health Statistics, Chapter IV: Leading health indicators, *Healthy People 2020 Midcourse Review,* Hyattsville, MD, 2016, www.cdc.gov/nchs/data/hpdata2020/HP2020MCR-BO4-LHI.pdf.

13. American Cancer Society, *Cancer Prevention and Early Detection: Facts and Figures 2017–2018* (Atlanta, GA: American Cancer Society, 2017), pp. 17–34; D. Mozaffarian and coauthors, Heart disease and stroke statistics—2016 update: A report from the American Heart Association, *Circulation* 1133 (2016): e38–e360; M. A. H. Hendriksen and coauthors, Potential effect of salt reduction in processed foods on health, *American Journal of Clinical Nutrition* 99 (2014): 446–453; R. H. Eckel and coauthors, 2013 AHA/ ACC Guidelines on lifestyle management to reduce cardiovascular risk: A report of the American College of Cardiology/ American Heart Association Task Force on Practice Guidelines, *Circulation* 129 (2014): S76–S99; A. B. Evert and coauthors, Position statement: Nutrition therapy recommendations for the management of adults with diabetes, *Diabetes Care* 37 (2014): S120–S143; Position of the Academy of Nutrition and Dietetics: The role of nutrition in health promotion and chronic disease prevention, *Journal of the Academy of Nutrition and Dietetics* 113 (2013): 972–979.

14. Position of the Academy of Nutrition and Dietetics: Total diet approach to healthy eating, *Journal of the Academy of Nutrition and Dietetics* 113 (2013): 307–317.

15. Practice paper of the Academy of Nutrition and Dietetics: Selecting nutrient-dense foods for good health, *Journal of the Academy of Nutrition and Dietetics* 116 (2016): 1473–1479.

16. A. Drewnowski and V. L. Fulgoni, Nutrient density: Principles and evaluation tools, *American Journal of Clinical Nutrition* 99 (2014): 1223S–1228S.

17. G. Masset and coauthors, Can nutrient profiling help to identify foods which diet variety should be encouraged? Results from the Whitehall II cohort, *British Journal of Nutrition* 113 (2015): 1800–1809; Drewnowski and Fulgoni, 2014.

18. U. Ekelund and coauthors, Does physical activity attenuate, or even eliminate, the detrimental association of sitting time with mortality? A harmonised meta-analysis of data from more than 1 million men and women, *Lancet* 2016, doi:10.1016/S0140-6736(16)30370-1; D. Schmid and coauthors, Replacing sedentary time with physical activity in relation to mortality, *Medicine and Science in Sports and Exercise* 48 (2016): 1312–1319; C. Y. Wu and coauthors, The association of physical activity with all-cause, cardiovascular, and cancer mortality among older adults, *Preventive Medicine* 72 (2015): 23–29; U. Ekelund and coauthors, Physical activity and all-cause mortality across levels of overall and abdominal adiposity in European men and women: The European Prospective Investigation into Cancer and Nutrition Study (EPIC), *American Journal of Clinical Nutrition* 101 (2015): 613–621; H. Nakahara, S. Y. Ueda, and T. Miyamoto, Low-frequency severe-intensity interval training improves cardiorespiratory functions, *Medicine and Science in Sports and Exercise* 47 (2015): 789–798; P. T. Williams, Dose- response relationship between exercise and respiratory disease mortality, *Medicine and Science in Sports and Exercise* 46 (2014): 711–717.

19. Centers for Disease Control and Prevention, National Center for Health Statistics, *Exercise or physical activity*, www.cdc.gov/nchs/fastats/exercise.htm, updated January 20, 2017.

20. P. Ladenvall and coauthors, Low aerobic capacity in middle-aged men associated with increased mortality rates during 45 years of follow-up, *European Journal of Preventive Cardiology*, 2016, doi:10.1177/2047487316655466; S. C. Moore and coauthors, Association of leisure-time physical activity with risk of 26 types of cancer in 1.44 million adults, *JAMA Internal Medicine*, May 16, 2016, doi:10.1001/jamainternmed.2016.1548; R. Cannioto and coauthors, Chronic recreational physical inactivity and epithelial ovarian cancer risk: Evidence from the ovarian cancer association consortium, *Cancer, Epidemiology, Biomarkers, and Prevention* 25 (2016): 1114–1124; Wu and coauthors, 2015; S. W. Farrell and coauthors, Is there a gradient of mortality risk among men with low cardiorespiratory fitness? *Medicine and Science in Sports and Exercise* 47 (2015): 1825–1832; C. H. Lin and coauthors, Moderate physical activity level as a protective factor against metabolic syndrome in middle-aged and older women, *Journal of Clinical Nursing* 24 (2015): 1234–1245; J. P. Thyfault and coauthors, Physiology of sedentary behavior and its Relationship to health outcomes, *Medicine and Science in Sports and Exercise* 47 (2015): 1301–1305.

21. B. A. Ekelund and coauthors, 2016; A. Philipsen and coauthors, Associations of objectively measured physical activity and abdominal fat distribution, *Medicine and Science in Sports and Exercise* 47 (2015): 983–989; D. L. Swift and coauthors, The role of exercise and physical activity in weight loss and maintenance, *Progress in Cardiovascular Diseases* 56 (2014): 441–447; Larsen and coauthors, Associations of physical activity and sedentary behavior with regional fat deposition, *Medicine and Science in Sports and Exercise* 46 (2014): 520–528.

22. S. J. Warden and coauthors, Physical activity when young provides lifelong benefits to cortical bone size and strength in men, *Proceedings of the National Academy of Sciences of the United States of America* 111 (2014): 5337–5342.

23. Moore and coauthors, 2016; Cannioto and coauthors, 2016; Wu and coauthors, 2015; P. T. Williams, Reduced risk of incident kidney cancer from walking and running, *Medicine and Science in Sports and Exercise* 46 (2014): 312–317.

24. Wu and coauthors, 2015; Nakahara, Ueda, and Miyamoto, 2015; M. E. G. Armstrong and coauthors, Frequent physical activity may not reduce vascular disease risk as much as moderate activity: Large prospective study of UK women, *Circulation* 131 (2015): 721–729.

25. Philipsen and coauthors, 2015; V. Lévesque and coauthors, Targeting abdominal adiposity and cardiorespiratory fitness in the workplace, *Medicine and Science in Sports and Exercise* 47 (2015): 1342–1350; Lin and coauthors, 2015; J. H. Goedecke and L. K. Micklesfield, The effect of exercise on obesity, body fat distribution, and risk for type 2 diabetes, *Medicine and Science in Sports and Exercise* 60 (2014): 82–93.

26. S. Fan and coauthors, Physical activity level and incident type 2 diabetes among Chinese adults, *Medicine and Science in Sports and Exercise* 47 (2015): 751–756; D. T. Lackland and J. H. Voeks, Metabolic syndrome and hypertension: Regular exercise as part of lifestyle management, *Current Hypertension Reports* 16 (2014): 492; C. P. Earnest and coauthors, Aerobic and strength training in concomitant metabolic syndrome and type 2 diabetes, *Medicine and Science in Sports and Exercise* 46 (2014): 1293–1301.

27. D. Aune, M. Leitzmann, and L. J. Vatten, Physical activity and the risk of gallbladder disease: A systematic review and meta-analysis of cohort studies, *Journal of Physical Activity and Health*, 2016, doi:10.1123/jpah.2015-0456; R. J. Shephard, Physical activity and the biliary tract in health and disease, *Sports Medicine* 45 (2015): 1295–1309.

28. E. M. McMahon and coauthors, Physical activity in European adolescents and associations with anxiety, depression and well-being, *European Child and Adolescent Psychiatry*, 2016, doi:10.1007/s00787-016-0875-9; M. B. Powers, G. J. Asmundson, and J. A. J. Smits, Exercise for mood and anxiety disorders: The state-of-the-science, *Cognitive Behavior Therapy* 44 (2015): 237–239.

29. Ekelund and coauthors, 2016; Ladenvall and coauthors, 2016; L. M. León-Muñoz and coauthors, Continued sedentariness, change in sitting time and mortality in older adults, *Medicine and Science in Sports and Exercise* 45 (2013): 1501–1507.

30. H. Arem and coauthors, Leisure time physical activity and mortality: A detailed pooled analysis of the dose-response relationship, *JAMA Internal Medicine* 175 (2015): 959–967.

31. K. Uusi-Rasi and coauthors, Exercise and vitamin D in fall prevention among older women, *JAMA Internal Medicine* 175 (2015): 703–711; M. Pahor and coauthors, Effect of structured physical activity on prevention of major mobility disability in older adults, *Journal of the American Medical Association* 311 (2014): 2387–2396; L. Krist, F. Dimeo, and T. Keil, Can progressive resistance training twice a week improve mobility, muscle strength, and quality of life in very elderly nursing-home residents with impaired mobility? A pilot study, *Clinical Interventions in Aging* 8 (2013): 443–448.

32. American College of Sports Medicine position stand, Quantity and quality of exercise for developing and maintaining cardiorespiratory, musculoskeletal, and neuromotor fitness in apparently healthy adults: Guidance for prescribing exercise, *Medicine and Science in Sports and Exercise* 43 (2011): 1334–1359.

33. American College of Sports Medicine position stand, 2011.

34. U.S. Department of Agriculture, Vegetables: Peas and beans are unique foods, www.choosemyplate.gov/food-groups/vegetables-beans-peas.html, updated January 12, 2016.

35. Position of the Academy of Nutrition and Dietetics: Vegetarian diets, *Journal of the Academy of Nutrition and Dietetics* 115 (2015): 801–810.

36. S. H. Lee-Kwan and coauthors, Restaurant menu labeling use among adults—17 states, 2012, *Morbidity and Mortality Weekly Report* 63 (2014): 581–584; J. P. Block and C. A. Roberto, Potential benefits of calorie labeling in restaurants, *Journal of the American Medical Association* 312 (2014): 887–888.

37. U. S. Food and Drug Administration, Changes to the Nutrition Facts label, www.fda.gov/Food/GuidanceRegulation/GuidanceDocumentsRegulatoryInformation/LabelingNutrition/ucm385663.htm, updated April 25, 2017.

38. J. C. Hersey and coauthors, Effects of front-of-package and shelf nutrition labeling systems on consumers, *Nutrition Reviews* 71 (2013): 1–14.

39. M. S. Edge and coauthors, The impact of variations in a fact-based front-of-package nutrition labeling system on consumer comprehension, *Journal of the Academy of Nutrition and Dietetics* 114 (2014): 843–854.

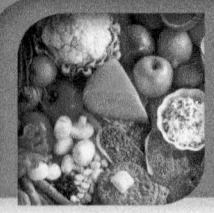

1.7 Nutrition in Practice
Finding the Truth about Nutrition

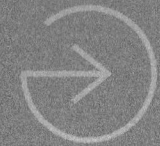

Nutrition and health receive so much attention on television, on the radio, in the popular press, and on the Internet that it is easy to be overwhelmed with inconsistent, unclear information.[1] More than two-thirds of U.S. consumers are interested in the relationship between nutrition and health, but for many of them, such information is often confusing and conflicting.[2] Determining whether nutrition information is accurate can be a challenging task. It is also an important task because nutrition affects a person both professionally and personally.

A person watches a nutrition report on television and then reads a conflicting report in the newspaper. Why do nutrition news reports and claims for nutrition products seem to contradict each other so often?

The problem of conflicting messages arises for several reasons:

- Popular media, often faced with tight deadlines and limited time or space to report new information, rush to present the latest "breakthrough" in a headline or a 60-second spot. They can hardly help omitting important facts about the study or studies that the "breakthrough" is based on. Biases influence choices and perceptions.[3]
- Despite tremendous advances in the past few decades, scientists still have much to learn about the human body and nutrition. Scientists themselves often disagree on their first tentative interpretations of new research findings, yet these are the very findings that the public hears most about.
- The popular media often broadcast preliminary findings in hopes of grabbing attention and boosting readership or television ratings.
- Commercial promoters turn preliminary findings into advertisements for products or supplements long before the findings have been validated—or disproved. The scientific process requires many experiments or trials to confirm a new finding. Seldom do promoters wait as long as they should to make their claims.
- Promoters are aware that consumers like to try new products or treatments even though they probably will not withstand the tests of time and scientific scrutiny.

So how can a person tell what claims to believe?

Valid nutrition information derives from scientific research, which has the following characteristics:

- Scientists test their ideas by conducting properly designed scientific experiments. They report their methods and procedures in detail so that other scientists can verify the findings through replication.
- Scientists recognize the inadequacy of personal testimonials.
- Scientists who use animals in their research do not apply their findings directly to human beings.
- Scientists may use specific segments of the population in their research. When they do, they are careful not to generalize the findings to all people.
- Scientists report their findings in respected scientific journals. Their work must survive a screening review by their peers before it is accepted for publication.

With each report from scientists, the field of nutrition changes a little—each finding contributes another piece to the whole body of knowledge. Table NP1-1 features nine

---

TABLE NP1-1 Warning Signs of Nutrition Quackery

1. *Quick and easy fixes.* Even proven treatments take time to be effective.
2. *Personal testimonials.* Hearsay is the weakest form of scientific validity.
3. *One product does it all.* No one product can treat every disease and condition.
4. *Natural.* Natural is not necessarily safer or better. Any product strong enough to be effective is strong enough to cause side effects.
5. *Time-tested or latest innovation.* Such findings would be widely publicized and accepted by health professionals.
6. *Satisfaction guaranteed.* Marketers of fraudulent products may make generous promises, but consumers won't be able to collect on them.
7. *Paranoid accusations.* These claims suggest that health professionals and legitimate drug manufacturers are conspiring with each other to promote drug companies' products for financial gain.
8. *Meaningless medical jargon.* Phony terms hide the lack of scientific proof.
9. *Too good to be true.* If it sounds too good to be true, it probably isn't true.

red flags of junk science to help consumers distinguish valid from misleading nutrition information.

Because nutrition misinformation harms the health and economic status of consumers, the **Academy of Nutrition and Dietetics** works with health care professionals and educators to present sound nutrition information to the public and to actively confront nutrition misinformation.[3] Table NP1-2 (p. 36) offers a list of credible sources of nutrition information.

What about nutrition and health information found on the Internet? How does a person know whether the websites are reliable?

With hundreds of millions of websites on the Internet, searching for nutrition and health information can be daunting. The Internet offers no guarantee of the accuracy of the information found there, and much of it is pure fiction. Websites must be evaluated for their accuracy, just like every other source. Table NP1-3 (p. 37) provides clues to identifying reliable nutrition information sites and lists some credible sites.

One of the most trustworthy sites used by scientists and others is the National Library of Medicine's PubMed (*www.ncbi.nlm.nih.gov/pubmed*), which provides free access to more than 25 million abstracts (short descriptions) of research papers published in scientific journals around the world. Many abstracts provide links to websites where full articles are available.

Promoters of fraudulent "health" products use the Internet as a primary means to sell their wares. Agencies such as the Food and Drug Administration (FDA) take action against fraudulent marketing of supplements and health products on the Internet.[4] The latest actions target unscrupulous companies that use the Internet to promote products to the most vulnerable consumers—those with diseases such as cancer or Alzheimer's. Of greatest concern are those products that not only make false promises but also are potentially dangerous. For example, herbal products touted as safe treatments for serious illnesses such as cancer may interact with and impair the effectiveness of medications. The FDA advises consumers to be suspicious of:

- Claims that a product is "natural" or "nontoxic." "Natural" or "nontoxic" does not always mean safe.
- Claims that a product is a "scientific breakthrough," "miraculous cure," "secret ingredient," or "ancient remedy."
- Claims that a product cures a wide range of illnesses.
- Claims that use impressive-sounding medical terms.
- Claims of a "money-back" guarantee.

Consumers with questions or suspicions about fraud can contact the FDA on the Internet at www.FDA.gov or by telephone at (888) INFO-FDA.

Everyone seems to be giving advice on nutrition. How can a person tell whom to listen to?

Registered dietitian nutritionists (RDNs) and nutrition professionals with advanced degrees (M.S., Ph.D.) are experts (see Box NP1-1). These professionals are in the best position to answer a person's nutrition questions. On the other hand, a "**nutritionist**" may be an expert or a quack, depending on the state in which the person practices. Some states require people who use this title to meet strict standards. In other states, a "nutritionist" may be any individual who claims a career connection with the nutrition field. There is no accepted national definition for the term nutritionist.

Other purveyors of nutrition information may also lack credentials. A health-food store owner may be in the nutrition business simply because it is a lucrative market. The owner may have a background in business or sales and no education in nutrition at all. Such a person is not

---

Box NP1-1 Glossary of Nutrition Experts

Academy of Nutrition and Dietetics: the professional organization of dietitians in the United States; formerly the Academy of Nutrition and Dietetics. The Canadian equivalent is Dietitians of Canada, which operates similarly.

dietetic technicians: persons who have completed a minimum of an associate's degree from an accredited college or university and an approved dietetic technician program that includes a supervised practice experience. A **dietetic technician, registered (DTR)** or a **nutrition and dietetics technician, registered (NDTR),** has also passed a national examination and maintains registration through continuing professional education.

dietetics: the application of nutrition principles to achieve and maintain optimal human health.

nutritionists: all registered dietitians are nutritionists, but not all nutritionists are registered dietitians. Some state licensing

boards set specific qualifications for holding the title. For states that regulate this title, the definition varies from state to state. To obtain some "nutritionist" credentials requires little more than a payment.

registered dietitian nutritionists (RDNs): food and nutrition experts who have earned a minimum of a bachelor's degree from an accredited university or college after completing a program of coursework approved by the Academy of Nutrition and Dietetics also called registered dietitians (RDs). The dietitians must serve in an approved, supervised practice program pass the registration examination, and maintain competency through continuing education. Many states require licensing for practicing dietitians. Licensed dietitians (LDs) have met all state requirements to offer nutrition advice.

Government agencies, volunteer associations, consumer groups, and professional organizations provide consumers with reliable health and nutrition information. Credible sources of nutrition information include:

- Nutrition and food science departments at a university or community college

- Local agencies such as the health department or County Cooperative Extension Service

- Government resources such as:
  - Centers for Disease Control and Prevention (CDC)
  - Department of Agriculture (USDA)
  - Department of Health and Human Services (DHHS)
  - Dietary Guidelines for Americans
  - Food and Drug Administration (FDA)
  - Health Canada
  - Healthy People
  - Let's Move!
  - MyPlate
  - National Institutes of Health
  - Physical Activity Guidelines for Americans

  - www.cdc.gov
  - www.usda.gov
  - www.hhs.gov
  - fnic.nal.usda.gov/dietary-guidance
  - www.fda.gov
  - www.hc-sc.gc.ca/fn-an/index-eng.php
  - www.healthypeople.gov
  - www.letsmove.gov
  - www.choosemyplate.gov
  - www.nih.gov
  - www.health.gov/paguidelines

- Volunteer health agencies such as:
  - American Cancer Society
  - American Diabetes Association
  - American Heart Association

  - www.cancer.org
  - www.diabetes.org
  - www.heart.org/HEARTORG

- Reputable consumer groups such as:
  - American Council on Science and Health
  - International Food Information Council

  - www.acsh.org
  - www.foodinsight.org

- Professional health organizations such as:
  - Academy of Nutrition and Dietetics
  - American Medical Association
  - Dietitians of Canada

  - www.eatright.org
  - www.ama-assn.org
  - www.dietitians.ca

- Journals such as:
  - *American Journal of Clinical Nutrition*
  - *Journal of the Academy of Nutrition and Dietetics*
  - *New England Journal of Medicine*
  - *Nutrition Reviews*

  - ajcn.nutrition.org
  - www.andjrnl.org
  - www.nejm.org
  - www.ilsi.org

qualified to provide nutrition information to customers. For accurate nutrition information, seek out a trained professional with a college education in nutrition—an expert in the field of **dietetics**.

What are some of the job responsibilities of dietitians?

Dietitians perform a multitude of duties in many settings in most communities. They work in the food industry, pharmaceutical companies, home health agencies, long-term care facilities, private practice, public health departments, research centers, education settings, fitness centers, and hospitals. Depending on their work settings, dietitians can assume a number of different job responsibilities and positions. For example, in hospitals, administrative dietitians manage the foodservice system; clinical dietitians provide client care, and nutrition support team dietitians coordinate nutrition care with other health care professionals. Recent rulings now allow qualified dietitians to order therapeutic diets and nutrition-related lab tests without the supervision or approval of a physician, thus improving the nutritional diagnosis and treatment plans of hospitalized patients.[5]

What about nurses and other health care professionals?

All members of the health care team share responsibility for helping each client to achieve optimal health, but the registered dietitian nutritionist is usually the primary nutrition expert. Each of the other team members has a related specialty. Some physicians are specialists in clinical nutrition and thus are also experts in the field. Other physicians, nurses, and **dietetic technicians** often assist

TABLE NP1-3 Evaluating the Reliability of Websites

To determine whether an Internet site offers reliable nutrition information, answer the following questions.

- **Who is responsible for the site?** Clues can be found in the three letters that follow the dot in the site's name. For example, "gov" and "edu" indicate government and university sites, respectively, which are usually reliable sources of information.

- **Do the names and credentials of information providers appear?** Is an editorial board identified? Many legitimate sources provide e-mail addresses or other ways to obtain more information about the site and the information providers behind it.

- **Are links with other reliable information sites provided?** Reputable organizations almost always provide links with other similar sites because they want you to know of other experts in their area of knowledge. Caution is needed when you evaluate a site by its links, however. Anyone, even a quack, can link a web page to a reputable site without the organization's permission. Doing so may give the quack's site the appearance of legitimacy, just the effect for which the quack is hoping.

- **Is the site updated regularly?** Nutrition information changes rapidly, and sites should be updated often.

- **Is the site selling a product or service?** Commercial sites may provide accurate information, but they also may not. Their profit motive increases the risk of bias.

- **Does the site charge a fee to gain access to it?** Many academic and government sites offer the best information, usually for free. Some legitimate sites do charge fees, but before paying up, check the free sites. Chances are good you will find what you are looking for without paying.

dietitians in providing nutrition information and may help to administer direct nutrition care. Nurses play central roles in client care management and client relationships. Visiting nurses and home health care nurses may become intimately involved in clients' nutrition care at home, teaching them both theory and cooking techniques. Physical therapists can provide individualized exercise programs related to nutrition—for example, to help control obesity. Social workers may provide practical and emotional support.

What roles might these other health care professionals play in nutrition care?

Some of the responsibilities of the health care professional might be:

- Helping people understand why nutrition is important to them.
- Answering questions about food and diet.
- Explaining to clients how modified diets work.
- Collecting information about clients that may influence their nutritional health.
- Identifying clients at risk for poor nutrition status (see Chapter 13) and recommending or taking appropriate action.

- Recognizing when clients need extra help with nutrition problems (in such cases, the problems should be referred to a registered dietitian nutritionist or physician).

Health care professionals may routinely perform these nutrition-related tasks:

- Obtaining diet histories.
- Taking weight and height measurements.
- Feeding clients who cannot feed themselves.
- Recording what clients eat or drink.
- Observing clients' responses and reactions to foods.
- Helping clients mark menus.
- Monitoring weight changes.
- Monitoring food and drug interactions.
- Encouraging clients to eat.
- Assisting clients at home in planning their diets and managing their kitchen chores.
- Alerting the physician or dietitian when nutrition problems are identified.
- Charting actions taken and communicating on these matters with other professionals as needed.

Thus, although the registered dietitian nutritionist assumes the primary role as the nutrition expert on a health care team, other health care professionals play important roles in administering nutrition care.

Notes

1. S. B. Rowe and N. Alexander, Communicating nutrition and other science: A reality check, *Nutrition Today* 51 (2016): 29–32; D. Quagliani and M. Hermann, Practice paper of the Academy of Nutrition and Dietetics: Communicating accurate food and nutrition information, *Journal of the Academy of Nutrition and Dietetics* 112 (2012): 759.
2. A. C. Sylvetsky and W. H. Dietz, Nutrient-content claims—guidance or cause for confusion, *New England Journal of Medicine* 371 (2014): 195–198.
3. S. Rowe and N. Alexander, Conflicted science: Can nutrition communicators be biased too? *Nutrition Today* 50 (2015): 8–11.
4. Food and Drug Administration, 6 tip-offs to rip-offs: Don't fall for health fraud scams, www.fda.gov/forconsumers/consumerupdates/ucm341344.htm, updated April 21, 2017.
5. B. Boyce, CMS final rule on therapeutic diet orders means new opportunities for RDNs, *Journal of the Academy of Nutrition and Dietetics* 114 (2014): 1326–1328.

Digestion and Absorption

Chapter Sections and Learning Objectives (LOs)

chapter
2

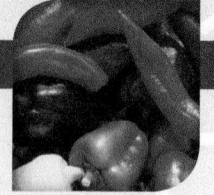

THE BODY'S ABILITY TO TRANSFORM THE FOODS A PERSON EATS INTO THE

nutrients that fuel the body's work is quite remarkable. Yet most people probably give little, if any, thought to all the body does with food once it is eaten. This chapter offers the reader the opportunity to learn how the body digests, absorbs, and transports the nutrients and how it excretes the unwanted substances in foods.

One of the beauties of the digestive tract is that it is selective. Materials that are nutritive for the body are broken down into particles that can be absorbed into the bloodstream. Most of the nonnutritive materials are left undigested and pass out the other end of the digestive tract.

2.1 Anatomy of the Digestive Tract

The **gastrointestinal (GI) tract** is a flexible muscular tube extending from the mouth to the anus. Figure 2-1 illustrates the digestive tract and associated organs. Box 2-1 defines GI anatomical terms. In a sense, the human body surrounds the GI tract. Only when a nutrient or other substance passes through the cells of the digestive tract wall does it actually enter the body.

The Digestive Organs

The process of **digestion** begins in the **mouth**. As you chew, your teeth crush and soften the food, while saliva mixes with the food mass and moistens it for comfortable swallowing. Saliva also helps dissolve the food so that you can taste it; only particles in solution can react with taste buds.

> **gastrointestinal (GI) tract:** the digestive tract. The principal organs are the stomach and intestines.
>
> *gastro* = stomach
>
> **digestion:** the process by which complex food particles are broken down to smaller absorbable particles.

Box 2-1   **Glossary of GI Anatomy Terms**

These terms are listed in order from start to end of the digestive system.

mouth: the oral cavity containing the tongue and teeth.

pharynx (FAIR-inks): the passageway leading from the nose and mouth to the larynx and esophagus, respectively.

epiglottis (epp-ih-GLOTT-iss): cartilage in the throat that guards the entrance to the trachea and prevents fluid or food from entering it when a person swallows.

- *epi* = upon (over)
- *glottis* = back of tongue

esophagus (ee-SOFF-ah-gus): the food pipe; the conduit from the mouth to the stomach.

sphincter (SFINK-ter): a circular muscle surrounding, and able to close, a body opening. Sphincters are found at specific points along the GI tract and regulate the flow of food particles.

- *sphincter* = band (binder)

esophageal (ee-SOF-a-GEE-al) sphincter: a sphincter muscle at the upper or lower end of the esophagus. The *lower esophageal sphincter* is also called the *cardiac sphincter*.

stomach: a muscular, elastic, saclike portion of the digestive tract that grinds and churns swallowed food, mixing it with acid and enzymes to form chyme.

pyloric (pie-LORE-ic) sphincter: the circular muscle that separates the stomach from the small intestine and regulates the flow of partially digested food into the small intestine; also called *pylorus or pyloric valve*.

- *pylorus* = gatekeeper

small intestine: a 10-foot length of small-diameter intestine that is the major site of digestion of food and absorption of nutrients. Its segments are the duodenum, jejunum, and ileum.

duodenum (doo-oh-DEEN-um, doo-ODD-num): the top portion of the small intestine (about "12 fingers' breadth long" in ancient terminology).

- *duodecim* = twelve

jejunum (je-JOON-um): the first two-fifths of the small intestine beyond the duodenum.

ileum (ILL-ee-um): the last segment of the small intestine.

gallbladder: the organ that stores and concentrates bile. When it receives the signal that fat is present in the duodenum, the gallbladder contracts and squirts bile through the bile duct into the duodenum.

pancreas: a gland that secretes digestive enzymes and juices into the duodenum. (The pancreas also secretes hormones that help to maintain glucose homeostasis into the blood.)

ileocecal (ill-ee-oh-SEEK-ul) valve: the sphincter separating the small and large intestines.

large intestine or colon (COAL-un): the lower portion of intestine that completes the digestive process. Its segments are the ascending colon, the transverse colon, the descending colon, and the sigmoid colon.

- *sigmoid* = shaped like the letter S (sigma in Greek)

appendix: a narrow blind sac extending from the beginning of the colon that stores lymph cells.

rectum: the muscular terminal part of the intestine, extending from the sigmoid colon to the anus.

anus (AY-nus): the terminal outlet of the GI tract.

The tongue allows you not only to taste food but also to move food around the mouth, facilitating chewing and swallowing. When you swallow a mouthful of food, it passes through the **pharynx**, a short tube that is shared by both the **digestive system** and the respiratory system.

Mouth to the Esophagus Once a mouthful of food has been chewed and swallowed, it is called a **bolus**. Each bolus first slides across your **epiglottis**, bypassing the entrance to your lungs. During each swallow, the epiglottis closes off your trachea, the air passageway to the lungs, so that you do not choke.

Esophagus to the Stomach The **esophagus** has a **sphincter** muscle at each end. During a swallow, the upper **esophageal sphincter** opens. The bolus then slides down the esophagus, which conducts it through the diaphragm to the **stomach**. The lower

---

FIGURE 2-1 The Gastrointestinal Tract

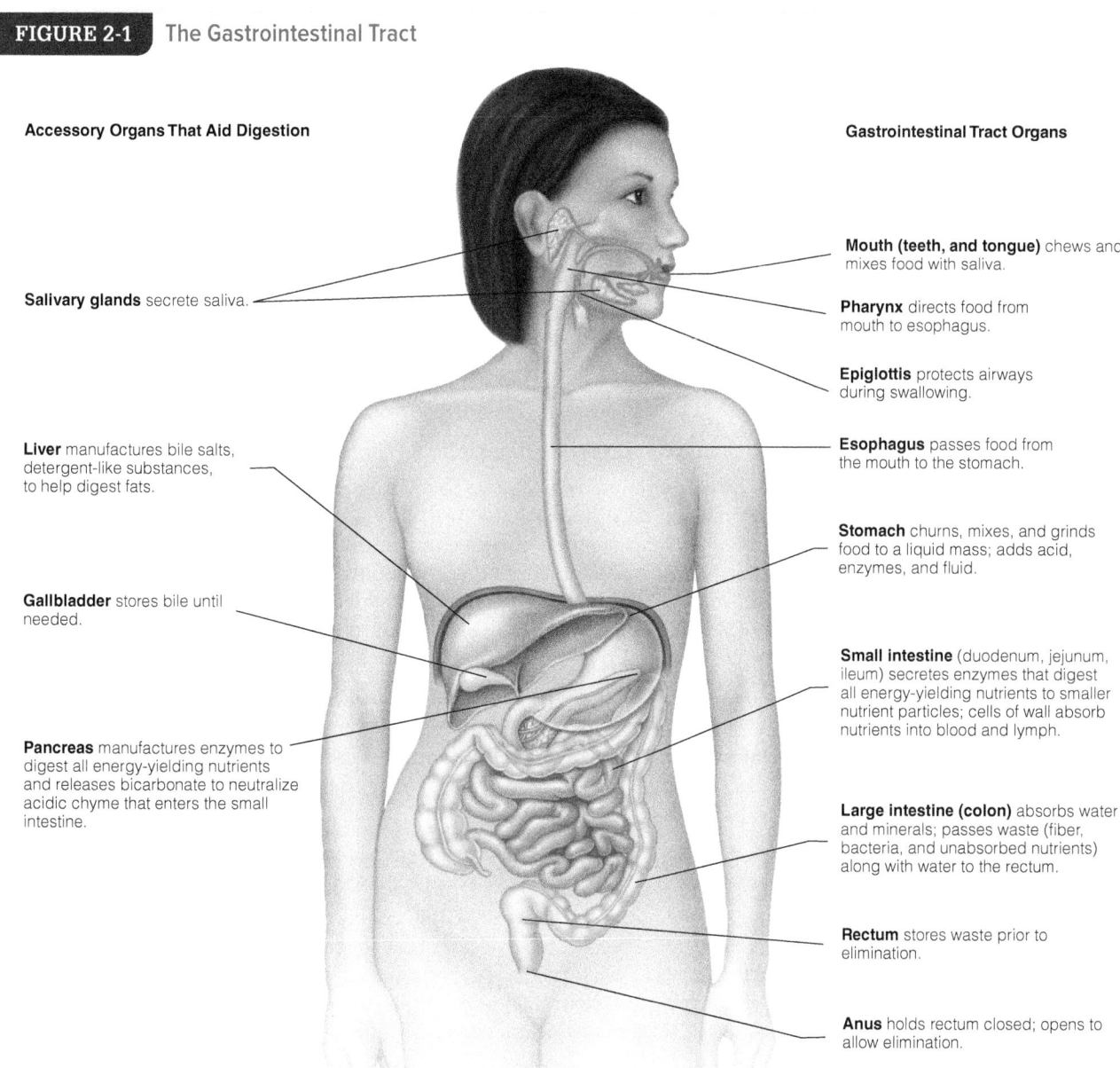

Accessory Organs That Aid Digestion

Salivary glands secrete saliva.

Liver manufactures bile salts, detergent-like substances, to help digest fats.

Gallbladder stores bile until needed.

Pancreas manufactures enzymes to digest all energy-yielding nutrients and releases bicarbonate to neutralize acidic chyme that enters the small intestine.

Gastrointestinal Tract Organs

Mouth (teeth, and tongue) chews and mixes food with saliva.

Pharynx directs food from mouth to esophagus.

Epiglottis protects airways during swallowing.

Esophagus passes food from the mouth to the stomach.

Stomach churns, mixes, and grinds food to a liquid mass; adds acid, enzymes, and fluid.

Small intestine (duodenum, jejunum, ileum) secretes enzymes that digest all energy-yielding nutrients to smaller nutrient particles; cells of wall absorb nutrients into blood and lymph.

Large intestine (colon) absorbs water and minerals; passes waste (fiber, bacteria, and unabsorbed nutrients) along with water to the rectum.

Rectum stores waste prior to elimination.

Anus holds rectum closed; opens to allow elimination.

esophageal sphincter closes behind the bolus so that it cannot slip back. The stomach retains the bolus for a while, adds juices to it (gastric juices are discussed on pp. 45–46), and transforms it into a semiliquid mass called **chyme**. Then, bit by bit, the stomach releases the chyme through another sphincter, the **pyloric sphincter**, which opens into the **small intestine** and then closes after the chyme passes through.

The Small Intestine At the beginning of the small intestine, the chyme passes by an opening from the common bile duct, which secretes digestive fluids into the small intestine from two organs outside the GI tract—the **gallbladder** and the **pancreas**. The chyme travels on down the small intestine through its three segments—the **duodenum**, the **jejunum**, and the **ileum**. Together, the segments amount to a total of about 10 feet of tubing coiled within the abdomen.* Digestion is completed within the small intestine.

The Large Intestine (Colon) Having traveled the length of the small intestine, what remains of the intestinal contents passes through another sphincter, the **ileocecal valve**, into the beginning of the **large intestine (colon)** in the lower right-hand side of the abdomen. Upon entering the colon, the contents pass another opening: the one leading to the **appendix**, a blind sac about the size of your little finger. Normally, the contents bypass this opening, however, and travel up the right-hand side of the abdomen, across the front to the left-hand side, down to the lower left-hand side, and finally below the other folds of the intestines to the back side of the body above the **rectum**.

The Rectum As the intestinal contents pass to the rectum, the colon withdraws water, leaving semisolid waste. The strong muscles of the rectum hold back this waste until it is time to defecate. Then the rectal muscles relax, and the last sphincter in the system, the **anus**, opens to allow the wastes to pass. Thus, food travels through the digestive tract in this order: mouth, esophagus, lower esophageal sphincter (or cardiac sphincter), stomach, pyloric sphincter, duodenum (common bile duct enters here), jejunum, ileum, ileocecal valve, large intestine (colon), rectum, and anus.

The Involuntary Muscles and the Glands

You are usually unaware of all the activity that goes on between the time you swallow and the time you defecate. As is the case with so much else that happens in the body, the muscles and **glands** of the digestive tract meet internal needs without your having to exert any conscious effort to get the work done.

People consciously chew and swallow, but even in the mouth there are some processes over which you have no control. The salivary glands secrete just enough saliva to moisten each mouthful of food so that it can pass easily down your esophagus.

Gastrointestinal Motility Once you have swallowed, materials are moved through the rest of the GI tract by involuntary muscular contractions. This motion, known as **gastrointestinal motility**, consists of two types of movement, peristalsis and segmentation (see Figure 2-2). Peristalsis propels, or pushes; segmentation mixes, with more gradual pushing.

Peristalsis **Peristalsis** begins when the bolus enters the esophagus. The entire GI tract is ringed with circular muscles, which are surrounded by longitudinal muscles. When the rings tighten and the long muscles relax, the tube is constricted. When the rings relax and the long muscles tighten, the tube bulges. These actions alternate continually and push the intestinal contents along. If you have ever watched a bolus of food pass along the body of a snake, you have a good picture of how these muscles work. The waves of contraction ripple through the GI tract at varying rates and intensities depending on the part of the GI tract and on whether food is present. Peristalsis, aided by the sphincter muscles located at key places, keeps things moving along. However, factors such as stress, medicines, and medical conditions may interfere with normal GI tract contractions.[1]

chyme (KIME): the semiliquid mass of partly digested food expelled by the stomach into the duodenum (the top portion of the small intestine).

gastrointestinal motility: spontaneous motion in the digestive tract accomplished by involuntary muscular contractions.

peristalsis (peri-STALL-sis): successive waves of involuntary muscular contractions passing along the walls of the GI tract that push the contents along.

  peri = around
  stellein = wrap

---

*The small intestine is almost two and a half times shorter in living adults than it is at death, when muscles are relaxed and elongated.

FIGURE 2-2 Peristalsis and Segmentation

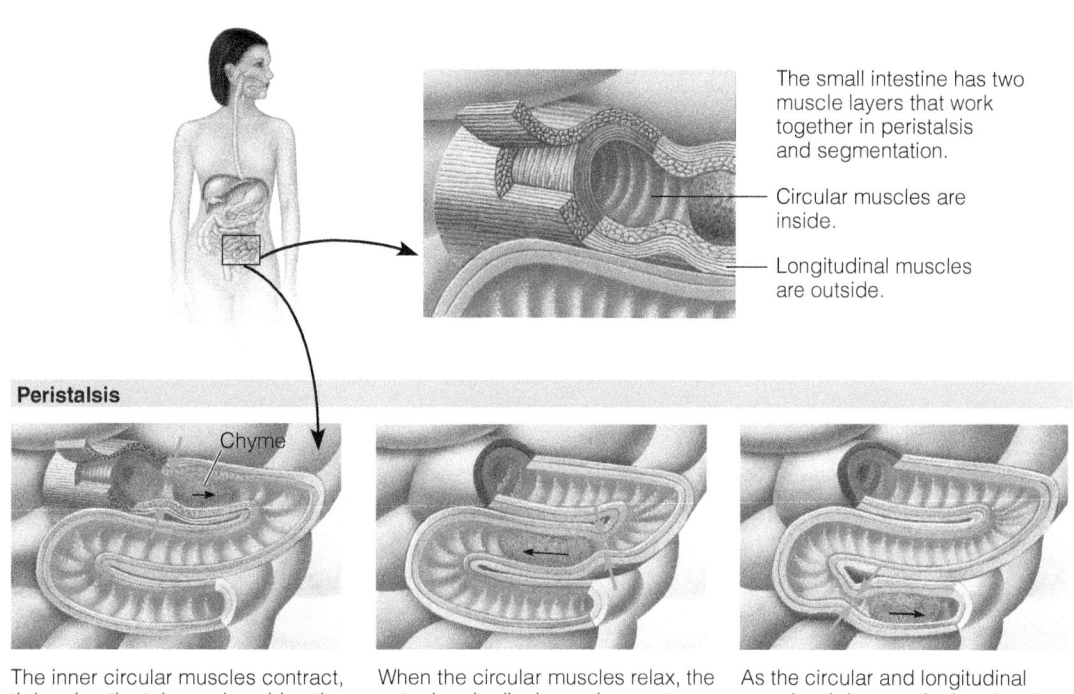

The small intestine has two muscle layers that work together in peristalsis and segmentation.

Circular muscles are inside.

Longitudinal muscles are outside.

Peristalsis

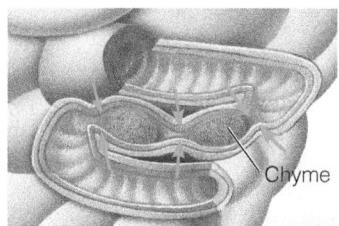

Chyme

The inner circular muscles contract, tightening the tube and pushing the food forward in the intestine.

When the circular muscles relax, the outer longitudinal muscles contract, and the intestinal tube is loose.

As the circular and longitudinal muscles tighten and relax, the chyme moves ahead of the constriction.

Segmentation

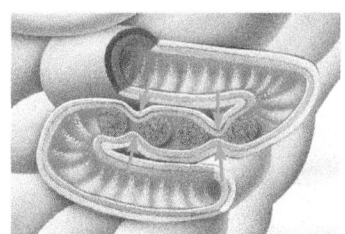

Chyme

Circular muscles contract, creating segments within the intestine.

As each set of circular muscles relaxes and contracts, the chyme is broken up and mixed with digestive juices.

These alternating contractions, occurring 12 to 16 times per minute, continue to mix the chyme and bring the nutrients into contact with the intestinal lining for absorption.

Segmentation The intestines not only push but also periodically squeeze their contents as if a string tied around the intestines were being pulled tight. This motion, called **segmentation**, forces the contents back a few inches, mixing them and promoting close contact with the digestive juices and the absorbing cells of the intestinal walls before letting the contents slowly move along again.

Liquefying Process Besides forcing the intestinal contents along, the muscles of the GI tract help to liquefy them to chyme so that the digestive juices will have access to all their nutrients. The mouth initiates this liquefying process by chewing, adding saliva, and stirring with the tongue to reduce the food to a coarse mash suitable for swallowing. The stomach then further mixes and kneads the food.

Stomach Action The stomach has the thickest walls and strongest muscles of all the GI tract organs. In addition to circular and longitudinal muscles, the stomach has a third layer of diagonal muscles that also alternately contract and relax (see Figure 2-3).

segmentation: periodic squeezing or partitioning of the intestine by its circular muscles that both mixes and slowly pushes the contents along.

FIGURE 2-3 Stomach Muscles

The stomach has three layers of muscles.

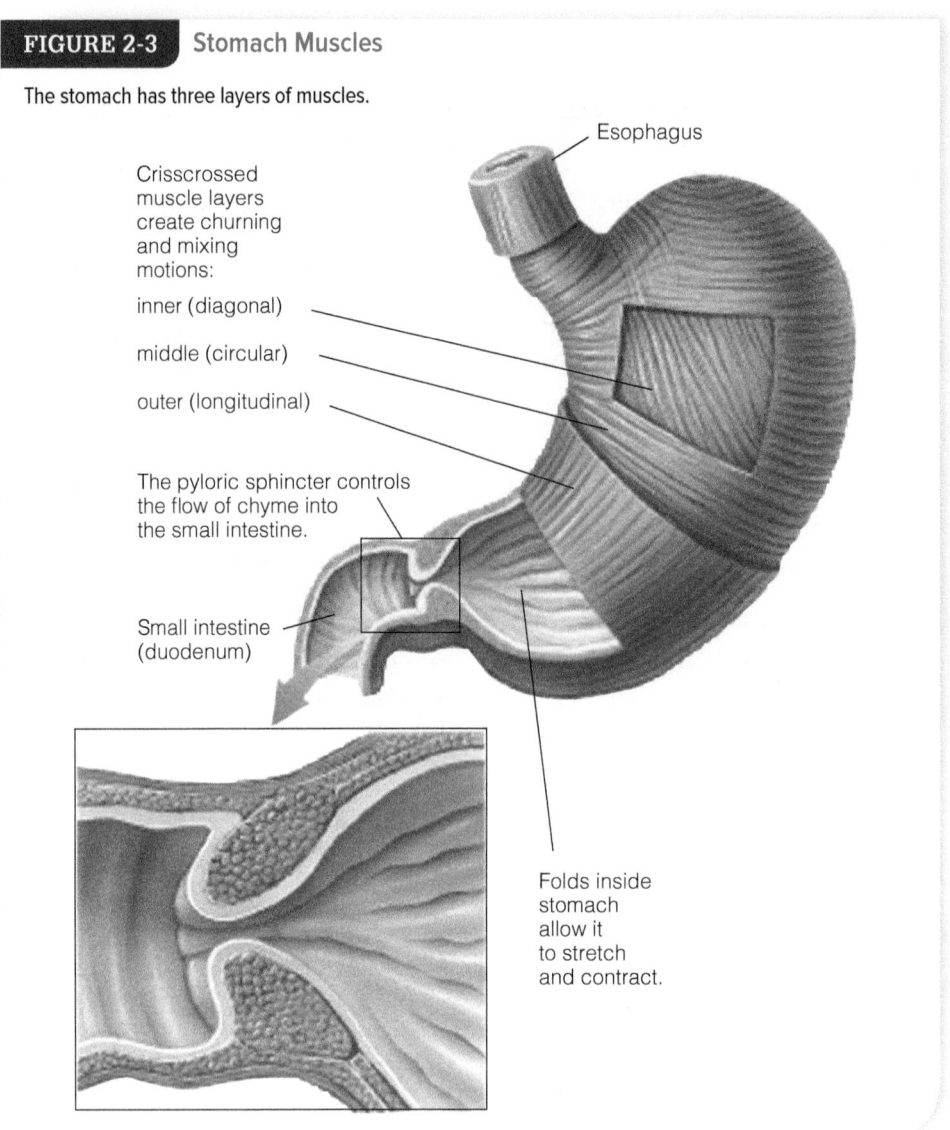

Esophagus

Crisscrossed muscle layers create churning and mixing motions:

inner (diagonal)

middle (circular)

outer (longitudinal)

The pyloric sphincter controls the flow of chyme into the small intestine.

Small intestine (duodenum)

Folds inside stomach allow it to stretch and contract.

These three sets of muscles work to force the chyme downward, but the pyloric sphincter usually remains tightly closed so that the stomach's contents are thoroughly mixed and squeezed before being released. Meanwhile, the gastric glands are adding juices. When the chyme is thoroughly liquefied, the pyloric sphincter opens briefly, about three times a minute, to allow small portions through. At this point, the intestinal contents no longer resemble food in the least.

Review Notes

- Food enters the mouth and travels down the esophagus and through the lower esophageal sphincter to the stomach, then through the pyloric sphincter to the small intestine, on through the ileocecal valve to the large intestine, and past the appendix to the rectum, exiting through the anus.
- The wavelike contractions of peristalsis and the periodic squeezing of segmentation keep things moving at a reasonable pace.
- The mouth begins the process of liquefying food by chewing and adding saliva to reduce food to a coarse mash for swallowing. The stomach then further mixes and kneads the food.

2.2 The Process of Digestion

One person eats nothing but vegetables, fruit, and nuts; another, nothing but meat, milk, and potatoes. How is it that both people wind up with essentially the same body composition? It all comes down to the body rendering food—whatever it is to start with—into the basic units that make up carbohydrate, fat, and protein. The body absorbs these units and builds its tissues from them.

To digest food, five different body organs secrete digestive juices: the salivary glands, the stomach, the small intestine, the liver (via the gallbladder), and the pancreas. These secretions enter the GI tract at various points along the way, bringing an abundance of water and a variety of **enzymes**. Each of the juices has a turn to mix with the food and promote its breakdown to small units that can be absorbed into the body. Box 2-2 defines some of the digestive glands and their juices.

Digestion in the Mouth

Digestion of carbohydrate begins in the mouth, where the **salivary glands** secrete **saliva**, which contains water, salts, and enzymes (including salivary **amylase**) that break the bonds in the chains of starch. Saliva also protects the tooth surfaces and linings of the mouth, esophagus, and stomach from attack by molecules that might harm them. The enzymes in the mouth do not, for the most part, affect the fats, proteins, vitamins, minerals, and fiber that are present in the foods people eat.

Box 2-2   Glossary of Digestive Glands and Their Secretions

amylase (AM-uh-lace): an enzyme that splits amylose (a form of starch).

-ase (ACE): a suffix denoting an enzyme. The root of the word often identifies the compound the enzyme works on. Examples include:

- *carbohydrase* (car-boe-HIGH-drase), any of a number of enzymes that break the chemical bonds of carbohydrates.
- *lipase* (LYE-pase), any of a number of enzymes that break the chemical bonds of lipids (fats).
- *protease* (PRO-tee-ase), any of a number of enzymes that break the chemical bonds of proteins.

bicarbonate: an alkaline secretion of the pancreas; part of the pancreatic juice. (Bicarbonate also occurs widely in all cell fluids.)

bile: an emulsifier that prepares fats and oils for digestion; made by the liver, stored in the gallbladder, and released into the small intestine when needed.

gastric glands: exocrine glands in the stomach wall that secrete gastric juice into the stomach.

- *gastro* = stomach

gastric juice: the digestive secretion of the gastric glands containing a mixture of water, hydrochloric acid, and enzymes. The principal enzymes are pepsin (acts on proteins) and lipase (acts on emulsified fats).

glands: cells or groups of cells that secrete materials for special uses in the body. Glands may be *exocrine* (EKS-oh-crin) *glands*, secreting their materials "out" (into the digestive tract or onto the surface of the skin), or *endocrine* (EN-doe-crin) *glands*, secreting their materials "in" (into the blood).

- *exo* = outside
- *endo* = inside
- *krine* = to separate

hydrochloric acid (HCl): an acid composed of hydrogen and chloride atoms; normally produced by the gastric glands.

intestinal juice: the secretion of the intestinal glands; contains enzymes for the digestion of carbohydrate and protein and a minor enzyme for fat digestion.

liver: the organ that manufactures bile. (The liver's other functions are described in Chapter 19.)

mucus (MYOO-cuss): a mucopolysaccharide (a relative of carbohydrate) secreted by cells of the stomach wall that protects the cells from exposure to digestive juices (and other destructive agents). The cellular lining of the stomach wall with its coat of mucus is known as the *mucous membrane*. (The noun is *mucus*; the adjective is *mucous*.)

pancreatic (pank-ree-AT-ic) juice: the exocrine secretion of the pancreas, containing enzymes for the digestion of carbohydrate, fat, and protein. Juice flows from the pancreas into the small intestine through the pancreatic duct. The pancreas also has an endocrine function, the secretion of insulin and other hormones.

pepsin: a protein-digesting enzyme (gastric protease) in the stomach. It circulates as a precursor, pepsinogen, and is converted to pepsin by the action of stomach acid.

saliva: the secretion of the salivary glands. The principal enzyme is salivary amylase.

salivary glands: exocrine glands that secrete saliva into the mouth.

Digestion in the Stomach

Gastric juice, secreted by the **gastric glands**, is composed of water, enzymes, and **hydrochloric acid**. The acid is so strong that it burns the throat if it happens to reflux into the upper esophagus and mouth. The strong acidity of the stomach prevents bacterial growth and kills most bacteria that enter the body with food. You might expect that the stomach's acid would attack the stomach itself, but the cells of the stomach wall secrete **mucus**, a thick, slimy, white polysaccharide that coats and protects the stomach's lining.

The major digestive event in the stomach is the initial breakdown of proteins. Other than being crushed and mixed with saliva in the mouth, nothing happens to protein until it comes in contact with the gastric juices in the stomach. There, the acid helps to uncoil (denature) the protein's tangled strands so that the stomach enzymes can attack the bonds. Both the enzyme **pepsin** and the stomach acid itself act as catalysts in the process. Minor events are the digestion of some fat by a gastric lipase, the digestion of sucrose (to a very small extent) by the stomach acid, and the attachment of a protein carrier to vitamin B_{12}.

The stomach enzymes work most efficiently in the stomach's strong acid, but salivary amylase, which is swallowed with food, does not work in acid this strong. Consequently, the digestion of starch gradually ceases as the acid penetrates the bolus. In fact, salivary amylase becomes just another protein to be digested.

Digestion in the Small and Large Intestines

By the time food leaves the stomach, digestion of all three energy-yielding nutrients has begun, but the process gains momentum in the small intestine. There, the pancreas and the liver contribute additional digestive juices through the duct leading into the duodenum, and the small intestine adds **intestinal juice**. These juices contain digestive enzymes, bicarbonate, and bile.

Digestive Enzymes **Pancreatic juice** contributes enzymes that digest fats, proteins, and carbohydrates. Glands in the intestinal wall also secrete digestive enzymes. (Review Box 2-2 for details.)

Bicarbonate The pancreatic juice also contains sodium **bicarbonate**, which neutralizes the acidic chyme as it enters the small intestine. From this point on, the contents of the digestive tract are neutral or slightly alkaline. The enzymes from both the intestine and the pancreas work best in this environment.

Bile **Bile** is secreted continuously by the liver and is concentrated and stored in the gallbladder. The gallbladder squirts bile into the duodenum whenever fat arrives there. Bile is not an enzyme but an **emulsifier** that brings fats into suspension in water (see Figure 2-4).* After the fats are emulsified, enzymes can work on them, and they can be absorbed. Thanks to all these secretions, all three energy-yielding nutrients are digested in the small intestine.

The Rate of Digestion The rate of digestion of the energy nutrients depends on the contents of the meal. If the meal is high in simple sugars, digestion proceeds fairly rapidly. On the other hand, if the meal is rich in fat, digestion is slower.

The Final Stage The story of how food is broken down into nutrients that can be absorbed is now nearly complete. The three energy-yielding nutrients—carbohydrate, fat, and protein—are disassembled to basic building blocks before they are absorbed. Most of the other nutrients—vitamins, minerals, and water—are absorbed as they are.

emulsifier: a substance that mixes with both fat and water and that disperses the fat in the water, forming an emulsion.

---

*Mayonnaise, made from vinegar and oil, would separate as other vinegar-and-oil salad dressings do if food chemists did not blend in a third ingredient—an emulsifier. The emulsifier mixes well with the fatty oil and the watery vinegar. In the case of mayonnaise, the emulsifier is lecithin from egg yolks.

FIGURE 2-4 Emulsification of Fat by Bile

Like bile, detergents are emulsifiers and work the same way, which is why they are effective at removing grease spots from clothes. Molecule by molecule, the grease is dissolved out of the spot and suspended in water, where it can be rinsed away.

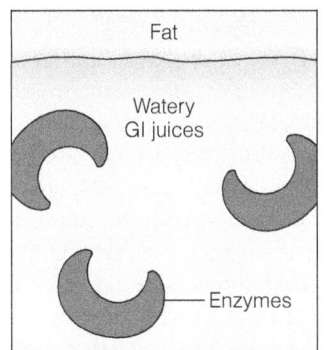 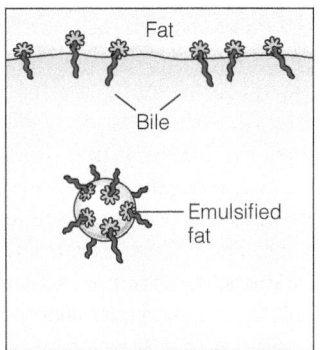 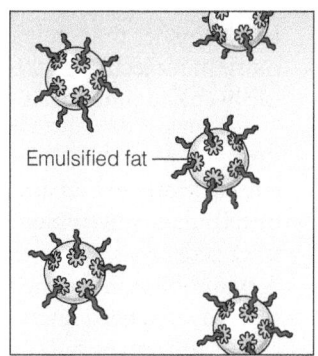 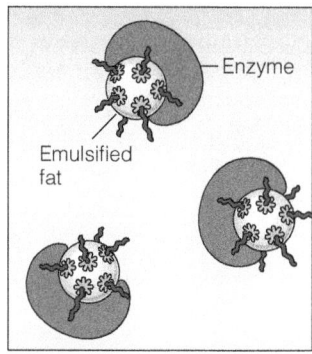

In the stomach, the fat and watery GI juices tend to separate. The enzymes are in the water and can't get at the fat.

When fat enters the small intestine, the gallbladder secretes bile. Bile has an affinity for both fat and water, so it can bring the fat into the water.

Bile's emulsifying action converts large fat globules into small droplets that repel each other.

After emulsification, the enzymes have easy access to the fat droplets.

Undigested residues, such as some fibers, are not absorbed but continue through the digestive tract as a semisolid mass that stimulates the tract's muscles, helping them remain strong and able to perform peristalsis efficiently. Fiber also retains water, keeping the stools soft, and carries some bile acids, sterols, and fat out of the body. Drinking plenty of water in conjunction with eating foods high in fiber supplies fluid for the fiber to take up. This is the basis for the recommendation to drink water and eat fiber-rich foods to relieve constipation.

The process of absorbing the nutrients into the body is discussed in the next section. For the moment, let us assume that the digested nutrients simply disappear from the GI tract as they are ready. Virtually all nutrients are gone by the time the contents of the GI tract reach the end of the small intestine. Little remains but water, a few salts and body secretions, and undigested materials such as fiber. These enter the large intestine (colon).

In the colon, intestinal bacteria degrade some of the fiber to simpler compounds. The colon itself retrieves from its contents the materials that the body is designed to recycle—water and dissolved salts. The waste that is finally excreted has little or nothing of value left in it. The body has extracted all that it can use from the food.

Review Notes

- Digestive enzymes secreted by the salivary glands, stomach, pancreas, and small intestine break down macronutrients into absorbable components.
- Bile produced by the liver and delivered by the gallbladder emulsifies fats to prepare them for digestion.

2.3 The Absorptive System

Within three or four hours after you have eaten a meal, your body must find a way to absorb millions of molecules one by one. The absorptive system is ingeniously designed to accomplish this task.

The Small Intestine

Most absorption takes place in the small intestine. The small intestine is a tube about 10 feet long and about an inch across, yet it provides a surface comparable in area to a small studio apartment (100 to 130 square feet).[2] This may sound quite large, but it is much smaller than previous estimates based on older measurement techniques. When nutrient molecules make contact with this surface, they are absorbed and carried off to the liver and other parts of the body.

Villi and Microvilli How does the intestine manage to provide such a large absorptive surface area? Its inner surface looks smooth, but viewed through a microscope, it turns out to be wrinkled into hundreds of folds. Each fold is covered with thousands of fingerlike projections called **villi**. The villi are as numerous as the hairs on velvet fabric. A single villus, magnified still more, turns out to be composed of several hundred cells, each covered with microscopic hairs called **microvilli** (see Figure 2-5).

The villi are in constant motion. A thin sheet of muscle lines each villus so that it can wave, squirm, and wiggle like the tentacles of a sea anemone. Any nutrient molecule small enough to be absorbed is trapped among the microvilli and drawn into a cell beneath them. Some partially digested nutrients are caught in the microvilli, digested further by enzymes there, and then absorbed into the cells.

Specialization in the Intestinal Tract As you can see, the intestinal tract is beautifully designed to perform its functions. A further refinement of the system is that the cells of

FIGURE 2-5 The Small Intestinal Villi

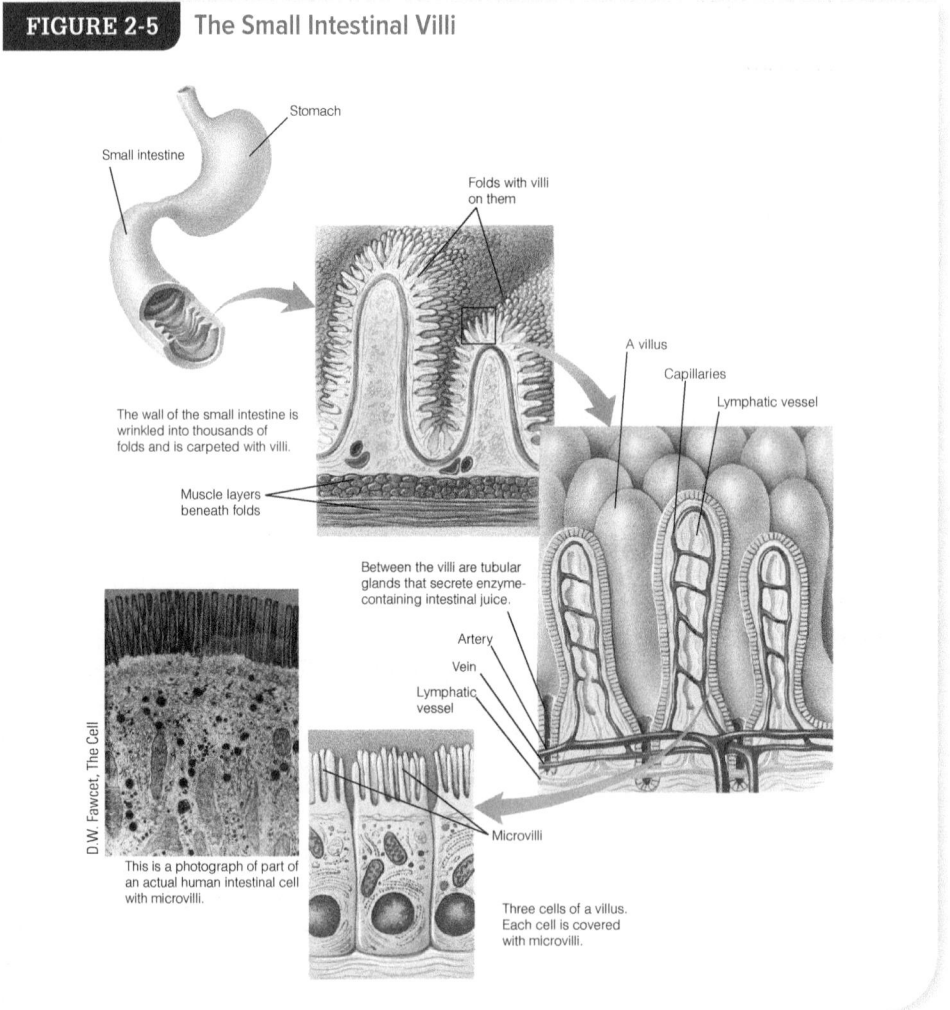

Stomach

Small intestine

Folds with villi on them

The wall of the small intestine is wrinkled into thousands of folds and is carpeted with villi.

Muscle layers beneath folds

A villus

Capillaries

Lymphatic vessel

Between the villi are tubular glands that secrete enzyme-containing intestinal juice.

Artery

Vein

Lymphatic vessel

D.W. Fawcet, The Cell

This is a photograph of part of an actual human intestinal cell with microvilli.

Microvilli

Three cells of a villus. Each cell is covered with microvilli.

successive portions of the tract are specialized to absorb different nutrients. The nutrients that are ready for absorption early are absorbed near the top of the tract; those that take longer to be digested are absorbed farther down. The rate at which the nutrients travel through the GI tract is finely adjusted to maximize their availability to the appropriate absorptive segment of the tract when they are ready. The lowly "gut" turns out to be one of the most elegantly designed organ systems in the body.

The Myth of "Food Combining" Some popular fad diets advocate the idea that people should not eat certain food combinations (for example, fruit and meat) at the same meal because the digestive system cannot handle more than one task at a time. This is a myth. The art of "food combining" (which actually emphasizes "food separating") is based on this idea, and it represents faulty logic and a gross underestimation of the body's capabilities. In fact, the opposite is often true: foods eaten together can enhance each other's use by the body. For example, vitamin C in a pineapple or citrus fruit can enhance the absorption of iron from a meal of chicken and rice or other iron-containing foods. Many other instances of mutually beneficial interactions are presented in later chapters.

Absorption of Nutrients

Once a molecule has entered a cell in a villus, the next step is to transmit it to a destination elsewhere in the body by way of the body's two transport systems—the bloodstream and the **lymphatic system**. As Figure 2-5 shows, both systems supply vessels to each villus. Through these vessels, the nutrients leave the cell and enter either the **lymph** or the blood. In either case, the nutrients end up in the blood, at least for a while. The water-soluble nutrients (and the smaller products of fat digestion) are released directly into the bloodstream by way of the capillaries, but the larger fats and the fat-soluble vitamins find direct access into the capillaries impossible because these nutrients are insoluble in water (and blood is mostly water). They require some packaging before they are released.

The intestinal cells assemble the products of fat digestion into larger molecules called triglycerides. These **triglycerides**, fat-soluble vitamins (when present), and other large lipids (cholesterol and the phospholipids) are then packaged for transport. They cluster together with special proteins to form **chylomicrons**, one kind of lipoproteins (**lipoproteins** are described beginning on p. 51). Finally, the cells release the chylomicrons into the lymphatic system. They can then glide through the lymph spaces until they arrive at a point of entry into the bloodstream near the heart. Thus, some materials from the GI tract initially enter the lymphatic system but soon reach the bloodstream.

lymphatic system: a loosely organized system of vessels and ducts that conveys the products of digestion toward the heart.

lymph (LIMF): the body fluid found in lymphatic vessels. Lymph consists of all the constituents of blood except red blood cells.

triglycerides (try-GLISS-er-rides): one of the main classes of lipids; the chief form of fat in foods and the major storage form of fat in the body; composed of glycerol with three fatty acids attached.

tri = three
glyceride = a compound of glycerol

chylomicrons (kye-lo-MY-crons): the lipoproteins that transport lipids from the intestinal cells into the body. The cells of the body remove the lipids they need from the chylomicrons, leaving chylomicron remnants to be picked up by the liver cells.

lipoproteins: clusters of lipids associated with proteins that serve as transport vehicles for lipids in the lymph and blood.

Review Notes

- The many folds and villi of the small intestine dramatically increase its surface area, facilitating nutrient absorption.
- Nutrients pass through the cells of the villi and enter either the blood (if they are water soluble or small fat fragments) or the lymph (if they are fat soluble).

2.4 Transport of Nutrients

Once a nutrient has entered the bloodstream or the lymphatic system, it may be transported to any part of the body, from the tips of the toes to the roots of the hair, where it becomes available to any of the cells. The circulatory systems are arranged to deliver nutrients wherever they are needed.

The Vascular System

The vascular or blood circulatory system is a closed system of vessels through which blood flows continuously in a figure eight, with the heart serving as a pump at the crossover point. On each loop of the figure eight, blood travels a simple route: heart to arteries to capillaries to veins to heart.

The routing of the blood through the digestive system is different, however. The blood is carried to the digestive system (as it is to all organs) by way of an **artery**, which (as in all organs) branches into **capillaries** to reach every cell. Blood leaving the digestive system, however, goes by way of a **vein**. The **hepatic portal vein** directs blood not back to the heart but to another organ—the liver. This vein branches into a network of small blood vessels (*sinusoids*) so that every cell of the liver has access to the newly absorbed nutrients that the blood is carrying. Blood leaving the liver then *again* collects into a vein, called the **hepatic vein**, which returns the blood to the heart. The route is thus heart to arteries to capillaries (in intestines) to hepatic portal vein to sinusoids (in liver) to hepatic vein to heart.

An anatomist studying this system knows there must be a reason for this special arrangement. The liver is located in the circulation system at the point where it will have the first chance at most of the materials absorbed from the GI tract. In fact, the liver is the body's major metabolic organ (see Figure 2-6) and must prepare the absorbed

---

FIGURE 2-6 The Liver and Its Circulatory System

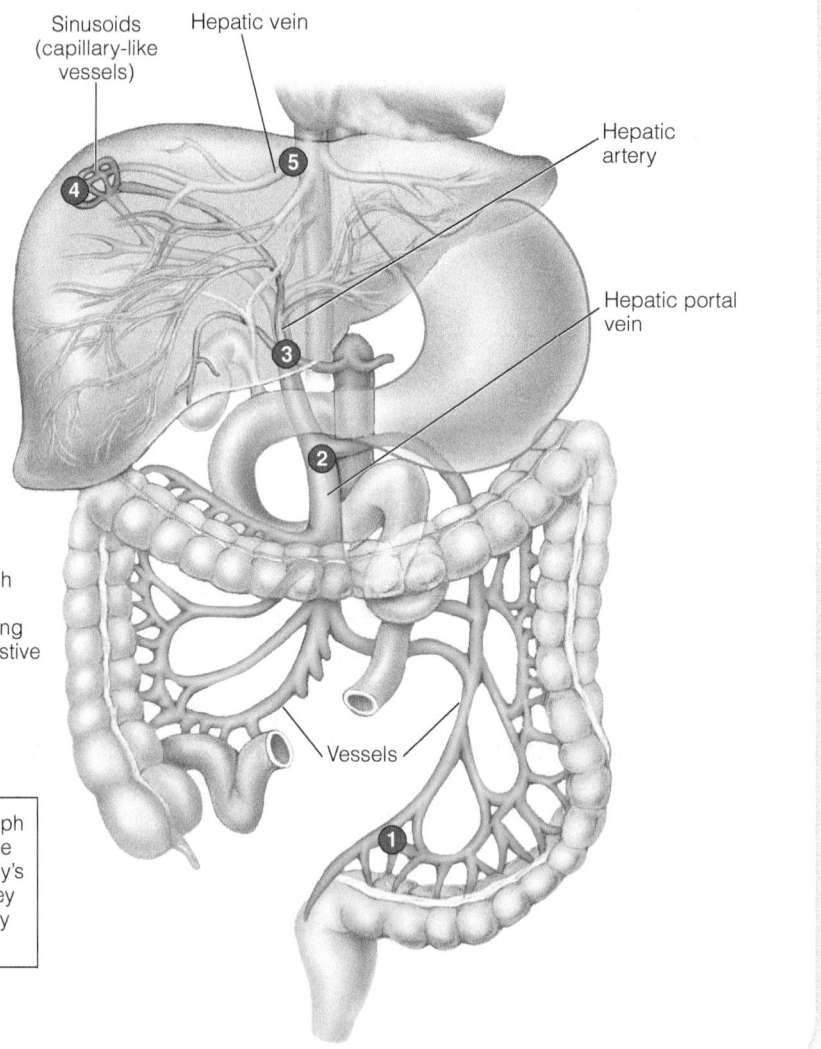

① Vessels gather up nutrients and reabsorbed water and salts from all over the digestive tract.

Not shown here:
Parallel to these vessels (veins) are other vessels (arteries) that carry oxygen-rich blood from the heart to the intestines.

② The vessels merge into the hepatic portal vein, which conducts all absorbed materials to the liver.

③ The hepatic artery brings a supply of freshly oxygenated blood (not loaded with nutrients) from the lungs to supply oxygen to the liver's own cells.

④ Capillary-like vessels (sinusoids) branch all over the liver, making nutrients and oxygen available to all its cells and giving the cells access to blood from the digestive system.

⑤ The hepatic vein gathers up blood in the liver and returns it to the heart.

In contrast, nutrients absorbed into lymph do not go to the liver first. They go to the heart, which pumps them to all the body's cells. The cells remove the nutrients they need, and the liver then has to deal only with the remnants.

Sinusoids (capillary-like vessels)
Hepatic vein
Hepatic artery
Hepatic portal vein
Vessels

nutrients for use by the rest of the body. Furthermore, the liver stands as a gatekeeper to waylay intruders that might otherwise harm the heart or brain. Chapter 19 offers more information about this crucial organ.

The Lymphatic System

The lymphatic system is a one-way route for fluids to travel from tissue spaces into the blood. The lymphatic system has no pump; instead, lymph is squeezed from one portion of the body to another like water in a sponge, as muscles contract and create pressure here and there. Ultimately, the lymph flows into the thoracic duct, a large duct behind the heart. This duct terminates in the subclavian vein, which conducts the lymph into the right upper chamber of the heart. In this way, fat-soluble nutrients absorbed into the lymphatic system from the GI tract finally enter the bloodstream.

Transport of Lipids: Lipoproteins

Within the circulatory system, lipids always travel from place to place bundled with protein, that is, as lipoproteins. When physicians measure a person's blood lipid profile, they are interested in both the types of fat present (such as triglycerides and cholesterol) and the types of lipoproteins that carry them.

VLDL, LDL, and HDL As mentioned earlier, chylomicrons transport newly absorbed (*diet-derived*) lipids from the intestinal cells to the rest of the body. As chylomicrons circulate through the body, cells remove their lipid contents, so the chylomicrons get smaller and smaller. The liver picks up these chylomicron remnants. When necessary, the liver can assemble different lipoproteins, which are known as **very-low-density lipoproteins (VLDL)**. As the body's cells remove triglycerides from the VLDL, the proportions of their lipid and protein contents shift. As this occurs, VLDL become cholesterol-rich **low-density lipoproteins (LDL)**. Cholesterol returning to the liver for metabolism or excretion from other parts of the body is packaged in lipoproteins known as **high-density lipoproteins (HDL)**. HDL are synthesized primarily in the liver.

The density of lipoproteins varies according to the proportion of lipids and protein they contain. The more lipids in the lipoprotein molecule, the lower the density; the more protein, the higher the density. Both LDL and HDL carry lipids around in the blood, but LDL are larger, lighter, and filled with more lipid; HDL are smaller, denser, and packaged with more protein. LDL deliver cholesterol and triglycerides from the liver to the tissues; HDL scavenge excess cholesterol from the tissues and return it to the liver for metabolism or disposal. These different functions explain why some people refer to LDL as "bad" cholesterol and HDL as "good" cholesterol. Keep in mind, though, that there is only one kind of cholesterol molecule; the differences between LDL and HDL reflect proportions of lipids and proteins within them—not the type of cholesterol. Figure 2-7 shows the relative sizes and compositions of the lipoproteins.

Health Implications of LDL and HDL The distinction between LDL and HDL has implications for the health of the heart and blood vessels. High concentrations of LDL in the blood are associated with an increased risk of heart disease, as are low concentrations of HDL.[3] Factors that lower LDL concentrations and raise HDL concentrations include:

- Weight management (see Chapter 7).
- Polyunsaturated or monounsaturated, instead of saturated, fatty acids in the diet (see Chapter 4).
- Soluble fibers (see Chapter 3).
- Physical activity.

Lipoproteins and heart disease are discussed in Chapter 21.

very-low-density lipoproteins (VLDL): the type of lipoproteins made primarily by liver cells to transport lipids to various tissues in the body; composed primarily of triglycerides.

low-density lipoproteins (LDL): the type of lipoproteins derived from VLDL as cells remove triglycerides from them. LDL carry cholesterol and triglycerides from the liver to the cells of the body and are composed primarily of cholesterol.

high-density lipoproteins (HDL): the type of lipoproteins that transport cholesterol back to the liver from peripheral cells; composed primarily of protein.

FIGURE 2-7 The Lipoproteins

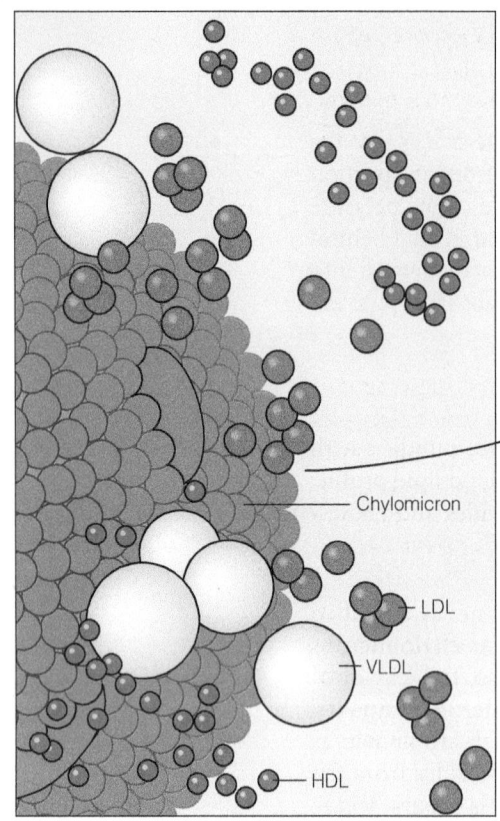

This solar system of lipoproteins shows their relative sizes. Notice how large the fat-filled chylomicron is compared with the others and how the others get progressively smaller as their proportion of fat declines and protein increases.

Chylomicrons contain so little protein and so much triglyceride that they are the lowest in density.

Very-low-density lipoproteins (VLDL) are half triglycerides, accounting for their low density.

Low-density lipoproteins (LDL) are half cholesterol, accounting for their implication in heart disease.

High-density lipoproteins (HDL) are half protein, accounting for their high density.

A typical lipoprotein contains an interior of triglycerides and cholesterol surrounded by phospholipids. The phospholipids' fatty acid "tails" point toward the interior, where the lipids are. Proteins near the outer ends of the phospholipids cover the structure. This arrangement of hydrophobic molecules on the inside and hydrophilic molecules on the outside allows lipids to travel through the watery fluids of the blood.

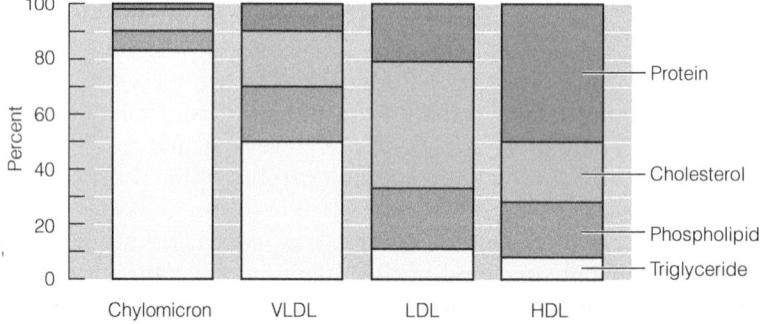

Review Notes

- Nutrients leaving the digestive system via the blood are routed directly to the liver before being transported to the body's cells. Those leaving via the lymphatic system eventually enter the vascular system but bypass the liver at first.
- Within the circulatory system, lipids travel bundled with proteins as lipoproteins. Different types of lipoproteins include chylomicrons, very-low-density lipoproteins (VLDL), low-density lipoproteins (LDL), and high-density lipoproteins (HDL).
- High blood concentrations of LDL and low blood concentrations of HDL are associated with an increased risk of heart disease.

2.5 The Health and Regulation of the GI Tract

This section offers a brief description of the hormonal and nerve regulation of a healthy GI tract as well as bacterial conditions, but many factors influence normal GI function. For example, older adults often experience constipation, in part because the intestinal wall loses strength and elasticity with age, which slows GI motility. Diseases and medications can also interfere with digestion and absorption and often lead to malnutrition. Lack of nourishment, in general, and lack of certain dietary constituents such as fiber, in particular, alter the structure and function of GI cells. Quite simply, GI tract health depends on adequate nutrition.

Gastrointestinal Hormones and Nerve Pathways

The ability of the digestive tract to handle its ever-changing contents illustrates an important physiological principle that governs the way all living things function—the principle of **homeostasis**. Simply stated, survival depends on body conditions staying about the same; if they deviate too far from the norm, the body must "do something" to bring them back to normal. The body's regulation of digestion is one example of homeostatic regulation. The body also regulates it temperature, its blood pressure, and all other aspects of its blood chemistry in similar ways.

Two intricate and sensitive systems coordinate all the digestive and absorptive processes of the GI tract: the hormonal (or endocrine) system and the nervous system. Even before the first bite of food is taken, the mere thought, sight, or smell of food can trigger a response from these systems. Then, as food travels through the GI tract, it either stimulates or inhibits digestive secretions and motility by way of messages that are carried from organ to another by both **hormones** and nerve pathways.

For example, food entering the stomach stimulates cells in the stomach wall to release the hormone gastrin. **Gastrin**, in turn, stimulates the stomach glands to secrete the components of hydrochloric acid. When the appropriate stomach acidity is reached, the acid itself turns off the gastrin-producing cells; they stop releasing gastrin, and the glands stop producing hydrochloric acid.

Nerve receptors in the stomach wall also respond to the presence of food and stimulate the gastric glands to secrete juices and the muscles to contract. As the stomach empties, the receptors are no longer stimulated, the flow of juices slows, and the stomach quiets down. Hormonal and nervous mechanisms like the one just described account for much of the GI tract's ability and the entire body's ability, to adapt to changing conditions.

Gastrin is one of the most-studied GI hormones, but the GI tract releases more than 50 hormones. In addition to assisting with digestion and absorption, many of these hormones regulate food intake and influence satiation—the feeling of satisfaction and fullness that occurs during a meal and halts eating. Current research is focusing on the roles these hormones may play in the development of obesity and its treatments (Chapter 7 provides more details).

Gastrointestinal Microbes

A healthy GI tract is home to a vibrant community of some 100 trillion **microbes**—bacteria, viruses, fungi, protozoa, and other microorganisms, collectively known as the **GI microbiota**. The prevalence of different microbes in various parts of the GI tract depends on such factors as **pH**, peristalsis, diet, and other microbes. Relatively few microbes can live in the low pH of the stomach with its somewhat rapid peristalsis, whereas the neutral pH and slower peristalsis of the lower small intestine and the large intestine permit the growth of a diverse and abundant population.

homeostasis (HOME-ee-oh-STAY-sis): the maintenance of constant internal conditions (such as blood chemistry, temperature, and blood pressure) by the body's control systems.

homeo = like, similar
stasis = staying

hormones: chemical messengers. Hormones are secreted by a variety of glands in response to altered conditions in the body. Each hormone travels to one or more specific target tissues or organs, where it elicits a specific response to maintain homeostasis. The study of hormones and their actions is called *endocrinology*.

gastrin: a hormone secreted by cells in the stomach wall. Target organ: the glands of the stomach. Response: secretion of gastric acid.

microbes (MY-krobes): microscopically small organisms including bacteria, viruses, fungi, and protozoa; also called microorganisms.

mikros = small

GI microbiota: the collection of microbes found in the GI tract, sometimes called the *microflora* or *gut flora*. The collection of genes and genomes of the microbiota is called the *microbiome*.

pH: the concentration of hydrogen ions. The lower the pH, the stronger the acid. Thus, pH 2 is a strong acid; pH 6 is a weak acid; pH 7 is neutral; and a pH above 7 is alkaline.

Recent research has revealed that the GI microbiota may play a critical role in health.[4] Changes in the microbiota composition and activity are associated with dozens of common diseases, such as irritable bowel syndrome and obesity.[5] Ongoing research is trying to determine exactly how the GI microbiota might contribute to the development of obesity and other metabolic diseases.[6] The GI microbiota changes in response to diet—both in the short term (daily meals) and in the long term (habitual diet patterns.)[7] In fact, one of the ways diet may help manage diseases is by changing the microbiota.[8] Consider, for example, that the most recommended diet strategy to improve health—plant-based eating patterns—promotes the most favorable changes in the GI microbiota.[9] Such diets are high in fibers that cannot be digested by the human body but can provide a major source of energy for bacteria, fostering their growth. As GI bacteria digest and metabolize fibers, they produce short fragment of fat, which influence metabolism, inflammation, and disease.[10] These actions may help to explain how dietary fiber protects against colon cancer.[11]

Fiber and some other food components are called prebiotics because they encourage the growth and activity of bacteria. Research suggests that **prebiotics** may reduce the risk of GI infections, inflammation, and disorders; increase the bioavailability of nutrients; and regulate appetite and satiety.[12]

Some foods contain probiotics, live microbes that change the conditions in the GI tract in ways that seem to benefit health. For example, yogurt, with its live bacteria strains, has been used for thousands of years for health-promoting properties.[13] The influence of probiotics on intestinal health is the topic of Nutrition in Practice 18. Research studies continue to explore how diet influences GI bacteria and which foods—with their prebiotics and probiotics—affect GI health. In addition, research studies are beginning to reveal several health benefits beyond the GI tract—such as lowering blood cholesterol, blood pressure, and inflammation.[14]

Bacteria in the GI tract also produce several vitamins, including biotin, folate, pantothenic acid, riboflavin, thiamin, vitamin B_6, vitamin B_{12}, and vitamin K. Because the amount produced is insufficient to meet the body's needs fully, these vitamins are considered essential nutrients and must be provided by the diet.

The System at Its Best

The GI tract is the first organ in the body to deal with the nutrients that will ultimately maintain the health and nutrition status of the whole body. The intricate architecture of the GI tract makes it sensitive and responsive to conditions in its environment. One condition indispensable to its performance is its own good health. Such lifestyle factors as sleep, physical activity, state of mind, and nutrition affect GI tract health. Adequate sleep allows for repair and maintenance of tissue. Physical activity promotes healthy muscle tone and may protect against cancer of the colon.[15] Mental state profoundly affects digestion and absorption through the activity of nerves and hormones that help regulate these processes. A relaxed, peaceful attitude during a meal enhances digestion and absorption.

Review Notes

- The regulation of GI tract function depends on the coordinated efforts of the hormonal system and the nervous system.
- A diverse and abundant microbiome supports GI health.
- To function properly, a healthy GI tract needs adequate sleep, regular physical activity, and adequate nutrition.

1. Once food is swallowed, it travels through the digestive tract in this order:
   a. esophagus, stomach, large intestine, liver.
   b. esophagus, stomach, small intestine, large intestine.
   c. small intestine, stomach, esophagus, large intestine.
   d. small intestine, large intestine, stomach, esophagus.

2. Once chyme travels the length of the small intestine, it passes through the ileocecal valve at the beginning of the:
   a. large intestine.
   b. stomach.
   c. esophagus.
   d. jejunum.

3. The periodic squeezing or partitioning of the intestine by its circular muscles that both mixes and slowly pushes the contents along is known as:
   a. secretion.
   b. absorption.
   c. peristalsis.
   d. segmentation.

4. An enzyme in saliva begins the digestion of:
   a. starch.
   b. vitamins.
   c. protein.
   d. minerals.

5. Bile is:
   a. an enzyme that splits starch.
   b. an alkaline secretion of the pancreas.
   c. an emulsifier made by the liver that prepares fats and oils for digestion.
   d. a stomach secretion containing water, hydrochloric acid, and the enzymes pepsin and lipase.

6. Which nutrient passes through the large intestine mostly unabsorbed?
   a. Fiber
   b. Vitamins
   c. Minerals
   d. Starch

7. The two major nutrient transport systems in the body are:
   a. LDL and HDL.
   b. digestion and absorption.
   c. lipoproteins and chylomicrons.
   d. the vascular and lymphatic systems.

8. Within the circulatory system, lipids always travel from place to place bundled with proteins as:
   a. microvilli.
   b. chylomicrons.
   c. lipoproteins.
   d. phospholipids.

9. Elevated LDL concentrations in the blood are associated with:
   a. a high-protein diet.
   b. a low risk of diabetes.
   c. too much physical activity.
   d. an increased risk of heart disease.

10. Three factors that lower the concentration of LDL and raise the concentration of HDL in the blood are:
    a. polyunsaturated fat, rest, and dietary HDL.
    b. antioxidants, insoluble fibers, and dietary HDL.
    c. saturated fat, antioxidants, and insoluble fibers.
    d. weight control, soluble fibers, and physical activity.

Answers: 1. b, 2. a, 3. d, 4. a, 5. c, 6. a, 7. d, 8. c, 9. d, 10. d

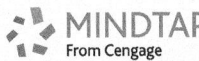 **MINDTAP** From Cengage   For more chapter resources visit **www.cengage.com** to access MindTap, a complete digital course.

Clinical Applications

1. People who experience malabsorption frequently have the most difficulty digesting fat. Considering the differences in fat, carbohydrate, and protein digestion and absorption, can you offer an explanation?

2. How might you explain the importance of dietary fiber to a client who frequently experiences constipation?

Notes

1. C. Stasi and coauthors, Serotonin receptors and their role in the Pathophysiology and therapy of irritable bowel syndrome, *Techniques in Coloproctology* 18 (2014): 613–621.

2. H. F. Helander and L. Fändriks, Surface area of the digestive tract—revisited, *Scandinavian Journal of Gastroenterology* 49 (2014): 681–689.

3. D. Mozaffarian and coauthors, Heart disease and stroke statistics—2016 update: A report from the American Heart Association, *Circulation* 133 (2016): e38-360.

4. S. V. Lynch and O. Pedersen, The human intestinal microbiome in health and disease, *New England Journal of Medicine* 375 (2016): 2369–2379; D. S. Spasova and C. D. Surh, Blowing on embers: Commensal microbiota and our immune system, *Frontiers in Immunology* 5 (2014): 1–20.

5. D. A. Relman, The human microbiome and the future practice of medicine, *Journal of the American Medical Association* 314 (2015): 1127–1128; C. M. Ferreira and coauthors, The central role of the gut microbiota in chronic inflammatory diseases, *Journal of Immunology Research* 2014 (2014): 689492.

6. I. Moreno-Indias and coauthors, Impact of the gut microbiota on the development of obesity and type 2 diabetes mellitus, *Frontiers in Microbiology* 5 (2014): 1–10.

7. L. A. David and coauthors, Diet rapidly and reproducibly alters the human gut microbiome, *Nature* 505 (2014): 559–563; N. Voreades, A. Kozil, and T. L. Weir, Diet and the development of the human intestinal microbiome, *Frontiers in Microbiology*, 5 (2014): 1–9.

8. T. Patel, P. Bhattacharya, and S. Das, Gut microbiota: An indicator to gastrointestinal tract diseases, *Journal of Gastrointestinal Cancer* 47 (2016): 232–238; O. O. Erejuwa, S. A. Sulaiman, and M. S. Ab Wahab, Modulation of gut microbiota in the management of metabolic disorders: The prospects and challenges, International *Journal of Molecular Sciences* 15 (2014): 4158–4188.

9. V. A. do Rosario, R. Fernandes, and E. B. S. de M. Trindade, Vegetarian diets and gut microbiota: Important shifts in markers of metabolism and cardiovascular disease, *Nutrition Reviews* 74 (2016): 444–454; J. M. W. Wong, Gut microbiota and cardiometabolic outcomes: Influence of dietary patterns and their associated components, *American Journal of Clinical Nutrition* 100 (2014): 369S–377S.

10. J. Tan and coauthors, The role of short-chain fatty acids in health and disease, *Advances in Immunology* 121 (2014): 91–119.

11. H. Zeng, D. L. lazarova, M. Bordonaro, Mechanisms linking dietary fiber, gut microbiota and colon cancer prevention, *World Journal of Gastrointestinal Oncology* 6 (2014): 41–51.

12. J. R. Marchesi and coauthors, The gut microbiota and host health: A new clinical frontier, Gut 65 (2016): 330–339; J. Breton and coauthors, Gut commensal *E. coli* proteins activate host satiety pathways following nutrient-induced bacterial growth, *Cell Metabolism* 23 (2016): 324–334; A. Perez-Cornago and coauthors, Prebiotic consumption and the incidence of overweight in a Mediterranean cohort: The Seguimiento Universidad de navarra Project, *American Journal of Clinical Nutrition* 102 (2015): 1554–1562.

13. M. Fisberg and R. Machado, History of yogurt and current patterns of consumption, *Nutrition Reviews* 73 (2015): 4–7.

14. Marchesi and coauthors, 2016; D. B. DiRienzo, Effect of probiotics on biomarkers of cardiovascular disease: Implications for heart-healthy diets, *Nutrition Reviews* 72 (2014): 18–29.

15. F. T. Bosman, Colorectal cancer, in *World Cancer Report* 2014, eds., B. W. Stewart and C. P. Wild (Geneva, Switzerland, International Agency for Research on Cancer, 2014), pp. 392–402.

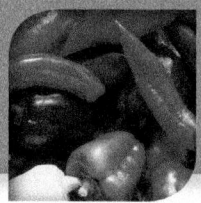

2.6 Nutrition in Practice
Food Safety

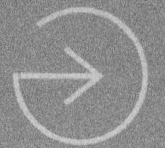

The Food and Drug Administration (FDA) lists **foodborne illness** as the leading food safety concern in the United States because **outbreaks** of food poisoning far outnumber episodes of any other kind of food contamination. The **CDC (Centers for Disease Control and Prevention)** estimates that 48 million cases of foodborne illnesses occur each year in the United States.[1] An estimated 128,000 people become so sick as to need hospitalization. For some 3000 people each year, the symptoms (Table NP2-1) are so severe as to cause death. Most vulnerable are pregnant women; very young, very old, sick, or malnourished people; and those with an immune system weakened by disease or medical treatment.[2] By taking the proper precautions, people can minimize their chances of contracting foodborne illnesses. Box NP2-1 defines related terms.

What is foodborne illness?

Foodborne illness can be caused by either an infection or an intoxication. Table NP2-2 summarizes the **pathogens** responsible for 90 percent of foodborne illnesses, related hospitalizations, and deaths, along with food sources, general symptoms, and prevention methods.

What is the difference between foodborne infections and food intoxications?

Foodborne infections are caused by eating foods contaminated by infectious microbes. Among foodborne infections, *Salmonella* is the leading cause of illnesses

TABLE NP2-1	Symptoms of Foodborne Illness

GET MEDICAL HELP WHEN THESE SYMPTOMS OCCUR:

- Bloody diarrhea
- Diarrhea lasting more than three days
- Prolonged vomiting that prevents keeping liquids down and can lead to dehydration
- Difficulty breathing
- Difficulty swallowing
- Double vision
- Fever lasting more than 24 hours
- Headache accompanied by muscle stiffness and fever
- Numbness, muscle weakness, and tingling sensations in the skin
- Rapid heart rate, fainting, and dizziness

and hospitalizations; *Listeria* is responsible for the most deaths.[3] Pathogens commonly enter the GI tract in contaminated foods such as undercooked poultry and unpasteurized milk. Symptoms generally include abdominal cramps, fever, vomiting, and diarrhea.

Food intoxications are caused by eating foods containing natural toxins or, more likely, microbes that produce toxins. The most common food toxin is produced by *Staphylococcus aureus*; it affects more than 1 million people each year. Less common, but more infamous, is

Box NP2-1 Glossary

CDC (Centers for Disease Control and Prevention): a branch of the Department of Health and Human Services that is responsible for, among other things, identifying, monitoring, and reporting foodborne illnesses and outbreaks (www.cdc.gov).

cross-contamination: the contamination of food by bacteria that occurs when the food comes into contact with surfaces previously touched by raw meat, poultry, or seafood.

foodborne illness: illness transmitted to human beings through food and water, caused by either an infectious agent (foodborne infection) or a poisonous substance (foodborne intoxication); commonly known as food poisoning.

Hazard Analysis Critical Control Points (HACCP): a systematic plan to identify and correct potential microbial hazards in the manufacturing, distribution, and commercial use of food products; commonly referred to as "HASS-ip."

outbreaks: two or more cases of a similar illness resulting from the ingestion of a common food.

pasteurization: heat processing of food that inactivates some, but not all, microorganisms in the food; not a sterilization process. Bacteria that cause spoilage are still present.

pathogens (PATH-oh-jens): microorganisms capable of producing disease.

sushi: vinegar-flavored rice and seafood, typically wrapped in seaweed and stuffed with colorful vegetables. Some sushi is stuffed with raw fish; other varieties contain cooked seafood.

traveler's diarrhea: nausea, vomiting, and diarrhea caused by consuming food or water contaminated by any of several organisms, most commonly *Escherichia coli, Shigella, Campylobacter jejuni,* and *Salmonella.*

TABLE NP2-2 The Major Microbes of Foodborne Illnesses

ORGANISM NAME	MOST FREQUENT FOOD SOURCES	ONSET AND GENERAL SYMPTOMS	PREVENTION METHODS[a]
FOODBORNE INFECTIONS			
Campylobacter (KAM-pee-loh-BAK-ter) bacterium	Raw and undercooked poultry, unpasteurized milk, contaminated water	Onset: 2 to 5 days. Diarrhea, vomiting, abdominal cramps, fever; sometimes bloody stools; lasts 2 to 10 days.	Cook foods thoroughly; use pasteurized milk; use sanitary food-handling methods.
Clostridium (claw-STRID-ee-um) *perfringens* (per-FRINGE-enz) bacterium	Meats and meat products stored at between 120°F and 130°F	Onset: 8 to 16 hours. Abdominal pain, diarrhea, nausea; lasts 1 to 2 days.	Use sanitary food-handling methods; use pasteurized milk; cook foods thoroughly; refrigerate foods promptly and properly.
Escherichia (esh-uh-REEK-ee-uh) *coli* (KOH-lye) bacterium (including shiga toxin-producing strains)[b]	Undercooked ground beef, unpasteurized milk and juices, raw fruit and vegetables, contaminated water, and person-to-person contact	Onset: 1 to 8 days. Severe bloody diarrhea, abdominal cramps, vomiting; lasts 5 to 10 days.	Cook ground beef thoroughly; use pasteurized milk; use sanitary food-handling methods; use treated, boiled, or bottled water.
Listeria (lis-TER-ee-AH) bacterium	Unpasteurized milk; fresh soft cheeses; luncheon meats, hot dogs	Onset: 1 to 21 days. Fever, muscle aches, nausea, vomiting, blood poisoning, complications in pregnancy, and meningitis (stiff neck, severe headache, and fever).	Use sanitary food-handling methods; cook foods thoroughly; use pasteurized milk.
Norovirus	Person-to-person contact; raw foods, salads, sandwiches	Onset: 1 to 2 days. Vomiting, diarrhea, abdominal pain; lasts 1 to 3 days.	Use sanitary food-handling methods.
Salmonella (sal-moh-NEL-ah) bacteria (2300 types)	Raw or undercooked eggs, meats, poultry, raw milk and other dairy products, shrimp, frog legs, yeast, coconut, pasta, and chocolate	Onset: 1 to 3 days. Fever, vomiting, abdominal cramps, diarrhea; lasts 4 to 7 days; can be fatal.	Use sanitary food-handling methods; use pasteurized milk; cook foods thoroughly; refrigerate foods promptly and properly.
Toxoplasma (TOK-so-PLAZ-ma) gondii parasite	Raw or undercooked meat; contaminated water; unpasteurized goat's milk; contact with infected cat feces	Onset: 7 to 21 days. Swollen glands, fever, headache, muscle pain, stiff neck.	Use sanitary food-handling methods; cook foods thoroughly.
FOODBORNE INTOXICATIONS			
Clostridium (claw-STRID-ee-um) *botulinum* (bot-chew-LINE-um) bacterium produces botulin toxin, responsible for causing botulism	Anaerobic environment of low acidity (canned corn, peppers, green beans, soups, beets, asparagus, mushrooms, ripe olives, spinach, tuna, chicken, chicken liver, liver pâté, luncheon meats, ham, sausage, stuffed eggplant, lobster, and smoked and salted fish)	Onset: 4 to 36 hours. Nervous system symptoms, including double vision, inability to swallow, speech difficulty, and progressive paralysis of the respiratory system; often fatal; leaves prolonged symptoms in survivors.	Use proper canning methods for low-acid foods; refrigerate homemade garlic and herb oils; avoid commercially prepared foods with leaky seals or with bent, bulging, or broken cans. Do not give infants honey because it may contain spores of *Clostridium botulinum*, which is a common source of infection for infants.
Staphylococcus (STAF-il-oh-KOK-us) *aureus* bacterium produces staphylococcal toxin	Toxin produced in improperly refrigerated meats; egg, tuna, potato, and macaroni salads; cream-filled pastries	Onset: 1 to 6 hours. Diarrhea, nausea, vomiting, abdominal cramps, fever; lasts 1 to 2 days.	Use sanitary food-handling methods; cook food thoroughly; refrigerate foods promptly and properly; use proper home-canning methods.

[a]Table NP2-3 on pp. 61–62 provides more details on the proper handling, cooking, and refrigeration of foods.
[b]O157, O145, and other Shiga toxin-producing strains.

Note: Travelers' diarrhea is most commonly caused by *E. coli, Campylobacter jejuni, Shigella*, and *Salmonella*.

Clostridium botulinum, an organism that produces a deadly toxin in anaerobic (without oxygen) conditions such as improperly canned (especially home-canned) foods and homemade garlic or herb-flavored oils stored at room temperature. The botulism toxin paralyzes muscles, making it difficult to see, speak, swallow, and breathe. Because death can occur within 24 hours of onset, botulism demands immediate medical attention. Even then, survivors may suffer the effects for months or years.

How do people get foodborne illness?

Transmission of foodborne illness has changed as our food supply and lifestyles have changed.[4] In the past, foodborne illness was caused by one person's error in a small setting, such as improperly refrigerated egg salad at a family picnic, and affected only a few victims. Today, we are eating more foods grown, processed, transported, prepared, and packaged by others. Consequently, when a food manufacturer or restaurant chef makes an error, foodborne illness can quickly affect many people. An estimated 80 percent of reported foodborne illnesses are caused by errors in a commercial setting, such as the improper **pasteurization** of milk at a large dairy.

The Dietary Guidelines for Americans recommend that consumers should increase their intakes of fruit and vegetables but be aware that, if contaminated, some raw produce may pose a risk of illness. For example, packaged salads were recalled when *Listeria* poisoning caused one death and sickened 18 people across nine states. Other kinds of produce, and even peanut butter, have been responsible for transmitting dangerous foodborne illnesses to consumers. These incidents and others focus the national spotlight on two important safety issues: disease-causing organisms are commonly found in a variety of foods, and safe food-handling practices can minimize harm from most of these foodborne pathogens.

What kinds of programs are in place to help keep foods safe?

To improve the safety of the U.S. food supply, the Food Safety Modernization Act (FSMA) was signed into law. The law has been called "historic" because it shifts the focus of FDA activities from reacting after people become ill to preventing foodborne illness in the first place. The law stresses prevention at food-processing facilities; provides the FDA with greater enforcement, inspection, and recall authorities; and affords the FDA greater oversight of imported foods.[5] U.S. Food and Drug Administration, Five ways new FDA rules will make your foods safer, www.fda .gov/ForConsumers/ConsumerUpdates/ucm459072.htm, updated November 3, 2015.

In addition, the U.S. Department of Agriculture (USDA), the FDA, and the food-processing industries have developed and implemented programs to control foodborne illness.*

For example, USDA inspectors examine meat-processing plants every day to ensure that these facilities meet government standards. Seafood, egg, produce, and processed food facilities are inspected less often, but all food producers must use a **Hazard Analysis Critical Control Points (HACCP)** plan to help prevent foodborne illnesses at their source. Each slaughterhouse, packer, distributor, and transporter of susceptible foods must identify "critical control points" that pose a risk of contamination and implement verifiable procedures to eliminate or minimize the risk. The HACCP system has proved a remarkable success for domestic products, but such programs do not apply to imported foods.

An estimated $2 trillion worth of products are imported into the United States from more than 150 countries each year. Many countries cooperate with the FDA and have adopted many of the safe food-handling practices used in the United States, but some imported foods come from countries with little or no regulatory oversight. To help consumers distinguish between imported and domestic foods, certain foods—including fish, shellfish, fruit, vegetables, and some nuts—must display a Country of Origin Label specifying where they were produced.[6]

Importantly, the implementation of the FSMA strengthens the FDA's ability to safeguard imported foods. Under the FSMA, the FDA is permitted to inspect foreign facilities. If a food producer in another country does not allow the FDA to inspect its facility, the FDA can refuse to allow food from that facility into the United States. The FSMA also requires importers to verify the food safety practices of their suppliers and adds new checks on imported foods.*

Are foods bought in grocery stores and foods eaten in restaurants safe?

Canned and packaged foods sold in grocery stores are easily controlled, but rare accidents do happen. Batch numbering makes it possible to recall contaminated foods through public announcements via the Internet, newspapers, television, and radio. In the grocery store, consumers can buy items before the "sell by" date and inspect the safety seals and wrappers of packages. A broken seal, bulging can lid, or mangled package fails to protect the consumer against microbes, insects, spoilage, or even vandalism.

State and local health regulations provide guidelines on the cleanliness of facilities and the safe preparation of foods for restaurants, cafeterias, and fast-food establishments. Even so, consumers should take these actions to help prevent foodborne illnesses when dining out:

- Wash hands with hot, soapy water before meals.
- Expect clean tabletops, dinnerware, utensils, and food preparation areas.
- Expect cooked foods to be served piping hot and salads to be fresh and cold.

---

*In addition to HACCP, other programs initiated under the Food Safety Initiative include FoodNet, PulseNet, the Environmental Health Specialists Network (EHS-Net), and Fight BAC!

- Refrigerate take-home items within two hours and use leftovers within three to four days.

   Improper handling of foods can occur anywhere along the line from commercial manufacturers to large supermarkets to small restaurants to private homes. Maintaining a safe food supply requires everyone's efforts.

What can people do to protect themselves from foodborne illness?

Whether microbes multiply and cause illness depends, in part, on a few key food-handling behaviors in the kitchen—whether the kitchen is in your home, a school cafeteria, a gourmet restaurant, or a canned goods manufacturer. Figure NP2-1 summarizes the four simple things that can help most to prevent foodborne illness:

- *Clean*. Keep a clean, safe kitchen by washing hands and surfaces often. Wash countertops, cutting boards, sponges, and utensils in hot, soapy water before and after each step of food preparation. To reduce bacterial contamination on hands, wash hands with soap and water (Figure NP2-2); if soap and water are not available, use an alcohol-based sanitizing gel.[7]
- *Separate*. Avoid cross-contamination by keeping raw eggs, meat, poultry, and seafood separate from other foods at every step of food handling, from purchase to preparation to serving. Wash all utensils and surfaces (such as cutting boards or platters) that have been in contact with these foods with hot, soapy water before using them again. Bacteria inevitably left on the surfaces from the raw meat can recontaminate the cooked meat or other foods—a problem known as **cross-contamination**. Washing raw eggs, meat, and poultry is not recommended as the extra handling increases the risk of cross-contamination.
- *Cook*. Keep hot foods hot by cooking to proper temperatures. Foods need to cook long enough to reach internal temperatures that will kill microbes, and maintain adequate temperatures to prevent bacterial growth until the foods are served.
- *Chill*. Keep cold foods cold by refrigerating promptly. Go directly home upon leaving the grocery store and immediately unpack foods into the refrigerator or freezer upon arrival. After a meal, refrigerate any leftovers immediately.

   Unfortunately, consumers commonly fail to follow these simple food-handling recommendations. See Table NP2-3 for additional food safety tips.

What precautions need to be taken when preparing meat and poultry?

Figure NP2-3 presents label instructions for the safe handling of meat and poultry. Meats and poultry contain bacteria and provide a moist, nutrient-rich environment that favors

Four ways to keep food safe. The Fight Bac! website is at www.fightbac.org.

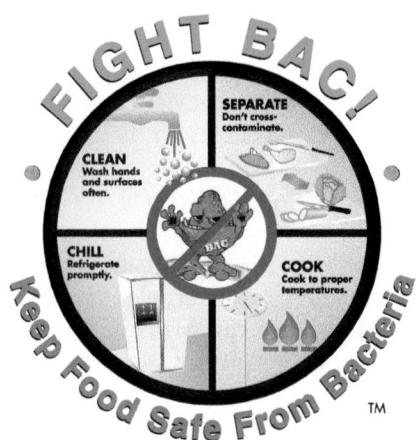

You can avoid many illnesses by following these hand washing procedures before, during, and after food preparation; before eating; after using the bathroom, blowing your nose, or touching your hair; after handling animals or their waste; or when your hands are dirty.

1. Wet your hands with clean, running water (warm or cold), turn off the tap, and apply soap.
2. Lather your hands by rubbing them together with the soap. Be sure to lather the backs of your hands, between your fingers, and under your nails.
3. Scrub your hands for at least 20 seconds.
4. Rinse your hands well under clean, running water.
5. Dry your hands using a clean towel or air dry them.

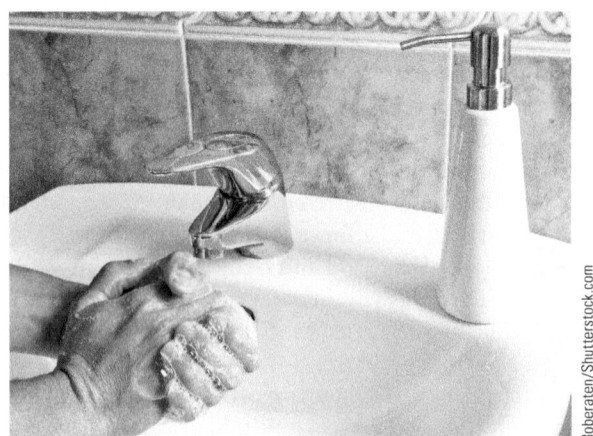

Source: Handwashing: Clean hands save lives (2014), www.cdc.gov/handwashing.

Most foodborne illnesses can be prevented by following four simple rules: clean, separate, cook, and chill.

CLEAN

- Wash fruit and vegetables in a clean sink with a scrub brush and warm water; store washed and unwashed produce separately.
- Use hot, soapy water to wash hands, utensils, dishes, nonporous cutting boards, and countertops before handling food and between tasks when working with different foods. Use a bleach solution on cutting boards (one capful per gallon of water).
- Cover cuts with clean bandages before food preparation; dirty bandages carry harmful microorganisms.
- Mix foods with utensils, not hands; keep hands and utensils away from mouth, nose, and hair.
- Anyone may be a carrier of bacteria and should avoid coughing or sneezing over food. A person with a skin infection or infectious disease should not prepare food.
- Wash or replace sponges and towels regularly.
- Clean up food spills and crumb-filled crevices.

SEPARATE

- Wash all surfaces that have been in contact with raw meats, poultry, eggs, fish, and shellfish before reusing.
- Serve cooked foods on a clean plate with a clean utensil. Separate raw foods from those that have been cooked.
- Don't use marinade that was in contact with raw meat for basting or sauces.

COOK

- When cooking meats or poultry, use a thermometer to test the internal temperature. Insert the thermometer between the thigh and the body of a turkey or into the thickest part of other meats, making sure the tip of the thermometer is not in contact with bone or the pan. Cook to the temperature indicated for that particular meat (see Figure NP2-4 on p. 63); cook hamburgers to at least medium well done. If you have safety questions, call the USDA Meat and Poultry Hotline: (800) 535-4555.
- Cook stuffing separately, or stuff poultry just prior to cooking.
- Do not cook large cuts of meat or turkey in a microwave oven; it leaves some parts undercooked while overcooking others.
- Cook eggs before eating them (soft-boiled for at least 3½ minutes; scrambled until set, not runny; fried for at least 3 minutes on one side and 1 minute on the other).
- Cook seafood thoroughly. If you have safety questions about seafood, call the FDA hotline: (800) FDA-4010.
- When serving foods, maintain temperatures at 140°F or higher.
- Heat leftovers thoroughly to at least 165°F.

CHILL

- When running errands, stop at the grocery store last. When you get home, refrigerate the perishable groceries (such as meats and dairy products) immediately. Do not leave perishables in the car any longer than it takes for ice cream to melt.
- Put packages of raw meat, fish, or poultry on a plate before refrigerating to prevent juices from dripping on food stored below.
- Buy only foods that are solidly frozen in store freezers.
- Keep cold foods at 40°F or less; keep frozen foods at 0°F or less (keep a thermometer in the refrigerator).
- Marinate meats in the refrigerator, not on the counter.
- Look for "Keep Refrigerated" or "Refrigerate After Opening" on food labels.
- Refrigerate leftovers promptly; use shallow containers to cool foods faster; use leftovers within 3 to 4 days.
- Thaw meats or poultry in the refrigerator, not at room temperature. If you must hasten thawing, use cool water (changed every 30 minutes) or a microwave oven.
- Freeze meat, fish, or poultry immediately if not planning to use within a few days.

IN GENERAL

- Do not reuse disposable containers; use nondisposable containers or recycle instead.
- Do not taste food that is suspect. "If in doubt, throw it out."
- Throw out foods with danger-signaling odors. Be aware, though, that most food-poisoning bacteria are odorless, colorless, and tasteless.
- Do not buy or use items that have broken seals or mangled packaging; such containers cannot protect against microbes, insects,
- spoilage, or even vandalism. Check safety seals, buttons, and expiration dates.
- Follow label instructions for storing and preparing packaged and frozen foods; throw out foods that have been thawed or refrozen.
- Discard foods that are discolored, moldy, or decayed or that have been contaminated by insects or rodents.

(Continued)

FOR SPECIFIC FOOD ITEMS

- **Canned goods.** Carefully discard food from cans that leak or bulge so that other people and animals will not accidentally ingest it; before canning, seek professional advice from the USDA National Institute of Food and Agriculture (online at *nifa.usda.gov*).
- *Milk and cheeses.* Use only pasteurized milk and milk products. Aged cheeses, such as cheddar and Swiss, do well for an hour or two without refrigeration, but they should be refrigerated or stored in an ice chest for longer periods.
- *Eggs.* Use clean eggs with intact shells. Do not eat eggs, even pasteurized eggs, raw; raw eggs are commonly found in Caesar salad dressing, eggnog, cookie dough, hollandaise sauce, and key lime pie. Cook eggs until whites are firmly set and yolks begin to thicken.
- *Honey.* Honey may contain dormant bacterial spores, which can awaken in the human body to produce botulism. In adults, this poses little hazard, but infants younger than 1 year of age should never be fed honey. Honey can accumulate enough toxin to kill an infant; it has been implicated in several cases of sudden infant death. (Honey can also be contaminated with environmental pollutants picked up by the bees.)
- *Mayonnaise.* Commercial mayonnaise may actually help a food to resist spoilage because of the acid content. Still, keep it refrigerated after opening.
- *Mixed salads.* Mixed salads of chopped ingredients spoil easily because they have extensive surface area for bacteria to invade, and they have been in contact with cutting boards, hands, and kitchen utensils that easily transmit bacteria to food (regardless of their mayonnaise content). Chill them well before, during, and after serving.
- *Picnic foods.* Choose foods that last without refrigeration, such as fresh fruit and vegetables, breads and crackers, and canned spreads and cheeses that can be opened and used immediately. Pack foods cold, layer ice between foods, and keep foods out of water.
- *Seafood.* Buy only fresh seafood that has been properly refrigerated or iced. Cooked seafood should be stored separately from raw seafood to avoid cross-contamination.

Note: Learn more about food safety at www.HomeFoodSafety.org or by downloading Is My Food Safe?, a free phone app sponsored by the Academy of Nutrition and Dietetics.

FIGURE NP2-3   Meat and Poultry Safety

The USDA requires that safe handling instructions appear on all packages of meat and poultry. Consumers can help to prevent foodborne illnesses by following the safe handling instructions.

Safe Handling Instructions

THIS PRODUCT WAS PREPARED FROM INSPECTED AND PASSED MEAT AND/OR POULTRY. SOME FOOD PRODUCTS MAY CONTAIN BACTERIA THAT CAN CAUSE ILLNESS IF THE PRODUCT IS MISHANDLED OR COOKED IMPROPERLY. FOR YOUR PROTECTION, FOLLOW THESE SAFE HANDLING INSTRUCTIONS.

 KEEP REFRIGERATED OR FROZEN. THAW IN REFRIGERATOR OR MICROWAVE.

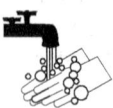 KEEP RAW MEAT AND POULTRY SEPARATE FROM OTHER FOODS. WASH WORKING SURFACES (INCLUDING CUTTING BOARDS), UTENSILS, AND HANDS AFTER TOUCHING RAW MEAT OR POULTRY.

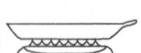 COOK THOROUGHLY. KEEP HOT FOODS HOT. REFRIGERATE LEFTOVERS IMMEDIATELY OR DISCARD.

microbial growth. Ground meat is especially susceptible because it receives more handling than other kinds of meat and has more surface exposed to bacterial contamination. Consumers cannot detect the harmful bacteria in or on meat. For safety's sake, cook meat thoroughly, using a thermometer to test the internal temperature (see Photo NP2-1 and Figure NP2-4).

How can a person enjoy seafood safely?

Most seafood available in the United States and Canada is safe, but eating it undercooked or raw (Photo NP2-2) can cause severe illnesses—hepatitis, worms, parasites, viral intestinal disorders, and other diseases.* Rumor has it that freezing fish will make it safe to eat raw, but this is only partly true. Commercial freezing will kill mature parasitic worms, but only cooking can kill all worm eggs and other microorganisms that can cause illness. For safety's sake, all seafood should be cooked until it is opaque. Even

*Diseases caused by toxins from the sea include ciguatera poisoning, scombroid poisoning, and paralytic and neurotoxic shellfish poisoning.

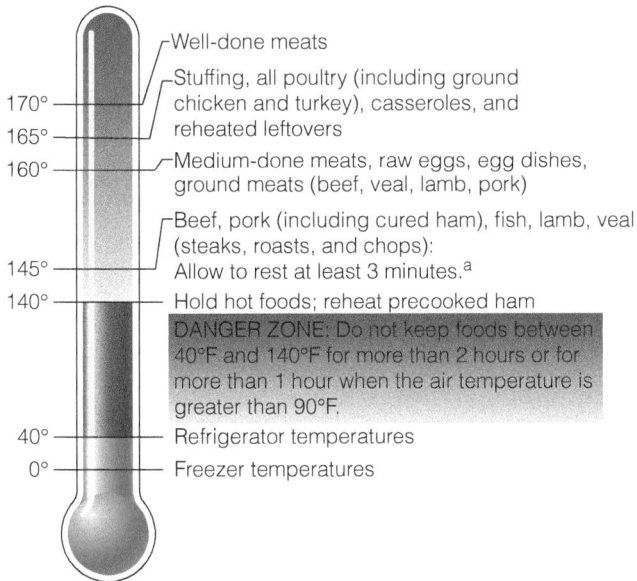

Cook hamburgers to 160°F; color alone cannot determine doneness. Some burgers will turn brown before reaching 160°F, whereas others may retain some pink color, even when cooked to 175°F.

FIGURE NP2-4 Recommended Safe Temperatures (Fahrenheit)

Bacteria multiply rapidly at temperatures in the danger zone—between 40°F and 140°F. Cook foods to the temperatures shown on this thermometer and hold them at 140°F or higher.

170° — Well-done meats

— Stuffing, all poultry (including ground chicken and turkey), casseroles, and reheated leftovers

165° —

160° — Medium-done meats, raw eggs, egg dishes, ground meats (beef, veal, lamb, pork)

— Beef, pork (including cured ham), fish, lamb, veal (steaks, roasts, and chops):

145° — Allow to rest at least 3 minutes.[a]

140° — Hold hot foods; reheat precooked ham

DANGER ZONE: Do not keep foods between 40°F and 140°F for more than 2 hours or for more than 1 hour when the air temperature is greater than 90°F.

40° — Refrigerator temperatures

0° — Freezer temperatures

[a] During the 3 minutes after meat is removed from the heat source, its temperature remains constant or continues to rise, which destroys pathogens.

sushi can be safe to eat when chefs combine cooked seafood and other ingredients into delicacies.

Eating raw oysters can be dangerous for anyone, but people with liver disease and weakened immune systems are most vulnerable. At least 10 species of bacteria found

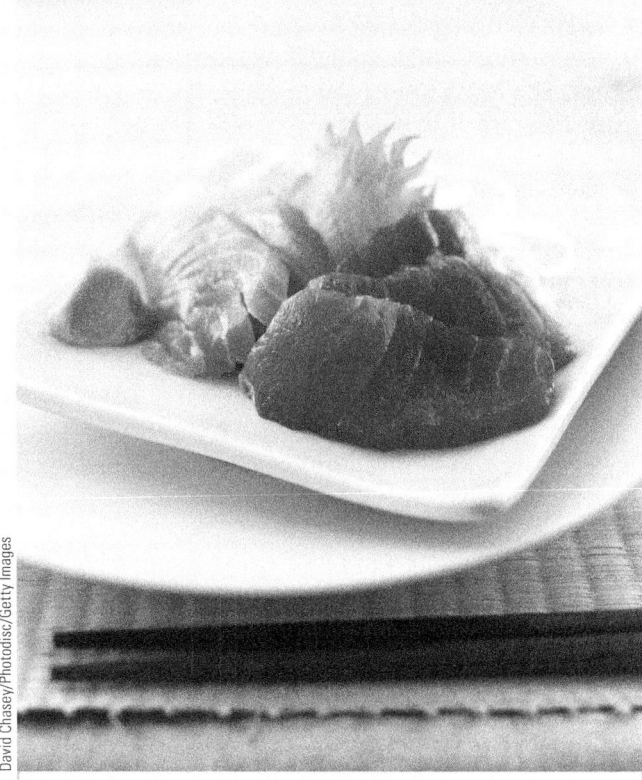

Eating raw seafood is a risky proposition.

in raw oysters can cause serious illness and even death. Raw oysters may also carry the hepatitis A virus, which can cause liver disease. Some hot sauces can kill many of these bacteria but not the virus; alcohol may also protect some people against some oyster-borne illnesses but not enough to guarantee safety (or to recommend drinking alcohol). Pasteurization of raw oysters—holding them at a specified temperature for a specified time—holds promise for killing bacteria without cooking the oyster or altering its texture or flavor.

As population density increases along the shores of seafood-harvesting waters, pollution inevitably invades the sea life there. Preventing seafood-borne illness is in large part a task of controlling water pollution. To help ensure a safe seafood market, the FDA requires processors to adopt food safety practices based on the HACCP system mentioned earlier.

Chemical pollution and microbial contamination lurk not only in the water but also in the boats and warehouses where seafood is cleaned, prepared, and refrigerated. Seafood is one of the most perishable foods: time and temperature are critical to its freshness and flavor. To keep seafood as fresh as possible, people in the industry "keep it cold, keep it clean, and keep it moving." Wise consumers eat it cooked.

Do foods that are unsafe to eat smell bad?

Fresh food generally smells fresh. Not all types of food poisoning are detectable by odor, but some bacterial wastes produce "off" odors. Food with an abnormal odor is spoiled. Throw it out or, if it was recently purchased, return it to the grocery store. Do not taste it. Table NP2-4 lists safe refrigerator storage times for selected foods.

Local health departments and the USDA Extension Service can provide additional information about food safety. Should precautions fail and mild foodborne illness develop, drink clear liquids to replace fluids lost through vomiting and diarrhea. If serious foodborne illness is suspected, first call a physician. Then wrap the remainder of the suspected food and label the container so that the food cannot be mistakenly eaten, place it in the refrigerator, and hold it for possible inspection by health authorities.

How can a person defend against foodborne illness when traveling to foreign countries?

People who travel to other countries have a 50-50 chance of contracting a foodborne illness, commonly described as **traveler's diarrhea**. Like many other foodborne illnesses, traveler's diarrhea is a sometimes serious, always annoying

TABLE NP2-4 Refrigerator Home Storage (at 40°F or below)

If product has a "use-by" date, follow that date. If product has a "sell-by" date or no date, cook or freeze the product by the time on the following chart.

FRESH OR UNCOOKED PRODUCTS

PRODUCT	STORAGE TIMES AFTER PURCHASE
Poultry	1 or 2 days
Beef, veal, pork, and lamb	3 to 5 days
Ground meat and ground poultry	1 or 2 days
Fresh variety meats (liver, tongue, brain, kidneys, heart, chitterlings)	1 or 2 days
Cured ham, cook-before-eating	5 to 7 days
Sausage from pork, beef, or turkey (uncooked)	1 or 2 days
Eggs	3 to 5 weeks

SEALED PROCESSED PRODUCTS

PROCESSED PRODUCT	UNOPENED, AFTER PURCHASE	AFTER OPENING
Cooked poultry	3 to 4 days	3 to 4 days
Cooked sausage	3 to 4 days	3 to 4 days
Sausage, hard/dry, shelf-stable	6 weeks/pantry	3 weeks
Corned beef, uncooked, in pouch with pickling juices	5 to 7 days	3 to 4 days
Vacuum-packed dinners, commercial brand with USDA seal	2 weeks	3 to 4 days
Bacon	2 weeks	7 days
Hot dogs	2 weeks	1 week
Luncheon meat	2 weeks	3 to 5 days
Ham, fully cooked	7 days	slices, 3 days; whole, 7 days
Ham, canned, labeled "keep refrigerated"	9 months	3 to 4 days
Ham, canned, shelf-stable	2 years/pantry	3 to 5 days
Canned meat and poultry, shelf-stable	2 to 5 years/pantry	3 to 4 days

bacterial infection of the digestive tract. The risk is high because some countries' cleanliness standards for food and water may be lower than those in the United States and Canada. Also, every region's microbes are different, and while people are immune to those in their own neighborhoods, they have had no chance to develop immunity to the pathogens in places they are visiting for the first time. In addition to the food safety tips outlined previously (on pp. 61–62), precautions while traveling include:

- Wash hands frequently with soap and hot water, especially before handling food or eating. Use sanitizing gel or hand wipes regularly.

- Eat only well-cooked and hot or canned foods. Eat raw fruit or vegetables only if washed in purified water and peeled with clean hands.
- Use purified, bottled water for drinking, making ice cubes, and brushing teeth. Alternatively, use disinfecting tablets or boil water.
- Refuse dairy products that have not been pasteurized and refrigerated properly.
- Travel with antidiarrheal medication in case efforts to avoid illness fail.

To sum up these recommendations, "Boil it, cook it, peel it, or forget it."

Notes

1. Centers for Disease Control and Prevention, Estimates of foodborne illness in the United States, Burden of foodborne illness: Overview, www.cdc.gov/foodborneburden/estimates-overview.html, updated July 15, 2016.
2. U.S. Food and Drug Administration, Food safety: It's especially important for at-risk groups, www.fda.gov/Food/FoodborneIllnessContimanants/PeopleAtRisk/htm, updated April 6, 2016; Position of the Academy of Nutrition and Dietetics: Food and water safety, *Journal of the Academy of Nutrition and Dietetics* 114 (2014): 1819–1829.
3. S. J. Crowe and coauthors, Vital signs: Multistate foodborne outbreaks—United States, 2010–2014, *Morbidity and Mortality Weekly Report* 64 (2015): 1221–1225.
4. Position of the Academy of Nutrition and Dietetics, 2014.
5. U.S. Food and Drug Administration, Five ways new FDA rules will make your foods safer, www.fda.gov/ForConsumers/ConsumerUpdates/ucm459072.htm, updated November 3, 2015.
6. USDA Agricultural Marketing Service, Country of Origin Labeling, 2014, www.ams.usda.gov/AMSv1.0/cool.
7. Centers for Disease Control and Prevention, Handwashing: Clean hands save lives, www.cdc.gov/handwashing, updated January 27, 2016.

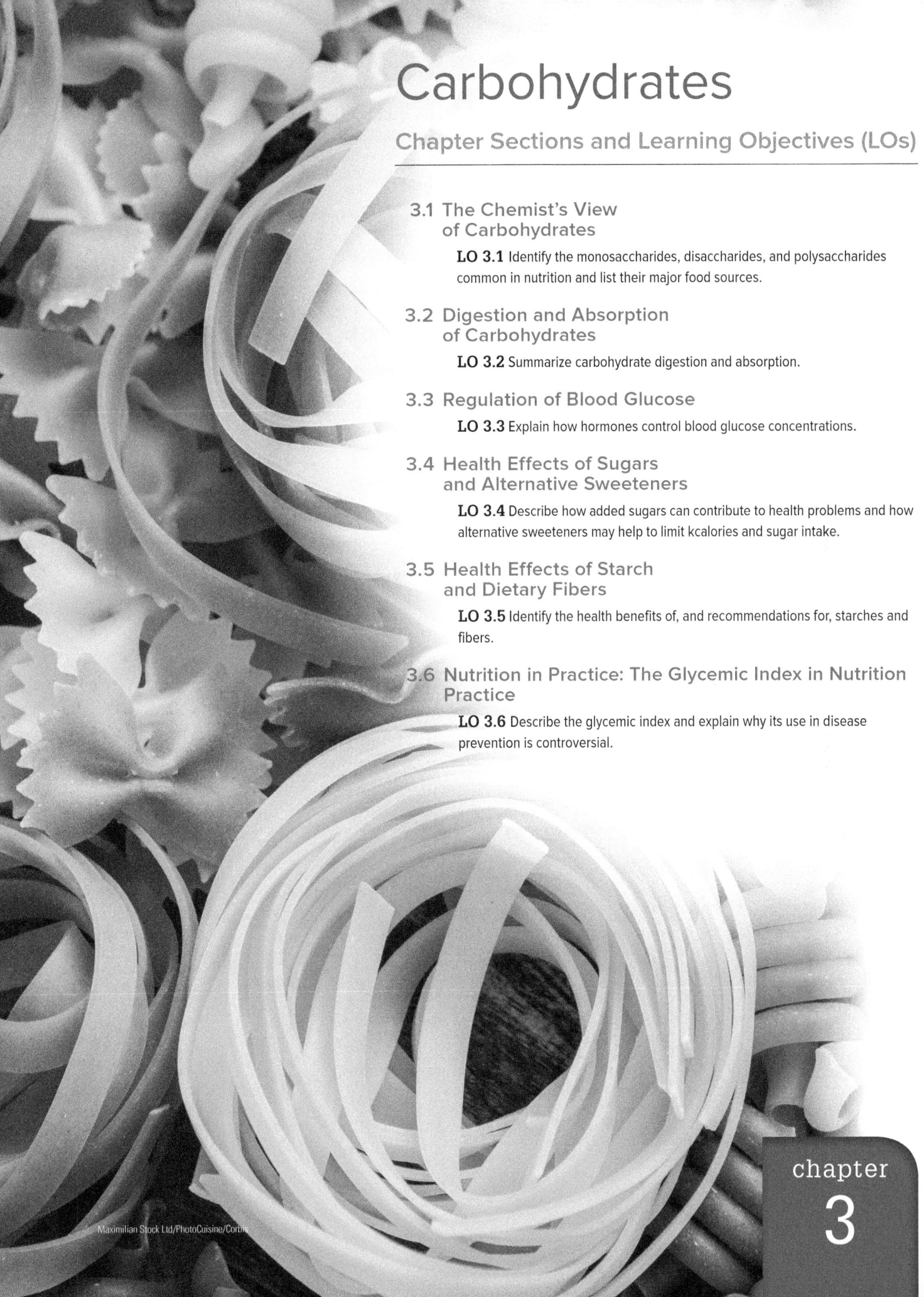

Carbohydrates

Chapter Sections and Learning Objectives (LOs)

Maximilian Stock Ltd/PhotoCuisine/Corbis

chapter

3

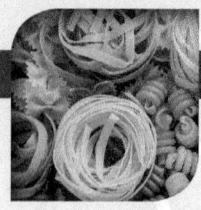
secret of feeling good is replenishing the body's energy supply with food. Carbohydrate is the preferred energy source for many of the body's functions. As long as carbohydrate is available, the human brain depends exclusively on it as an energy source. Athletes eat a "high-carb" diet to store as much muscle fuel as possible, and dietary recommendations urge people to eat carbohydrate-rich foods for better health. Some people, however, mistakenly think of carbohydrate-rich foods as "fattening" and avoid them when trying to lose weight. This strategy may be helpful if the carbohydrates are the concentrated sugars of soft drinks, candies, and cookies, but it is counterproductive if the carbohydrates are from whole grains, vegetables, legumes, and fruit (see Photo 3-1). These plant foods provide carbohydrate and fiber with little or no fat. Milk is the only animal-derived food that contains significant amounts of carbohydrate. Thus, people who wish to lose fat, maintain lean tissue, and stay healthy can best do so by being physically active, paying close attention to portion sizes, and designing an eating pattern based on foods that supply fiber-rich carbohydrate in balance with other energy nutrients.

This chapter on carbohydrates is the first of three on the energy-yielding nutrients. Fats are the topic of Chapter 4 and protein is featured in Chapter 5. Nutrition in Practice 19 addresses one other contributor of energy to the human diet, alcohol. Alcohol, of course, has well-known undesirable side effects when used in excess.

carbohydrates: energy nutrients composed of monosaccharides.

carbo = carbon
hydrate = water

monosaccharides (mon-oh-SACK-uh-rides): single sugar units.

mono = one
saccharide = sugar

disaccharides (dye-SACK-uh-rides): pairs of sugar units bonded together.

di = two

polysaccharides: long chains of monosaccharide units arranged as starch, glycogen, or fiber.

poly = many

3.1 The Chemist's View of Carbohydrates

The dietary **carbohydrates** include the sugars, starch, and fiber. Chemists describe the sugars as:

- **Monosaccharides** (single sugars)
- **Disaccharides** (double sugars)

Starch and fiber are:*

- **Polysaccharides**—chains of monosaccharide units

All of these carbohydrates are composed of the single sugar **glucose** and other compounds that are much like glucose in composition and structure. Figure 3-1 shows the chemical structure of glucose.

Monosaccharides

Three monosaccharides are important in nutrition: glucose, **fructose**, and **galactose**. All three monosaccharides have the same number and kinds of atoms but in different arrangements.

Glucose Most cells depend on glucose for their fuel to some extent, and the cells of the brain and the rest of the nervous system depend almost exclusively on glucose for their energy. The body can obtain this glucose from carbohydrates. To function optimally, the body must maintain blood glucose within limits that allow the cells to nourish themselves. A later section describes blood glucose regulation.

Fructose Fructose is the sweetest of the sugars. Fructose occurs naturally in fruit, in honey, and as part of table sugar. However, most fructose is consumed in sweet beverages such as soft drinks, in ready-to-eat cereals, and in other products sweetened with **high-fructose corn syrup** or other **added sugars**. Glucose and fructose are the most common monosaccharides in nature.

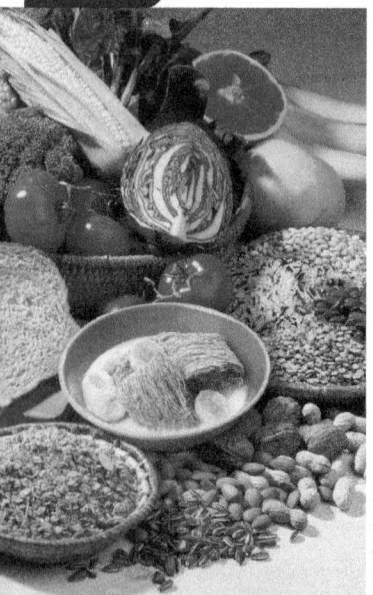

Photo 3-1

Grains, vegetables, legumes, fruit, and milk offer ample carbohydrate.

---

*Monosaccharides and disaccharides (sugars) are sometimes called *simple carbohydrates*, and the polysaccharides (starch and fiber) are sometimes called *complex carbohydrates*.

Galactose The third single sugar, galactose, occurs mostly as part of lactose, a disaccharide also known as milk sugar. During digestion, galactose is freed as a single sugar.

Disaccharides

In disaccharides, pairs of single sugars are linked together. Three disaccharides are important in nutrition: maltose, sucrose, and lactose. All three contain glucose as one of their single sugars. As Table 3-1 shows, the other monosaccharide is either another glucose (in maltose), fructose (in sucrose), or galactose (in lactose). The shapes of the sugars in Table 3-1 reflect their chemical structures as drawn on paper.

Sucrose **Sucrose** (table, or white, sugar) is the most familiar of the three disaccharides and is what people mean when they speak of "sugar." This sugar is usually obtained by refining the juice from sugar beets or sugarcane to provide the brown, white, and powdered sugars available in the supermarket, but it occurs naturally in many fruits and vegetables. When a person eats a food containing sucrose, enzymes in the digestive tract split the sucrose into its glucose and fructose components.

Lactose **Lactose** is the principal carbohydrate of milk. Most human infants are born with the digestive enzymes necessary to split lactose into its two monosaccharide parts, glucose and galactose, so as to absorb it. Breast milk thus provides a simple, easily digested carbohydrate that meets an infant's energy needs; many formulas do, too, because they are made from milk. Many people lose the ability to digest lactose after infancy. This condition, known as *lactose intolerance*, is discussed in Chapter 18.

Maltose The third disaccharide, **maltose**, is a plant sugar that consists of two glucose units. Maltose is produced whenever starch breaks down—as happens in plants when they break down their stored starch for energy and start to sprout and in human beings during carbohydrate digestion.

Polysaccharides

Unlike the sugars, which contain the three monosaccharides—glucose, fructose, and galactose—in different combinations, the polysaccharides are composed almost entirely of glucose (and, in some cases, other monosaccharides). Three types of polysaccharides are important in nutrition: glycogen, starch, and fibers.

   Glycogen is a storage form of energy for human beings and animals; starch plays that role in plants; and fibers provide structure in stems, trunks, roots, leaves, and skins of plants. Both glycogen and starch are built entirely of glucose units; fibers are composed of a variety of monosaccharides and other carbohydrate derivatives.

Glycogen **Glycogen** molecules are made of chains of glucose that are more highly branched than those of starch molecules (see the left side of Figure 3-2 on p. 70). Glycogen is found in meats only to a limited extent and not at all in plants.* For this reason, glycogen

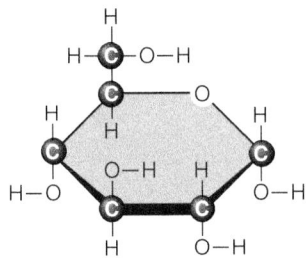

FIGURE 3-1 Chemical Structure of Glucose

On paper, the structure of glucose has to be drawn flat, but in nature the five carbons and oxygen are roughly in a plane, with the H, OH, and CH₂OH extending out above and below it.

glucose: a monosaccharide; the sugar common to all disaccharides and polysaccharides; also called *blood sugar* or *dextrose*.

fructose: a monosaccharide; sometimes known as *fruit sugar*.

   fruct = fruit

galactose: a monosaccharide; part of the disaccharide lactose.

high-fructose corn syrup: a widely used commercial kcaloric sweetener made by adding enzymes to cornstarch to convert a portion of its glucose molecules into sweet-tasting fructose.

added sugars: sugars, syrups, and other kcaloric sweeteners that are added to foods during processing or preparation or at the table. Added sugars do not include the naturally occurring sugars found in fruit and in milk products. Also called *carbohydrate sweeteners*, they include glucose, fructose, high-fructose corn syrup, concentrated fruit juice, and other sweet carbohydrates. Also defined in Chapter 1.

sucrose: a disaccharide composed of glucose and fructose; commonly known as *table sugar*, *beet sugar*, or *cane sugar*.

   sucro = sugar

lactose: a disaccharide composed of glucose and galactose; commonly known as *milk sugar*.

   lact = milk

maltose: a disaccharide composed of two glucose units; sometimes known as *malt sugar*.

TABLE 3-1	The Major Sugars		
MONOSACCHARIDES		**DISACCHARIDES**	
Glucose		Sucrose (glucose + fructose)	
Fructose		Lactose (glucose + galactose)	
Galactose (found mostly as part of lactose)		Maltose (glucose + glucose)	

*Glycogen in animal muscles rapidly breaks down after slaughter.

FIGURE 3-2 Glycogen and Starch Compared

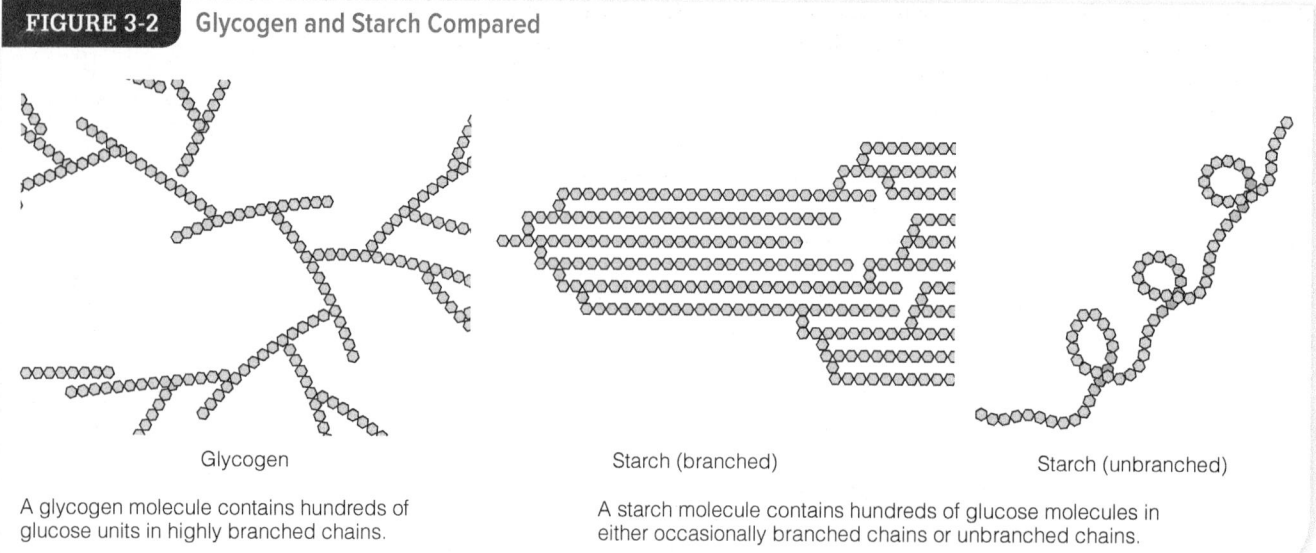

Glycogen

Starch (branched)

Starch (unbranched)

A glycogen molecule contains hundreds of glucose units in highly branched chains.

A starch molecule contains hundreds of glucose molecules in either occasionally branched chains or unbranched chains.

is not a significant food source of carbohydrate, but it does play an important role in the body. The human body stores much of its glucose as glycogen in the liver and muscles.

Starch **Starch** is a long, straight or branched chain of hundreds or thousands of glucose units linked together (see the middle and right side of Figure 3-2). These giant molecules are packed side by side in grains such as rice or wheat, in root crops and tubers such as yams and potatoes, and in legumes such as peas and beans. When a person eats the plant, the body splits the starch into glucose units and uses the glucose for energy.*

All starchy foods come from plants. Grains are the richest food source of starch. In most human societies, people depend on a staple grain for much of their food energy: rice in Asia; wheat in Canada, the United States, and Europe; corn in much of Central and South America; and millet, rye, barley, and oats elsewhere. A second important source of starch is the legume (bean and pea) family. Legumes include peanuts and "dry" beans such as butter beans, kidney beans, "baked" beans, black-eyed peas (cowpeas), chickpeas (garbanzo beans), and soybeans. Root vegetables (tubers) such as potatoes and yams are a third major source of starch, and in many non-Western societies, they are the primary starch sources. Grains, legumes, and tubers not only are rich in starch but may also contain abundant dietary fiber, protein, and other nutrients.

Fibers **Dietary fibers** are the structural parts of plants and thus are found in all plant-derived foods—vegetables, fruit, **whole grains**, and legumes (see Photo 3-2). Most dietary fibers are polysaccharides—chains of sugars—just as starch is, but in fibers the sugar units are held together by bonds that human digestive enzymes cannot break. Consequently, most dietary fibers pass through the body, providing little or no energy for its use. Figure 3-3 illustrates

glycogen (GLY-co-gen): a polysaccharide composed of glucose, made and stored by liver and muscle tissues of human beings and animals as a storage form of glucose. Glycogen is not a significant food source of carbohydrate and is not counted as one of the polysaccharides in foods.

starch: a plant polysaccharide composed of glucose and digestible by human beings.

dietary fibers: a general term denoting in plant foods the polysaccharides cellulose, hemicellulose, pectins, gums, and mucilages, as well as the nonpolysaccharide lignins, which are not digested by human digestive enzymes, although some are digested by GI tract bacteria.

whole grains: grains or foods made from them that contain all the essential parts and naturally occurring nutrients of the entire grain seed (except the inedible husk).

FIGURE 3-3 The Bonds of Starch and Cellulose Molecules Compared (Small Segments)

Human enzymes can digest starch, but they cannot digest cellulose because the bonds that link the glucose units together in cellulose are different.

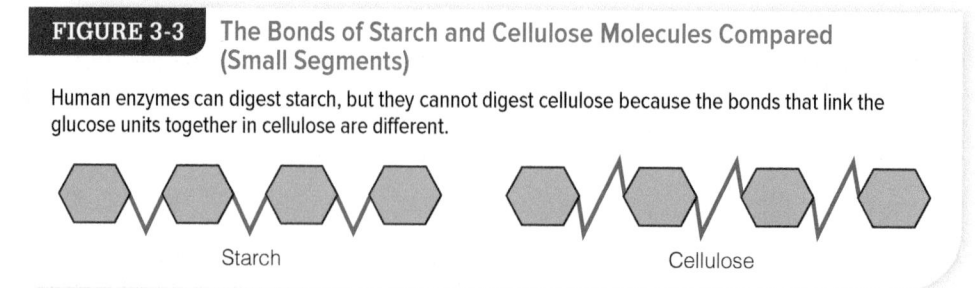

Starch

Cellulose

---

*The short chains of glucose units that result from the breakdown of starch are known as *dextrins*. The word sometimes appears on food labels because dextrins can be used as thickening agents in foods.

the difference in the bonds that link glucose molecules together in starch and those found in the plant fiber cellulose. In addition to cellulose, fibers include the polysaccharides hemicellulose, pectins, gums, and mucilages, as well as the nonpolysaccharide lignins.

Cellulose is the main constituent of plant cell walls, so it is found in all vegetables, fruit, and legumes. Hemicellulose is the main constituent of cereal fibers. Pectins are abundant in vegetables and fruit, especially citrus fruit and apples. The food industry uses pectins to thicken jelly and keep salad dressing from separating. Gums and mucilages have similar structures and are used as additives or stabilizers by the food industry. Lignins are the tough, woody parts of plants; few foods people eat contain much lignin.

A few starches are classified as fibers. Known as **resistant starches**, these starches escape digestion and absorption in the small intestine. Starch may resist digestion for several reasons, including the individual's efficiency in digesting starches and the food's physical properties. Resistant starch is common in whole or partially milled grains, legumes, raw potatoes, intact seeds and kernels, and unripe bananas. Cooked potatoes, pasta, and rice that have been chilled also contain resistant starch. Similar to some fibers, resistant starch may support a healthy colon.[1]

Although cellulose and other dietary fibers are not broken down by human enzymes, some fibers can be digested by bacteria in the human digestive tract. Bacterial **fermentation** of fibers can generate some absorbable products that can yield energy when metabolized. Food fibers, therefore, can contribute some energy (1.5 to 2.5 kcalories per gram), depending on the extent to which they break down in the body. Fibers are often divided into two general groups by their chemical and physical properties.* In the first group are fibers that dissolve in water (**soluble fibers**). In foods, soluble fibers add a pleasing consistency; for example, pectin puts the gel in jelly, and gums are added to salad dressings or other foods to thicken them.

In the body, some soluble fibers form gels (are **viscous**) and are more readily digested by bacteria in the human large intestine (are easily fermented). Commonly found in barley, legumes, fruit, oats, and vegetables, these fibers are often associated with lower risks of chronic diseases (as discussed in a later section). In addition to food sources, extracted single soluble fiber preparations are used as medications or as food additives.[†]

Other fibers do not dissolve in water (**insoluble fibers**), do not form gels (are not viscous), and are less readily fermented. Insoluble fibers, such as cellulose and many hemicelluloses, are found in the outer layers of whole grains (bran), the strings of celery, the hulls of seeds, and the skins of corn kernels. These fibers retain their structure and rough texture even after hours of cooking. In the body, they aid the digestive system by easing elimination.[2]

Photo 3-2

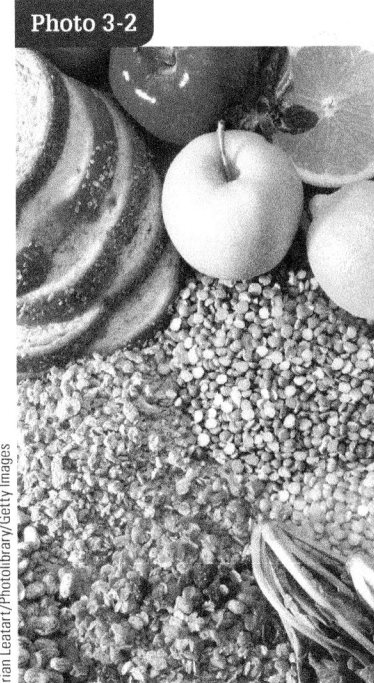

Brian Leatart/Photolibrary/Getty Images

Starch- and fiber-rich foods are the foods to emphasize.

resistant starches: starches that escape digestion and absorption in the small intestine of healthy people.

fermentation: the anaerobic (without oxygen) breakdown of carbohydrates by microorganisms that releases small organic compounds along with carbon dioxide and energy.

soluble fibers: indigestible food components that readily dissolve in water and often impart gummy or gel-like characteristics to foods. An example is pectin from fruit, which is used to thicken jellies.

viscous: having a gel-like consistency.

insoluble fibers: the tough, fibrous structures of fruit, vegetables, and grains; indigestible food components that do not dissolve in water.

Review Notes

- Carbohydrate is the body's preferred energy source. Six sugars are important in nutrition: the three monosaccharides (glucose, fructose, and galactose) and the three disaccharides (sucrose, lactose, and maltose).
- The three disaccharides are pairs of monosaccharides; each contains glucose paired with one of the three monosaccharides. The polysaccharides (chains of monosaccharides) are glycogen, starches, and fibers.
- Both glycogen and starch are storage forms of glucose—glycogen in the body and starch in plants—and both yield energy for human use.
- The dietary fibers also contain glucose (and other monosaccharides), but their bonds cannot be broken by human digestive enzymes, so they yield little, if any, energy.

*The DRI committee has proposed these fiber definitions: the term *dietary fibers* refers to naturally occurring fibers in intact foods, and *functional fibers* refers to added fibers that have health benefits; *total fiber* refers to the sum of fibers from both sources.

†Examples are pills of the fibers psyllium or methylcellulose used to relieve constipation; inulin, a slightly sweet-tasting fiber, is added to increase fiber in foods and reduce kcalories.

3.2 Digestion and Absorption of Carbohydrates

The ultimate goal of digestion and absorption of sugars and starches is to break them down into small molecules—chiefly glucose—that the body can absorb and use. The large starch molecules require extensive breakdown; the disaccharides need only be broken once and the monosaccharides not at all. Most fiber passes intact through the small intestine to the large intestine. There, bacteria digest many soluble fibers to produce short-chain fatty acids, which are rapidly absorbed by the large intestine. Table 3-2 provides the details.

3.3 Regulation of Blood Glucose

If blood glucose falls below normal, a person may become dizzy and weak; if it rises substantially above normal, the person may become fatigued. **Diabetes**, a disorder characterized by elevated blood glucose, is the topic of Chapter 20. Left untreated, fluctuations to the extremes—either high or low—can be fatal. Blood glucose homeostasis

diabetes (DYE-uh-BEE-teez): a group of metabolic disorders characterized by elevated blood glucose resulting from insufficient insulin, ineffective insulin, or both; the complete medical term is *diabetes mellitus* (MELL-ih-tus or mell-EYE-tus).

TABLE 3-2 Carbohydrate Digestion and Absorption

SUGAR AND STARCH	FIBER
MOUTH AND SALIVARY GLANDS	**MOUTH**
The salivary glands secrete saliva into the mouth to moisten the food. The salivary enzyme amylase begins digestion:	The mechanical action of the mouth crushes and tears fiber in food and mixes it with saliva to moisten it for swallowing.
Starch $\xrightarrow{\text{Amylase}}$ Small polysaccharides, maltose	
STOMACH	**STOMACH**
Stomach acid inactivates salivary enzymes, halting starch digestion.	Fiber is not digested, and it delays gastric emptying.
SMALL INTESTINE AND PANCREAS	**SMALL INTESTINE**
The pancreas produces an amylase that is released through the pancreatic duct into the small intestine:	Fiber is not digested but passes intact through to the large intestine. It delays absorption of some nutrients.
Starch $\xrightarrow{\text{Pancreatic amylase}}$ Small polysaccharides, maltose	
Then disaccharidase enzymes on the surface of the small intestinal cells hydrolyze the disaccharides into monosaccharides:	**LARGE INTESTINE**
Maltose $\xrightarrow{\text{Maltase}}$ Glucose + Glucose	Bacterial enzymes digest many soluble fibers, producing short-chain fatty acids that are preferentially and immediately absorbed by the large intestine.
Sucrose $\xrightarrow{\text{Sucrase}}$ Fructose + Glucose	Soluble fibers $\xrightarrow{\text{Bacterial enzymes}}$ Short-chain fatty acids, gas
Lactose $\xrightarrow{\text{Lactase}}$ Galactose + Glucose	Most insoluble fibers remain intact, retain some water, and bind substances such as bile, cholesterol, and some minerals, carrying them out of the body.
Intestinal cells absorb these monosaccharides.	

is regulated primarily by two hormones: **insulin**, which moves glucose from the blood into the cells, and **glucagon**, which brings glucose out of storage when blood glucose falls (as occurs between meals).

Insulin   After a meal, as blood glucose rises, the pancreas is the first organ to respond. It releases the hormone insulin, which signals body tissues to take up surplus glucose. Muscle tissue responds to insulin by taking up excess blood glucose and using it to make glycogen. The liver takes up excess blood glucose, too, but it needs no help from insulin to do so. Instead, the liver cells respond to insulin by speeding up their glycogen production. Adipose (fat) tissue also responds to insulin by both taking up blood glucose and slowing its release of the fat stored within its cells. Simply put, insulin regulates blood glucose by:

- Facilitating blood glucose uptake by the muscles and adipose tissue.
- Stimulating glycogen synthesis in the liver.

The muscles hoard two-thirds of the body's total glycogen to ensure that glucose, a critical fuel for physical activity, is available for muscular work. The brain stores a tiny fraction of the total, thought to provide an emergency glucose reserve sufficient to fuel the brain for an hour or two in severe glucose deprivation. The liver stores the remainder and is generous with its glycogen, making it available as blood glucose for the brain or other tissues when the supply runs low. Without carbohydrate from food to replenish it, the liver glycogen stores can be depleted in less than a day. Balanced meals and snacks, eaten on a regular schedule, help the body to maintain its blood glucose. Meals with starch and soluble fiber combined with some protein and a little fat slow digestion so that glucose enters the blood gradually at an ongoing, steady rate.

The Release of Glucose from Glycogen   The glycogen molecule is highly branched with hundreds of ends bristling from each molecule's surface (review this structure in Figure 3-2). When blood glucose starts to fall too low, the hormone glucagon is released into the bloodstream and triggers the breakdown of liver glycogen to single glucose molecules. Enzymes in liver cells respond to glucagon by attacking a multitude of glycogen ends simultaneously to release a surge of glucose into the blood for use by all the body's cells. Thus, the highly branched structure of glycogen uniquely suits the purpose of releasing glucose on demand.

Review Notes

- Blood glucose concentrations are regulated primarily by two hormones: insulin, which moves glucose from the blood into the cells, and glucagon, which brings glucose out of storage when blood glucose falls.

3.4 Health Effects of Sugars and Alternative Sweeteners

Fiber-rich carbohydrate foods such as vegetables, whole grains, legumes, and fruit should predominate in people's diets; the **naturally occurring sugars** in these foods and in milk are acceptable because they are accompanied by many nutrients. In contrast, concentrated sweets such as candy, cola beverages and other soft drinks, cookies, pies, cakes, and other foods with added sugars add kcalories, but few, if any, other nutrients or fiber. The Dietary Guidelines for Americans offer clear advice on added sugars: reduce intake.[3] People who want to limit their use of sugar may choose from two sets of alternative sweeteners: sugar alcohols and nonnutritive sweeteners.

insulin: a hormone secreted by the pancreas in response to (among other things) high blood glucose. It promotes cellular glucose uptake for use or storage.

glucagon (GLOO-ka-gon): a hormone that is secreted by special cells in the pancreas in response to low blood glucose concentration and that elicits release of glucose from storage.

naturally occurring sugars: sugars that are not added to a food but are present as its original constituents, such as the sugars of fruit or milk.

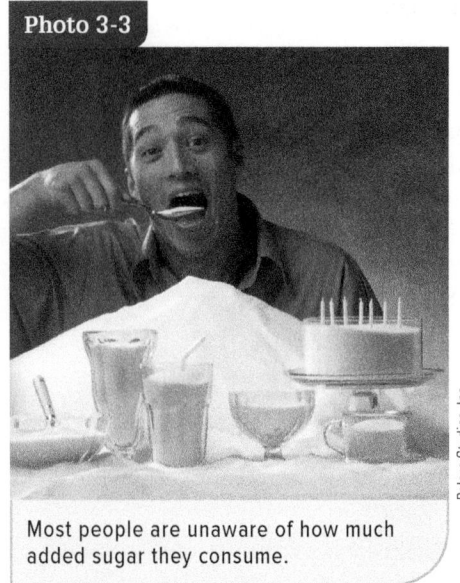

Most people are unaware of how much added sugar they consume.

Sugars

Recent decades have seen a dramatic upward trend in consumption of added sugars. Sugary foods and beverages taste delicious, cost little money, and are readily available, making overconsumption extremely likely. Though people are adding less sugar in the kitchen, food manufacturers are adding plenty to foods during processing. Soft drinks and other sugar-sweetened beverages are a major source of added sugars in the diets of U.S. consumers.[4] As Chapter 1 describes, these beverages and other products manufactured by the food industry (cakes, cookies, pies, other sweet desserts, powders for juice drinks, frozen and shelf-stable meals, cereal bars, fish sticks and chicken nuggets, and other products) are examples of ultra-processed foods. Findings from one large U.S. study revealed that ultra-processed foods contribute about 60 percent of total energy intake and nearly 90 percent of added sugar intake.[5] Thus, replacing ultra-processed products with minimally processed or whole foods such as milk, lean meats, legumes, nuts, fruit, vegetables, and whole grains will not only reduce added sugar intake but will provide health benefits beyond those of decreasing sugar intake. On average, U.S. adults consume almost 15 percent of their daily energy intake from added sugars.[6] Most people can afford only a little (less than 10 percent) added sugar in their diets if they are to meet nutrient needs within kcalorie limits.

The increase in sugar consumption has raised many questions about sugar's effects on health. In moderate amounts, sugars may add pleasure to meals without harming health. In excess, however, sugars can be detrimental, and the average American diet currently delivers excessive amounts (see Photo 3-3). Mounting evidence links high intakes of added sugars with obesity and other chronic diseases.[7] Sugars can also contribute to nutrient deficiencies by supplying energy (kcalories) without providing nutrients and to tooth decay, or **dental caries**.

Sugar and Obesity Over the past several decades, as obesity rates increased sharply, consumption of added sugars reached an all-time high—largely because high-fructose corn syrup use, especially in beverages, surged. High-fructose corn syrup is composed of fructose and glucose in a ratio of about 50:50. Compared with sucrose, high-fructose corn syrup is less expensive, easier to use, and more stable. In addition to being used in beverages, high-fructose corn syrup sweetens candies, baked goods, and hundreds of other foods. The use of high-fructose corn syrup sweetener parallels unprecedented increases in the incidence of obesity, but does this mean that sugar intakes are responsible for the increase in body fat and its associated health problems?[8] Excess sugar in the diet may be associated with more fat on the body.[9] When they are eaten in excess of need, energy from added sugars contributes to body fat stores, raising the risk of weight gain.[10] When total energy intake is controlled, however, *moderate* amounts of sugar do not *cause* obesity. Thus, to the extent that sugar contributes to an excessive energy intake, it can play a role in the development of obesity.

Because swallowing liquids requires little effort, the liquid form of sugar in soft drinks makes it especially easy to overconsume kcalories. Sugar-sweetened beverages are energy-dense, providing more than 150 kcalories per 12-ounce can, and many people drink several cans a day. The sugar kcalories of sweet beverages also cost less than many other energy sources, and they are widely available. The convenience, economy, availability, and flavors of sugary foods and beverages encourage overconsumption.

Limiting selections of foods and beverages high in added sugars can be an effective weight-loss strategy, especially for people whose excess kcalories come primarily from added sugars. For this reason, researchers suggest replacing sugar-sweetened beverages with water, and the American Heart Association recommends limiting added sugars to no more than 100 kcalories per day for women and 150 kcalories

dental caries: the gradual decay and disintegration of a tooth.

per day for men (which is about 5 percent of a 2000- and 2500-kcalorie diet, respectively).[11]

Sugar and Heart Disease Some research suggests that excess added sugars, and excess fructose in particular, favor the fat-making pathways and impair the fat-clearing pathways in the liver.[12] The resulting blood lipid profile increases the risk of heart disease.[13]

Researchers who reviewed 15 studies of fructose intakes from added sugars observed that people with higher fructose intakes had blood lipid values indicating an increased risk of heart disease.[14] In another study, children and adolescents who consumed more than 10 percent of their kcalories from added sugars had lower blood HDL cholesterol over 10 years' time than those consuming less (low HDL is undesirable for heart health).[15] As little as the equivalent of one or two high-fructose corn syrup-sweetened soft drinks a day consumed for only a few weeks significantly changes blood lipids in ways that may pose risks to the heart and arteries.[16]

Sugar and Type 2 Diabetes Since diabetes involves blood sugar, it was once believed that eating sugar *caused* diabetes by overworking the pancreas. We now know that this is not the case. Excess body fatness is more closely related to type 2 diabetes than is diet composition.[17]

Nevertheless, the incidence of type 2 diabetes often rises in populations as they take in more added sugars. A striking example is the profound increase in diabetes observed among some Native Americans when added sugars and refined flour replaced traditional roots, gourds, whole corn, and seeds as staple foods in their diets.[18] No simple cause-and-effect conclusion about sugar is possible, however, because at the same time, these people ate more processed meats and fats, increased total kcalorie intakes, and gained weight, too. Also, when *kcalorie* intakes do not exceed daily needs, links between sugar intakes and obesity, and sugar and type 2 diabetes, diminish.[19]

Several large review studies do show that increased consumption of sugar-sweetened beverages such as soft drinks is consistently linked to a greater risk of type 2 diabetes, however.[20] Some, but not all, of the risk is attenuated when BMI is factored in.

Thus, it is impossible to say, given this evidence alone, whether or not sugar causes diabetes—the evidence is observational and therefore circumstantial. The best conclusion may be that a healthy body weight and an eating pattern based on the Dietary Guidelines reduce diabetes risk; in addition, the person who is physically active, limits alcohol, and doesn't smoke reduces those risks dramatically.

Nutrient Deficiencies Added sugars contribute to nutrient deficiencies by displacing nutrients. Empty-kcalorie foods that contain lots of added sugars such as cakes, candies, and sodas provide the body with glucose and energy, but few, if any, other nutrients. By comparison, foods such as whole grains, vegetables, legumes, and fruit that contain some natural sugars and lots of starches and fibers also provide protein, vitamins, minerals, and phytochemicals.

A person spending 200 kcalories of a day's energy allowance on a 16-ounce soda gets little of value for those kcalories. In contrast, a person using 200 kcalories on three slices of whole-wheat bread gets 9 grams of protein, 6 grams of fiber, plus several B vitamins and minerals with those kcalories. For the person who wants something sweet, a reasonable compromise might be two slices of bread with a teaspoon of jam on each. For nutrition's sake, the appropriate attitude to take is not that sugar is "bad" and must be avoided, but that nutritious foods must come first. If nutritious foods crowd sugar out of the diet, that is fine—but not the other way around.

Sugar and Dental Caries Does sugar contribute to dental caries? The evidence says yes. Any carbohydrate-containing food, including bread, bananas, or milk, as well as sugar, can support bacterial growth in the mouth. These bacteria produce the acid that eats away tooth enamel. Of major importance is the length of time the food stays in the mouth. This, in turn, depends on the composition of the food, how sticky the food is, how often a person eats the food, and especially whether the teeth are brushed afterward. Total sugar intake still plays a major role in caries incidence; populations whose diets provide no more than 10 percent of kcalories from sugar have a low prevalence of dental caries. The Academy of Nutrition and Dietetics recommends a combined approach to prevent dental caries—practicing good oral hygiene, drinking fluoridated water, and reducing the amount of time sugars and starches are in the mouth.[21] Nutrition in Practice 17 discusses nutrition and oral health.

Recommended Sugar Intakes Moderate sugar intakes are not harmful and may make eating more enjoyable, but the average U.S. intake is well above moderate. These added sugar kcalories (and those from solid fats and alcohol) are considered empty kcalories—and most people need to limit their intake.

The DRI committee did not set a Tolerable Upper Intake Level for added sugars, but as discussed earlier, excessive intakes can interfere with sound nutrition and good health. Few people can eat lots of sugary treats and still meet all of their nutrient needs without exceeding their kcalorie allowance. For this reason, the *Dietary Guidelines for Americans* urges consumers to limit intake to less than 10 percent of total kcalories from added sugars per day. For most people, this means reducing their intake of kcalories from added sugars (and those from solid fats as well). By reducing the intake of foods and beverages with added sugars, consumers can lower the kcalorie content of the diet without compromising the nutrient content. Box 3-1 provides strategies for reducing the intake of added sugars. People who successfully reduce their intake of added sugars seem to adapt over time, perceiving sugar more intensely and preferring less sugar in their foods and beverages, making it a habit that is relatively easy to maintain.[22] The World Health Organization agrees, recommending no more than 10 percent of total energy from added sugars, with greater benefits expected from an intake of less than 5 percent.

Recognizing Sugars People often fail to recognize sugar in all its forms and so do not realize how much they consume. To help your clients estimate their sugar intakes, tell them to treat all of the following concentrated sweets as equivalent to 1 teaspoon of white sugar (4 grams of carbohydrate):

- 1 teaspoon brown sugar, candy, jam, jelly, any corn sweetener, syrup, honey, molasses, or maple sugar or syrup
- 1 tablespoon ketchup
- 1½ ounces carbonated soft drink

Box 3-1 **_HOW TO_ Reduce Intakes of Added Sugars**[a]

Use less table sugar when preparing meals and at the table.

- Use your sugar kcalories to sweeten nutrient-dense foods (such as oatmeal) instead of consuming empty-kcalorie foods and beverages (such as candy and soda).
- Replace empty-kcalorie-rich regular sodas, sports drinks, energy drinks, and fruit drinks with water, fat-free milk, 100% fruit juice, or unsweetened tea or coffee.
- Use sweet spices such as cinnamon, nutmeg, allspice, or clove.
- Select fruit for dessert. Eat less cake, cookies, ice cream, other desserts, and candy. If you do eat these foods, have a small portion.

- Warm up sweet foods before serving (heat enhances sweet tastes).
- Read the Nutrition Facts on labels to choose foods with less sugar. Select the unsweetened version of a food (such as corn flakes) instead of the sweetened version (such as frosted corn flakes) to reduce the quantity of added sugars in the diet.
- Read the ingredients list to identify foods with little or no added sugars. A food is likely to be high in added sugars if its ingredient list starts with any of the sugars named in Box 3-2, or if it includes several of them.

[a]As Chapter 1 described, once the updated Nutrition Facts panel is displayed on labels, added sugars will be listed separately.

Box 3-2   Glossary of Added Sugars

brown sugar: refined white sugar with molasses added; 95 percent pure sucrose.

concentrated fruit juice sweetener: a concentrated sugar syrup made from dehydrated, deflavored fruit juice, commonly grape juice; used to sweeten products that can then claim to be "all fruit."

confectioners' sugar: finely powdered sucrose; 99.9 percent pure.

corn sweeteners: corn syrup and sugar solutions derived from corn.

corn syrup: a syrup, mostly glucose, partly maltose, produced by the action of enzymes on cornstarch. It may be dried and used as *corn syrup solids*.

dextrose, anhydrous dextrose: forms of glucose.

evaporated cane juice: raw sugar from which impurities have been removed.

granulated sugar: white sugar.

high-fructose corn syrup (HFCS): a widely used commercial kcaloric sweetener made by adding enzymes to cornstarch to convert a portion of its glucose molecules into sweet-tasting fructose.

honey: a concentrated solution primarily composed of glucose and fructose; produced by enzymatic digestion of the sucrose in nectar by bees.

invert sugar: a mixture of glucose and fructose formed by the splitting of sucrose in an industrial process. Sold only in liquid form and sweeter than sucrose, invert sugar forms during certain cooking procedures and works to prevent crystallization of sucrose in soft candies and sweets.

malt syrup: a sweetener made from sprouted barley.

maple syrup: a concentrated solution of sucrose derived from the sap of the sugar maple tree, mostly sucrose. This sugar was once common but is now usually replaced by sucrose and artificial maple flavoring.

molasses: a thick, brown syrup left over from the refining of sucrose from sugarcane. The major nutrient in molasses is iron, a contaminant from the machinery used in processing it.

raw sugar: the first crop of crystals harvested during sugar processing. Raw sugar cannot be sold in the United States because it contains too much filth (dirt, insect fragments, and the like). Sugar sold as "raw sugar" is actually evaporated cane juice.

turbinado (ter-bih-NOD-oh) sugar: raw sugar from which the filth has been washed; legal to sell in the United States.

white sugar: granulated sucrose or "table sugar," produced by dissolving, concentrating, and recrystallizing raw sugar; 99.9 percent pure.

These portions of sugar all provide about the same number of kcalories. Some are closer to 10 kcalories (for example, 14 kcalories for molasses), whereas some are more than 20 kcalories (22 kcalories for honey), so an average figure of 16 kcalories is an acceptable approximation. Box 3-2 presents the multitude of names that denote sugar on food labels.

People often ask: Is honey, by virtue of being natural, more nutritious than white sugar? Honey, like white sugar, contains glucose and fructose. The difference is that, in white sugar, the glucose and fructose are bonded together in pairs, whereas in honey some of them are paired and some are free single sugars. When you eat either white sugar or honey, though, your body breaks all of the sugars apart into single sugars. It ultimately makes no difference, then, whether you eat single sugars linked together, as in white sugar, or the same sugars unlinked, as in honey; they will end up as single sugars in your body.

Honey does contain a few vitamins and minerals but not many. Honey is denser than crystalline sugar, too, so it provides more energy per spoonful. Table 3-3 (p. 78) shows that honey and white sugar are similar nutritionally—and both fall short of milk, legumes, fruit, grains, and vegetables. Honey may offer some health benefits, however: it seems to relieve nighttime coughing in children and reduce the severity of mouth ulcers in cancer patients undergoing chemotherapy or radiation.

Some sugar sources are more nutritious than others, though (see Photo 3-4). Consider a fruit such as an orange. The orange provides the same sugars and about the same energy as a tablespoon of sugar or honey, but the packaging makes a big difference in nutrient density. The sugars of the orange are diluted in a large volume of fluid that contains valuable vitamins and minerals, and the flesh and skin of the orange are supported by fibers that also offer health benefits. A tablespoon of honey offers no such bonuses.

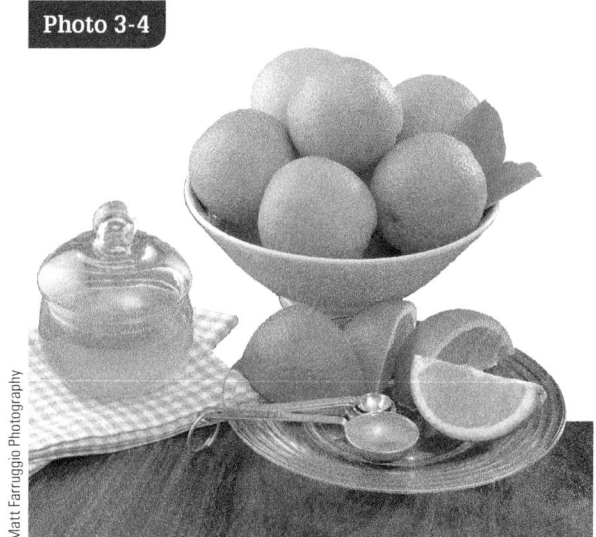

Photo 3-4

Matt Farruggio Photography

You receive about the same amount and kinds of sugars from an orange as from a tablespoon of honey, but the packaging makes a big nutrition difference.

TABLE 3-3 Sample Nutrients in Sugars and Other Foods

The indicated portion of any of these foods provides approximately 100 kcalories. Notice that—for a similar number of kcalories and grams of carbohydrate—milk, legumes, fruit, grains, and vegetables offer more of the other nutrients than do the sugars.

	SIZE OF 100 KCAL PORTION	CARBOHYDRATE (g)	PROTEIN (g)	CALCIUM (mg)	IRON (mg)	VITAMIN A (µg)	VITAMIN C (mg)
FOODS							
Milk, 1% low-fat	1 c	12	8	300	0.1	144	2
Kidney beans	½ C	20	7	30	1.6	0	2
Apricots	6	24	2	30	1.1	554	22
Bread, whole wheat	1½ slices	20	4	30	1.9	0	0
Broccoli, cooked	2 c	20	12	188	2.2	696	148
SUGARS							
Sugar, white	2 tbs	24	0	trace	trace	0	0
Molasses, blackstrap	2½ tbs	28	0	343	12.6	0	0.1
Cola beverage	1 c	26	0	6	trace	0	0
Honey	1½ tbs	26	trace	2	0.2	0	trace

Review Notes

- In moderation, sugars pose no major health threat except for an increased risk of dental caries.
- Excessive sugar intakes may displace needed nutrients and fiber and may contribute to obesity, heart disease, and type 2 diabetes.
- A person deciding to limit daily sugar intake should recognize that it is the added sugars in concentrated sweets, which are high in kcalories and relatively lacking in other nutrients, that should be restricted. Sugars that occur naturally in fruit, vegetables, and milk are acceptable.

Alternative Sweeteners: Sugar Alcohols

sugar alcohols: sugarlike compounds in the chemical family *alcohol* derived from fruit or manufactured from carbohydrates; sugar alcohols are absorbed more slowly than other sugars, are metabolized differently, and do not elevate the risk of dental caries. Examples are erythritol, maltitol, mannitol, sorbitol, isomalt, lactitol, and xylitol.

nutritive sweeteners: sweeteners that yield energy, including both the sugars and the sugar alcohols.

The **sugar alcohols** are carbohydrates, but they trigger a lower glycemic response and yield slightly less energy (2 to 3 kcalories per gram) than sucrose (4 kcalories per gram) because they are not absorbed completely. The sugar alcohols are sometimes called **nutritive sweeteners** because they do yield some energy. One exception, erythritol, cannot be metabolized by human enzymes and so is kcalorie free. Most sugar alcohols are slightly less sweet than sucrose; maltitol and xylitol are about as sweet as sucrose.

The sugar alcohols occur naturally in fruit and vegetables; they are also used by manufacturers to provide sweetness and bulk to cookies, sugarless gum, hard candies, and jams and jellies. Unlike sucrose, sugar alcohols are fermented in the large intestine by intestinal bacteria. Consequently, side effects such as gas, abdominal discomfort, and diarrhea make the sugar alcohols less attractive than the nonnutritive sweeteners.

The advantage of using sugar alcohols is that they do not contribute to dental caries. Bacteria in the mouth metabolize sugar alcohols much more slowly than sucrose, thereby inhibiting the production of acids that promote caries formation. They are therefore valuable in chewing gums, breath mints, and other products that people keep in their mouths awhile. The Food and Drug Administration (FDA) allows food labels to carry a health claim about the relationship between sugar alcohols and the nonpromotion of dental caries as long as certain FDA criteria, including those for sugar-free status, are met. Figure 3-4 presents labeling information for products using sugar alternatives.

Alternative Sweeteners: Nonnutritive Sweeteners

The **nonnutritive sweeteners** sweeten with minimal or no carbohydrate or energy. The human taste buds perceive many of them as extremely sweet, so just tiny amounts are added to foods to achieve the desired sweet taste. The FDA endorses nonnutritive sweeteners as safe for use over a lifetime within **Acceptable Daily Intake (ADI)** levels. Like the sugar alcohols, nonnutritive sweeteners make foods taste sweet without promoting tooth decay. Table 3-4 (p. 80) offers details about nonnutritive sweeteners, including ADI levels.

Nonnutritive Sweeteners and Weight Management Whether the use of nonnutritive sweeteners promotes weight loss or improves health by reducing total kcalorie intakes is not known with certainty. A rigorous, large analysis of research, however, does suggest that substituting nonnutritive sweeteners for sugar results in modest weight loss and may be helpful in improving compliance with weight-loss or weight-maintenance plans.[23] Earlier research suggesting that the use of nonnutritive sweeteners may *promote* weight gain through unknown mechanisms is not supported by more recent findings.[24]

When people reduce their energy intakes by replacing sugar in their diets with nonnutritive sweeteners and then compensate for the reduced energy at later meals, energy intake may stay the same or increase. Using nonnutritive sweeteners will not automatically lower energy intake; to successfully control energy intake, a person needs to make informed diet and activity decisions throughout the day.

nonnutritive sweeteners: synthetic or natural food additives that offer sweet flavor but with negligible or no kcalories per serving; also called *artificial sweeteners, intense sweeteners, noncaloric sweeteners,* and *very-low-calorie sweeteners.*

Acceptable Daily Intake (ADI): the amount of a nonnutritive sweetener that individuals can safely consume each day over the course of a lifetime without adverse effect. It includes a 100-fold safety factor.

FIGURE 3-4 Sugar Alternatives on Food Labels

Products containing sugar replacers may claim to "not promote tooth decay" if they meet FDA criteria for dental plaque activity.

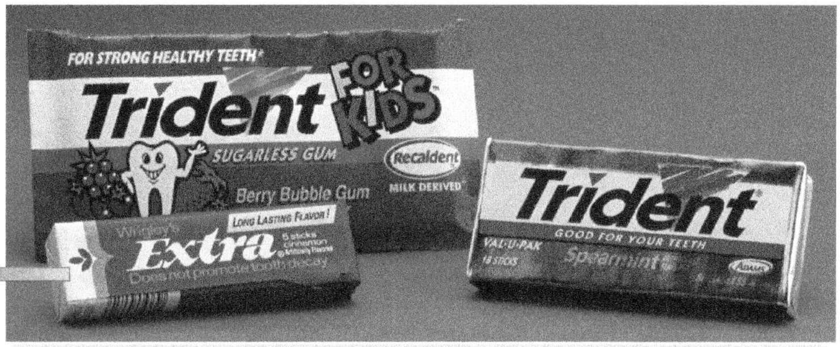

Products containing aspartame must carry a warning for people with phenylketonuria.

This ingredient list includes both sugar alcohols and nonnutritive sweeteners.

INGREDIENTS: SORBITOL, MALTITOL, GUM BASE, MANNITOL, ARTIFICIAL AND NATURAL FLAVORING, ACACIA, SOFTENERS, TITANIUM DIOXIDE (COLOR), ASPARTAME, ACESULFAME POTASSIUM AND CANDELILLA WAX. PHENYLKETONURICS: CONTAINS PHENYLALANINE.

35% FEWER CALORIES THAN SUGARED GUM

Nutrition Facts

Serving Size 2 pieces (3g)
Servings 6
Calories 5

Amount per serving	% DV*
Total Fat 0g	0%
Sodium 0mg	0%
Total Carb. 2g	1%
Sugars 0g	
Added Sugars 0g	0%
Sugar Alcohol 2g	
Protein 0g	

*Percent Daily Values (DV) are based on a 2000-calorie diet. Not a significant source of other nutrients.

Products containing less than 0.5 g of sugar per serving can claim to be "sugarless" or "sugar-free."

Products that claim to be "reduced kcalories" must provide at least 25% fewer kcalories per serving than the comparison item.

Craig M. Moore Photography

TABLE 3-4   U.S.-Approved Nonnutritive Sweeteners

SWEETENER	CHEMICAL COMPOSITION	BODY'S RESPONSE	RELATIVE SWEETNESS[a]	ENERGY (kcal/g)	ADI (mg/kg BODY WEIGHT) AND ESTIMATED EQUIVALENT[b]	COMMENTS
Acesulfame potassium or AceK[c] (AY-sul-fame)	Potassium salt	Not digested or absorbed	200	0	15 (23 packets of sweetener)	Approved as a sweetener and flavor enhancer in foods (except in meat and poultry)
Advantame (ad-VAN-tame)	Aspartame derivative, similar to neotame	Rapidly, but poorly absorbed	20,000	0	32.8 (4920 packets of sweetener)	Approved as a sweetener and flavor enhancer in foods (except in meat and poultry)
Aspartame[e] (ah-SPAR-tame or ASS-par-tame)	Amino acids (phenylalanine and aspartic acid) and a methyl group	Digested and absorbed	200	4[f]	50[g] (75 packets of sweetener)	Approved as a sweetener and flavor enhancer in foods
Luo han guo[h]	Cucurbitane glycosides extracts from Siraitia grosvenorii swingle fruit (also known as monk fruit)	Digested and absorbed	175	1	Not determined	GRAS[i]
Neotame (NEE-oh-tame)	Aspartame with an additional side group attached	Not digested or absorbed	10,000	0	0.3 (23 packets of sweetener)	Approved as a sweetener and flavor enhancer in foods (except in meat and poultry)
Saccharin[j] (SAK-ah-ren)	Benzoic sulfimide	Rapidly absorbed and excreted	400	0	15 (45 packets of sweetener)	Approved as a sweetener only in certain special dietary foods and as an additive used for certain technological purposes
Stevia[k] (STEE-vee-ah)	Glycosides found in the leaves of the Stevia rebaudiana herb	Digested and absorbed	300	0	4 (9 packets of sweetener)	GRAS[i]
Sucralose[l] (SUE-kra-lose)	Sucrose with Cl atoms instead of OH groups	Not digested or absorbed	600	0	5 (23 packets of sweetener)	Approved as a sweetener in foods

[a]Relative sweetness is determined by comparing the approximate sweetness of a sugar substitute with the sweetness of pure sucrose, which has been defined as 1.0. Chemical structure, temperature, acidity, and other flavors of the foods in which the substance occurs all influence relative sweetness.

[b]The Acceptable Daily Intake (ADI) is the estimated amount of a sweetener that individuals can safely consume each day over the course of a lifetime without adverse effects. The Estimated Equivalent is the number of packets of sweetener a person needs to consume to reach the ADI based on a person weighing 60 kg (132 lb).

[c]Marketed under the trade names Sunett and Sweet One.

[d]Recommendations from the WHO limit acesulfame K intake to 9 mg per kilogram of body weight per day.

[e]Marketed under the trade names NutraSweet, Equal, and Sugar Twin.

[f]Aspartame provides 4 kcal per gram, as does protein, but because so little is used, its energy contribution is negligible. In powdered form, it is sometimes mixed with lactose, however, so a 1-g packet may provide 4 kcal.

[g]Recommendations from the WHO and in Europe and Canada limit aspartame intake to 40 mg per kilogram of body weight per day.

[h]Marketed under the trade name Fruit-Sweetness.

[i]GRAS = generally recognized as safe. The GRAS list is subject to revision as new facts become known. For stevia, only one highly refined extract (known as Rebaudioside A) has been granted GRAS status; whole-leaf stevia and other extracts have not been approved.

[j]Marketed under the trade names Sweet'N Low, Sweet Twin, and Necta Sweet.

[k]Marketed under the trade names SweetLeaf, Purevia, Truvia, and Honey Leaf.

[l]Marketed under the trade name Splenda.

Safety of Nonnutritive Sweeteners Through the years, questions have emerged about the safety of nonnutritive sweeteners, but these issues have since been resolved. For example, early research indicating that large quantities of saccharin caused bladder tumors in laboratory animals was later shown to be inapplicable to humans. Common sense dictates that consuming large amounts of saccharin is probably not safe, but consuming moderate amounts poses no known hazard.

Aspartame, a sweetener made from two amino acids (phenylalanine and aspartic acid), is one of the most thoroughly studied food additives ever approved, and no scientific evidence supports the Internet stories that accuse it of causing disease. However, aspartame's phenylalanine base poses a threat to those with the inherited disease phenylketonuria (PKU). People with PKU cannot dispose of phenylalanine efficiently (see Nutrition in Practice 15). Food labels warn people with PKU of the presence of phenylalanine in aspartame-sweetened foods (see Figure 3-4). In addition, foods and drinks containing nonnutritive sweeteners have no place in the diets of even healthy infants or toddlers.

Review Notes

- Two types of alternative sweeteners are sugar alcohols and nonnutritive sweeteners.
- Sugar alcohols are carbohydrates, but they yield slightly less energy than sucrose.
- Sugar alcohols do not contribute to dental caries.
- The FDA endorses the use of nonnutritive sweeteners within ADI levels as safe over a lifetime.
- The nonnutritive sweeteners sweeten with minimal or no carbohydrate and energy.
- Like the sugar alcohols, nonnutritive sweeteners do not promote tooth decay.

3.5 Health Effects of Starch and Dietary Fibers

For health's sake, most people should increase their intakes of carbohydrate-rich foods such as whole grains, vegetables, legumes, and fruit—foods noted for their starch, fiber, and naturally occurring sugars.[25] In addition, most people should also limit their intakes of foods high in added sugars and the types of fats associated with heart disease (see Chapter 4). A diet that emphasizes whole grains, vegetables, legumes, and fruit is almost invariably moderate in food energy, low in fats that can harm health, and high in dietary fiber, vitamins, and minerals. All these factors working together can help reduce the risks of obesity, cancer, cardiovascular disease, diabetes, dental caries, gastrointestinal disorders, and malnutrition.

Carbohydrates: Disease Prevention and Recommendations

Fiber-rich carbohydrate foods benefit health in many ways. Foods such as whole grains, legumes, vegetables, and fruit supply valuable vitamins, minerals, and phytochemicals, along with abundant dietary fiber and little or no fat. The following paragraphs describe some of the health benefits of diets that emphasize a variety of these foods each day.

Heart Disease Diets rich in whole grains, legumes, and vegetables, especially those rich in whole grains, may protect against heart disease and stroke by lowering blood pressure, improving blood lipids, and reducing inflammation.[26] Such diets are generally low in saturated fat and *trans* fat, and high in dietary fibers, nutrients, and phytochemicals—all factors associated with a lower risk of heart disease (see also Chapter 4 and Nutrition in Practice 8). Foods rich in gel-forming soluble fibers (such as oat bran, barley, and legumes) lower blood cholesterol by binding bile, which contains cholesterol. Normally, much of this bile would be reabsorbed from the intestine for reuse, but the fiber carries some of it out with the feces.[27] Bile is needed in digestion, so the liver responds to its loss by drawing on blood cholesterol stores to synthesize more bile.

Diabetes High-fiber foods—and especially whole grains—play a key role in reducing the risk of **type 2 diabetes** (see Chapter 20).[28] The soluble fibers of foods such as oats and legumes can help regulate blood glucose following a carbohydrate-rich meal.[29] Soluble fibers trap nutrients and delay their transit through the digestive tract, slowing glucose absorption and preventing the glucose surge and rebound often associated with diabetes onset.

The term **glycemic response** refers to how quickly glucose is absorbed after a person eats, how high blood glucose rises, and how quickly it returns to normal. Slow absorption, a modest rise in blood glucose, and a smooth return to normal are desirable (a low glycemic response). Fast absorption, a surge in blood glucose, and an overreaction that plunges glucose below normal are less desirable (a high glycemic response). Different foods have different effects on blood glucose. The **glycemic index**, a method of classifying foods according to their potential to raise blood glucose, is the topic of Nutrition in Practice 3.

GI Health Soluble and insoluble fibers, along with ample fluid intake, enhance the health of the large intestine. Fermentable, soluble fibers of whole foods are of special importance in this regard.[30] Although human enzymes cannot digest these fibers, colonic bacteria readily ferment them, deriving sustenance that allows beneficial colonies to multiply and flourish.[31]

Makers of soluble fiber supplements choose specially manufactured unfermentable soluble fibers.* These fibers do not feed the colonic bacteria but remain intact in the digestive tract, swelling with water, softening and giving weight to fecal matter and facilitating elimination. Insoluble fibers such as cellulose (in wheat bran and other cereal brans, fruit, and vegetables) also remain intact in the colon. Coarse insoluble fibers stimulate the tissue linings of the colon to secrete water and mucus, which enlarge and soften the stools, easing their passage out of the body. Thus, both soluble and insoluble fibers help to alleviate or prevent constipation.

Large, soft stools ease the task of elimination. Pressure in the lower colon is then reduced, making it less likely that the rectal veins will swell (causing hemorrhoids). Fiber prevents compaction of the intestinal contents, which could obstruct the appendix and permit bacteria to invade and infect it. In addition, many people suffer from a weakness in the wall of the large intestine that leads portions of the wall to bulge out into pouches, as occurs in diverticulosis. Recommendations typically suggest increasing fiber to protect against diverticular disease, but research findings are inconsistent.[32]

Cancer Many studies show that, as people increase their dietary fiber intakes, their risk for colon cancer declines.[33] Importantly, findings support dietary fiber and not fiber supplements, which lack valuable nutrients and phytochemicals that also help protect against cancer.

All plant foods—vegetables, fruit, and whole-grain products—have attributes that may reduce the risks of colon and rectal cancers. Their fiber dilutes, binds, and rapidly removes potential cancer-causing agents from the colon. In addition, small fatlike molecules arising from bacterial fermentation lower the **pH**. These small fatlike molecules activate cancer-killing enzymes and inhibit inflammation in the colon.[34]

Other processes may also be at work. As research progresses, cancer experts recommend that fiber in the diet come from adequate amounts of vegetables and fruit daily, along with generous portions of whole grains and legumes.

---

*The unfermentable manufactured fibers are methylcellulose (from wood pulp) and psyllium (from seed husk).

Weight Management Fiber-rich foods tend to be low in solid fats, added sugars, and kcalories and can therefore help to prevent weight gain and promote weight loss by delivering less energy per bite. In addition, fibers absorb water from the digestive juices; as they swell, they create feelings of fullness, delay hunger, and reduce food intake. Fermentable fibers may be especially useful for appetite control. The small fats formed during fiber fermentation may shift the body's hormones in ways that promote feelings of fullness.[35] By whatever mechanism, as populations eat more refined, low-fiber foods and concentrated sweets, body fat stores creep up. In contrast, people who eat three or more ounces of whole-grain foods each day tend to have lower body and abdominal fatness over time.

Commercial weight-loss products often contain bulk-inducing fibers such as methylcellulose, but pure fiber compounds are not advised. High-fiber foods not only add bulk to the diet but are economical, are nutritious, and supply health-promoting phytochemicals—benefits that no purified fiber preparation can match. Figure 3-5 summarizes fibers and their health benefits.

Harmful Effects of Excessive Fiber Intake Despite fiber's benefits to health, when too much fiber is consumed, some minerals may bind to it and be excreted with it without becoming available for the body to use. When mineral intake is adequate, however, a reasonable intake of high-fiber foods does not seem to compromise mineral balance.

People with marginal food intakes who eat mostly high-fiber foods may not be able to take in enough food to meet energy or nutrient needs. Those who are malnourished, older adults, and young children adhering to all-plant (vegan) diets are especially vulnerable

---

FIGURE 3-5 Characteristics, Sources, and Health Effects of Fibers

People who eat these foods...	obtain these types of fibers...	with these actions in the body...	and receive these probable health benefits.
	Viscous, soluble, often fermentable and gel-forming		
• Barley, oats, oat bran, rye, fruit (apples, citrus), legumes (especially young green peas and black-eyed peas), seaweeds, seeds and many vegetables, fibers used as food additives[b]	• Beta-glucans • Gums • Inulin[a] • Pectins • Psyllium[b] • Some hemicellulose	• Reduce blood cholesterol by binding bile • Slow glucose absorption • Slow transit of food through upper GI tract; delay nutrient absorption • Hold moisture in stools, softening them (less fermentable soluble fibers) • Nourish beneficial bacterial colonies in the colon • Yield small fat molecules after fermentation that the colon can use for energy • Increase satiety	• Alleviate constipation (less fermentable soluble fibers) • Lower risk of heart disease • Lower risk of diabetes • Lower risk of colon and rectal cancer • Increase satiety (weight management)
	Nonviscous, insoluble, mostly non-fermentable		
• Brown rice, fruit, legumes, seeds, vegetables (cabbage, carrots, brussels sprouts), wheat bran, whole grains, extracted fibers used as food additives	• Cellulose • Lignins • Resistant starch • Hemicellulose	• Stimulate colon lining, increase fecal weight, and speed fecal passage through colon • Provide bulk and feelings of fullness	• Alleviate constipation • Lower risk of hemorrhoids and appendicitis • Reduce complications from diverticulosis • Lower risk of colon and rectal cancer

[a] Inulin, a soluble and fermentable but nonviscous fiber, is found naturally in a few vegetables, but is also purified from chicory root for use as a food additive.
[b] Psyllium, a soluble fiber derived from seed husks, is used as a laxative and food additive.

Sources: Information from J. W. McRorie, Evidence-based approach to fiber supplements and clinically meaningful health benefits, part 1, *Nutrition Today* 50 (2015): 82–89; J. W. McRorie, Evidence-based approach to fiber supplements and clinically meaningful health benefits, part 2, *Nutrition Today* 50 (2015): 90–97.

to this problem. Fibers also carry water out of the body and can cause dehydration. Advise clients to add an extra glass or two of water to go along with the fiber added to their diets. Athletes may want to avoid bulky, fiber-rich foods just prior to competition.

Recommended Intakes of Starches and Fibers The DRI committee advises that carbohydrates should contribute about half (45 to 65 percent) of the energy requirement. A person consuming 2000 kcalories a day should therefore obtain 900 to 1300 kcalories' worth of carbohydrate, or between 225 and 325 grams. This amount is more than adequate to meet the RDA for carbohydrate, which is set at 130 grams per day based on the average minimum amount of glucose used by the brain.

When it established the Daily Values that appear on food labels, the FDA used a guideline of 55 percent of kcalories in setting the Daily Value for carbohydrate at 275 grams per day. For most people, this means increasing total carbohydrate intake. To this end, the Dietary Guidelines for Americans encourage people to choose fiber-rich whole grains, vegetables, fruit, and legumes daily.

Recommendations for fiber encourage the same foods just mentioned: whole grains, vegetables, fruit, and legumes, which also provide vitamins, minerals, and phytochemicals. The FDA set the Daily Value for fiber at 28 grams for a 2000-kcalorie intake. This is based on the DRI recommendation of 14 grams per 1000-kcalorie intake—roughly 25 to 35 grams of dietary fiber daily. These recommendations are almost two times higher than the usual intake in the United States.[36]

As health care professionals, you can advise your clients that an effective way to add dietary fiber while lowering fat is to substitute plant sources of proteins (legumes) for some of the animal sources of protein (meats and cheeses) in the diet. Another way to add fiber is to encourage clients to consume the recommended amounts of fruit and vegetables each day. People choosing high-fiber foods are wise to seek out a variety of fiber sources and to drink extra fluids to help the fiber do its job. Many foods provide fiber in varying amounts, as Figure 3-6 shows.

As mentioned earlier, too much fiber is no better than too little. The World Health Organization recommends an upper limit of 40 grams of dietary fiber a day.

Review Notes

- A diet rich in starches and dietary fibers helps prevent heart disease, diabetes, GI disorders, and possibly some types of cancer. It also supports efforts to manage body weight.
- For these reasons, recommendations urge people to eat plenty of whole grains, vegetables, legumes, and fruit—enough to provide 45 to 65 percent of the daily energy from carbohydrate and 14 grams of fiber per 1000 kcalories.

Carbohydrates: Food Sources

A day's meals based on the USDA Healthy U.S.-Style Food Patterns not only meet carbohydrate recommendations but provide abundant fiber, too. Grains, vegetables, fruit, and legumes deliver dietary fiber and are noted for their valuable energy-yielding starches and dilute sugars. Each class of foods makes its own typical carbohydrate contribution. The USDA Food Groups and Subgroups on pp. 20–21 in Chapter 1 can help you and your clients choose carbohydrate-rich foods.

Grains Most foods in this group—a slice of whole-wheat bread, half an English muffin or bagel, a 6-inch tortilla, or ½ cup of rice, pasta, or cooked cereal—provide about 15 grams of carbohydrate per ounce equivalent, mostly as starch.* Be aware that

---

*Gram values in this section are adapted from *Choose Your Foods: Food Lists for Diabetes.*

FIGURE 3-6 Fiber in Selected Foods

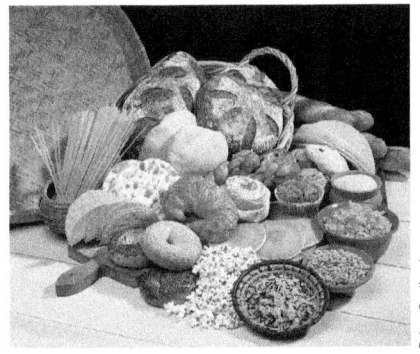

Grains

Whole-grain products provide 1 to 2 g of fiber or more per serving:

- 1 slice whole-wheat or rye bread (1 g).
- 1 slice pumpernickel bread (2 g).
- 1 oz ready-to-eat cereal (100% bran cereals contain 10 g or more).
- ½ c cooked barley, bulgur, grits, oatmeal (2 to 3 g).

Tips to increase fiber intake:

- Eat whole-grain breads that contain ≥3 g fiber per serving.
- Eat whole-grain cereals that contain ≥5 g fiber per serving.

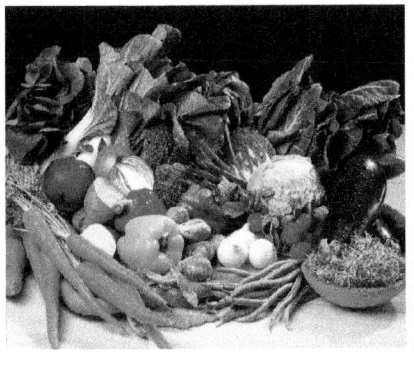

Vegetables

Most vegetables contain 2 to 3 g of fiber per serving:

- 1 c raw bean sprouts.
- ½ c cooked broccoli, brussels sprouts, cabbage, carrots, cauliflower, collards, corn, eggplant, green beans, green peas, kale, mushrooms, okra, parsnips, potatoes, pumpkin, spinach, sweet potatoes, swiss chard, winter squash.
- ½ c chopped raw carrots, peppers.

Tips to increase fiber intake:

- Eat raw vegetables.
- Eat vegetables (such as potatoes and zucchini) with their skins.

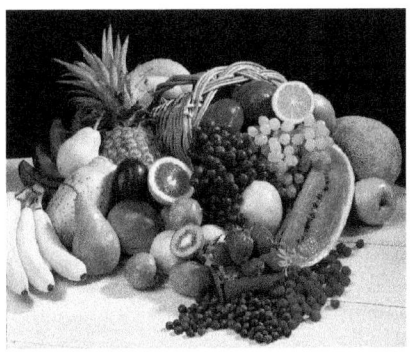

Fruit

Fresh, frozen, and dried fruits have about 2 g of fiber per serving:

- 1 medium apple, banana, kiwi, nectarine, orange, pear.
- ½ c applesauce, blackberries, blueberries, raspberries, strawberries.
- Fruit juices contain very little fiber.

Tips to increase fiber intake:

- Eat fresh and dried fruit for snacks.
- Eat fruit (such as apples and pears) with their skins.

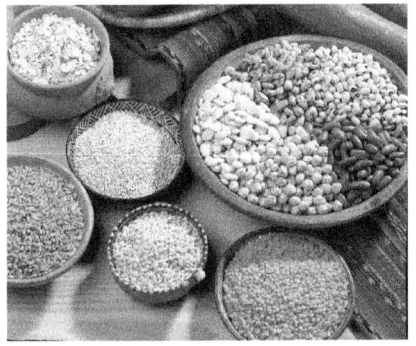

Legumes and Nuts

Many legumes provide about 8 g of fiber per serving:

- ½ c cooked baked beans, black beans, black-eyed peas, kidney beans, navy beans, pinto beans.

Some legumes provide about 5 g of fiber per serving:

- ½ c cooked garbanzo beans, great northern beans, lentils, lima beans, split peas.

Most nuts and seeds provide 1 to 3 g of fiber per serving:

- 1 oz almonds, cashews, hazelnuts, peanuts, pecans, pumpkin seeds, sunflower seeds.

Tip to increase fiber intake:

- Add legumes to soups, salads, and casseroles.

some foods in this group, especially snack crackers and baked goods such as biscuits, croissants, and muffins, contain added sugars, solid fats, and sodium. When selecting from the grain group, limit refined grains and be sure at least half of the foods chosen are whole-grain products. People who eat more whole grains tend to have healthier diets.[37]

Vegetables Some vegetables are major contributors of starch in the diet. Just a small white or sweet potato or ½ cup of cooked dry beans, corn, peas, plantain, or winter squash provides 15 grams of carbohydrate, as much as in a slice of bread, though as a mixture of sugars and starch. One-half cup of carrots, okra, onions, tomatoes, cooked greens, or most other nonstarchy vegetables or a cup of salad greens provides about 5 grams as a mixture of starch and sugars. Each of these foods also contributes a little protein, some fiber, and no fat.

Fruit A half-cup equivalent of fruit contains an average of about 15 grams of carbohydrate, mostly as sugars, including the fruit sugar fructose. The amount of fruit equivalent to a half-cup varies depending on the form of the fruit: ½ cup of juice; a small banana, apple, or orange; ½ cup of most canned or fresh fruit; or ¼ cup of dried fruit. Fruit varies greatly in its water and fiber contents; therefore, its sugar concentrations vary also. No more than one-half of the day's fruit should come from juice. With the exception of avocado, which is high in fat, fruit contains insignificant amounts of fat and protein.

Milk and Milk Products One cup of milk or yogurt or the equivalent (1 cup of buttermilk, ⅓ cup of dry milk powder, or ½ cup of evaporated milk) provides a generous 12 grams of carbohydrate. Among cheeses, cottage cheese provides about 6 grams of carbohydrate per cup, whereas most other types contain little, if any, carbohydrate. These foods also contribute high-quality protein as well as several important vitamins and minerals. Calcium-fortified soy beverages are options for providing calcium and about the same amount of carbohydrate as milk. All milk products vary in fat content, an important consideration in choosing among them; Chapter 4 provides the details.

Cream and butter, although dairy products, are not equivalent to milk because they contain little or no carbohydrate and insignificant amounts of the other nutrients important in milk. They are appropriately classified as solid fats.

Protein Foods With two exceptions, foods of this group provide almost no carbohydrate to the diet. The exceptions are nuts, which provide a little starch and fiber along with their abundant fat, and dry beans, which are excellent sources of both starch and fiber. Just ½ cup of beans provides 15 grams of carbohydrate, an amount equal to the richest carbohydrate sources. Among sources of fiber, beans and other legumes are outstanding, providing as much as 8 grams in ½ cup. The carbohydrate content of a diet can be determined by using the food list system described in Chapter 20, or a computer diet analysis program.

Carbohydrates: Food Labels and Health Claims

Food labels list the amount, in grams, of total carbohydrate—including starch, fibers, and sugars—per serving. Grams of fiber and sugars (and added sugars) are listed separately. (With this information, consumers can calculate starch grams by subtracting the grams of fibers and sugars from the total carbohydrate.) Total carbohydrate and dietary fiber are also expressed as "% Daily Values" for a person consuming 2000 kcalories; there is no Daily Value for sugars.

The FDA authorizes four health claims on food labels concerning fiber-rich carbohydrate foods. One is for "fiber-containing grain products, fruits, and vegetables and reduced risk of cancer." Another is for "fruits, vegetables, and grain products that contain fiber, and reduced risk of coronary heart disease." A third is for "soluble fiber from whole oats and from psyllium seed husk and reduced risk of coronary heart disease," and a fourth is for "whole grains and reduced risk of heart disease and certain cancers."

Review Notes

- Grains, vegetables, fruit, and legumes contribute dietary fiber and energy-yielding starches and dilute sugars to people's diets. One cup of milk or yogurt or the equivalent contributes a generous 12 grams of carbohydrate as well as protein and other important nutrients.
- Food labels list grams of total carbohydrate and also provide separate listings of grams of fiber and sugar.

Self Check

1. Which of the following foods is *not* a good source of carbohydrates?
   a. Plain yogurt
   b. Steak
   c. Brown rice
   d. Green peas

2. Polysaccharides include:
   a. galactose, starch, and glycogen.
   b. starch, glycogen, and fiber.
   c. lactose, maltose, and glycogen.
   d. sucrose, fructose, and glucose.

3. The chief energy source of the body is:
   a. sucrose.
   b. starch.
   c. glucose.
   d. fructose.

4. The primary form of stored glucose in animals is:
   a. glycogen.
   b. cellulose.
   c. starch.
   d. lactose.

5. The polysaccharide that helps form the cell walls of plants is:
   a. cellulose.
   b. starch.
   c. glycogen.
   d. lactose.

6. Which of the following terms on a food label may denote sugar?
   a. Corn syrup
   b. Aspartame
   c. Xylitol
   d. Cellulose

7. The two types of alternative sweeteners are:
   a. saccharin and cyclamate.
   b. sugar alcohols and nonnutritive sweeteners.
   c. sorbitol and xylitol.
   d. sucrose and fructose.

8. A diet high in carbohydrate-rich foods such as whole grains, vegetables, fruit, and legumes is:
   a. most likely low in fat.
   b. most likely low in fiber.
   c. most likely poor in vitamins and minerals.
   d. most likely disease promoting.

9. A fiber-rich diet may help to prevent or control:
   a. diabetes.
   b. heart disease.
   c. constipation.
   d. all of the above.

10. The DRI fiber recommendation is:
    a. 10 grams per 1000 kcalories.
    b. 15 to 25 grams per day.
    c. 14 grams per 1000 kcalories.
    d. 40 to 55 grams per day.

Answers: 1.b, 2.b, 3.c, 4.a, 5.a, 6.a, 7.b, 8.a, 9.d, 10.c

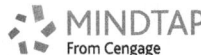 **MINDTAP** From Cengage   For more chapter resources visit **www.cengage.com** to access MindTap, a complete digital course.

Clinical Applications

1. Considering the health benefits of carbohydrate-rich foods, especially those that provide starch and fiber, what suggestions would you offer to a client who reports the following:

   - Eats only 3 ounces of refined, sugary breads or cereals each day.
   - Eats 1 cup of vegetables (usually french fries) each day.
   - Drinks fruit juice once a day but never eats fruit.
   - Eats cheese at least twice a day but does not drink milk.
   - Eats large portions of meat at least twice a day.
   - Eats hard candy two or three times a day.

Notes

1. M. J. Keenan and coauthors, Role of resistant starch in improving gut health, adiposity, and insulin resistance, *Advances in Nutrition* 6 (2015): 198–205; D. F. Birt and coauthors, Resistant starch: Promise for improving human health, *Advances in Nutrition* 4 (2013): 587–601.

2. Position of the Academy of Nutrition and Dietetics: Health Implications of dietary fiber, *Journal of the Academy of Nutrition and Dietetics* 115 (2015): 1861–1870; A. Dilzer, J. M. Jones, and M. E. Latulippe, The family of dietary fibers: Dietary variety for maximum health benefit, *Nutrition Today* 48 (2013): 108–118.

3. U.S. Department of Health and Human Services and U.S. Department of Agriculture, *2015–2020 Dietary Guidelines for Americans*, 8th ed., 2015, health.gov/dietaryguidelines/2015/guidelines.

4. American Heart Association, Sugar 101, www.heart.org/HEARTORG /HealthyLiving/HealthyEating/Nutrition/Sugar- 101_UCM_306024 _Article.jsp#.WUAcd2jyuzd, 2017; S. Park and coauthors, Prevalence of sugar-sweetened beverage intake among adults—23 states and the District of Columbia, 2013, *Morbidity and Mortality Weekly Report* 65 (2016): 169–174.

5. E. M. Steele and coauthors, Ultra-processed foods and added sugars in the US diet: Evidence from a nationally representative cross-sectional study, *BMJ Open* 6 (20016): e009892.

6. U.S. Department of Health and Human Services and U.S. Department of Agriculture, *2015–2020 Dietary Guidelines for Americans*, 8th ed., 2015, health.gov/dietaryguidelines/2015/guidelines.

7. B. M. Appelhans and coauthors, Beverage intake and metabolic syndrome risk over 14 years: The Study of Women's Health Across the Nation, *Journal of the Academy of Nutrition and Dietetics* 117 (2017): 554–562; B. Xi and coauthors, Sugar-sweetened beverages and risk of hypertension and CVD: A dose-response meta-analysis, *British Journal of Nutrition* 113 (2015): 709–717; K. L. Stanhope and coauthors, A dose-response study of consuming high-fructose corn syrup-sweetened beverages on lipid/lipoprotein risk factors for cardiovascular disease in young adults, *American Journal of Clinical Nutrition* 101 (2015): 1144–1154; K. R. Saab and coauthors, New insights on the risk for cardiovascular disease in African Americans: The role of added sugars, *Journal of the American Society of Nephrology* 26 (2015): 247–257; R. Kelishadi, M. Mansourian, and M. Heidari-Beni, Association of fructose consumption and components of metabolic syndrome in human studies: A systematic review and meta-analysis, *Nutrition* 30 (2014): 503–510; G. A. Bray, Energy and fructose from beverages sweetened with sugar or highfructose corn syrup pose a health risk for some people, *Advances in Nutrition* 4 (2013): 220–225; G. L. Ambrosini and coauthors, Prospective associations between sugarsweetened beverage intakes and cardiometabolic risk factors in adolescents, *American Journal of Clinical Nutrition* 98 (2013): 327–334; V. S. Malik and coauthors, Sugarsweetened beverages and weight gain in children and adults: A systematic review and meta-analysis, *American Journal of Clinical Nutrition* 98 (2013): 1084–1102.

8. S. D. Poppitt, Beverage consumption: Are alcoholic and sugary drinks tipping the balance towards overweight and obesity? *Nutrients* 7 (2015): 6700-6718; G. A. Bray and B. M. Popkin, Dietary sugar and body weight: Have we reached a crisis in the epidemic of obesity and diabetes? *Diabetes Care* 37 (2014): 950–956; F. B. Hu, Resolved: There is sufficient scientific evidence that decreasing sugar-sweetened beverage consumption will reduce the prevalence of obesity and obesity-related diseases, *Obesity Reviews* 14 (2013): 606–619; Malik and coauthors, 2013.

9. M. Siervo and coauthors, Sugar consumption and global prevalence of obesity and hypertension: An ecological analysis, *Public Health Nutrition* 17 (2014): 587–596; S. C. Bundrick and coauthors, Soda consumption during ad libitum food intake predicts weight change, *Journal of the Academy of Nutrition and Dietetics* 114 (2014): 444–449; Hu, 2013; Malik and coauthors, 2013.

10. L. Tappy and K. A. Le, Health effects of fructose and fructose-containing caloric sweeteners: Where do we stand 10 years after the initial whistle blowings? *Current Diabetes Reports* 15 (2015): 54; Bray and Popkin, 2014; Hu, 2013; Bray, 2013.

11. American Heart Association, *Sugar 101*. www.heart.org /HEARTORG/HealthyLiving/HealthyEating/Nutrition/Sugar-101 _UCM_306024_Article.jsp#.WUAcd2jyuzd; M. Zheng and coauthors, Substitution of sugar-sweetened beverages with other beverage alternatives: A review of long-term health outcomes, *Journal of the Academy of Nutrition and Dietetics* 115 (2015): 767–779.

12. J. Ma and coauthors, Potential link between excess added sugar intake and ectopic fat: A systematic review of randomized controlled trials, *Nutrition Reviews* 74 (2016): 18–32; A. Kolderup and B. Svihus, Fructose metabolism and relation to atherosclerosis, type 2 diabetes, and obesity, *Journal of Nutrition and Metabolism*, 2015, dx.doi.org /10.1155/2015/823081; J. Ma and coauthors, Sugar-sweetened beverage, diet soda, and fatty liver disease in the Framingham Heart Study cohorts, *Journal of Hepatology* 63 (2015): 462–469; S. Chiu and coauthors, Effect of fructose on markers of non-alcoholic fatty liver disease (NAFLD): A systematic review and meta-analysis of controlled feeding trials, *European Journal of Clinical Nutrition* 68 (2014): 416–423; R. H. Lustig, Fructose: It's "alcohol without the buzz," *Advances in Nutrition* 4 (2013): 226–235.

13. L. Chiavaroli and coauthors, Effect of fructose on established lipid targets: A systematic review and meta-analysis of controlled feeding trials, *Journal of the American Heart Association* 4 (2015): e001700; Kolderup and Svihus, 2015; D. David Wang and coauthors, Effect of fructose on postprandial triglycerides: A systematic review and metaanalysis of controlled feeding trials, *Atherosclerosis* 232 (2014): 125–133.

14. Kelishadi, Mansourian, and Heidari-Beni, 2014.

15. A. K. Lee and coauthors, Consumption of less than 10% of total energy from added sugars is associated with increasing HDL in females during adolescence: A longitudinal analysis, *Journal of the American Heart Association* 3 (2014): e000615.

16. K. L. Stanhope and coauthors, A dose-response study of consuming high-fructose corn syrup-sweetened beverages on lipid/lipoprotein risk factors for cardiovascular disease in young adults, *American Journal of Clinical Nutrition* 101 (2015): 1144–1154.

17. American Diabetes Association, Classification and diagnosis of diabetes, *Diabetes Care* 40 (2017): S11–S24; A. Abbasi and coauthors, Body mass index and incident type 1 and type 2 diabetes in children and young adults: A retrospective cohort study, *Journal of the Endocrine Society* 1 (2017): 524–537; A. Fardet and Y. Boirie, Associations between dietrelated diseases and impaired physiological mechanisms: A holistic approach based on meta-analyses to identify targets for preventive nutrition, *Nutrition Reviews* 71 (2013): 643–656.

18. N. I. Toufel-Shone and coauthors, Demographic characteristics and food choices of participants in the Special Diabetes Program for American Indians Diabetes Prevention Demonstration Project, *Ethnicity and Health* 20 (2015): 327–340.

19. J. L. Sievenpiper and R. J. de Souza, Are sugar-sweetened beverages the whole story? *American Journal of Clinical Nutrition* 98 (2013): 261–263.

20. V. S. Malik and F. B. Hu, Fructose and cardiometabolic health: What the evidence from sugar-sweetened beverages tells us, *Journal of the American College of Cardiology* 66 (2015): 1615–1624; D. C. Greenwood and coauthors, Association between sugarsweetened and artificially sweetened soft drinks and type 2 diabetes: Systematic review and dose-response meta-analysis of prospective studies, *British Journal of Nutrition* 112 (2014): 725–734; B. Xi and coauthors, Intake of fruit juice and incidence of type 2 diabetes: A systematic review and meta-analysis, *PLos One* 9 (2014): e93471, doi: 10.1371/journal.pone.009347; D. Romaguera and coauthors, Consumption of sweet beverages and type 2 diabetes incidence in European adults: Results from EPIC-InterAct, *Diabetologia* 56 (2013): 1520–1530.

21. Position of the Academy of Nutrition and Dietetics: Oral health and nutrition, *Journal of the Academy of Nutrition and Dietetics* 113 (2013): 693–701.

22. P. M. Wise and coauthors, Reduced dietary intake of simple sugars alters perceived sweet taste intensity but not perceived pleasantness, *American Journal of Clinical Nutrition* 103 (2016): 50–60.

23. P. E. Miller and V. Perez, Low-calorie sweeteners and body weight and composition: A meta-analysis of randomized controlled trials and prospective cohort studies, *American Journal of Clinical Nutrition* 100 (2014): 765–777.

24. C. Piernas and coauthors, Does diet-beverage intake affect dietary consumption patterns? Results from the Choose Healthy Options Consciously Everyday (CHOICE) randomized clinical trial, *American Journal of Clinical Nutrition* 97 (2013): 604–611.

25. Position of the Academy of Nutrition and Dietetics, 2015; P. Buil-Cosiales and coauthors, Fiber intake and all-cause mortality in the Prevención con Dieta Mediterránea (PREDIMED) study, *American Journal of Clinical Nutrition* 100 (2014): 498–507; O. Oyebode and coauthors, Fruit and vegetable consumption and all-cause, cancer and CVD mortality: Analysis of Health Survey for England data, *Journal of Epidemiology and Community Health* 68 (2014): 856–862.

26. H. Wu and coauthors, Association between dietary whole grain intake and risk of mortality: Two large prospective studies in US men and women, *JAMA Internal Medicine* 175 (2015): 373–384; R.H. Eckel and coauthors, 2013 AHA/ACC guidelines on lifestyle management to reduce cardiovascular risk: A report of the American College of Cardiology/ American Heart Association Task Force on Practice Guidelines, *Circulation* 129 (2014): S76–S99; D. E. Threapleton and coauthors, Dietary fibre intake and risk of cardiovascular disease: Systematic review and meta-analysis, *BMJ* 347 (2013): f6879.

27. J. W. McRorie, Evidence-based approach to fiber supplements and clinically meaningful health benefits, part 1, *Nutrition Today* 50 (2015): 82–89.

28. B. Yao and coauthors, Dietary fiber intake and risk of type 2 diabetes: A dose-response analysis of prospective studies, *European Journal of Epidemiology* 29 (2014): 79–88; S. S. Cho and coauthors, Consumption of cereal fiber, mixtures of whole grains and bran, and whole grains and risk reduction in type 2 diabetes, obesity, and cardiovascular disease, *American Journal of Clinical Nutrition* 98 (2013): 594–619; T. Wirström and coauthors, Consumption of whole grain reduces risk of deteriorating glucose tolerance, including progression to prediabetes, *American Journal of Clinical Nutrition* 97 (2013): 179–187.

29. F. M. Silva and coauthors, Fiber intake and glycemic control in patients with type 2 diabetes mellitus: A systematic review with meta-analysis of randomized controlled trials, *Nutrition Reviews* 71 (2013): 790–801.

30. J. Tan and coauthors, The role of short-chain fatty acids in health and disease, *Advances in Immunology* 121 (2014): 91–119.

31. J. R. Marchesi and coauthors, The gut microbiota and host health: A new clinical frontier, *Gut* 65 (2016): 330–339; J. Slavin, Fiber and prebiotics: Mechanisms and health benefits, *Nutrients* 5 (2013): 1417–1435.

32. J. D. Feuerstein and D. R. Falchuk, Diverticulosis and diverticulitis, *Mayo Clinic Proceedings* 91 (2016): 1094–1104; F. L. Crowe and coauthors, Source of dietary fibre and diverticular disease incidence: A prospective study of UK women, *Gut* 63 (2014): 1450–1456; A. F. Peery and coauthors, Constipation and a low-fiber diet are not associated with diverticulosis, *Clinical Gastroenterology and Hepatology* 11 (2013): 1622–1627; A. W. Templeton and L. L. Strate, Updates in Diverticular disease, *Current Gastroenterology Reports* 15 (2013): 339.

33. A. T. Kunzmann and coauthors, Dietary fiber intake and risk of colorectal cancer and incident and recurrent adenoma in the Prostate, Lung, Colorectal, and Ovarian Cancer Screening Trial, *American Journal of Clinical Nutrition* 102 (2015): 881–890; D. H. Zeng, D. L. Lazarova, and M. Bordonaro, Mechanisms linking dietary fiber, gut microbiota and colon cancer prevention, *World Journal of Gastrointestinal Oncology* 6 (2014): 41–51.

34. Marchesi and coauthors, 2016; Slavin, 2013; H.M. Chen and coauthors, Decreased dietary fiber intake and structural alteration of gut microbiota in patients with advanced colorectal adenoma, *American Journal of Clinical Nutrition* 97 (2013): 1044–1052.

35. Tan and coauthors, 2014.

36. Position of the Academy of Nutrition and Dietetics, 2015.

37. C. J. Seal and I. A. Brownlee, Whole grains, dietary fibre and grain-derived phytochemicals, *Proceedings of the Nutrition Society* 74 (2015): 313–319; G. Tang and coauthors, Meta-analysis of the association between whole grain intake and coronary heart disease risk, *American Journal of Cardiology* 115 (2015): 625–629; P. L. B. Hollænder, A. B. Ross, and M. Kristensen, Whole-grain and blood lipid changes in apparently healthy adults: A systematic review and meta-analysis of randomized controlled studies, *American Journal of Clinical Nutrition* 102 (2015): 556–572S; S. Cho and coauthors, Consumption of cereal fiber, mixtures of whole drains and bran, and whole grains and risk reduction in type 2 diabetes, obesity, and cardiovascular disease, *American Journal of Clinical Nutrition* 98 (2013): 594–619.

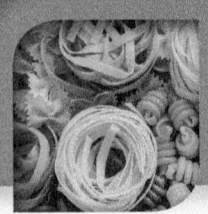

3.6 Nutrition in Practice

The Glycemic Index in Nutrition Practice

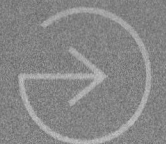

Carbohydrate-rich foods vary in the degree to which they elevate both blood glucose and insulin concentrations. Chapter 3 introduced the *glycemic index (GI)*, a ranking of carbohydrate foods based on their glycemic effect after ingestion. The glycemic index may be of interest to people with diabetes who must regulate their blood glucose to protect their health. In diabetes treatment, however, the total amount of carbohydrate is more important than the type of carbohydrate consumed.[1] Thus, dietetics experts have debated the usefulness of the glycemic index for diabetes treatment. Despite some controversy, however, the American Diabetes Association encourages low-glycemic foods that are rich in fiber and other nutrients.[2] Furthermore, because some recent research shows that a low-glycemic index diet can improve blood glucose control in type 2 diabetes, the use of low-glycemic diets for this purpose may be gaining credibility.[3]

Researchers are also trying to determine whether low-GI diets may be helpful for improving risk factors for a number of other chronic diseases.[4] This Nutrition in Practice describes the factors that contribute to a food's glycemic effect and the results of research studies that have examined the potential benefits of selecting mainly low-GI foods.

How is the glycemic index measured?

The glycemic index is essentially a measure of how quickly the carbohydrate in a food is digested and absorbed. Although testing methods vary to some degree, the most common protocol is to feed the test food—which contains a measured quantity of digestible carbohydrate—to research subjects and then measure blood glucose levels for two or three hours after the feeding. The increase in blood glucose over the two- or three-hour period is then compared to the blood glucose rise after an identical amount of digestible carbohydrate is ingested from a reference food such as pure glucose or white bread. Figure NP3-1 illustrates the difference in the blood glucose response to a low-GI food and a high-GI food. The blood glucose curve displays the surge in blood glucose above normal fasting levels after the food is consumed and the subsequent fall over several hours. Table NP3-1 lists the GIs of various carbohydrate-containing foods, arranged from highest to lowest within each food group listed.

The *amount* of carbohydrate consumed also influences the glycemic response. A food's total glycemic effect—expressed as the *glycemic load (GL)*—is the product of its GI and the amount of available carbohydrate from the portion consumed, divided by 100. For example, if the GI of

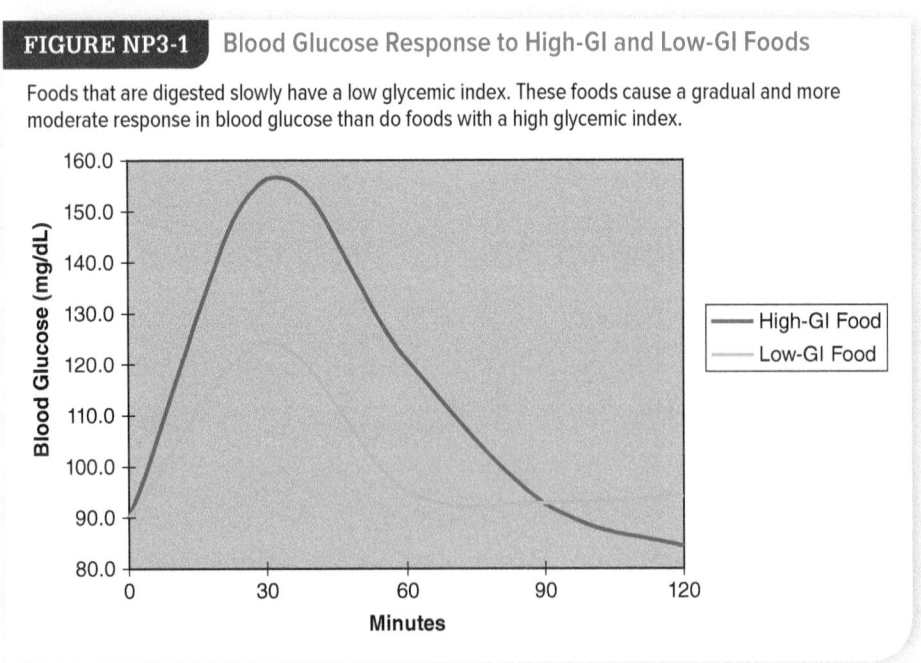

FIGURE NP3-1 Blood Glucose Response to High-GI and Low-GI Foods

Foods that are digested slowly have a low glycemic index. These foods cause a gradual and more moderate response in blood glucose than do foods with a high glycemic index.

VALUE	GI
High	≥70
Medium	56–69
Low	≤55

FOOD ITEM	GLYCEMIC INDEX
GRAINS	
• Cornflakes	81
• Instant oatmeal, cooked	79
• White bread, enriched	75
• Whole wheat bread	74
• White rice	73
• Bagel, white	69
• Brown rice	68
• Couscous	65
• Popcorn	65
• Bran flakes	63
• Oatmeal, cooked	55
• Spaghetti, white, boiled	49
• Spaghetti, whole meal, boiled	48
• Corn tortilla	46
• Oat bran bread; 50% oat bran	44
• Barley	28
MILK PRODUCTS	
• Ice cream	51
• Yogurt, fruit	41
• Whole milk	39
• Nonfat milk	37
• Soy milk	34
LEGUMES	
• Lentils	32
• Garbanzo beans	28
• Kidney beans	24
• Soy beans	16

FOOD ITEM	GLYCEMIC INDEX
VEGETABLES	
• Russet potato, baked	111
• Potato, instant mash	87
• Potato, boiled	78
• Pumpkin, boiled	64
• Potato, french fries	63
• Sweet potato, boiled	63
• Taro	53
• Sweet corn	52
• Green peas, boiled	51
• Carrots, boiled	39
FRUIT	
• Watermelon	76
• Pineapple	59
• Bananas	51
• Mangoes	51
• Orange juice	50
• Oranges	43
• Apple juice	41
• Apples	36
SNACK FOODS/BEVERAGES	
• Fruit punch	67
• Soft drink/soda	59
• Chocolate	56
• Potato chips	40
SUGARS	
• Sucrose	65
• Honey	61
• Fructose	15

[a]Reference food: glucose = 100

Source: F. S. Atkinson, K. Foster-Powell, and J. C. Brand-Miller, International tables of glycemic index and glycemic load values: 2008, *Diabetes Care* (2008): 2281–2283.

sweet potato is 60, a 100-gram serving containing about 20 grams of carbohydrates would have a GL of 12. The GL is used to standardize GI values to the carbohydrate content and portion size of a food or a meal.

What factors influence a food's glycemic effect?

Table NP3-1 shows that starchy foods such as bread and potatoes tend to have high GI values, whereas many fruits and legumes have low GI values. The main factors that influence the GI value of a food include the following:

- *Starch structure.* Starch is present in foods as either a straight chain or branched chain of glucose molecules. Whereas digestion of the branched form tends to release glucose quickly, the straight chain is resistant to digestion. Thus, foods that contain mainly the branched form of starch tend to raise blood glucose levels more quickly and have a high GI value. Due to the subtle differences in starch among foods, different species of the same foods can have substantially different GI values; for example, current GI values for rice range from low (38 for parboiled white rice) to high (85 for Japanese sushi-style white rice).[5]
- *Fiber content.* Certain types of dietary fibers (primarily soluble fibers) increase the viscosity of chyme, slowing the passage of food in the stomach and upper intestine and making it more difficult for enzymes to digest the food. Therefore, foods such as oats, barley, beans, fruit, and vegetables, which contain soluble fibers, tend to have lower GI values.[6]
- *Presence of fat and protein.* The fat in foods tends to slow stomach emptying, thus reducing the rate of digestion and absorption; hence, the presence of fat usually reduces a food's GI value.[7] The protein in foods can also influence the GI because protein promotes insulin secretion, increasing the rate at which glucose is taken up from the blood.[8]
- *Food processing.* The manner in which a food is processed and cooked influences the interactions among starch, protein, and fiber and thus affects the final GI value. For example, both pasta and bread are prepared from wheat flour, but pasta (cooked *al dente*) has a lower GI because the starch granules in pasta are surrounded by a sturdy protein barrier that hampers starch digestion (see Photo NP3-1). Cooking the pasta for longer periods can break down its structure and raise the GI value. As another example, the GI values for oatmeal vary according to the size and thickness of the oats used to prepare it: oatmeal prepared from steel-cut oats has a lower GI value than oatmeal prepared from quick oats. This is because the steel-cut oats are solid particles of grain, whereas "quick oats" are small, thin flakes.

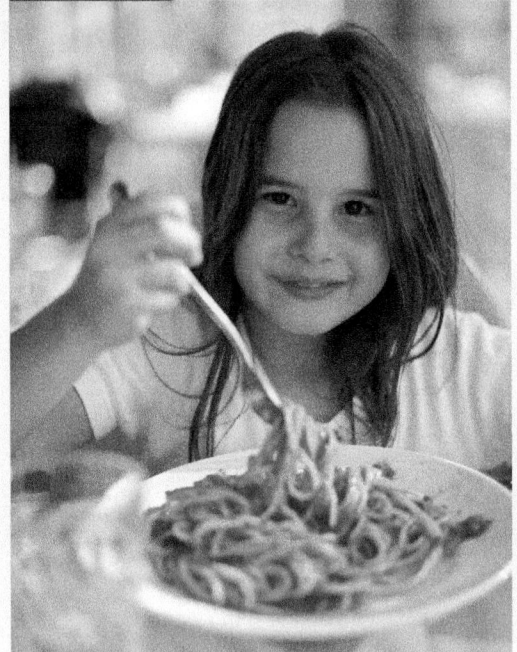

Photo NP3-1

Pasta cooked *al dente* has a lower glycemic index than many other starchy foods.

Noam Armonn/Shutterstock.com

- *Mixture of foods in a meal.* Because foods are rarely consumed in isolation, the GI value of an individual food may be less important than the combination of foods consumed at a meal. For example, in a cheese sandwich, the high GI of the bread is lowered by the addition of fat and protein in the cheese.
- *Individual glucose tolerance.* Cellular responses to insulin vary; thus, individual variability affects the glycemic response to foods. Factors such as genetics, physical activity, blood pressure, and sleep patterns as well as an individual's gastrointestinal microbiota influence blood glucose responses to food.[9]
- People with diabetes or prediabetes exhibit higher blood glucose levels after ingesting carbohydrate foods than do healthy individuals.[10]

What evidence suggests that a low-GI diet may influence chronic disease risk?

Some research shows that low-GI diets may reduce the risks of developing diabetes, heart disease, and obesity and help individuals lose weight.[11] Other studies, however, do not support such findings.[12] Studies are often difficult to interpret because low-GI foods often provide abundant soluble fiber, and some soluble fibers slow glucose absorption, sustain feelings of fullness, and improve blood lipids. Therefore, it could be that soluble fiber, and not the low-GI diet, is responsible for any reported effects. Because of mixed findings so far, health practitioners do not routinely recommend that patients consume low-GI diets to prevent or treat disease. An abundance of ongoing research to reveal specific relationships between low-GI diets and chronic disease risk, however, may change such thinking. Examples of research include the following:

- *Diabetes prevention.* Some researchers have proposed that a high glycemic load can increase the body's demand for insulin and eventually reduce pancreatic function, resulting in inadequate insulin secretion. Indeed, results of several studies suggest that low-GI diets might prevent or delay the onset of type 2 diabetes in those at risk or help with glycemic control in those who already have the disease.[13]
- *Heart disease risk.* Although some research suggests that low-GI diets may improve blood lipids, other research shows no consistent effects of low-GI diets on heart disease risk.[14]
- *Weight management.* Some research suggests low GI-diets may help with weight loss, but more research is needed to confirm these findings.[15]

Given the mixed results of research studies on chronic disease prevention, are there any benefits associated with consuming low-GI foods?

Yes, if the low-GI foods are nutrient-dense, high-fiber foods. Not all low-GI foods meet these criteria: note that cakes, cookies, and candy bars may have a low GI due to their high fat content. Thus, a food's GI should be considered along with other nutrient criteria when assessing the health benefits.

The GI can be a helpful tool for choosing the most healthful food from a food group. For example, low-GI breakfast cereals tend to be high in fiber and low in added sugars, whereas high-GI cereals tend to be those that contain refined flours and significant amounts of added sugars. In other words, low-GI foods are often wholesome foods that have been minimally processed.

In general, should people avoid consuming high-GI foods?

Some people assume that starchy foods such as breads and potatoes should be avoided due to their high GI values. As mentioned earlier, these foods are rarely consumed in isolation, and their GI values are reduced in a mixed meal. For example, breads often have a GI greater than 70, but adding cheese or peanut butter reduces the GI to 55 or 59, respectively. Also worth considering is that GI values often vary considerably. For example, published values for white potatoes range from 24 to 101, and many samples have values in the mid-50s.[16] For these reasons and others, more studies are needed to confirm whether the GI is practical or beneficial for healthy people.

Given the complexity of the GI, what are the current recommendations?

The potential benefits associated with consuming low-GI diets are still under investigation. As discussed earlier, people with type 2 diabetes may benefit from limiting high-GI foods—those that produce too great a rise, or too sudden a fall, in blood glucose. Additional research is needed to justify the use of diets based on the GI for preventing or treating diseases such as heart disease, obesity, or other medical problems.

At present, many nutrition scientists advocate consuming a plant-based diet that contains minimally processed grains, legumes, vegetables, and fruit. Such a diet would include abundant fiber and limited amounts of solid fats and added sugars. Undoubtedly, meals consisting of these foods would tend to have low or medium GI values.

Notes

1. A. B. Evert and coauthors, American Diabetes Association, Position statement: Nutrition therapy recommendations for the management of adults with diabetes, *Diabetes Care* 37 (2014): S120–S143.
2. American Diabetes Association, Standards of medical care in diabetes—2015, *Diabetes Care* 38 (2015): S1–S93; Evert and coauthors, American Diabetes Association, 2013.
3. J. Tay, C. H. Thompson, and G. D. Brinkworth, Glycemic variability: Assessing glycemia differently and implications for dietary management of diabetes, *Annual Review of Nutrition* 35 (2015): 389–424; Evert and coauthors, American Diabetes Association, 2013; O. Ajala, P. English, and J. Pinkney, Systematic review and meta-analysis of different dietary approaches to the management of type 2 diabetes, *American Journal of Clinical Nutrition* 97 (2013): 505–516.

4. C. E. L. Evans and coauthors, Glycemic index, glycemic load, and blood pressure: A systematic review and meta-analysis of randomized controlled trials, *American Journal of Clinical Nutrition* 105 (2017): 1176–1190; D. Yu and coauthors, Dietary glycemic index, glycemic load, and refined carbohydrates are associated with risk of stroke: A prospective cohort study in urban Chinese women, *American Journal of Clinical Nutrition* 104 (2016): 1345–1351; E. V. Pereira, J. A. Costa, and C. R. Alfensas, Effect of glycemic index on obesity control, *Archives of Endocrinology and Metabolism* 59 (2015): 245–251; F. M. Sacks and coauthors, Effects of high vs low glycemic index of dietary carbohydrate on cardiovascular disease risk factors and insulin sensitivity, The OMNICARB Randomized Clinical Trial, *Journal of the American Medical Association* 312 (2014): 2531–2541; A. S. Kristo, N. R. Matthan, and A. H. Lichtenstein, Effect of diets differing in glycemic

index and glycemic load on cardiovascular risk factors: Review of randomized controlled- feeding trials, *Nutrients* 5 (2013): 1071–1080; S. Sieri and coauthors, Dietary glycemic load and glycemic index and risk of cerebrovascular disease in the EPICOR Cohort, *PLoS One* 8 (2013): e62625; J. M. Jones, Glycemic index: The state of the science, part 3—Role in cardiovascular disease and blood lipids, *Nutrition Today* 48 (2013): 61–67; J. M. Jones, Glycemic index: The state of the science, part 4—Roles in inflammation, insulin resistance, and metabolic syndrome, *Nutrition Today* 48 (2013): 101–107.

5. F. S. Atkinson, K. Foster-Powell, and J. C. Brand-Miller, International tables of glycemic index and glycemic load values: 2008, *Diabetes Care* 31 (2008): 2281–2283.

6. J. W. McRorie, Evidence-based approach to fiber supplements and clinically meaningful health benefits, part 1, *Nutrition Today* 50 (2015): 82–89.

7. L. Sun and coauthors, Effect of chicken, fat, and vegetable on glycaemia and insulinaemia to a white rice-based meal in healthy adults, *European Journal of Nutrition* 53 (2014): 1719–1726.

8. R. George, A. L. Garcia, and C. A. Edwards, Glycaemic responses of staple South Asian foods alone and combined with curried chicken as a mixed meal, *Journal of Human Nutrition and Dietetics* 28 (2015): 283–291; Sun and coauthors, 2014.

9. N. R. Matthan and coauthors, Estimating the reliability of glycemic index values and potential sources of methodological and biological variability, *American Journal of Clinical Nutrition* 104 (2016): 1004–1013; D. Zeevi and coauthors, Personalized nutrition by prediction of glycemic responses, *Cell* 163 (2015): 1079–1094.

10. American Diabetes Association, Classification and diagnosis of diabetes, *Diabetes Care* 40 (2017): S10–S24.

11. Evans and coauthors, 2017; Yu and coauthors, 2016; Pereira, Costa, and Alfenas, 2015; A. E. Buyken and coauthors, Association between carbohydrate quality and inflammatory markers: Systematic review of observational and interventional studies, *American Journal of Clinical Nutrition* 99 (2014): 813–833; M. Juanola-Falgarona and coauthors, Effect of the glycemic index of the diet on weight loss, modulation of satiety, inflammation, and other metabolic risk factors: A randomized controlled trial, *American Journal of Clinical Nutrition* 100 (2014): 27–35; S. N. Bhupathiraju and coauthors, Glycemic index, glycemic load, and risk of type 2 diabetes: Results from 3 large US cohorts and updated meta-analysis, *American Journal of Clinical Nutrition* 100 (2014): 218–232; L. M. Goff and coauthors, Low glycaemic index diets and blood lipids: A systematic review and meta-analysis of randomized controlled trials, *Nutrition, Metabolism, and Cardiovascular Diseases* 23 (2013): 1–10; G. Livesey and coauthors, Is there a dose- response relation of dietary glycemic load to risk of type 2 diabetes?: Meta-analysis of prospective cohort studies, *American Journal of Clinical Nutrition* 97 (2013): 584–596.

12. Sacks and coauthors, 2014; A. Mirrahimi and coauthors, The role of Glycemic index and glycemic load in cardiovascular disease and its risk factors: A review of the recent literature, *Current Atherosclerosis Reports* 16 (2014): 381; Kristo, Matthan, and Lichtenstein, 2013; I. Sluijs and coauthors, Dietary glycemic index, glycemic load, and digestible carbohydrate intake are not associated with risk of type 2 diabetes in eight European countries, *Journal of Nutrition* 143 (2013): 93–99.

13. Bhupathiraju and coauthors, 2014; M. L. Wang and coauthors, Decrease in glycemic index associated with improved glycemic control among Latinos with type 2 diabetes, *Journal of the Academy of Nutrition and Dietetics*, 115 (2015): 898–906; Livesey and coauthors, 2013.

14. Sacks and coauthors, 2014; Kristo, Matthan, and Lichtenstein, 2013; Goff and coauthors, 2013.

15. Pereira, Costa, and Alfenas, 2015; Juanola-Falgarona and coauthors, 2014; J. M. Jones, Glycemic index: the state of the science, part 2—Roles in weight, weight loss, and satiety, *Nutrition Today* 48 (2013): 61–67.

16. Atkinson, Foster-Powell, and Brand-Miller, 2008.

Lipids

Chapter Sections and Learning Objectives (LOs)

Age fotostock/Superstock

chapter
4

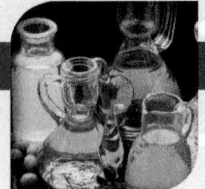

of fat, in the diet imposes health risks, but they may be surprised to learn that too little does, too. People in the United States, however, are more likely to eat too much fat than too little.

Fat is a member of the class of compounds called **lipids**. The lipids in foods and in the human body include triglycerides (**fats** and **oils**), phospholipids, and sterols.

4.1 Roles of Body Fat

lipids: a family of compounds that includes triglycerides (fats and oils), phospholipids, and sterols. Lipids are characterized by their insolubility in water.

fats: lipids that are solid at room temperature (70°F or 21°C).

oils: lipids that are liquid at room temperature (70°F or 21°C).

adipose tissue: the body's fat, which consists of masses of fat-storing cells called adipose cells.

Lipids perform many tasks in the body, but, most importantly, they provide energy. A constant flow of energy is so vital to life that, in a pinch, any other function is sacrificed to maintain it. Chapter 3 described one safeguard against such an emergency—the stores of glycogen in the liver that provide glucose to the blood whenever the supply runs short. The body's stores of glycogen are limited, however. In contrast, the body's capacity to store fat for energy is virtually unlimited due to the fat-storing cells of the **adipose tissue**. The fat cells of the adipose tissue readily take up and store fat, growing in size as they do so. Fat cells are more than just storage depots, however; fat cells secrete hormones that help to regulate the appetite and influence other body functions.[1] Figure 4-1 shows a fat cell.

The fat stored in fat cells supplies 60 percent of the body's ongoing energy needs during rest. The fat embedded in muscle tissue shares with muscle glycogen the task of providing energy when the muscles are active (see Photo 4-1). During some types

---

FIGURE 4-1 A Fat Cell

Within the fat, or adipose, cell, lipid is stored in a droplet. This droplet can greatly enlarge, and the fat cell membrane will expand to accommodate its swollen contents.

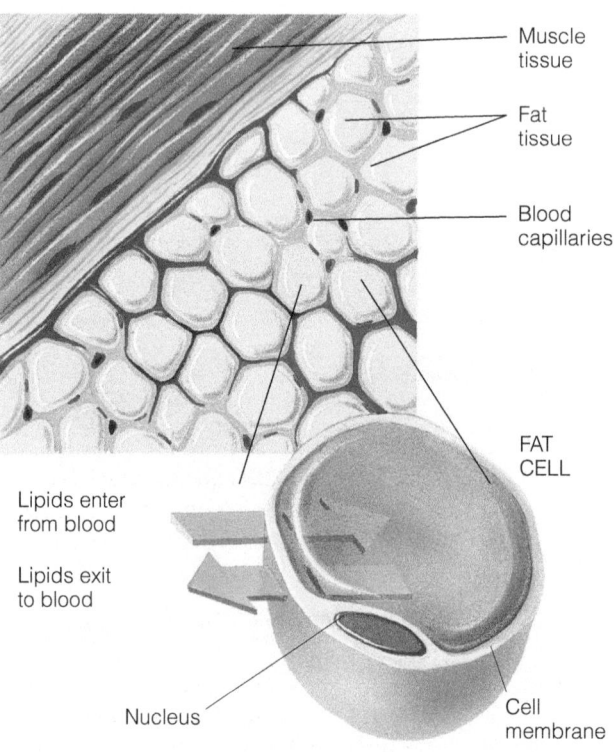

Muscle tissue

Fat tissue

Blood capillaries

FAT CELL

Lipids enter from blood

Lipids exit to blood

Nucleus

Cell membrane

TABLE 4-1	The Functions of Fats in the Body

- *Energy stores.* Fats are the body's chief form of stored energy.

- *Muscle fuel.* Fats provide much of the energy to fuel muscular work.

- *Padding.* Fat pads inside the body cavity protect the internal organs from shock.

- *Insulation.* Fats insulate against temperature extremes by forming a fat layer under the skin.

- *Cell membranes.* Fats form the major material of cell membranes.

- *Raw materials.* Fats are converted to other compounds, such as hormones, bile, and vitamin D, as needed.

Photo 4-1

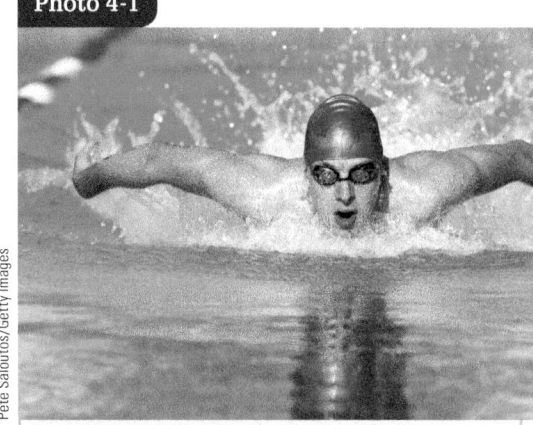

Pete Saloutos/Getty Images

Body fat supplies much of the fuel that muscles need to do their work.

of physical activity or prolonged periods of food deprivation, fat stores may make an even greater energy contribution. The brain and nerves, however, need their energy as glucose, and, as explained in Chapter 6, fat is an inefficient source of glucose. After a long period of glucose deprivation (during fasting or starvation), brain and nerve cells develop the ability to derive about half of their energy from a special form of fat known as **ketones**, but they still require glucose as well. This means that people wanting to lose weight need to eat a certain minimum amount of carbohydrate to meet their energy needs, even when they are limiting their food intakes.

In addition to supplying energy, fat serves other roles in the body. Natural oils in the skin provide a radiant complexion; in the scalp, they help nourish the hair and make it glossy. The layer of fat beneath the skin insulates the body from extremes of temperature. A pad of hard fat beneath each kidney protects it from being jarred and damaged, even during a motorcycle ride on a bumpy road. The soft fat in a woman's breasts protects her mammary glands from heat and cold and cushions them against shock. The phospholipids and the sterol cholesterol are cell membrane constituents that help maintain the structure and health of all cells. Table 4-1 summarizes the major functions of fats in the body.

ketones (KEY-tones): acidic, water-soluble compounds produced by the liver during the breakdown of fat when carbohydrate is not available; technically known as *ketone bodies.*

Review Notes

- Lipids in the body not only serve as energy reserves but also protect the body from temperature extremes, cushion the vital organs, and provide the major material of cell membranes.

4.2 The Chemist's View of Lipids

The diverse and vital functions that lipids perform in the body reveal why eating too little fat can be harmful. As mentioned earlier, though, too much fat in the diet seems to be the greater problem for most people. To understand both the beneficial and harmful effects that fats exert on the body, a closer look at the structure and function of members of the lipid family is in order.

Triglycerides

When people talk about fat—for example, "I'm too fat" or "That meat is fatty"—they are usually referring to triglycerides. Among lipids, **triglycerides** predominate—both in the diet and in the body. The name *triglyceride* almost explains itself: three (*tri*)

triglycerides (try-GLISS-er-rides): one of the main classes of lipids; the chief form of fat in foods and the major storage form of fat in the body; composed of glycerol with three fatty acids attached.

tri = three
glyceride = a compound of glycerol

FIGURE 4-2 Triglyceride Formation

Glycerol, a small, water-soluble compound, plus three fatty acids, equals a triglyceride.

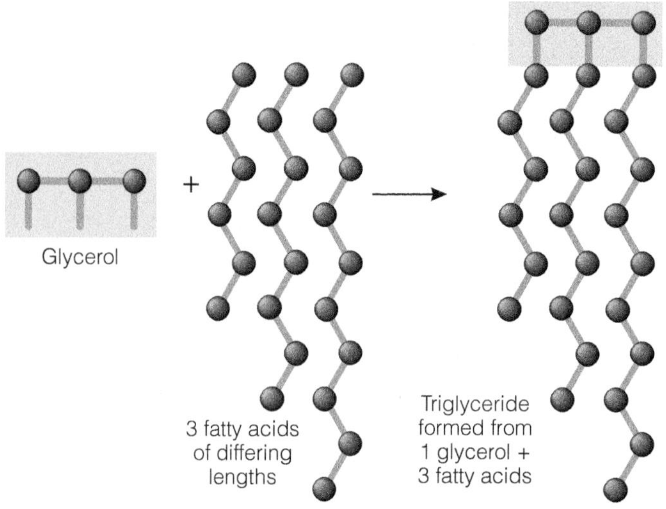

Glycerol

+

3 fatty acids of differing lengths

Triglyceride formed from 1 glycerol + 3 fatty acids

fatty acids: organic compounds
composed of a chain of carbon atoms
with hydrogen atoms attached and an
acid group at one end.

glycerol (GLISS-er-ol): an organic
compound, three carbons long,
that can form the backbone of
triglycerides and phospholipids.

saturated fatty acid: a fatty acid
carrying the maximum possible
number of hydrogen atoms (having no
points of unsaturation).

unsaturated fatty acid: a
fatty acid with one or more
points of unsaturation where
hydrogen atoms are missing
(includes monounsaturated and
polyunsaturated fatty acids).

monounsaturated fatty acid
(MUFA): a fatty acid that has one
point of unsaturation; for example,
the oleic acid found in olive oil.

polyunsaturated fatty acid (PUFA):
fatty acids with two or more points
of unsaturation. For example,
linoleic acid has two such points,
and linolenic acid has three. Thus,
polyunsaturated *fat* is composed
of triglycerides containing a high
percentage of PUFA.

fatty acids attached to a **glycerol** "backbone." Figure 4-2 shows how three fatty acids combine with glycerol to make a triglyceride.

Fatty Acids

When energy from any energy-yielding nutrient is to be stored as fat, the nutrient is first broken into small fragments. Then the fragments are linked together into chains known as fatty acids. The fatty acids are then packaged, three at a time, with glycerol to make triglycerides.

Chain Length and Saturation Fatty acids may differ from one another in two ways—in chain length and in degree of saturation. The chain length refers to the number of carbons in a fatty acid. Saturation also refers to its chemical structure—specifically, to the number of hydrogen atoms the carbons in the fatty acid are holding. If every available carbon is filled to capacity with hydrogen atoms, the chain is called a **saturated fatty acid**. A saturated fatty acid is fully loaded with hydrogen atoms and has only single bonds between the carbons. The first zigzag structure in Figure 4-3 represents a saturated fatty acid.

Unsaturated Fatty Acids In some fatty acids, including most of those in plants and fish, hydrogen atoms are missing from the fatty acid chains. The places where the hydrogen atoms are missing are called points of unsaturation, and a chain containing such points is called an **unsaturated fatty acid**. An unsaturated fatty acid has at least one double bond between its carbons. If there is one point of unsaturation, the chain is a **monounsaturated fatty acid**. The second structure in Figure 4-3 is an example. If there are two or more points of unsaturation, then the fatty acid is a **polyunsaturated fatty acid** (see the third structure in Figure 4-3).

Hard and Soft Fat A triglyceride can contain any combination of fatty acids—long chain or short chain and saturated, monounsaturated, or polyunsaturated. The degree of saturation of the fatty acids in a fat influences the health of the body (discussed in a later section) and the characteristics of foods. Fats that contain the shorter-chain or the more unsaturated fatty acids are softer at room temperature and melt more readily. A comparison of three fats—lard (which comes from pork), chicken fat, and safflower oil—illustrates these differences: lard is the most saturated and the hardest; chicken fat is less saturated and somewhat soft; and safflower oil, which is the most unsaturated, is a liquid at room temperature.

FIGURE 4-3 Three Types of Fatty Acids

The more carbon atoms in a fatty acid, the longer it is. The more hydrogen atoms attached to those carbons, the more saturated the fatty acid is.

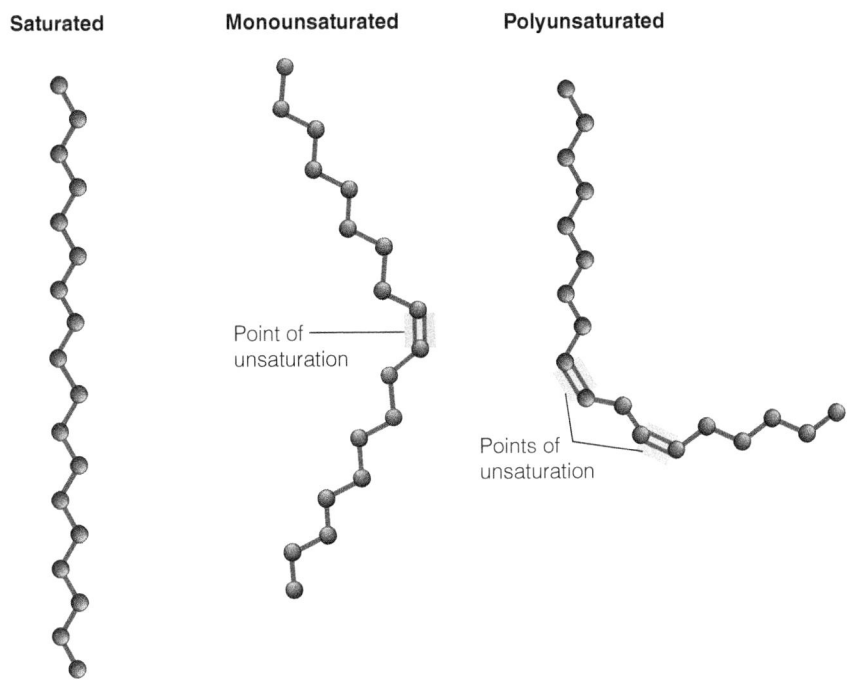

Saturated   **Monounsaturated**   **Polyunsaturated**

Point of unsaturation

Points of unsaturation

Stability Saturation also influences stability. Fats can become **rancid** when exposed to oxygen. Polyunsaturated fatty acids spoil most readily because their double bonds are unstable. The **oxidation** of unsaturated fats produces a variety of compounds that smell and taste rancid; saturated fats are more resistant to oxidation and thus less likely to become rancid. Other types of spoilage can occur due to microbial growth, however.

Manufacturers can protect fat-containing products against rancidity in three ways—none of them perfect. First, products may be sealed airtight and refrigerated—an expensive and inconvenient storage system. Second, manufacturers may add **antioxidants** to compete for the oxygen and thus protect the oil (examples are the additives **BHA** and **BHT** and vitamins C and E).* Third, manufacturers may saturate some or all of the points of unsaturation by adding hydrogen atoms—a process known as *hydrogenation*.

Hydrogenation **Hydrogenation** offers two advantages: it protects against oxidation (thereby prolonging shelf-life) and also alters the texture of foods by increasing the solidity of fats. When partially hydrogenated, vegetable oils become spreadable margarine. Hydrogenated fats make piecrusts flaky and puddings creamy. A disadvantage is that hydrogenation makes polyunsaturated fats more saturated. Consequently, any health advantages of using polyunsaturated fats instead of saturated fats are lost with hydrogenation.

Trans-**Fatty Acids** Another disadvantage of hydrogenation is that some of the molecules that remain unsaturated after processing change shape from *cis* to *trans*. In nature, most unsaturated fatty acids are *cis*-fatty acids—meaning that the hydrogen atoms next to the double bonds are on the same side of the carbon chain. Only a few fatty acids in nature (notably a small percentage of those found in milk and meat products) are

rancid: the term used to describe fats when they have deteriorated, usually by oxidation. Rancid fats often have an "off" odor.

oxidation (OKS-ee-day-shun): the process of a substance combining with oxygen.

antioxidants: as a food additive, preservatives that delay or prevent rancidity of foods and other damage to food caused by oxygen.

BHA, BHT: preservatives commonly used to slow the development of "off" flavors, odors, and color changes caused by oxidation.

hydrogenation (high-dro-gen-AY-shun): a chemical process by which hydrogen atoms are added to monounsaturated or polyunsaturated fats to reduce the number of double bonds, making the fats more saturated (solid) and more resistant to oxidation (protecting against rancidity). Hydrogenation produces *trans*-fatty acids.

---

*BHA is butylated hydroxyanisole; BHT is butylated hydroxytoluene.

FIGURE 4-4 *Cis*- and *Trans*-Fatty Acids Compared

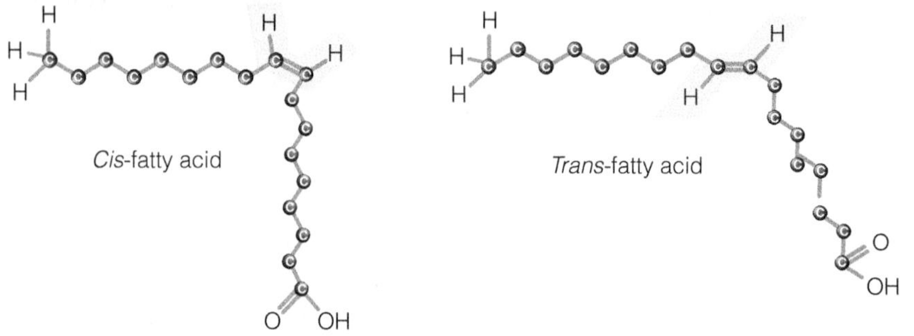

Cis-fatty acid

Trans-fatty acid

trans-fatty acids—meaning that the hydrogen atoms next to the double bonds are on opposite sides of the carbon chain (see Figure 4-4). These arrangements result in different configurations for the fatty acids, and this difference affects function: in the body, *trans*-fatty acids behave more like saturated fats, increasing blood cholesterol and the risk of heart disease (as a later section describes).[2]

Researchers are trying to determine whether the health effects of naturally occurring *trans* fats differ from those of commercially created *trans* fats.[3] In any case, the important distinction is that intake of naturally occurring *trans*-fatty acids is typically low. At current levels of consumption, naturally occurring *trans* fats are unlikely to have adverse effects on blood lipids. The naturally occurring *trans*-fatty acid **conjugated linoleic acid** may even have health benefits.[4]

Essential Fatty Acids Using carbohydrate, fat, or protein, the human body can synthesize all the fatty acids it needs except for two—**linoleic acid** and **linolenic acid**. Both linoleic acid and linolenic acid are polyunsaturated fatty acids. Because they cannot be made from other substances in the body, they must be obtained from food and are therefore called **essential fatty acids**. Linoleic acid and linolenic acid are found in small amounts in plant oils, and the body readily stores them, making deficiencies unlikely. From both of these essential fatty acids, the body makes important substances that help regulate a wide range of body functions: blood pressure, clot formation, blood lipid concentration, the immune response, the inflammatory response to injury, and many others.[5] These two essential nutrients also serve as structural components of cell membranes.

Linoleic Acid: An Omega-6 Fatty Acid Linoleic acid is an **omega-6 fatty acid**, found in the seeds of plants and in the oils produced from the seeds. Any diet that contains vegetable oils, seeds, nuts, and whole-grain foods provides enough linoleic acid to meet the body's needs. Researchers have long known and appreciated the importance of the omega-6 fatty acid family.

Linolenic Acid and Other Omega-3 Fatty Acids Linolenic acid belongs to a family of polyunsaturated fatty acids known as **omega-3 fatty acids**, a family that also includes **EPA** and **DHA**. EPA and DHA are found primarily in fish oils. As mentioned, the human body cannot make linolenic acid, but given dietary linolenic acid, it can make EPA and DHA, although the process is slow.

The importance of omega-3 fatty acids has been recognized since the 1980s, and research continues to unveil impressive roles for EPA and DHA in metabolism and disease prevention. The brain has a high content of DHA, and both EPA and DHA are needed for normal brain development.[6] DHA is also especially active in the rods and cones of the retina of the eye. Today, researchers know that these omega-3 fatty acids are essential for normal growth and development and that they may play an important role in the prevention and treatment of heart disease.[7]

Phospholipids

Up to now, this discussion has focused on one class of lipids, the triglycerides (fats and oils), and their component parts, the fatty acids (see Table 4-2). Two other classes of lipids, the **phospholipids** and sterols, make up only 5 percent of the lipids in the diet, but they are nevertheless worthy of attention. Among the phospholipids, the lecithins are of particular interest.

Structure of Phospholipids Like the triglycerides, the **lecithins** and other phospholipids have a backbone of glycerol; they differ from the triglycerides in having only two fatty acids attached to the glycerol. In place of the third fatty acid, they have a phosphate group (a phosphorus-containing acid) and a molecule of **choline** or a similar compound. The fatty acids make the phospholipids soluble in fat; the phosphate group enables them to dissolve in water. Such versatility benefits the food industry, which uses phospholipids as **emulsifiers** to mix fats with water in such products as mayonnaise and candy bars.

Phospholipids in Foods In addition to the phospholipids used by the food industry as emulsifiers, phospholipids are also found naturally in foods. The richest food sources of lecithin are eggs, liver, soybeans, wheat germ, and peanuts.

Roles of Phospholipids Lecithins and other phospholipids are important constituents of cell membranes. They also act as emulsifiers in the body, helping to keep other fats in solution in the watery blood and body fluids. In addition, some phospholipids generate signals inside the cells in response to hormones, such as insulin, to help alter body conditions.

Sterols

Sterols are large, complex molecules consisting of interconnected rings of carbon. Cholesterol is the most familiar sterol, but others, such as vitamin D and the sex hormones (for example, testosterone), are important, too.

Sterols in Foods Foods derived from both plants and animals contain sterols, but only those from animals—meats, eggs, fish, poultry, and dairy products—contain significant amounts of cholesterol. Organ meats, such as liver and kidneys, and eggs, are richest in cholesterol; cheeses and meats have less. Shellfish contain many sterols but much less cholesterol than was previously thought.

Sterols other than cholesterol are naturally found in plants. Being structurally similar to cholesterol, plant sterols interfere with cholesterol absorption. Food manufacturers have fortified foods such as margarine with plant sterols, creating a functional food that helps to reduce blood cholesterol.

Cholesterol Synthesis Like the lecithins, cholesterol can be made by the body, so it is not an essential nutrient. Right now, as you read, your liver is manufacturing cholesterol from fragments of carbohydrate, protein, and fat. Most of the body's cholesterol ends up in the membranes of cells, where it performs vital structural and metabolic functions.

Cholesterol's Two Routes in the Body After it is made, cholesterol leaves the liver by two routes:

1. It may be incorporated into bile, stored in the gallbladder, and delivered to the intestine.
2. It may travel, via the bloodstream, to all the body's cells.

The bile that is made from cholesterol in the liver is released into the intestine to aid in the digestion and absorption of fat. After bile does its job, most of it is absorbed and reused by the body; the rest is excreted in the feces.

TABLE 4-2 The Lipid Family

Triglycerides (fats and oils)

- Glycerol (1 per triglyceride)
- Fatty acids (3 per triglyceride)
  Saturated
  Monounsaturated
  Polyunsaturated
    Omega-6
    Omega-3

Phospholipids (such as the lecithins)

Sterols (such as cholesterol)

phospholipids: one of the three main classes of lipids; compounds that are similar to triglycerides but have *choline* (or another compound) and a phosphorus-containing acid in place of one of the fatty acids.

lecithins: one type of phospholipid.

choline: a nutrient that can be made in the body from an amino acid.

emulsifiers: substances that mix with both fat and water and that disperse the fat in the water, forming an emulsion.

sterols: one of the main classes of lipids; includes cholesterol, vitamin D, and the sex hormones (such as testosterone).

Cholesterol Excreted While bile is in the intestine, some of it may be trapped by soluble fibers or by some medications, which carry it out of the body in feces. The excretion of bile reduces the total amount of cholesterol remaining in the body.

Cholesterol Transport As Chapter 2 describes, some cholesterol, packaged with other lipids and protein, leaves the liver via the arteries and is transported to the body tissues by the blood. These packages of lipids and proteins are called **lipoproteins**. As the lipoproteins travel through the body, tissues can extract lipids from them. Cholesterol can be harmful to the body when it forms deposits in the artery walls. These deposits contribute to **atherosclerosis**, a disease that can cause heart attacks and strokes.

Review Notes

- Table 4-2 summarizes the members of the lipid family.
- The predominant lipids both in foods and in the body are triglycerides, which have glycerol backbones with three fatty acids attached.
- Fatty acids vary in the length of their carbon chains and their degree of saturation. Those that are fully loaded with hydrogen atoms are saturated; those that are missing hydrogen atoms and therefore have double bonds are unsaturated (monounsaturated or polyunsaturated).
- Most triglycerides contain more than one type of fatty acid.
- Fatty acid saturation affects the physical characteristics and storage properties of fats.
- Hydrogenation, which makes polyunsaturated fats more saturated, gives rise to *trans*-fatty acids, altered fatty acids that may have health effects similar to those of saturated fatty acids.
- Linoleic acid and linolenic acid are essential nutrients. In addition to serving as structural parts of cell membranes, they make powerful substances that help regulate blood pressure, blood clot formation, and the immune response.
- Phospholipids, including the lecithins, have a unique chemical structure that allows them to be soluble in both water and fat.
- In the body, phospholipids are major constituents of cell membranes; the food industry uses phospholipids as emulsifiers.
- Sterols include cholesterol, bile, vitamin D, and the sex hormones.
- Only animal-derived foods contain significant amounts of cholesterol.

4.3 Digestion and Absorption of Lipids

The goal of fat digestion is to dismantle triglycerides into small molecules that the body can absorb and use—namely **monoglycerides**, fatty acids, and glycerol. Table 4-3 provides the details.

4.4 Health Effects and Recommended Intakes of Fats

Some fats in the diet are essential for good health, but others can be harmful.[8] For this reason, recommendations focus both on the *quantity* and the *quality* of the fat in the diet.[9] The person who chooses a diet too high in saturated fats or *trans* fats invites the risk of **cardiovascular disease (CVD)**, and heart disease is the number one killer of adults in the United States and Canada. As for cancer, evidence is less compelling than

| TABLE 4-3 | Fat Digestion and Absorption |

MOUTH AND SALIVARY GLANDS

Some hard fats begin to melt as they reach body temperature. The sublingual salivary gland in the base of the tongue secretes lingual lipase. The degree of hydrolysis by lingual lipase is slight for most fats but may be appreciable for milk fats.

STOMACH

The stomach's churning action mixes fat with water and acid. A gastric lipase accesses and hydrolyzes (only a very small amount of) fat.

SMALL INTESTINE AND PANCREAS

Cholecystokinin (CCK) signals the gallbladder to release bile (via the common bile duct):

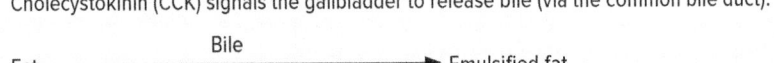

Fat ——— Bile ———▶ Emulsified fat

Pancreatic lipase flows in from the pancreas (via the pancreatic duct):

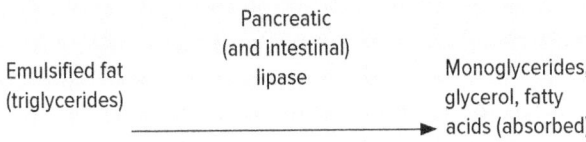

Emulsified fat (triglycerides) ——— Pancreatic (and intestinal) lipase ———▶ Monoglycerides, glycerol, fatty acids (absorbed)

LARGE INTESTINE

Some fat and cholesterol, trapped in fiber, exit in feces.

for heart disease, but it does suggest that a diet high in certain kinds of fat is associated with a greater-than-average risk of developing some types of cancer.[10] Conversely, some research suggests that omega-3 fatty acids from fish may protect against some cancers.[11] Nutrition and cancer is a topic of Chapter 23.

The links between diet and disease are the focus of much research. Some points about fats and heart health are presented here because they underlie dietary recommendations concerning fats. Nutrition and heart disease is the topic of Chapter 21.

Fats and Heart Health

As noted earlier, cholesterol travels in the blood within lipoproteins. Two of the lipoproteins, LDL and HDL, play major roles with regard to heart health and are the focus of most recommendations made for reducing the risk of heart disease. A high blood LDL cholesterol concentration is a predictor of the likelihood of suffering a fatal heart attack or stroke, and the higher the LDL, the earlier the episode is expected to occur. A *low* blood concentration of HDL cholesterol also signifies a higher disease risk.[12]

Most people realize that elevated blood cholesterol is an important risk factor for heart disease. Most people may not realize, though, that cholesterol in *food* is not a major influential factor in raising *blood* cholesterol.

Saturated Fats and Blood Cholesterol The main dietary factors associated with elevated blood LDL cholesterol are high saturated fat and high *trans* fat intakes.*[13] High LDL cholesterol levels increase the risk of heart disease because high LDL concentrations promote the uptake of cholesterol in the blood vessel walls. Nutrition in Practice 4 examines various types of fats and their roles in supporting or harming heart health.

---

*It should be noted that not all saturated fatty acids have the same cholesterol-raising effect. Stearic acid, an 18-carbon fatty acid, does not seem to raise blood cholesterol.

solid fats: fats that are not usually liquid at room temperature; commonly found in most foods derived from animals and vegetable oils that have been hydrogenated. Solid fats typically contain more saturated and *trans* fats than most oils. Also defined in Chapter 1.

Solid fats, introduced in Chapter 1, are foods or ingredients in foods (such as shortening in cakes or pies) that provide abundant saturated fat and *trans* fat, as well as many kcalories. The current American diet delivers excessive amounts of solid fats. The easiest way to lower saturated fat, then, is to limit solid fats in the diet. Grain-based desserts, pizza, cheese, and processed and fatty meats are major providers of solid fats. Solid fats from animal sources contribute a great deal of the saturated fat in most people's diets. Some vegetable fats (coconut oil, palm kernel oil, and palm oil) and hydrogenated fats such as shortening or stick margarine provide smaller amounts of saturated fats.

Importantly, replacing dietary saturated fats with added sugars and refined starches is counterproductive.[14] The best dietary pattern for health not only replaces saturated fats with polyunsaturated and monounsaturated oils (as discussed in a later section), but also is adequate, balanced, kcalorie controlled, and based on mostly nutrient-dense whole foods. Table 4-4 summarizes which foods provide which fats.

Trans-Fatty Acids and Blood Cholesterol Consuming commercially derived *trans* fat poses a risk to the health of the heart and arteries by raising LDL and lowering HDL cholesterol, and by producing inflammation.[15] Commercially derived *trans* fats are found in the partially hydrogenated oils used in some margarines, snack foods, and prepared desserts. The risk to heart health from *trans* fats is similar to or slightly greater than that from saturated fat, so the American Heart Association (AHA) advises people to keep *trans* fat intake as low as possible.[16] Limiting the intake of *trans* fats can improve blood cholesterol and lower the risk of heart disease. To that end, many restaurants and food manufacturers have taken steps to eliminate or greatly reduce *trans* fats in foods.[17]

For example, margarine makers have reformulated their products to contain much less *trans* fat. Soft or liquid varieties are made from unhydrogenated oils, which are mostly unsaturated and so are less likely to elevate blood cholesterol than the saturated

TABLE 4-4 Major Sources of Various Lipids

HEALTHFUL FATTY ACIDS

MONOUNSATURATED	OMEGA-6 POLYUNSATURATED	OMEGA-3 POLYUNSATURATED
• Avocado • Oils (canola, olive, peanut, sesame) • Nuts (almonds, cashews, filberts, hazelnuts, macadamia nuts, peanuts, pecans, pistachios) • Olives • Peanut butter • Seeds (sesame)	• Margarine (nonhydrogenated) • Oils (corn, cottonseed, safflower, soybean) • Nuts (pine nuts, walnuts) • Mayonnaise • Salad dressing • Seeds (pumpkin, sunflower)	• Fatty fish (herring, mackerel, salmon, tuna) • Flaxseed, chia seed • Marine algae • Nuts (walnuts) • Oils (canola, flaxseed, soybean, walnut) • Yeast

HARMFUL FATTY ACIDS

SATURATED *TRANS*	*TRANS*
• Bacon, butter, lard • Cheese, whole milk products • Chocolate, coconut • Cream, half-and-half, cream cheese, sour cream • Meats • Oil (coconut, palm, palm kernel) • Shortening	• Fried foods (hydrogenated shortening) • Margarine (hydrogenated or partially hydrogenated) • Nondairy creamers • Many fast foods • Shortening • Commercial baked goods (including doughnuts, cakes, cookies) • Many snack foods (including microwave popcorn, chips, crackers)

fats of butter. Some margarines contain olive oil, omega-3 fatty acids, or plant sterols (mentioned earlier), making these products preferable to butter and other margarines for the heart.* The words *hydrogenated vegetable oil* or *shortening* in an ingredients list indicate *trans*-fatty acids in the product.

In the past, most commercially fried foods, from doughnuts to chicken, delivered a sizeable amount of *trans* fats to consumers. Today, newly formulated commercial oils and fats perform the same tasks as the previously used hydrogenated fats but with fewer *trans*-fatty acids. Some manufacturers, however, merely substitute saturated fats— which pose well-established risks to heart health—for *trans* fats. When reformulating their products, food companies must consider not only the fat composition, but also the taste, texture, cost, and availability of materials. No health benefits can be expected when saturated fats replace *trans* fats in the diet.

Dietary Cholesterol and Blood Cholesterol Unlike saturated fat and *trans* fat, dietary cholesterol seems to have little or no effect on the blood cholesterol levels of most people.[18] Older recommendations limited dietary cholesterol to less than 300 milligrams per day for healthy people (less than 200 milligrams for some people with or at high risk of heart disease). However, the AHA concludes there is insufficient evidence to determine whether lowering dietary cholesterol reduces blood levels of LDL cholesterol.[19] On average, women take in about 240 milligrams a day and men take in about 350 milligrams. Foods providing the greatest share of cholesterol to the U.S. diet are eggs and egg dishes, chicken and chicken dishes, beef and beef dishes, and all types of beef burgers.

In healthy people, evidence suggests no association between consuming one egg per day and increased risk of heart disease.[20] The cholesterol content of one egg is about 210 milligrams.

Monounsaturated Fatty Acids and Blood Cholesterol Replacing saturated and *trans* fats with monounsaturated fat such as olive oil may be an effective dietary strategy to prevent heart disease. The lower rates of heart disease among people in the Mediterranean region of the world are often attributed to their liberal use of olive oil, a rich source of monounsaturated fatty acids.[21] Olive oil also delivers valuable phytochemicals that help to protect against heart disease.[22] Nutrition in Practice 4 examines the role of olive oil and other fats in supporting or harming heart health.

Polyunsaturated Fatty Acids, Blood Cholesterol, and Heart Disease Risk Polyunsaturated fatty acids (PUFA) of the omega-3 families are potent protectors against heart disease. The omega-3 fatty acids EPA and DHA, which are found mainly in fatty fish, exert their beneficial effects by influencing the function of both the heart and blood vessels. Specifically, EPA and DHA protect heart health by:[23]

- Lowering blood triglycerides.
- Preventing blood clots.
- Protecting against irregular heartbeats.
- Lowering blood pressure.
- Defending against inflammation.

The primary member of the omega-3 family, linolenic acid, may benefit heart health as well, but evidence for this effect is much less certain than for EPA and DHA. Table 4-4 names sources of omega-6 and omega-3 fatty acids, and Table 4-5 (p. 106) lists fish and seafood by their quantity of omega-3 fatty acids.

The AHA recommends including at least two 3.5-ounce servings of fish each week in a heart-healthy eating pattern. Greater heart health benefits can be expected when fish is grilled, baked (see Photo 4-2), or broiled, partly because the varieties prepared this way often contain more EPA and DHA than species used for fried fish in fast-food restaurants and frozen products. Additionally, benefits are attained by avoiding

---

*Two brand names of margarines with plant sterols currently on the market are *Benecol* and *Promise activ.*

TABLE 4-5	Omega-3 Fatty Acids in Fish and Seafood (3.5-oz Serving)
500 mg	European sea bass (bronzini), herring (Atlantic and Pacific), mackerel, oysters (Pacific wild), salmon (wild and farmed), sardines, toothfish (includes Chilean sea bass), trout (wild and farmed)
150–500 mg	Black bass, catfish (wild and farmed), clams, cod (Atlantic), crab (Alaskan king), croakers, flounder, haddock, hake, halibut, oysters (eastern and farmed), perch, scallops, shrimp (mixed varieties), sole, swordfish, tilapia (farmed)
<150 mg	Cod (Pacific), grouper, lobster, mahimahi, monkfish, red snapper, skate, triggerfish, tuna, wahoo

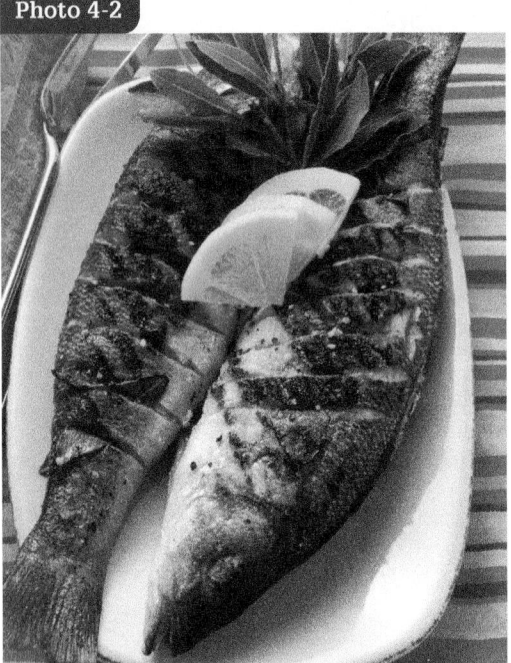

Photo 4-2

Stockfood

Grilling or broiling fish, instead of frying it, preserves its beneficial omega-3 fatty acids while adding little or no saturated fat.

commercial frying fats, which may be laden with *trans* fat and saturated fat. Further benefits arise when fish replaces high-fat meats or other foods rich in saturated fats in several meals each week.

Some species of fish and shellfish, however, may contain significant levels of mercury or other environmental contaminants. Most healthy people can safely consume most species of ocean fish several times a week, but for some, the risks are greater. Women who may become pregnant, pregnant and lactating women, and children are more sensitive to contaminants than others, but even they can benefit from consuming safer fish varieties within recommended limits (see Chapter 10 for details).

For everyone, consuming a variety of different types of fish to minimize exposure to any single toxin that may accumulate in a favored species is a good idea. The fish most heavily contaminated with mercury are king mackerel, shark, swordfish, and tilefish (also called golden bass or golden snapper). Those lower in mercury are catfish, pollock, salmon, sardines, and canned light tuna. Canned albacore ("white") tuna generally contains more mercury than light tuna. Consumers should check local advisories to determine the safety of freshwater fish caught by family and friends.

Omega-3 Supplements Fish, not fish oil supplements, is the preferred source of omega-3 fatty acids. High intakes of omega-3 polyunsaturated fatty acids may increase bleeding time, interfere with wound healing, raise LDL cholesterol, and suppress immune function.[24] People with heart disease, however, may benefit from doses greater than can be achieved through diet alone. This paradox reminds us that dietary advice to lower the risk of heart disease may differ from dietary advice to treat patients with heart disease.[25] Because supplements pose risks, such as excessive bleeding, those taking daily fish oil supplements need medical supervision. The benefits and risks from EPA and DHA illustrate an important concept in nutrition: too much of a nutrient is often as harmful as too little.

Recommendations

Some fat in the diet is essential for good health. The Dietary Guidelines for Americans recommend that a portion of each day's total fat intake come from a few teaspoons of raw oil, such as that found in nuts, avocados, and seafood. In addition, many commonly used oils such as olive, peanut, safflower, soybean, and sunflower oils are extracted from plants. When choosing oils, alternate among the various types to obtain the benefits different oils offer. Peanut and safflower oils are especially rich in vitamin E. Olive oil contributes naturally occurring antioxidant phytochemicals with potential heart benefits (see Nutrition in Practice 4), and canola oil is rich in monounsaturated and essential fatty acids. An adequate intake of the needed fat-soluble nutrients can be ensured by a small daily intake of oil: 27 grams (6 tsp) for a 2000-kcalorie diet, for example (see Table 1-6 (p. 21) for recommendations for other kcalorie levels).

Defining the exact amount of fat, saturated fat, or cholesterol that benefits health or begins to harm health, however, is not possible. For this reason, no RDA or UL has been set. Instead, the DRI suggests a diet that is low in saturated fat and *trans* fat and provides 20 to 35 percent of the daily energy intake from fat. These recommendations recognize that diets with up to 35 percent of kcalories from fat can be compatible with good health if energy intake is reasonable and saturated and *trans* fat intakes are low. When total fat intake exceeds 35 percent of kcalories, saturated fat intakes increase to unhealthy levels. For a 2000-kcalorie diet, 20 to 35 percent represents 400 to 700 kcalories from fat (roughly 45 to 75 grams). Fat and oil intakes below 20 percent of kcalories increase the risk of inadequate essential fatty acid intakes. The FDA established Daily Values for food labels using 35 percent of energy intake as the guideline for fat.

Part of the allowance for total fat provides for the essential fatty acids—linoleic acid and linolenic acid—and Adequate Intakes (AI) have been established for these two fatty acids (see the inside front cover). The DRI suggest that linoleic acid provide 5 to 10 percent of the daily energy intake and linolenic acid, 0.6 to 1.2 percent.

Recommendations urge people to eat diets that are low in saturated fat and *trans* fat. Specifically, consume less than 10 percent of total kcalories from saturated fat, and keep *trans* fat intakes as low as possible.[26] To help consumers meet these goals, the FDA established Daily Values for food labels using 10 percent of energy intake for saturated fat; the Daily Value for cholesterol is 300 milligrams, regardless of energy intake. There is no Daily Value for *trans* fat.

Review Notes

- High intakes of saturated or *trans* fats contribute to heart disease, obesity, and other health problems.
- High blood cholesterol, specifically, poses a risk of heart disease, and high intakes of saturated fat and *trans* fat contribute most to high blood cholesterol. Cholesterol in foods presents little or no risk.
- When monounsaturated fat such as olive oil replaces saturated and *trans* fats in the diet, the risk of heart disease may be lessened.
- Polyunsaturated fatty acids of the omega-6 and omega-3 families protect against heart disease.
- Though some fat in the diet is necessary, health authorities recommend a diet moderate in total fat and low in saturated fat and *trans* fat.

4.5 Fats in Foods

Fats are important in foods as well as in the body. Many of the compounds that give foods their flavors and aromas are found in fats and oils. The delicious aromas associated with sizzling bacon, onions being sautéed, and vegetables in a stir-fry come from fats. Fats also influence the texture of many foods, enhancing smoothness, creaminess, moistness, or crispness. In addition, four vitamins—A, D, E, and K—are soluble in fat. When the fat is removed from a food, many fat-soluble compounds, including these vitamins, are also removed. Table 4-6 (p. 108) summarizes the roles of fats in foods.

Fats are also an important part of most people's ethnic or national cuisines. Each culture has its own favorite food sources of fats and oils. In Canada, canola oil (also known

TABLE 4-6	The Functions of Fats in Foods

- *Nutrient.* Food fats provide essential fatty acids and other raw materials.

- *Energy.* Food fats provide a concentrated energy source.

- *Transport.* Fats carry fat-soluble vitamins A, D, E, and K along with some phytochemicals and assist in their absorption.

- *Sensory appeal.* Fats contribute to the taste and smell of foods.

- *Appetite.* Fats stimulate the appetite.

- *Satiety.* Fats contribute to feelings of fullness.

- *Texture.* Fats make fried foods crisp and other foods tender.

as rapeseed oil) is widely used. In the Mediterranean area, Greeks, Italians, and Spaniards rely heavily on olive oil. Both canola oil and olive oil are rich sources of monounsaturated fatty acids. Asians use the polyunsaturated oil of soybeans. Jewish people traditionally employ chicken fat. Everywhere in North America, butter and margarine are widely used.

Finding the Fats in Foods

The remainder of this chapter and the Nutrition in Practice show you how to choose fats wisely with the goals of providing optimal health and pleasure in eating. To achieve such goals, you need to know which foods offer unsaturated oils that provide the essential fatty acids and which foods are loaded with solid fats—the saturated and *trans* fats. Also important for many people is learning to control portion sizes, particularly portions of fatty foods that can pack hundreds of kcalories into just a few bites.

Keep in mind that, whether solid or liquid, essential or nonessential, all fats bring the same abundant kcalories to the diet and excesses contribute to body fat stores. No benefits can be expected when oil is added to an already fat-rich eating pattern. The following amounts of these fats contain about 5 grams of pure fat, providing 45 kcalories and negligible protein and carbohydrate:

- 1 teaspoon of oil or shortening
- 1½ teaspoons of mayonnaise, butter, or margarine
- 1 tablespoon of regular salad dressing, cream cheese, or heavy cream
- 1½ tablespoons of sour cream

The solid fat of some foods, such as the rim of fat on a steak, is visible (and therefore identifiable and removable). Other solid fats, such as those in candy, cheeses, coconut, hamburger, homogenized milk, and lunch meats, are invisible (and therefore easily missed or ignored). Equally hidden are the solid fats blended into biscuits, cakes, cookies, chip dips, ice cream, mixed dishes, pastries, sauces, and creamy soups and in fried foods. Invisible fats supply the majority of solid fats in the U.S. diet.

Milk and Milk Products Milk products go by different names that reflect their varying fat contents (see Table 4-7). A cup of homogenized whole milk contains the protein

TABLE 4-7	Fat Options among Milk and Milk Products
Fat-free and low-fat options	Fat-free (skim) or 1% (low-fat) milk or yogurt (plain)
Reduced-fat options	2% milk or yogurt (plain)
High-fat options	Whole milk, yogurt Most cheeses

and carbohydrate of fat-free milk, but in addition it contains about 80 extra kcalories from butterfat, a solid fat. A cup of reduced-fat (2 percent fat) milk falls between whole milk and fat-free, with 45 kcalories from fat.

Note that cream and butter do not appear in the milk and milk products group. Milk and yogurt are rich in calcium and protein, but cream and butter are not. Cream and butter are solid fats, as are whipped cream, sour cream, and cream cheese. Other cheeses, grouped with milk products, vary in their fat contents and are major contributors of saturated fat in people's diets.

Protein Foods Meats conceal a good deal of the fat—and much of the solid fat—that people consume. To help "see" the fat in meats, it is useful to think of them in three categories according to their fat contents: lean, medium-fat, and high-fat meats (as the Food Lists for Diabetes in Appendix C do). Meats in all three categories contain about equal amounts of protein, but their fat, saturated fat, and kcalorie amounts vary significantly. Table 1-11 (pp. 28 and 29) in Chapter 1 provides definitions for common terms used to describe the fat contents of meats.

The USDA eating patterns suggest that most adults limit their intake of protein foods to about 5 to 7 ounces per day. For comparison, the smallest fast-food hamburger weighs about 3 ounces. A steak served in a restaurant often runs 8, 12, or 16 ounces, more than a whole day's meat allowance. You may have to weigh a serving or two of meat to see how much you are eating.

People think of meat as a protein food, but calculation of its nutrient content reveals a surprising fact. A big (4-ounce) fast-food hamburger sandwich contains 24 grams of protein and 18 grams of fat, 7 of them saturated fat. Because protein offers 4 kcalories per gram and fat offers 9, the sandwich provides 96 kcalories from protein but 162 kcalories from fat. Hot dogs, fried chicken sandwiches, and fried fish sandwiches also provide hundreds of fat kcalories, mostly from invisible solid fat. Because so much meat fat is hidden from view, meat eaters can easily and unknowingly consume a great many grams of solid fat from this source.

When choosing beef or pork, look for lean cuts named *loin* or *round* from which the fat can be trimmed, and eat small portions. Chicken and turkey flesh are naturally lean, but commercial processing and frying add solid fats, especially in "patties," "nuggets," "fingers," and "wings." Chicken wings are mostly skin, and a chicken stores most of its fat just under its skin. The tastiest wing snacks have also been fried in cooking fat (often a hydrogenated, saturated type with *trans*-fatty acids); smothered with a buttery, spicy sauce; and then dipped in blue cheese dressing, making wings an extraordinarily high-fat snack. People who snack on wings may want to plan on eating low-fat foods at several other meals to balance them out.

Vegetables, Fruit, and Grains Choosing vegetables, fruit, whole grains, and legumes helps lower the saturated fat and total fat content of the diet. Most vegetables and fruit naturally contain little or no fat; avocados and olives are exceptions, but most of their fat is unsaturated, which is not harmful to heart health. Most grains contain only small amounts of fat. Some refined grain *products* such as fried taco shells, croissants, and biscuits are high in saturated fat, so consumers need to read food labels. Similarly, many people add butter, margarine, or cheese sauce to grains and vegetables, which raises their saturated and *trans* fat contents. Because fruit is often eaten without added fat, a diet that includes several servings of fruit daily can help a person meet the dietary recommendations for fat.

A diet rich in vegetables, fruit, whole grains, and legumes offers abundant vitamin C, folate, vitamin A, vitamin E, and dietary fiber—all important in supporting health. Consequently, such a diet protects against disease both by reducing saturated fat and total fat and by increasing nutrients. It also provides valuable phytochemicals that help defend against heart disease.

TABLE 4-8	Solid Fat Ingredients Listed on Food Labels

- Beef fat (tallow)
- Butter
- Chicken fat
- Coconut oil
- Cream
- Hydrogenated oil
- Milk fat
- Palm kernel oil; palm oil
- Partially hydrogenated oil
- Pork fat (lard)
- Shortening
- Stick margarine

Source: U.S. Department of Agriculture and U.S. Department of Health and Human Services, *Scientific Report of the 2015 Dietary Guidelines Advisory Committee* (2015), www.heath.gov.

Cutting Solid Fats and Choosing Unsaturated Fats

Meeting today's lipid guidelines can be challenging. Reducing intakes of saturated and *trans*-fatty acids, for example, involves identifying food sources of these fatty acids—that is, foods that contain solid fats. Then, replacing them appropriately involves identifying unsaturated oils. To help simplify these tasks:

1. Select the most nutrient-dense foods from all food groups. Solid fats and high-kcalorie choices can be found in every food group.
2. Consume fewer and smaller portions of foods and beverages that contain solid fats.
3. Replace solid fats with liquid oils whenever possible.
4. Check Nutrition Facts labels and select foods with little saturated fat and no *trans* fat.

Such advice is easily dispensed but not easily followed. The first step in doing so is learning which foods contain heavy doses of solid fats. Table 4-8 lists some terms that indicate solid fats in a food label ingredients list.

Box 4-1 offers strategies for making heart-healthy choices, food group by food group. The best diet for heart health is also rich in fruit, vegetables, nuts, and whole grains that offer many health advantages by supplying abundant nutrients, fiber, and phytochemicals.

Fats and kCalories Removing fat from food also removes energy, as Figure 4-5 shows. A pork chop with the fat trimmed to within a half-inch of the lean

---

Box 4-1	*HOW TO* Make Heart-Healthy Choices—by Food Group

In General

- Select the most nutrient-dense foods from all food groups.
- Consume fewer and smaller portions of foods and beverages that contain solid fats.
- Check the Nutrition Facts label to choose foods with little or no saturated fat and no *trans* fat.

Breads and Cereals

- Select whole-grain breads, cereals, and crackers that are low in saturated and *trans* fat (for example, bagels instead of croissants).
- Prepare pasta with a tomato sauce instead of a cheese or cream sauce.
- Limit intake of cookies, doughnuts, pastries, and croissants.

Vegetables and Fruit

- Enjoy the natural flavor of steamed vegetables (without butter) for dinner and fruits for dessert.
- Eat at least two vegetables (in addition to a salad) with dinner.
- Snack on raw vegetables or fruit instead of high-fat items like potato chips.
- Buy frozen vegetables without sauce.

Milk and Milk Products

- Switch from whole milk to reduced-fat, from reduced-fat to low-fat, and from low-fat to fat-free (nonfat).
- Use fat-free and low-fat cheeses (such as part-skim ricotta and low-fat mozzarella) instead of regular cheeses.

- Use fat-free or low-fat yogurt or sour cream instead of regular sour cream.
- Use evaporated fat-free milk instead of cream.
- Enjoy fat-free frozen yogurt, sherbet, or ice milk instead of ice cream.

Protein Foods

- Fat adds up quickly, even with lean meat; limit intake to about 6 ounces (cooked weight) daily.
- Eat at least two servings of fish per week (particularly fish such as mackerel, lake trout, herring, sardines, and salmon).
- Choose fish, poultry, or lean cuts of pork or beef; look for unmarbled cuts named *round* or *loin* (eye of round, top round, bottom round, round tip, tenderloin, sirloin, center loin, and top loin).
- Trim the fat from pork and beef; remove the skin from poultry.
- Grill, roast, broil, bake, stir-fry, stew, or braise meats; don't fry. When possible, place food on a rack so that fat can drain.
- Use lean ground turkey or lean ground beef in recipes; brown ground meats without added fat, then drain off fat.
- Select tuna, sardines, and other canned meats packed in water; rinse oil-packed items with hot water to remove much of the fat.
- Fill kabob skewers with lots of vegetables and slivers of meat; create main dishes and casseroles by combining a little meat, fish, or poultry with whole-grain pasta or brown rice and generous amounts of vegetables.

(Continued)

Box 4-1 | **HOW TO** Make Heart-Healthy Choices—by Food Group (*continued*)

- Use legumes often.
- Eat a meatless meal or two daily.
- Use egg substitutes in recipes instead of whole eggs, or use two egg whites in place of each whole egg.

Fats and Oils

- Use small amounts of vegetable oils in place of solid fats.
- Use butter or stick margarine sparingly; select soft margarines instead of hard margarines.
- Use fruit butters, reduced-kcalorie margarines, or butter replacers instead of butter.
- Use low-fat or fat-free mayonnaise and salad dressing instead of regular.
- Limit use of lard and meat fat.
- Limit use of products made with coconut oil, palm kernel oil, and palm oil (read labels on bakery goods, processed foods, microwave popcorn, and nondairy creamers).
- Reduce use of hydrogenated shortenings and stick margarines and products that contain them (read labels on crackers, cookies, and other commercially prepared baked goods); use vegetable oils instead.

Miscellaneous

- Use a nonstick pan, or coat the pan lightly with vegetable oil.
- Refrigerate soups and stews; when the fat solidifies, remove it before reheating.
- Use wine; lemon, orange, or tomato juice; herbs; spices; fruit; or broth instead of butter or margarine when cooking.
- Stir-fry in a small amount of oil; add moisture and flavor with broth, tomato juice, or wine.
- Use variety to enhance enjoyment of the meal: vary colors, textures, and temperatures—hot, cooked versus cool, raw foods—and use garnishes to complement food.
- Omit high-fat meat gravies and cheese sauces.
- Order pizzas with lots of vegetables, a little lean meat, and half the cheese.

FIGURE 4-5 | Cutting Fat Cuts kCalories—and Saturated Fat

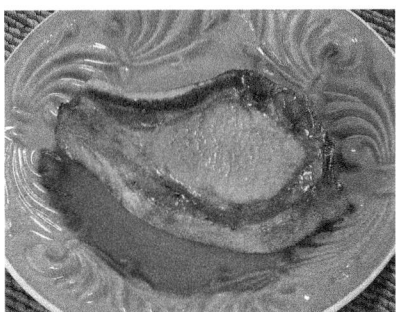

Pork chop with fat (290 kcal, 24 g fat, 9 g saturated fat)

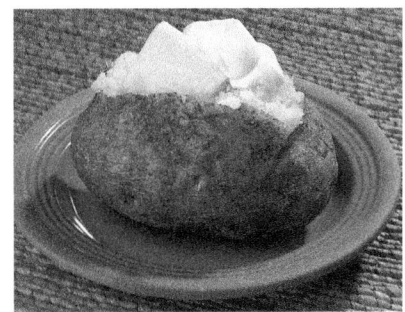

Potato with 1 tbs butter and 1 tbs sour cream (315 kcal, 14 g fat, 9 g saturated fat)

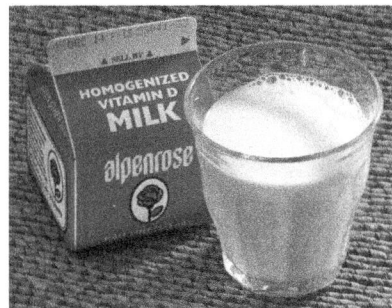

Whole milk, 1 c (150 kcal, 8 g fat, 5 g saturated fat)

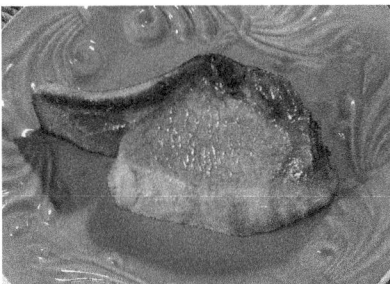

Pork chop with fat trimmed off (174 kcal, 8 g fat, 3 g saturated fat)

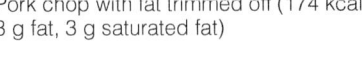

Savings:
116 kcal, 16 g fat, 6 g saturated fat

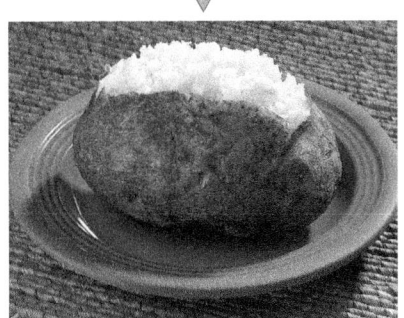

Plain potato (188 kcal, <1 g fat, 0 g saturated fat)

Savings:
127 kcal, 13 g fat, 9 g saturated fat

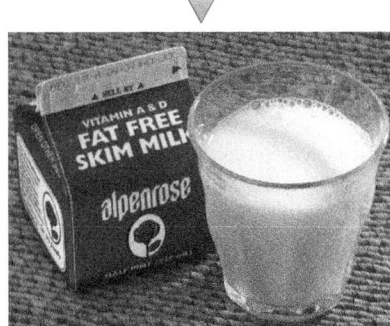

Fat-free milk, 1 c (90 kcal, <1 g fat, <1 g saturated fat)

Savings:
60 kcal, 7 g fat, 4 g saturated fat

Polara Studios, Inc.

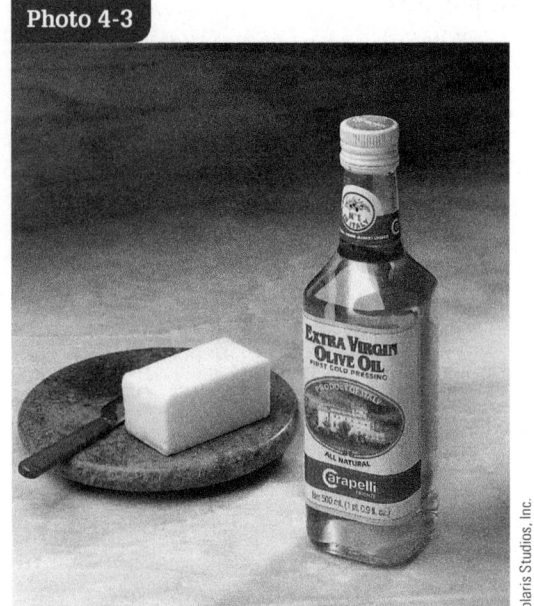

Photo 4-3

At room temperature, unsaturated fats (such as those found in oil) are usually liquid, whereas saturated fats (such as those found in butter) are solid.

provides 290 kcalories; with the fat trimmed off completely, it supplies 174 kcalories. A baked potato with butter and sour cream (1 tablespoon each) has 315 kcalories; a plain baked potato has 188 kcalories. The single most effective step you can take to reduce the energy value of a food is to eat it with less fat.

Choosing Unsaturated Fats When a person does eat fats, those to choose are the unsaturated ones. Remember, the softer a fat is, the more unsaturated it is (see Photo 4-3). Generally speaking, vegetable and fish oils are rich in polyunsaturates, olive oil and canola oil are rich in monounsaturates, and the harder fats—animal fats—are more saturated (see Figure 4-6). Remember, however, that vegetable fat or vegetable oil doesn't always mean unsaturated fat. Both coconut oil and palm oil, for example, which are often used in nondairy creamers, are saturated fats, and both raise blood cholesterol.

Don't Overdo Fat Restriction Some people actually manage to eat too *little* fat—to their detriment. Among them are young women and men with eating disorders, described in Nutrition in Practice 6. As a practical guideline, it is wise to include the equivalent of at least a teaspoon of fat in every meal.

FIGURE 4-6 Comparison of Dietary Fats

Most fats are a mixture of saturated, monounsaturated, and polyunsaturated fatty acids.

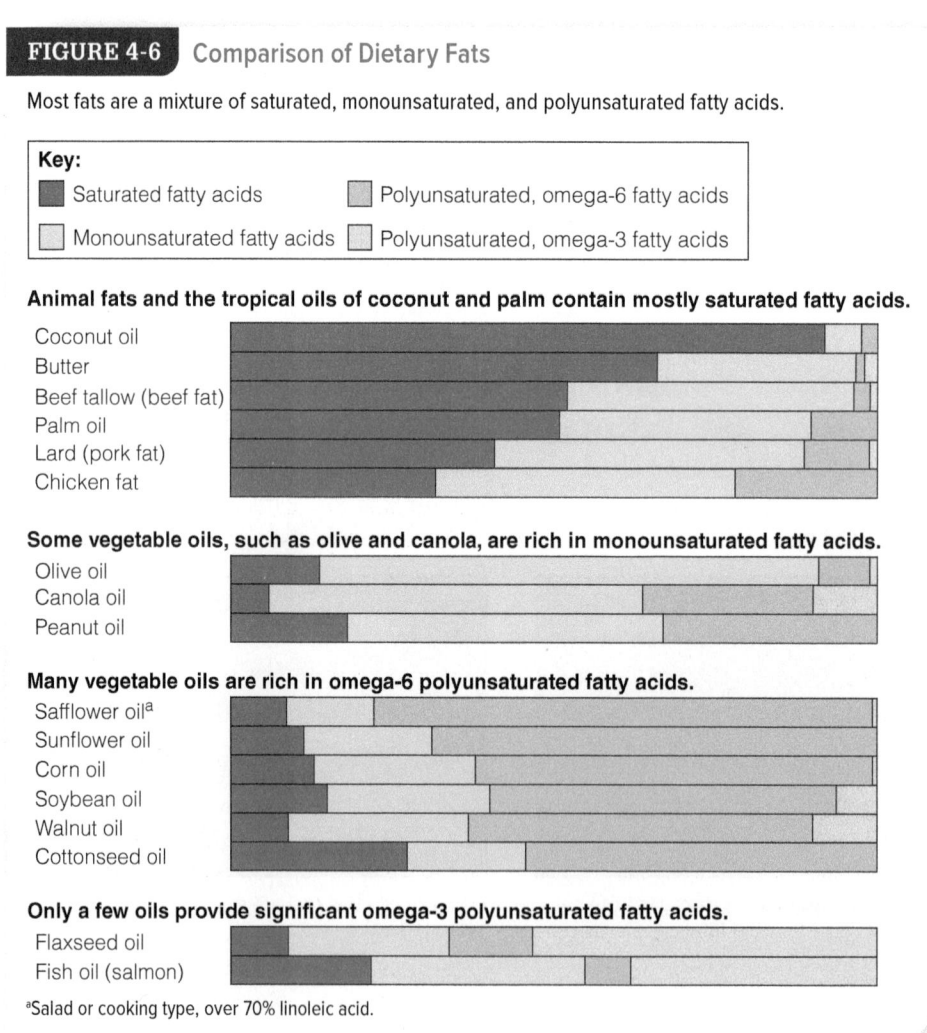

Key:
- Saturated fatty acids
- Monounsaturated fatty acids
- Polyunsaturated, omega-6 fatty acids
- Polyunsaturated, omega-3 fatty acids

Animal fats and the tropical oils of coconut and palm contain mostly saturated fatty acids.

Coconut oil
Butter
Beef tallow (beef fat)
Palm oil
Lard (pork fat)
Chicken fat

Some vegetable oils, such as olive and canola, are rich in monounsaturated fatty acids.

Olive oil
Canola oil
Peanut oil

Many vegetable oils are rich in omega-6 polyunsaturated fatty acids.

Safflower oil[a]
Sunflower oil
Corn oil
Soybean oil
Walnut oil
Cottonseed oil

Only a few oils provide significant omega-3 polyunsaturated fatty acids.

Flaxseed oil
Fish oil (salmon)

[a]Salad or cooking type, over 70% linoleic acid.

Fat Replacers Today, consumers can choose from thousands of fat-reduced products. Many bakery goods, lunch meats, cheeses, spreads, frozen desserts, and other products made with **fat replacers** offer less than half a gram of fat, saturated fat, and *trans* fat in a serving. Some of these products contain **artificial fats**, and others use conventional ingredients in unconventional ways to reduce fats and kcalories. Among the latter, manufacturers can:

- Add water or whip air into foods.
- Add fat-free milk to creamy foods.
- Use lean meats and soy protein to replace high-fat meats.
- Bake foods instead of frying them.

Common food ingredients such as fibers, sugars, or proteins can also take the place of fats in some foods. Products made from sugars or proteins still provide kcalories but far fewer kcalories from fats. Manufactured fat replacers consist of chemical derivatives of carbohydrate, protein, or fat, or modified versions of foods rich in those constituents.

A familiar example of an artificial fat that has been approved for use in snack foods such as potato chips, crackers, and tortilla chips is **olestra**. Olestra's chemical structure is similar to that of a regular fat (a triglyceride) but with important differences. A triglyceride is composed of a glycerol molecule with three fatty acids attached, whereas olestra is made of a sucrose molecule with six to eight fatty acids attached. Enzymes in the digestive tract cannot break the bonds of olestra, so unlike sucrose or fatty acids, olestra passes through the system unabsorbed.

The FDA's evaluation of olestra's safety addressed two questions. First, is olestra toxic? Research on both animals and humans supports the safety of olestra as a partial replacement for dietary fats and oils, with no reports of cancer or birth defects. Second, does olestra affect either nutrient absorption or the health of the digestive tract? When olestra passes through the digestive tract unabsorbed, it binds with the fat-soluble vitamins A, D, E, and K and carries them out of the body, robbing the person of these valuable nutrients. To compensate for these losses, the FDA requires the manufacturer to fortify olestra with vitamins A, D, E, and K. Saturating olestra with these vitamins does not make the product a good source of vitamins, but it does block olestra's ability to bind with the vitamins from other foods. An asterisk in the ingredients list informs consumers that these added vitamins are "dietarily insignificant."

Consumers need to keep in mind that low-fat and fat-free foods still deliver kcalories. Decades ago, consumers hailed the arrival of artificial sweeteners as a weight-loss wonder, but in reality, kcalories saved by using artificial sweeteners were readily replaced by kcalories from other foods. Alternatives to fat can help to lower energy intake and support weight loss only when they actually *replace* fat and energy in the diet.

Read Food Labels Labels list total fat, saturated fat, *trans* fat, and cholesterol contents of foods. Because each package provides information for a single serving and serving sizes are standardized, consumers can easily compare similar products.

fat replacers: ingredients that replace some or all of the functions of fat in foods and may or may not provide energy.

artificial fats: zero-energy fat replacers that are chemically synthesized to mimic the sensory and cooking qualities of naturally occurring fats but are totally or partially resistant to digestion.

olestra: a synthetic fat made from sucrose and fatty acids that provides zero kcalories per gram; also known as *sucrose polyester*.

Review Notes

- Fats in foods contribute to sensory appeal—enhancing the flavor, aroma, and texture of foods.
- Fats in foods deliver fat-soluble vitamins, energy, and essential fatty acids.
- While some fat in the diet is necessary, limiting intakes of saturated fat and *trans* fat is advised.
- Fats added to foods during preparation or at the table are a major source of fat in the diet.
- The choice between whole and fat-free milk products can make a big difference to the fat, saturated fat, and cholesterol content of an eating pattern.
- Meats account for a large proportion of hidden solid fats in many people's diets.

(Continued)

- Most people consume more meat than is recommended.
- Most vegetables and fruit naturally contain little or no fat.
- Grain products such as croissants and biscuits can be high in saturated fat, so consumers need to read food labels to learn which foods in this group contain fats.
- Consumers today can choose from an array of fat-reduced products, and many bakery goods and other foods made with fat replacers offer less than half a gram of fat, saturated fat, and *trans* fat in a serving.
- Some products use artificial fats such as olestra, while others use conventional ingredients such as water or fat-free milk to reduce fat and kcalories.
- Food labels list total fat, saturated fat, cholesterol, and *trans* fat.

Chapters 3 and 4 have looked briefly at the two major energy fuels in the body—carbohydrate and fat. When used for energy, each has desirable characteristics. The glucose derived from carbohydrate is needed by the brain and nerve tissues and is easily used for energy in other cells. Fat is a particularly useful fuel because the body stores it efficiently and in generous amounts. Chapter 5 looks at protein, a nutrient that can be used as fuel, but whose primary role is to provide machinery for getting things done.

Self Check

1. Three classes of lipids in the body are:
   a. triglycerides, fatty acids, and cholesterol.
   b. triglycerides, phospholipids, and sterols.
   c. fatty acids, phospholipids, and cholesterol.
   d. glycerol, fatty acids, and triglycerides.

2. A triglyceride consists of:
   a. three glycerols attached to a lipid.
   b. three fatty acids attached to a glucose.
   c. three fatty acids attached to a glycerol.
   d. three phospholipids attached to a cholesterol.

3. A fatty acid that has the maximum possible number of hydrogen atoms is known as a(n):
   a. saturated fatty acid.
   b. monounsaturated fatty acid.
   c. PUFA.
   d. essential fatty acid.

4. The difference between *cis-* and *trans*-fatty acids is:
   a. the number of double bonds.
   b. the length of their carbon chains.
   c. the location of the first double bond.
   d. the configuration around the double bond.

5. Essential fatty acids:
   a. are used to make substances that regulate blood pressure, among other functions.
   b. can be made from carbohydrates.
   c. include lecithin and cholesterol.
   d. cannot be found in commonly eaten foods.

6. Lecithins and other phospholipids in the body function as:
   a. emulsifiers.
   b. enzymes.
   c. temperature regulators.
   d. shock absorbers.

7. To minimize saturated fat intake and lower the risk of heart disease, most people need to:
   a. eat less meat.
   b. select fat-free milk.
   c. use nonhydrogenated margarines and cooking oils such as olive oil or canola oil.
   d. All of the above

8. To include omega-3 fatty acids in the diet, the American Heart Association recommends eating:
   a. cholesterol-free margarine.
   b. fish oil supplements.
   c. hydrogenated margarine.
   d. at least two 3.5-ounce portions of seafood per week.

9. Some examples of foods with hidden solid fats are:
   a. cheese, lettuce, and fruit juices.
   b. fried foods, sauces, dips, and lunch meats.
   c. fish, rice, and nuts.
   d. baked potatoes, vegetables, and fruit.

10. Generally speaking, vegetable and fish oils are rich in:
    a. polyunsaturated fat.
    b. saturated fat.
    c. cholesterol.
    d. *trans*-fatty acids.

Answers: 1. b, 2. c, 3. a, 4. d, 5. a, 6. a, 7. d, 8. d, 9. b, 10. a

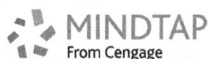 MINDTAP
From Cengage   For more chapter resources visit **www.cengage.com** to access MindTap, a complete digital course:

Clinical Applications

1. The connection between the overconsumption of saturated and *trans* fats and chronic diseases (obesity, diabetes, cancer, and cardiovascular disease) underscores the importance of being alert to a client's fat intake. What advice would you offer a client who reports the following?
   • Eats more than 12 ounces of meat each day.
   • Drinks whole milk and eats regular cheddar cheese each day.
   • Eats the following breads and cereals each day: a bagel with cream cheese for breakfast, a bologna sandwich on white bread for lunch, and biscuits or cornbread with butter to accompany dinner.
   • Eats less than the equivalent of a cup of fruit each day and eats vegetables only on occasion.

2. Make a list of foods, beverages, and seasonings that your client can substitute for foods high in saturated fat.

Notes

1. M. Blüher and C. S. Mantzoros, From leptin to other adipokines in health and disease: Facts and expectations at the beginning of the 21st century, *Metabolism* 64 (2015): 131–145; H. Cao, Adipocytokines in obesity and metabolic disease, *Journal of Endocrinology* 220 (2014): T47–T59.

2. F. M. Sacks and coauthors, Dietary fats and cardiovascular disease: A Presidential Advisory from the American Heart Association, *Circulation* 136 (2017): e195 Position of the Academy of Nutrition and Dietetics: Dietary fatty acids for healthy adults, *Journal of the Academy of Nutrition and Dietetics* 114 (2014): 136–153.

3. S. K. Gebauer and coauthors, Vaccenic acid and *trans* fatty acid isomers from partially hydrogenated oil both adversely affect LDL cholesterol: A double-blind, randomized controlled trial, *American Journal of Clinical Nutrition* 102 (2015): 1339–1346; R. Ganguly and G. N. Pierce, The toxicity of dietary *trans* fats, *Food and Chemical Toxicology* 78 (2015): 170–176; P. Nestel, Trans fatty acids: Are its cardiovascular risks fully appreciated? *Clinical Therapeutics* 36 (2014): 315–321; A. H. Lichtenstein, Dietary *trans* fatty acids and cardiovascular disease risk: Past and present, *Current Atherosclerosis Reports* 16 (2014): 433.

4. T. Wang and H. G. Lee, Advances in research on cis-9, *trans*-11 conjugated linoleic acid: A major functional conjugated linoleic acid isomer, *Critical Reviews in Food Science and Nutrition* 55 (2015): 720–731; H. S. Moon, Biological effects of conjugated linoleic acid on obesity-related cancers, *Chemico-Biological Interactions* 224 (2014): 189–195.

5. Position of the American Academy of Nutrition and Dietetics, Dietary fatty acids for healthy adults, 2014; T. A. Mori, Conference on "Dietary strategies for the management of cardiovascular risk," Dietary n-3 PUFA

and CVD: A review of the evidence, *Proceedings of the Nutrition Society* 73 (2014): 57–64; K. Takada and coauthors, Effects of eicosapentaenoic acid on platelet function in patients taking long-term aspirin following coronary stent implantation, *International Heart Journal* 55 (2014): 228–233; M. van Bilsen and A. Planavila, Fatty acids and cardiac disease: Fuel carrying a message, *Acta Physiologica* 211 (2014): 476–490.

6. W. Stonehouse, Does consumption of LC omega-3 PUFA enhance cognitive performance in healthy school-aged children and throughout adulthood? Evidence from clinical trials, *Nutrients* 6 (2014): 2730–2758; J. Jiao and coauthors, Effect of n-3 PUFA supplementation on cognitive function throughout the life span from infancy to old age: A systematic review and meta-analysis of randomized controlled trials, *American Journal of Clinical Nutrition* 100 (2014): 1422–1436.

7. L. C. Del Gobbo and coauthors, ω-3 polyunsaturated fatty acid biomarkers and coronary heart disease, *JAMA Internal Medicine* 176 (2016): 1155–1166; D. Kromhout and J. de Goede, Update on cardiometabolic health effects of ω-3 fatty acids, *Current Opinion in Lipidology* 25 (2014): 85–90; O. A. Khawaja, J. M. Gaziano, and L. Djoussé, N-3 fatty acids for prevention of cardiovascular disease, *Current Atherosclerosis Reports* 16 (2014): 450; Mori, 2014.

8. T. Ulven and E. Christiansen, Dietary fatty acids and their potential for controlling metabolic diseases through activation of FFA4/GPR120, *Annual Review of Nutrition* 35 (2015): 239–263.

9. Position of the American Academy of Nutrition and Dietetics, Dietary fatty acids for healthy adults, 2014.

10. M.S. Farvid and coauthors, Adolescent meat intake and breast cancer risk, *International Journal of Cancer* 136 (2015): 1909–1920; S. Sieri and coauthors, Dietary fat intake and development of specific breast cancer subtypes, *Journal of the National Cancer Institute*, April 9, 2014, doi: 10.1093/jnci/dju068.

11. T. M. Brasky and coauthors, Long-chain v-3 fatty acid intake and Endometrial cancer risk in the Women's Health Initiative, *American Journal of Clinical Nutrition* 101 (2015): 824–834; E. D. Kantor and coauthors, Long-chain omega-3 polyunsaturated fatty acid intake and risk of colorectal cancer, *Nutrition and Cancer* 66 (2014): 716–727.

12. Sacks and coauthors, 2017.

13. Sacks and coauthors, 2017; R. H. Eckel and coauthors, 2013 AHA/ACC guideline on lifestyle Management to reduce cardiovascular risk: A report of the American College of Cardiology/American Heart Association Task Force on Practice Guidelines, *Circulation* 129 (2014): S76–S99; Nestel, 2014.

14. Sacks and coauthors, 2017.

15. Sacks and coauthors, 2017; Position of the Academy of Nutrition and Dietetics, Dietary fatty acids for healthy adults, 2014; Nestel, 2014.

16. Eckel and coauthors, 2014.

17. K. D. Brownell and J. L. Pomeranz, The Trans-fat ban—Food regulation and long-term health, *New England Journal of Medicine* 370 (2014): 1773–1775.

18. D. Mozaffarian, Dietary and public policy priorities for cardiovascular disease, diabetes, and obesity, *Circulation* 133 (2016): 187–225; D. J. McNamara, Dietary cholesterol, heart disease risk and cognitive dissonance, *Proceedings of the Nutrition Society*, 73 (2014): 161–166.

19. Eckel and coauthors, 2014.

20. D. D. Alexander and coauthors, Meta-analysis of egg consumption and risk of coronary heart disease and stroke, *Journal of the American College of Nutrition* 35 (2016): 704–716.

21. A. Hernáez and coauthors, Olive oil polyphenols decrease LDL concentrations and LDL atherogenicity in men in a randomized controlled trial, *Journal of Nutrition* 145 (2015): 1692–1697; A. Medina-Remón and coauthors, Effects of total dietary polyphenols on plasma nitric oxide and blood pressure in a high cardiovascular risk cohort. The PREDIMED randomized trial, *Nutrition, Metabolism, and Cardiovascular Disease* 25 (2015): 60–67; A. Hernáez and coauthors, Olive oil polyphenols enhance high-density lipoprotein function in humans: A randomized controlled trial, *Atherosclerosis, Thrombosis, and Vascular Biology* 34 (2014): 2115–2119; S. Bulotta and coauthors, Beneficial effects of the olive oil phenolic Components oleuropein and hydroxytyroso: Focus on protection against cardiovascular and metabolic diseases, *Journal of Translational Medicine* 12 (2014): 219.

22. Bulotta and coauthors, 2014.

23. Mozaffarian, 2016; Khawaja, Gaziano, and Djoussé, 2014; Kromhout and de Goede, 2014.

24. Fish oil supplements, *Journal of the American Medical Association* 312 (2014): 839.

25. B. Heydari and coauthors, Effect of omega-3 acid ethyl esters on left ventricular remodeling after acute myocardial infarction, *Circulation* 134 (2016): 378–391; M. van Bilsen and A. Planavila, Fatty acids and cardiac disease: Fuel carrying a message, *Acta Physiologica* 211 (2014): 476–490.

26. U.S. Department of Health and Human Services and U.S. Department of Agriculture, *2015–2020 Dietary Guidelines for Americans*, 8th ed. (2015), health.gov/dietaryguidelines/2015/guidelines.

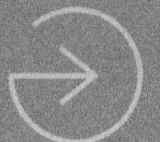

4.6 Nutrition in Practice
Figuring Out Fats

To consumers, advice about dietary fat appears to change almost daily. "Eat less fat." "Eat more fatty fish." "Give up butter—use margarine instead." "Give up margarine—replace it with olive oil." "Steer clear of saturated fats." "Seek out omega-3." "Stay away from *trans* fats." "Stick with mono- and polyunsaturated fats." No wonder some people feel confused about dietary fat. This Nutrition in Practice begins with the dietary guidelines for, and health consequences of, fat intake. Then it presents the Mediterranean diet, an example of an eating pattern that embraces the heart-healthy fats. It closes with the current opinion that, while specific lipids are associated with disease risks, a person's repetitive daily food choices—that is, his or her entire eating pattern—seems to have the greatest impact.

Why do today's fat messages seem to change constantly and become more confusing?

The confusion stems in part from the complexities of fat and in part from the nature of guidelines. As Chapter 4 explains, "dietary fat" refers to several kinds of fats; some fats support health, whereas others damage it, and foods typically provide a mixture of fats in varying proportions. It has taken researchers decades to sort through the relationships among the various kinds of fat and their roles in supporting or harming health. Translating these research findings into dietary recommendations is a challenging process. Too little information can mislead consumers, but too much detail can overwhelm them. As scientific understanding has grown, guidelines have evolved to become less general and more specific. Guidelines may seem to "change constantly and become more confusing," but in fact they are becoming more meaningful.

How exactly have dietary guidelines for fat changed to become more meaningful for consumers?

Dietary guidelines for fat have shifted away from limiting total fat, in general, to lowering saturated and *trans* fats, specifically, along with a greater emphasis on kcalorie control to maintain a healthy body weight.[1] For decades, health experts urged consumers to limit total fat intake to 30 percent or less of energy intake. This advice was straightforward—cut the fat and improve your health. Health experts recognized that saturated fats and *trans* fats are the ones that raise blood cholesterol, but they reasoned that when total fat was limited, saturated and *trans* fat

intake would decline as well. People were simply advised to cut back on all fat so that they would cut back on saturated and *trans* fat. Such advice may have oversimplified the message and unnecessarily restricted total fat.

But low-fat diets have been recommended for years to help people manage weight and reduce the risk of heart disease. Are you saying that low-fat diets are no longer recommended?

Low-fat diets remain a key recommendation in treatment plans for people with elevated blood lipids or heart disease and therefore are important in nutrition.[2] As for healthy people, evidence from around the world has led researchers to change population-wide recommendations from a "low-fat" to a "wise-fat" approach. Several problems accompany low-fat diets. First, many people find low-fat diets difficult to maintain over time. Second, low-fat diets are not necessarily low-kcalorie diets; if energy intake exceeds energy needs, weight gain follows, and obesity brings a host of health problems, including heart disease. Third, diets high in refined carbohydrates, even if low in fat, can cause blood triglycerides to rise and HDL to fall, a deleterious combination for heart health.[3] Finally, taken to the extreme, a low-fat diet may exclude fatty fish, nuts, seeds, and vegetable oils—all valuable sources of many essential fatty acids, phytochemicals, vitamins, and minerals. Importantly, the fats from these sources protect against heart disease, as later sections explain.

How have today's guidelines for fat been revised?

Today, health experts have revised guidelines to acknowledge that not all fats have damaging health consequences.[4] In fact, higher intakes of some kinds of fats (for example, the omega-3 fatty acids) support good health. Instead of urging people to cut back on all fats, current recommendations suggest carefully replacing the "bad" saturated and *trans* fats with the "good" unsaturated fats and enjoying these fats within kcalorie limits. The goal is to create an overall dietary pattern moderate in kcalories that provides enough of the fats that support good health, but not too much of those that harm health. (Turn to pp. 102–106 for a review of the health consequences of each type of fat.)

With these findings and goals in mind, the committee writing the *Dietary Guidelines for Americans 2015–2020* concluded that a healthy dietary pattern is higher in vegetables, fruit, whole grains, low-fat or nonfat dairy, seafood, legumes, and nuts; moderate in alcohol (among adults); lower in red and processed meat; and low in sugar-sweetened foods and drinks and refined grains.

How can people distinguish between the fats in foods that support health and those that might harm it?

Asking consumers to limit their total fat intake was less than perfect advice, but it was straightforward—find the fat and cut back. Asking consumers to keep their intakes of saturated fats and *trans* fats low and to use monoun-saturated and polyunsaturated fats instead may be more on target with heart health, but it also makes diet planning more complicated. To make appropriate selections, consumers must first learn which foods contain which fats. For example, avocados, bacon, walnuts, potato chips, and mackerel are all high-fat foods, yet some of these foods have detrimental effects on heart health when consumed in excess, and others seem neutral or even beneficial.

Is there evidence to clarify why some high-fat foods are compatible with a heart-healthy diet and others are not?

Yes. The traditional diets of Greece and other countries in the Mediterranean region are exemplary in their use of "good" fats, especially olives and olive oil. A classic study of the world's people, the Seven Countries Study, found that death rates from heart disease were strongly associated with diets high in saturated fats, but only weakly linked with total fat.[5] In fact, the two countries with the highest fat intakes, Finland and the Greek island of Crete, had the highest (Finland) and lowest (Crete) rates of heart disease deaths. In both countries, people consumed 40 percent or more of their kcalories from fat. Clearly, a high-fat diet was not the primary problem. When researchers refocused their attention on the *type* of fat, they found that the Cretes ate diets high in olive oil but low in saturated fat (less than 10 percent of kcalories), an eating pattern still linked with relatively low risks of heart disease today. Many studies that followed yielded similar results—people who follow "Mediterranean-style" eating patterns have low rates of heart disease, some cancers, and other chronic diseases, and their life expectancy is high.[6]

When olive oil replaces saturated fats, such as those of butter, coconut oil or palm oil, hydrogenated stick margarine, lard, or shortening, it may offer numerous health benefits.[7] Olive oil helps to protect against heart disease by lowering blood-clotting factors, blood pressure, and total and LDL cholesterol (but not HDL cholesterol);

Photo NP4-1

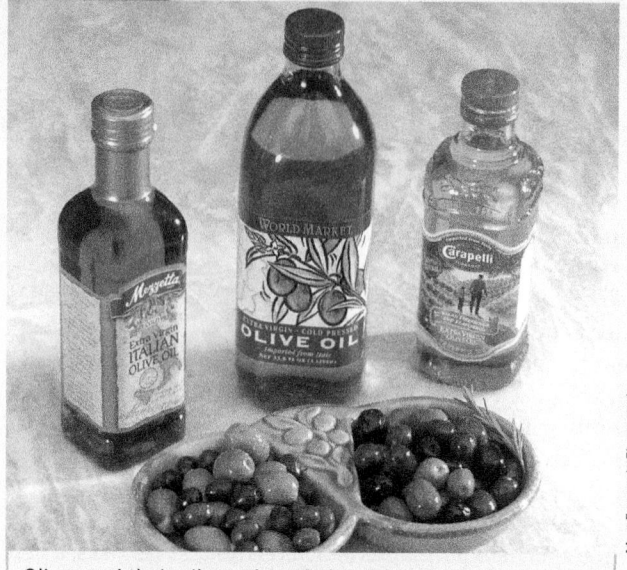

Matt Farruggio Photography

Olives and their oil may benefit heart health.

reducing LDL susceptibility to oxidation; interfering with the inflammatory response; and providing antimicrobial actions (see Photo NP4-1).[8]

The phytochemicals of olives captured in extra virgin olive oil, and not its monounsaturated fatty acids, seem responsible for these potential effects.[9] When processors lighten olive oils to make them more appealing to consumers, they strip away the intensely flavored phytochemicals of the olives, thus diminishing not only the bitter flavor of the oils, but also their potential for protecting the health of the heart.

Importantly, olive oil is not a magic potion; drizzling it on foods does not make them healthier. Like other fats, olive oil delivers 9 kcalories per gram, which can contribute to weight gain in people who fail to balance their energy intake with their energy output. Its role in a healthy diet is to *replace* the saturated fats.

Other vegetable oils, such as canola oil or safflower oil, in their liquid unhydrogenated states are also generally low in saturated fats and high in unsaturated fats. Such oils, when they replace solid, saturated fats in the diet, may help to preserve heart health.

Good, olive oil may help protect against heart disease; are there other food fats that may also be protective?

Possibly so. People who eat an ounce or so of nuts on several days a week appear to have lower risks of chronic diseases such as heart disease and diabetes than those consuming no nuts.[10]

The nuts under study are those commonly eaten in the United States: almonds, Brazil nuts, cashews, hazelnuts, macadamia nuts, pecans, pistachios, walnuts, and even peanuts. On average, these nuts contain mostly mono-unsaturated fat (59 percent), some polyunsaturated fat (27 percent), and little saturated fat (14 percent).

Research has shown a benefit from walnuts and almonds in particular. In study after study, walnuts, when substituted for other fats in the diet, produce favorable effects on blood lipids—even in people with elevated total and LDL cholesterol.[11] Results are similar for almonds.[12]

Studies on peanuts, macadamia nuts, pecans, and pistachios follow suit, indicating that including nuts may be a wise strategy against heart disease. Nuts may protect against heart disease because they provide:

- Monounsaturated and polyunsaturated fats in abundance but few saturated fats.
- Fiber, vegetable protein, essential fatty acids, and other valuable nutrients, including the antioxidant vitamin E.
- Phytochemicals that act as antioxidants (see Nutrition in Practice 8).
- Plant sterols.

Tree nuts and peanuts once had no place in a low-fat or low-kcalorie diet. Nuts provide up to 80 percent of their kcalories from fat, and a quarter cup (about an ounce) of mixed nuts provides more than 200 kcalories. Despite this, people who regularly eat nuts tend to be leaner, not fatter, and generally have smaller waistlines than others.[13] No one can yet say, however, whether nut eaters owe their leaner physiques to an overall health-conscious lifestyle or whether nuts might be extra satiating and thus reduce food and kcalorie intake at other meals. In any case, replacing potato chips or chocolate candy snacks with nuts certainly improves nutrition by reducing intakes of saturated fats and increasing intakes of vitamin E and other nutrients.

When designing a test diet, researchers must carefully use nuts *instead of*, not in addition to, other fat sources to keep kcalories constant. If you decide to snack on nuts, you should probably do the same thing and use them to replace other fats in your diet. Remember that nuts, although not associated with obesity or weight gain in research, provide substantially more kcalories per bite than crunchy raw vegetables, for example (see Photo NP4-2).

What about fish? I have a friend whose doctor told her that eating fish is good for the heart. Is this true?

Yes. The preceding chapter made clear that fish oils hold the potential to improve health, and particularly the health of the heart. Because increasing omega-3 fatty acids in the diet supports heart health and lowers the

Photo NP4-2

Stay mindful of kcalories when snacking on nuts.

risk of death from heart disease, the American Heart Association and other authorities recommend including fish in a heart-healthy diet.[14] Consumers in the United States currently receive only about one-third of the 8-ounce weekly recommendation of seafood. People who eat some fish each week can lower their risks of heart attack and stroke (see Photo NP4-3 on p. 120).

Fish is the best source of EPA and DHA in the diet, but it is also a major source of mercury and other environmental contaminants. Most fish contain at least trace amounts of mercury, but tilefish, swordfish, king mackerel, and shark have especially high levels. Freshwater fish may contain PCBs and other pollutants, so local advisories warn sport fishers of species that can pose problems. The chapter listed safer species of fish. To minimize risks while obtaining fish benefits, vary your choices among fatty fish species often.

If olive oil, nuts, and fatty fish are protective against heart disease, which fats are harmful?

A main dietary determinant of LDL cholesterol is saturated fat. Importantly, however, the effects of reduced saturated fat consumption on heart health vary based on which nutrients or foods replace it in a person's eating pattern.[15] As noted in Chapter 4, replacing dietary saturated fat with added sugars and refined starches can be detrimental to heart health. Replacing dietary saturated fat with fiber-rich carbohydrate foods such as whole grains, legumes, vegetables, and fruit, along with foods rich in monounsaturated and polyunsaturated fatty acids such as fish, nuts, and vegetable oils, reduces the risk of heart disease.[16] *Trans* fats, of course, also raise heart disease risk by elevating LDL cholesterol.

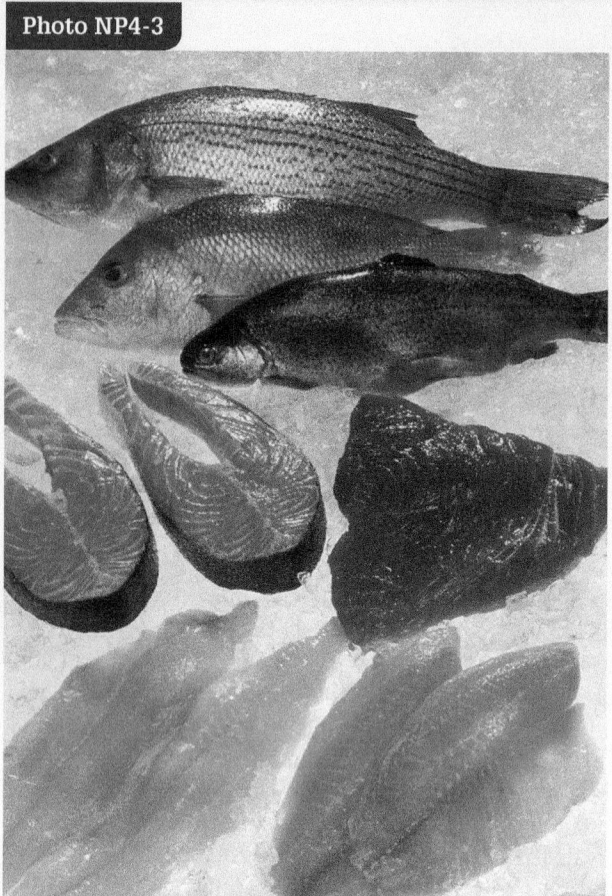

Fish is a good source of the omega-3 fatty acids.

Comstock

Which foods are highest in saturated and *trans* fats?

The major sources of saturated fats in the U.S. diet are fatty meats, whole-milk products, tropical oils, and products made from any of these foods. To limit saturated fat intake, consumers must choose carefully among these high-fat foods. More than a third of the fat in most meats is saturated. Similarly, more than half of the fat is saturated in whole milk and other high-fat dairy products, such as cheese, butter, cream, half-and-half, cream cheese, sour cream, and ice cream. Consumers rarely use the tropical oils of palm, palm kernel, and coconut in the kitchen, but these oils are used heavily by food manufacturers and so are commonly found in many commercially prepared foods.

When choosing meats, milk products, and commercially prepared foods, look for those lowest in saturated fat. Labels help consumers to compare products.

Even with careful selections, a nutritionally adequate diet will provide some saturated fat. Zero saturated fat is not possible even when experts design menus with the mission to minimize saturated fat. Eating patterns based on fruit, vegetables, legumes, nuts, soy products, and whole grains can, and often do, deliver less saturated fat than diets that depend heavily on animal-derived foods, however.

As for *trans* fats, Chapter 4 explained that solid shortening and margarine are made from vegetable oil that has been hardened through hydrogenation. This process both saturates some of the unsaturated fatty acids and introduces *trans*-fatty acids. Many convenience foods contain *trans* fats. Table 4-4 (p. 104) summarizes which foods provide which fats. Substituting unsaturated fats for saturated fats at each meal and snack can help protect against heart disease. Figure NP4-1 compares two meals and shows how such substitutions can lower saturated fat and raise unsaturated fat—even when total fat and kcalories remain the same.

Tell me more about the Mediterranean-style eating pattern mentioned earlier with regards to olive oil. Are there other features of the Mediterranean eating pattern that can be credited with reducing disease risks?

Yes, although each of the many countries that border the Mediterranean Sea has its own culture, traditions, and dietary habits, their similarities are much greater than the use of olive oil alone. In fact, no one factor alone can be credited with reducing disease risks—the association holds true only when the overall eating pattern is present. Apparently, each of the foods contributes small benefits that harmonize to produce either a substantial cumulative or synergistic effect.

The Mediterranean eating pattern features fresh, whole foods. The people select crusty breads, whole grains, potatoes, and pastas; a variety of vegetables (including wild greens) and legumes; feta and mozzarella cheeses and yogurt; nuts; and fruit (especially grapes and figs). They eat some fish, other seafood, poultry, a few eggs, and little meat. Along with olives and olive oil, their principal sources of fat are nuts and fish; they rarely use butter or encounter hydrogenated fats. They commonly use herbs and spices instead of salt. Consequently, traditional Mediterranean diets are low in saturated fat and very low in *trans* fat.

Furthermore, Mediterranean diets are rich in monounsaturated and polyunsaturated fat, starch- and fiber-rich carbohydrates, and nutrients and phytochemicals that support good health.[17] As a result, lipid profiles improve, blood pressure lowers, plaque stabilizes, inflammation diminishes, and the risk of heart disease declines.[18]

People following the traditional Mediterranean diet can receive as much as 40 percent of a day's kcalories from fat, but their limited consumption of milk and milk products and meats provides less than 10 percent from saturated fats. In addition, because the animals in the Mediterranean region pasture-graze, the meat, milk and milk products, and eggs are richer in omega-3 fatty acids than those from

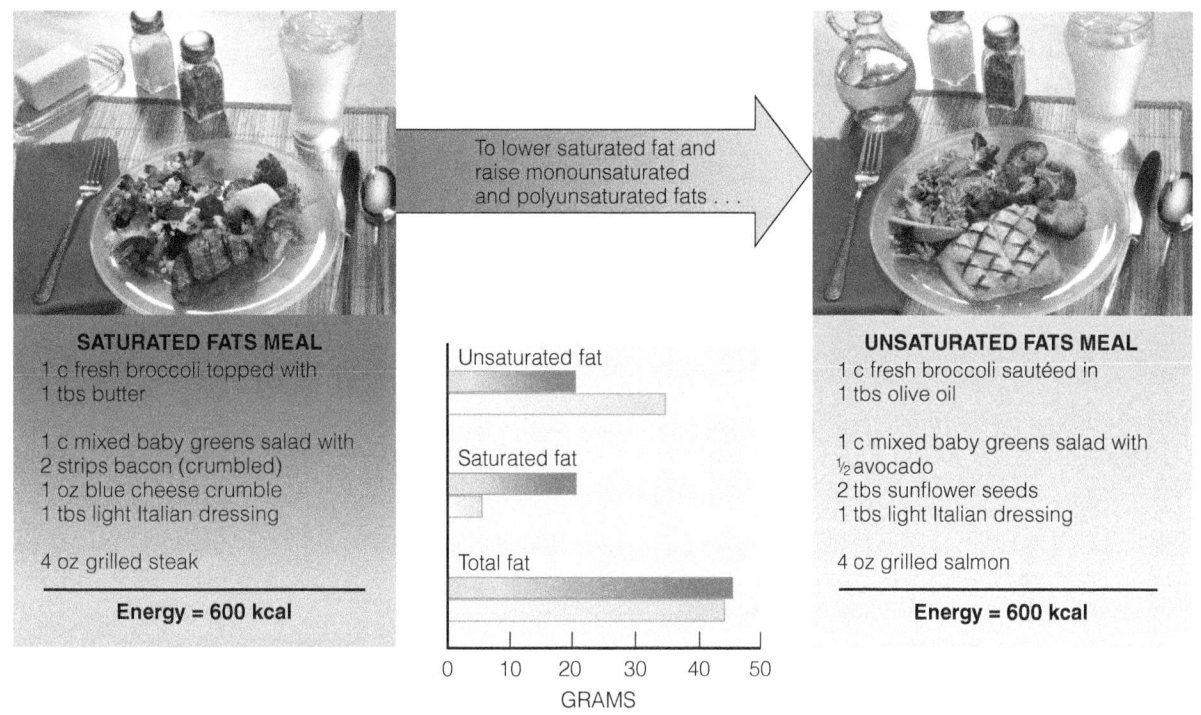

FIGURE NP4-1 Two Meals Compared: Replacing Saturated Fat with Unsaturated Fat

Examples of ways to replace saturated fats with unsaturated fats include sautéing vegetables in olive oil instead of butter, garnishing salads with avocado and sunflower seeds instead of bacon and blue cheese, and eating salmon instead of steak. Each of these meals provides roughly the same number of kcalories and grams of fat, but the one on the left has almost four times as much saturated fat and only half as many omega-3 fatty acids.

To lower saturated fat and raise monounsaturated and polyunsaturated fats . . .

SATURATED FATS MEAL
1 c fresh broccoli topped with
1 tbs butter

1 c mixed baby greens salad with
2 strips bacon (crumbled)
1 oz blue cheese crumble
1 tbs light Italian dressing

4 oz grilled steak

Energy = 600 kcal

Unsaturated fat

Saturated fat

Total fat

0 10 20 30 40 50
GRAMS

UNSATURATED FATS MEAL
1 c fresh broccoli sautéed in
1 tbs olive oil

1 c mixed baby greens salad with
½ avocado
2 tbs sunflower seeds
1 tbs light Italian dressing

4 oz grilled salmon

Energy = 600 kcal

Both photos: Matt Farruggio Photography

animals fed grain. All in all, the traditional Mediterranean diet has earned a reputation for its health benefits as well as delicious flavors. Consumers need to be aware that the typical Mediterranean-style cuisine available in U.S. restaurants, however, has been adjusted to popular tastes. Quite often, these meals are much higher in saturated fats and meats—and much lower in the polyunsaturated fats and vegetables—than the traditional fare. Table NP4-1 (p. 122) presents the USDA Healthy Mediterranean Eating Pattern, which has more fruit and seafood and fewer milk and milk products than the Healthy U.S.-Style Eating Pattern that Chapter 1 introduced.

So it seems that some fats are "good" and others are "bad" from the body's point of view. Is that right?

The saturated and *trans* fats do indeed seem mostly bad for the health of the heart. Aside from providing energy, which unsaturated fats can do equally well, saturated and *trans* fats bring no indispensable benefits to the body. Furthermore, no harm can come from consuming diets low in them. In contrast, the unsaturated fats are mostly good for the health of the heart when consumed in moderation.

When judging foods by their fatty acids, keep in mind that the fat in foods is a mixture of both saturated and unsaturated fatty acids. Even predominantly monounsaturated olive oil delivers some saturated fat. Consequently, even when a person chooses foods with mostly unsaturated fats, saturated fat can still add up if total fat is high. For this reason, fat must be kept below 35 percent of total kcalories if the diet is to be moderate in saturated fat.

Consumers who focus solely on saturated fats may not necessarily improve their overall diet quality, and it is overall diet quality that improves heart health. Striving instead for a dietary pattern that follows the Dietary Guidelines described in Chapter 1 can improve health markedly. The components of such a diet work in harmony to improve health beyond the effects of fats alone. To further protect health, you may want to choose small portions of meats, fish, and poultry; and include fresh foods from all the groups each day. Take care to select portion sizes that will best meet your energy needs. Also, be physically active each day.

USDA Food Patterns: Healthy Mediterranean Eating Pattern

The table first lists recommended amounts from each food group per day and then shows the amounts for vegetables and protein foods dispersed among subgroups per week. The rows highlighted in tan indicate which food groups and serving sizes differ from the Healthy U.S.-Style Eating Pattern (see Tables 1-6 and 1-8 on pp. 19 and 22).

RECOMMENDED DAILY AMOUNTS FROM EACH FOOD GROUP

FOOD GROUP	1600 kcal	1800 kcal	2000 kcal	2200 kcal	2400 kcal	2600 kcal	2800 kcal	3000 kcal
Fruit	2 c	2 c	2½ c	2½ c	2½ c	2½ c	3 c	3 c
Vegetables	2 c	2½ c	2½ c	3 c	3 c	3½ c	3½ c	4 c
Grains	5 oz	6 oz	6 oz	7 oz	8 oz	9 oz	10 oz	10 oz
Protein foods	5½ oz	6 oz	6½ oz	7 oz	7½ oz	7½ oz	8 oz	8 oz
Milk and milk products	2 c	2 c	2 c	2 c	2½ c	2½ c	2½ c	2½ c
Oils	5 tsp	5 tsp	6 tsp	6 tsp	7 tsp	8 tsp	8 tsp	10 tsp
Limit on kcalories available for other uses[a]	140 kcal	160 kcal	260 kcal	270 kcal	300 kcal	330 kcal	350 kcal	430 kcal

RECOMMENDED WEEKLY AMOUNTS FROM SUBGROUPS

	1600 kcal	1800 kcal	2000 kcal	2200 kcal	2400 kcal	2600 kcal	2800 kcal	3000 kcal
VEGETABLES SUBGROUPS								
Dark green	1½ c	1½ c	1½ c	2 c	2 c	2½ c	2½ c	2½ c
Red and orange	4 c	5½ c	5½ c	6 c	6 c	7 c	7 c	7½ c
Legumes	1 c	1½ c	1½ c	2 c	2 c	2½ c	2½ c	3 c
Starchy	4 c	5 c	5 c	6 c	6 c	7 c	7 c	8 c
Other	3½ c	4 c	4 c	5 c	5 c	5½ c	5½ c	7 c
PROTEIN FOODS SUBGROUPS								
Seafood	11 oz	15 oz	15 oz	16 oz	16 oz	17 oz	17 oz	17 oz
Meats, poultry, eggs	23 oz	23 oz	26 oz	28 oz	31 oz	31 oz	33 oz	33 oz
Nuts, seeds, soy products	4 oz	4 oz	5 oz	5 oz	5 oz	5 oz	6 oz	6 oz

[a]The limit on kcalories for other uses describes how many kcalories are available for foods that are not in nutrient-dense forms; these kcalories may also be referred to as discretionary kcalories (discussed on p. 22).

Source: U.S. Department of Health and Human Services and U.S. Department of Agriculture. *2015–2020 Dietary Guidelines for Americans*, 8th ed. December 2015. Available at health.gov /dietaryguidelines/2015/guidelines/.

Notes

1. U.S. Department of Health and Human Services and U.S. Department of Agriculture, *2015–2020 Dietary Guidelines for Americans*, 8th ed. (2015), health.gov/dietaryguidelines/2015/guidelines/.

2. R. H. Eckel and coauthors, 2013 AHA/ACC guidelines on lifestyle Management to reduce cardiovascular risk: A report of the American College of Cardiology/American Health Association Task Force on Practice Guidelines, *Circulation*, 129 (2014): S76–S99.

3. F. M. Sacks and coauthors, Dietary fats and cardiovascular disease: A Presidential Advisory from the American Heart Association, *Circulation*, 136 (2017): e195.

4. Sacks and coauthors, 2017; Eckel and coauthors, 2014.

5. A. Keys, *Seven Countries: A Multivariate Analysis of Death and Coronary Heart Disease* (Cambridge, MA: Harvard University Press, 1980).

6. C. R. Davis and coauthors, A Mediterranean diet lowers blood pressure and improves endothelial function: Results from the MedLey randomized intervention trial, *American Journal of Clinical Nutrition* 105 (2017): 1305–1313; M. Garcia and coauthors, The effect of the traditional Mediterranean-style diet on metabolic risk factors: A meta-analysis, *Nutrients* 8 (2016): 168; T. Y. N. Tong and coauthors, Prospective association of the Mediterranean diet with cardiovascular disease incidence and mortality and it population impact in a non-Mediterranean population: The EPIC-Norfolk Study, *BMC Medicine* 14 (2016): 135; J. Shen and coauthors, Mediterranean dietary patterns and cardiovascular health, *Annual Review of Nutrition* 35 (2015): 425–449; E. Lopez-Garcia and coauthors, The Mediterranean-style dietary pattern and mortality among men and women with cardiovascular disease, *American Journal of Clinical Nutrition* 99 (2014): 172–180; M. L. Bertoia and coauthors, Mediterranean and Dietary Approaches to Stop Hypertension Dietary patterns and risk of sudden cardiac death in postmenopausal women, *American Journal of Clinical Nutrition* 99 (2014): 344–351.

7. S. Bulotta and coauthors, Beneficial effects of the olive oil phenolic components oleuropein and hydroxytyroso: Focus on protection against cardiovascular and metabolic diseases, *Journal of Translational Medicine* 12 (2014): 219.

8. A. Hernáez and coauthors, Olive oil polyphenols decrease LDL concentrations and LDL atherogenicity in men in a randomized controlled trial, *Journal of Nutrition* 145 (2015): 1692–1697; A. Medina-Remón and coauthors, Effects of total dietary polyphenols on plasma nitric oxide and blood pressure in a high cardiovascular risk cohort. The PREDIMED randomized trial, *Nutrition, Metabolism, and Cardiovascular Disease* 25 (2015): 60–67; M. Fitó and coauthors, Effect of the Mediterranean diet on heart failure biomarkers: A randomized sample from the PREDIMED trial, *European Journal of Heart Failure* 16 (2014): 543–550; A. Hernáez and coauthors, Olive oil polyphenols enhance high-density lipoprotein function in humans: A randomized controlled trial, *Atherosclerosis, Thrombosis, and Vascular Biology* 34 (2014): 2115–2119.

9. M. I. Covas, R. de la Torre, and M. Fitó, Virgin olive oil: A key food for cardiovascular risk protection, *British Journal of Nutrition* 113 (2015): S19–S28; M. A. Martinez-González and coauthors, Benefits of the Mediterranean diet: Insights from the PREDIMED Study, *Progress in Cardiovascular Disease* 58 (2015): 50–60; Hernáez and coauthors, 2015; Hernáez and coauthors, 2014; Bulotta and coauthors, 2014.

10. H. N. Luu and coauthors, Prospective evaluation of the association of nut/peanut consumption with total and cause-specific mortality, *JAMA Internal Medicine* 175 (2015): 755–766; G. Grosso and coauthors, Nut consumption on all-cause, cardiovascular, and cancer mortality risk: A systematic reviewe and meta-analysis of epidemiologic studies, *American Journal of Clinical Nutrition* 101 (2015): 783–793; P. A. van den Brandt and L. J. Schouten, Relationship of tree nut, peanut and peanut butter intake with total and cause-specific mortality: A cohort study and meta-analysis, *International Journal of Epidemiology* 44 (2015): 1038–1049; T. T. Hshieh and coauthors, Nut consumption and risk of mortality in the Physicians' Health Study, *American Journal of Clinical Nutrition* 101 (2015): 407–412; R. G. M. Souza and coauthors, Nuts and legume seeds for cardiovascular risk reduction: Scientific evidence and mechanisms of action, *Nutrition Reviews* 73 (2015): 335–347; C. Luo and coauthors, Nut consumption and risk of type 2 diabetes, cardiovascular disease, and all-cause mortality: A systematic review and meta-analysis, *American Journal of Clinical Nutrition* 100 (2014): 256–269; A. Afshin and coauthors, Consumption of nuts and legumes and risk of incident ischemic heart disease, stroke, and diabetes: A systematic review and meta-analysis, *American Journal of Clinical Nutrition* 100 (2014): 278–288.

11. C. Sánchez-González and coauthors, Health benefits of walnut polyphenols: An exploration beyond their lipid profile, *Critical Reviews in Food Science and Nutrition* 57 (2017): 3373–3383; B. Burns-Whitmore and coauthors, Effects of supplementing n-3 fatty acid enriched eggs and walnuts on cardiovascular disease risk markers in healthy free-living lacto-ovo-vegetarians: A randomized, crossover, free-living intervention study, *Nutrition Journal* 13 (2014): 29; P. M. Kris-Etherton, Walnuts decrease risk of cardiovascular disease: A summary of efficacy and biologic mechanisms, *Journal of Nutrition* 144 (2014): 547S–554S.

12. C. E. Berryman and coauthors, Effects of daily almond consumption on cardiometabolic risk and abdominal adiposity in healthy adults with elevated LDL-cholesterol: A randomized controlled trial, *Journal of the American Heart Association* 5 (2015): e000993.

13. S. Y. Tan, J. Dhillon, and R. D. Mattes, A review of the effects of nuts on appetite, food intake, metabolism, and body weight, *American Journal of Clinical Nutrition* 100 (2014): 412S–422S; C. L. Jackson and F. B. Hu, Long-term associations of nut consumption with body weight, *American Journal of Clinical Nutrition* 100 (2014): 408S–411S.

14. L. C. Del Gobbo and coauthors, ω-3 polyunsaturated fatty acid biomarkers and coronary heart disease, *JAMA Internal Medicine* 176 (2016): 1155–1166; D. Kromhout and J. de Goede, Update on cardiometabolic health effects of ω-3 fatty acids, *Current Opinion in Lipidology* 25 (2014): 85–90.

15. Sacks and coauthors, 2017; Position of the Academy of Nutrition and Dietetics, Dietary fatty acids for healthy adults, *Journal of the Academy of Nutrition and Dietetics* 114 (2014): 136–153.

16. Sacks and coauthors, 2017.

17. I. Castro-Quezada, B. Román-Viñas, and L. Serra-Majem, The Mediterranean diet and nutritional adequacy: A review, *Nutrients* 6 (2014): 231–248.

18. Tong and coauthors, 2016; Shen and coauthors, 2015; M. Bonaccio and coauthors, Adherence to the Mediterranean diet is associated with lower platelet and leukocyte counts: Results from the Molisani study, *Blood* 123 (2014): 3037–3044; E. Ros and coauthors, Mediterranean diet and cardiovascular health: Teachings of the PREDIMED study, *Advances in Nutrition* 5 (2014): 330S–336S; R. Casas and coauthors, The effects of the Mediterranean diet on biomarkers of vascular wall inflammation and plaque vulnerability in subjects with high risk for cardiovascular disease: A randomized trial, *PLoS One* 9 (2014): e100084; H. Gardener and coauthors, Mediterranean diet and carotid atherosclerosis in the Northern Manhattan Study, *Atherosclerosis* 234 (2014): 303–310.

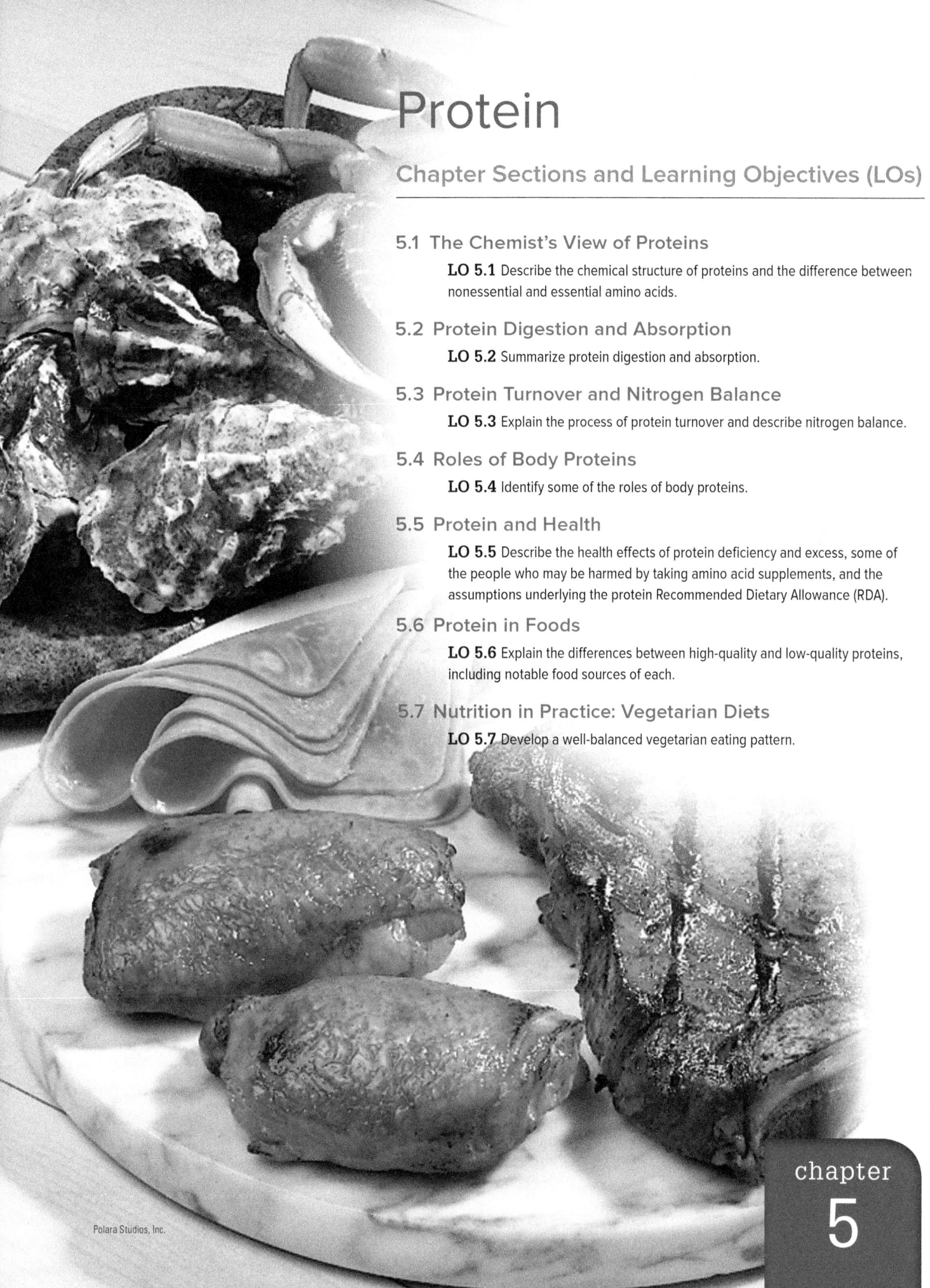

Protein

Chapter Sections and Learning Objectives (LOs)

Polara Studios, Inc.

chapter

5

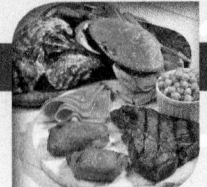

help your muscles to contract, your blood to clot, and your eyes to see. They keep you alive and well by facilitating chemical reactions and defending against infections. Without them, your bones, skin, and hair would have no structure. No new living tissue can be built without them. No wonder they were named proteins, *meaning* "of prime importance."

5.1 The Chemist's View of Proteins

Proteins are chemical compounds that contain the same atoms as carbohydrates and lipids—carbon (C), hydrogen (H), and oxygen (O)—but proteins are different in that they also contain nitrogen (N) atoms. These nitrogen atoms give the name *amino* (nitrogen containing) to the amino acids that form the links in the chains we call proteins.

The Structure of Proteins

About 20 different **amino acids** may appear in proteins.* All amino acids share a common chemical backbone consisting of a single carbon atom with both an amino group and an acid group attached to it. It is these backbones that are linked together to form proteins. Each amino acid also carries a side group, which varies from one amino acid to another (see Figure 5-1). The side group makes the amino acids differ in size, shape, and electrical charge. The side groups on amino acids are what make proteins so varied in comparison with either carbohydrates or lipids.

Protein Chains The 20 amino acids can be linked end to end in a virtually infinite variety of sequences to form proteins. When two amino acids bond together, the resulting structure is known as a **dipeptide**. Three amino acids bonded together form a **tripeptide**. As additional amino acids join the chain, the structure becomes a **polypeptide**. Most proteins are a few dozen to several hundred amino acids long.

Protein Shapes Polypeptide chains twist into complex shapes. Each amino acid has special characteristics that attract it to, or repel it from, the surrounding fluids and other amino acids. Because of these interactions, polypeptide chains fold and intertwine into intricate coils (see Figure 5-2) and other shapes. The amino acid sequence of a protein determines the specific way the chain will fold.

proteins: compounds made from strands of amino acids composed of carbon, hydrogen, oxygen, and nitrogen atoms. Some amino acids also contain sulfur atoms.

amino acids: building blocks of protein. Each contains an amino group, an acid group, a hydrogen atom, and a distinctive side group, all attached to a central carbon atom.

amino = containing nitrogen

dipeptide: two amino acids bonded together.

di = two
peptide = amino acid

tripeptide: three amino acids bonded together.

tri = three

polypeptide: 10 or more amino acids bonded together. An intermediate strand of between 4 and 10 amino acids is an *oligopeptide*.

poly = many
oligo = few

FIGURE 5-1 Amino Acid Structure and Examples of Amino Acids

All amino acids have a "backbone" made of an amino acid group (which contains nitrogen) and an acid group. The side group varies from one amino acid to the next. Note that the side group is a unique structure that differentiates one amino acid from another.

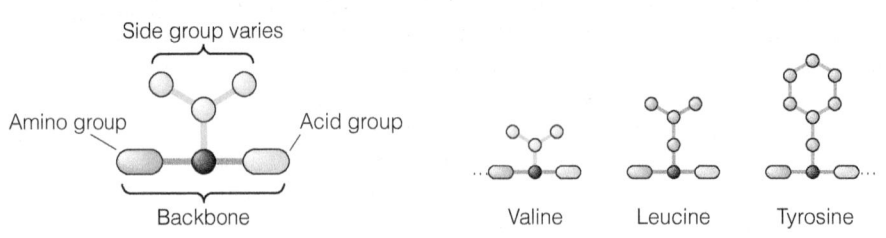

---

*Besides the 20 common amino acids, which can all be components of proteins, others occur individually (for example, ornithine).

FIGURE 5-2   The Coiling and Folding of a Protein Molecule

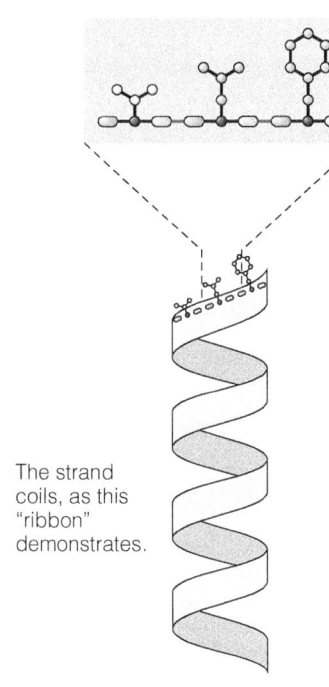

A portion of a strand of amino acids.

The strand coils, as this "ribbon" demonstrates.

The strand of amino acids takes on a springlike shape as their side groups variously attract and repel each other.

The completed protein.

Once coiled and folded, the protein may be functional as is, or it may need to join with other proteins or add a vitamin or mineral to become active.

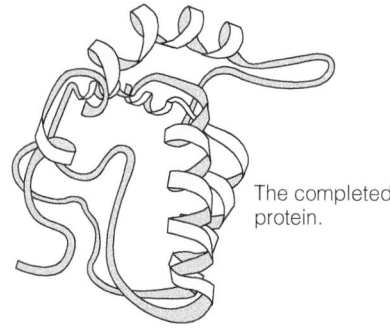

nonessential amino acids: amino acids that the body can synthesize.

essential amino acids: amino acids that the body cannot synthesize in amounts sufficient to meet physiological needs. Nine amino acids are known to be essential for human adults:

histidine (HISS-tuh-deen)
isoleucine (eye-so-LOO-seen)
leucine (LOO-seen)
lysine (LYE-seen)
methionine (meh-THIGH-oh-neen)
phenylalanine (fen-il-AL-uh-neen)
threonine (THREE-oh-neen)
tryptophan (TRIP-toe-fane, TRIP-toe-fan)
valine (VAY-leen)

conditionally essential amino acid: an amino acid that is normally nonessential but must be supplied by the diet in special circumstances when the need for it becomes greater than the body's ability to produce it.

Protein Functions The dramatically different shapes of proteins enable them to perform different tasks in the body. Some, such as hemoglobin in the blood (see Figure 5-3), are globular in shape; some are hollow balls that can carry and store materials within them; and some, such as those that form tendons, are more than 10 times as long as they are wide, forming stiff, sturdy, rodlike structures.

Nonessential and Essential Amino Acids

More than half of the amino acids are **nonessential amino acids**, meaning that the body can make them for itself. Proteins in foods usually deliver these amino acids, but it is not essential that they do so. There are other amino acids that the body cannot make at all, however, and some that it cannot make fast enough to meet its needs. The proteins in foods must supply these nine amino acids to the body; they are therefore called **essential amino acids**. (Some researchers refer to essential amino acids as *indispensable* and to nonessential amino acids as *dispensable*.)

Under special circumstances, a nonessential amino acid can become essential. For example, the body normally makes tyrosine (a nonessential amino acid) from the essential amino acid phenylalanine. If the diet fails to supply enough phenylalanine or if the body cannot make the conversion for some reason (as happens in the inherited disease phenylketonuria), then tyrosine becomes a **conditionally essential amino acid**.

FIGURE 5-3   The Structure of Hemoglobin

Four highly folded polypeptide chains form the globular hemoglobin protein.

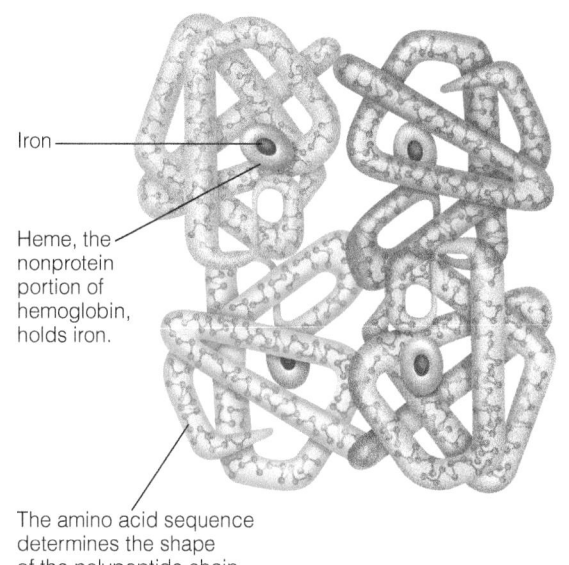

Iron

Heme, the nonprotein portion of hemoglobin, holds iron.

The amino acid sequence determines the shape of the polypeptide chain.

5.2 Protein Digestion and Absorption

Proteins in foods do not become body proteins directly. Instead, foods supply the amino acids from which the body makes its own proteins. When a person eats foods containing protein, enzymes break the long polypeptides into tripeptides and dipeptides and, finally, the tripeptides and dipeptides into amino acids. Table 5-1 provides the details.

5.3 Protein Turnover and Nitrogen Balance

Within each cell of the body, proteins are continually being made and broken down, a process known as **protein turnover**. Amino acids must be continuously available to build the proteins of new tissues. The new tissues may be in an embryo, in the muscles of an athlete in training, in a growing child, in the scar tissue that heals wounds, or in new hair and nails.

Less obvious is the protein that helps replace worn-out cells and internal cell structures. For example, the millions of cells that line the intestinal tract live for three to five days; they are constantly being shed and must be replaced. The cells of the skin die and rub off, and new ones grow from underneath.

TABLE 5-1 Protein Digestion and Absorption

MOUTH AND SALIVARY GLANDS

Chewing and crushing moisten protein-rich foods and mix them with saliva to be swallowed.

STOMACH

Hydrochloric acid (HCl) uncoils protein strands and activates stomach enzymes:

$$\text{Protein} \xrightarrow{\text{Pepsin, HCl}} \text{Smaller polypeptides}$$

SMALL INTESTINE AND PANCREAS

Pancreatic and small intestinal enzymes split polypeptides further:

$$\text{Polypeptides} \xrightarrow{\text{Pancreatic and intestinal proteases}} \text{Tripeptides, dipeptides, amino acids}$$

Then enzymes on the surface of the small intestinal cells hydrolyze these peptides and the cells absorb them:

$$\text{Peptides} \xrightarrow{\text{Intestinal tripeptidases and dipeptidases}} \text{Amino acids (absorbed)}$$

protein turnover: the continuous breakdown and synthesis of body proteins involving the recycling of amino acids.

Protein Turnover

When proteins break down, their component amino acids are liberated within the cells or released into the bloodstream. Some of these amino acids are promptly recycled into other proteins. By reusing amino acids to build proteins, the body conserves and recycles a valuable commodity. Other amino acids are stripped of their nitrogen and used for energy. Each day, about a quarter of the body's available amino acids are irretrievably broken down and used for energy. For this reason, amino acids from food are needed each day to support the new growth and maintenance of cells.

Nitrogen Balance

Researchers use **nitrogen balance** studies to estimate protein requirements. In healthy adults, protein synthesis balances with protein degradation, and nitrogen intake from protein in food balances with nitrogen excretion in the urine, feces, and sweat. When nitrogen intake equals nitrogen output, a person is in nitrogen equilibrium, or zero nitrogen balance.

If the body synthesizes more than it degrades and adds protein, nitrogen status becomes positive. Nitrogen status is positive in growing infants, children, and adolescents; pregnant women; and people recovering from protein deficiency or illness; their nitrogen intake exceeds their nitrogen output (see Photo 5-1). They are retaining protein in new tissues as they add blood, bone, skin, and muscle to their bodies.

If the body degrades more than it synthesizes and loses protein, nitrogen status becomes negative. Nitrogen status is negative in people who are starving or suffering other severe stresses such as burns, injuries, infections, and fever; their nitrogen output exceeds their nitrogen intake. During these times, the body loses nitrogen as it breaks down muscle and other body proteins for energy.

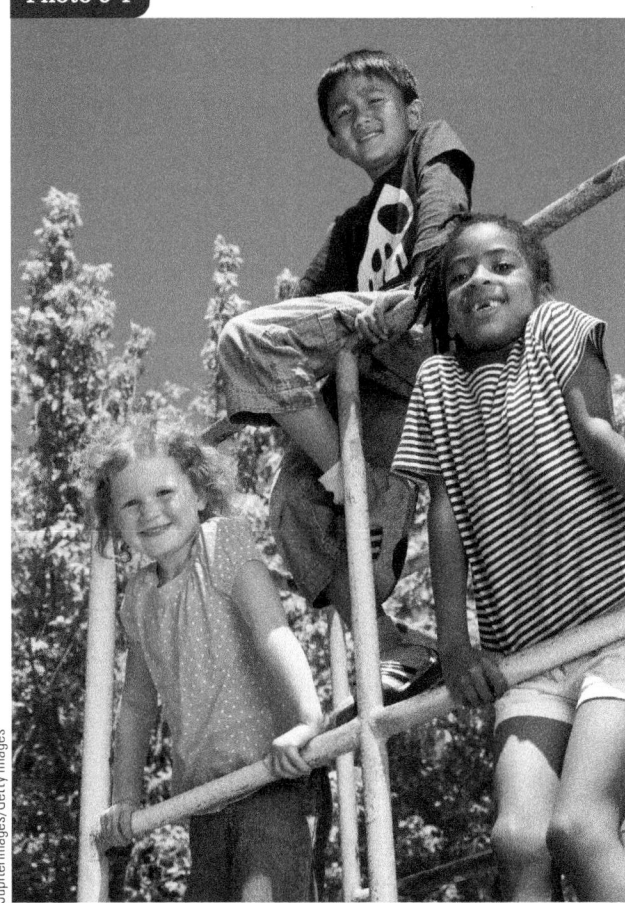

Photo 5-1

Jupiterimages/Getty Images

Growing children end each day with more bone, blood, muscle, and skin cells than they had at the beginning of the day.

Review Notes

- The process by which proteins are continually being made and broken down is known as protein turnover.
- The body needs dietary amino acids to grow new cells and to replace worn-out ones.
- When nitrogen intake equals nitrogen output, a person is in nitrogen equilibrium, or zero nitrogen balance.

nitrogen balance: the amount of nitrogen consumed (N in) as compared with the amount of nitrogen excreted (N out) in a given period of time. The laboratory scientist can estimate the protein in a sample of food, body tissue, or excreta by measuring the nitrogen in it.

5.4 Roles of Body Proteins

What distinguishes you chemically from any other human being are minute differences in your particular body proteins (enzymes, antibodies, and others). These differences are determined by your proteins' amino acid sequences, which are written into the genes you inherited from your parents and ancestors. The genes direct the making of all the body's proteins.

The human body has more than 20,000 genes that code for hundreds of thousands of proteins.[1] Relatively few proteins have been studied in detail, although this number is growing rapidly with the surge in knowledge gained from sequencing the

human genome. Only a few of the many roles proteins play are described here, but these should serve to illustrate proteins' versatility, uniqueness, and importance.

As Structural Components A great deal of the body's protein is found in muscle tissue, which allows the body to move. The amino acids of muscle protein can also be released when the need is dire, as in starvation. These amino acids are integral parts of the muscle structure, and their loss exacts a cost in functional protein, as a later section makes clear.

Other structural proteins confer shape and strength on bones, teeth, tendons, cartilage, blood vessels, and other tissues. These proteins exist in a stable form and are more resistant to breakdown than are the proteins of muscles.

As Enzymes **Enzymes** are catalysts that are essential to all life processes. Enzymes in the cells of plants or animals put together the pairs of sugars that make disaccharides and the long strands of sugars that make starch, cellulose, and glycogen. Enzymes also dismantle these compounds to free their constituent parts and release energy. Enzymes also assemble and disassemble lipids, assemble all other compounds that the body makes, and disassemble all compounds that the body can use for building tissue and other metabolic work. It is enzymes that put amino acids together to make needed proteins, too. In other words, these proteins can even make other proteins. As Figure 5-4 shows, enzymes themselves are not altered by the reactions they facilitate.

The protein story moves in a circle. To follow the circle in nutrition, start with a person eating food proteins. The food proteins are broken down by digestive enzymes, proteins themselves, into amino acids. The amino acids enter the cells of the body, where other proteins (enzymes) put the amino acids together in long chains whose sequences are specified by the genes. The chains fold and twist back on themselves to form proteins, and some of these proteins become enzymes themselves. Some of these enzymes break apart compounds; others put compounds together. Day by day, in billions of reactions, these processes repeat themselves, and life goes on. Only living systems can achieve such self-renewal. A toaster cannot produce another toaster; a car cannot fix a broken-down car. Only living creatures and the parts they are composed of—the cells—can duplicate and repair themselves.

As Transporters A large group of proteins specialize in transporting other substances, such as lipids, vitamins, and minerals, around the body. To do their jobs, those substances must move from place to place within the blood, into and out of cells, or around the cellular interiors. Two familiar examples: the protein hemoglobin transports oxygen from the lungs to the cells, and the lipoproteins transport lipids in the watery blood.

As Regulators of Fluid and Electrolyte Balance Proteins help maintain the body's **fluid and electrolyte balance.** As Figure 5-5 shows, the body's fluids are contained in three major body compartments: (1) the spaces inside the blood vessels, (2) the

---

human genome (GEE-nome): the complete set of genetic material (DNA) in a human being. (Nutritional genomics is the topic of Nutrition in Practice 13.)

enzymes: protein catalysts. A catalyst is a compound that facilitates chemical reactions without itself being changed in the process.

fluid and electrolyte balance: maintenance of the necessary amounts and types of fluid and minerals in each compartment of the body fluids.

edema (eh-DEEM-uh): the swelling of body tissue caused by leakage of fluid from the blood vessels and accumulation of the fluid in the interstitial spaces.

acids: compounds that release hydrogen ions in a solution.

bases: compounds that accept hydrogen ions in a solution.

acid–base balance: the balance maintained between acid and base concentrations in the blood and body fluids.

pH: the concentration of hydrogen ions. The lower the pH, the stronger the acid. Thus, pH 2 is a strong acid; pH 6 is a weak acid; pH 7 is neutral; and a pH above 7 is alkaline.

denaturation (dee-nay-cher-AY-shun): the change in a protein's shape brought about by heat, acid, or other agents. Past a certain point, denaturation is irreversible.

acidosis: acid accumulation in the blood and body fluids; depresses the central nervous system and can lead to disorientation and, eventually, coma.

FIGURE 5-4 Enzyme Action

Each enzyme facilitates a specific chemical reaction. In this diagram, an enzyme enables two compounds to make a more complex structure, but the enzyme itself remains unchanged.

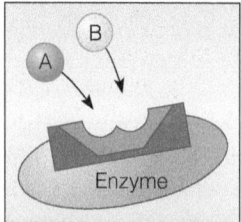

The separate compounds, A and B, are attracted to the enzyme's active site, making a reaction likely.

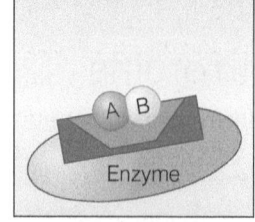

The enzyme forms a complex with A and B.

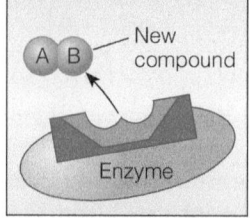

The enzyme is unchanged, but A and B have formed a new compound, AB.

spaces within the cells, and (3) the spaces between the cells (the interstitial spaces outside the blood vessels). Fluids flow back and forth between these compartments, and proteins in the fluids, together with minerals, help to maintain the needed distribution of these fluids.*

Proteins are able to help determine the distribution of fluids in living systems for two reasons: first, proteins cannot pass freely across the membranes that separate the body compartments and, second, they are attracted to water. A cell that "wants" a certain amount of water in its interior space cannot move the water around directly, but it can manufacture proteins, and these proteins will hold water. Thus, the cell can use proteins to help regulate the distribution of water indirectly. Similarly, the body makes proteins for the blood and the interstitial (intercellular) spaces. These proteins help maintain the fluid volume in those spaces. Excess fluid accumulation in the interstitial spaces is called **edema**.

Not only is the quantity of the body fluids vital to life, but so is their composition. Special transport proteins in the membranes of cells continuously transfer substances into and out of cells to maintain balance. For example, sodium is concentrated outside the cells, and potassium is concentrated inside. The balance of these two minerals is critical to nerve transmission and muscle contraction. Any disturbance in this balance triggers a major medical emergency. Such imbalances can cause irregular heartbeats, kidney failure, muscular weakness, and even death.

As Regulators of Acid–Base Balance Proteins also help maintain the balance between **acids** and **bases** within the body's fluids. Normal body processes continually produce acids and bases, which must be carried by the blood to the kidneys and lungs for excretion. The blood must do this without upsetting its own **acid–base balance**. Blood **pH** is one of the most tightly controlled conditions in the body. If the blood becomes too acidic, vital proteins may undergo **denaturation**, losing their shape and ability to function. A similar situation arises when there is an excess of base. These imbalances are known as **acidosis** and **alkalosis**, respectively, and both can be fatal.

Proteins such as albumin in blood help to prevent acid–base imbalances. In a sense, the proteins protect one another by gathering up extra acid (hydrogen) ions when there are too many in the surrounding medium and by releasing them when there are too few. By accepting and releasing hydrogen ions, proteins act as **buffers**, maintaining the acid–base balance of the blood and body fluids.

As Antibodies Proteins also defend the body against disease. A virus—whether it is one that causes flu, smallpox, measles, or the common cold—enters the cells and multiplies there. One virus may produce 100 replicas of itself within an hour or so. Each replica can then burst out and invade 100 different cells, soon yielding 10,000 viruses, which invade 10,000 cells. Left free to do their worst, they will soon overwhelm the body with disease.

Fortunately, when the body detects these invading **antigens**, it manufactures **antibodies**, giant protein molecules designed specifically to combat them. The antibodies work so swiftly and efficiently that in a healthy individual, most diseases never get started. Without sufficient protein, though, the body cannot maintain its army of antibodies to resist infectious diseases.

Each antibody is designed to destroy a specific antigen. Once the body has manufactured antibodies against a particular antigen (such as the measles virus), it "remembers" how to make them. Consequently, the next time the body encounters that same antigen, it produces antibodies even more quickly. In other words, the body develops a molecular memory, known as **immunity**. (Chapter 11 describes food allergies—the immune system's response to food antigens.)

As Hormones The blood also carries messenger molecules known as **hormones**, and *some* hormones are proteins. (Recall that some hormones are sterols, members of the

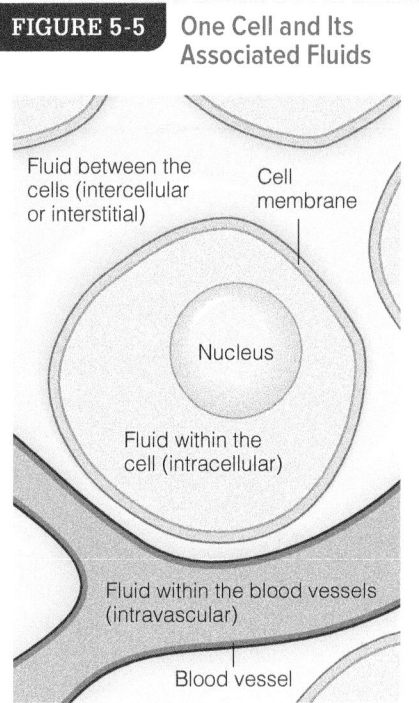

FIGURE 5-5 One Cell and Its Associated Fluids

Fluid between the cells (intercellular or interstitial)

Cell membrane

Nucleus

Fluid within the cell (intracellular)

Fluid within the blood vessels (intravascular)

Blood vessel

alkalosis: excessive base in the blood and body fluids.

buffers: compounds that can reversibly combine with hydrogen ions to help keep a solution's acidity or alkalinity constant.

antigens: substances that elicit the formation of antibodies or an inflammation reaction from the immune system. A bacterium, a virus, a toxin, and a protein in food that causes allergy are all examples of antigens.

antibodies: large proteins of the blood and body fluids, produced in response to invasion of the body by unfamiliar molecules (mostly proteins) called *antigens*. Antibodies inactivate the invaders and so protect the body.

anti = against

immunity: the body's ability to defend itself against diseases.

hormones: chemical messengers. Hormones are secreted by a variety of glands in the body in response to altered conditions. Each travels to one or more target tissues or organs and elicits specific responses to restore normal conditions.

---

*Minerals are helper nutrients. The attraction of protein and mineral particles to water is due to osmotic pressure (see Chapter 9).

Roles of Body Proteins 131

TABLE 5-2 Summary of Functions of Proteins

Structural components. Proteins form integral parts of most body tissues and confer shape and strength on bones, skin, tendons, and other tissues. Structural proteins of muscles allow movement.

Enzymes. Proteins facilitate chemical reactions.

Transporters. Proteins transport substances such as lipids, vitamins, minerals, and oxygen around the body.

Fluid and electrolyte balance. Proteins help to maintain the distribution and composition of various body fluids.

Acid–base balance. Proteins help maintain the acid–base balance of body fluids by acting as buffers.

Antibodies. Proteins inactivate disease-causing agents, thus protecting the body.

Hormones. Proteins regulate body processes. Some, but not all, hormones are proteins.

Energy and glucose. Proteins provide some fuel, and glucose if needed, for the body's energy needs.

Other. The protein fibrin creates blood clots; the protein collagen forms scars; the protein opsin participates in vision.

lipid family.) Among the proteins that act as hormones are glucagon and insulin. Hormones have many profound effects, which will become evident in subsequent chapters.

As a Source of Energy and Glucose Without energy, cells die; without glucose, the brain and nervous system falter. Even though amino acids are needed to do the work that only they can perform—build vital proteins—they will be sacrificed to provide energy and glucose during times of starvation or insufficient carbohydrate intake. When glucose or fatty acids are limited, cells are forced to use amino acids for energy and glucose. When amino acids are degraded for energy or converted into glucose, their nitrogen-containing amine groups are stripped off and used elsewhere or are incorporated by the liver into **urea** and sent to the kidneys for excretion in the urine. The fragments that remain are composed of carbon, hydrogen, and oxygen, as are carbohydrate and fat, and can be used to build glucose or fatty acids or can be metabolized like them.

The body does not make a specialized storage form of protein as it does for carbohydrate and fat. Glucose is stored as glycogen in the liver and muscles, fat as triglycerides in the adipose tissue, but body protein is available only as the working and structural components of the tissues. When the need arises, the body dismantles its tissue proteins and uses them for energy. Thus, over time, energy deprivation (starvation) always incurs wasting of lean body tissue as well as fat loss.

Review Notes

- The major functions of proteins are summarized in Table 5-2. This list, though by no means exhaustive, highlights the immense variety of proteins and their importance in the body.

5.5 Protein and Health

No nutrient has been more intensely scrutinized than protein. As you know by now, it is indispensable to life. And it should come as no surprise that protein deficiency can have devastating effects on people's health. But, as with the other nutrients, overconsumption of protein can be harmful, too, so this section also discusses the consequences of protein excess.

Protein Deficiency

In protein deficiency, when the diet supplies too little protein or lacks a specific essential amino acid relative to the others (a limiting amino acid), the body slows its synthesis of proteins while increasing its breakdown of body tissue protein to liberate the amino acids it needs to build other proteins of critical importance. When these proteins are not available to perform their roles, many of the body's life-sustaining activities come to a halt. The most recognizable consequences of protein deficiency include slow growth in children, impaired brain and kidney functions, weakened immune defenses, and impaired nutrient absorption from the digestive tract.

Malnutrition

In clinical settings, the term *protein-energy malnutrition (PEM)* has traditionally been used to describe the condition that develops when the diet delivers too little protein, too little energy, or both. PEM can be a consequence of many different conditions. PEM has been recognized in people with many chronic diseases such as cancer and AIDS and in those experiencing severe stresses such as burns or extensive infections (see Chapter 16).

The causes and consequences of PEM are complex, but clearly, such malnutrition reflects insufficient food intake. Importantly, not only are protein and energy inadequate, but so are many, if not all, of the vitamins and minerals. For this reason, the term **severe acute malnutrition (SAM)** is now used to describe severely malnourished infants and children. SAM most often occurs when food suddenly becomes unavailable, such as in drought or war. Less immediately deadly but still damaging to health is **chronic malnutrition**, the unrelenting, chronic food deprivation that occurs in areas where food supplies are usually meager and food quality is low. Table 5-3 compares key features of SAM with those of chronic malnutrition.

Each year, 6.3 million children younger than age 5 die—and 45 percent of these deaths are linked to malnutrition.[2] Most of these children do not starve to death—they die from the diarrhea and dehydration that accompany infections.

Severe Acute Malnutrition About 10 percent of the world's children suffer from the most severe form of SAM, often identified by their degree of **wasting**. In this form of SAM, called **marasmus**, lean and fat tissues have wasted away, broken down to provide energy to sustain life. These children weigh too little for their height and their upper arm circumference is smaller than normal.[3] Metabolism slows, so the child often feels cold and is obviously ill. As the photo on the left in Figure 5-6 shows, marasmic children look like little old people—just skin and bones.

severe acute malnutrition (SAM): malnutrition caused by recent severe food restriction; characterized in children by underweight for height (wasting).

chronic malnutrition: malnutrition caused by long-term food deprivation; characterized in children by short height for age (stunting).

wasting: in malnutrition, thinness for height, indicating recent rapid weight loss, often from severe, acute malnutrition.

marasmus (ma-RAZZ-mus): severe malnutrition characterized by poor growth, dramatic weight loss, loss of body fat and muscle, and apathy.

FIGURE 5-6 Malnourished Children

In the photo on the left, the extreme loss of muscle and fat characteristic of marasmus is apparent in the child's matchstick arms. In contrast, the edema characteristic of kwashiorkor is apparent in the child's swollen belly in the photo on the right.

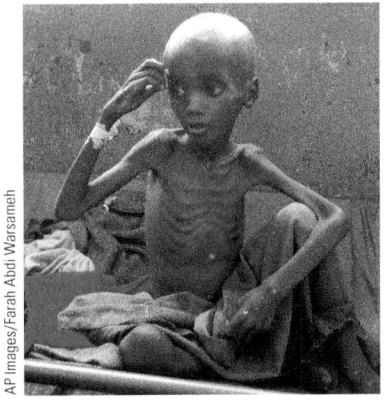
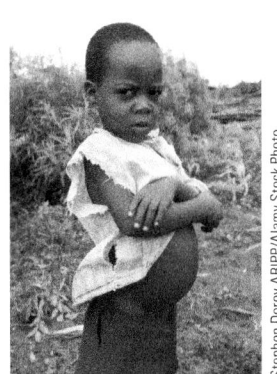

AP Images/Farah Abdi Warsameh

Stephen Dorey ABIPP/Alamy Stock Photo

TABLE 5-3 Severe Acute Malnutrition and Chronic Malnutrition Compared

	SEVERE ACUTE MALNUTRITION	CHRONIC MALNUTRITION
Food deprivation	Current or recent	Long term
Physical features	Rapid weight loss	Stunting (low height for age)
	Wasting (underweight for height; small upper arm circumference; marasmus)	
	Edema (kwashiorkor)	

Note: Vitamin and mineral deficiencies are common in both of these types of malnutrition.

Sometimes the starving child faces this threat to life by engaging in as little activity as possible—not even crying for food. Other children cry inconsolably. All of the muscles, including the heart muscle, weaken and deteriorate. Enzymes are in short supply, and the digestive tract lining deteriorates. Consequently, what little food is eaten often cannot be absorbed.

Marasmus reflects a severe, unrelenting deprivation of food observed in children living in war-torn, overpopulated, and impoverished nations. Children living in such severe poverty simply do not have enough food to protect body tissues from being degraded for energy.

A less common form of SAM is **kwashiorkor**. As the photo on the right in Figure 5-6 shows, the distinguishing feature of kwashiorkor is edema, in which fluids shift out of the blood and into the tissues, causing swelling.[4] Other common symptoms include loss of hair color and the development of patchy, scaly skin, often with sores that fail to heal. In a dangerous combination condition—**marasmic kwashiorkor**—muscles waste, but the wasting may not be apparent because the child's face, limbs, and abdomen are swollen with edema. Historically, kwashiorkor was attributed to too little protein in the diet, but today, researchers recognize that the sparse diets of children with the various forms of SAM do not differ much—all lack protein and many other nutrients.[5]

Chronic Malnutrition   A much greater number of children live with chronic malnutrition. They subsist on diluted cereal drinks that supply little energy and even less protein; such food allows them to survive but not to thrive. Intestinal parasites rob them of ingested nutrients as well.[6] These children are short for their age—they stop growing because they chronically lack the nutrients required for normal growth (described as **stunting**). Though they may appear normal because their bodies are proportionate, these stunted children may be no larger at age 4 than at age 2 and they often suffer the miseries of malnutrition: increased risks of infection and diarrhea along with vitamin and mineral deficiencies.

A fully nourished developing brain usually grows to almost its full adult size within the first two years of life. When malnutrition occurs during these years, it can impair brain development and learning ability, sometimes irreversibly.

Rehabilitation   Ideally, optimal breastfeeding and improved complementary feedings would prevent malnutrition and save the lives of children. Once a child becomes malnourished, however, loss of appetite and impaired food assimilation interfere with attempts to provide nourishment. To restore metabolic balance and promote physical growth, mental development, and recovery from illnesses, malnourished children need specially formulated fluids and foods. SAM demands hospitalization, including intensive nursing care, medical nutrition therapy, and medication, particularly when complications develop.

Experts assure us that we possess the knowledge, technology, and resources to end the hunger that leads to SAM. Programs that have involved the local people in the process of identifying the problem and devising its solution have met with some success. Until those who have the food, technology, and resources make fighting hunger a priority, however, the war on hunger will not be won.

Protein Excess

While many of the world's people struggle to obtain enough food and enough protein to survive, in the developed nations protein is so abundant that problems of protein excess are observed. Overconsumption of protein offers no benefits and may pose a health risk for people with chronic kidney disease.[7]

Heart Disease   Protein itself is not known to contribute to heart disease and mortality but some of its food sources may do so. Selecting too many animal-derived protein foods—such as fatty red meats, processed meats, and fat-containing milk products—adds a burden of saturated fat to the diet and crowds out fruit, vegetables, legumes, nuts, and whole grains. Consequently, it is not surprising that people who eat substantial amounts of animal protein, particularly **processed meat** such as lunch

kwashiorkor: severe malnutrition characterized by failure to grow and develop, edema, changes in the pigmentation of the hair and skin, fatty liver, anemia, and apathy.

marasmic kwashiorkor: a particularly lethal form of SAM, in which a child's dangerous loss of lean tissue (wasting) is masked by edema, making it harder to detect.

stunting: low height for age, indicating restriction of potential growth in children.

processed meat: meat that has been preserved or flavored by additives, curing, salting, or smoking. Examples include bacon, ham, hot dogs, jerky, luncheon meats, salami, and other sausages.

meats and hot dogs—have higher body weights and a greater risk of obesity, heart disease, and diabetes than those who eat less.[8] As the Nutrition in Practice points out, people who substitute vegetable protein for animal protein may improve risk factors for chronic diseases and mortality.[9]

Kidney Disease Excretion of the end products of protein metabolism depends, in part, on an adequate fluid intake and healthy kidneys. A high protein intake increases the work of the kidneys but does not appear to damage healthy kidneys or cause kidney disease.[10] In people with chronic kidney disease, however, a high-protein diet may accelerate the kidneys' decline. For people with established kidney problems, a moderately lower protein intake often improves the symptoms of their disease (see Chapter 22).[11]

Review Notes

- Children suffering from severe acute malnutrition (SAM) may be underweight for their height (due to wasting), while those experiencing chronic malnutrition are short for their age (known as stunting).
- Kwashiorkor and marasmus are two forms of SAM.
- Excesses of protein offer no advantage; in fact, overconsumption of certain protein-rich foods may contribute to health problems.

Protein and Amino Acid Supplements

Why do people take protein or amino acid supplements? Athletes often take them when trying to build muscle. Dieters may take them to spare their bodies' protein while losing weight. Some women take them to strengthen their fingernails. People take individual amino acid supplements, too—to cure herpes, to improve sleep, to lose weight, and to relieve pain and depression. Do protein and amino acid supplements really do these things? Probably not. Are they safe? Not always.

Protein Supplements Though protein supplements are popular with athletes, well-fed athletes do not need them. Dietary protein is necessary for building muscle tissue, and consuming protein in conjunction with resistance exercise helps muscles build new proteins.[12] Protein supplements, however, do not improve athletic performance beyond the gains from well-timed meals of ordinary foods.

Weight-loss dieters may benefit from consistently consuming protein-rich foods because protein often satisfies the appetite. Research is ongoing to determine whether sufficient protein content of a meal may help to prolong feelings of fullness or delay the urge to eat.[13] However, extra protein from powders, pills, or beverages is unlikely to dampen the appetite further, although it contributes unneeded kcalories—the wrong effect for weight loss. Evidence does not support taking protein supplements for weight loss, and common sense opposes it.

Amino Acid Supplements Enthusiastic popular reports have led to widespread use of individual amino acids. One such amino acid is lysine, promoted to prevent or relieve the infections that cause herpes sores on the mouth or genital organs. Lysine does not cure herpes infections.[14] Whether it reduces outbreaks or even whether it is safe is unknown because scientific studies are lacking.

Tryptophan supplements are advertised to relieve pain, depression, and insomnia. Tryptophan plays a role as a precursor for the brain neurotransmitter serotonin, an important regulator of sleep, appetite, mood, and sensory perception. The DRI committee concludes that high doses of tryptophan may induce sleepiness, but they may also cause nausea and other unpleasant side effects.

TABLE 5-4 **People Most Likely to Be Harmed by Amino Acid Supplements**

Growth or altered metabolism makes these people especially likely to be harmed by self-prescribed amino acid supplements.

- All women of childbearing age
- Pregnant or lactating women
- Infants, children, and adolescents
- Older adults
- People with inborn errors of metabolism that affect their bodies' handling of amino acids
- Smokers
- People on low-protein diets
- People with chronic or acute mental or physical illnesses who take amino acids without medical supervision

The body is designed to handle whole proteins best. It breaks them into manageable pieces (dipeptides and tripeptides) and then splits these, a few at a time, simultaneously releasing them into the blood. This slow bit-by-bit assimilation is ideal because groups of chemically similar amino acids compete for the carriers that absorb them into the blood. An excess of one amino acid can produce such a demand for a carrier that it limits the absorption of another amino acid, creating a temporary imbalance.

The DRI committee reviewed the available research on amino acids, but with next to no safety research in existence, the committee was unable to set Tolerable Upper Intake Levels for supplemental doses. Until research becomes available, no level of amino acid supplementation can be assumed to be safe for all people (see Table 5-4). A known side effect of these products is digestive disturbances: amino acids in concentrated supplements cause excess water to flow into the digestive tract, causing diarrhea. Anyone considering taking amino acid supplements should be cautious not to exceed levels normally found in foods.

Protein Recommendations and Intakes

The committee that established the RDA states that a generous daily protein allowance for a healthy adult is 0.8 gram per kilogram (2.2 pounds) of healthy body weight. The RDA covers the needs for replacing worn-out tissue, so it increases for larger people; it also covers the needs for building new tissue during growth, so it is slightly higher for infants, children, and pregnant and lactating women. Box 5-1 describes how to calculate your RDA for protein.

In setting the RDA, the committee assumes that the protein eaten will be of good quality, that it will be consumed together with adequate energy from carbohydrate and fat, and that other nutrients in the diet will be adequate. The committee also assumes that the RDA will be applied only to healthy individuals with no unusual alteration of protein metabolism.

Most people assume that Americans eat too much protein. Research demonstrates that the average protein intake for U.S. adult males is about 16 percent of total kcalories, an amount that falls directly within the DRI suggested range of between 10 and 35 percent of kcalories. Women, children, and some older adults may typically take in less protein—13 to 15 percent. A small percentage of adolescent girls and elderly women consume insufficient protein or barely enough to meet their needs.

Box 5-1 ***HOW TO* Calculate Recommended Protein Intakes**

To calculate your protein RDA:

- Look up the healthy weight for a person of your height (inside back cover). If your present weight falls within that range, use it for the following calculations. If your present weight falls outside the range, use the midpoint of the healthy weight range as your reference weight.

- Convert pounds to kilograms, if necessary (pounds divided by 2.2 equals kilograms).

- Multiply kilograms by 0.8 to get your RDA in grams per day. (Teens 14 to 18 years old, multiply by 0.85.)

    Example:
    Weight = 150 lb
    150 lb ÷ 2.2 lb/kg = 68 kg
    68 kg × 0.8 g/kg = 54 g protein (rounded off)

Review Notes

- Normal, healthy people do not need amino acid or protein supplements.
- Optimally, an adult's diet will be adequate in energy from carbohydrate and fat and will deliver at least 0.8 grams of protein per kilogram of healthy body weight each day.

5.6 Protein in Foods

In the United States and Canada, where nutritious foods are abundant, most people easily obtain enough protein to receive all the amino acids that they need. In countries where food is scarce and the people eat only marginal amounts of protein-rich foods, however, the *quality* of the protein becomes crucial.

Protein Quality

The protein quality of the diet determines, in large part, how well children grow and how well adults maintain their health. Put simply, **high-quality proteins** provide enough of all the essential amino acids needed to support the body's work, and low-quality proteins don't. Two factors influence protein quality: the protein's digestibility and its amino acid composition.

Digestibility As explained earlier, proteins must be digested before they can provide amino acids. **Protein digestibility** depends on such factors as the protein's source and the other foods eaten with it. The digestibility of most animal proteins is high (90 to 99 percent); plant proteins are less digestible (70 to 90 percent for most, but more than 90 percent for soy).

Amino Acid Composition To make proteins, cells must have all the needed amino acids available simultaneously. The liver can produce any nonessential amino acid that may be in short supply so that the cells can continue linking amino acids into protein strands. If an essential amino acid is missing, however, a cell must dismantle its own proteins to obtain it. Therefore, to prevent protein breakdown, dietary protein must supply at least the nine essential amino acids plus enough nitrogen-containing amino groups and energy for the synthesis of the others. If the diet supplies too little of any essential amino acid, protein synthesis will be limited. The body makes whole proteins only; if one amino acid is missing, the others cannot form a "partial" protein. An essential amino acid that is available in the shortest supply relative to the amount needed to support protein synthesis is called a **limiting amino acid**.

High-Quality Proteins A high-quality protein contains all the essential amino acids in amounts adequate for human use; it may or may not contain all the others. Generally, proteins derived from animal foods (meat, seafood, poultry, cheese, eggs, and milk and milk products) are high quality, although gelatin is an exception. Proteins derived from plant foods (legumes, grains, nuts, seeds, and vegetables) tend to be limiting in one or more essential amino acids. Some plant proteins are notoriously low quality—for example, corn protein. Others are high quality—for example, soy protein. As discussed in Nutrition in Practice 5, the educated vegetarian can design a diet that is adequate in protein by choosing a variety of legumes, whole grains, nuts, and vegetables (see Photo 5-2). Table 5-5 lists the protein contents of foods based on the USDA food groups presented in Chapter 1. Fruit is not included in Table 5-5 because it contributes only small amounts of protein.

Complementary Proteins If the body does not receive all the essential amino acids it needs, the supply of essential amino acids will dwindle until body organs are compromised. Obtaining enough essential amino acids presents no problem to people who regularly eat high-quality proteins, such as those of meat, seafood, poultry, cheese, eggs, milk, and many soybean products. The proteins of these foods contain ample amounts of all the essential amino acids. An equally

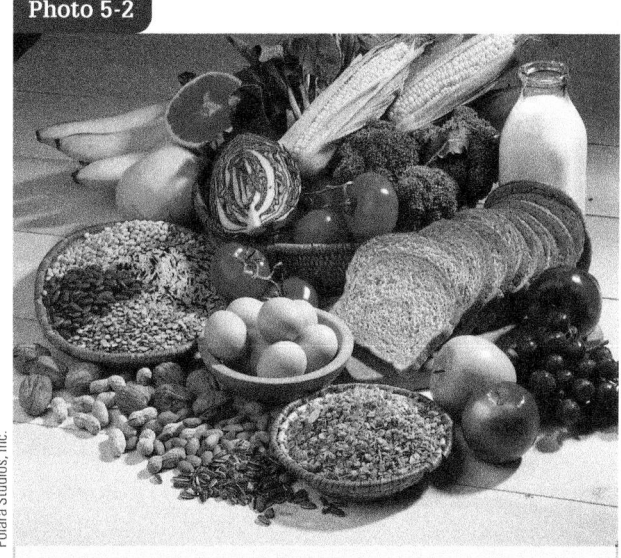

Photo 5-2

Vegetarians obtain their protein from whole grains, legumes, nuts, vegetables, and, in some cases, eggs and milk products.

Polara Studios, Inc.

TABLE 5-5 Protein-Containing Foods

MILK AND MILK PRODUCTS

Each of the following provides about 8 g of protein:
- 1 c milk, buttermilk, or yogurt (choose low-fat or fat-free)
- 1 oz regular cheese (for example, cheddar or Swiss; choose low-fat)
- ¼ c cottage cheese (choose low-fat or fat-free)

PROTEIN FOODS

Each of the following provides about 7 g of protein:
- 1 oz meat, poultry, or fish (choose lean meats to limit saturated fat intake)
- ½ c legumes (navy beans, pinto beans, black beans, lentils, soybeans, and other dried beans and peas)
- 1 egg
- ½ c tofu (soybean curd)
- 2 tbs peanut butter
- 1 to 2 oz nuts or seeds

GRAINS

Each of the following provides about 3 g of protein:
- 1 slice of bread
- ½ c cooked rice, pasta, cereals, or other grain foods

VEGETABLES

Each of the following provides about 2 g of protein:
- ½ c cooked vegetables
- 1 c raw vegetables

FIGURE 5-7 Complementary Proteins

In general, legumes provide plenty of isoleucine (Ile) and lysine (Lys) but fall short in methionine (Met) and tryptophan (Trp). Grains have the opposite strengths and weaknesses, making them a perfect match for legumes.

	Ile	Lys	Met	Trp
Legumes	✓	✓		
Grains			✓	✓
Together	✓	✓	✓	✓

complementary proteins: two or more proteins whose amino acid assortments complement each other in such a way that the essential amino acids missing from one are supplied by the other.

sound choice is to eat two different protein foods from plants so that each supplies the amino acids missing in the other. In this strategy, the two protein-rich foods are combined to yield **complementary proteins** (see Figure 5-7)—proteins containing all the essential amino acids in amounts sufficient to support health. The two proteins need not even be eaten together, as long as the day's meals supply them both, and the diet provides enough energy and total protein from a variety of sources.

Protein Sparing

Dietary protein—no matter how high the quality—will not be used efficiently and will not support growth when energy from carbohydrate and fat is lacking. The body assigns top priority to meeting its energy need and, if necessary, will break down protein to meet this need. After stripping off and excreting the nitrogen from the amino acids, the body will use the remaining carbon skeletons in much the same way it uses those from glucose or fat. A major reason why people must have ample carbohydrate and fat in the diet is to prevent this wasting of protein. Carbohydrate and fat allow amino acids to be used to build body proteins. This is known as the *protein-sparing effect* of carbohydrate and fat.

Protein on Food Labels

All food labels must state the *quantity* of protein in grams. The "percent Daily Value" for protein is not mandatory on all labels, but it is required whenever a food makes a protein claim or is intended for consumption by children younger than age four. Whenever the Daily Value percentage is declared, researchers must determine the *quality* of the protein. Thus, when a % Daily Value is stated for protein, it reflects both quantity and quality.

Review Notes

- A diet inadequate in any of the essential amino acids limits protein synthesis.
- The best guarantee of amino acid adequacy is to eat foods containing high-quality proteins or combinations of foods containing complementary proteins so that each can supply the amino acids missing in the other.
- Vegetarians who consume no foods of animal origin can meet their protein needs by eating a variety of whole grains, legumes, seeds, nuts, and vegetables.
- Ample carbohydrate and fat in the diet allow amino acids to be used to build body proteins.
- All food labels must state the quantity of protein in grams.

Self Check

1. Proteins are chemically different from carbohydrates and fats because they also contain:
   a. iron.
   b. sodium.
   c. nitrogen.
   d. phosphorus.

2. The basic building blocks for protein are:
   a. side groups.
   b. amino acids.
   c. glucose units.
   d. saturated bonds.

3. Enzymes are proteins that, among other things:
   a. defend the body against disease.
   b. regulate fluid and electrolyte balance.
   c. facilitate chemical reactions by changing themselves.
   d. help assemble disaccharides into starch, cellulose, or glycogen.

4. Functions of proteins in the body include:
   a. supplying omega-3 fatty acids for growth, lowering serum cholesterol, and helping with weight control.
   b. supplying fiber to aid digestion, digesting cellulose, and providing the main fuel source for muscles.
   c. protecting organs against shock, helping the body use carbohydrate efficiently, and providing triglycerides.
   d. serving as structural components, supplying hormones to regulate body processes, and maintaining fluid and electrolyte balance.

5. The swelling of body tissue caused by the leakage of fluid from the blood vessels into the interstitial spaces is called:
   a. edema.
   b. anemia.
   c. acidosis.
   d. sickle-cell anemia.

6. Major proteins in the blood that protect against bacteria and other disease agents are called:
   a. acids.
   b. buffers.
   c. antigens.
   d. antibodies.

7. Marasmus can be distinguished from kwashiorkor because in marasmus:
   a. only adults are victims.
   b. the cause is usually an infection.
   c. severe wasting of body fat and muscle are evident.
   d. the limbs, face, and belly swell with edema.

8. The RDA for protein for a healthy adult is ____ gram(s) per kilogram of appropriate body weight for height.
   a. 0.5
   b. 0.8
   c. 1.1
   d. 1.4

9. Generally speaking, from which of the following foods are complete proteins derived?
   a. Milk, gelatin, and soy
   b. Rice, potatoes, and eggs
   c. Meats, fish, and poultry
   d. Vegetables, grains, and fruit

10. An incomplete protein lacks one or more:
    a. hydrogen bonds.
    b. essential fatty acids.
    c. dispensable amino acids.
    d. essential amino acids.

Answers: 1. c, 2. b, 3. d, 4. d, 5. a, 6. d, 7. c, 8. b, 9. c, 10. d

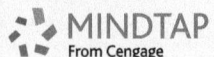
Clinical Applications

1. Considering the health effects of too little dietary protein, what suggestions would you have for a teenage girl who reports the following information about her food intake?

   - She never eats any meat or other animal-derived foods because she is a vegan. On a typical day, she consumes toast and juice for breakfast; chips, a soft drink, and a piece of fruit for lunch; and a small amount of plain pasta with tomato sauce or steamed vegetables for dinner, along with a glass of water or tea.

   - She takes amino acid supplements because a friend told her that the only way to get amino acids if she doesn't eat meat is to take them as supplements.

2. Considering the health effects of excess dietary protein, what advice would you have for a college athlete who tells you he wants to bulk up his muscles and reports the following information about his food intake?

   - He eats large portions of meat (usually red meat) at least twice a day. He drinks whole milk two or three times a day and eats eggs and bacon for breakfast almost every day.

   - He avoids breads, cereals, and pasta in order to save room for protein-rich foods such as meat, milk, and eggs.

   - He eats a piece of fruit once in a while but seldom eats vegetables because they are too time consuming to prepare.

Notes

1. Position of the Academy of Nutrition and Dietetics: Nutritional genomics, *Journal of the Academy of Nutrition and Dietetics* 114 (2014): 299–312.
2. World Health Organization, Fact sheet on child mortality, www.who.int /mediacentre/factsheets/fs178/en/, updated September 2016.
3. P. J. Becker and coauthors, Consensus statement of the Academy of Nutrition and Dietetics/American Society for Parenteral and Enteral Nutrition: Indicators recommended for the identification and Documentation of pediatric malnutrition (undernutrition), *Journal of the Academy of Nutrition and Dietetics* 114 (2014): 1988–2000.
4. I. Trehan and M. J. Manary, Management of severe acute malnutrition in low-income and middle-income countries, *Archives of Disease in Childhood* 100 (2015): 283–287.
5. R. L. Bailey, K. P. West, and R. E. Black, The epidemiology of global micronutrient deficiencies, *Annals of Nutrition and Metabolism* 66 (2015): 22–33.
6. B. de Gier and coauthors, Helminth infections and micronutrients in school-age children: A systematic review and meta-analysis, *American Journal of Clinical Nutrition* 99 (2014): 1499–1509.
7. M. Cuenca-Sánchez, D. Navas-Carrillo, and E. Orenes-Piñero, Controversies surrounding high-protein diet intake: Satiating effect and kidney and bone health, *Advances in Nutrition* 6 (2015): 260–266; E. Kanda and coauthors, Dietary acid intake and kidney disease progression in the elderly, *American Journal of Nephrology* 39 (2014): 145–152.
8. A. Etemadi and coauthors, Mortality from different causes associated with meat, heme iron, nitrates, and nitrites in the NIH-AARP Diet and Health Study: Population based cohort study, *BMJ* 357 (2017): j1957; X. Wang and coauthors, Red and processed meat consumption and mortality: Dose-response meta-analysis of prospective cohort studies, *Public Health Nutrition* 19 (2016): 893–905; P. Hernández-Alonso and coauthors, High dietary protein intake is associated with an increased body weight and total death risk, *Clinical Nutrition* 35 (2016): 496–506.
9. A. Satija and coauthors, Plant-based dietary patterns and incidence of type 2 diabetes in US men and women: Results from three prospective cohort studies, *PLos Medicine* 2016, dx.doi.org/10.137/journal. pmed.1002039; P. Tuso, S. R. Stoll, and W. W. Li, A plant-based diet,

atherogenesis, and coronary artery disease prevention, *Permanente Journal* 19 (2015):62–67; M. J. Orlich and coauthors, Vegetarian dietary patterns and the risk of colorectal cancers, *JAMA Internal Medicine* 175 (2015): 767–776; G. M. Turner-McGrievy and coauthors, Comparative effectiveness of plant-based diets for weight loss: A randomized controlled trial of five different diets, *Nutrition* 31 (2015): 350–358; P. N. Appleby and T. J. Key, The long-term health of vegetarians and vegans, *Proceedings of the Nutrition Society* 28 (2015): 1–7; Y. Yokoyama and coauthors, Vegetarian diets and blood pressure, *JAMA Internal Medicine* 174 (2014): 577–587.
10. Cuenca-Sánchz, Navas-Carrillo, and Orenes-Piñero, 2015.
11. J. A. Beto, W. E. Ramirez, and V. K. Bansal, Medical nutrition therapy in adults with chronic kidney disease: Integrating evidence and consensus into practice for the generalist Registered Dietitian Nutritionist, *Journal of the Academy of Nutrition and Dietetics* 114 (2014): 1077–1087; M. Giordano and coauthors, Long-term effects of moderate protein diet on renal function and low-grade inflammation in older adults with type 2 diabetes and chronic kidney disease, *Nutrition* 30 (2014): 1045–1049.
12. D. M. Camera and coauthors, Protein ingestion increases myofibrillar protein synthesis after concurrent exercise, *Medicine and Science in Sports and Exercise* 47 (2015): 82–91; C. Rosenbloom, Protein power, *Nutrition Today* 50 (2015): 72–77; O. C. Witard and coauthors, Myofibrillar muscle protein synthesis rates subsequent to a meal in response to increasing doses of whey protein at rest and after resistance exercise, *American Journal of Clinical Nutrition* 99 (2014): 86–95; J. L. Areta and coauthors, Timing and distribution of protein ingestion during prolonged recovery from resistance exercise alters myofibrillar protein synthesis, *Journal of Physiology* 591 (2013): 2319–2331.
13. S. M. Phillips, S. Chevalier, and H. J. Leidy, Protein "requirements" beyond the RDA: Implications for optimizing health, *Applied Physiology, Nutrition, and Metabolism* 41 (2016): 565-572; Cuenca-Sánchez, Navas-Carrillo, and Orenes-Piñero, 2015; D. H. Pesta and V. T. Samuel, A high-protein diet for reducing body fat: Mechanisms and possible caveats, *Nutrition and Metabolism* 11 (2014): 53.
14. C. C. Chi and coauthors, Interventions for prevention of herpes simplex labialis (cold sores on the lips), *Cochrane Database of Systematic Reviews* 8 (2015): CD010095.

5.7 Nutrition in Practice
Vegetarian Diets

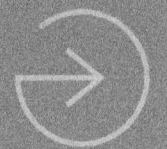

The quality of the diet depends not on whether it consists of all plant foods or centers on meat but on whether the eater's food choices are based on sound nutrition principles: adequacy of nutrient intakes, balance and variety of foods chosen, appropriate energy intake, and moderation in intakes of substances such as saturated fat, *trans* fat, added sugars, sodium, and alcohol that are harmful when consumed in excess.

The health benefits of a primarily **vegetarian diet** seem to have encouraged many people to reduce their consumption of meat and to eat more plant-based meals. The popular press sometimes refers to individuals who eat small amounts of meat, seafood, or poultry from time to time as "flexitarians."

People who choose to exclude meat and other animal-derived foods from their diets today do so for many of the same reasons the Greek philosopher Pythagoras cited in the 6th century B.C.: physical health, ecological responsibility, and philosophical concerns. Whatever their reasons, vegetarians and health professionals who work with them should be aware of the nutrition and health implications of vegetarian diets.

Vegetarian diets generally are categorized not by a person's motivation but by the foods that are excluded (see Box NP5-1). Because vegetarian diets vary in both the types and the amounts of animal-derived foods they include, these differences must be considered when evaluating the health status of vegetarians.

Are vegetarian diets nutritionally sound?

The Academy of Nutrition and Dietetics takes the position that well-planned vegetarian (and vegan) dietary patterns offer nutrition and health benefits to adults in general.[1]

Research suggests that meat-eating adults who switch to vegetarian eating patterns reduce their risks of heart disease, hypertension, diabetes, some types of cancer, and obesity.[2] Eating patterns that include very little, if any, meat are associated with a lower rate of death from all causes.[3]

What should be my main concerns when planning a nutritionally sound vegetarian diet?

A vegetarian diet planner faces the same task as other diet planners—obtaining a variety of foods that provide all the needed nutrients within an energy allowance that maintains a healthy body weight. The challenge is to do so without the use of some or all animal-derived foods. Because all vegetarians omit meat and some omit other animal-derived foods, protein—the nutrient that meat is famous for—merits some discussion here.

Isn't protein a problem in vegetarian diets?

No, protein is not the problem it was once thought to be in vegetarian eating patterns. People who include animal-derived foods such as milk and eggs in their diets need not worry at all about protein deficiency. Even for those who choose a **vegan diet**—which includes only plant-based foods—protein intakes are usually satisfactory as long as energy intakes are adequate and protein sources are varied.[4] A mixture of proteins from whole grains, legumes, seeds, nuts, and vegetables can provide adequate amounts of high-quality protein. An advantage of many vegetarian sources of protein is that they are generally lower in saturated fat than meat and are often high in fiber and richer in some vitamins and minerals.

Box NP5-1 Glossary

lacto-ovo vegetarian diet: an eating pattern that includes milk, milk products, eggs, vegetables, grains, legumes, fruit, and nuts; excludes meat, poultry, and seafood.

lacto-vegetarian diet: an eating pattern that includes milk, milk products, vegetables, grains, legumes, fruit, and nuts; excludes meat, poultry, seafood, and eggs.

macrobiotic diet: a philosophical eating pattern based on mostly plant foods such as whole grains, legumes, and certain vegetables, with small amounts of fish, fruit, nuts, and seeds.

ovo-vegetarian diet: an eating pattern that includes eggs, vegetables, grains, legumes, fruit, and nuts; excludes meat, poultry, seafood, and milk and milk products.

partial vegetarian diet: a term sometimes used to describe an eating pattern that includes seafood, poultry, eggs, milk and milk products, vegetables, grains, legumes, fruit, and nuts; excludes or strictly limits certain meats, such as red meat. Also called *semi-vegetarian.*

vegan diet: an eating pattern that includes only plant-based foods: vegetables, grains, legumes, fruit, seeds, and nuts; excludes all animal-derived foods. Also called *strict vegetarian, pure vegetarian,* or *total vegetarian.*

vegetarian diet: a general term used to describe an eating pattern that includes plant-based foods and eliminates some or all animal-derived foods.

Some vegetarians may use meat replacements made of textured vegetable protein (soy protein). These foods are formulated to look and taste like meat, fish, or poultry. Many of these products are fortified to provide the vitamins and minerals found in animal sources of protein. Some products, however, may fall short of providing the nutrients of meat, and they may be high in salt, sugar, or other additives. Labels list all of the ingredients in such foods. A wise vegetarian learns to use a variety of whole, unrefined foods often and commercially prepared foods less frequently. Vegetarians may also use soybeans in other forms, such as plain tofu (soybean curd), edamame (cooked green soybeans), or soy flour, to bolster protein intake without consuming unwanted salt, sugar, or other additives.

Do vegetarian diets provide appropriate food energy?

Researchers find that vegetarians as a group are closer to a healthy body weight than nonvegetarians.[5] Because obesity impairs health in a number of ways, vegetarians therefore have a health advantage. In general, vegetarian dietary patterns tend to be nutrient-dense and consistent with recommendations for weight management.

Not all vegetarians fit the average pattern, though. Obesity can be a concern for vegetarians who include whole milk, eggs, and cheese in their diets. They can easily consume excess saturated fat and food energy and so must be careful to select fat-free and low-fat milk and milk products and to avoid relying too heavily on these foods in general.

In contrast, eating patterns that exclude all animal-derived foods (vegan diets) may not provide *enough* food energy. This is especially true for children. Vegan diets can fail to provide food energy sufficient to support the growth of a child within a bulk of food small enough for the child to eat. Frequent meals of fortified breads, cereals, or pastas with legumes, nuts, nut butters, and sources of unsaturated fats can help to meet protein and energy needs in a smaller volume at each sitting. The MyPlate resources, introduced in Chapter 1, include tips for planning vegetarian diets.

How can vegetarians and health professionals who plan vegetarian meals best apply the USDA Food Patterns?

The Healthy Vegetarian Eating Pattern is flexible enough that a variety of people can use it: people who have adopted various vegetarian diets, those who want to make the transition to a vegetarian diet, and those who simply want to reduce their meat intake and include more plant-based meals in their diets. The Healthy Vegetarian Eating Pattern is similar to the Healthy U.S.-Style Eating Pattern presented in Chapter 1, with a slight increase in grain

servings and notable differences in the protein foods quantities and subgroups, as shown in Table NP5-1. Figure NP5-1 focuses on selections from the milk and milk products group and from the protein foods group because these groups are the focus of meal planning to ensure adequate nutrient intakes for vegetarians. For example, the protein foods group emphasizes legumes, nuts, seeds, and soy products in place of meat, poultry, and seafood, while the milk group features fortified soy milks for those who do not use milk, cheese, or yogurt.

When selecting from the vegetable and fruit groups, vegetarians may want to emphasize particularly good sources of calcium and iron, respectively. Some green leafy vegetables, for example, provide almost five times as much calcium per serving as other vegetables. Similarly, dried fruit deserves special notice in the fruit group because it delivers six times as much iron as other fruit.

Most vegetarians easily obtain large quantities of the nutrients that are abundant in plant foods: carbohydrate, fiber, thiamin, folate, vitamin B_6, vitamin C, vitamin A, and vitamin E. Well-planned vegetarian eating patterns help to ensure adequate intakes of the main nutrients vegetarian diets might otherwise lack: protein, iron, zinc, calcium, vitamin B_{12}, vitamin D, and omega-3 fatty acids. Table NP5-2 presents good vegetarian sources of these key nutrients. For example, the use of vegetable oils rich in unsaturated fats provides essential omega-3 fatty acids. To ensure adequate intakes of vitamin B_{12}, vitamin D, and calcium, vegetarians need to select fortified foods or use supplements daily.

Tell me about vitamins and minerals. Does a person eating a vegetarian diet need to take vitamin supplements?

That depends on the kind of vegetarian diet. The **lacto-ovo vegetarian diet** can be adequate in all vitamins, but for those who choose a vegan diet, several vitamins may be a problem. One such vitamin is B_{12}. Because vitamin B_{12} occurs only in animal-derived foods, regular use of either vitamin B_{12}–fortified foods—such as fortified soy and rice beverages, some breakfast cereals, and meat replacements—or supplements is necessary to prevent deficiency.[6] Women who have adhered to all-plant diets for many years are especially likely to have low vitamin B_{12} stores. Pregnant vegan women, whose needs for vitamin B_{12} are especially high, find it virtually impossible to maintain adequate vitamin B_{12} status without taking supplements or including a reliable food source of the nutrient.

People who stop eating animal-derived foods containing vitamin B_{12} may take several years to develop deficiency symptoms because the body recycles much of its vitamin B_{12}, reabsorbing it over and over again. Even when the body fails to absorb vitamin B_{12}, deficiency may take up to

USDA Food Patterns: Healthy Vegetarian Eating Pattern

The table first lists recommended amounts from each food group per day and then shows the amounts for vegetables and protein foods dispersed among subgroups per week. The rows highlighted in tan indicate which food groups and serving sizes differ from the Healthy U.S.-Style Eating Pattern (see Table 1-6 on p. 19, and Table 1-8 on p. 22).

RECOMMENDED DAILY AMOUNTS FROM EACH FOOD GROUP

FOOD GROUP	1600 kcal	1800 kcal	2000 kcal	2200 kcal	2400 kcal	2600 kcal	2800 kcal	3000 kcal
Fruit	1½ c	1½ c	2 c	2 c	2 c	2 c	2½ c	2½ c
Vegetables	2 c	2½ c	2½ c	3 c	3 c	3½ c	3½ c	4 c
Grains	5½ oz	6½ oz	6½ oz	7½ oz	8½ oz	9½ oz	10½ oz	10½ oz
Protein foods	2½ oz	3 oz	3½ oz	3½ oz	4 oz	4½ oz	5 oz	5½ oz
Milk and milk products	3 c	3 c	3 c	3 c	3 c	3 c	3 c	3 c
Oils	5 tsp	5 tsp	6 tsp	6 tsp	7 tsp	8 tsp	8 tsp	10 tsp
Limit on kcalories available for other uses[a]	180 kcal	190 kcal	290 kcal	330 kcal	390 kcal	390 kcal	400 kcal	440 kcal

RECOMMENDED WEEKLY AMOUNTS FROM EACH FOOD GROUP

	1600 kcal	1800 kcal	2000 kcal	2200 kcal	2400 kcal	2600 kcal	2800 kcal	3000 kcal
VEGETABLES SUBGROUPS								
Dark green	1½ c	1½ c	1½ c	2 c	2 c	2½ c	2½ c	2½ c
Red and orange	4 c	5½ c	5½ c	6 c	6 c	7 c	7 c	7½ c
Legumes	1 c	1½ c	1½ c	2 c	2 c	2½ c	2½ c	3 c
Starchy	4 c	5 c	5 c	6 c	6 c	7 c	7 c	8 c
Other	3½ c	4 c	4 c	5 c	5 c	5½ c	5½ c	7 c
PROTEIN FOODS SUBGROUPS								
Eggs	3 oz	3 oz	3 oz	3 oz	3 oz	3 oz	4 oz	4 oz
Legumes[b]	4 oz	6 oz	6 oz	6 oz	8 oz	9 oz	10 oz	11 oz
Soy products	6 oz	6 oz	8 oz	8 oz	9 oz	10 oz	11 oz	12 oz
Nuts and seeds	5 oz	6 oz	7 oz	7 oz	8 oz	9 oz	10 oz	12 oz

[a]The limit on kcalories for other uses describes how many kcalories are available for foods that are not in nutrient-dense forms, discussed on p. 22.

[b]About half of total legumes are listed as vegetables (measured in cup-equivalents) and half as protein foods (measured in ounce-equivalents); an ounce-equivalent of legumes in the protein foods subgroup is equal to ¼ cup. To convert legumes from the protein foods subgroup from ounce-equivalents to cups, divide by 4. Using the 1600-kcalorie recommendations for an example, the total legumes would be 2 cups—1 cup from the vegetable subgroup and the 1 cup from the protein foods subgroup (1 oz = ¼ cup; therefore, 4 oz = 1 cup).

Note: Milk and eggs are included in the Healthy Vegetarian Eating Pattern because they are commonly consumed as part of most vegetarian diets. To plan vegan diets, use fortified soy beverages (soymilk) or other plant-based dairy substitutes instead of milk and milk products and replace eggs with legumes, soy products, and nuts and seeds.

Source: U.S. Department of Health and Human Services and U.S. Department of Agriculture. *2015–2020 Dietary Guidelines for Americans*, 8th ed. (December 2015), health.gov/dietaryguidelines/2015/guidelines/.

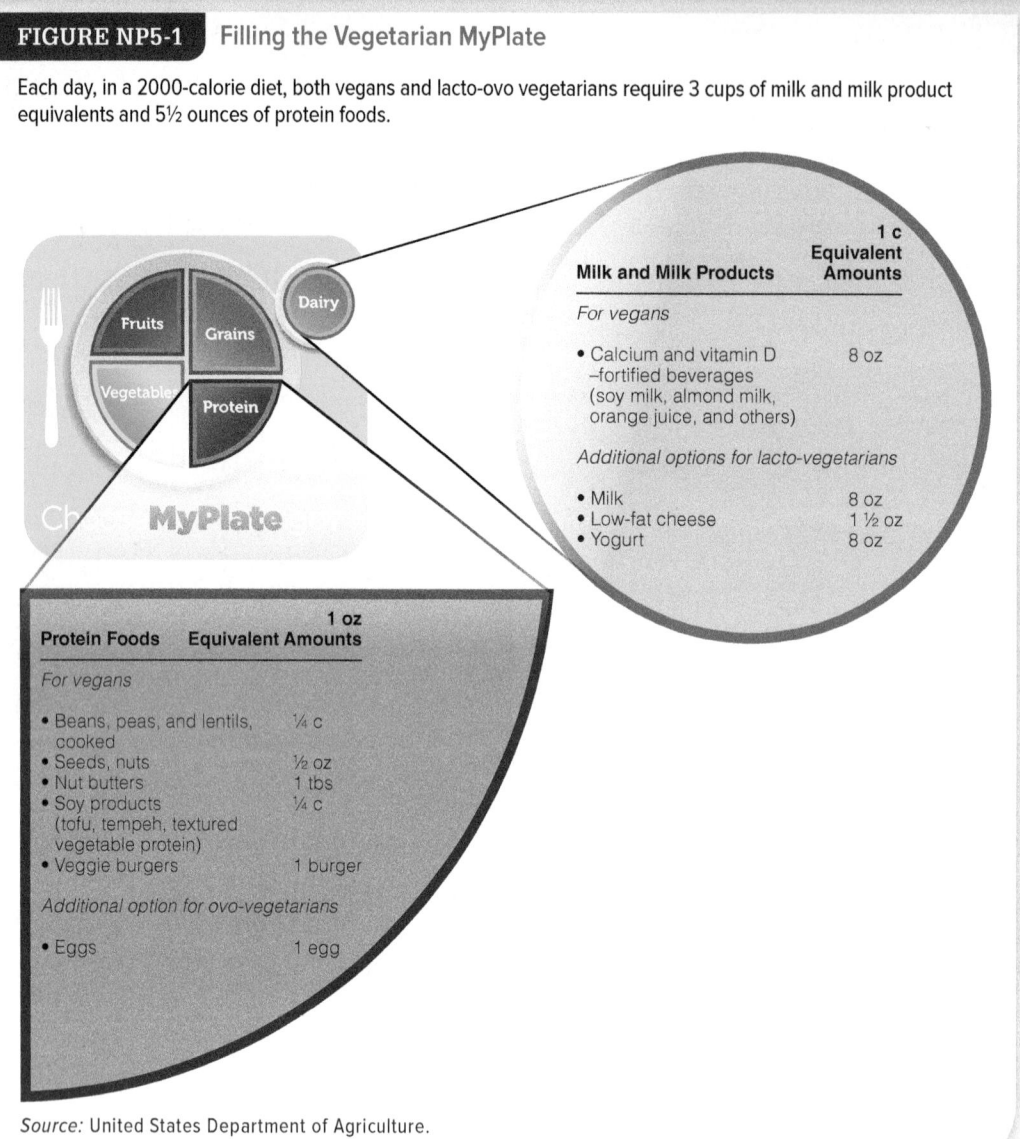

FIGURE NP5-1 Filling the Vegetarian MyPlate

Each day, in a 2000-calorie diet, both vegans and lacto-ovo vegetarians require 3 cups of milk and milk product equivalents and 5½ ounces of protein foods.

Milk and Milk Products	1 c Equivalent Amounts
For vegans	
• Calcium and vitamin D –fortified beverages (soy milk, almond milk, orange juice, and others)	8 oz
Additional options for lacto-vegetarians	
• Milk	8 oz
• Low-fat cheese	1 ½ oz
• Yogurt	8 oz

Protein Foods Equivalent Amounts	1 oz
For vegans	
• Beans, peas, and lentils, cooked	¼ c
• Seeds, nuts	½ oz
• Nut butters	1 tbs
• Soy products (tofu, tempeh, textured vegetable protein)	¼ c
• Veggie burgers	1 burger
Additional option for ovo-vegetarians	
• Eggs	1 egg

Source: United States Department of Agriculture.

three years to develop because the body conserves its supply. For pregnant and lactating women, obtaining vitamin B₁₂ is critical to prevent serious deficiency-related disorders that develop in infants who do not receive sufficient vitamin B₁₂. All vegan mothers must be sure to take the appropriate supplements or to use vitamin B₁₂–fortified products.

Do vegans, who do not drink vitamin D–fortified cow's milk, get enough vitamin D?

Overall, vegetarians are similar to nonvegetarians in their vitamin D status; factors such as taking supplements, skin color, and sun exposure have a greater influence on vitamin D than diet. People who do not use vitamin D–fortified foods and do not receive enough exposure to sunlight to synthesize adequate vitamin D may need

supplements to fend off bone loss. Of particular concern are infants, children, and older adults in northern climates during winter months.

So, on a vegan diet, vitamin B₁₂ and vitamin D can be problems if a person is not careful. What about minerals?

For *all* vegetarians, not just vegans, two minerals may be of concern: iron and zinc. The iron in plant foods such as legumes, dark green leafy vegetables, iron-fortified cereals, and whole-grain breads and cereals is not as absorbable as that in meat. For this reason, the iron recommendation for adult vegetarian men, premenopausal women, and adolescent girls is almost double the recommendation for meat eaters of the same gender and age.

FOOD GROUPS

Nutrients	Grains	Vegetables	Fruit	Protein-Rich Foods	Milk or Soy milk	Oils
Protein	Whole grains[a]			Legumes, seeds, nuts, nut butters, soy products (tempeh, tofu, veggie burgers)[a] Eggs (for ovo-vegetarians)	Milk, cheese, yogurt (for lacto-vegetarians) Soy milk, soy yogurt, soy cheeses	
Iron	Fortified cereals, enriched and whole grains	Dark green leafy vegetables (spinach, turnip greens)	Dried fruit (apricots, prunes, raisins)	Legumes (black-eyed peas, kidney beans, lentils), soy products		
Zinc	Fortified cereals, whole grains			Legumes (garbanzo beans, kidney beans, navy beans), nuts, seeds (pumpkin seeds)	Milk, cheese, yogurt (for lacto-vegetarians) Soy milk, soy yogurt, soy cheeses	
Calcium	Fortified cereals	Dark green leafy vegetables (bok choy, broccoli, collard greens, kale, mustard greens, turnip greens, watercress)	Fortified juices, figs	Fortified soy products, nuts (almonds), seeds (sesame seeds)	Milk, cheese, yogurt (for lacto-vegetarians) Fortified soy milk, fortified soy yogurt, fortified soy cheese	
Vitamin B$_{12}$	Fortified cereals			Eggs (for ovo-vegetarians) Fortified soy products	Milk, cheese, yogurt (for lacto-vegetarians) Fortified soy milk, fortified soy yogurt, fortified soy cheese	
Vitamin D	Fortified cereals				Milk, cheese, yogurt (for lacto-vegetarians) Fortified soy milk, fortified soy yogurt, fortified soy cheese	
Omega-3 Fatty Acids		Marine algae and its oils		Flaxseed, walnuts, soybeans Fortified margarine Fortified eggs (for ovo-vegetarians)	Fortified soy milk	Flaxseed oil, walnut oil, soybean oil

[a] As Chapter 5 explains, many plant proteins do not contain all the essential amino acids in the amounts and proportions needed by human beings. To improve protein quality, vegetarians can eat grains and legumes together, for example, although it is not necessary if protein intake is varied and energy intake is sufficient.

Fortunately, the body seems to adapt to a vegetarian diet by absorbing iron more efficiently. Furthermore, iron absorption is enhanced by vitamin C, and vegetarians typically eat many vitamin C–rich fruit and vegetables. Consequently, vegetarians suffer no more iron deficiency than other people do.

Zinc is similar to iron in that meat is its richest food source, and zinc from plant sources is not as well absorbed. In addition, phytates, fiber, and calcium, which are common in vegetarian diets, interfere with zinc absorption. The zinc needs of vegetarians and the effects of mineral binders are subjects of intensive study at the present time. While research continues, vegetarians are advised to eat varied diets that include legumes such as navy beans and kidney beans, zinc-enriched cereals, and whole-grain breads well leavened with yeast, which improves the availability of their minerals.

What about calcium for the vegan?

Good thinking. Yes, calcium is of concern. The milk-drinking vegetarian is protected from deficiency, but the vegan must find other sources of calcium. Some good calcium sources are regular and ample servings of dark green leafy vegetables such as kale and collard; legumes; calcium-fortified foods such as breakfast cereals, soy milk, and orange juice; some nuts such as almonds; and certain seeds such as sesame seeds. The choices should be varied because binders in some of these foods may hinder calcium absorption. The vegan is urged to use calcium-fortified soy milk in ample quantities regularly. This is especially important for children. Infant formula based on soy is fortified with calcium and can easily be used in food preparation, even for adults.

Do vegetarian diets provide adequate amounts of the essential fatty acids?

Vegetarian diets typically provide enough of the essential fatty acids linoleic acid and linolenic acid, but they lack a dietary source of EPA and DHA. Fatty fish and DHA-fortified eggs and other products can provide EPA and DHA, but fortified sources that ultimately derive from fish are unacceptable for vegans. Alternatively, certain marine algae and their oils provide DHA, and vegans can select foods fortified with such oils, which are listed among the ingredients on a food's label. A vegetarian's daily diet should include small amounts of flaxseed, walnuts, and their oils, as well as soybeans and canola oil to provide essential fatty acids.

Are there any other health advantages to the vegetarian diet?

Yes. Vegetarian protein foods are often higher in fiber, richer in certain vitamins and minerals, and lower in fat—especially saturated fat—than meats. Vegetarians can enjoy a nutritious diet low in saturated fat provided that they limit foods such as butter, cream cheese, and sour cream. If vegetarians follow the guidelines presented here and plan carefully, they can support their health as well as, or perhaps better than, nonvegetarians.

Abundant evidence supports the idea that vegetarians may actually be healthier than meat eaters. Informed vegetarians are not only more likely to be at the desired weights for their heights, but they are also more likely to have lower blood cholesterol levels, lower rates of certain kinds of cancer, better digestive function, and more. Even among people who are health conscious, generally vegetarians experience fewer deaths from cardiovascular disease than meat eaters do. Because many vegetarians also abstain from smoking and the consumption of alcohol, dietary practices alone probably do not account for all the aspects of improved health. Clearly, however, they contribute significantly to it.

Notes

1. Position of the Academy of Nutrition and Dietetics: Vegetarian diets, *Journal of the Academy of Nutrition and Dietetics* 116 (2016): 1970–1980.
2. A. Satija and coauthors, Plant-based dietary patterns and incidence of type 2 diabetes in US men and women: Results from three prospective cohort studies, *PLos Medicine* 2016, dx.doi.org/10.137/journal.pmed.1002039; P. Tuso, S. R. Stoll, and W. W. Li, A plantbased diet, atherogenesis, and coronary artery disease prevention, *Permanente Journal* 19 (2015): 62–67; M. J. Orlich and coauthors, Vegetarian dietary patterns and the risk of colorectal cancers, *JAMA Internal Medicine* 175 (2015): 767–776; G. M. Turner-McGrievy and coauthors, Comparative effectiveness of plant-based diets for weight loss: A randomized controlled trial of five different diets, *Nutrition* 31 (2015): 350–358; P. N. Appleby and T. J. Key, The long-term health of vegetarians and vegans, *Proceedings of the Nutrition Society* 28 (2015): 1–7; Y. Yokoyama and coauthors, Vegetarian diets and blood pressure, *JAMA Internal Medicine* 174 (2014): 577–587.
3. M. Song and coauthors, Association of animal and plant protein intake with all-cause and causespecific mortality, *JAMA Internal Medicine* 176 (2016): 1453–1463; M. A. Martínez-González and coauthors, A provegetarian food pattern and reduction in total mortality in the Prevención con Dieta Mediterránea (PREDIMED) study, *American Journal of Clinical Nutrition* 100 (2014): 320S–328S.
4. Position of the Academy of Nutrition and Dietetics, 2016.
5. Position of the Academy of Nutrition and Dietetics, 2016.
6. R. Pawlak, S.E. Lester, and T. Babatunde, The prevalence of cobalamin deficiency among vegetarians assessed by serum vitamin B12: A review of literature, *European Journal of Clinical Nutrition* 68 (2014): 541–548.

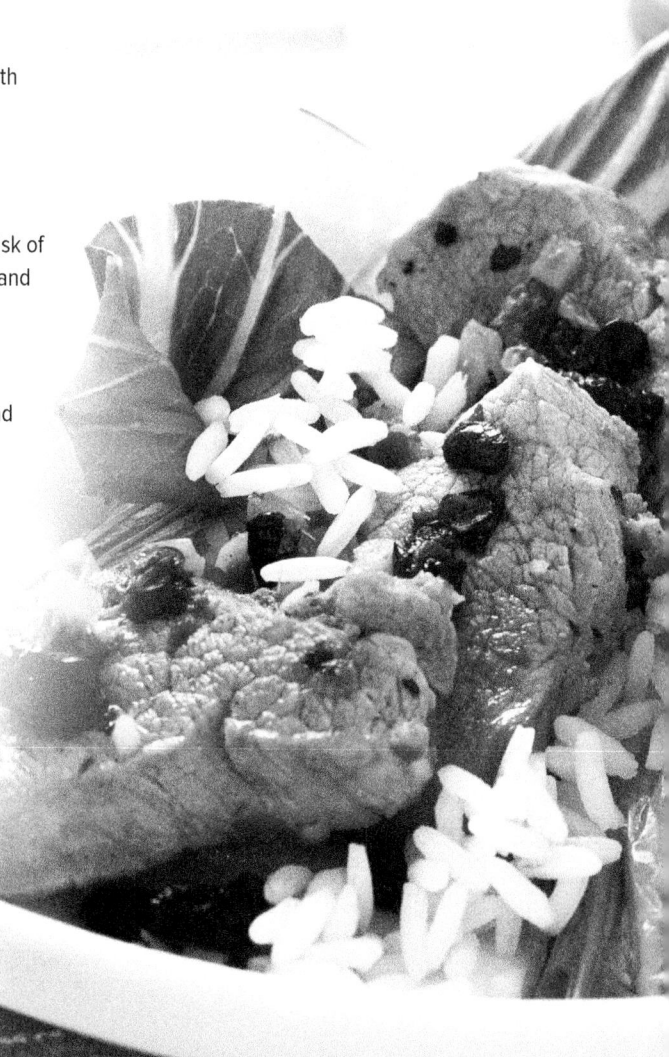

Energy Balance and Body Composition

Chapter Sections and Learning Objectives (LOs)

Envision/Corbis Documentary/Getty Images

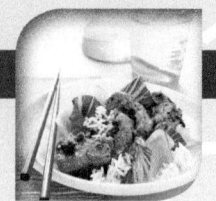

Consider that many people maintain their weight within about a 10- to 20-pound range throughout their lives. How do they do this? How does the body manage excess energy? And how does it manage to do without food for prolonged periods—as when someone is starving or fasting? The answers to these questions lie in our understanding of how the body adapts to energy imbalances, the focus of the first part of this chapter. The chapter then describes energy balance, body composition, and the health risks associated with too much or too little body fat. The next chapter offers strategies toward solving the problems of too much or too little body fat.

6.1 Energy Imbalance

When a person is maintaining weight, energy in equals energy out. In other words, the body's energy is in balance. Many people, however, eat too much or exercise too little and get fat; others eat too little or exercise too much and get thin. This section examines the two extremes of energy imbalance: feasting and fasting.

Feasting

When people consume more energy than they expend, much of the excess is stored as body fat. Excess energy from fat, carbohydrate, or protein can lead to weight gain. In addition, excess energy from alcohol is also stored as fat. Alcohol has also been shown to slow down the body's use of fat for fuel, causing more fat to be stored, much of it as abdominal fat tissue.[1] Alcohol therefore is fattening, both through the kcalories it provides and through its effects on fat metabolism. The fat cells of the adipose tissue enlarge as they fill with fat, as Figure 6-1 shows.

Excess Carbohydrate Surplus carbohydrate (glucose) is first stored as glycogen in the liver and muscles, but the glycogen-storing cells have a limited capacity. Once glycogen stores are filled, excess glucose can be converted to fat, but this conversion is not energy-efficient. Excess carbohydrate may also be burned for energy, displacing the body's use of fat for energy and allowing body fat to accumulate. Thus, excess carbohydrate can contribute to obesity.

Excess Fat Surplus dietary fat contributes more directly to the body's fat stores. After a meal, fat is routed to the body's adipose tissue, where it is stored until needed for energy. Thus, excess fat from food easily adds to body fat.

FIGURE 6-1 Fat Cell Enlargement

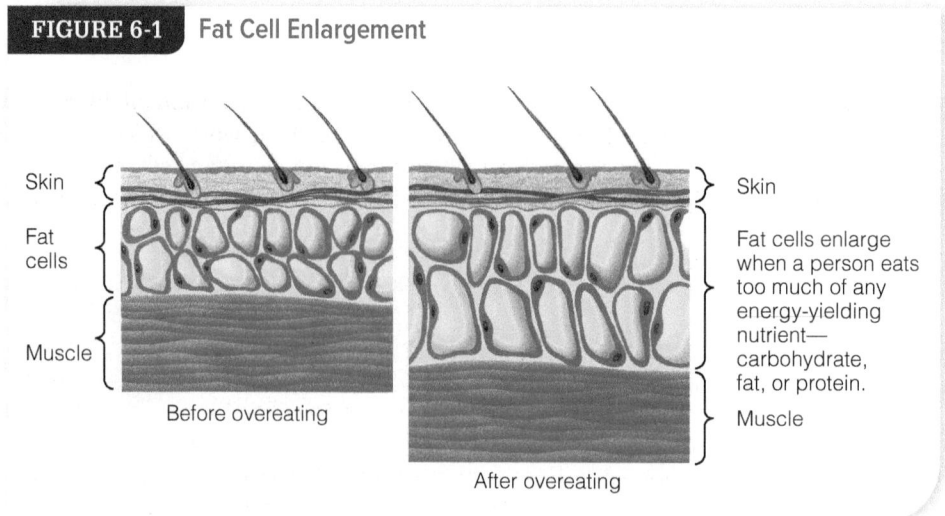

Skin

Fat cells

Muscle

Before overeating

Skin

Fat cells enlarge when a person eats too much of any energy-yielding nutrient—carbohydrate, fat, or protein.

Muscle

After overeating

FIGURE 6-2 Feasting

When people overeat, they store energy.

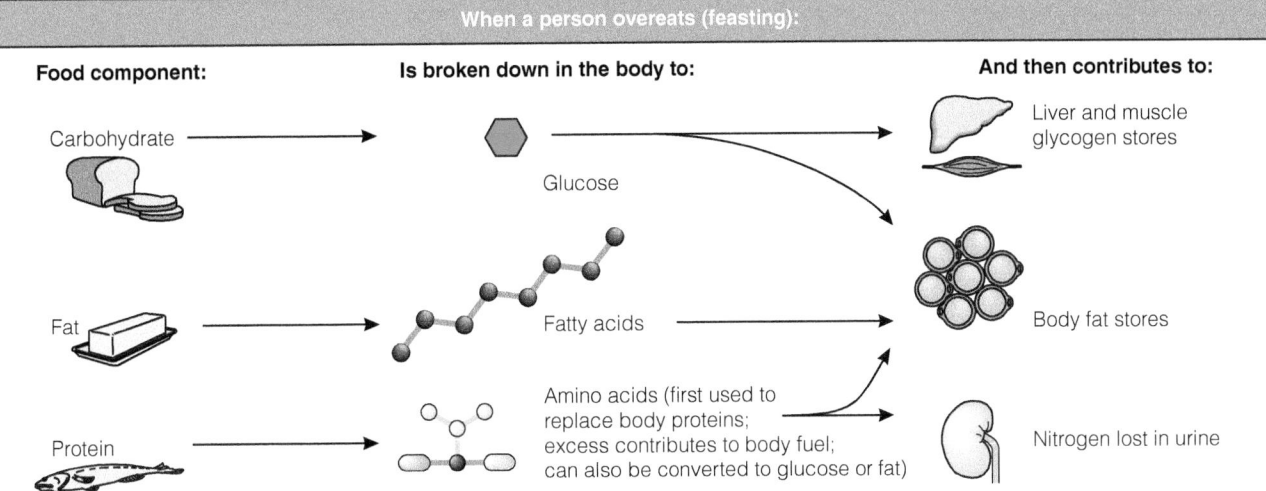

Excess Protein Although the body possesses enzymes to convert excess protein to body fat, this process is far less efficient than converting excess carbohydrate, and especially excess fat, to body fat. Researchers are investigating the degree to which it occurs under normal conditions.[2] Figure 6-2 shows the metabolic events of feasting.

Review Notes

- Too much food, too little physical activity, or both encourage body fat accumulation.
- A net excess of energy is almost all stored in the body as fat in adipose (fat) tissue.
- Alcohol both delivers kcalories and encourages storage of body fat.
- Once glycogen stores are filled, excess carbohydrate may be converted to fat or used for energy, displacing the body's use of fat for energy and allowing fat to accumulate.
- Fat from food is particularly easy for the body to store as adipose tissue.
- The body possesses enzymes to convert excess protein to fat, but researchers are investigating the degree to which this occurs under normal conditions.

The Economics of Fasting

The body expends energy all the time. Even when a person is asleep and totally relaxed, the cells of many organs are hard at work. In fact, this cellular work, which maintains all life processes, represents about two-thirds of the total energy a sedentary person expends in a day. (The other one-third is the work that a person's muscles do voluntarily during waking hours.)

Energy Deficit The body's top priority is to meet the energy needs for this ongoing cellular activity. Its normal way of doing so is by periodic refueling, that is, by eating several times a day. When food is not available, the body uses fuel reserves from its own tissues. If people voluntarily choose not to eat, we say they are fasting; if they have no choice (as in a famine), we say they are starving. The body, however, makes no distinction between the two—metabolically, fasting and starving are identical. In either case, the body is forced to switch to a wasting metabolism, drawing on its stores of carbohydrate and fat and, within a day or so, on its vital protein tissues as well.

Glycogen Used First As fasting begins, glucose from the liver's glycogen stores and fatty acids from the body's adipose tissue flow into the cells to fuel their work. Within a day, liver glycogen is exhausted, and most of the glucose is used up. Low blood glucose concentrations serve as a signal to promote further fat breakdown.

Glucose Needed for the Brain At this point, a few hours into a fast, most cells depend on fatty acids to continue providing fuel. But the nervous system (brain and nerves) and red blood cells cannot use fatty acids; they still need glucose. Even if other energy sources are available, glucose has to be present to permit the brain's energy-metabolizing machinery to work. Normally, the nervous system consumes a little more than half of the total glucose used each day—about 400 to 600 kcalories' worth.

Protein Breakdown and Ketosis Because fat stores cannot provide the glucose needed by the brain and nerves, body protein tissues (such as liver and muscle) always break down to some extent during fasting. In the first few days of a fast, body protein provides about 90 percent of the needed glucose, and glycerol provides about 10 percent. If body protein losses were to continue at this rate, death would ensue within weeks. As the fast continues, however, the body finds a way to use its fat to fuel the brain. It adapts by condensing together fragments derived from fatty acids to produce **ketone bodies**, which can serve as fuel for some brain cells. Ketone body production rises until, after several weeks of fasting, it is meeting much of the nervous system's energy needs. Still, many areas of the brain rely exclusively on glucose, and body protein continues to be sacrificed to produce it. Thus, in fasting, muscle and lean tissues give up protein to supply amino acids for conversion to glucose. This glucose, with ketone bodies produced from fat, fuels the brain's activities. Figure 6-3 shows the metabolic events that occur during fasting.

FIGURE 6-3 Fasting

When people are fasting, they draw on stored energy.

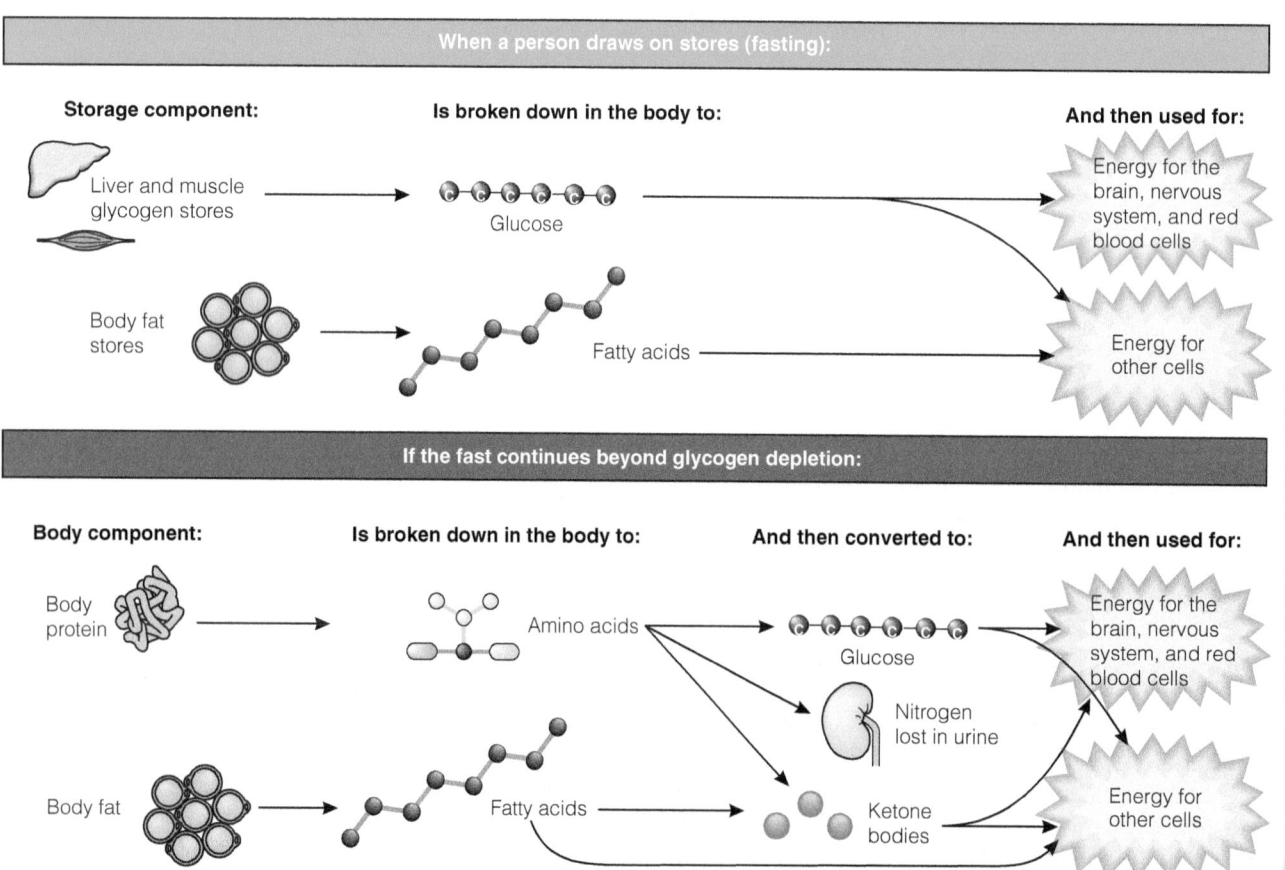

CHAPTER 6   Energy Balance and Body Composition

Slowed Metabolism As fasting continues and the nervous system shifts to partial dependence on ketone bodies for energy, the body simultaneously reduces its energy output (metabolic rate) and conserves both fat and lean tissue. Because of the slowed metabolism, energy use falls to a bare minimum.

Hazards of Fasting The body's adaptations to fasting are sufficient to maintain life for a long period. Mental alertness need not be diminished. Even physical energy may remain unimpaired for a surprisingly long time. Still, fasting is not without its hazards. Among the many changes that take place in the body are:

- Wasting of lean tissues.
- Impairment of disease resistance.
- Lowering of body temperature.
- Disturbances of the body's fluid and electrolyte balances.

For the person who wants to lose weight, fasting is not the best way to go. The body's lean tissue continues to be degraded, sometimes amounting to as much as 50 percent of the weight lost over the first week. Over the long term, a diet only moderately restricted in energy promotes primarily *fat* loss and the retention of more lean tissue than a severely restrictive fast.

Intermittent Fasting Intermittent fasting has gained renewed interest in recent years. Some people practice alternate day fasting in which they alternate days of consuming no energy-containing foods or beverages with days of eating and drinking whatever they like. Others practice modified fasting in which they consume only 20 to 25 percent of their energy needs a couple of nonconsecutive days each week. These eating patterns result in some weight loss, although no more than typically occurs with standard energy-restricted weight-loss diet plans.[3] Little evidence suggests that intermittent fasting is harmful physically or mentally, and a few studies even suggest some health benefits.[4]

Review Notes

- When fasting, the body makes a number of adaptations: increasing the breakdown of fat to provide energy for most of the cells, using glycerol and amino acids to make glucose for the red blood cells and central nervous system, producing ketones to fuel the brain, and slowing metabolism.
- All of these measures conserve energy and minimize losses.
- Over the long term, a diet moderately restricted in energy promotes primarily fat loss and the retention of lean tissue.

6.2 Energy Balance

If a person maintains a healthy weight over time, the person is in energy balance. Food energy intake equals energy expenditure: deposits of fat made at one time have been compensated for by withdrawals made at another. In other words, the body uses fat as a savings account for energy. But, unlike money, having more fat is not better; there is an optimum.

A day's energy balance can be stated like this: change in energy stores equals the food energy taken in (kcalories) minus the energy spent on metabolism and physical activities (kcalories). More simply:

Change in energy stores = energy in (kcalories) − energy out (kcalories)

Energy In

The energy in food and beverages is the only contributor to the "energy in" side of the energy balance equation. Before you can decide how much food will supply the energy you or one of your clients needs in a day, you must first become familiar with the amounts of energy in foods and beverages. Computer programs such as the USDA Food Composition Database (ndb.nal.usda.gov) can readily provide this information.

Food composition data would reveal that an apple provides about 70 kcalories from carbohydrate and a candy bar supplies about 250 kcalories, mostly from fat and carbohydrate. You may have heard that for each 3500 kcalories you eat in excess of expenditures, you store 1 pound of body fat—a general rule that has previously been used for mathematical estimations. Keep in mind, however, that this number can vary widely with individual metabolic tendencies and efficiencies of nutrient digestion and absorption. The dynamics of energy storage is a topic of current scientific investigation.[5] The fat stores of even a healthy-weight adult represent an ample reserve of energy—50,000 to 200,000 kcalories.

Energy Out

The body expends energy in two major ways: to fuel its **basal metabolism** and to fuel its **voluntary activities**. People can change their voluntary activities to expend more or less energy in a day, and over time they can also change their basal metabolism by building up the body's metabolically active lean tissue, as explained in Chapter 7.

Basal Metabolism Basal metabolism supports the body's work that goes on all the time without the person's conscious awareness. The beating of the heart, the inhalation and exhalation of air, the maintenance of body temperature, and the transmission of nerve and hormonal messages to direct these activities are the basal processes that maintain life. As Figure 6-4 shows, basal metabolism represents about two-thirds of the total energy a sedentary person expends in a day. In practical terms, a person whose total energy needs are 2000 kcalories per day may expend 1000 to 1300 of them to support basal metabolism.

The **basal metabolic rate (BMR)** is the rate at which the body expends energy for these life-sustaining activities. This rate varies from person to person and may vary for an individual with a change in circumstance or physical condition. The rate is slowest when a person is sleeping undisturbed, but it is usually measured when the person is awake, but lying still, in a room with a comfortable temperature after a restful sleep and an overnight (12- to 14-hour) fast. A similar measure of energy output—called the **resting metabolic rate (RMR)**—is slightly higher than the BMR because its criteria for recent food intake and physical activity are not as strict.

Table 6-1 summarizes the factors that raise and lower the BMR. For the most part, the BMR is highest in people who are growing (children, adolescents, and pregnant women) and in those with considerable lean body mass (physically fit people and males). One way to increase the BMR, then, is to maximize lean body tissue by participating regularly in endurance and strength-building activities. The BMR is also fast in people who are tall and so have a large surface area for their weight, in people with fever or under stress, in people taking certain medications, and in people with highly active thyroid glands. The BMR slows down with a loss of lean body mass and during fasting and malnutrition.

Energy for Physical Activities The number of kcalories spent on voluntary activities depends on three factors: muscle mass, body weight, and activity. The larger the muscle mass required for the activity and the heavier the weight of the body part being moved, the more kcalories are spent. The activity's duration, frequency, and intensity also influence energy costs: the longer, the more frequent, and the more intense the activity, the more kcalories are expended. Table 6-2 lists average energy expenditures for various activities.

FIGURE 6-4 Components of Energy Expenditure

The amount of energy expended in a day differs for each individual, but, in general, basal metabolism is the largest component of energy expenditure, and the thermic effect of food is the smallest. The amount expended in voluntary physical activities has the greatest variability, depending on a person's activity patterns. For a sedentary person, physical activities may account for less than half as much energy as basal metabolism, whereas an extremely active person may expend as much on activity as for basal metabolism.

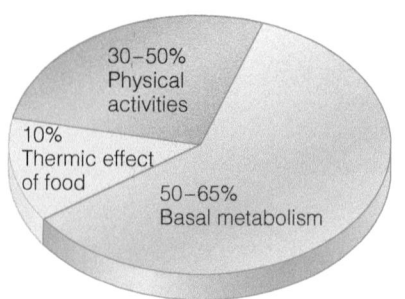

TABLE 6-1 Factors That Affect the BMR

FACTOR	EFFECT ON BMR
Age	Lean body mass diminishes with age, slowing the BMR.[a]
Height	In tall, thin people, the BMR is higher.[b]
Growth	In children, adolescents, and pregnant women, the BMR is higher.
Body composition (gender)	The more lean tissue, the higher the BMR (which is why males usually have a higher BMR than females). The more fat tissue, the lower the BMR.
Fever	Fever raises the BMR.[c]
Stresses	Stresses (including many diseases and certain drugs) raise the BMR.
Environmental temperature	Both heat and cold raise the BMR.
Fasting/starvation	Fasting/starvation lowers the BMR.[d]
Malnutrition	Malnutrition lowers the BMR.
Hormones (gender)	The thyroid hormone thyroxin, for example, can speed up or slow down the BMR.[e] Premenstrual hormones slightly raise the BMR.
Smoking	Nicotine increases energy expenditure.
Caffeine	Caffeine increases energy expenditure.
Sleep	BMR is lowest when sleeping.

[a]The BMR begins to decrease in early adulthood (after growth and development cease) at a rate of about 2 percent a decade. A simultaneous reduction in voluntary activity brings the total decline in energy expenditure to 5 percent a decade.
[b]If two people weigh the same, the taller, thinner person will have the faster metabolic rate, reflecting the greater skin surface, through which heat is lost by radiation, in proportion to the body's volume.
[c]Fever raises the BMR by 7 percent for each degree Fahrenheit.
[d]Prolonged starvation reduces the total amount of metabolically active lean tissue in the body, although the decline occurs sooner and to a greater extent than body losses alone can explain. More likely, the neural and hormonal changes that accompany fasting are responsible for changes in the BMR.
[e]The thyroid gland releases hormones that travel to the cells and influence cellular metabolism. Thyroid hormone activity can speed up or slow down the rate of metabolism by as much as 50 percent.

TABLE 6-2 Energy Spent on Various Activities

The values listed in this table reflect both the energy spent in physical activity and the amount used for BMR.

ACTIVITY	kcal/lb/min[a]
Aerobic dance (vigorous)	0.062
Basketball (vigorous, full court)	0.097
Bicycling	
13 mph	0.045
15 mph	0.049
17 mph	0.057
19 mph	0.076
21 mph	0.090
23 mph	0.109
25 mph	0.139

(Continued)

TABLE 6-2 Energy Spent on Various Activities (*continued*)

ACTIVITY	kcal/lb/min[a]
Canoeing, flat water, moderate pace	0.045
Cross-country skiing	
8 mph	0.104
Golf (carrying clubs)	0.045
Handball	0.078
Horseback riding (trot)	0.052
Rowing (vigorous)	0.097
Running	
5 mph	0.061
6 mph	0.074
7.5 mph	0.094
9 mph	0.103
10 mph	0.114
11 mph	0.131
Soccer (vigorous)	0.097
Studying	0.011
Swimming	
20 yd/min	0.032
45 yd/min	0.058
50 yd/min	0.070
Table tennis (skilled)	0.045
Tennis (beginner)	0.032
Walking (brisk pace)	
3.5 mph	0.035
4.5 mph	0.048
Weight lifting	
light-to-moderate effort	0.024
vigorous effort	0.048
Wheelchair basketball	0.084
Wheeling self in wheelchair	0.030
Wii games	
bowling	0.021
boxing	0.021
tennis	0.022

[a]To calculate kcalories spent per minute of activity for your own body weight, multiply kcal/lb/min by your exact weight and then multiply that number by the number of minutes spent in the activity. For example, if you weigh 142 pounds, and you want to know how many kcalories you spent doing 30 minutes of vigorous aerobic dance: $0.062 \times 142 = 8.8$ kcalories per minute; 8.8×30 (minutes) $= 264$ total kcalories spent.

Energy to Manage Food When food is taken into the body, many cells that have been dormant become active. The muscles that move the food through the intestinal tract speed up their rhythmic contractions, and the cells that manufacture and secrete digestive juices begin their tasks. All these and other cells need extra energy as they participate in the digestion, absorption, and metabolism of food. This cellular activity produces heat and is known as the **thermic effect of food**. The thermic effect of food is generally thought to represent about 10 percent of the total food energy taken in. For purposes of rough estimates, though, the thermic effect of food is not always included.

Estimating Energy Requirements

In estimating energy requirements, the DRI committee developed equations that consider how the following factors influence energy expenditure:*

- *Gender.* Women generally have a lower BMR than men, in large part because men typically have more lean body mass. In addition, menstrual hormones influence the BMR in women, raising it just prior to menstruation. Two sets of energy equations—one for men and one for women—were developed to accommodate the influence of gender on energy expenditure.
- *Growth.* The BMR is high in people who are growing. For this reason, pregnant and lactating women, infants, children, and adolescents have their own sets of energy equations.
- *Age.* The BMR declines during adulthood as lean body mass diminishes. Physical activities tend to decline as well, bringing the average reduction in energy expenditure to about 5 percent per decade. The decline in the BMR that occurs when a person becomes less active reflects the loss of lean body mass and may be prevented with ongoing physical activity (see Photo 6-1). Because age influences energy expenditure, it is also factored into the energy equations.
- *Physical activity.* Using individual values for various physical activities (as in Table 6-2) is time consuming and impractical for estimating the energy needs of a population. Instead, various activities are clustered according to the typical intensity of a day's efforts (Appendix D provides details).
- *Body composition and body size.* The BMR is high in people who are tall and so have a large surface area. Similarly, the more a person weighs, the more energy is expended on basal metabolism. For these reasons, the energy equations include a factor for both height and weight.

As just explained, energy needs vary among individuals depending on such factors as gender, growth, age, physical activity, and body composition. Even when two people are similarly matched, however, their energy needs will still differ because of genetic differences. Perhaps one day genetic research will reveal how to estimate requirements for each individual. For now, Box 6-1 provides instructions on calculating estimated energy requirements using the DRI equations and physical activity factors.† Appendix D presents tables that provide a shortcut to estimating total energy expenditure.

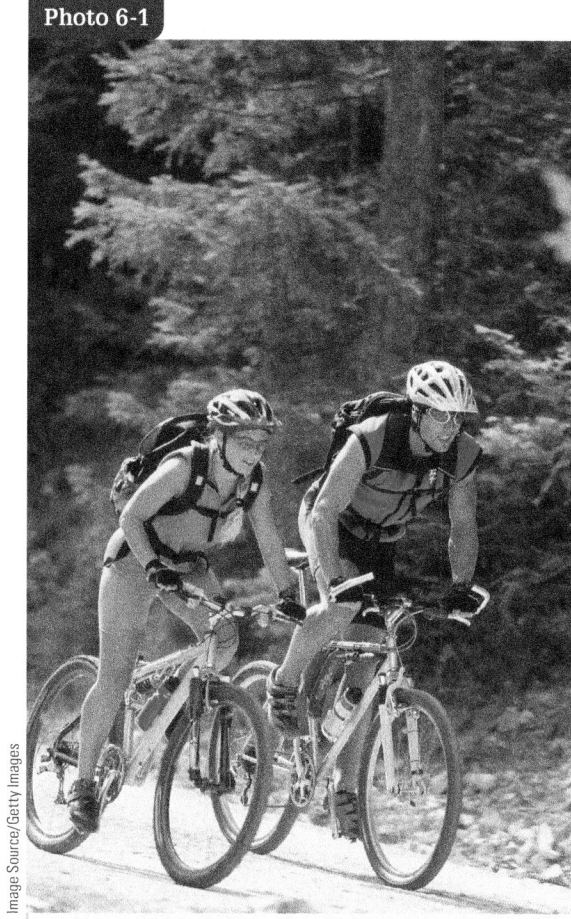

Image Source/Getty Images

Physical activity expends energy and benefits health in many ways.

*Note that Table 6-1 listed these factors among those that influence BMR and, consequently, energy expenditure.

†For *most* people, the energy requirement falls within these ranges: (Men) EER ±200 kcal; (Women) EER ±160 kcal. For almost all people, the actual energy requirement falls within these larger ranges: (Men) EER ±400 kcal; (Women) EER ±320 kcal.

thermic effect of food: an estimation of the energy required to process food (digest, absorb, transport, metabolize, and store ingested nutrients).

| Box 6-1 | *HOW TO* Estimate Energy Requirements |

To determine your estimated energy requirements (EER), use the appropriate equation (of the two options below), inserting your age in years, weight (wt) in kilograms, height (ht) in meters, and physical activity (PA) factor from the accompanying table. (To convert pounds to kilograms, divide by 2.2; to convert inches to meters, divide by 39.37.)

- For men 19 years and older:

$$EER = [662 - (9.53 \times age)] + PA \times [(15.91 \times wt) + (539.6 \times ht)]$$

- For women 19 years and older:

$$EER = [354 - (6.91 \times age)] + PA \times [(9.36 \times wt) + (726 \times ht)]$$

For example, consider an active 30-year-old male who is 5 feet 11 inches tall and weighs 178 pounds. First, he converts his weight from pounds to kilograms and his height from inches to meters, if necessary:

$$178 \text{ lb} \div 2.2 = 80.9 \text{ kg}$$
$$1 \text{ in} \div 39.37 = 1.8 \text{ m}$$

Next, he considers his level of daily physical activity and selects the appropriate PA factor from the accompanying table (in this example, 1.25 for an active male). Then, he inserts his age, PA factor, weight, and height into the appropriate equation:

$$EER = [662 - (9.53 \times 30)] + 1.25 \times [(15.91 \times 80.9) + (539.6 \times 1.8)]$$

(A reminder: do calculations within the parentheses first, and multiply before adding or subtracting.) He calculates

$$EER = [662 - (9.53 \times 30)] + 1.25 \times (1287 + 971)$$
$$EER = [662 - (9.53 \times 30)] + (1.25 \times 2258)$$
$$EER = 662 - 286 + 2823$$
$$EER = 3199$$

The estimated energy requirement for an active 30-year-old male who is 5 feet 11 inches tall and weighs 178 pounds is about 3200 kcalories/day. His actual requirement probably falls within a range of 200 kcalories above and below this estimate.

Physical Activity (PA) Factors for EER Equations

	Men	Women	Physical Activity
Sedentary	1.0	1.0	Typical daily living activities
Low active	1.11	1.12	Plus 30 to 60 minutes moderate activity
Active	1.25	1.27	Plus >60 minutes moderate activity
Very active	1.48	1.45	Plus >60 minutes moderate activity and 60 minutes vigorous activity or 120 minutes moderate activity

Note: Moderate activity is equivalent to walking at 3½ to 4½ miles per hour.

Review Notes

- A person takes in energy from food and, on average, expends most of it on basal metabolic activities, some of it on physical activities, and about 10 percent on the thermic effect of food.
- Because energy requirements vary from person to person, such factors as age, gender, and weight must be considered when calculating energy expended on basal metabolism, and the intensity and duration of the activity must be taken into account when calculating expenditures on physical activities.

6.3 Body Weight and Body Composition

The body's weight reflects its composition—the proportions of its bone, muscle, fat, fluid, and other tissue. All of these body components can vary in quantity and quality: the bones can be dense or porous, the muscles can be well developed or underdeveloped, fat can be abundant or scarce, and so on. By far the most variable tissue, though, is body fat. For health's sake, weight management efforts should focus on eating and activity habits to improve body composition.

Defining Healthy Body Weight

How much should a person weigh? How can a person know if her weight is appropriate for her height and age? How can a person know if his weight is jeopardizing his health? Questions such as these seem so simple, yet the answers can be complex—and different depending on whom you ask.

The Criterion of Fashion When asking the question, "What is an ideal body weight?" people often mistakenly turn to fashion for the answer. Without a doubt, our society sets unrealistic ideals for body weight, especially for women.[6] The Internet, social media, magazines, movies, and television all convey the message that to be thin is to be beautiful and happy. As a result, the Internet and media have a great influence on the weight concerns and dieting patterns of people of all ages but most tragically on young, impressionable children and adolescents.

Importantly, perceived body image has little to do with actual body weight or size. People of all shapes, sizes, and ages—including extremely thin fashion models with anorexia nervosa and fitness instructors with ideal body composition—have learned to be unhappy with their "overweight" bodies. Such dissatisfaction can lead to damaging behaviors, such as starvation diets, diet pill abuse, and failure to seek health care. The first step toward making healthy changes may be self-acceptance. Keep in mind that fashion is fickle; the body shapes that our society values change with time and, furthermore, differ from those valued by other societies. The standards defining "ideal" are subjective and frequently have little in common with health. Table 6-3 offers some tips for adopting health as an ideal.

The Criterion of Health Even if our society were to accept fat as beautiful, obesity would still be a major risk factor for several life-threatening diseases, as discussed later in the chapter. For this reason, the most important criterion for determining how much a person should weigh and how much body fat a person needs is not appearance but good health and longevity. A range of healthy body weights has been identified using a common measure of weight and height—the body mass index.

Body Mass Index The **body mass index (BMI)** describes relative weight for height:

$$\text{BMI} = \frac{\text{weight (kg)}}{\text{height (m)}^2} \text{ or } \frac{\text{weight (lb)}}{\text{height (in)}^2} \times 703$$

To convert pounds to kilograms, divide by 2.2. To convert inches to meters, divide by 39.37.

body mass index (BMI): an index of a person's weight in relation to height; determined by dividing the weight (in kilograms) by the square of the height (in meters).

TABLE 6-3 Tips for Accepting a Healthy Body Weight

- Value yourself and others for human attributes other than body weight. Realize that prejudging people by weight is as harmful as prejudging them by race, religion, or gender.

- Use positive, nonjudgmental descriptions of your body.

- Accept positive comments from others.

- Focus on your whole self, including your intelligence, social grace, and professional and scholastic achievements.

- Accept that no magic diet exists.

- Stop dieting to lose weight. Adopt a lifestyle of healthy eating and physical activity permanently.

- Follow the USDA Food Patterns. Never restrict food intake below the minimum levels that meet nutrient needs.

- Become physically active, not because it will help you get thin but because it will make you feel good and enhance your health.

- Seek support from loved ones. Tell them of your plan for a healthy life in the body you have been given.

- Seek professional counseling, *not* from a weight-loss counselor but from someone who can help you make gains in self-esteem without weight as a factor.

Weight classifications based on BMI are presented in the table on the inside back cover. Notice that a healthy weight falls between a BMI of 18.5 and 24.9, with **underweight** below 18.5, **overweight** above 25, and **obese** above 30. Figure 6-5 presents body shapes associated with various BMI values. Most people with a BMI within the healthy weight range have few of the health risks typically associated with too-low or too-high body weight. Risks increase as BMI falls below 18.5 or rises above 24.9 (see Figure 6-6), reflecting the reality that both underweight and overweight impair health status.

The BMI values are most accurate in assessing degrees of obesity and are less useful for evaluating nonobese people's body fatness. BMI values fail to provide two valuable

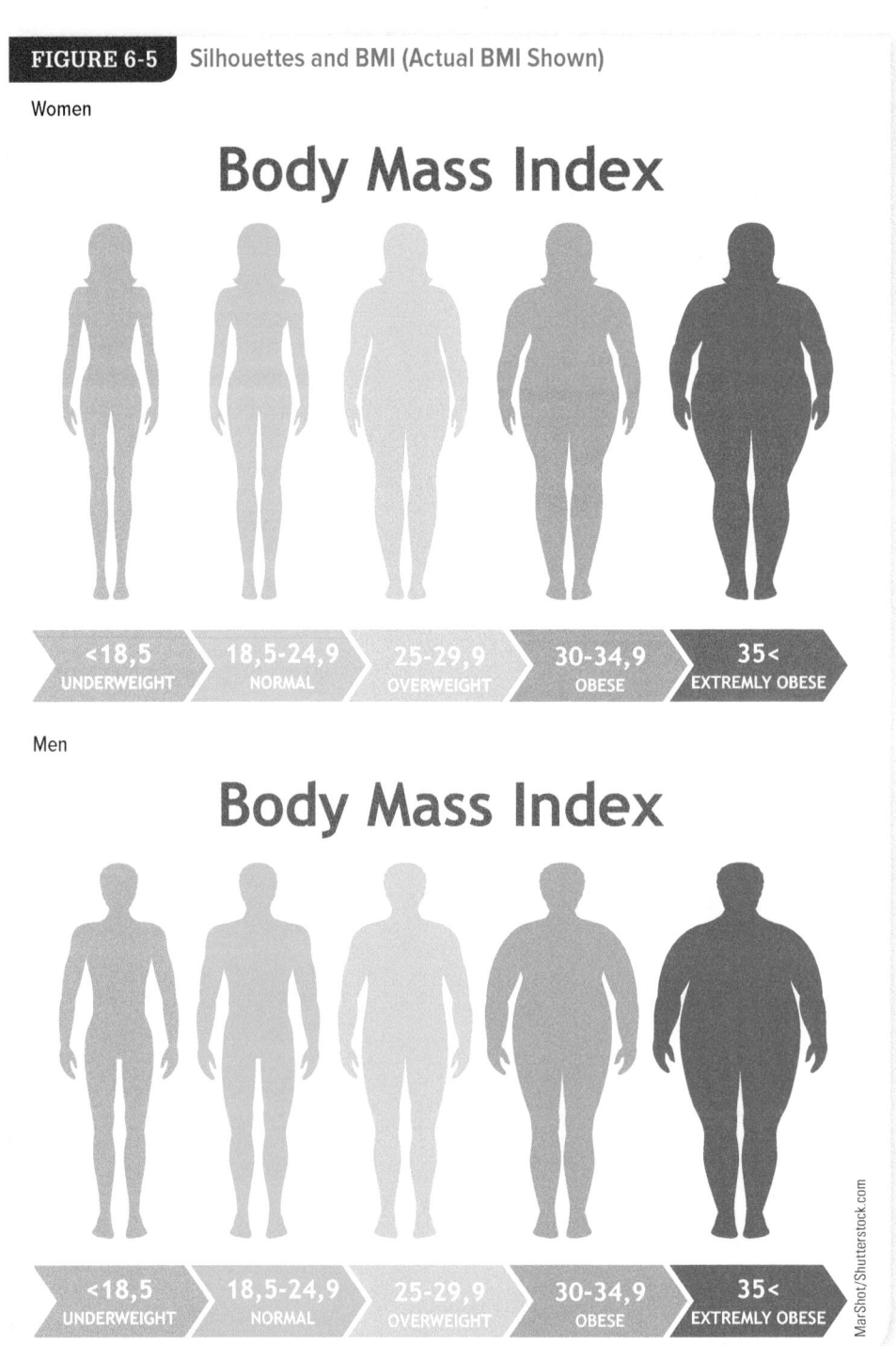

FIGURE 6-5 Silhouettes and BMI (Actual BMI Shown)

underweight: body weight lower than the weight range that is considered healthy; BMI below 18.5.

overweight: body weight greater than the weight range that is considered healthy; BMI 25.0 to 29.9.

obese: having too much body fat with adverse health effects; BMI 30 or more.

pieces of information used in assessing disease risk: they don't reveal how much of the weight is fat, and they don't indicate where the fat is located. To obtain these data, measures of body composition are needed.

Body Composition

For many people, being overweight compared with the standard means that they are over*fat*. This is not the case, though, for athletes with dense bones and well-developed muscles; they may be over*weight* but carry little body fat. Conversely, inactive people may seem to have acceptable weights but still carry too much body fat for health. In addition, among some racial and ethnic groups, BMI values may not precisely identify overweight and obesity. Thus, a diagnosis of obesity or overweight requires a BMI value *plus* some measure of body composition and fat distribution. In other words, although BMI can be used to estimate body fatness, it falls short as a predictor of health. Because obesity can have many adverse effects on health related to the quantity, distribution, and function of adipose tissue, a new medical term for obesity has been established: **adiposity-based chronic disease**.[7]

Central Obesity The distribution of fat on the body may influence health as much as, or more than, the total amount of fat alone. **Visceral fat** that is stored deep within the central abdominal area of the body is referred to as **central obesity** or upper body fat (see Figure 6-7). Much research supports

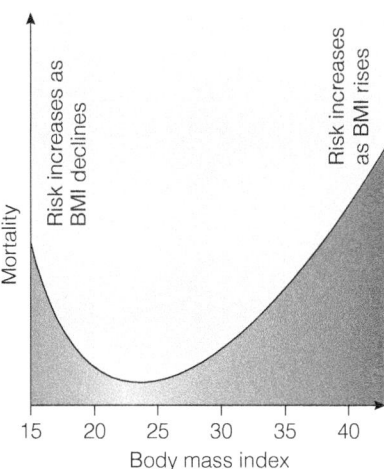

FIGURE 6-6 Body Mass Index and Mortality

This J-shaped curve describes the relationship between body mass index (BMI) and mortality and shows that both underweight and overweight present risks of a premature death.

FIGURE 6-7 Abdominal Fat

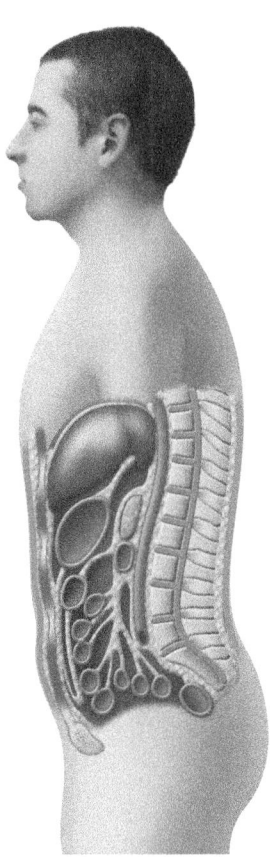

In healthy-weight people, some fat is stored around the organs of the abdomen.

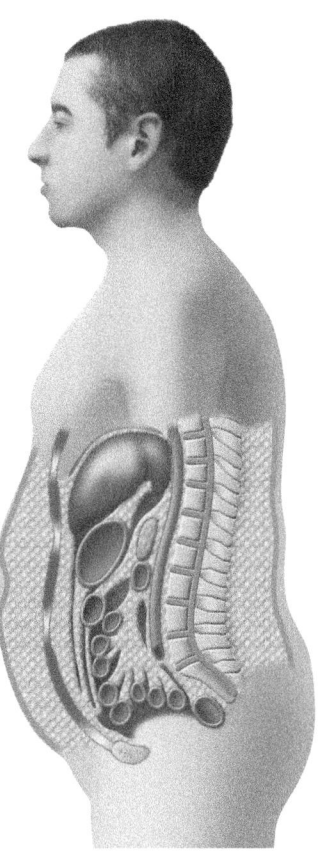

In overweight people, excess abdominal fat increases the risks of diseases.

adiposity-based chronic disease: a medical name for obesity. *Adiposity* refers to fat cells and tissues and identifies them as the source of the disease.

visceral fat: fat stored within the abdominal cavity in association with the internal abdominal organs, as opposed to fat stored directly under the skin (subcutaneous fat); also called *intra-abdominal fat*.

central obesity: excess fat around the trunk of the body; also called *abdominal fat* or *upper-body fat*.

FIGURE 6-8   "Apple" and "Pear" Body
Shapes Compared

Popular articles sometimes call bodies with upper-body fat "apples" and those with lower-body fat "pears."

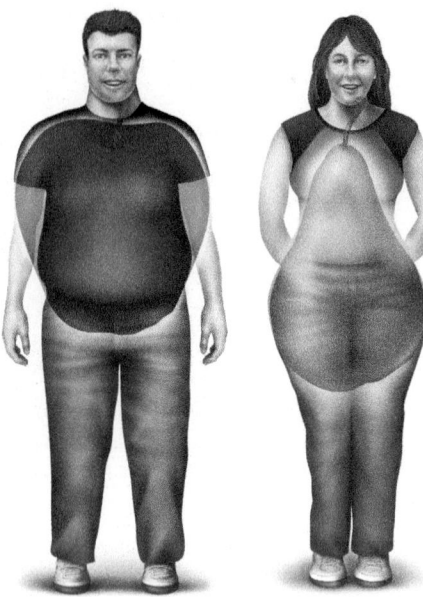

Upper-body fat is more common in men than in women and is closely associated with heart disease, stroke, diabetes, hypertension, and some types of cancer.

Lower-body fat is more common in women than in men and is not usually associated with chronic diseases.

the widely held belief that central obesity—significantly and independently of BMI—contributes to heart disease, cancers, diabetes, and related deaths.[8]

One possible explanation for why fat in the abdomen may increase the risk of disease involves **adipokines**, hormones released by adipose tissue. Adipokines help to regulate **inflammation** and energy metabolism in the tissues.[9] The inflammatory response is described in detail in Chapter 16.

In central obesity, a shift occurs in the balance of adipokines, favoring those that increase both inflammation and insulin resistance of tissues.[10] The resulting chronic inflammation and insulin resistance contribute to diabetes, atherosclerosis (a cause of heart disease), and other chronic diseases. Insulin resistance is a central feature of metabolic syndrome, which is discussed in Nutrition in Practice 20.

Visceral fat creates the "apple" profile of central obesity. **Subcutaneous fat** around the hips and thighs creates more of a "pear" profile (see Figure 6-8). Visceral fat is common in women past menopause and even more common in men. Even when total body fat is similar, men have more visceral fat than either premenopausal or postmenopausal women. For those women with visceral fat, the risks of cardiovascular disease and mortality are increased, just as they are for men. Interestingly, smokers tend to have more visceral fat than nonsmokers even though they typically have a lower BMI. Two other factors that may affect body fat distribution are intakes of alcohol and physical activity. Moderate-to-high alcohol consumption may favor central obesity. In contrast, regular physical activity seems to prevent visceral fat accumulation.[11]

Waist Circumference   A person's **waist circumference** is a good indicator of fat distribution and central obesity (see Appendix E). In general, women with a waist circumference greater than 35 inches and men with a waist circumference greater than 40 inches have a high risk of central obesity–related health problems.

Skinfold Measures   Skinfold measurements provide an accurate estimate of total body fat and a fair assessment of the fat's location. About half of the fat in the body lies directly beneath the skin, so the thickness of this subcutaneous fat is assumed to reflect total body fat. Measures taken from central-body sites (around the abdomen) better reflect changes in fatness than those taken from upper sites (arm and back). A skilled assessor can obtain an accurate **skinfold measure** and then compare the measurement with standards (see Appendix E).

How Much Body Fat Is Too Much?

People often ask exactly how much fat is too fat for health. Ideally, a person has enough fat to meet basic needs but not so much as to incur health risks. The ideal amount of body fat depends partly on the person. A man with a BMI within the recommended range may have between 18 and 24 percent body fat; a woman, because of her greater quantity of essential fat, 23 to 31 percent.

Many athletes have a lower percentage of body fat—just enough fat to provide fuel, insulate and protect the body, assist in nerve impulse transmissions, and support normal hormone activity, but not so much as to burden the muscles (see Photo 6-2). For athletes, then, body fat might be 5 to 10 percent for men and 15 to 20 percent for women.

adipokines (AD-ih-poh-kynz): protein hormones made and released by adipose tissue (fat) cells.

inflammation: an immunological response to cellular injury characterized by an increase in white blood cells.

subcutaneous fat: fat stored directly under the skin.

   sub = beneath
   cutaneous = skin

waist circumference: a measurement used to assess a person's abdominal fat.

skinfold measure: a clinical estimate of total body fatness in which the thickness of a fold of skin on the back of the arm (over the triceps muscle), below the shoulder blade (subscapular), or in other places is measured with a caliper.

For an Alaskan fisherman, a higher-than-average percentage of body fat is probably beneficial because fat helps prevent heat loss in cold weather. A woman starting a pregnancy needs sufficient body fat to support conception and fetal growth. Below a certain threshold for body fat, individuals may become infertile, develop depression, experience abnormal hunger regulation, or be unable to keep warm. These thresholds differ for each function and for each individual; much remains to be learned about them.

Photo 6-2

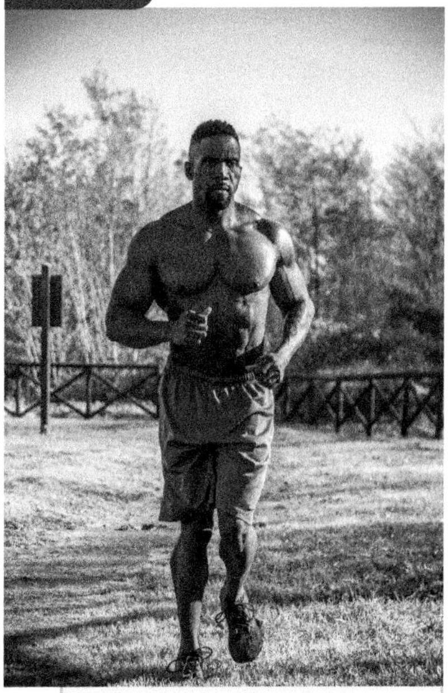

At 6 feet 4 inches tall and 250 pounds, this runner would be considered overweight by most standards. Yet he is clearly not overfat.

Review Notes

- Clearly, the most important criterion of appropriate fatness is health.
- Current standards for body weight are based on the body mass index (BMI), which describes a person's weight in relation to height.
- Health risks increase with a BMI below 18.5 or above 24.9.
- Central obesity, in which excess fat is distributed around the trunk of the body, may present greater health risks than excess fat distributed on the lower body.
- Researchers use a number of techniques to assess body composition, including waist circumference and skinfold measures.

6.4 Health Risks of Underweight and Obesity

As mentioned earlier and shown in Figure 6-6, health risks increase as BMI falls below 18.5 or rises above 24.9. People who are extremely underweight or extremely obese carry higher risks of early death than those whose weights fall within the healthy, or even the slightly overweight, range.[12] These mortality risks decline with age. Independently of BMI, factors such as smoking habits raise health risks, and physical fitness lowers them.

Health Risks of Underweight

Some underweight people enjoy an active, healthy life, but others are underweight because of malnutrition, smoking habits, substance abuse, or illnesses. Weight and fat measures alone would not reveal these underlying causes, but a complete assessment that includes a diet and medical history, physical examination, and biochemical analysis would.

Underweight people, especially older adults, may be unable to preserve lean tissue when fighting a wasting disease such as cancer. Overly thin people are also at a disadvantage in the hospital, where nutrient status can easily deteriorate if they have to go without food for an extended time while undergoing tests or surgery. Underweight women often develop menstrual irregularities and become infertile. Underweight and significant weight loss are also associated with osteoporosis and bone fractures. For all these reasons, underweight people may benefit from enough of a weight gain to provide an energy reserve and protective amounts of all the nutrients that can be stored.

An extreme underweight condition known as anorexia nervosa is sometimes seen in young people who exercise unreasonable self-denial in order to control their weight. Anorexia nervosa is a major eating disorder seen in our society today. Eating disorders are the subject of Nutrition in Practice 6.

FIGURE 6-9

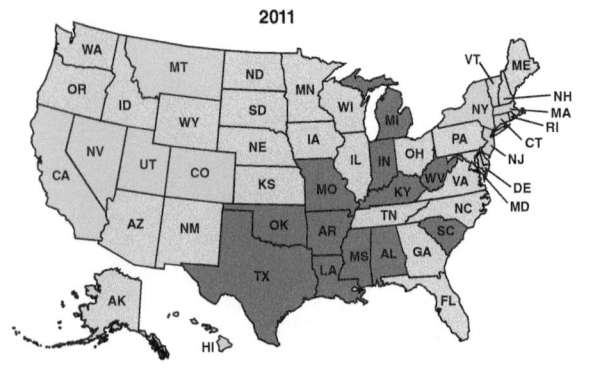

2011

<20%	20% to 24.9%	25% to 29.9%	30% to 34.9%	≥35%
0 states	11 states	27 states	12 states	0 states

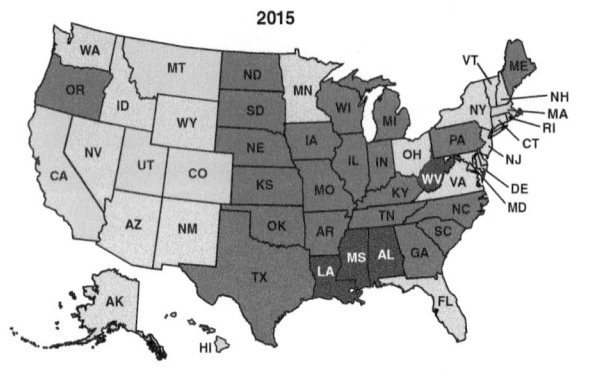

2015

<20%	20% to 24.9%	25% to 29.9%	30% to 34.9%	≥35%
0 states	6 states	19 states	21 states	4 states

insulin resistance: the condition in which a normal amount of insulin produces a subnormal effect in muscle, adipose, and liver cells, resulting in an elevated fasting glucose; a metabolic consequence of obesity that precedes type 2 diabetes.

Health Risks of Overweight and Obesity

Despite our nation's preoccupation with body image and weight loss, the prevalence of overweight and obesity continues to be high.[13] The maps in Figure 6-9 show the increases in obesity prevalence over a recent 5-year time period alone. Over the past five *decades*, obesity has soared in every state, in both genders, and across all ages, races, and educational levels. An estimated 71 percent of U.S. adults are overweight (BMI of 25 or greater) or dangerously obese (BMI of 30 or greater).[14] Even among children and adolescents, 18 percent are obese and many more are overweight. The United States is caught in a global obesity epidemic that is harming the health of people of all ages, in urban and rural areas alike.[15] Nevertheless, U.S. efforts to curb domestic obesity may be paying off, especially among low-income children, women, and girls; their rates of newly diagnosed obesity are showing signs of slowing.[16] Among men and boys, however, rates of obesity are still on the rise, and more people fall into the severely obese category than ever before.

The high prevalence of overweight and obesity is a matter of concern because both conditions present risks to health. Indeed, the health risks of obesity are so numerous that it has been declared a chronic disease. Excess weight contributes to up to half of all cases of hypertension, thereby increasing the risk of heart attack and stroke. Obesity raises blood pressure in part by altering kidney function, increasing blood volume, and promoting blood vessel damage through insulin resistance. Often weight loss alone can normalize the blood pressure of an overweight person.

Excess body weight also increases the risk of type 2 diabetes. Most adults with type 2 diabetes are overweight or obese, and obesity itself can directly cause some degree of **insulin resistance**.[17] Diabetes (type 2) is far more likely to develop in an obese person than in a nonobese person.[18] Furthermore, the person with type 2 diabetes often has central obesity.[19] Central-body fat cells appear to be larger and more insulin resistant than lower-body fat cells.

In addition to diabetes and hypertension, other risks threaten obese adults. Among them are high blood lipids, cardiovascular disease, sleep apnea (abnormal cessation of breathing during sleep), osteoarthritis, abdominal hernias, some cancers, varicose veins, gout, gallbladder disease, kidney stones, respiratory problems (including Pickwickian syndrome, a breathing blockage linked with sudden death), nonalcoholic fatty liver disease, complications in pregnancy and surgery, flat feet, and even a high accident rate.[20] Each year these obesity-related illnesses cost our nation billions of dollars. The cost in terms of lives is also great.[21] In fact, obesity is second only to tobacco use as the most significant cause of preventable death.

Some obese people, however, have been described as "healthy obese" or metabolically normal obese"; they have normal blood pressure, blood glucose, and blood lipids.[22] Most notable is that they maintain their sensitivity to insulin.[23] Compared with insulin-resistant obese people, insulin-sensitive obese people tend to have less central obesity and inflammation, characteristics that, among others, seem to protect them from type 2 diabetes and heart disease—at least for a short while. Over the long term, metabolically healthy obese people may be at increased risk for inflammation and other adverse health outcomes, compared with metabolically healthy normal-weight people.[24] To help in identifying those most at risk, obesity experts have developed guidelines for health practitioners, described next.

Guidelines for Identifying Those at Risk from Obesity

The guidelines for identifying and evaluating the risks to health from overweight and obesity rely on three indicators. The first indicator is a person's BMI. As a general guideline, overweight for adults is defined as BMI of 25.0 through 29.9, and obesity is defined as BMI equal to or greater than 30.

The second indicator is waist circumference, which, as discussed earlier, reflects the degree of abdominal fatness in proportion to body fatness. People in the "overweight" BMI range of 25–29.9 or those in the "obese" BMI range of 30–34.9 often face a greater risk of heart disease and mortality if their waist measurement is more than 35 inches for women and 40 inches for men. For people with a BMI above 35, waist circumference is less meaningful because their degree of obesity incurs a high risk for health problems and mortality, regardless of their waist measurement.[25]

The third indicator is the person's disease risk profile. The disease risk profile takes into account life-threatening diseases, family history, and risk factors for heart disease (such as blood lipid profile). The higher the BMI, the greater the waist circumference, and the more risk factors, the greater the urgency to treat obesity. People who are obese or those who are overweight and have one or more indicators of increased risk of heart disease (diabetes, prediabetes, hypertension, abnormal lipid profile, or elevated waist circumference) have a high risk for disease complications and mortality that requires treatment to manage the disease or modify the risk factors.[26]

Other Risks of Obesity

Although some obese people seem to escape health problems, few in our society can avoid the social and economic handicaps. Our society places enormous value on thinness. Obese people are less sought after for romance, less often hired, and less often admitted to college. They pay higher insurance premiums and more for clothing. This is especially true for women. In contrast, people with other chronic conditions such as asthma, diabetes, and epilepsy do not differ socially or economically from healthy nonoverweight people.

Prejudice defines people by their appearance rather than by their abilities and characters. Obese people suffer emotional pain when others treat them with insensitivity, hostility, and contempt, and they may internalize a sense of guilt and self-deprecation. Health care professionals, even dietitians, can be among the offenders without realizing it. To free our society of its obsession with body fatness and prejudice against obese people, activists are promoting respect for individuals of all body weights.

Review Notes

- The health risks of underweight include infertility (women), bone loss, and inability to preserve lean tissue when fighting a wasting disease such as cancer; risks of obesity include chronic diseases such as hypertension, type 2 diabetes, and heart disease. Both underweight and obesity increase the risk of premature death.
- Guidelines for identifying the health risks of overweight and obesity are based on a person's BMI, waist circumference, and disease risk profile.
- Obesity also incurs social, economic, and psychological risks.

Self Check

1. As carbohydrate and fat stores are depleted during fasting or starvation, the body then uses _____ as its fuel source.
   a. alcohol
   b. protein
   c. glucose
   d. triglycerides

2. When carbohydrate is not available to provide energy for the brain, as in starvation, the body produces ketone bodies from:
   a. glucose.
   b. glycerol.
   c. fatty acid fragments.
   d. amino acids.

3. Three hazards of fasting are:
   a. water weight loss, decrease in mental alertness, and wasting of lean tissue.
   b. water weight gain, impairment of disease resistance, and lowering of body temperature.
   c. water weight gain, decrease in mental alertness, and impairment of disease resistance.
   d. wasting of lean tissue, impairment of disease resistance, and disturbances of the body's salt and water balance.

4. Two activities that contribute to the basal metabolic rate are:
   a. walking and running.
   b. maintenance of heartbeat and running.
   c. maintenance of body temperature and walking.
   d. maintenance of heartbeat and body temperature.

5. Three factors that affect the body's basal metabolic rate are:
   a. height, weight, and energy intake.
   b. age, body composition, and height.
   c. fever, body composition, and altitude.
   d. weight, fever, and environmental temperature.

6. The largest component of energy expenditure is:
   a. basal metabolism.
   b. physical activity.
   c. indirect calorimetry.
   d. thermic effect of food.

7. Which of the following reflects height and weight?
   a. Body mass index
   b. Central obesity
   c. Waist circumference
   d. Body composition

8. The BMI range that correlates with the fewest health risks is:
   a. 16.5 to 20.9.
   b. 18.5 to 24.9.
   c. 25.5 to 30.9.
   d. 30.5 to 34.9.

9. The profile of central obesity is sometimes referred to as a(n):
   a. beer.
   b. pear.
   c. apple.
   d. potato.

10. Which of the following health risks is *not* associated with being overweight?
    a. Hypertension
    b. Heart disease
    c. Type 1 diabetes
    d. Gallbladder disease

Answers: 1. b, 2. c, 3. d, 4. d, 5. b, 6. a, 7. a, 8. b, 9. c, 10. c

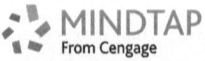 **MINDTAP** From Cengage   For more chapter resources visit **www.cengage.com** to access MindTap, a complete digital course.

Clinical Applications

1. Compare the energy a person might spend on various physical activities. Refer to Table 6-2 on pp. 153–154, and compute how much energy a person who weighs 142 pounds would spend doing each of the following activities. An example using aerobic dance has been provided for you. You may want to compare various activities based on your own weight.

   30 minutes of vigorous aerobic dance:
   0.062 kcal/lb/min × 142 lb = 8.8 kcal/min

   8.8 kcal/min × 30 min = 264 kcal

   a. 2 hours of golf, carrying clubs.
   b. 20 minutes running at 9 mph.
   c. 45 minutes of swimming at 20 yd/min.
   d. 1 hour of walking at 3.5 mph.

2. Using Box 6-1 on p. 156 as a guide, determine your Estimated Energy Requirement (EER).

Answers: 1. (a) 0.045 kcal/lb/min × 142 lb = 6.4 kcal/min, 6.4 kcal/min × 120 min = 768 kcal;
(b) 0.103 kcal/lb/min × 142 lb = 14.6 kcal/min, 14.6 kcal/min × 20 min = 292 kcal;
(c) 0.032 kcal/lb/min × 142 lb = 4.5 kcal/min, 4.5 kcal/min × 45 = 202.5 kcal;
(d) 0.035 kcal/lb/min × 142 lb = 5 kcal/min, 5 kcal/min × 60 min = 300 kcal

Notes

1. G. Traversy and J. P. Chaput, Alcohol consumption and obesity: An update, *Current Obesity Reports* 4 (2015): 122–130; T. Kondoh and coauthors, Association of dietary factors with abdominal subcutaneous and visceral adiposity in Japanese men, *Obesity Research and Clinical Practice* 8 (2014): e16–25.

2. R. Jäger and coauthors, International Society of Sports Nutrition Position Stand: Protein and exercise, *Journal of the International Society of Sports Nutrition* 14 (2017): 20; D. H. Pesta and V. T. Samuel, A high-protein diet for reducing body fat: Mechanisms and possible caveats, *Nutrition and Metabolism* 11 (2014): 11.

3. R. E. Patterson and coauthors, Intermittent fasting and human metabolic health, *Journal of the Academy of Nutrition and Dietetics* 115 (2015): 1203–1212.

4. B. D. Horne, J. B. Muhlestein, and J. L. Anderson, Health effects of intermittent fasting: Hormesis or harm? A systematic review, *American Journal of Clinical Nutrition* 102 (2015): 464–470; G. M. Tinsley and P. M. LaBounty, Effects of intermittent fasting on body composition and clinical health markers in humans, *Nutrition Reviews* 73 (2015): 661–674.

5. D. M. Thomas and coauthors, Time to correctly predict the amount of weight loss with dieting, *Journal of the Academy of Nutrition and Dietetics* 114 (2014): 857–861.

6. S. A. McLean, S. J. Paxton, and E. H. Wertheim, The role of media literacy in body dissatisfaction and disordered eating: A systematic review, *Body Image* 19 (2016): 9–23; L. Das, R. Mohan, and T. Makaya, The bid to lose weight: Impact of social media on weight perceptions, weight control and diabetes, *Current Diabetes Reviews* 10 (2014): 291–297; L. P. MacNeill and L. A. Best, Perceived current and ideal body size in female undergraduates, *Eating Behaviors* 18 (2015): 71–75.

7. J. I. Mechanick, D. L. Hurley, and W. T. Garvey, Adiposity-based chronic disease as a new diagnostic term: The American Association of Clinical Endocrinologists and American College of Endocrinology Position Statement, *Endocrine Practice* 23 (2017): 372–378.

8. S. Sharma and coauthors, Normal-weight central obesity and mortality risk in older adults with coronary artery disease, *Mayo Clinic Proceedings* 91 (2016): 343–351; K. R. Sahakyan and coauthors, Normal-weight central obesity: Implications for total and cardiovascular mortality, *Annals of Internal Medicine* 163 (2015): 827–835; A. Steffen and coauthors, General and abdominal obesity and risk of esophageal and gastric adenocarcinoma in the European Prospective Investigation into Cancer and Nutrition, *International Journal of Cancer* 137 (2015): 646–657; M. Bastien and coauthors, Overview of epidemiology and contribution of obesity to cardiovascular disease, *Progress in Cardiovascular Diseases* 56 (2014): 369–381; J. R. Cerhan and coauthors, A pooled analysis of waist circumference and mortality in 650,000 adults, *Mayo Clinic Proceedings* 89 (2014): 335–345.

9. Mechanick, Hurley, and Garvey, 2017; J. I. Mechanick, S. Zhao, and W. T. Garvey, The adipokines-cardiovascular-lifestyle network: Translation to clinical practice, *Journal of the American College of Cardiology* 68 (2016): 1785–1803; F. Molica and coauthors, Adipokines at the crossroad between obesity and cardiovascular disease, *Thrombosis and Haemostasis* 113 (2015): 553–566; Bastien and coauthors, 2014.

10. Molica and coauthors, 2015; Bastien and coauthors, 2014.

11. S. Ada Garcez and coauthors, Physical activity in adolescence and Abdominal obesity in adulthood: A case-control study among women shift workers, *Women Health* 55 (2015): 419–431.

12. D. K. Tobias and coauthors, Body-mass index and mortality among adults with incident type 2 diabetes, *New England Journal of Medicine* 370 (2014): 233–244; D. W. Gord and coauthors, Body mass index, poor diet quality, and health-related quality of life are associated with mortality in rural older adults, *Journal of Nutrition in Gerontology and Geriatrics* 33 (2014): 23–34.

13. C. L. Ogden, M. D. Carroll, and K. M. Flegal, Prevalence of childhood and adult obesity in the United States, 2011–2012, *Journal of the American Medical Association* 311 (2014): 806–814; S. A. Cunningham, M. R. Kramer, and K. M. Venkat Narayan, Incidence of childhood obesity in the United States, *New England Journal of Medicine* 370 (2014): 403–411.

14. Centers for Disease Control and Prevention, Fast Stats: Obesity and Overweight, www.cdc.gov/nchs/fastats/obesity-overweight.htm, updated May 3, 2017.

15. J. C. Seidell and J. Halberstadt, The global burden of obesity and the challenges of prevention, *Annals of Nutrition and Metabolism* 66 (2015): 7–12; M. Ng and coauthors, Global, regional, and national prevalence of Overweight and obesity in children and adults during 1980–2013: A systematic analysis for the Global Burden of Disease Study 2013, *Lancet* 384 (2014): 766–781.

16. W. Dietz, Current epidemiology of obesity in the United States, in *The Current State of Obesity Solutions in the United States* (Washington, D.C.: National Academies Press, 2014), pp. 5–14.

17. American Diabetes Association, Classification and diagnosis of diabetes, *Diabetes Care* 40 (2017): S11–S24.

18. P. Nordström and coauthors, Risks of myocardial infarction, death, and diabetes in identical twin pairs with different body mass indexes, *JAMA Internal Medicine* 176 (2016): 1522–1529.

19. U. Smith, Abdominal obesity: A marker of ectopic fat accumulation, *Journal of Clinical Investigation* 125 (2015): 1790–1792; H. Cederberg and coauthors, Family history of type 2 diabetes increases the risk of both obesity and its complications: Is type 2 diabetes a disease of inappropriate lipid storage? *Journal of Internal Medicine* 277 (2015): 540–551; J. H. Goedecke and L. K. Micklesfield, The effect of exercise on obesity, body fat distribution and risk for type 2 diabetes, *Medicine and Sport Science* 60 (2014): 82–93.

20. E. J. Benjamin and coauthors, Heart disease and stroke statistics—2017 update: A report from the American Heart Association, *Circulation* 135 (2017): e146–e608; C. Nunez and coauthors, Obesity, physical activity and cancer risks: Results from the Cancer, Lifestyle and Evaluations of Risk Study (CLEAR), *Cancer Epidemiology* 47 (2017): 56–63; K. B. Smith and M.S. Smith, Obesity statistics, *Primary Care* 43 (2016): 121–135; P. Manna and S. K. Jain, Obesity, oxidative stress, adipose tissue dysfunction, and the associated health risks: Causes and therapeutic strategies, *Metabolic Syndrome and Related Disorders* 13 (2015): 423–444; Bastien and coauthors, 2014; J. A. Ligibel and coauthors, American Society of Clinical Oncology position statement on obesity and cancer, *Journal of Clinical Oncology* 32 (2014): 3568–3574.

21. S. A. Grover and coauthors, Years of life lost and healthy life-years lost from diabetes and cardiovascular disease in overweight and obese people: A modeling study, *Lancet: Diabetes and Endocrinology* 3 (2015): 114–122.

22. E. Fabbrini and coauthors, Metabolically normal obese people are protected from adverse effects following weight gain, *Journal of Clinical Investigation* 125 (2015): 787–795; E. Navarro and coauthors, Can metabolically healthy obesity be explained by diet, genetics, and inflammation? *Molecular Nutrition and Food Research* 59 (2015): 75–93.

23. T. F. S. Teixeira and coauthors, Main characteristics of metabolically obese normal weight and metabolically healthy obese phenotypes, *Nutrition Reviews* 73 (2015): 175–190.

24. C. Lassale and coauthors, Separate and combined associations of obesity and metabolic health with coronary heart disease: A pan-European case-cohort analysis, *European Heat Journal,* 2017, doi.org/10.1093/eurheart/ehx448; A. Muñoz-Garach, I. Cornejo-Pareja, and F. J. Tinahones, Does metabolically healthy obesity exist? *Nutrients* 8 (2016): 320.

25. M. D. Jensen and coauthors, 2013 AHA/ACC/TOS guideline for the Management of overweight and obesity in adults: A report of the American College of Cardiology/American Heart Association Task Force on Practice Guidelines and The Obesity Society, *Circulation* 22 (2014): S5–S39.

26. Jensen and coauthors, 2014.

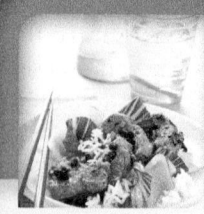

6.5 Nutrition in Practice
Eating Disorders

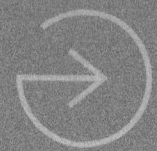

The exact number of people in the United States afflicted with some form of **eating disorder** (see Box NP6-1 for the relevant terms) is unknown because many such individuals do not seek treatment, so their cases are never reported. An estimated 6 percent of females and 3 percent of males have **anorexia nervosa**, **bulimia nervosa**, or **binge eating disorder**. Many more suffer from other unspecified eating disorders that do not meet the strict diagnostic criteria for anorexia nervosa, bulimia nervosa, or binge eating disorder but still imperil a person's well-being. Characteristics of **disordered eating**—such as restrained eating, binge eating, purging, fear of fatness, and distortion of body image—are common, especially among young middle-class girls. The incidence and prevalence of eating disorders in young people has increased steadily over recent decades.[1] Most alarming is the rising prevalence of eating disorders at progressively younger ages. In most other societies, these behaviors and attitudes are much less prevalent.

Why do so many young people in our society suffer from eating disorders?

Most experts agree that the causes are multifactorial: sociocultural, psychological, genetic, and probably also neurochemical.[2] However, excessive pressure to be thin in our society is at least partly to blame. When low body weight becomes an important goal, people begin to view normal, healthy body weight as too fat. Healthy people then take unhealthy actions to lose weight. Severe restriction of food intake can create intense stress and extreme hunger that leads to binges. Many adolescents diet to lose weight and choose unhealthy behaviors associated with disordered eating. Energy restriction followed by bingeing can set in motion a pattern of **weight cycling**, which may make weight loss and maintenance more difficult over time. Importantly, healthful dieting and physical activity in overweight adolescents do not appear to trigger eating disorders.

People who attempt extreme weight loss are dissatisfied with their bodies to begin with; they may also be depressed

---

Box NP6-1 Glossary

amenorrhea (ay-MEN-oh-RE-ah): the absence of or cessation of menstruation. Primary amenorrhea is menarche delayed beyond 16 years of age. Secondary amenorrhea is the absence of three to six consecutive menstrual cycles.

anorexia nervosa: an eating disorder characterized by restriction of energy intake relative to requirements, leading to a significantly low body weight, and a disturbed perception of body weight and shape; seen (usually) in adolescent girls and young women.

> *anorexia* = without appetite
> *nervosa* = of nervous origin

binge eating disorder: an eating disorder characterized by recurring episodes of eating a significant amount of food in a short period of time with marked feelings of lack of control.

bulimia (byoo-LEM-ee-uh) nervosa: an eating disorder characterized by repeated episodes of binge eating combined with a fear of becoming fat, usually followed by self-induced vomiting, misuse of laxatives or diuretics, fasting, or excessive exercise.

cathartic: a strong laxative.

cognitive behavioral therapy: psychological therapy aimed at changing undesirable behaviors by changing the underlying thought processes contributing to these behaviors. In anorexia nervosa, a goal is to replace false beliefs about body weight, eating, and self-worth with health-promoting beliefs.

disordered eating: eating behaviors that are neither normal nor healthy, including restrained eating, fasting, binge eating, and purging.

eating disorder: a disturbance in eating behavior that jeopardizes a person's physical and psychological health.

emetic (em-ET-ic): an agent that causes vomiting.

female athlete triad: a potentially fatal triad of medical problems seen in female athletes: low energy availability (with or without disordered eating), menstrual dysfunction, and low bone mineral density.

RED-S (relative energy deficiency in sport): a syndrome of impaired physiological function including, but not limited to, metabolic rate, menstrual function, bone health, immunity, protein synthesis, and cardiovascular health caused by relative energy deficiency.

stress fractures: bone damage or breaks caused by stress on bone surfaces during exercise.

weight cycling: repeated rounds of weight loss and subsequent regain, with reduced ability to lose weight with each attempt; also called *yo-yo dieting*.

or suffer social anxiety.[3] As weight loss becomes increasingly difficult, psychological problems worsen, and the likelihood of developing full-blown eating disorders increases.

People with anorexia nervosa suffer from an extreme preoccupation with weight loss that seriously endangers their health and even their lives. People with bulimia engage in episodes of binge eating alternating with periods of severe dieting or self-starvation. Some bulimics also follow binge eating with self-induced vomiting, laxative abuse, or diuretic abuse in an attempt to undo the perceived damage caused by the binge.

Are there other groups, besides girls and young women, who are vulnerable to anorexia nervosa and bulimia nervosa?

Yes. Athletes and dancers are at special risk for eating disorders.[4] They may severely restrict energy intakes in an attempt to enhance performance or appearance or to meet weight guidelines of a sport. In reality, severe energy restriction causes a loss of lean tissue that impairs physical performance and imposes a risk of eating disorders. Risk factors for eating disorders among athletes include:

- Young age (adolescence)
- Pressure to excel in a sport
- Focus on achieving or maintaining an "ideal" body weight or body fat percentage
- Participation in sports or competitions that judge performance on aesthetic appeal such as gymnastics, figure skating, or dance
- Unhealthy, unsupervised weight-loss dieting at an early age

Female athletes are most vulnerable, but males—especially dancers, swimmers, divers, wrestlers, skaters, jockeys, and gymnasts—suffer from eating disorders, too, and their numbers may be increasing.[5]

Male athletes and dancers with eating disorders often deny having them because they mistakenly believe that such disorders afflict only women. Under the same pressures as female athletes, males may also develop eating disorders. They skip meals, restrict fluids, practice in plastic suits, or train in heated rooms to lose a quick 4 to 7 pounds.[6] Wrestlers, especially, must "make weight" to compete in the lowest possible weight class to face smaller opponents. Conversely, male athletes may suffer weight-*gain* problems. When young men with low self-esteem internalize unrealistically bulky male body images, they can become dissatisfied with their own healthy bodies and practice unhealthy behaviors, even steroid drug abuse.

Even among athletes, however, women are most susceptible to developing eating disorders, and the term **female athlete triad** is used to refer to the syndrome characterized by low energy availability (with or without disordered eating), menstrual dysfunction (including **amenorrhea**), and low bone mineral density observed in these women.[7] Because the problems reach beyond these three components and male athletes are also affected, some, but not all, researchers use a more comprehensive term, **relative energy deficiency in sport (RED-S)**.[8]

How does the female athlete triad develop?

The underlying problem of the female athlete triad (and RED-S) is an energy deficiency—too little energy intake for the energy expenditure needed to support health and the activities of daily living, growth, and sporting activities. This energy imbalance disrupts the body's normal hormonal, metabolic, and functional activities. Disordered eating underlies many cases of low energy availability, but other situations such as rapid, unsupervised weight loss or failure to eat enough during times of extreme exercise may also play a part.

Many athletic women and men engage in self-destructive eating behaviors (disordered eating) because they and their coaches have adopted unsuitable weight standards. An athlete's body must be heavier for height than a nonathlete's body because the athlete's bones and muscles are denser. Weight standards that may be appropriate for others are inappropriate for athletes. Techniques such as skinfold measures yield more useful information about body composition.

As for amenorrhea a common type of menstrual dysfunction in young female athletes, its prevalence among premenopausal women in the United States is about 2 to 5 percent overall, but among female athletes it may be as high as 54 percent. Amenorrhea is *not* a normal adaptation to strenuous physical training: it is a symptom of something going wrong. Amenorrhea is characterized by low blood estrogen, infertility, and often bone mineral losses.

In general, weight-bearing physical activity, dietary calcium, and the hormone estrogen protect against the bone loss of osteoporosis, but in women with disordered eating and amenorrhea, strenuous activity may impair bone health.[9] As noted above, vigorous training combined with low food energy intakes disrupts metabolic and hormonal balances. These disturbances compromise bone health, greatly increasing the risks of **stress fractures**.[10] Stress fractures, a serious form of bone injury, commonly occur among dancers and other competitive athletes with amenorrhea, low calcium intakes, and disordered eating. Many underweight young athletes have bones like those of postmenopausal women, and they may never recover their lost bone even after diagnosis and treatment—which makes prevention critical. Young athletes should be encouraged to consume at least 1300 milligrams of calcium each day, to eat nutrient-dense foods, and to obtain enough food energy to support weight gain and the energy expended in physical activity. Nutrition is critical to bone recovery.

| **TABLE NP6-1** | Strategies to Combat Eating Disorders |

TABLE NP6-1   Strategies to Combat Eating Disorders

The following guidelines may be useful in combating eating disorders:

- Never restrict food intakes to below the amounts suggested for adequacy by the USDA Food Patterns (see Table 1-6 , p. 19).
- Eat frequently. Include healthy snacks between meals. The person who eats regularly throughout the day never gets so hungry as to allow hunger to dictate food choices.
- If not at a healthy weight, establish a reasonable weight goal based on a healthy body composition.
- Allow a reasonable time to achieve the goal. A reasonable loss of excess fat can be achieved at the rate of about 10 percent of body weight in 6 months.
- Learn to recognize media image biases, and reject ultra-thin standards for beauty. Shift focus to health, competencies, and human interactions; bring behaviors in line with those beliefs.

Specific guidelines for athletes and dancers:

- Replace weight-based goals with performance-based goals.
- Remember that eating disorders impair physical performance. Seek confidential help in obtaining treatment if needed.
- Restrict weight-loss activities to the off-season.
- Focus on proper nutrition as an important facet of your training—as important as proper technique.

What can be done to prevent eating disorders in athletes and dancers?

To prevent eating disorders in athletes and dancers, both the performers and their coaches must be educated about links between inappropriate body weight ideals, improper weight-loss techniques, eating disorder development, adequate nutrition, and safe weight-management strategies. Coaches and dance instructors should never encourage unhealthy weight loss to qualify for competition or to conform with distorted artistic ideals. Frequent weighings can push young people who are striving to lose weight into a cycle of starving to confront the scale and then bingeing uncontrollably afterward. The erosion of self-esteem that accompanies these events can interfere with the normal psychological development of the teen years and set the stage for serious problems later on.

Table NP6-1 provides some suggestions to help athletes and dancers protect themselves against developing eating disorders. The next sections describe eating disorders that anyone, athlete or nonathlete, may experience.

Who is at risk for anorexia nervosa?

Many anorexia nervosa victims are females who come from middle- or upper-class families. The person with anorexia nervosa is often a perfectionist who works hard to please her parents. She may identify so strongly with her parents' ideals and goals for her that she sometimes feels she has no identity of her own. She is respectful of authority but sometimes feels like a robot, and she may act that way, too: polite but controlled, rigid, and unspontaneous. She earnestly desires to control her own destiny, but she feels controlled by others. When she does not eat, she gains control.

How does a person know when dieting is going too far?

When a person loses weight to well below the average for her height, becoming too slim, and still doesn't stop, she has gone too far. Regardless of how thin she is, she looks in the mirror and sees herself as fat (see Photo NP6-1). Specific criteria for the diagnosis of anorexia nervosa include

Photo NP6-1

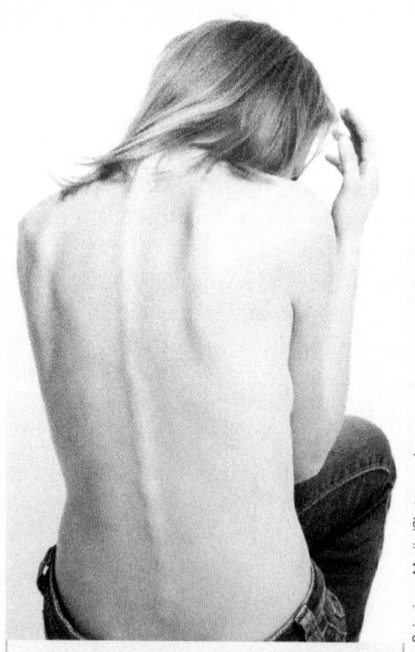

Sniegirova Mariia/Shutterstock.com

People with anorexia nervosa see themselves as fat, even when they are dangerously underweight.

significantly low body weight caused by persistent restriction of energy intake; an intense fear of gaining weight or becoming fat, or persistent behaviors that interfere with weight gains; and a disturbance in self-perceived weight or shape.[11] Central to the diagnosis of anorexia nervosa is a distorted body image that overestimates body fatness. Anorexia nervosa resembles an addiction. The characteristic behavior is obsessive and compulsive. Before drawing conclusions about someone who is extremely thin or who eats very little, remember that diagnosis of anorexia nervosa requires professional assessment.

What is the harm in being very thin?

Anorexia nervosa damages the body much as starvation does. In young people, growth ceases and normal development falters. They lose so much lean tissue that basal metabolic rate slows. Bones weaken, too—low bone density develops in adults and adolescents, male and female, with anorexia nervosa.[12] Additionally, the heart pumps inefficiently and irregularly, the heart muscle becomes weak and thin, the heart chambers diminish in size, and the blood pressure falls. Minerals that help to regulate the heartbeat become unbalanced. Many deaths in people with anorexia nervosa are due to heart failure.[13] The kidneys often fail as well.[14]

Starvation brings other physical consequences: loss of brain tissue, impaired immune response, anemia, and a loss of digestive function that worsens malnutrition. Digestive functioning becomes sluggish, the stomach empties slowly, and the lining of the intestinal tract shrinks. The ailing digestive tract fails to sufficiently digest any food the victim may eat. The pancreas slows its production of digestive enzymes. The person may suffer from diarrhea, further worsening malnutrition.

What kind of treatment helps people with anorexia nervosa?

Treatment of anorexia nervosa requires a multidisciplinary approach that addresses two sets of issues and behaviors: those relating to food and weight, and those involving relationships with oneself and others. Teams of physicians, nurses, psychiatrists, family therapists, and dietitians work together to treat people with anorexia nervosa. The expertise of a registered dietitian nutritionist is essential because an appropriate, individually crafted diet is crucial for normalizing body weight, and dietary counseling is indispensable. Seldom are clients willing to eat for themselves, but if they are, chances are they can recover without other interventions.

Professionals classify clients based on the risks posed by the degree of malnutrition present.* Clients with low risks may benefit from family counseling, **cognitive-behavioral therapy**, other psychotherapies, and

nutrition guidance; those with greater risks may also need supplemental formulas to provide extra nutrients and energy.

Sometimes, intensive behavior management treatment in a live-in facility can help to normalize food intake and exercise. When starvation leads to severe underweight (less than 75 percent of ideal body weight), high medical risks ensue, and patients require hospitalization. They must be stabilized and carefully fed to forestall death. However, involuntary feeding through a tube can cause psychological trauma and may not be necessary in all cases. Antidepressants and other drugs are commonly prescribed but rarely help.

Stopping weight loss is a first goal; establishing regular eating patterns is next. Because body weight is low and fear of weight gain is high, initial food intake may be small—1200 kcalories per day can be an achievement. A variety of high-energy foods and beverages can help deliver needed kcalories and nutrients. Even after recovery, however, energy intakes and eating behaviors may not fully return to normal.

Almost half of women who are treated can successfully maintain their body weight at just below a healthy weight; at that weight, many of them begin menstruating again. The other half have poor or fair treatment outcomes, relapse into abnormal eating behaviors, or die. Anorexia nervosa has one of the highest mortality rates among psychiatric disorders—most commonly from cardiac complications or by suicide.[15]

How does bulimia nervosa differ from anorexia nervosa?

Bulimia nervosa is distinct from anorexia nervosa and is more prevalent. More men suffer from bulimia nervosa than from anorexia, but bulimia is still more common in women. The secretive nature of bulimic behaviors makes recognition of the problem difficult, but once it is recognized, diagnosis is based on such criteria as number and frequency of binge eating episodes, inappropriate compensatory behaviors to prevent weight gain (such as self-induced vomiting or misuse of laxatives), and self-evaluation that is unduly influenced by body shape and weight.[16]

The typical person with bulimia is well educated, in her early twenties, and close to ideal body weight. She is a high achiever but emotionally insecure. She experiences considerable social anxiety and has difficulty establishing personal relationships. She is sometimes depressed and often exhibits impulsive behavior.

Like the person with anorexia nervosa, the person with bulimia spends much time thinking about her body weight and food. Her preoccupation with food manifests itself in secretive binge eating episodes followed by self-induced

---

*Indicators of malnutrition include a low percentage of body fat, low blood proteins, and impaired immune response.

vomiting, fasting, or the use of laxatives or diuretics. Such behaviors typically begin in late adolescence after a long series of various unsuccessful weight-reduction diets. People with bulimia commonly follow a pattern of restrictive dieting interspersed with bulimic behaviors and experience weight fluctuations of more than 10 pounds over short periods of time.

Unlike the person with anorexia nervosa, the person with bulimia is aware of the consequences of her behavior, feels that it is abnormal, and is deeply ashamed of it. She feels inadequate and unable to control her eating, so she tends to be passive and to look to others for confirmation of her sense of self-worth. When she is rejected, either in reality or in her imagination, her bulimia becomes worse. If her depression deepens, she may seek solace in drug or alcohol abuse or other addictive behaviors. Clinical depression is common in people with bulimia nervosa, and the rates of substance abuse are high.

What exactly is binge eating?

Binge eating is unlike normal eating, and the food is not consumed for its nutritional value. The binge eater has a compulsion to eat. A typical binge occurs periodically, is done in secret, usually at night, and lasts an hour or more. A binge frequently follows a period of rigid dieting, so the binge eating is accelerated by hunger. During a binge, the person with bulimia may consume a thousand kcalories or more. The food typically contains little fiber or water, has a smooth texture, and is high in sugar and fat, so it is easy to consume vast amounts rapidly with little chewing.

What are the consequences of binge eating and purging?

After a binge, the person may use a **cathartic**—a strong laxative that can injure the lower intestinal tract. Or the person may induce vomiting, using an **emetic**—a drug intended as first aid for poisoning.

On first glance, purging seems to offer a quick and easy solution to the problems of unwanted kcalories and body weight. Many people perceive such behavior as neutral or even positive, when, in fact, bingeing and purging have serious physical consequences. Fluid and electrolyte imbalances caused by vomiting or diarrhea can lead to abnormal heart rhythms and injury to the kidneys. Vomiting causes irritation and infection of the pharynx, esophagus, and salivary glands; erosion of the teeth; and dental caries. The esophagus may rupture or tear, as may the stomach. Overuse of emetics depletes potassium concentrations and can lead to death by heart failure.

What is the treatment for bulimia nervosa?

As for people with anorexia nervosa, a team approach provides the most effective treatment for people with bulimia nervosa. Bulimia nervosa is easier to treat than anorexia nervosa in many respects because people with bulimia know that their behavior is abnormal, and many are willing to try to cooperate.

The goal of the dietary plan to treat bulimia is to help the client gain control, establish regular eating patterns, and restore nutritional health. Energy intake should not be severely restricted—hunger can be a trigger for a binge. The person needs to learn to eat a quantity of nutritious food sufficient to nourish his or her body and to satisfy hunger (at least 1600 kcalories per day). Table NP6-2 offers some ways to begin correcting bulimia nervosa. Most people diagnosed with bulimia nervosa recover within 5 to 10 years, with or without treatment, but treatment probably speeds the recovery process.

Anorexia nervosa and bulimia nervosa are distinct eating disorders, yet they sometimes overlap. Anorexia victims may purge, and victims of both conditions share an overconcern with body weight and the tendency to drastically undereat. The two disorders can also appear in the same person, or one can lead to the other. Other people have eating disorders that fall short of anorexia nervosa or bulimia nervosa but share some of their features, such as fear of body fatness. One such condition is binge eating disorder.

How does binge eating disorder differ from bulimia nervosa?

Up to half of all people who restrict eating to lose weight periodically binge without purging, including about one-third of obese people. Obesity itself, however, does not constitute an eating disorder.

Clinicians note differences between people with bulimia nervosa and those with binge eating disorder. People with binge eating disorder consume less during a binge, rarely purge, and exert less restraint during times of dieting. Similarities also exist, including feeling out of control, disgusted, depressed, embarrassed, or guilty because of their self-perceived gluttony. Binge eating behavior responds more readily to treatment than other eating disorders, and resolving such behaviors can be a first step to authentic weight control. Successful treatment also improves physical health, mental health, and the chances of breaking the cycle of rapid weight losses and gains.

Chapter 6 describes how our society sets unrealistic ideals for body weight, especially in women, and devalues those who do not conform to them. Anorexia nervosa and bulimia nervosa are not a form of rebellion against these unreasonable expectations but rather the exaggerated acceptance of them. Body dissatisfaction is a primary factor in the development of eating disorders. Perhaps a person's best defense against these disorders is to learn to appreciate his or her own uniqueness.

PLANNING PRINCIPLES

- Plan meals and snacks; record plans in a food diary prior to eating.
- Plan meals and snacks that require eating at the table and using utensils.
- Refrain from finger foods.
- Refrain from fasting or skipping meals.

NUTRITION PRINCIPLES

- Eat a well-balanced diet and regularly timed meals consisting of a variety of foods.
- Include raw vegetables, salad, or raw fruit at meals to prolong eating times.
- Choose whole-grain, high-fiber breads, pasta, rice, and cereals to increase bulk.
- Consume adequate fluid, particularly water.

OTHER TIPS

- Choose foods that provide protein and fat for satiety and bulky, fiber-rich carbohydrates for immediate feelings of fullness.
- Try including soups and other water-rich foods for satiety.
- Choose portions that are appropriate for your energy needs according to the USDA Food Patterns (p. 18–19).
- For convenience (and to reduce temptation) select foods that naturally divide into portions. Select one potato, rather than rice or pasta that can be overloaded onto the plate; purchase yogurt and cottage cheese in individual containers; look for small packages of precut steak or chicken; choose frozen dinners with measured portions.
- Include 30 minutes of physical activity every day—exercise may be an important tool in defeating bulimia.

Notes

1. B. Herpertz-Dahlmann, Adolescent eating disorders: Update on definitions, symptomatology, epidemiology, and comorbidity, *Child and Adolescent Psychiatric Clinics of North America* 24 (2015): 177–196.
2. K. Campbell and R. Peebles, Eating disorders in children and adolescents: State of the art review, *Pediatrics* 134 (2014): 582–592.
3. I. Brechan and I.L. Kvalem, Relationship between body dissatisfaction and disordered eating: Mediating role of self-esteem and depression, *Eating Behaviors* 17 (2015): 49–58.
4. J. G. Robbeson, H. S. Kruger, and H. H. Wright, Disordered eating behavior, body image, and energy status of female student dancers, *International Journal of Sport Nutrition and Exercise Metabolism* 25 (2015): 344–352; M. Martinsen and coauthors, Preventing eating disorders among young elite athletes: A randomized controlled trial, *Medicine and Science in Sports and Exercise* 46 (2014): 435–447.
5. E. Joy, A. Kussman and A. Nattiv, 2016 update on eating disorders in athletes: A comprehensive narrative review with a focus on clinical assessment and management, *British Journal of Sports Medicine* 50 (2016): 154–162; A. Melin and coauthors, Disordered eating and eating disorders in aquatic sports, *International Journal of Sport Nutrition and Exercise Metabolism* 24 (2014): 450–459.
6. G. Wilson and coauthors, Weight-making strategies in professional jockeys: Implications for physical and mental health and well-being, *Sports Medicine* 44 (2014): 785–796.
7. A. K. Weiss Kelly and S. Hecht, AAP Council on Sports Medicine and Fitness, The female athlete triad, *Pediatrics* 138 (2016): 80–89.
8. M. Mountjoy and coauthors, Consensus statement: The IOC consensus statement: Beyond the female athlete triad—relative energy deficiency in sport (RED-S), *British Journal of Sports Medicine* 48 (2014): 491–497.
9. J. C. Gibbs and coauthors, Low bone density risk is higher in exercising women with multiple triad risk factors, *Medicine and Science in Sports and Exercise* 46 (2014): 167–176; M. J. de Souza and coauthors, 2014 Female Athlete Triad Coalition Consensus Statement on treatment and return to play of the Female Athlete Triad, *British Journal of Sports Medicine* 48 (2014): 289; M. Payne and J. T. Kirchner, Should you suspect the female athlete triad? *Journal of Family Practice* 63 (2014): 187–192.
10. M. J. Hilibrand and coauthors, Common injuries and ailments of the female athlete: Pathophysiology, treatment and prevention, *The Physician and Sportsmedicine* 43 (2015): dx.doi.org/10.1080/00913847.2015.1092856; M. T. Barrack and coauthors, Higher incidence of bone stress injuries with increasing female athlete triad-related risk factors: A prospective multisite study of exercising girls and women, *American Journal of Sports Medicine* 42 (2014): 949–958.
11. Herpertz-Dahlmann, 2015; American Psychiatric Association, *Diagnostic and Statistical Manual of Mental Disorders* (Washington, D.C.: American Psychiatric Publishing, 2013).
12. Herpertz-Dalmann, 2015; M. Misra and A. Klibanski, Anorexia nervosa and bone, *Journal of Endocrinology* 221 (2014): R163–R176.
13. G. Di Cola and coauthors, Cardiovascular disorders in anorexia nervosa and potential therapeutic targets, *Internal and Emergency Medicine* 9 (2014): 717–721.
14. C. Stheneur, S. Bergeron, and A. L. Lapeyraque, Renal complications in anorexia nervosa, *Eating and Weight Disorders* 19 (2014): 455–460.
15. M. M. Fichter and N. Quadflieg, Mortality in eating disorders—results of a large prospective clinical longitudinal study, *International Journal of Eating Disorders* 49 (2016): 391–401; A. Keshaviah and coauthors, Re-examining premature mortality in anorexia nervosa: A meta-analysis redux, *Comprehensive Psychiatry* 55 (2014): 1773–1784; Di Cola and coauthors, 2014.
16. American Psychiatric Association, 2013.

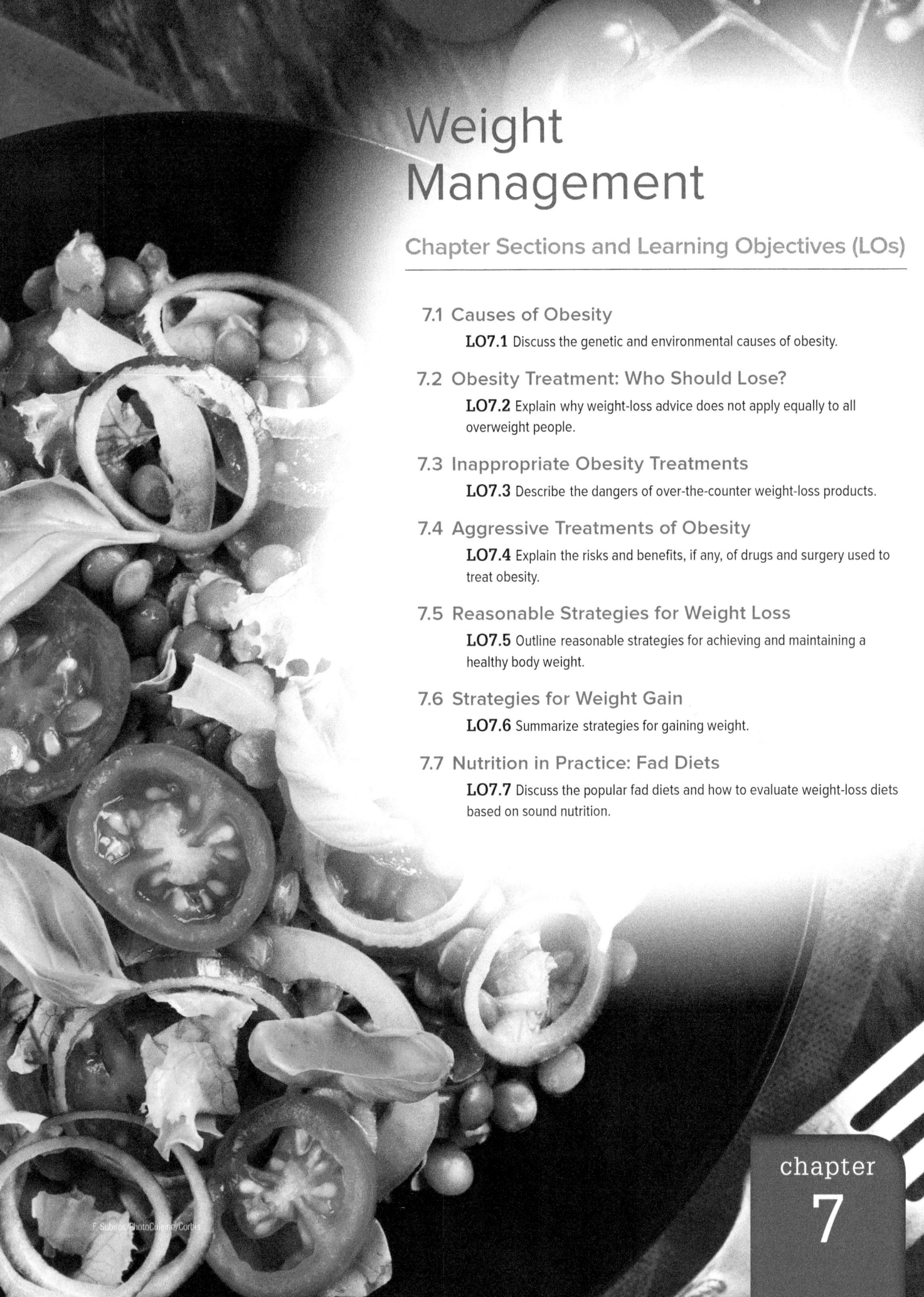

Weight Management

Chapter Sections and Learning Objectives (LOs)

7.1 Causes of Obesity
LO7.1 Discuss the genetic and environmental causes of obesity.

7.2 Obesity Treatment: Who Should Lose?
LO7.2 Explain why weight-loss advice does not apply equally to all overweight people.

7.3 Inappropriate Obesity Treatments
LO7.3 Describe the dangers of over-the-counter weight-loss products.

7.4 Aggressive Treatments of Obesity
LO7.4 Explain the risks and benefits, if any, of drugs and surgery used to treat obesity.

7.5 Reasonable Strategies for Weight Loss
LO7.5 Outline reasonable strategies for achieving and maintaining a healthy body weight.

7.6 Strategies for Weight Gain
LO7.6 Summarize strategies for gaining weight.

7.7 Nutrition in Practice: Fad Diets
LO7.7 Discuss the popular fad diets and how to evaluate weight-loss diets based on sound nutrition.

chapter

7

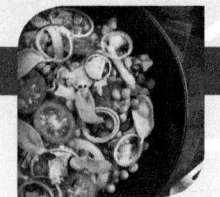
you are a rare individual. Nearly all people in our society think they should weigh more or less (mostly less) than they do. Usually, their primary reason is appearance, but they often perceive, correctly, that their weight is also related to physical health. Chapter 6 addressed the health risks of being overweight or underweight.

Overweight and underweight both result from energy imbalance. The simple picture is as follows. Overweight people have consumed more food energy than they have expended and have banked the surplus in their body fat. To reduce body fat, overweight people need to expend more energy than they take in from food. In contrast, underweight people have consumed too little food energy to support their activities and so have depleted their bodies' fat stores and possibly some of their lean tissues as well. To gain weight, they need to take in more food energy than they expend.

This chapter's missions are to present strategies for solving the problems of excessive and deficient body fatness and to point out how appropriate body composition, once achieved, can be maintained. The chapter emphasizes overweight and obesity, partly because they have been more intensively studied and partly because they represent a major health problem in the United States and a growing concern worldwide.

7.1 Causes of Obesity

Henceforth, this chapter will use the term *obesity* to refer to excess body fat. Excess body fat accumulates when people take in more food energy than they expend. Why do they do this? Is it genetic? Metabolic? Psychological? Behavioral? All of these? Most likely, obesity has many interrelated causes. This section reviews the two major contributing and interacting factors: genetics and the environment.[1]

Genetics and Weight

A person's genetic makeup influences the body's tendency to consume or store too much energy or to expend too little.[2] Evidence that genes influence eating behavior and body composition comes from family, twin, and adoption studies. Adopted children tend to be more similar in weight to their biological parents than to their adoptive parents.[3] Studies of twins yield similar findings: compared with fraternal twins, identical twins are far more likely to weigh the same. Genes clearly influence a person's tendency to gain weight or stay lean.[4] For someone with at least one obese parent, the chance of becoming obese is estimated to fall between 30 and 70 percent. Despite such findings, however, only 1 to 5 percent of obesity cases can be explained by a single gene mutation. Furthermore, although genomics researchers have identified hundreds of genes with possible roles in obesity development, they have not yet identified a single genetic cause of common obesity.

Exceptionally complex relationships exist among the many genes related to energy metabolism and obesity, and they each interact with environmental factors, too. Although an individual's genetic inheritance may make obesity likely, it will not necessarily develop unless given a push by environmental factors that encourage energy consumption and discourage energy expenditure. High-fat diets, sugar-sweetened beverages, and low physical activity, for example, can accentuate the genetic influences on obesity.[5] Likewise, physical activity can minimize the genetic influences on BMI. The following sections describe research involving proteins that might help explain appetite control, energy regulation, and obesity development.

lipoprotein lipase (LPL): an enzyme mounted on the surface of fat cells (and other cells) that hydrolyzes triglycerides in the blood into fatty acids and glycerol for absorption into the cells. There they are metabolized or reassembled for storage.

Lipoprotein Lipase Some of the research investigating genetic influence on obesity focuses on the enzyme **lipoprotein lipase (LPL)**, which promotes fat storage in fat cells and muscle cells. People with high LPL activity are especially efficient at storing fat. Obese people generally have much more LPL activity in their fat cells than lean people do (their muscle cell LPL activity is similar, though). This high LPL activity makes fat storage especially efficient. Consequently, even modest excesses in energy intake have a more dramatic impact on obese people than on lean people.

Leptin Researchers have identified a gene in humans called the obesity (*ob*) gene. The obesity gene codes for the protein **leptin**. Leptin is a hormone primarily produced and secreted by the fat cells in proportion to the amount of fat stored. A gain in body fatness stimulates the production of leptin, which, by way of the **hypothalamus**, suppresses the appetite, increases energy expenditure, and produces fat loss.[6] Fat loss produces the opposite effect— suppression of leptin production, increased appetite, and decreased energy expenditure. As Figure 7-1 shows, mice with a defective obesity gene do not produce leptin and can weigh up to three times as much as normal mice. When injected with leptin, the mice lose weight. (Because leptin is a protein, it would be destroyed during digestion if given orally; consequently, it must be given by injection.)

Courtesy Amgen, Inc. Photo © John Sholtis/The Rockefeller University

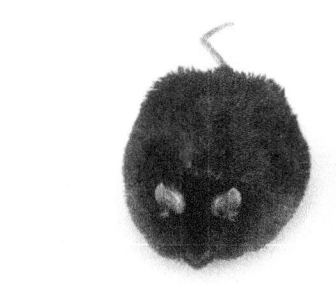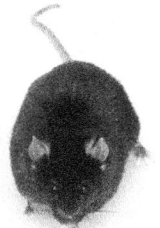

FIGURE 7-1 Mice with and without Leptin Compared

The mouse on the left is genetically obese—it lacks the gene for producing leptin. The mouse on the right is also genetically obese, but because it receives leptin, it eats less, expends more energy, and is less obese than it would be had it not received the leptin.

Although it is extremely rare, researchers have identified a genetic deficiency of leptin in human beings as well. An error in the gene that codes for leptin was discovered in two extremely obese children whose blood levels of leptin were barely detectable. Without leptin, the children had little appetite control; they were constantly hungry and ate considerably more than their siblings or peers. Given daily injections of leptin, these children lost a substantial amount of weight, confirming leptin's role in regulating appetite and body weight.

Most obese people do not have leptin deficiency, however. In fact, most obese people produce plenty of leptin, but they fail to respond to it, a condition called *leptin resistance*.[7] Researchers speculate that blood leptin rises in an effort to suppress appetite and inhibit fat storage when fat cells are ample. Obese people with elevated leptin concentrations may be resistant to its satiating effect. The absence of or resistance to leptin in obesity parallels the scenario of insulin in diabetes: some people have an insulin deficiency (type 1), whereas many others have elevated insulin but are resistant to its glucose-storing effect (type 2).

Ghrelin Another protein known as **ghrelin** works in the opposite direction of leptin. Ghrelin is synthesized and secreted primarily by the stomach cells but works in the hypothalamus to promote a positive energy balance by increasing smell sensitivity, stimulating appetite, and promoting efficient energy storage.[8] The role ghrelin plays in regulating food intake and body weight is the subject of much intense research. Pharmaceutical companies are eager to develop products that mimic ghrelin to treat wasting conditions, as well as products that oppose ghrelin's action to treat obesity.[9]

Ghrelin powerfully triggers the desire to eat. Blood levels of ghrelin typically rise before and fall after a meal—reflecting the hunger and satiety that precede and follow eating. In general, fasting blood levels correlate inversely with body weight: Lean people have high ghrelin levels and obese people have low levels.

Ghrelin fights to maintain a stable body weight. On average, ghrelin levels are high whenever the body is in negative energy balance, as occurs during low-kcalorie diets, for example. This response may help explain why weight loss is so difficult to maintain. Ghrelin levels decline again whenever the body is in positive energy balance, as occurs with weight gains.

Interestingly, research suggests an association between ghrelin and sleep duration. A lack of sleep increases levels of ghrelin, which may help to explain the associations between inadequate sleep, higher energy intakes and weight gain.[10]

leptin: a hormone produced by fat cells under the direction of the (*ob*) gene. It decreases appetite and increases energy expenditure.

leptos = thin

hypothalamus (high-po-THAL-ah-mus)**:** a brain center that controls activities such as maintenance of water balance, regulation of body temperature, and control of appetite.

ghrelin (GRELL-in)**:** a hormone produced primarily by the stomach cells. It signals the hypothalamus of the brain to stimulate appetite and food intake.

FIGURE 7-2 Fat Cell Development

Fat cells are capable of increasing their size by 20-fold and their number by several thousand-fold.

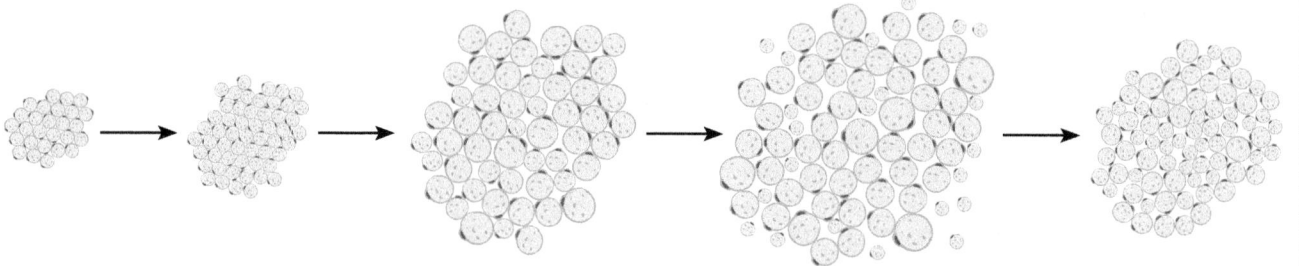

During growth, fat cells increase in number.

When energy intake exceeds expenditure, fat cells increase in size.

When fat cells have enlarged and energy intake continues to exceed energy expenditure, fat cells increase in number again.

With fat loss, the size of the fat cells shrinks, but not the number.

Fat Cell Development When "energy in" exceeds "energy out," much of the excess energy is stored in the fat cells of adipose tissue. The amount of fat in adipose tissue reflects both the *number* and the *size* of the fat cells.* Thus, obesity develops when a person's fat cells increase in number, in size, or quite often both. The number of fat cells increases most rapidly during the growing years of late childhood and early puberty. After growth ceases, fat cell number may continue to increase whenever energy balance is positive. Fat cells can also expand in size. After they reach their maximum size, more cells can develop to store more fat. Obese people have more fat cells than healthy-weight people; their fat cells are also larger. Figure 7-2 illustrates fat cell development.

With fat loss, the size of the fat cells shrinks, but their number cannot. For this reason, people with extra fat cells may tend to regain lost weight rapidly. Prevention of obesity is most critical, then, during the growing years of childhood and adolescence when fat cells increase in number most profoundly.

As mentioned, excess fat first fills the body's natural storage site—adipose tissue. If fat is still abundant, the excess is deposited in organs such as the heart and liver and plays a key role in the development of heart failure and fatty liver, respectively.[11] As adipose tissue produces adipokines, metabolic changes that indicate disease risk—such as insulin resistance—become apparent and chronic inflammation develops.[12]

Set-Point Theory One popular theory of why a person may store too much fat is the **set-point theory**. The set-point theory proposes that body weight, like body temperature, is physiologically regulated.[13] Researchers have noted that many people who lose weight quickly regain it all. This suggests that somehow the body chooses a preferred weight and defends that weight by regulating eating behaviors and hormonal actions. After weight losses, the body reduces its metabolic rate. The decrease in metabolic rate after weight loss is greater than would be expected based on body composition alone.[14] This adaptation helps to explain why it can be difficult for an overweight person to maintain weight losses. While set point answers some questions regarding the biology of energy balance, it fails to explain the many other influences contributing to the population's obesity epidemic.

Intestinal Bacteria As noted in Chapters 2 and 3, certain remnants of food, largely fibers, not digested by human enzymes in the small intestine are often broken down by billions of living inhabitants (primarily bacteria) in the colon, collectively called the **microbiota**. These intestinal bacteria may affect many body systems. They generate compounds that communicate with such diverse tissues as muscle, adipose tissue, and

set-point theory: the theory that the body tends to maintain a certain weight by means of its own internal controls.

microbiota: the mix of microbial species of a community; for example, all of the bacterium, fungi, and viruses present in the human digestive tract.

*Obesity due to an increase in the *number* of fat cells is *hyperplastic obesity.* Obesity due to an increase in the *size* of fat cells is *hypertrophic obesity.*

even the brain, in ways that alter the body's use and storage of energy. The bacteria also deliver messages to the immune system, affecting health and disease.[15] Research suggests that when the mix of bacterial species fall out of balance, potentially harmful bacteria proliferate, producing substances that increase inflammation and that are associated with obesity, diabetes, several intestinal conditions, fatty liver disease, certain cancers, and even asthma.[16]

Changes in the makeup of the intestinal microbiota are known to accompany changes in body weight. Mechanisms by which the intestinal microbiota may influence energy balance include regulation of energy availability and storage, interaction with signaling molecules involved in metabolism, modification of intestinal permeability, release of intestinal hormones, and low-grade, chronic inflammation.[17] Determining whether certain bacteria might be the cause or consequence of weight change is difficult, however, because the colonies quickly grow or diminish with changes in diet.[18]

Environmental Stimuli

As discussed earlier, genetic factors play a partial role in determining a person's susceptibility to obesity, but they do not fully explain obesity. Obesity rates have risen dramatically during recent decades, but the human gene pool has remained unchanged. The environment must therefore play a role as well. Obesity reflects the interaction between genes and the environment.[19] An **obesogenic environment** includes all of the circumstances that people encounter daily that push them toward fatness. Over past decades, the demand for physical activity has decreased as the abundance of food has increased.

Overeating People may overeat in response to stimuli in their surroundings—primarily, the availability of many delectable foods. Most people in the United States find high-kcalorie foods readily available, relatively inexpensive, heavily advertised, and reasonably tasty—thanks largely to fast food. With around-the-clock access to rich palatable foods, we eat more meals more frequently than in decades past—and energy intakes have risen accordingly. By comparison, simply eating meals at regularly scheduled times can be helpful in managing weight.[20]

Most alarming are the extraordinarily large serving sizes and ready-to-go meals offered in supersize combinations. Eating large portion sizes multiple times a day accounts for much of the weight increase seen over the decades. People buy the large sizes and combinations, perceiving them to be a good value, but then they eat more than they need. Research suggests that people eat more if they're served more.[21] Portion sizes of virtually all foods and beverages (and even sizes of plates, glasses, and utensils) have increased markedly in past decades, most notably at fast-food restaurants. The increase in portion sizes parallels the growing prevalence of overweight and obesity in the United States, beginning in the 1970s, rising sharply in the 1980s, and continuing today.

Restaurant food, especially fast food, contributes significantly to the development of obesity. Fast food is often energy-dense food, which increases energy intake, BMI, and body fatness.[22] The combination of large portions and energy-dense foods strikes a double blow. Reducing portion sizes is helpful, but the real kcalorie savings come from lowering the energy density. Satisfying portions of foods with low energy density such as fruit and vegetables can help with weight loss.[23]

Consumers' health would benefit from restaurants providing appropriate portion sizes and offering more fruit, vegetables, legumes, and whole grains. In an effort to help consumers make healthier choices, the FDA requires chain restaurants with 20 or more locations, including fast-food restaurants, to provide kcalorie information on menus and menu boards for each standard menu item. In local, nonchain restaurants, where such helpful information may be lacking, people must learn to judge portions on their own.

Learned Behavior Psychological stimuli also trigger inappropriate eating behaviors in some people. Appropriate eating behavior is a response to **hunger**. Hunger is a drive programmed into people by their heredity. **Appetite**, in contrast, is learned and can lead

obesogenic (oh- BES-oh-JEN-ick) environment: all the factors surrounding a person that promote weight gain, such as an increased food intake—especially of unhealthy choices—and decreased physical activity.

hunger: the physiological need to eat, experienced as a drive to obtain food; an unpleasant sensation that demands relief.

appetite: the psychological desire to eat; a learned motivation that is experienced as a pleasant sensation that accompanies the sight, smell, or thought of appealing foods.

Photo 7-1

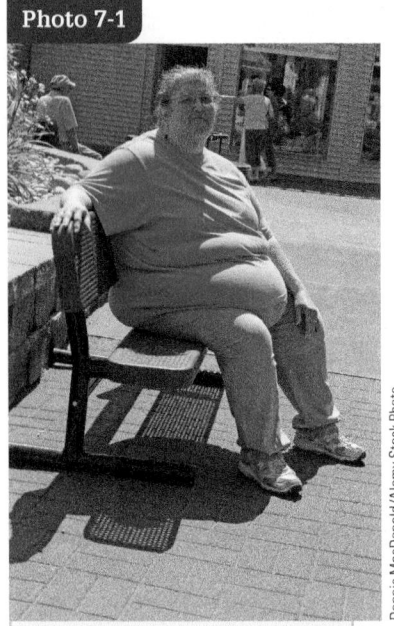

Lack of physical activity fosters obesity.

Dennis MacDonald/Alamy Stock Photo

people to ignore hunger or to overrespond to it. Hunger is physiological, whereas appetite is psychological, and the two do not always coincide.

During the course of a meal, as food enters the GI tract and hunger diminishes, **satiation** occurs. As receptors in the stomach stretch and hormones become active, the person begins to feel full. The response is satiation, which prompts the person to stop eating.

After a meal, the feeling of **satiety** continues to suppress hunger and allow a person to not eat again for a while. Whereas *satiation* tells us to "stop eating," *satiety* reminds us to "not start eating again." As mentioned above, people can override these signals, especially when presented with favorite foods or stressful situations.

Food behavior is intimately connected to deep emotional needs such as the primitive fear of starvation. Yearnings, cravings, and addictions with profound psychological significance can express themselves in people's eating behavior. An emotionally insecure person might eat rather than call a friend and risk rejection. Another person might eat to relieve boredom or to ward off depression.

Physical Inactivity The possible causes of obesity mentioned so far all relate to the input side of the energy equation. What about output? People may be obese, not because they eat too much, but because they move too little—both in purposeful exercise and in the activities of daily life.[24] Obese people observed closely are often seen to eat less than lean people, but they are sometimes so extraordinarily inactive that they still manage to accumulate an energy surplus (see Photo 7-1). Reducing their food intake further would jeopardize health and incur nutrient deficiencies. Physical activity, then, is a necessary component of nutritional health. People must be physically active if they are to eat enough food to deliver all the nutrients needed without unhealthy weight gain.

Our environment, however, fosters inactivity. In turn, inactivity contributes to obesity and poor health.[25] Sedentary **screen time** has all but replaced outdoor activity for many people. In addition, most people work at sedentary jobs. One hundred years ago, 30 percent of the energy used in farm and factory work came from muscle power; today, only 1 percent does. Modern technology has replaced physical activity at home, at work, at school, and in transportation. The more time spent sitting still, the higher the risk of dying from heart disease and other causes.[26]

Health experts urge people to "take the stairs instead of the elevator" or "walk or bike to work." These are excellent suggestions: Climbing stairs provides an impromptu workout, and people who walk or ride a bicycle for transportation most often meet their needs for physical activity. Physical activity strategies for weight loss and weight maintenance are offered in a later section of this chapter.

Neighborhood Obstacles to Physical Activity and Healthy Foods Some aspects of the **built environment**, including buildings, sidewalks, and transportation opportunities, can discourage physical activity. For example, many stairwells of modern buildings are inconvenient, isolated, and unsafe. Roadways often lack sidewalks, crosswalks, or lanes marked for bicycles. The air on roadways can be dangerously high in carbon monoxide gas and other pollutants from gasoline engine emissions. Hot and cold weather also pose hazards for outdoor commuters. In contrast, those with access to health-promoting foods and built environments more easily make healthy choices.[27] Safe, affordable biking and walking areas and public exercise facilities help maintain health and body leanness.

In addition, residents of many low-income urban and rural areas lack access to even a single supermarket. Often overweight and lacking transportation, residents of these so-called **food deserts** have limited access to the affordable, fresh, nutrient-dense foods they need. Instead, they shop at local convenience stores and fast-food places, where they purchase mostly refined packaged sweets and starches, sugary soft drinks, fatty canned meats, or fast foods, and have eating patterns that predict high rates of obesity and chronic diseases. Still unknown is whether efforts to increase access to healthy foods will improve people's odds of escaping these ills.[28]

satiation (say-she-AY-shun): the feeling of satisfaction and fullness that occurs during a meal and halts eating. Satiation determines how much food is consumed during a meal.

satiety: the feeling of fullness and satisfaction that occurs after a meal and inhibits eating until the next meal. Satiety determines how much time passes between meals.

screen time: sedentary time spent using an electronic device, such as a television, computer, or video-game player.

built environment: the buildings, roads, utilities, homes, fixtures, parks, and all other manufactured entities that form the physical characteristics of a community.

food deserts: urban and rural low-income areas with limited access to affordable and nutritious foods.

The prestigious National Academies' Institute of Medicine has put forth the national goals in Table 7-1 as most likely to slow or reverse the obesity epidemic and improve the nation's health. Such changes require leaders at all levels and citizenry across all sectors of society to work toward one goal: improving the health of the nation.

TABLE 7-1	National Goals to Combat Obesity

- Make physical activity an integral and routine part of American life.
- Make healthy foods and beverages available everywhere.
- Create food and beverage environments to make healthy food and beverage choices the routine, easy choice.
- Advertise and market what matters for a healthy life.
- Engage employers and healthcare professionals.
- Strengthen schools as centers that promote fitness and health.

Source: Adapted from: Institute of Medicine (U.S.) Committee on Accelerating Progress in Obesity Prevention, *Accelerating Progress in Obesity Prevention: Solving the Weight of the Nation* (Washington, D.C.: National Academies Press, 2012), available at www.nap.edu.

Review Notes

- Genetics, fat cell development, set point, intestinal microbiota, overeating, and inactivity all offer possible, but still incomplete, explanations of obesity.
- Most likely, obesity has not one cause but different causes and combinations of causes in different people.
- The easy availability of large portions of energy-dense foods is a major environmental factor thought to be contributing to the obesity epidemic.
- Built environments that lack opportunities for safe physical activity and access to fresh, nutrient-dense foods are also linked with obesity.

7.2 Obesity Treatment: Who Should Lose?

Millions of U.S. adults are trying to lose weight at any given time. Some of these people do not even need to lose weight. Others may benefit from weight loss but are not successful. Relatively few people succeed in losing weight, and even fewer succeed permanently.

Many people assume that every overweight person can achieve slenderness and should pursue that goal. Consider, however, that most overweight people cannot become slender. People vary in their weight tendencies just as they vary in their potentials for height and degrees of health. The question of whether a person should lose weight depends on many factors: the extent of overweight, age, health, and genetics, to name a few. Weight-loss advice, then, does not apply equally to all overweight people. Some people may risk more in the process of losing weight than in remaining overweight. Others may reap significant health benefits with even modest weight loss.

Review Notes

- Weight-loss advice does not apply equally to all overweight people.
- Some people may risk more through misguided efforts to lose weight than by remaining overweight, whereas others may benefit from even a modest weight loss.

7.3 Inappropriate Obesity Treatments

The risks people incur in attempting to lose weight often depend on how they go about it. Weight-loss plans and obesity treatments abound—some are adequate, but many are ineffective and possibly dangerous. Fad diets are the topic of Nutrition in Practice 7. This section addresses other inappropriate obesity interventions. Aggressive treatment approaches for obese people who face high risks of medical problems and must lose weight rapidly are discussed in the next section. Reasonable approaches to overweight for those seeking safe, gradual weight losses are saved for the last part of the obesity treatment discussion.

Over-the-Counter Weight-Loss Products

Millions of people in the United States, even some who are not overweight, use over-the-counter (OTC) weight-loss products, believing them to be safe. Promoters and marketers of weight-loss products make all kinds of claims for their products with only one intention—profit. Such claims as "eat all you want and lose weight," "take three pills before bedtime and watch the fat disappear," "blocks carbs," "blocks fat," and many more lure people into believing that maybe this time a product will really work.

OTC weight-loss pills, powders, herbs, and other "dietary supplements" are not associated with successful weight loss and maintenance, and they may not be safe. In fact, the FDA has found an alarming number of products that illegally contain prescription medications. Strong diuretics, unproven experimental drugs, psychotropic drugs used to treat mental illnesses, and even drugs deemed unsafe and so banned from U.S. markets have been identified and all pose serious health risks.[29]

Nutrition in Practice 15 explores the possible benefits and potential dangers of herbal products and other alternative therapies. Anyone using dietary supplements for weight loss should first consult a physician.

Other Gimmicks

Other gimmicks don't help with weight loss either. Hot baths do not speed up metabolism so that pounds can be lost in hours. Steam and sauna baths do not melt the fat off the body, although they may dehydrate people so that they lose water weight. Brushes, sponges, wraps, creams, and massages intended to move, burn, or break up fat do nothing of the kind.

Review Notes

- Efforts to lose weight via unwise techniques, such as use of over-the-counter supplements and herbal products, can be physically and psychologically damaging.

7.4 Aggressive Treatments of Obesity

For some obese people, the medical problems caused by obesity demand treatment approaches that may, themselves, incur some risks. The health benefits to be gained by weight loss, however, may make these risks worth taking.

Obesity Drugs

Several prescription medications for weight loss have been tried over the years. When used as part of a long-term, comprehensive weight-loss program, medications can help with modest weight loss.[30] Drugs may be an option for people who are unable to achieve adequate weight loss with diet and exercise; have a BMI ≥30 (or ≥27 with weight-related health problems); and have no medical contraindications. Because weight regain commonly occurs with the discontinuation of drug therapy, treatment is long term—and the long-term use of medications poses risks. Medical experts do not yet know whether a person would benefit more from maintaining a 50-pound excess or from taking a medication for a decade to keep the 50 pounds off.

The challenge, then, is to develop an effective drug—or more likely, a combination of drugs—that can be used over time without adverse side effects or the potential for abuse. Weight-loss drugs should be prescribed in tandem with a healthy diet and physical activity program. Table 7-2 presents the drugs to treat obesity that meet the FDA mandate that "benefits must exceed risks."

TABLE 7-2 FDA-Approved Drugs for Weight Loss

PRODUCT	ACTION	SIDE EFFECTS
Liraglutide (LIR-a-GLOO-tide), trade name: Saxenda (sax-EN-dah)	Daily injection stimulates insulin production and the release of glucagon and suppresses appetite	Nausea, diarrhea, constipation, vomiting, low blood glucose, inflammation of the pancreas, gallbladder disease, reduced kidney function, suicidal thoughts, increased heart rate; should not be used by people taking certain diabetes drugs
Lorcaserin hydrochloride, trade name: Belviq (BELL-veek)	Interacts with brain serotonin receptors to increase satiety	Headache, dizziness, fatigue, nausea, dry mouth, and constipation; low blood glucose in people with diabetes; serotonin syndrome, including agitation, confusion, fever, loss of coordination, rapid or irregular heart rate, shivering, seizures, and unconsciousness; cannot be safely used by pregnant or lactating women or people with heart valve problems; high doses cause hallucinations
Naltrexone (NAL-trex-OWN) hydrochloride (used to treat alcohol and drug dependence) and Bupropion (byu-PRO-pee-on) hydrochloride (an antidepressant used in smoking cessation) combination, trade name: Contrave (CON-trave)	Suppresses appetite	Nausea, constipation, headache, vomiting, dizziness, insomnia, dry mouth, and diarrhea; increased blood pressure, accelerated heart rate, suicidal thoughts, serious neuropsychiatric events, seizures; should not be used by pregnant women or women trying to become pregnant
Orlistat (OR-leh-stat), trade names: Alli, Xenical	Inhibits pancreatic lipase activity in the GI tract, thus blocking digestion and absorption of dietary fat and limiting energy intake	Cramping, diarrhea, gas, frequent bowel movements, reduced absorption of fat-soluble vitamins; rare cases of liver injury
Phentermine (an appetite suppressant) and topiramate (a seizure/migraine medication) combination, trade name: Qsymia (kyoo-sim-EE-uh)	Enhances the release of the neurotransmitter norepinephrine, which suppresses appetite and increases feelings of fullness, making foods taste less appealing	Increased heart rate; can cause birth defects if taken in the first weeks or months of pregnancy; may worsen glaucoma or hyperthyroidism; may interact with other medications

Note: Weight-loss drugs are most effective when taken as directed and used in combination with a reduced-kcalorie diet and increased physical activity.

Surgery

The U.S. prevalence of **clinically severe obesity** is estimated at 8 percent.[31] At this level of obesity, lifestyle changes and modest weight losses can improve disease risks a little, but the most effective treatment is surgery.[32] Three procedures, gastric bypass, gastric banding, and sleeve gastrectomy have gained wide acceptance. Each procedure limits food intake by effectively reducing the capacity of the stomach. In addition, gastric bypass suppresses hunger by changing production of gastrointestinal hormones.[33] Changes in appetite, food preferences, and GI microbiota may also influence weight losses.[34] The results are significant: depending on the type of surgery, 20 to 30 percent of the excess weight remains lost after 10 years.[35] More long-term studies are needed, but surgery with weight loss often brings immediate and lasting improvements in blood lipids, diabetes, sleep apnea, heart disease, and hypertension.[36]

Review Notes

- Obese people with high risks of medical problems may need aggressive treatment, including drugs or surgery.

clinically severe obesity: a BMI of 40 or greater, or a BMI of 35 or greater with one or more serious conditions such as hypertension. Another term used to describe the same condition is *morbid obesity*.

Photo 7-2

A healthy body contains enough lean tissue to support health and the right amount of fat to meet body needs.

7.5 Reasonable Strategies for Weight Loss

As noted at the beginning of this chapter, the factors contributing to obesity are numerous and complex. Efforts to combat obesity must integrate healthy eating patterns, physical activities, supportive environments, and psychosocial support; such interventions can be effective, even when genetic factors are in play.[37] Successful weight-loss strategies embrace small changes; moderate, sustained losses; and reasonable goals. People who consistently choose nutrient-dense foods and engage in regular physical activity can reap substantial health benefits. A modest, sustained weight loss of 3 to 5 percent, even when a person is still overweight, can reduce blood glucose and improve control of diabetes as well as reduce the risk of heart disease by lowering blood triglycerides.[38] Greater weight loss reduces blood pressure, improves levels of low-density and high-density lipoproteins, and further reduces levels of blood triglycerides and blood glucose.

Of course, the same eating and activity habits that improve health often lead to a healthier body weight and composition as well (see Photo 7-2). Successful weight loss, then, is defined not by pounds lost but by health gained. People less concerned with disease risks may prefer to set goals for personal fitness, such as being able to play with children or climb stairs without becoming short of breath.

Whether the goal is health or fitness, weight-loss expectations need to be reasonable. Unreachable targets ensure frustration and failure. Setting reasonable goals helps to achieve the desired result in managing weight. For example, obese people who must reduce their weight to lower their disease risks might set three broad goals:

1. Reduce body weight by about 5 to 10 percent over half a year's time.
2. Maintain a lower body weight over the long term.
3. At a minimum, prevent further weight gain.

Such goals may be achieved or even exceeded, providing a sense of accomplishment instead of disappointment.

After all, excess weight takes years to accumulate. Losing excess body fat also takes time, along with patience and perseverance. The person must adopt healthy eating patterns, engage in physical activity, create a supportive environment, and seek out behavioral and social support; continue these behaviors for at least six months for initial weight loss; and then continue all of it for a lifetime to maintain the losses.[39] Setbacks are a given, and according to recent evidence, the size of the kcalorie deficit required to lose a pound of weight initially may be smaller than that required later on. In other words, weight loss is hard at first, and then it may get harder.

A Healthful Eating Plan

Contrary to the claims of many fad diets, no particular eating plan is magical, and no specific food must be either included or avoided for weight management. In designing an eating pattern, people need only consider foods that they like or can learn to like, that are available, and that are within their means.

A Realistic Energy Intake The main characteristic of a weight-loss diet is that it provides less energy than the person needs to maintain present body weight. If food energy is restricted too severely, dieters may not receive sufficient nutrients and may lose lean tissue. Rapid weight loss usually means excessive loss of lean tissue, a lower BMR, and a rapid weight regain to follow. Restrictive eating may also set in motion the unhealthy behaviors of eating disorders (described in Nutrition in Practice 6).

Obesity experts recommend that reductions in energy intake should be based on a person's BMI.[40] Overweight (BMI of 25 or greater) and obese (BMI of 30 or greater) people are encouraged to reduce their usual daily kcalorie intakes by about 500 to 750 kcalories to produce a weight loss of about 1 to 2 pounds per week while retaining lean tissue.

Weight loss may proceed rapidly for some weeks or months but will eventually slow down. The following factors contribute to a decline in the rate of loss:

- Metabolism may slow in response to a lower kcalorie intake and loss of metabolically active lean tissue.
- Less energy may be expended in physical activity as body weight diminishes.

In addition, the composition of weight loss itself may affect the rate of loss. Body weight lost early in dieting may be composed of a greater percentage of water and lean tissue, which contains fewer kcalories per pound as compared with later losses that appear to be composed mostly of fat. This may mean that dieters should expect a slowdown in weight loss as they progress past the initial phase.

Most people can lose weight safely on an eating pattern providing approximately 1200 to 1500 kcalories per day for women and 1500 to 1800 kcalories per day for men. Table 7-3 suggests daily food amounts from which to build balanced 1200- to 1800-kcalorie diets.

Nutritional Adequacy Nutritional adequacy is difficult to achieve on fewer than 1200 kcalories a day, and most healthy adults need never consume any less than that. A plan that provides an adequate intake supports a healthier and more successful weight loss than a restrictive plan that creates feelings of starvation and deprivation, which can lead to an irresistible urge to binge.

Take a look at the 1200-kcalorie diet in Table 7-3. Such an intake would allow most people to lose weight and still meet their nutrient needs with careful, low-kcalorie, nutrient-dense food selections. Healthy eating patterns for weight loss should provide all of the needed nutrients from:

- Fruit and vegetables
- Legumes
- Fish
- Whole grains
- Moderate amounts of unsaturated oils and low-fat or nonfat dairy products

They should also be lower in total meat and refined grains and low in saturated fat, sodium, and sugar-sweetened foods and drinks.[41] Such patterns, including vegetarian and Mediterranean patterns, provide nutrient adequacy and are generally associated with leanness.

Choose fats sensibly by avoiding most solid fats and by including enough unsaturated oils (details in Nutrition in Practice 4) to support health but not so much as to oversupply kcalories. People who regularly eat nuts often maintain a healthy body weight.[42] Lean meats or other low-fat protein sources also play important roles in weight loss and provide satiety. Sufficient protein foods may also help to preserve lean tissue, including muscle tissue, during weight loss.[43]

A dietary supplement providing vitamins and minerals—especially iron and calcium for women—at or below 100 percent of the Daily Values can help people following low-kcalorie eating patterns to achieve nutrient adequacy. A person who plans resolutely to include all of the foods from each group needed each day will be satisfied and well nourished, and have little appetite left for high-kcalorie treats.

Small Portions As mentioned earlier, large portion sizes increase energy intakes, and the huge helpings served by restaurants and sold in packages are the enemies of people striving to manage their weight. Similarly, big bowls, plates, utensils, and

TABLE 7-3 Daily Amounts from Each Food Group for 1200- to 1800-kcalorie Diets

FOOD GROUP	1200 kcal	1400 kcal	1600 kcal	1800 kcal
Fruit	1 c	1½ c	1½ c	1½ c
Vegetables	1½ c	1½ c	2 c	2½ c
Grains	4 oz	5 oz	5 oz	6 oz
Protein foods	3 oz	4 oz	5 oz	5 oz
Milk	2½ c	2½ c	3 c	3 c
Oils	4 tsp	4 tsp	5 tsp	5 tsp

drinking glasses may encourage people to take and consume larger portions. Small plates and bowls, tall and thin drinking glasses, and luncheon-sized plates may have the opposite effect.

For health's sake, overweight people may need to learn to eat less food at each meal—one piece of chicken for dinner instead of two, a teaspoon of butter on vegetables instead of a tablespoon, and one cookie for dessert instead of six. Chew foods slowly and thoroughly. The goal is to eat enough food for energy, nutrients, and pleasure, but not more. This amount should leave a person feeling satisfied—not necessarily full.

People who have difficulty making low-kcalorie selections or controlling portion sizes may find it easier to use prepared meal plans. Prepared meals that provide low-kcalorie, nutritious meals or snacks can support weight loss while easing the task of diet planning. Ideally, those using a prepared meal plan will also receive counsel from a registered dietitian nutritionist to learn how to select appropriately from conventional food choices as well.

Lower Energy Density As discussed earlier, to lower energy intake, people can choose smaller portion sizes, or they can reduce the energy density of the foods they eat. In general, foods high in fat or low in water, such as fatty meats, cookies, or chips, rank high in energy density: foods high in water and fiber, such as fruits and vegetables, rank lower. Foods with lower energy density are bulkier, providing more bites for fewer kcalories, and thus may be more satisfying (see Figure 7-3). The Clinical Applications feature at the end of this chapter describes how to calculate the energy density of foods.

Energy density may be more important in some cultures than in others. Energy-dense olive oil, olives, and nuts, when consumed in a Mediterranean-style eating pattern, appear to be compatible with a healthy body weight.[44] This pattern is also rich in vegetables, fruit, and seafood, with few or none of the choices that abound in the United States. As noted earlier, even here, consumption of tree nuts, such as almonds, walnuts, and pecans, is associated with a lower BMI and smaller waist circumference compared with people who do not eat nuts.[45]

Sugar and Alcohol A person trying to achieve or maintain a healthy weight needs to limit intakes of added sugars and alcohol, as well as solid fats. Including them for pleasure on occasion is compatible with health as long as most daily choices are of nutrient-dense foods.

FIGURE 7-3 Energy Density

Decreasing the energy density (kcal/g) of foods allows a person to eat satisfying portions while still reducing energy intake. To lower energy density, select foods high in water or fiber and low in fat.

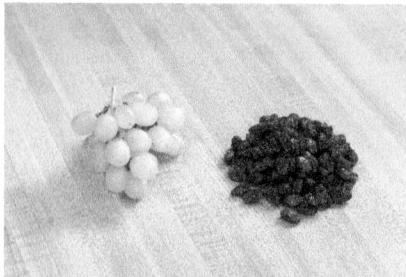

Selecting grapes with their high water content instead of raisins increases the volume and cuts the energy intake in half.

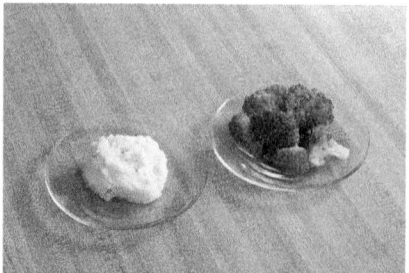

Even at the same weight and similar serving sizes, the fiber-rich broccoli delivers twice the fiber of the potatoes for about one-fourth the energy.

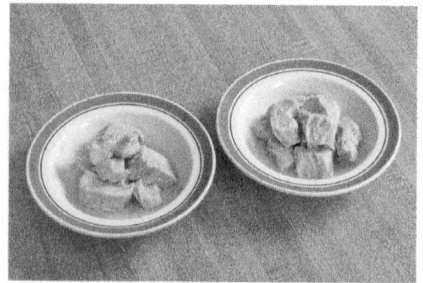

By selecting the water-packed tuna (on the right) instead of the oil-packed tuna, a person can enjoy the same amount for fewer kcalories.

Matthew Farruggio (all)

Meal Spacing Three meals a day is standard in our society, but no law says you can't have four or five—just be sure they are smaller, of course. People who eat small, frequent meals can be as successful at weight loss and maintenance as those who eat three. Make sure that mild hunger, not appetite, is prompting you to eat. Eat regularly, and eat before you become extremely hungry.[46]

Adequate Water In addition to lowering the energy density of foods, water seems to help those who are trying to lose or maintain weight. Drinking a large glass of water before a meal may ease hunger, fill the stomach, and reduce energy intake. Importantly, water adds no kcalories. On average, sugar-sweetened beverages contribute about 135 kcalories a day. Simply replacing nutrient-poor, energy-dense beverages with water can help a person lower energy intake by at least 5 percent.[47] Water also helps the GI tract adapt to a high-fiber diet.

Physical Activity

The best approach to weight management includes physical activity.[48] Either energy restriction or physical activity alone can produce some weight loss. Clearly, however, the combination is most effective. People who combine diet and physical activity are more likely to lose more fat, retain more muscle, and regain less weight than those who only diet. Table 7-4 presents physical activity strategies from the American College of Sports Medicine developed specifically to prevent weight gain and promote at least modest weight loss.

Even without weight loss, physical activity may also help counteract some of the negative effects of excess body weight on health.[49] For example, physical activity reduces abdominal obesity, and this change improves blood pressure, insulin resistance, and fitness of the heart and lungs, even without weight loss.[50]

Energy Expenditure Physical activity directly increases energy output by the muscles and cardiovascular system. Table 6-2 in Chapter 6 (pp. 153–154) shows how much energy each of several activities uses. The number of kcalories spent in an activity depends on body weight, intensity, and duration. For example, a 150-pound person who walks 3.5 miles in 60 minutes expends about 315 kcalories. That same person running 3 miles in 30 minutes uses a similar amount. By comparison, a 200-pound person running 3 miles in 30 minutes expends an additional 125 kcalories or so (about 444 kcalories total). The goal is to expend as much energy as time allows. The greater the energy deficit created by physical activity, the greater the fat loss. A word of caution, however: People who reward themselves with high-kcalorie foods for "good behavior" can easily negate any kcalorie deficits incurred with physical activity.

Basal Metabolic Rate (BMR) The BMR is elevated in the hours after vigorous physical activity, but this effect requires a sustained high-intensity workout beyond the level achievable by most weight-loss seekers. Over the long term, however, a person who engages in daily vigorous activity gradually develops more lean tissue, which is more active metabolically than fat tissue. Metabolic rate rises accordingly, and this makes a contribution toward continued weight loss or maintenance.

Appetite Control Physical activity also helps to control appetite. Some people think that being active will make them want to eat. Active people do have healthy appetites, but physical activity helps to heighten feelings of satiation, delaying the onset of hunger.[51] The reasons are unclear, but physical activity may help to control appetite by altering the levels of appetite-regulating hormones.[52]

TABLE 7-4 Physical Activity Strategies for Weight Management

A negative energy balance incurred through physical activity will result in weight loss, and the larger the negative energy balance, the greater the weight loss.

- Weight gain prevention and augmented weight loss occur with at least 2 hours and 30 minutes (150 minutes) per week of at least moderate-intensity physical activity.
- Greater weight loss and improved weight maintenance after weight loss occur with more than 4 hours and 10 minutes (>250 minutes) per week of at least moderate-intensity physical activity.
- Both aerobic (endurance) and muscle-strengthening (resistance) physical activities are beneficial, but kcalorie restriction must accompany resistance training to achieve weight loss.

Source: Adapted from American College of Sports Medicine, Position stand: Appropriate physical activity intervention strategies for weight loss and prevention of weight regain for adults, *Medicine and Science in Sports and Exercise* 41 (2009): 459–471.

- Improved body composition
- Favorable effects on disease risks
- Short-term increase in energy expenditure (from exercise and from a slight rise in BMR)
- Long-term increase (slight) in BMR (from an increase in lean tissue)
- Appetite control
- Stress reduction and control of stress eating
- Physical, and therefore psychological, well-being
- Improved self-esteem

Psychological Benefits Physical activity helps especially to curb the inappropriate appetite that prompts a person to eat when bored, anxious, or depressed. Weight-management programs encourage people to go out and be active when they're tempted to eat but are not really hungry.

Physical activity also helps to reduce stress. Because stress itself is a cue to inappropriate eating behavior for many people, activity can help here, too. In addition, physical activity helps to improve body image and separate the connections between body weight and self-worth.[53] A physically active person begins to look and feel healthy, and, as a result, gains self-esteem. High self-esteem tends to support a person's resolve to persist in a weight-control effort, rounding out a beneficial cycle. Table 7-5 and Chapter 1 present the benefits of physical activity.

Choosing Activities What kind of physical activity is best? For health, a combination of moderate to vigorous aerobic physical activity along with **resistance training** at a safe level provides benefits. However, any physical activity is better than being sedentary.

People seeking to lose weight should choose activities that they enjoy and are willing to do regularly. Health care professionals frequently advise people who want to manage their body weight and lose fat to engage in activities of low-to-moderate intensity for a long duration, such as an hour-long fast-paced walk. The reasoning behind such advice is that people exercising at low to moderate intensity are likely to stick with their activity for longer times and are less likely to injure themselves. People who regularly engage in more *vigorous* physical activities (fast bicycling or endurance running, for example), however, have less body fat than those who engage in moderately intense activities. The conditioned body that is adapted to strenuous and prolonged aerobic activity uses more fat all day long, not just during activity. The bottom line on physical activity and weight and/or fat loss seems to be that total energy expenditure is the main factor, regardless of how a person does it.

In addition to activities such as walking or cycling, there are hundreds of ways to incorporate energy-expending activities into daily routines: take the stairs instead of the elevator, walk to a neighbor's house instead of making a phone call, and rake the leaves instead of using a blower. These activities burn only a few kcalories each, but over a year's time they become significant.

Spot Reducing People sometimes ask about "spot reducing." Unfortunately, no one part of the body gives up fat in preference to another. Fat cells all over the body release fat in response to demand, and the fat is then used by whatever muscles are active. No exercise can remove the fat from any one particular area—and, incidentally, neither can a massage machine that claims to break up fat on trouble spots.

Physical activity can help with trouble spots in another way, though. Strengthening muscles in a trouble area can help to improve their tone; stretching to gain flexibility can help with posture problems. Thus, cardiorespiratory endurance, strength, and flexibility workouts all have a place in fitness programs.

Behavior and Attitude

Behavior modification provides ways to overcome barriers to making dietary changes and increasing physical activity. Behavior-modification does more than help people decide which behaviors to change: it also teaches them how to change. Behavior and attitude are important supporting factors in achieving and maintaining appropriate body weight and composition. Changing the behaviors of overeating and underexercising that lead to, and perpetuate, obesity requires time and effort. A person must commit to take action.

Becoming Aware of Behaviors A person who is aware of all the behaviors that create a problem has a head start on developing a solution. Keeping a record will help identify eating and activity behaviors that may need changing. Such self-monitoring raises awareness, establishes a baseline against which to measure future progress, and improves compliance.[54]

resistance training: the use of free weights or weight machines to provide resistance for developing muscle strength, power, and endurance; also called *weight training*. A person's own body weight may also be used to provide resistance, as when a person does push-ups, pull-ups, or abdominal crunches.

behavior-modification: the changing of behavior by the manipulation of *antecedents* (cues or environmental factors that trigger behavior), the behavior itself, and *consequences* (the penalties or rewards attached to behavior).

One of the most common ways to self-monitor eating and activity behaviors has been the use of pen and paper to keep a food and activity diary. The diary includes the time and place of meals and snacks, the type and amount of foods eaten, the people present when food is eaten, and a description of the individual's feelings when eating. The record also includes information about physical activities: the kind, the intensity level, the duration, and the person's feeling about the activities. Although the pen and paper method has been shown to improve weight loss outcomes, it can be time consuming and does not provide immediate feedback to support and motivate the person.

In this era of technology, many companies have developed weight-loss applications for smartphones and other mobile devices to help users manage their daily food and physical activity behaviors.* Applications include diet analysis tools that can track eating habits, scanning devices that can quickly enter food data, customized activity and meal plans that can be sent to users, and support programs that deliver encouraging messages and helpful tips. Social media sites allow users to upload progress reports and receive texts. Using these applications can help a person become more aware of behaviors that lead to weight gains and losses.

Making Small Changes Behavior modification strategies focus on learning desired eating and exercise behaviors and eliminating unwanted behaviors. With so many possible behavior changes, a person can feel overwhelmed. Start with small time-specific goals for each behavior—for example, "I'm going to take a 30-minute walk after dinner every evening" instead of "I'm going to run a marathon someday." Practice desired behaviors until they become routine. Using a reward system seems to effectively support weight-loss efforts. Box 7-1 describes behavioral strategies to support weight management. A particularly attractive feature of these strategies is that they do not involve blaming oneself or putting oneself down—an important element in fostering self-esteem.

Box 7-1 | *HOW TO* Apply Behavior Modification to Manage Body Fatness

1. Eliminate inappropriate cues:
   - Do not buy problem foods.
   - Eat only in one place at the designated time.
   - Shop when not hungry.
   - Replace large plates, cups, and utensils with smaller ones.
   - Avoid vending machines, fast-food restaurants, and convenience stores.
   - Measure out appropriate snack portions to eat during entertainment.

2. Suppress the cues you cannot eliminate:
   - Serve individual plates; do not serve "family style."
   - Remove food from the table after eating a meal.
   - Create obstacles to consuming problem foods—wrap them and freeze them, making them less quickly accessible.
   - Control deprivation; plan and eat regular meals.
   - Plan the time spent in sedentary activities, such as watching television or using a computer—do not use these activities just to fill time.

3. Strengthen cues to appropriate behaviors:
   - Choose to dine with companions who make appropriate food choices.
   - Learn appropriate portion sizes.
   - Plan appropriate snacks and keep them handy.

   - Keep sports and play equipment by the door.

4. Repeat desired behaviors:
   - Slow down eating—always use utensils and put them down between bites.
   - Leave some food on your plate.
   - Move more—shake a leg, pace, stretch often.
   - Join groups of active people and participate.

5. Arrange negative consequences for negative behavior:
   - Ask that others respond neutrally to your deviations (make no comments—even negative attention is a reward).
   - If you slip, do not punish yourself.

6. Reward yourself personally and immediately for positive behaviors:
   - Buy tickets to sports events, movies, concerts, or other nonfood amusement.
   - Indulge in a new small purchase.
   - Get a massage; buy some flowers.
   - Take a hot bath; read a good book.
   - Treat yourself to a lesson in a new active pursuit such as horseback riding, handball, or tennis.
   - Praise yourself; visit friends.

---

*Reliable reviews of food and nutrition apps are available at *www.eatright.org/appreviews*.

Cognitive Skills Behavior therapists often teach **cognitive skills**, or new ways of thinking, to help overweight people solve problems and correct false thinking that can undermine healthy eating behaviors. Thinking habits are as important for achieving a healthy body weight as eating and activity habits, and they can be changed. A paradox of making a change is that it takes belief in oneself and honoring of oneself to lay the foundation for changing that self. That is, self-acceptance predicts success, while self-loathing predicts failure. "Positive self-talk" is a concept worth cultivating—many people succeed because their mental dialogue supports, rather than degrades, their efforts. Negative thoughts ("I'm not getting thin anyway, so what is the use of continuing?") should be viewed in light of empirical evidence ("My starting weight: 174 pounds; today's weight: 163 pounds").

Take credit for new behaviors; be aware of any physical improvements, too, such as lower blood pressure, or less painful knees, even without a noticeable change in pant size. Finally, remember to enjoy your emerging fit and healthy self.

Personal Attitude For many people, overeating and being overweight may have become an integral part of their identity. Changing diet and activity behaviors without attention to a person's self-concept invites failure.

Many people overeat to cope with the stresses of life. To break out of that pattern, they must first identify the particular stressors that trigger their urges to overeat. Then, when faced with these situations, they must learn to practice problem-solving skills. When the problems that trigger the urge to overeat are dealt with in alternative ways, people may find that they eat less. The message is that sound emotional health supports the ability to take care of health in all ways—including nutrition, weight management, and fitness.

Weight Maintenance

Finally, be aware that it can be hard to maintain weight loss. Millions of people have experienced the frustration of achieving a desired change in weight only to see their hard work visibly slip away in a seemingly never-ending cycle of weight loss and weight regain. Disappointment, frustration, and self-condemnation are common in people who have slipped back to their original weight or even higher.

A key to weight maintenance is accepting it as a lifelong endeavor and not a goal to be achieved and then forgotten. People who maintain their weight loss continue to employ the behaviors that reduced their weight in the first place (see Table 7-6). They cultivate habits of people who maintain a healthy weight, such as eating low-kcalorie meals (averaging 1800 kcalories per day) and being physically active. They must also control susceptibility to overeating regardless of the initial weight-loss method.

TABLE 7-6 Behaviors to Maintain Weight Loss

Those who maintain weight losses over time:

- Believe they have the ability to control their weight, an attribute known as **self-efficacy**.
- Eat breakfast every day.
- Average about one hour of physical activity per day.
- Monitor body weight about once a week.
- Maintain consistent lower-kcalorie eating patterns.
- Quickly address small **lapses** to prevent small gains from turning into major ones.
- Watch less than 10 hours of television per week.
- Eat high-fiber food, particularly whole grains, vegetables, and fruit, and consume sufficient water each day.
- Cultivate and honor realistic expectations regarding body size and shape.

---

cognitive skills: as taught in behavior therapy, changes to conscious thoughts with the goal of improving adherence to lifestyle modifications; examples are problem-solving skills or the correction of false-negative thoughts, termed *cognitive restructuring.*

self-efficacy: a person's belief in his or her ability to succeed in an undertaking.

lapses: periods of returning to old habits.

Review Notes

- A person who adopts a lifelong "eating plan for good health" rather than a "diet for weight loss" will be more likely to keep the lost weight off. Table 7-7 offers strategies for successful weight management.
- Reducing daily energy intake, choosing foods of low energy density, and eating smaller portions are important dietary strategies for weight management.
- Physical activity should be an integral part of a weight-management program.
- Physical activity can increase energy expenditure, improve body composition, help control appetite, reduce stress and stress eating, and enhance physical and psychological well-being.
- Behavior modification provides ways to overcome barriers to successful weight management.

TABLE 7-7	Weight-Loss Strategies	
FOOD	**ACTIVITIES**
• To maintain weight, consume foods and drinks to meet, not exceed, kcalorie needs. To lose weight, energy out should exceed energy in by about 500 kcalories/day.	• Limit screen time.
• Emphasize foods with a low energy density and a high nutrient density; make legumes, whole grains, vegetables, and fruit central to your eating pattern.	• Increase physical activity.
• Eat slowly.	• Choose moderate- or vigorous-intensity physical activities.
• Drink water before you eat and while you eat; drink plenty of water throughout the day.	• Avoid inactivity. Some physical activity is better than none.
• Track food and kcalorie intake.	• Slowly build up the amount of physical activity you choose.
• Plan ahead to make better food choices.	
• Limit kcalorie intake from solid fats and added sugars.	
• Reduce portions, especially of high-kcalorie foods.	
• Cook and eat more meals at home, instead of eating out. When eating out, think about choosing healthy options.	

7.6 Strategies for Weight Gain

Underweight is far less prevalent than overweight, affecting about 2 percent of U.S. adults.[55] Whether the underweight person needs to gain weight is a question of health and, like weight loss, a highly individual matter. People who are healthy at their present weight may stay there; there are no compelling reasons to try to gain weight. Those who are thin because of malnourishment or illness, however, might benefit from a diet that supports weight gain. Medical advice can help make the distinction. Eating disorders are the subject of Nutrition in Practice 6.

Some people are unalterably thin by reasons of genetics or early physical influences. Those who wish to gain weight for appearance's sake or to improve athletic performance should be aware that a healthful weight can be achieved only through physical activity, particularly strength training, combined with a high energy intake. Eating many high-kcalorie foods can bring about weight gain, but it will be mostly fat, and this can be as detrimental to health as being slightly underweight. In an athlete, such a weight gain can impair performance. Therefore, in weight gain, as in weight loss, physical activity and energy intake are essential components of a sound plan.

Physical Activity to Build Muscles The person who wants to gain weight should use resistance training primarily. As activity is increased, energy intake must be increased to support that activity. Eating extra food will then support a gain of both muscle and fat.

Energy-Dense Foods Energy-dense foods (the very ones eliminated from a successful weight-loss diet) hold the key to weight gain. Pick the highest-kcalorie items from each food group—that is, milkshakes instead of fat-free milk, peanut butter instead of lean meat, avocados instead of cucumbers, and whole-wheat muffins instead of whole-wheat bread. Because fat contains more than twice as many kcalories per teaspoon as sugar does, fat adds kcalories without adding much bulk.

Be aware that health experts recommend a moderate-fat diet for the general U.S. population because the general population is overweight and at risk for heart disease. Consumption of excessive fat is not healthy for most people, of course, but may be essential for an underweight individual who needs to gain weight. An underweight person who is physically active and eating a nutritionally adequate diet can afford a few extra kcalories from fat. For health's sake, it is wise to select foods with monounsaturated and polyunsaturated fats instead of those with saturated or *trans* fats; for example, sautéing vegetables in olive oil instead of butter or hydrogenated margarine.

Three Meals Daily People wanting to gain weight should eat at least three healthy meals a day. Many people who are underweight have simply been too busy (sometimes for months) to eat enough to gain or maintain weight. Therefore, they need to make meals a priority and plan them in advance. Taking time to prepare and eat each meal can help, as can learning to eat more food within the first 20 minutes of a meal before you begin to feel full. Another suggestion is to eat meaty appetizers or the main course first and leave the soup or salad until later.

Large Portions It is also important for the underweight person to learn to eat more food at each meal: have two sandwiches for lunch instead of one, drink milk from a larger glass, and eat cereal from a larger bowl. Expect to feel full. Most underweight individuals are accustomed to small quantities of food. When they begin eating significantly more, they feel uncomfortable. This is normal and passes over time.

Extra Snacks Because a substantially higher energy intake is needed each day, in addition to eating more food at each meal, it is necessary to eat more frequently. Between-meal snacking offers a solution. For example, a student might make three sandwiches in the morning and eat them between classes in addition to the day's three regular meals.

Juice and Milk Beverages provide an easy way to increase energy intake. Consider that 6 cups of cranberry juice add almost 1000 kcalories to the day's intake. kCalories can be added to milk by mixing in powdered milk or packets of instant breakfast.

For people who are underweight due to illness, concentrated liquid formulas are often recommended because a weak person can swallow them easily. A registered dietitian nutritionist can recommend high-protein, high-kcalorie formulas to help the underweight person maintain or gain weight. Used in addition to regular meals, these formulas can help considerably.

Review Notes

- Both the incidence of underweight and the health problems associated with it are less prevalent than overweight and its associated problems.
- To gain weight, a person must train physically and increase energy intake by selecting energy-dense foods, eating regular meals, taking larger portions, and consuming extra snacks and beverages. Table 7-8 offers a summary of weight-gain strategies.

TABLE 7-8 Weight-Gain Strategies

IN GENERAL:
- Eat enough to store more energy than you expend—at least 500 extra kcalories a day.
- Exercise to build muscle.
- Be patient. Weight gain takes time (1 pound per month would be reasonable).
- Choose energy-dense foods most often.
- Eat at least three meals a day, and add snacks between meals.
- Choose large portions and expect to feel full.
- Drink kcaloric fluids—juice, chocolate milk, sweet coffee drinks, sweet iced tea.

IN ADDITION:
- Cook and bake often—delicious cooking aromas whet the appetite.
- Invite others to the table—companionship often boosts eating.
- Make meals interesting—try new vegetables and a variety of fruits, add crunchy nuts or creamy avocado, and explore the flavors of herbs and spices.
- Keep a supply of favorite snacks, such as trail mix or granola bars, handy for grabbing.
- Control stress and relax. Enjoy your food.

Self Check

1. Two causes of obesity in humans are:
   a. set-point theory and BMI.
   b. genetics and physical inactivity.
   c. genetics and low-carbohydrate diets.
   d. mineral imbalances and fat cell imbalance.

2. The protein produced by the fat cells under the direction of the *ob* gene is called:
   a. leptin.
   b. orlistat.
   c. sibutramine.
   d. lipoprotein lipase.

3. All of the following describe the behavior of fat cells *except:*
   a. the number decreases when fat is lost from the body.
   b. the storage capacity for fat depends on both cell number and cell size.
   c. the size is larger in obese people than in normal-weight people.
   d. the number increases most rapidly during the growth years and tapers off when adult status is reached.

4. The obesity theory that suggests the body chooses to be at a specific weight is the:
   a. fat cell theory.
   b. enzyme theory.
   c. set-point theory.
   d. external cue theory.

5. The biggest problem associated with the use of prescription drugs in the treatment of obesity is:
   a. cost.
   b. the necessity for long-term use.
   c. ineffectiveness.
   d. adverse side effects.

6. A nutritionally sound weight-loss diet might restrict daily energy intake to create a:
   a. 1000-kcalorie-per-month deficit.
   b. 500-kcalorie-per-month deficit.
   c. 500-kcalorie-per-day deficit.
   d. 3500-kcalorie-per-day deficit.

7. What is the best approach to weight loss?
   a. Avoid foods containing carbohydrates.
   b. Eliminate all fats from the diet and decrease water intake.
   c. Greatly increase protein intake to prevent body protein loss.
   d. Reduce daily energy intake and increase energy expenditure.

8. Physical activity does *not* help a person to:
   a. lose weight.
   b. lose fat in trouble spots.
   c. retain muscle.
   d. maintain weight loss.

9. Which of these behaviors will best support successful weight management?
   a. Shop only when hungry.
   b. Eat in front of the television for distraction.
   c. Learn appropriate portion sizes.
   d. Eat quickly.

10. Which strategy would *not* help an underweight person to gain weight?
    a. Exercise.
    b. Drink plenty of water.
    c. Eat snacks between meals.
    d. Eat large portions of foods.

Answers: 1. b, 2. a, 3. a, 4. c, 5. b, 6. c, 7. d, 8. b, 9. c, 10. b

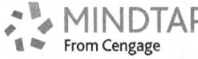 **MINDTAP** From Cengage   For more chapter resources visit **www.cengage.com** to access MindTap, a complete digital course.

Clinical Applications

1. Chapter 1 discussed the nutrient density of foods—their nutrient contribution per kcalorie. Another way to evaluate foods is to consider their energy density—their energy contribution per gram:
   - A carrot weighing 72 grams delivers 31 kcalories.
   - To calculate the energy density, divide kcalories by grams: 31 kcalories divided by 72 grams = 0.43 kcalories per gram.

2. Do the same for french fries weighing 50 grams and contributing 167 kcalories: 167 kcalories divided by 50 grams = _____ kcalories per gram.

   - The more kcalories per gram, the greater the energy density.
   - Which food is more energy dense? The conclusion is no surprise, but understanding the mathematics may offer valuable insight into the concept of energy density.
   - French fries are more energy dense, providing 3.34 kcalories per gram. They provide more energy per gram—and per bite.

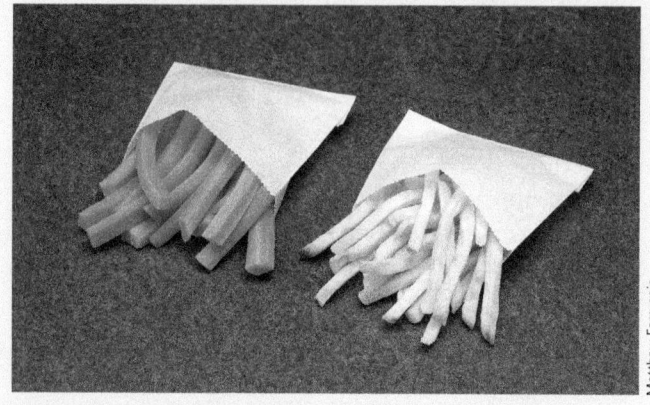

Matthew Farruggio

3. Considering a food's energy density is especially useful in planning diets for weight management. Foods with a high energy density can help with weight gain, whereas those with a low energy density can help with weight loss. Give some examples of foods that you might suggest for a client who wants to gain weight and some that might be appropriate for a client who is trying to lose weight.

Notes

1. K. Silventoinen and coauthors, Genetic and environmental effects on body mass index from infancy to the onset of adulthood: An individual-based pooled analysis of 45 twin cohorts participating in the Collaborative project of Development of Anthropometrical measures in Twins (CODATwins) study, *American Journal of Clinical Nutrition* 104 (2016): 371–379; M. Claussnitzer and coauthors, *FTO* obesity variant circuitry and adipocyte browning in humans, *New England Journal of Medicine* 373 (2015): 895–907; T. Huang and F. B. Hu, Gene-environment interactions and obesity: Recent developments and future directions, *BMC Medical Genomics* 15 (2015): S2.

2. Claussnitzer and coauthors, 2015; A. E. Locke and coauthors, Genetic studies of body mass index yield new insights for obesity biology, *Nature* 518 (2015): 197–206; B. Fontaine-Bisson and coauthors, Melanin-concentrating hormone receptor 1 polymorphisms are associated with components of energy balance in the Complex Diseases in the Newfoundland Population: Environment and Genetics (CODING) study, *American Journal of Clinical Nutrition* 99 (2014): 384–391; L. Goni and coauthors, Single-nucleotide Polymorphisms and DNA methylation markers associated with central obesity and regulation of body weight, *Nutrition Reviews* 72 (2014): 673–690.

3. C. Jou, The biology and genetics of obesity—a century of inquiries, *New England Journal of Medicine* 370 (2014): 1874–1877.

4. Silventoinen and coauthors, 2016; Claussnitzer and coauthors, 2015; Locke and coauthors, 2015; Fontaine-Bisson and coauthors, 2014; Goni and coauthors, 2014.

5. L. Brunkwall and coauthors, Sugar-sweetened beverage consumption and genetic predisposition to obesity in 2 Swedish cohorts, *American Journal of Clinical Nutrition* 104 (2016): 809–815.

6. A. B. Crujeiras and coauthors, Leptin resistance in obesity: An epigenetic landscape, *Life Sciences* 140 (2015): 57–63; H. Pan, J. Guo, and Z. Su, Advances in understanding the interrelations between leptin resistance and obesity, *Physiology and Behavior* 130 (2014): 157–169.

7. Crujeiras and coauthors, 2015; Pan, Guo, and Su, 2014.

8. L. Mihalache and coauthors, Effects of ghrelin in energy balance and body weight homeostasis, *Hormones (Athens)* 15 (2016): 186–196; A. Rodriquez, Novel molecular aspects of ghrelin and leptin in the control of adipobiology and the cardiovascular system, *Obesity Facts* 7 (2014): 82–95.

9. O. Al Massadi and coauthors, What is the real relevance of endogenous ghrelin? *Peptides* 70 (2015): 1–6; A. Molfino and coauthors, Ghrelin: From discovery to cancer cachexia therapy, *Current Opinion in Clinical Nutrition and Metabolic Care* 17 (2014): 471–476.

10. J. L. Broussard and coauthors, Elevated ghrelin predicts food intake during experimental sleep restriction, *Obesity* 24 (2016): 132–138; H. S. Dashti and coauthors, Short sleep duration and dietary intake: Epidemiologic evidence, mechanisms, and health implications, *Advances in Nutrition* 6 (2015): 648–659; H. S. Dashti and coauthors, Habitual sleep duration is associated with BMI and macronutrient intake and may be modified by *CLOCK* genetic variants, *American Journal of Clinical Nutrition* 101 (2015): 135–143.

11. E. Fabbrini and coauthors, Metabolically normal obese people are Protected from adverse effects following weight gain, *Journal of Clinical Investigation* 125 (2015): 787–795; M. Bastien, and coauthors, Overview of epidemiology and contribution of obesity to cardiovascular disease, *Progress in Cardiovascular Diseases* 56 (2014): 369–381; V. G. Giby and T. A. Ajith, Role of adipokines and peroxisome proliferator-activated receptors in nonalcoholic fatty liver diseases, *World Journal of Hepatology* 6 (2014): 570–579.

12. A. Rodríguez and coauthors, Revisiting the adipocyte: A model for integration of cytokine signaling in the regulation of energy metabolism, *American Journal of Physiology, Endocrinology, and Metabolism* 309 (2015): E691–E714; T. F. S. Teixeira and coauthors, Main characteristics of metabolically obese normal weight and metabolically healthy obese phenotypes, *Nutrition Reviews* 73 (2015): 175–190; Giby and Ajith, 2014; Bastien and coauthors, 2014.

13. E. Ferrannini, M. Rosenbaum, and R. O. Leibel, The threshold shift Paradigm of obesity: evidence from surgically induced weight loss, *American Journal of Clinical Nutrition* 100 (2014): 996–1002.

14. F. L. Greenway, Physiological adaptations to weight loss and factors favouring weight regain, *International Journal of Obesity* 39 (2015): 1188–1196.

15. D. S. Spasova and C. D. Surh, Blowing on embers: Commensal microbiota and our immune system, *Frontiers in Immunology* 5 (2014), 318.

16. J. R. DiSpirito and D. Mathis, Immunological contributions to adipose tissue homeostasis, *Seminars in Immunology* 27 (2015): 315–321; C. M. Ferreira and coauthors, The central role of the gut microbiota in chronic inflammatory diseases, *Journal of Immunology Research* (2014), epub, doi:10.1155/2014/689492; Y. J. Lee and K. S. Park, Irritable bowel syndrome: Emerging paradigm in pathophysiology, *World Journal of Gastroenterology* 20 (2014): 2456–2469; H. Zeng, D. L. Lazarova, and M. Bordonaro, Mechanisms linking dietary fiber, gut microbiota and colon cancer prevention, *World Journal of Gastrointestinal Oncology* 6 (2014): 41–51; I. Moreno-Indias and coauthors, Impact of the gut microbiota on the development of obesity and type 2 diabetes mellitus, *Frontiers in Microbiology* 5 (2014), epub, doi:10.3389/fmicb.2014.00190.

17. M. J. Khan and coauthors, Role of gut microbiota in the aetiology of obesity: Proposed mechanisms and review of the literature, *Journal of Obesity* 2016, dx.doi.org/10.1155/2016/7353642; C. D. Davis, The gut

microbiome and its role in obesity, *Nutrition Today* 51 (2016): 167–174; C. Graham, A. Mullen, and K. Whelan, Obesity and the gastrointestinal microbiota: A review of associations and mechanisms, *Nutrition Reviews* 73 (2015): 376–385.

18. Davis, 2016; Graham, Mullen, and Whelan, 2015; M. J. Khan and coauthors, Unraveling the role of the gut microbiota in obesity; cause or effect? *Proceedings of the Nutrition Society* 73 (2014), epub, doi. org/10.1017/S0029665114000329.

19. T. Huang and F. B. Hu, Gene-environment interactions and obesity: Recent developments and future directions, *BMC Medical Genomics* 8 (2015): S2; Fontaine-Bisson and coauthors, 2014.

20. M. H. Alhussain, I. A. McDonald, and M. A. Taylor, Irregular meal-pattern effects on energy expenditure, metabolism, and appetite regulation: A randomized controlled trial in healthy normal-weight women, *American Journal of Clinical Nutrition* 104 (2016): 21–32.

21. G. J. Hollands and coauthors, Portion, package or tableware size for changing selection and consumption of food, alcohol and tobacco, *Cochrane Database of Systematic Reviews,* 2015, doi: 10.1002/14651858. CD011045.pub2; C. Berg and H. B. Forslund, The influence of portion size and timing of meals on weight balance and obesity, *Current Obesity Reports* 4 (2015): 11–18; B. J. Rolls, What is the role of portion control in weight management? *International Journal of Obesity* 38 (2014): S1–S8; M. B. Livingstone and L. K. Pourshahidi, Portion size and obesity, *Advances in Nutrition* 5 (2014): 829–834.

22. M. H. Rouhani and coauthors, Associations between dietary energy density and obesity: A systematic review and meta-analysis of observational studies, *Nutrition* 32 (2016): 1037–1047.

23. Position of the Academy of Nutrition and Dietetics: Interventions for the treatment of overweight and obesity in adults, *Journal of the Academy of Nutrition and Dietetics* 116 (2016): 129–147.

24. K. M. Whitaker and coauthors, Sedentary behavior, physical activity, and abdominal adipose tissue deposition, *Medicine and Science in Sports and Exercise* 49 (2017): 450–458; N. S. A. Hawari and coauthors, Frequency of breaks in sedentary time and postprandial metabolic responses, *Medicine and Science in Sports and Exercise* 48 (2016): 2495–2502; A. Philipsen and coauthors, Associations of objectively measured physical activity and abdominal fat distribution, *Medicine and Science in Sports and Exercise* 47 (2015): 983–989.

25. Whitaker and coauthors, 2017; B. J. Howard and coauthors, Associations of overall sitting time and TV viewing time with fibrinogen and C reactive protein: The AusDiab study, *British Journal of Sports Medicine* 49 (2015): 255–258; J. Y. Chau and coauthors, Cross-sectional associations of total sitting and leisure screen time with cardiometabolic risk in adults: Results from the HUNT Study, Norway, *Journal of Science and Medicine in Sport* 17 (2014): 78–84.

26. S. K. Keadle and coauthors, Targeting reductions in sitting time to increase physical activity and improve health, *Medicine and Science in Sports and Exercise* 49 (2017): 1572–1582; C. E. Matthews and coauthors, Mortality benefits for replacing sitting time with different physical activities, *Medicine and Science in Sports and Exercise* 47 (2015): 1833–1840; A. Biswas and coauthors, Sedentary time and its association with risk for disease incidence, mortality, and hospitalization in adults: A systematic review and meta-analysis, *Annals of Internal Medicine* 162 (2015): 123–132.

27. E. Cerin and coauthors, Neighborhood environments and objectively measured physical activity in 11 countries, *Medicine and Science in Sports and Exercise* 46 (2014): 2253–2264.

28. D. Stern and coauthors, Where people shop is not associated with the nutrient quality of packaged foods for any racial-ethnic group in the United States, *American Journal of Clinical Nutrition* 103 (2016): 1125–1134; T. Dubowitz and coauthors, Healthy food access for urban food desert residents: Examination of the food environment, food purchasing practices, diet, and BMI, *Public Health Nutrition* 18 (2015): 2220–2230.

29. FDA, Tainted weight loss products, www.fda.gov/drugs/resourcesforyou /consumers/buyingusingmedicinesafely/medicationhealthfraud/ ucm234592.htm, updated August 31, 2017.

30. R. Khera and coauthors, Association of pharmacological treatments for obesity with weight loss and adverse events: A systematic review and meta-analysis, *Journal of the American Medical Association* 315 (2016): 2424–2434; S. Z. Yanovski and J. A. Yanovski, Long-term drug treatment for obesity: A systematic and clinical review, *Journal of the American Medical Association* 311 (2014): 74–86.

31. K. M. Flegal and coauthors, Trends in obesity among adults in the United States, 2005 to 2014, *Journal of the American Medical Association* 315 (2016): 2284–2291.

32. S. H. Chang and coauthors, Effectiveness and risks of bariatric surgery: An updated systematic review and meta-analysis, 2003–2012, *JAMA Surgery* 19 (2014): 275–287; A. P. Courcoulas and coauthors, Weight change and health outcomes at 3 years after bariatric surgery among individuals with severe obesity, *Journal of the American Medical Association* 310 (2014): 2416–2425; C. S. Kwok and coauthors, Bariatric surgery and its impact on cardiovascular disease and mortality: A systematic review and meta-analysis, *International Journal of Cardiology* 173 (2014): 20–28.

33. T. Reinehr and C. L. Roth, The gut sensor as regulator of body weight, *Endocrine* 49 (2015): 35–50; J. B. Dixon, E. A. Lambert, and G.W. Lambert, Neuroendocrine adaptations to bariatric surgery, *Molecular and Cellular Endocrinology* 418 (2015): 143–152; S. Barja-Fernandez and coauthors, Peripheral signals mediate the beneficial effects of gastric surgery in obesity, *Gastroenterology Research and Practice* 2015, doi: 10.1155/2015/560938.

34. V. Tremaroli and coauthors, Roux-en-Y gastric bypass and vertical banded gastroplasty induce long-term changes on the human gut microbiome contributing to fat mass regulation, *Cell Metabolism* 22 (2015): 228–238; L. Graham, G. Murty, and D. J. Bowrey, Taste, smell and appetite change after Roux-en-Y gastric bypass surgery, *Obesity Surgery* 24 (2014): 1463–1468.

35. T. D. Adams and coauthors, Weight and metabolic outcomes 12 years after gastric bypass, *New England Journal of Medicine* 377 (2017): 1143–1155; M. L. Maciejewski and coauthors, Bariatric surgery and long-term durability of weight loss, *JAMA Surgery* (2016): doi 10.1001/ jamasurg.2016.2317.

36. J. Hoffstedt and coauthors, Long-term protective changes in adipose tissue after gastric bypass, *Diabetes Care* 40 (2017): 77–84; D. Arterburn and D. McCulloch, Bariatric surgery for type 2 diabetes getting closer to the long-term goal, *JAMA Surgery* 150 (2015): 931–940; Kwok and coauthors, 2014; L. Sjöström and coauthors, Association of bariatric surgery with long-term remission of type 2 diabetes and with microvascular and macrovascular complications *Journal of the American Medical Association* 311 (2014): 2297–2304; N. Puzziferri and coauthors, Long term follow-up after bariatric surgery: A systematic review, *Journal of the American Medical Association* 312 (2014): 934–942.

37. B. Y. Lee and coauthors, A systems approach to obesity, *Nutrition Reviews* 75 (2017): 94–106; Position of the Academy of Nutrition and Dietetics: Interventions for the treatment of overweight and obesity in adults, *Journal of the Academy of Nutrition and Dietetics* 116 (2016): 129–147; K. M. Livingstone and coauthors, FTO genotype and weight loss: Systematic review and meta-analysis of 9563 individual participant data from eight randomised controlled trials, *British Medical Journal* 354 (2016): i4707.

38. M. D. Jensen and coauthors, 2013 AHA/ACC/TOS guideline for the Management of overweight and obesity in adults: A report of the American College of Cardiology/American Heart Association Task Force on Practice Guidelines and the Obesity Society, *Circulation* 22 (2014): S5–S39.

39. Greenway, 2015.

40. Jensen and coauthors, 2013 AHA/ACC/TOS guidelines for the management of overweight and obesity in adults, 2014.

41. U.S. Department of Agriculture and U.S. Department of Health and Human Services, *Scientific Report of the 2015 Dietary Guidelines Advisory Committee*, 2015, D-2:43, www.health.gov; U.S. Department of Agriculture, Evidence Analysis Library Division, A series of systematic reviews on the relationship between dietary patterns and health outcomes (2014), www.nel.gov/vault/2440/web/files/DietaryPatterns /DPRptFullFinal.pdf; N. D. Barnard, S. M. Levin, and Y. Yokovarma, A systematic review and meta-analysis of changes in body weight in clinical trials of vegetarian diets, *Journal of the Academy of Nutrition and Dietetics* 115 (2015): 954–969.

42. C. E. O'Neil, V. L. Fulgoni, and T. A. Nicklas, Tree nut consumption is associated with better adiposity measures and cardiovascular and metabolic syndrome health risk factors in U.S. adults: NHANES 2005–2010, *Nutrition Journal* 14 (2015): 64; C. L. Jackson and F. B. Hu, Long-term associations of nut consumption with body weight and obesity, *American Journal of Clinical Nutrition* 100 (2014): 408S–411S; S. Y. Tan, J. Dhillon, and R. D. Mattes, A review of the effects of nuts on appetite, food intake, metabolism, and body weight, *American Journal of Clinical Nutrition* 100 (2014): 412S–422S.

43. S. M. Phillips, S. Chevalier, and H. J. Leidy, Protein "requirements" beyond the RDA: Implications for optimizing health, *Applied Physiology, Nutrition, and Metabolism* 41 (2016): 565–572; Leidy and coauthors, 2015. D. L. Layman and coauthors, Defining meal requirements for protein to optimize metabolic roles of amino acids, *American Journal of Clinical Nutrition* 101 (2015): 1330S–1338S.

44. R. Estruch and coauthors, Effect of a high-fat Mediterranean diet on bodyweight and waist circumference: A prespecified secondary outcomes analysis of the PREDIMED randomised controlled trial, *Lancet Diabetes and Endocrinology* (2016), epub ahead of print, DOI: dx.doi.org/10.1016/S2213-8587(16)30085-7; M. Garcia and coauthors, The effect of the traditional Mediterranean-style diet on metabolic risk factors: A meta-analysis, *Nutrients* (2016), epub, doi: 10.3390/nu8030168.

45. O'Neil, Fulgone, and Nicklas, 2015.

46. M. H. Alhussain, I. A. Macdonald, and M. A. Taylor, Irregular meal-pattern effects on energy expenditure, metabolism, and appetite regulation: A randomized controlled trial in healthy normal-weight women, *American College of Clinical Nutrition* 104 (2016): 21–32.

47. K. J. Duffey and J. Poti, Modeling the effect of replacing sugar-sweetened beverage consumption with water on energy intake, HBI score, and obesity prevalence, *Nutrients* 8 (2016): 395.

48. R. J. Verheggen and coauthors, A systematic review and meta-analysis on the effects of exercise training versus hypocaloric diet: Distinct effects on body weight and visceral adipose tissue, *Obesity Reviews* 17 (2016): 664–690; Position of the Academy of Nutrition and Dietetics, 2016; D. J. Johns and coauthors, Diet or exercise interventions vs combined behavioral weight management programs: A systematic review and meta-analysis of direct comparisons, *Journal of the Academy of Nutrition and Dietetics* 114 (2014): 1557–1568; D. L. Swift and coauthors, The role of exercise and physical activity in weight loss and maintenance, *Progress in Cardiovascular Diseases* 56 (2014): 441–447.

49. Verheggen and coauthors, 2016; Swift and coauthors, 2014.

50. F. M. Schmidt and coauthors, Inflammatory cytokines in general and central obesity and modulating effects of physical activity, *PLoS One* 10 (2015): e0121971; U. Ecklund and coauthors, Physical activity and all-cause mortality across levels of overall and abdominal adiposity in European men and women: the European Prospective Investigation into Cancer and Nutrition Study (EPIC), *American Journal of Clinical Nutrition* 101 (2015): 613–621.

51. K. Deighton and D. J. Stensel, Creating an acute energy deficit without stimulating compensatory increases in appetite: Is there an optimal exercise protocol? *Proceedings of the Nutrition Society* 73 (2014): 352–358.

52. J. E. Blundell and coauthors, Appetite control and energy balance: Impact of exercise, *Obesity Reviews* 16 (2015): 67–76; M. M. Schubert and coauthors, Acute exercise and hormones related to appetite regulation: A meta-analysis, *Sports Medicine* 44 (2014): 387–403.

53. R. Bassett-Gunter, D. McEwan, and A. Kamarhie, Physical activity and body image among men and boys: A meta-analysis, *Body Image* 22 (2017): 114–128.

54. Z. Yu, C. Sealey-Potts, and J. Rodriquez, Dietary self-monitoring in weight management: Current evidence on efficacy and adherence, *Journal of the Academy of Nutrition and Dietetics* 115 (2015): 1931–1938.

55. C. D. Fryar, M. D. Carroll, and C. L. Ogden, Prevalence of underweight among adults aged 20 and over: United States, 1960–1962 through 2013–2014, www.cdc.gov/nchs/data/hestat/underweight_adult_13_14/underweight_adult_13_14.htm, updated July 18, 2016.

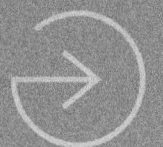

7.7 Nutrition in Practice

Fad Diets

To paraphrase William Shakespeare, "a fad diet by any other name would still be a fad diet." Year after year, "new and improved" diets appear on bookstore shelves and circulate among friends.* People of all sizes eagerly try the best diet on the market, hoping that this one will really work. Sometimes the diets seem to work for a while, but more often than not, their success is short-lived. Then another fad diet takes the spotlight. Here's how Dr. Kelly Brownell, an obesity researcher, describes this phenomenon: "When I get calls about the latest diet fad, I imagine a trick birthday cake candle that keeps lighting up and we have to keep blowing it out."

Why don't health professionals speak out against the relentless promotion of fad diets?

Realizing that many fad diets do not offer a safe and effective plan for weight loss, health professionals speak out, but they never get the candle blown out permanently. New fad diets can keep making outrageous claims because no one requires their advocates to prove what they say. Fad diet promoters do not have to conduct credible research on the benefits or dangers of their diets. They can simply make recommendations and then later, if questioned, search for bits and pieces of research that support the conclusions they have already reached. That's backward. Diet and health recommendations should *follow* years of sound research that has been reviewed by panels of scientists *before* being offered to the public.

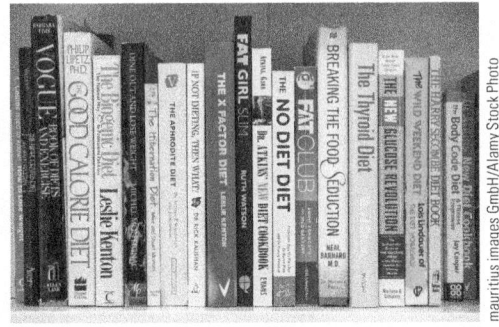

How can the promoters of fad diets get away with exaggerated claims?

Because anyone can publish anything—in books or on the Internet—peddlers of fad diets can make unsubstantiated statements that fall far short of the truth but sound impressive to the uninformed. They often offer distorted bits of legitimate research. They may start with one or more actual facts but then leap from one erroneous conclusion to the next. Anyone who wants to believe these claims has to wonder how the thousands of scientists working on obesity research over the past century could possibly have missed such obvious connections.

Each popular diet features a unique way to make losing weight fast and easy. Which one works best?

Fad diets come in almost as many shapes and sizes as the people who search them out. Some restrict fats or carbohydrates, some limit portion sizes, some focus on food combinations, some claim that a person's genetic type or blood type determines the foods best suited to manage weight, and others advocate taking unproven "weight-loss dietary supplements." A lack of scientific evidence just doesn't seem to stop the advertised claims made for fad diets.[1] Despite claims that each new diet is "unique" in its approach to weight loss, most fad diets are designed to ensure a low energy intake. The "magic feature" that best supports weight loss is to limit energy intake to less than energy expenditure. Most of the sample menu plans, especially in the early stages, deliver an average of 1200 kcalories per day. Total kcalories tend to be low simply because food intake is so limited.

What is the appeal of fad diets?

Probably the greatest appeal of some fad diets is that they tend to ignore current diet recommendations. Foods such as meats and milk products that need to be selected carefully to limit saturated fat can now be eaten with abandon. Whole grains, legumes, vegetables, and fruit that should be eaten in abundance can now be bypassed. For some people, this is a dream come true: steaks without

---

*The Academy of Nutrition and Dietetics offers reviews of popular diet books on their website at *www.eatrightpro.org/resources/media/trends-and-reviews/book-reviews.*

the potatoes, ribs without the coleslaw, and meatballs without the pasta. Who can resist the promise of weight loss while eating freely from a list of favorite foods?

Dieters are also lured into fad diets by sophisticated— yet often erroneous—explanations of the metabolic consequences of eating certain foods. Terms such as *eicosanoids* or *adipokines* are scattered about, often intimidating readers into believing that the authors must be right given their brilliance in understanding the body.

With over half of our nation's adults overweight and many more concerned about their weight, weight-loss services and products are a $60 billion-a-year business. Even a plan that offers only minimal weight-loss success easily attracts a following.

Are fad diets adequate?

When food choices are limited, nutrient intakes may be inadequate. To help shore up some of these inadequacies, fad diets often recommend a dietary supplement. Conveniently, many of the companies selling fad diets also sell these supplements, often at an inflated price. As Nutrition in Practice 9 explains, however, foods offer many more health benefits than any supplement can provide. Quite simply, if the diet is inadequate, it needs to be improved, not supplemented.

Are the diets effective?

If fad diets were entirely ineffective, consumers would eventually stop pursuing them. Obviously, this is not the case. Similarly, if the diets were especially effective, then consumers who tried them would lose weight, and the obesity problem would be solved. Clearly, this is not happening either. As mentioned earlier, most fad diets succeed in contriving ways to limit kcalorie intakes, and so produce weight loss for some people for a short time, but they fail to produce long-lasting results for most people.

For example, low-carbohydrate, high-protein diets produce a little more weight loss than balanced diets during the first few months of dieting. Over time, however, low-carbohydrate diets perform no better than others. Also, diets with less than 45 percent of kcalories from carbohydrate are difficult to maintain over time and may be less safe.[2] Still, it makes good nutritional sense to cut kcalories by cutting down on added sugars and starch-based ultraprocessed foods, such as soft drinks, snack cakes, and chips.

Protein nutrition during kcalorie restriction deserves attention. A meal with too little protein may not produce enough satiety, the satisfaction of feeling full after a meal, to prevent between-meal hunger, although research is not consistent on this point.[3] Also, high-quality protein, along with performing muscle-building resistance exercise, may help to minimize muscle tissue loss, an unwelcome side effect of kcalorie restriction and fat loss.[4]

Most people in the United States take in about 1.2 to 1.5 grams of protein per kilogram of body weight, or about 16 percent of kcalories as protein.[5] While this amount exceeds the RDA of 0.8 grams per kilogram of body weight, it is well below the upper boundary of 35 percent of energy as protein mentioned earlier. Some research suggests that a little extra protein (1.2 to 1.6 grams per kilogram body weight) may turn out to be useful for weight loss as long as the dieter can adhere to a kcalorie-reduced diet over time.[6] However, protein sources matter, too. In one well-controlled, long-term study, weight *gain*, not loss, was associated with higher intakes of full fat cheeses, chicken with skin, and processed and red meats (particularly hamburger).[7] In contrast, plain yogurt, peanut butter, walnuts, other nuts, chicken without skin, low-fat cheese, and seafood were associated with weight loss, an effect sometimes magnified when the diet was also rich in whole grains, fruit, and vegetables.

Many people seem confused about what kinds of dietary changes they need to make to lose weight. Isn't it helpful to follow a plan?

Yes. Most people need specific instructions and examples to make dietary changes. Popular diets offer dieters a plan. The user doesn't have to decide what foods to eat, how to prepare them, or how much to eat. Unfortunately, these instructions serve short-term weight-loss needs only. Over the long run, people tire of the monotony of diet plans, and most revert to their previous patterns.

By now you can see that the major drawback of most fad weight-loss schemes is that they fail to create lifestyle changes needed to support long-term weight maintenance and improve health. For that, people must do the hard work of learning the facts about nutrition and weight loss, setting their own realistic goals and then devising a lifestyle plan that can achieve them. A balanced, kcalorie-restricted diet with sufficient physical activity to support it may not be the shortcut that most people wish for, but it ensures nutrient adequacy and provides the best chance of long-term success.

Some currently popular diet plans offer a sensible approach to weight loss and healthy eating. The challenge is sorting the fad diets from the healthy options. Table NP7-1 presents some tips for identifying fad diets and weight-loss scams.

Chapter 7 describes reasonable approaches to weight management and concludes that the ideal diet is one you can live with for the rest of your life. Keep that criterion in mind when you evaluate the next "latest and greatest weight-loss diet" that comes along.

TABLE NP7-1 Tips for Identifying Fad Diets and Weight-Loss Scams

It may be a fad diet or weight-loss scam if it:

- Sounds too good to be true.
- Recommends using a single food consistently as the key to the program's success.
- Promises quick and easy weight loss with no effort ("Lose weight while you sleep!").
- Eliminates an entire food group such as grains or milk and milk products.
- Guarantees an unrealistic outcome in an unreasonable time period ("Lose 10 pounds in 2 days!").
- Bases evidence for its effectiveness on anecdotal stories or testimonials.
- Blames weight gain on a single nutrient, such as carbohydrate, or constituent, such as gluten.
- Requires that you buy special products that are not readily available in the marketplace at affordable prices.
- Specifies a proportion for the energy nutrients that falls outside the recommended ranges—carbohydrate (45 to 65 percent), fat (20 to 35 percent), and protein (10 to 35 percent).
- Claims to alter your genetic code or reset your metabolism.
- Fails to mention potential risks or additional costs.
- Promotes products or procedures that have not been proven safe and effective.
- Neglects plans for weight maintenance following weight loss.

Notes

1. L. E. Matarese and W. J. Pories, Adult weight loss diets: Metabolic effects and outcomes, *Nutrition in Clinical Practice* 29 (2014): 759–767.
2. U.S. Department of Health and Human Services, Scientific report of the 2015 Dietary Guidelines Advisory Committee, 2015, D-7, available at www.health.gov.
3. H. J. Leidy and coauthors, The role of protein in weight loss and maintenance, *American Journal of Clinical Nutrition* 101 (2015): 1320S–1329S; A. Astrup, A. Raben, and N. Gieker, The role of higher protein diets in weight control and obesity-related comorbidities, *International Journal of Obesity* 39 (2015): 721–726; E. A. Martens and M. S. Westerterp-Plantenga, Protein diets, body weight loss and weight maintenance, *Current Opinion in Clinical Nutrition and Metabolic Care* 17 (2014): 75–79; D. H. Pesta and V. T. Samuel, A high-protein diet for reducing body fat: Mechanisms and possible caveats, *Nutrition and Metabolism* 11 (2014): 53.
4. D. L. Layman and coauthors, Defining meal requirements for protein to optimize metabolic roles of amino acids, *American Journal of Clinical Nutrition* 101 (2015): 1330S–1338S; A. J. Hector and coauthors, Whey Protein supplementation preserves postprandial myofibrillar protein synthesis during short-term energy restriction in overweight and obese adults, *Journal of Nutrition* 145 (2015): 246–252.
5. N. R. Rodriguez and S. L. Miller, Effective translation of current dietary guidance: Understanding and communicating the concepts of minimal and optimal levels of dietary protein, *American Journal of Clinical Nutrition* 101 (2015): 1353S–1358S.
6. S. M. Phillips, S. Chevalier, and H. J. Leidy, Protein "requirements" beyond the RDA: Implications for optimizing health, *Applied Physiology, Nutrition, and Metabolism* 41 (2016): 565–572; Leidy and coauthors, 2015.
7. J. D. Smith and coauthors, Changes in intake of protein foods, carbohydrate amount and quality, and long-term weight change: Results from 3 prospective cohorts, *American Journal of Clinical Nutrition* 101 (2015): 1216–1224.

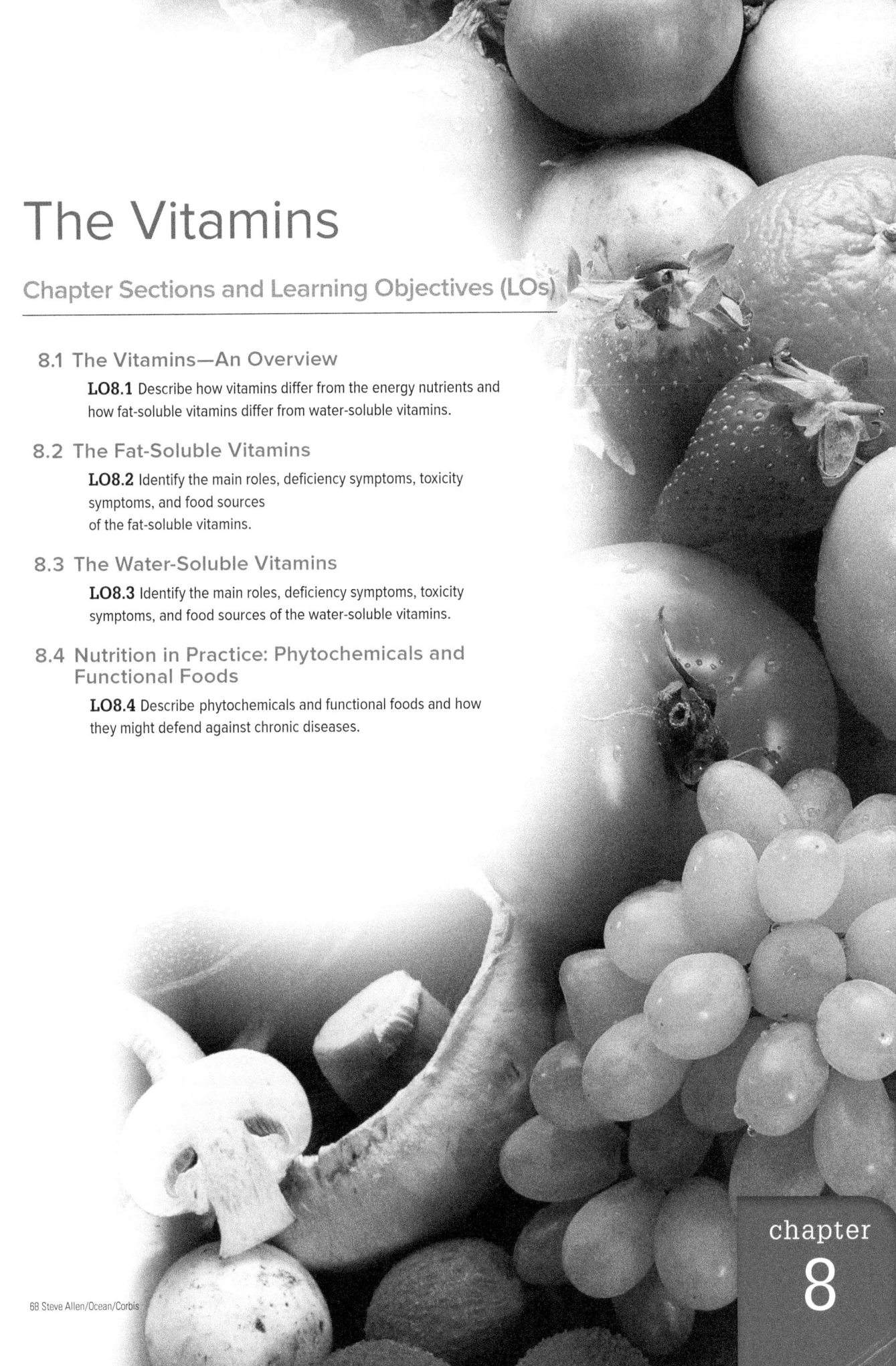

The Vitamins

Chapter Sections and Learning Objectives (LOs)

8.1 The Vitamins—An Overview

LO8.1 Describe how vitamins differ from the energy nutrients and how fat-soluble vitamins differ from water-soluble vitamins.

8.2 The Fat-Soluble Vitamins

LO8.2 Identify the main roles, deficiency symptoms, toxicity symptoms, and food sources of the fat-soluble vitamins.

8.3 The Water-Soluble Vitamins

LO8.3 Identify the main roles, deficiency symptoms, toxicity symptoms, and food sources of the water-soluble vitamins.

8.4 Nutrition in Practice: Phytochemicals and Functional Foods

LO8.4 Describe phytochemicals and functional foods and how they might defend against chronic diseases.

chapter

8

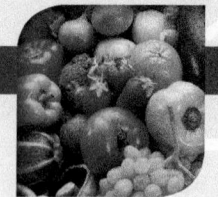

nutrients—carbohydrate, fat, and protein. This chapter and the next one discuss the nutrients everyone thinks of when nutrition is mentioned—the vitamins and minerals.

8.1 The Vitamins—An Overview

The **vitamins** occur in foods in much smaller quantities than do the energy-yielding nutrients, and they themselves contribute no energy to the body. Instead, they serve mostly as facilitators of body processes. They are a powerful group of substances, as their absence attests: Vitamin A deficiency can cause blindness, a lack of niacin can cause dementia, and a lack of vitamin D can retard bone growth. The consequences of deficiencies are so dire and the effects of restoring the needed nutrients so dramatic that people spend billions of dollars each year on **dietary supplements** to cure many different ailments. Vitamins certainly contribute to sound nutritional health, but supplements do not cure all ills. Furthermore, vitamin supplements do not offer the many benefits that come from vitamin-rich foods. The only disease a vitamin will *cure* is the one caused by a deficiency of that vitamin. The vitamins' roles in supporting optimal health extend far beyond preventing deficiency diseases, however. Emerging evidence supports the role of vitamin-rich *foods*, but not vitamin supplements, as protective against cancer and heart disease.[1] According to the Dietary Guidelines 2015 committee, today's intakes of the following vitamins may fall below recommended intakes:

- Vitamin A
- Vitamin D
- Vitamin E
- Vitamin C

These vitamins and others play critical roles in the body.

A child once defined vitamins as "what, if you don't eat, you get sick." The description is both insightful and accurate. A more prosaic definition is that vitamins are potent, essential, non-kcaloric, organic nutrients needed from foods in trace amounts to perform specific functions that promote growth, reproduction, and the maintenance of health and life. The vitamins differ from carbohydrates, fats, and proteins in the following ways:

- *Structure.* Vitamins are individual units; they are not linked together (as are molecules of glucose or amino acids).
- *Function.* Vitamins do not yield energy when metabolized; many of them do, however, assist the enzymes that participate in the release of energy from carbohydrate, fat, and proteins.
- *Dietary intakes.* The amounts of vitamins people ingest daily from foods and the amounts they require are measured in *micrograms* (µg) or *milligrams* (mg), rather than grams (g). For this reason, the vitamins are sometimes described as *micronutrients*.

The vitamins are similar to the energy-yielding nutrients, though, in that they are vital to life, organic, and available from foods.

As the individual vitamins were discovered, they were named or given letters, numbers, or both. This led to the confusion that still exists today. This chapter uses the names shown in Table 8-1; alternative names are given in Tables 8-4 and 8-5, which appear later in the chapter.

vitamins: essential, non-kcaloric, organic nutrients needed in tiny amounts in the diet.

dietary supplements: products that are added to the diet and contain any of the following ingredients: a vitamin, a mineral, an herb or other botanical, an amino acid, a metabolite, a constituent, or an extract.

Bioavailability The amount of vitamins available from foods depends on two factors: the quantity provided by a food and the amount absorbed and used by the body (the vitamin's **bioavailability**). Researchers analyze foods to determine their vitamin contents and publish the results in tables of food composition such as the USDA's Food Composition Databases. Determining the bioavailability of a vitamin is more difficult because it depends on many factors, including:

- Efficiency of digestion and time of transit through the GI tract.
- Previous nutrient intake and nutrition status.
- Other foods consumed at the same time.
- The method of food preparation (raw or cooked, for example).
- Source of the nutrient (naturally occurring, synthetic, or fortified)

This chapter and the next describe factors that inhibit or enhance the absorption of individual vitamins and minerals. Experts consider these factors when estimating recommended intakes.

Precursors Some of the vitamins are available from foods in inactive forms known as **precursors**, or provitamins. Once inside the body, the precursor is converted to the active form of the vitamin. Thus, in measuring a person's vitamin intake, it is important to count both the amount of the actual vitamin and the potential amount available from its precursors. Tables 8-4 and 8-5 later in the chapter specify which vitamins have precursors.

Organic Nature Fresh foods naturally contain vitamins, but because they are organic, vitamins can be readily destroyed during processing. Therefore, processed foods should be used sparingly, and fresh foods must be handled with care during storage and in cooking. Prolonged heating may destroy much of the thiamin in food. Because riboflavin can be destroyed by the ultraviolet rays of the sun or by fluorescent light, foods stored in transparent glass containers are most likely to lose riboflavin. Oxygen destroys vitamin C, so losses occur when foods are cut, processed, and stored. Table 8-2 summarizes ways to minimize nutrient losses in the kitchen.

Solubility Vitamins fall naturally into two classes—fat soluble and water soluble. The water-soluble vitamins are the B vitamins and vitamin C; the fat-soluble ones are

---

TABLE 8-1 Vitamin Names

FAT-SOLUBLE VITAMINS

Vitamin A
Vitamin D
Vitamin E
Vitamin K

WATER-SOLUBLE VITAMINS

B vitamins
 Thiamin
 Riboflavin
 Niacin
 Pantothenic acid
 Biotin
 Vitamin B_6
 Folate
 Vitamin B_{12}
Vitamin C

TABLE 8-2 Minimizing Nutrient Losses

Each of these tactics saves a small percentage of the vitamins in foods, but repeated each day this can add up to significant amounts in a year's time.

PREVENT ENZYMATIC DESTRUCTION

- Refrigerate most fruit, vegetables, and juices to slow breakdown of vitamins.

PROTECT FROM LIGHT AND AIR

- Store milk and enriched grain products in opaque containers to protect riboflavin.
- Store cut fruit and vegetables in the refrigerator in airtight wrappers; reseal opened juice containers before refrigerating.

PREVENT HEAT DESTRUCTION OR LOSSES IN WATER

- Wash intact fruit and vegetables before cutting or peeling to prevent vitamin losses during washing.
- Cook fruit and vegetables in a microwave oven, or quickly stir fry, or steam them over a small amount of water to preserve heat-sensitive vitamins and to prevent vitamin loss in cooking water. Recapture dissolved vitamins by using cooking water for soups, stews, or gravies.
- Avoid high temperatures and long cooking times.

bioavailability: the rate and extent to which a nutrient is absorbed and used.

precursors: compounds that can be converted into other compounds; with regard to vitamins, compounds that can be converted into active vitamins; also known as *provitamins*.

TABLE 8-3 Fat-Soluble and Water-Soluble Vitamins Compared

While each vitamin has unique functions and features, a few generalizations about the fat-soluble and water-soluble vitamins can aid understanding.

	FAT-SOLUBLE VITAMINS: VITAMINS A, D, E, AND K	WATER-SOLUBLE VITAMINS: B VITAMINS AND VITAMIN C
Absorption	Absorbed like fats, first into the lymph and then into the blood.	Absorbed directly into the blood.
Transport and storage	Must travel with protein carriers in watery body fluids; stored in the liver or fatty tissues.	Travel freely in watery fluids; most are not stored in the body.
Excretion	Not readily excreted; tend to build up in the tissues.	Readily excreted in the urine.
Toxicity	Toxicities are likely from supplements but occur rarely from food.	Toxicities are unlikely but possible with high doses from supplements.
Requirement	Needed in periodic doses (weekly or even monthly) depending on the extent of body stores.	Needed frequently (often daily) because the body does not store most of them to any extent.

vitamins A, D, E, and K. The solubility of a vitamin confers on it many characteristics and determines how it is absorbed, transported, stored, and excreted (see Table 8-3). This discussion of vitamins begins with the fat-soluble vitamins.

Review Notes

- Vitamins are essential, non-kcaloric, organic nutrients that are needed in trace amounts in the diet to help facilitate body processes.
- The amount of vitamins available from foods depends on the quantity provided by a food and the amount absorbed and used by the body—the vitamins' bioavailability.
- Vitamin precursors in foods are converted into active vitamins in the body.
- Vitamins can be readily destroyed during processing.
- The water-soluble vitamins are the B vitamins and vitamin C; the fat-soluble vitamins are vitamins A, D, E, and K.

8.2 The Fat-Soluble Vitamins

The fat-soluble vitamins—A, D, E, and K—usually occur together in the fats and oils of foods, and the body absorbs them in the same way it absorbs lipids. Therefore, any condition that interferes with fat absorption can precipitate a deficiency of the fat-soluble vitamins. Once absorbed, fat-soluble vitamins are stored in the liver and fatty tissues until the body needs them. They are not readily excreted, and, unlike most of the water-soluble vitamins, they can build up to toxic concentrations.

The capacity to store fat-soluble vitamins affords a person some flexibility in dietary intake. When blood concentrations begin to decline, the body can retrieve the vitamins from storage. Thus, a person need not eat a day's allowance of each fat-soluble vitamin every day but need only make sure that, over time, average daily intakes approximate recommended intakes. In contrast, most water-soluble vitamins must be consumed more regularly because the body does not store them to any great extent.

Vitamin A and Beta-Carotene

Vitamin A has the distinction of being the first fat-soluble vitamin to be recognized. More than a century later, vitamin A and its plant-derived precursor, **beta-carotene**, continue to intrigue researchers with their diverse roles and profound effects on health.

Vitamin A is a versatile vitamin, with roles in gene expression, vision, cell differentiation (thereby maintaining the health of body linings and skin), immunity, and reproduction and growth.[2] Three different forms of vitamin A are active in the body: retinol, retinal, and retinoic acid. Each form of vitamin A performs specific tasks. Retinol supports reproduction and is the major transport and storage form of the vitamin; the cells convert retinol to retinal or retinoic acid as needed. Retinal is active in vision, and retinoic acid acts as a hormone, regulating cell differentiation, growth, and embryonic development. A special transport protein, **retinol-binding protein (RBP)**, picks up retinol from the liver, where it is stored, and carries it in the blood.

Vitamin A's Role in Gene Expression Vitamin A exerts considerable influence on an array of body functions through its interaction with genes—hundreds of genes are regulated by the retinoic acid form of the vitamin.[3] Genes direct the synthesis of proteins, including enzymes, and enzymes perform the metabolic work of the tissues (see Chapter 5). Hence, factors that influence gene expression also affect the metabolic activities of the tissues and the health of the body.

Researchers have long known that simply possessing the genetic equipment needed to make a particular protein does not guarantee that the protein will be produced, any more than owning a car guarantees you a trip across town. To make the journey, you must also use the right key to trigger the events that start up its engine or turn it off at the appropriate time. Some dietary components, including the retinoic acid form of vitamin A, are now known to be such keys—they help to activate or deactivate certain genes and thus affect the production of specific proteins.[4]

Vitamin A's Role in Vision Vitamin A plays two indispensable roles in the eye. It helps maintain a healthy, crystal-clear outer window, the **cornea**; and it participates in light detection at the **retina**. Some of the photosensitive cells of the retina contain **pigment** molecules called **rhodopsin**; each rhodopsin molecule is composed of a protein called **opsin** bonded to a molecule of retinal, which plays a central role in vision. When light passes through the cornea of the eye and strikes the retina, rhodopsin responds by changing shape and becoming bleached. In turn, this initiates the signal that conveys the sensation of sight to the optic center in the brain. Figure 8-1 shows vitamin A's site of action inside the eye.

When vitamin A is lacking, the eye has difficulty adapting to changing light levels. At night, after the eye has adapted to darkness, a flash of bright light is followed by a brief delay before the eye can see again. This lag in the recovery of night vision is known as **night blindness**. Because night blindness is easy to test, it aids in the diagnosis of vitamin A deficiency. Night blindness is only a symptom, however, and may indicate a condition other than vitamin A deficiency.

Vitamin A's Role in Protein Synthesis and Cell Differentiation The role that vitamin A plays in vision is undeniably important, but only one-thousandth of the body's vitamin A is in the retina. Much more is in the skin and the linings of organs, where it works behind the scenes at the genetic level to promote protein synthesis and cell **differentiation**. The process of cell differentiation allows each type of cell to mature so that it is capable of performing a specific function.

vitamin A: a fat-soluble vitamin with three chemical forms: *retinol* (the alcohol form), *retinal* (the aldehyde form), and *retinoic acid* (the acid form).

beta-carotene: a vitamin A precursor made by plants and stored in human fat tissue; an orange pigment.

retinol-binding protein (RBP): the specific protein responsible for transporting retinol. Measurement of the blood concentration of RBP is a sensitive test of vitamin A status.

cornea (KOR-nee-uh): the hard, transparent membrane covering the outside of the eye.

retina (RET-in-uh): the layer of light-sensitive nerve cells lining the back of the inside of the eye; consists of rods and cones.

pigment: a molecule capable of absorbing certain wavelengths of light so that it reflects only those that we perceive as a certain color.

rhodopsin (ro-DOP-sin): a light-sensitive pigment of the retina; contains the retinal form of vitamin A and the protein opsin.

rhod = red (pigment)
opsin = visual protein

opsin (OP-sin): the protein portion of the visual pigment molecule.

night blindness: the slow recovery of vision after exposure to flashes of bright light at night; an early symptom of vitamin A deficiency.

differentiation: the development of specific functions different from those of the original.

FIGURE 8-1 Vitamin A's Role in Vision

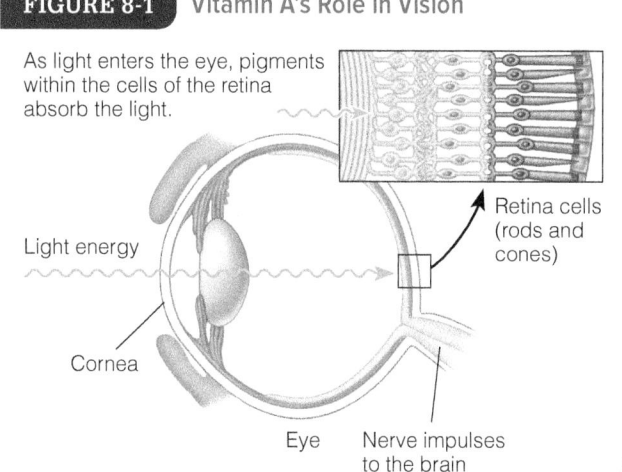

As light enters the eye, pigments within the cells of the retina absorb the light.

Light energy

Retina cells (rods and cones)

Cornea

Eye   Nerve impulses to the brain

All body surfaces, both inside and out, are covered by layers of cells known as **epithelial cells**. The **epithelial tissue** on the outside of the body is, of course, the skin—and vitamin A and beta-carotene help to protect against skin damage from the sunlight. In the eye, epithelial tissue covers the outermost layer of the cornea, where it blocks the passage of foreign materials such as dust, water, and bacteria. The epithelial tissues inside the body include the linings of the mouth, stomach, and intestines; the linings of the lungs and the passages leading to them; the lining of the bladder; the linings of the uterus and vagina; and the linings of the eyelids and sinus passageways. The epithelial tissues on the inside of the body must be kept smooth. To ensure that they are, the epithelial cells on their surfaces secrete a smooth, slippery substance (mucus) that coats the tissues and protects them from invasive microorganisms and other harmful particles. The **mucous membrane** that lines the stomach also shields its cells from digestion by gastric juices. Vitamin A, by way of its role in cell differentiation, helps to maintain the integrity of the epithelial cells.

Vitamin A's Role in Immunity Vitamin A has gained a reputation as an "anti-infective" vitamin because so many of the body's defenses against infection depend on an adequate supply. Much research supports the need for vitamin A in the regulation of the genes involved in immunity. Without sufficient vitamin A, these genetic interactions produce an altered response to infection that weakens the body's defenses.

Vitamin A's Role in Reproduction, Growth, and Development Vitamin A is crucial to normal reproduction and growth. In men, vitamin A participates in sperm development, and, in women, vitamin A promotes normal fetal growth and development.[5] During pregnancy, vitamin A is transferred to the fetus and is essential to the development of the nervous system, lungs, heart, kidneys, skeleton, eyes, and ears. (Nutrition during pregnancy is discussed in Chapter 10.)

Beta-Carotene's Role as an Antioxidant For many years scientists believed beta-carotene to be of interest solely as a vitamin A precursor. Eventually, though, researchers began to recognize that beta-carotene is an extremely effective **antioxidant** in the body. Antioxidants are compounds that protect other compounds (such as lipids in cell membranes) from attack by oxygen. Oxygen triggers the formation of compounds known as **free radicals** that can start chain reactions in cell membranes. If left uncontrolled, these chain reactions can damage cell structures and impair cell functions. Oxidative and free-radical damage to cells is suspected of instigating some early stages of cancer and heart disease.[6] Research has identified links between oxidative damage and the development of many other diseases, including age-related blindness, Alzheimer's disease, arthritis, cataracts, diabetes, and kidney disease.[7]

Studies of populations suggest that people whose diets are low in foods rich in beta-carotene have higher incidences of certain types of cancer than those whose diets contain generous amounts of such foods. Based on findings that beta-carotene in foods may protect against cancer, researchers designed a study to determine the effects of beta-carotene *supplements* on the incidence of lung cancer among smokers. The researchers expected to see a beneficial effect, but instead they found that smokers taking the beta-carotene supplements suffered a *greater* incidence of lung cancer than those taking placebos. Beta-carotene is one of many **dietary antioxidants** present in foods—others include vitamin E, vitamin C, the mineral selenium, and many phytochemicals. Dietary antioxidants are just one class of a complex array of constituents in whole foods that seem to benefit health synergistically. Until more is known, eating beta-carotene-rich foods, not supplements, is in the best interests of health. Based on research so far, the DRI committee has not established a recommended intake value for beta-carotene.

Vitamin A Deficiency Up to a year's supply of vitamin A can be stored in the body, 90 percent of it in the liver. If a healthy adult were to stop eating vitamin A–rich foods, deficiency symptoms would not begin to appear until after stores were depleted, which

epithelial cells (ep-i-THEE-lee-ul): cells on the surface of the skin and mucous membranes.

epithelial tissue: tissue composing the layers of the body that serve as selective barriers between the body's interior and the environment (examples are the cornea, the skin, the respiratory lining, and the lining of the digestive tract).

mucous membrane: membrane composed of mucus-secreting cells that lines the surfaces of body tissues. (Reminder: *Mucus* is the smooth, slippery substance secreted by these cells.)

antioxidant (anti-OX-ih-dant): a compound that protects other compounds from oxygen by itself reacting with oxygen. *Oxidation* is a potentially damaging effect of normal cell chemistry involving oxygen.

anti = against
oxy = oxygen

free radicals: highly reactive chemical forms that can cause destructive changes in nearby compounds, sometimes setting up a chain reaction.

dietary antioxidants: compounds typically found in plant foods that significantly decrease the adverse effects of oxidation on living tissues. The major antioxidant vitamins are vitamin E, vitamin C, and beta-carotene.

would take one to two years. Then, however, the consequences would be profound and severe. Table 8-4, later in this chapter, lists some of them.

In vitamin A deficiency, cell differentiation and maturation are impaired. The epithelial cells flatten and begin to produce **keratin**—the hard, inflexible protein of hair and nails. In the eye, this process leads to drying and hardening of the cornea, which may progress to permanent blindness. Vitamin A deficiency is the major cause of preventable blindness in children worldwide, causing as many as half a million children to lose their sight every year.[8] Blindness due to vitamin A deficiency, known as **xerophthalmia**, develops in stages. At first, the cornea becomes dry and hard because of inadequate mucus production—a condition known as **xerosis**. Then xerosis quickly progresses to **keratomalacia**, the softening of the cornea that leads to irreversible blindness. Many children worldwide endure less severe forms of vitamin A deficiency, making them vulnerable to infectious diseases. Routine vitamin A supplementation and food fortification can be lifesaving interventions.

All body surfaces, both inside and out, maintain their integrity with the help of vitamin A. When vitamin A is lacking, cells of the skin harden and flatten, making it dry, rough, scaly, and hard. An accumulation of keratin makes a lump around each hair **follicle** (keratinization).

In the mouth, a vitamin A deficiency results in drying and hardening of the salivary glands, making them susceptible to infection. Secretions of mucus in the stomach and intestines are reduced, hindering normal digestion and absorption of nutrients. Infections of other mucous membranes also become likely.

Vitamin A's role in maintaining the body's defensive barriers may partially explain the relationship between vitamin A deficiency and susceptibility to infection. In developing countries around the world, measles is a devastating infectious disease, killing an estimated 400 children each day.[9] Deaths are usually due to related infections such as pneumonia and severe diarrhea. Providing large doses of vitamin A reduces the risk of dying from these infections.

The evidence that vitamin A reduces the severity of measles and measles-related infections and diarrhea has prompted the World Health Organization (WHO) and the United Nations International Children's Emergency Fund (UNICEF) to make control of vitamin A deficiency a major goal in their quest to improve child survival throughout the developing world. They recommend routine vitamin A supplementation for all children with measles in areas where vitamin A deficiency is a problem or where the measles death rate is high.

Vitamin A Toxicity Vitamin A toxicity is a real possibility when people consume concentrated amounts of **preformed vitamin A** in foods derived from animals, fortified foods, or supplements. Plant foods contain the vitamin only as beta-carotene, its inactive precursor form. The precursor does not convert to active vitamin A rapidly enough to cause toxicity.

Overdoses of vitamin A damage the same body systems that exhibit symptoms in vitamin A deficiency (see Table 8-4 later in the chapter). Children are most vulnerable to vitamin A toxicity because they need less vitamin A and are more sensitive to overdoses. The availability of breakfast cereals, instant meals, fortified milk, and chewable candy-like vitamins, each containing 100 percent or more of the recommended daily intake of vitamin A, makes it possible for a well-meaning parent to provide several times the daily allowance of the vitamin to a child within a few hours.

Excessive vitamin A also poses a **teratogenic** risk. Excessive vitamin A during pregnancy can injure the spinal cord and other tissues of the developing fetus, increasing the risk of birth defects.[10] The Tolerable Upper Intake Level of 3000 micrograms for women of childbearing age is based on the teratogenic effect of vitamin A.

Multivitamin supplements typically provide 1500 micrograms—much more vitamin A than most people need. For perspective, the RDA for vitamin A is 700 micrograms for women and 900 micrograms for men.

keratin (KERR-uh-tin): a water-insoluble protein; the normal protein of hair and nails. Keratin-producing cells may replace mucus-producing cells in vitamin A deficiency.

xerophthalmia (zer-off-THAL-mee-uh): progressive blindness caused by inadequate mucus production due to severe vitamin A deficiency.

xero = dry
ophthalm = eye

xerosis (zee-ROW-sis): abnormal drying of the skin and mucous membranes; a sign of vitamin A deficiency

keratomalacia (KARE-ah-toe-ma-LAY-shuh): softening of the cornea that leads to irreversible blindness; a sign of severe vitamin A deficiency

follicle (FOLL-i-cul): a group of cells in the skin from which a hair grows.

preformed vitamin A: vitamin A in its active form.

teratogenic (ter-AT-oh-jen-ik): causing abnormal fetal development and birth defects.

terato = monster
genic = to produce

Certain vitamin A relatives are available by prescription as acne treatments. When applied directly to the skin surface, these preparations help relieve the symptoms of acne. Taking massive doses of vitamin A internally will *not* cure acne, however, and may cause the symptoms itemized in Table 8-4, later in the chapter. In most cases, foods are a better choice than supplements for needed nutrients. The best way to ensure a safe vitamin A intake is to eat generous servings of vitamin A–rich foods.

Beta-Carotene Conversion and Toxicity Nutrition scientists do not use micrograms to specify the quantity of beta-carotene in foods. Instead, they use a value known as **retinol activity equivalents (RAE)**, which express the amount of retinol the body actually derives from a plant food after conversion. One microgram of retinol counts as 1 RAE, as does 12 micrograms of dietary beta-carotene. This difference recognizes that beta-carotene's absorption and conversion are significantly less efficient than those of the retinoids.

As mentioned earlier, beta-carotene from plant foods is not converted to the active form of vitamin A rapidly enough to be hazardous. It has, however, been known to turn people bright yellow if they eat too much. Beta-carotene builds up in the fat just beneath the skin and imparts a yellowish cast (see Figure 8-2). Additionally, as discussed earlier, overconsumption of beta-carotene from *supplements* may be harmful, especially to smokers.

Vitamin A in Foods Preformed vitamin A is found only in foods of animal origin. The richest sources of vitamin A are liver and fish oil, but milk, cheese, and fortified cereals are also good sources. Healthy people can eat vitamin A–rich foods—with the possible exception of liver—in large amounts without risking toxicity. Eating liver once every week or so is enough. Butter and eggs also provide some vitamin A to the diet.

Because vitamin A is fat soluble, it is lost when milk is skimmed. To compensate, reduced-fat, low-fat, and fat-free milks are often fortified with vitamin A. Margarine is also usually fortified so as to provide the same amount of vitamin A as butter. Figure 8-3 shows a sampling of the richest food sources of both preformed vitamin A and beta-carotene.

FIGURE 8-2 Symptom of Beta-Carotene Excess—Discoloration of the Skin

The hand on the right shows the skin discoloration that occurs when blood levels of beta-carotene rise in response to a low-kcalorie diet that features carrots, pumpkins, and orange juice. (The hand on the left belongs to someone else and is shown here for comparison.)

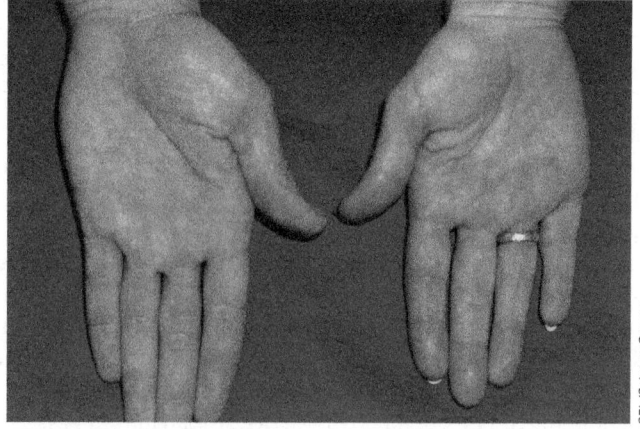

retinol activity equivalents (RAE): a measure of vitamin A activity; the amount of retinol that the body will derive from a food containing preformed retinol or its precursor beta-carotene.

FIGURE 8-3   Good Sources of Vitamin A and Beta-Carotene[a]

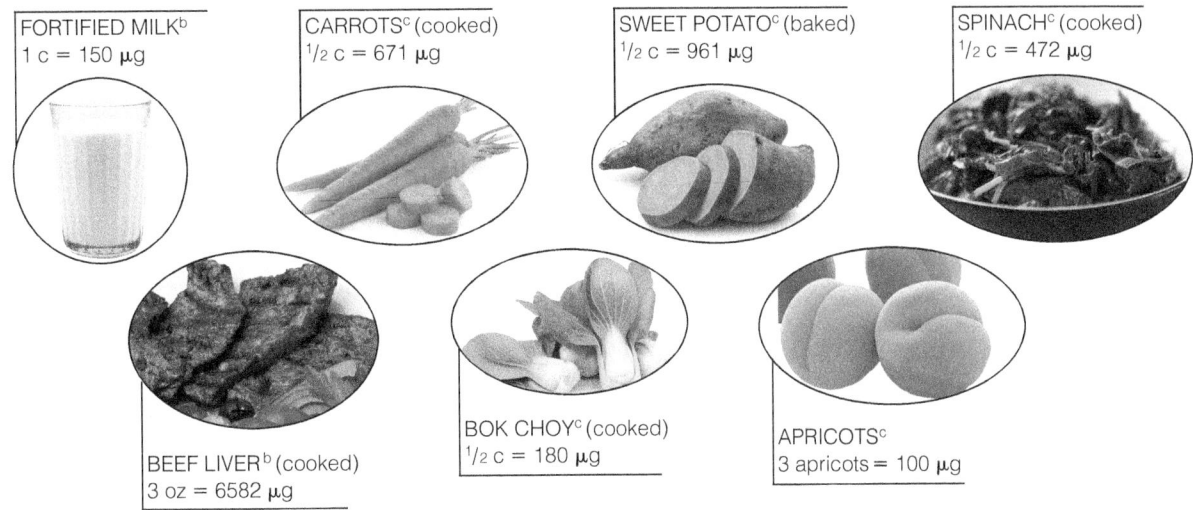

FORTIFIED MILK[b]
1 c = 150 μg

CARROTS[c] (cooked)
$1/2$ c = 671 μg

SWEET POTATO[c] (baked)
$1/2$ c = 961 μg

SPINACH[c] (cooked)
$1/2$ c = 472 μg

BEEF LIVER[b] (cooked)
3 oz = 6582 μg

BOK CHOY[c] (cooked)
$1/2$ c = 180 μg

APRICOTS[c]
3 apricots = 100 μg

[a]These foods provide 10 percent or more of the vitamin A Daily Value in a serving. For a 2000-kcalorie diet, the DV is 900 μg/day.
[b]This food contains preformed vitamin A.
[c]This food contains beta-carotene.

Fast-food meals often lack vitamin A. When fast-food restaurants offer salads with cheese, carrots, and other vitamin A–rich foods, the nutritional quality of their meals greatly improves.

Beta-Carotene in Foods Many foods from plants contain beta-carotene, the orange pigment responsible for the bold colors of many fruits and vegetables. Carrots, sweet potatoes, pumpkins, cantaloupe, and apricots are all rich sources, and their bright orange color enhances the eye appeal of the plate. Another colorful group, *dark* green vegetables, such as spinach, other greens, and broccoli, owe their color to both chlorophyll and beta-carotene. The orange and green pigments together impart a deep, murky green color to the vegetables. Other colorful vegetables, such as iceberg lettuce, beets, and sweet corn, can fool you into thinking they contain beta-carotene, but these foods derive their color from other pigments and are poor sources of beta-carotene. As for "white" plant foods such as rice and potatoes, they have little or none. Recommendations to eat *dark* green or *deep* orange vegetables and fruit at least every other day help people to meet their vitamin A needs.

Courtesy of Linda DeBruyne

Sunlight promotes vitamin D synthesis in the skin. Exposure to the sun should be moderate, however; excessive exposure may cause skin cancer.

Vitamin D

Vitamin D is different from all the other nutrients in that the body can synthesize it in significant quantities with the help of sunlight (see Photo 8-1). Therefore, in a sense, vitamin D is not an essential nutrient. Given enough sun, people need no vitamin D from foods.

Also known as **calciferol**, vitamin D comes in two major forms. **Vitamin D₂** derives primarily from plant foods in the diet. **Vitamin D₃** derives from animal foods in the diet and from synthesis in the skin. These two forms of vitamin D are similar and both must be activated before they become fully functional.

calciferol (kal-SIF-er-ol): vitamin D

vitamin D₂: vitamin D derived from plants in the diet; also called *ergocalciferol* (ER-go-kal-SIF-er-ol).

vitamin D₃: vitamin D derived from animals in the diet or made in the skin from 7-dehydrocholesterol, a precursor of cholesterol, with the help of sunlight; also called *cholecalciferol* (KO-lee-kal-SIF-er-ol).

Vitamin D's Metabolic Conversions The liver manufactures a vitamin D precursor, which migrates to the skin, where it is converted to a second precursor with the help of the sun's ultraviolet rays. Next, the liver and then the kidneys alter the second precursor to produce the active vitamin. Whether made from sunlight or obtained from food, vitamin D requires the same two conversions by the liver and kidneys to become active. The biological activity of the active vitamin is 500- to 1000-fold greater than that of its precursor. Diseases that affect either the liver or the kidneys may impair the transformations of precursor vitamin D to active vitamin D and therefore produce symptoms of vitamin D deficiency.

Vitamin D's Potential Roles in Health Although known as a vitamin, vitamin D is actually a hormone—a compound manufactured by one organ of the body that has effects on another. The best-known vitamin D target organs are the small intestine, the kidneys, and the bones, but scientists have discovered many other vitamin D target tissues. In many cases, vitamin D enhances or suppresses the activity of genes that regulate cell growth. Researchers are investigating an extensive list of effects on health. For example:

- In the brain and nerve cells, vitamin D may protect against cognitive decline and may have a connection with Parkinson disease.[11]
- Vitamin D in muscle cells encourages muscle strength and function in children and preserves strength in adults.[12]
- Vitamin D signals cells of the immune system to defend against infectious diseases.[13]

Vitamin D may also regulate the cells of the adipose tissue in ways that might contribute to obesity.[14] Conversely, obesity may be the *cause* of lower blood levels of vitamin D such that weight loss may help to correct an apparent deficiency.[15] Two mechanisms have been suggested to explain why lower vitamin D levels associate with overweight and obesity. First, fat-soluble vitamin D may be taken up and sequestered by adipose tissue, making it less available to the bloodstream.[16] Second, extra body tissue requires extra blood flow, so even with ample consumption, vitamin D may become diluted in the overweight person's greater blood volume.[17] More research is needed to address the relationships between vitamin D and obesity.

Research suggests that a deficit of vitamin D is also associated with an increased risk of high blood pressure; type 2 diabetes, cardiovascular diseases; some common cancers; infections such as tuberculosis; inflammatory conditions; autoimmune diseases such as type 1 diabetes, rheumatoid arthritis, macular degeneration, and multiple sclerosis; and even premature death.[18] Even so, evidence does not support taking vitamin D supplements to prevent diseases (except those caused by deficiency).[19] The well-established vitamin D roles, however, concern calcium balance and the bones during growth and throughout life, and these form the basis of the recommended intakes for vitamin D.

Vitamin D's Roles in Bone Growth Vitamin D is a member of a large, cooperative bone-making and maintenance team composed of nutrients and other compounds, including vitamins A, C, and K; the hormones parathormone (parathyroid hormone) and calcitonin; the protein collagen; and the minerals calcium, phosphorus, magnesium, and fluoride. Many of their interactions take place at the genetic level in ways that are under investigation. Vitamin D's special role in bone health is to assist in the absorption of calcium and phosphorus, thus helping to maintain blood concentrations of these minerals. The bones grow denser and stronger as they absorb and deposit these minerals. Details of calcium balance and mineral deposition appear in Chapter 9.

Vitamin D raises blood concentrations of bone minerals in three ways. When the diet is sufficient, vitamin D enhances their absorption from the GI tract. When the diet is insufficient, vitamin D provides the needed minerals from other sources: reabsorption by the kidneys and mobilization from the bones into the blood. The vitamin may work alone, as it does in the GI tract, or in combination with parathyroid hormone, as it does in the bones and kidneys.

Vitamin D Deficiency Overt signs of vitamin D deficiency are relatively rare, but vitamin D insufficiency is remarkably common. An estimated 16 percent of the U.S. population has low blood levels of vitamin D.[20] Factors that contribute to vitamin D deficiency include dark skin, breastfeeding without supplementation, lack of sunlight, and not using fortified milk.

Worldwide, the prevalence of the vitamin D–deficiency disease **rickets** is extremely high, affecting more than half of the children in some countries. In the United States, rickets is uncommon, but not unknown. To prevent rickets and support optimal bone health, the DRI committee recommends that all infants, children, and adolescents consume the recommended 15 micrograms of vitamin D each day. In rickets, the bones fail to calcify normally, causing growth retardation and skeletal abnormalities. The bones become so weak that they bend when they have to support the body's weight (see Figure 8-4). A child with rickets who is old enough to walk characteristically develops bowed legs, often the most obvious sign of the disease. Another sign is the beaded ribs that result from the poorly formed attachments of the bones to the cartilage.

Adolescents, who often abandon vitamin D–fortified milk in favor of soft drinks, may also prefer indoor pastimes such as computer games to outdoor activities during daylight hours. Such teens often lack vitamin D and so fail to develop the bone density needed to prevent bone loss in later life.

In adults, the poor mineralization of bone results in the painful bone disease **osteomalacia**. Any failure to synthesize adequate vitamin D or obtain enough from foods sets the stage for a loss of calcium from the bones, which can result in fractures secondary to **osteoporosis** (reduced bone density). Many older adults take vitamin D supplements to prevent bone fractures and falls. One recent study, however, suggests that vitamin D supplements, even in older women with low blood vitamin D concentrations, do not benefit bones or reduce the risk of falls.[21]

FIGURE 8-4 Vitamin D–Deficiency Symptoms: Bowed Legs and Beaded Ribs of Rickets

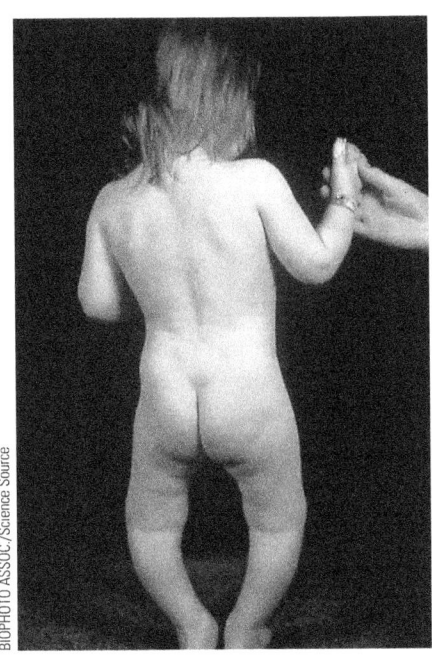

Bowed legs. In rickets, the poorly formed long bones of the legs bend outward as weight-bearing activities such as walking begin.

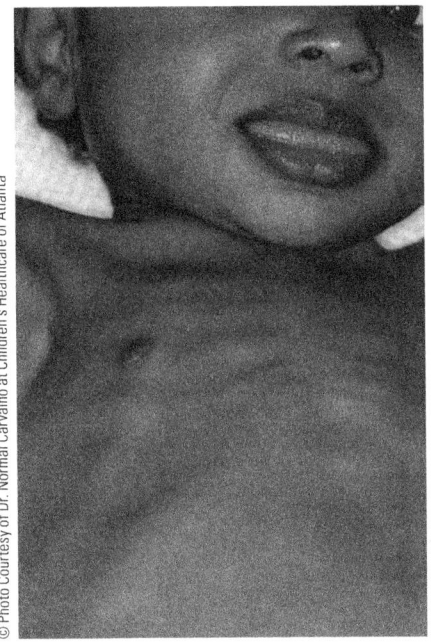

Beaded ribs. In rickets, a series of "beads" develop where the cartilages and bones attach.

rickets: the vitamin D–deficiency disease in children.

osteomalacia (os-tee-oh-mal-AY-shuh): a bone disease characterized by softening of the bones. Symptoms include bending of the spine and bowing of the legs. The disease occurs most often in adults with renal failure or malabsorption disorders.

osteo = bone
mal = bad (soft)

osteoporosis (os-tee-oh-pore-OH-sis): literally, porous bones; reduced density of the bones, also known as *adult bone loss*.

Vitamin D Toxicity Vitamin D clearly illustrates how optimal amounts of nutrients support health, but both inadequacies and excesses cause harm. Vitamin D is among the vitamins most likely to have toxic effects when consumed in excess. Excess vitamin D raises the concentration of blood calcium. Excess blood calcium tends to precipitate in the soft tissues and form stones, especially in the kidneys, where calcium is concentrated in an effort to excrete it. Calcification may also harden the blood vessels and is especially dangerous in the major arteries of the brain, heart, and lungs, where it can cause death.

The amounts of vitamin D made by the skin and found in foods are well within safe limits, but supplements containing the vitamin in concentrated form should be kept out of the reach of children and used cautiously, if at all, by adults. The DRI committee has set a Tolerable Upper Intake Level for vitamin D at 50 micrograms per day (2000 IU on supplement labels).

Vitamin D from the Sun Most of the world's population relies on natural exposure to sunlight to maintain adequate vitamin D nutrition. The sun imposes no risk of vitamin D toxicity. Prolonged exposure to sunlight degrades the vitamin D precursor in the skin, preventing its conversion to the active vitamin.

Prolonged exposure to sunlight has other undesirable consequences, however, such as premature wrinkling of the skin and skin cancers. Sunscreens help reduce the risks of these outcomes, but sunscreens with sun protection factors (SPF) of 8 and above also retard vitamin D synthesis. Still, even with an SPF 15–30 sunscreen, sufficient vitamin D synthesis can be obtained in 10 to 20 minutes of sun exposure. A strategy to avoid this dilemma is to apply sunscreen after enough time has elapsed to provide sufficient vitamin D. For most people, exposing hands, face, and arms on a clear summer day for 5 to 10 minutes, a few times a week, should be sufficient to maintain vitamin D nutrition. Dark-skinned people require longer exposure than light-skinned people, but by three hours, vitamin D synthesis in heavily pigmented skin arrives at the same plateau as in fair skin after 30 minutes.

Latitude, season, and time of day also have dramatic effects on vitamin D synthesis and status. Heavy cloud cover, smoke, or smog block the ultraviolet (UV) rays of the sun that promote vitamin D synthesis. Differences in skin pigmentation, latitude, and smog may account for the finding that African-American people, especially those in northern, smoggy cities, are most likely to be vitamin D deficient and develop rickets. Vitamin D deficiency is especially prevalent in the winter and in the Arctic and Antarctic regions of the world. To ensure an adequate vitamin D status, supplements may be needed. The body's vitamin D supplies from summer synthesis alone are insufficient to meet winter needs.

The ultraviolet rays from tanning lamps and tanning booths may also stimulate vitamin D synthesis, but the hazards outweigh any possible benefits. The Food and Drug Administration (FDA) warns that, if the lamps are not properly filtered, people using tanning booths risk burns, damage to the eyes and blood vessels, and skin cancer.

Vitamin D in Foods Only a few animal foods—notably, eggs, liver, butter, some fatty fish, and fortified milk—supply significant amounts of vitamin D. For those who use margarine in place of butter, fortified margarine is a significant source. Infant formulas are fortified with vitamin D in amounts adequate for daily intake as long as infants consume at least one liter (1000 milliliters) or one quart (32 ounces) of formula. Breast milk is low in vitamin D, so vitamin D supplements (10 micrograms daily) are recommended for infants who are breastfed exclusively and for those who do not receive at least 1000 milliliters of vitamin D–fortified formula per day. These sources, plus any exposure to the sun, provide infants with more than enough of this vitamin.

The fortification of milk with vitamin D is the best guarantee that children will meet their vitamin D needs and underscores the importance of milk in children's diets. Unlike milk, cheese and yogurt are not fortified with vitamin D. Vegans, and especially their children, may have low vitamin D intakes because few fortified plant sources exist. Exceptions include margarine and some soy milks. In the United States, breakfast cereals may be fortified with vitamin D, as their labels indicate.

Vitamin D Recommendations In setting the dietary recommendations, the DRI committee assumed that no vitamin D was available from skin synthesis. Advancing age increases the risk of vitamin D deficiency, so intake recommendations increase with age (see the inside front cover).

Vitamin E

Almost a century ago, researchers discovered a compound in vegetable oils necessary for reproduction in rats. The compound was named **tocopherol**, which means "offspring." Eventually, the compound was named vitamin E. When chemists isolated four tocopherol compounds, they designated them by the first four letters of the Greek alphabet: alpha, beta, gamma, and delta. Of these, alpha-tocopherol is the gold standard for vitamin E activity; recommended intakes are based on it. Four additional forms of vitamin E have also been identified and are of interest to researchers for potential roles in health.*[22] Table 8-4 later in the chapter summarizes important information about vitamin E.

Vitamin E as an Antioxidant Like beta-carotene, vitamin E is a fat-soluble antioxidant. It protects other substances from oxidation by being oxidized itself. If there is plenty of vitamin E in the membranes of cells exposed to an oxidant, chances are this vitamin will take the brunt of any oxidative attack, protecting the lipids and other vulnerable components of the membranes. Vitamin E is especially effective in preventing the oxidation of the polyunsaturated fatty acids (PUFA), but it protects all other lipids (for example, vitamin A) as well.

Vitamin E exerts an especially important antioxidant effect in the lungs, where the cells are exposed to high concentrations of oxygen. Vitamin E also protects the lungs from air pollutants that are strong oxidants.

Vitamin E may also offer protection against heart disease by protecting low-density lipoproteins (LDL) from oxidation and reducing inflammation.[23] The oxidation of LDL encourages the development of atherosclerosis; thus, in theory, halting LDL oxidation should reduce atherosclerosis. The results of controlled clinical studies in which human beings were given vitamin E supplements, however, have been disappointing. Several leading vitamin E researchers point out that clinical trials of vitamin E supplementation differ in many important ways, such as the selection of subjects, the source of the vitamin, the dose of the vitamin, and the outcomes studied. Such differences may partly explain the inconsistent findings. Further research that addresses such issues may clarify the relationship between vitamin E and heart disease. In the meantime, the American Heart Association supports the consumption of antioxidant-rich fruit and vegetables, as well as whole grains and nuts, to reduce the risk of heart disease.[24]

Vitamin E Deficiency When blood concentrations of vitamin E fall below a certain critical level, the red blood cells tend to break open and spill their contents, probably because the PUFA in their membranes oxidize. This classic vitamin E–deficiency symptom, known as **erythrocyte hemolysis**, is seen in premature infants born before the transfer of vitamin E from the mother to the fetus that takes place in the last weeks of pregnancy. Vitamin E treatment corrects **hemolytic anemia**.

The few symptoms of vitamin E deficiency that have been observed in adults include loss of muscle coordination and reflexes with impaired movement, vision, and speech. Vitamin E treatment corrects all of these symptoms.

In adults, vitamin E deficiency is usually associated with diseases, notably those that cause malabsorption of fat. These include diseases of the liver, gallbladder, and pancreas, as well as various hereditary diseases involving digestion and use of nutrients. (See Chapters 17, 18, and 19.) On rare occasions, vitamin E deficiencies develop in people without diseases. Most likely, such deficiencies occur after years of eating diets extremely low in fat; using fat substitutes, such as diet margarines and salad dressings,

tocopherol (tuh-KOFF-er-ol): a general term for several chemically related compounds, one of which has vitamin E activity.

erythrocyte (er-REETH-ro-cite) **hemolysis** (he-MOLL-uh-sis): rupture of the red blood cells, caused by vitamin E deficiency.

erythro = red
cyte = cell
hemo = blood
lysis = breaking

hemolytic (HE-moh-LIT-ick) **anemia:** the condition of having too few red blood cells as a result of erythrocyte hemolysis.

---

*The other forms of vitamin E are tocotrienols: alpha, beta, gamma, and delta.

FIGURE 8-5 Good Sources of Vitamin E

Vegetable oils, some nuts and seeds such as almonds and sunflower seeds, and wheat germ are rich in vitamin E.

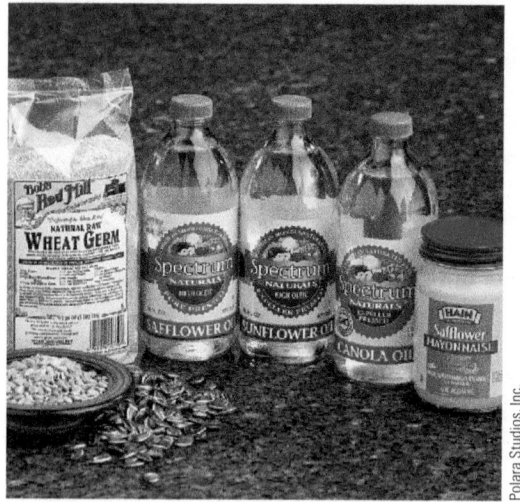

Polara Studios, Inc.

as the only sources of fat; or consuming diets composed of highly processed or convenience foods. Extensive heating in the processing of foods destroys vitamin E.

Vitamin E Toxicity Vitamin E in foods is safe to consume. Reports of vitamin E toxicity symptoms are rare across a broad range of intakes. Vitamin E supplement use has increased in recent years, however, as its antioxidant action against disease has been recognized. As a result, signs of toxicity are now known or suspected, although vitamin E toxicity is not nearly as common, and its effects are not as serious, as vitamin A or vitamin D toxicity. Extremely high doses of vitamin E interfere with the blood-clotting action of vitamin K and enhance the action of anticoagulant medications, leading to hemorrhage. The UL (1000 milligrams) for vitamin E is more than 65 times greater than the recommended intake for adults (15 milligrams).

Vitamin E in Foods Vitamin E is widespread in foods. Much of the vitamin E in the diet comes from vegetable oils and the products made from them, such as margarine, salad dressings, and shortenings (Figure 8-5). Wheat germ oil is especially rich in vitamin E. Other sources of the vitamin include whole grains, fruit, vegetables, and nuts. Because vitamin E is readily destroyed by heat processing and oxidation, fresh foods are the best sources of this vitamin.

FIGURE 8-6 Blood-Clotting Process

When blood is exposed to air, to foreign substances, or to secretions from injured tissues, platelets (small, cell-like structures in the blood) release a phospholipid known as thromboplastin. Thromboplastin catalyzes the conversion of the inactive protein prothrombin to the active enzyme thrombin. Thrombin then catalyzes the conversion of the precursor protein fibrinogen to the active protein fibrin that forms the clot.

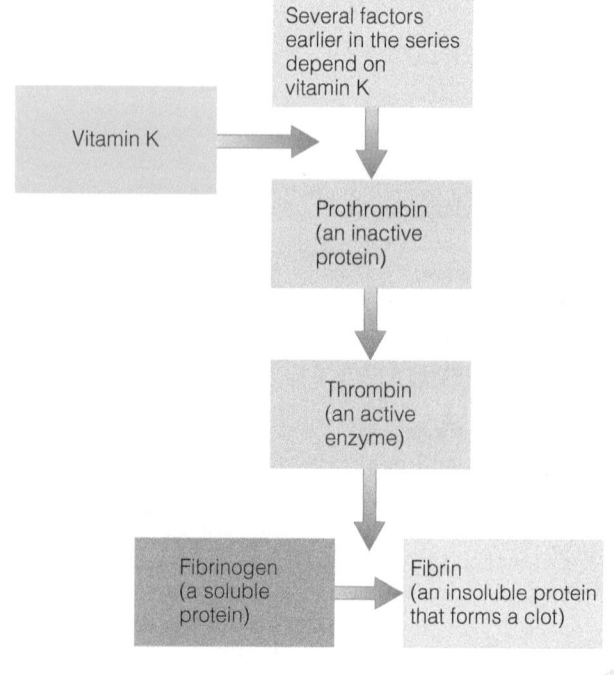

Vitamin K

Several factors earlier in the series depend on vitamin K

Prothrombin (an inactive protein)

Thrombin (an active enzyme)

Fibrinogen (a soluble protein)

Fibrin (an insoluble protein that forms a clot)

Vitamin K

Vitamin K has long been known for its role in blood clotting, where its presence can make the difference between life and death. Vitamin K appropriately gets its name from the Danish word *koagulation* (coagulation, or "clotting"). The vitamin also participates in the synthesis of several bone proteins. Without vitamin K, the bones produce an abnormal protein that cannot effectively bind to the minerals that normally form bones. An adequate intake of vitamin K helps to decrease bone turnover and protect against fractures.[25] Vitamin K supplements seem ineffective against bone loss, however, and more research is needed to clarify the links between vitamin K and bone health.[26]

Blood Clotting At least 13 different proteins and the mineral calcium are involved in making blood clots. Vitamin K is essential for the activation of several of these proteins, among them prothrombin, the precursor of the enzyme thrombin (see Figure 8-6). When any of the blood-clotting factors is lacking, **hemorrhagic disease** results. If an artery or vein is cut or broken, bleeding goes unchecked. Note, though, that hemorrhaging is not always caused by a vitamin K deficiency.

Intestinal Synthesis Like vitamin D, vitamin K can be obtained from a nonfood source. Bacteria in the intestinal tract synthesize vitamin K that the body can absorb, but people cannot depend on this source alone for their vitamin K.

Vitamin K Deficiency Vitamin K deficiency is rare, but it may occur in two circumstances. First, it may arise in conditions of fat malabsorption. Second, some medications interfere with vitamin K's synthesis and action in the body: antibiotics kill the vitamin K–producing bacteria in the intestine, and anticoagulant medications interfere with vitamin K metabolism and activity. When vitamin K deficiency does occur, it can be fatal.

Vitamin K for Newborns Newborn infants present a unique case of vitamin K nutrition. An infant is born with a **sterile** digestive tract, and some weeks pass before the vitamin K–producing bacteria become fully established in the infant's intestines. At the same time, plasma prothrombin concentrations are low (this helps prevent blood clotting during the stress of birth, which might otherwise be fatal). A single dose of vitamin K, usually in a water-soluble form, is given at birth to prevent hemorrhagic disease in the newborn.[27]

Vitamin K Toxicity Vitamin K toxicity is rare, and no adverse effects have been reported with high intakes. Therefore, a Tolerable Upper Intake Level has not been established. High doses of vitamin K can reduce the effectiveness of anticoagulant medications used to prevent blood clotting. People taking these medications should eat vitamin K–rich foods in moderation and keep their intakes consistent from day to day.

Vitamin K in Foods Many foods contain ample amounts of vitamin K, notably, green leafy vegetables, members of the cabbage family, and some vegetable oils (Figure 8-7). Other vegetables such as iceberg lettuce and green beans provide smaller amounts.

Table 8-4 offers a complete summary of the fat-soluble vitamins.

FIGURE 8-7 Good Sources of Vitamin K

Notable food sources of vitamin K include green vegetables such as collards, spinach, Bibb lettuce, brussels sprouts, and cabbage and vegetable oils such as soybean oil and canola oil.

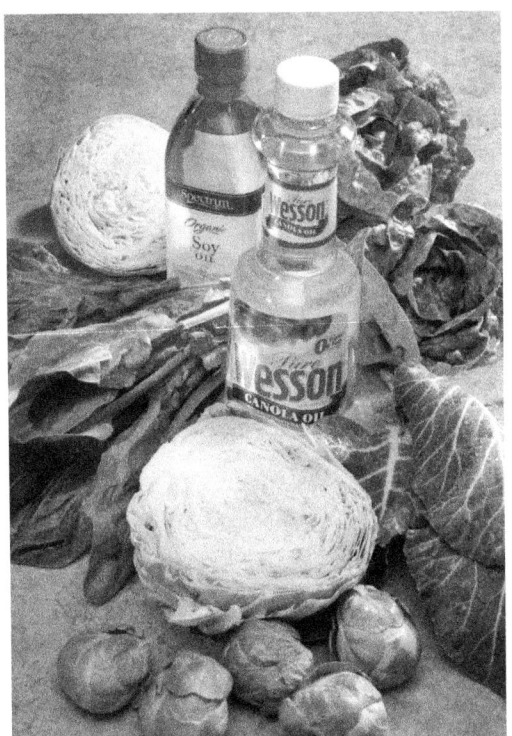

Matthew Farruggio Photography

Review Notes

- The fat-soluble vitamins are vitamins A, D, E, and K.
- Vitamin A is essential to gene expression, vision, cell differentiation and integrity of epithelial tissues, immunity, and reproduction and growth.
- Vitamin A deficiency can cause blindness, sickness, and death and is a major problem worldwide.
- Overdoses of vitamin A are possible and dangerous.
- Vitamin D raises calcium and phosphorus levels in the blood. A deficiency can cause rickets in children or osteomalacia in adults.
- Vitamin D is the most toxic of all the vitamins.
- People exposed to the sun make vitamin D in their skin; fortified milk is an important food source.
- Vitamin E acts as an antioxidant in cell membranes and is especially important in the lungs, where cells are exposed to high concentrations of oxygen.
- Vitamin E may protect against heart disease, but the evidence is not conclusive yet.
- Vitamin E deficiency is rare in healthy human beings. The vitamin is widely distributed in plant foods.
- Vitamin K is necessary for blood to clot and for bone health.
- The bacterial inhabitants of the digestive tract produce vitamin K, but people need vitamin K from foods as well.
- Dark green, leafy vegetables are good sources of vitamin K.

hemorrhagic (hem-oh-RAJ-ik) **disease:** the vitamin K–deficiency disease in which blood fails to clot.

sterile: free of microorganisms such as bacteria.

TABLE 8-4 The Fat-Soluble Vitamins: A Summary

VITAMIN NAME	CHIEF FUNCTIONS	DEFICIENCY SYMPTOMS	TOXICITY SYMPTOMS	SIGNIFICANT SOURCES
Vitamin A (Retinol, retinal, retinoic acid; main precursor is beta-carotene)	Vision, maintenance of cornea, epithelial cells, mucous membranes, skin; bone and tooth growth; reproduction; regulation of gene expression; immunity	Infectious diseases, night blindness, blindness (xerophthalmia), keratinization	*Chronic:* reduced bone mineral density, liver abnormalities, birth defects *Acute (single large dose or short term):* blurred vision, nausea, vomiting, vertigo; increase of pressure inside skull; headache; muscle incoordination	*Retinol:* milk and milk products; eggs; liver *Beta-carotene:* spinach and other dark, leafy greens; broccoli; deep orange fruit (apricots, cantaloupe) and vegetables (carrots, winter squashes, sweet potatoes, pumpkin)
Vitamin D (Calciferol, cholecalciferol, dihydroxy vitamin D; precursor is cholesterol)	Mineralization of bones (raises blood calcium and phosphorus by increasing absorption from digestive tract, withdrawing calcium from bones, stimulating retention by kidneys)	Rickets, osteomalacia	Calcium imbalance (calcification of soft tissues and formation of stones)	Synthesized in the body with the help of sunshine; fortified milk, margarine, butter, and cereals; eggs; liver; fatty fish (salmon, sardines)
Vitamin E (Alpha-tocopherol, tocopherol)	Antioxidant (stabilization of cell membranes, regulation of oxidation reactions, protection of polyunsaturated fatty acids [PUFA] and vitamin A)	Erythrocyte hemolysis, nerve damage	Hemorrhagic effects	Polyunsaturated plant oils (margarine, salad dressings, shortenings), green and leafy vegetables, wheat germ, whole-grain products, nuts, seeds
Vitamin K (Phylloquinone, menaquinone, naphthoquinone)	Synthesis of blood-clotting proteins and bone proteins	Hemorrhage	None known	Synthesized in the body by GI bacteria; green, leafy vegetables; cabbage-type vegetables; vegetable oils

8.3 The Water-Soluble Vitamins

The B vitamins and vitamin C are the water-soluble vitamins. These vitamins, found in the watery compartments of foods, are distributed into water-filled compartments of the body. They are easily absorbed into the bloodstream and are just as easily excreted if their blood concentrations rise too high. Thus, the water-soluble vitamins are less likely to reach toxic concentrations in the body than are the fat-soluble vitamins. Foods never deliver excessive amounts of the water-soluble vitamins, but the large doses concentrated in vitamin supplements can reach toxic levels.

The B Vitamins

Despite advertisements that claim otherwise, the B vitamins do not give people energy. Carbohydrate, fat, and protein—the *energy-yielding* nutrients—are used for fuel. The B vitamins *help* the body use that fuel but do not serve as fuel themselves.

coenzyme (co-EN-zime): a small molecule that works with an enzyme to promote the enzyme's activity. Many coenzymes contain B vitamins as part of their structure.

co = with

Coenzymes The eight B vitamins were listed in Table 8-1. Each is part of an enzyme helper known as a **coenzyme**. Some B vitamins have other important functions in the body as well, but the roles these vitamins play as parts of coenzymes are the best understood. A coenzyme is a small molecule that combines with an enzyme to make it active. With the coenzyme in place, a substance is attracted to the enzyme, and the reaction proceeds instantaneously. Figure 8-8 illustrates coenzyme action.

Active forms of five of the B vitamins—thiamin, riboflavin, niacin, pantothenic acid, and biotin—participate in the release of energy from carbohydrate, fat, and protein. A coenzyme containing vitamin B_6 assists enzymes that metabolize amino acids. Folate and vitamin B_{12} help cells to multiply. Among these cells are the red blood cells and the cells lining the GI tract—cells that deliver energy to all the others.

The eight B vitamins play many specific roles in helping the enzymes to perform thousands of different molecular conversions in the body. They must be present in every cell continuously for the cells to function as they should. As for vitamin C, its primary role, discussed later, is as an antioxidant.

B Vitamin Deficiencies In academic and clinical discussions of the vitamins, different sets of deficiency symptoms are ascribed to each individual vitamin. Such clear-cut symptoms, however, are found only in laboratory animals that have been fed contrived diets that lack just one nutrient. In reality, a deficiency of any single B vitamin seldom shows up in isolation because people do not eat nutrients one by one; they eat foods containing mixtures of many nutrients. If a major class of foods is missing from the diet, all of the nutrients delivered by those foods will be lacking to various extents.

In only two cases have dietary deficiencies associated with single B vitamins been observed on a large scale in human populations. Diseases have been named for these deficiency states. One of them, **beriberi**, was first observed in Southeast Asia when the custom of polishing rice became widespread. Rice contributed 80 percent of the energy intake of the people in these areas, and rice bran was their principal source of thiamin. When the bran was removed to make the rice whiter, beriberi spread like wildfire.

The niacin-deficiency disease, **pellagra**, became widespread in the southern United States in the early part of the 20th century among people who subsisted on a low-protein diet with corn as a staple grain. This diet was unusual in that it supplied neither enough niacin nor enough tryptophan, its amino acid precursor, to make the niacin intake adequate.

Even in the cases of beriberi and pellagra, the deficiencies were probably not pure. When foods were provided containing the one vitamin known to be needed, other vitamins that may have been in short supply came as part of the package.

Major deficiency diseases such as pellagra and beriberi seldom occur in the United States and Canada, but more subtle deficiencies of nutrients, including the B vitamins, are sometimes observed. When they do occur, it is usually in people whose food choices are poor because of poverty, ignorance, illness, or poor health habits such as alcohol abuse.

Interdependent Systems Table 8-5, at the end of this chapter, sums up a few of the better-established facts about B vitamin deficiencies. A look at the table will make another generalization possible. Different body systems depend on these vitamins to different extents. Processes in nerves and in their responding tissues, the muscles, depend heavily on glucose metabolism and hence on thiamin, so paralysis sets in when this vitamin is lacking. But thiamin is important in all cells, not just in nerves and muscles. Similarly, because the red blood cells and GI tract cells divide the most rapidly, two of the first symptoms of a deficiency of folate are a type of anemia and GI tract deterioration—but again, all systems depend on folate, not just these. The list of symptoms in Table 8-5, later in the chapter, is far from complete.

FIGURE 8-8   Coenzyme Action

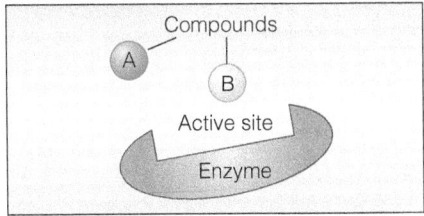

Without the coenzyme, compounds A and B do not respond to the enzyme.

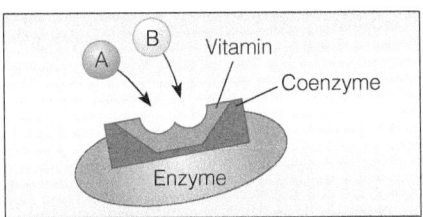

With the coenzyme in place, compounds A and B are attracted to the active site on the enzyme, and they react.

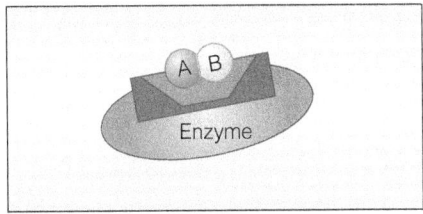

The reaction is completed with the formation of a new product. In this case the product is AB.

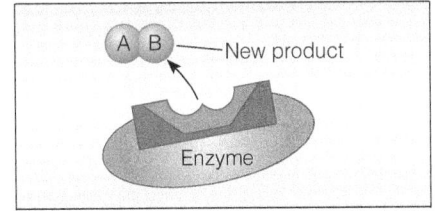

The product AB is released.

beriberi: the thiamin-deficiency disease; characterized by loss of sensation in the hands and feet, muscular weakness, advancing paralysis, and abnormal heart action.

pellagra (pell-AY-gra): the niacin-deficiency disease. Symptoms include the "4 Ds": diarrhea, dermatitis, dementia, and, ultimately, death.

pellis = skin
agra = seizure

B Vitamin Enrichment of Foods If the staple food of a region is made from **refined grain**, vitamin B deficiencies are especially likely. One way to protect people from deficiencies is to add nutrients to their staple food, a process known as **fortification** or **enrichment**. The enrichment of refined breads and cereals has drastically reduced the incidence of iron and B vitamin deficiencies.

The preceding discussion has shown both the great importance of the B vitamins in promoting normal, healthy functioning of all body systems and the severe consequences of deficiency. Now you may want to know how to be sure you and your clients are getting enough of these vital nutrients. The next sections present information on each B vitamin. While reading further, keep in mind that *foods* can provide all the needed nutrients and that supplements are a poor second choice. Some supplements are absurdly costly, but even if they are inexpensive, most people don't need them. Nutrition in Practice 9 discusses uses and choices of supplements in more detail.

Thiamin

All cells use thiamin, which plays a critical role in their energy metabolism. Thiamin also occupies a special site on nerve cell membranes. Consequently, as mentioned earlier, thiamin is critical to the normal functioning of the nerves and muscles.

Thiamin Deficiency and Toxicity People who fail to eat enough food to meet energy needs risk nutrient deficiencies, including thiamin deficiency. Inadequate thiamin intakes have been reported among the nation's malnourished and homeless people. Similarly, people risk thiamin deficiency when they derive most of their energy from empty-kcalorie foods and beverages. Alcohol is a good example. It contributes energy but provides few, if any, nutrients and often displaces food. In addition, alcohol impairs thiamin absorption and enhances thiamin excretion in the urine, doubling the risk of deficiency. Many alcoholics are thiamin deficient; some develop **Wernicke-Korsakoff syndrome**. No adverse effects have been associated with excesses of thiamin, and no UL has been determined.

FIGURE 8-9 Good Sources of Thiamin

Nutritious foods such as pork, legumes, sunflower seeds, and enriched and whole-grain breads are valuable sources of thiamin.

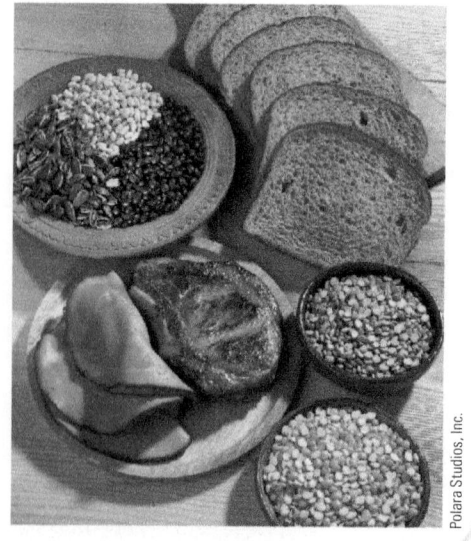

Polara Studios, Inc.

Thiamin in Foods Thiamin occurs in small quantities in virtually all nutritious foods, but it is concentrated in only a few foods, of which pork is the most commonly eaten (Figure 8-9). Generally, thiamin needs will be met if a person keeps empty-kcalorie foods to a minimum and eats enough nutritious foods to meet energy needs. Foods chosen from the bread and cereal group should be either whole grain or enriched. Thiamin is not stored in the body to any great extent, so daily intake is important.

Riboflavin

Like thiamin, riboflavin serves as a coenzyme in many reactions, most notably in energy metabolism. Women who are carrying more than one fetus or breastfeeding more than one infant may have increased needs for riboflavin. Individuals who are extremely physically active may also have increased riboflavin needs.

Riboflavin Deficiency and Toxicity When thiamin is deficient, riboflavin may be lacking too, but its deficiency symptoms, such as cracks at the corners of the mouth and sore throat, may go undetected because those of thiamin are more severe. A diet that remedies riboflavin deficiency invariably contains some thiamin and so clears up both deficiencies. Excesses of riboflavin appear to cause no harm, and no UL has been established.

Riboflavin in Foods Unlike thiamin, riboflavin is not evenly distributed among the food groups. The major contributors of riboflavin to people's diets are milk and milk products, followed by enriched breads, cereals, and other grain products (Figure 8-10). Green vegetables (broccoli, turnip greens, asparagus, and spinach) and meats are also contributors. The riboflavin richness of milk and milk products is a good reason to include these foods in every day's meals. No other commonly eaten food can make such a substantial contribution. People who omit milk and milk products from their diets can substitute generous servings of dark green, leafy vegetables. Among the meats, liver and heart are the richest sources, but all lean meats, as well as eggs, offer some riboflavin.

Effects of Light Riboflavin is light sensitive; the ultraviolet rays of the sun or of fluorescent lamps can destroy it, as can irradiation. For this reason, milk is often sold in cardboard or opaque plastic containers to protect the riboflavin in the milk from light. In contrast, riboflavin is heat stable, so ordinary cooking does not destroy it.

Niacin

Like thiamin and riboflavin, niacin participates in the energy metabolism of every body cell. Niacin is unique among the B vitamins in that the body can make it from protein. The amino acid tryptophan can be converted to niacin in the body: 60 milligrams of tryptophan yield 1 milligram of niacin. Recommended intakes are therefore stated in **niacin equivalents (NE)**. A food containing 1 mg of niacin and 60 mg of tryptophan contains the niacin equivalent of 2 mg, or 2 mg NE.

Niacin Deficiency and Toxicity The niacin deficiency disease pellagra, discussed earlier, is still common in parts of Africa and Asia. In the United States, the disease occurs among poorly nourished people living in urban slums and particularly among those with alcohol addiction.[28]

When a normal dose of a nutrient (levels commonly found in foods) provides a normal blood concentration, the nutrient is having a *physiological* effect. When a large dose (levels commonly available only from supplements) overwhelms the body and raises blood concentrations to abnormally high levels, the nutrient is acting like a drug and having a *pharmacological* effect.

Naturally occurring niacin from foods has a physiological effect that causes no harm. Certain forms of niacin supplements taken in doses three to four times the dietary recommendation or larger, however, produce pharmacological effects, most notably, "niacin flush." Niacin flush dilates the capillaries of the skin and causes a perceptible tingling that, if intense, can be painful. The Tolerable Upper Intake Level (35 milligrams NE) is based on flushing as the critical adverse effect.

Niacin in Foods Meat, poultry, fish, legumes, and enriched and whole grains contribute about half the niacin equivalents most people consume (Figure 8-11). Among the vegetables, mushrooms, asparagus, and potatoes are the richest niacin sources. Niacin is less vulnerable to losses during food preparation and storage than other water-soluble vitamins. Being fairly heat resistant, niacin can withstand reasonable cooking times, but like other water-soluble vitamins, it will leach into cooking water.

FIGURE 8-10 Good Sources of Riboflavin

Milk and milk products supply much (about 50 percent) of the riboflavin in people's diets, but meats, eggs, green vegetables, and enriched and whole-grain breads and cereals are good sources, too.

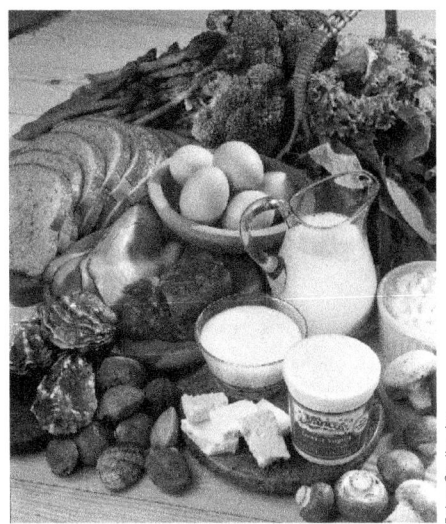

Polara Studios, Inc.

FIGURE 8-11 Good Sources of Niacin

Niacin-rich foods include meat, fish, poultry, and peanut butter, as well as enriched breads and cereals and a few vegetables.

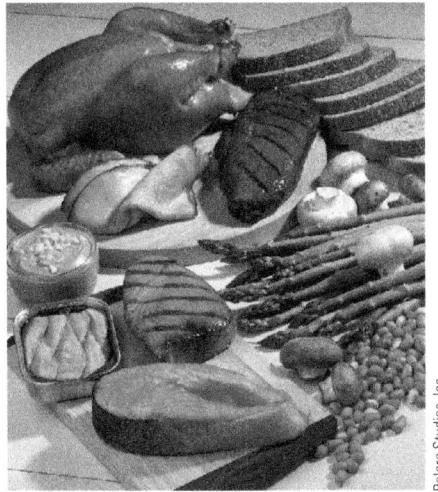

Polara Studios, Inc.

niacin equivalents (NE): the amount of niacin present in food, including the niacin that can theoretically be made from tryptophan, its precursor, present in the food.

Pantothenic Acid and Biotin

Two other B vitamins—pantothenic acid and biotin—are also important in energy metabolism. Pantothenic acid was first recognized as a substance that stimulates growth. It is a component of a key enzyme that makes possible the release of energy from the energy nutrients. Pantothenic acid is involved in more than 100 different steps in the synthesis of lipids, neurotransmitters, steroid hormones, and hemoglobin. Biotin plays an important role in metabolism as a coenzyme that carries carbon dioxide. Emerging evidence indicates that biotin participates in other processes such as gene expression and cell signaling and in the structure of DNA-binding proteins in the cell nucleus.[29]

Pantothenic Acid and Biotin in Foods Both pantothenic acid and biotin are more widespread in foods than the other vitamins discussed so far. There seems to be no danger that people who consume a variety of foods will suffer deficiencies. Claims that pantothenic acid and biotin are needed in pill form to prevent or cure disease conditions are at best unfounded and at worst intentionally misleading.

Biotin Deficiency Biotin deficiencies are rare but have been reported in adults fed artificially by vein without biotin supplementation. Researchers can induce biotin deficiency in animals or human beings by feeding them raw egg whites, which contain the protein avidin, which binds biotin and prevents its absorption.

Vitamin B_6

A surge of research interest in the past several decades has not only revealed new knowledge about vitamin B_6 but has also raised new questions. Most recently, research interest has centered on a possible role for vitamin B_6 in the treatment or prevention of disease.[30]

Metabolic Roles of Vitamin B_6 Vitamin B_6 has long been known to play roles in carbohydrate, fatty acid, and protein and amino acid metabolism. In the cells, vitamin B_6 helps convert one kind of amino acid, which the cells have in abundance, to other nonessential amino acids that the cells lack. It also aids in the conversion of the amino acid tryptophan to niacin and plays important roles in the synthesis of hemoglobin and neurotransmitters, the communication molecules of the brain. Vitamin B_6 also assists in releasing stored glucose from glycogen and thus contributes to the regulation of blood glucose.

Vitamin B_6 Deficiency Vitamin B_6 deficiency is expressed in general symptoms, such as weakness, depression, confusion, and irritability. Other symptoms include a greasy, flaky dermatitis; anemia; and, in advanced cases, convulsions. A shortage of vitamin B_6 may also weaken the immune response. Some evidence links low vitamin B_6 intakes with increased risk of some cancers and cardiovascular disease; more research is needed to clarify these associations.[31]

Vitamin B_6 Toxicity Years ago, it was believed that vitamin B_6, like other water-soluble vitamins, could not reach toxic concentrations in the body. Toxic effects of vitamin B_6 became known when a physician reported them in women who had been taking more than 2 *grams* of vitamin B_6 daily (20 times the current UL of 100 *milligrams*) for two months or more, attempting to cure premenstrual syndrome. The first symptom of toxicity was numb feet; then the women lost sensation in their hands; then they became unable to walk. The women recovered after they discontinued the supplements.

Vitamin B_6 Recommendations The RDA for vitamin B_6 is based on the amounts needed to maintain adequate levels of its coenzymes. Unlike other water-soluble vitamins, vitamin B_6 is stored extensively in muscle tissue. Research does not support claims that large doses of vitamin B_6 enhance muscle strength or physical endurance.

Vitamin B₆ in Foods The richest food sources of vitamin B_6 are protein-rich meat, fish, and poultry (Figure 8-12). Potatoes, a few other vegetables, and some types of fruits are good sources, too. Foods lose vitamin B_6 when heated.

Folate

The term *folate* refers to two forms of the B vitamin: the naturally occurring folates in foods and folic acid, which is the form used in dietary supplements and fortified foods. Folate is active in cell division. During periods of rapid growth and cell division, such as pregnancy and adolescence, folate needs increase, and deficiency is especially likely. When a deficiency occurs, the replacement of the rapidly dividing cells of the blood and the GI tract falters. Not surprisingly, then, two of the first symptoms of a folate deficiency are a type of anemia and GI tract deterioration (see Table 8-5 later in the chapter).

Folate, Alcohol, and Drugs Of all the vitamins, folate appears to be the most vulnerable to interactions with alcohol and other drugs. As Nutrition in Practice 20 describes, alcohol-addicted people risk folate deficiency because alcohol impairs folate's absorption and increases its excretion. Furthermore, as people's alcohol intakes rise, their folate intakes decline. Many medications, including aspirin, oral contraceptives, and anticonvulsants, also impair folate status. Smoking exerts a negative effect on folate status as well.

Folate and Neural Tube Defects Research studies confirm the importance of folate in preventing **neural tube defects (NTD)**. The brain and spinal cord develop from the neural tube, and defects in its orderly formation during the early weeks of pregnancy may result in various central nervous system disorders and death. Folate supplements taken before conception and continued throughout the first trimester of pregnancy can prevent NTD. For this reason, all women of childbearing age who are capable of becoming pregnant should consume 400 micrograms (0.4 milligrams) of folic acid daily from supplements, fortified foods, or both, *in addition* to eating folate-rich foods. Chapter 10 includes a figure of a neural tube defect and further discussion.

Folate status improves more with supplementation or fortification than with a dietary intake that meets recommendations. Neural tube defects arise early in pregnancy before most women realize they are pregnant, and most women eat too few fruits and vegetables to supply even half the folate needed to prevent NTD. For these reasons, the FDA mandated that enriched grain products (flour, cornmeal, pasta, and rice) be fortified with folic acid, which is an especially absorbable synthetic form of folate. Bread products, flour, corn grits, and pasta must be fortified with 140 μg folate per 100 g of food (about ½ c cooked food or 1 slice of bread).

Fortification has improved folate status in women of childbearing age and lowered the number of neural tube defects that occur each year.[32] Folate fortification also raises safety concerns, however. High doses of folate can complicate the diagnosis of vitamin B_{12} deficiency, as discussed later. The DRI committee set a Tolerable Upper Intake Level of 1000 micrograms per day from fortified foods or supplements. Except for individuals who take supplements with more than 400 micrograms of folic acid, few people (less than 3 percent of the U.S. population) exceed the Tolerable Upper Intake Level for folic acid. Thus, researchers conclude that the current level of fortification of the food supply appears to be safe.

Folate in Foods As Figure 8-13 shows, the best food sources of folate are liver, legumes, beets, and leafy green vegetables (the vitamin's name suggests the word

FIGURE 8-12 Good Sources of Vitamin B₆

Most protein-rich foods such as meat, fish, and poultry provide ample vitamin B₆; some vegetables and fruit are good sources, too.

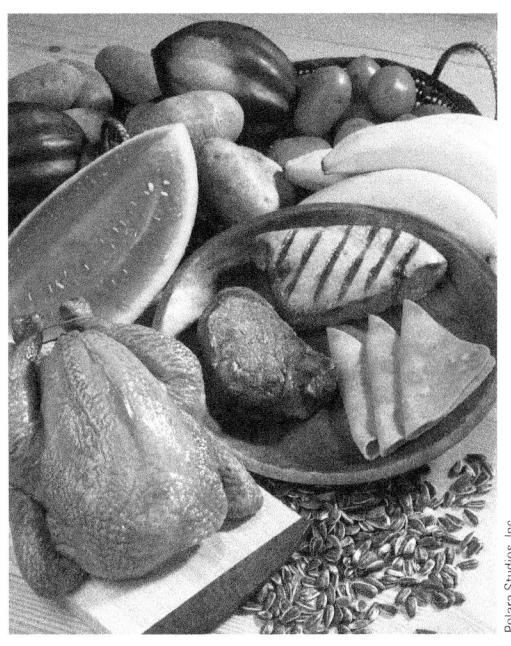

Polara Studios, Inc.

neural tube defects (NTD): malformations of the brain, spinal cord, or both that occur during embryonic development. The two main types of neural tube defects are *spina bifida* (literally, "split spine") and *anencephaly* ("no brain").

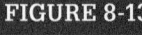

FIGURE 8-13 Good Sources of Folate[a]

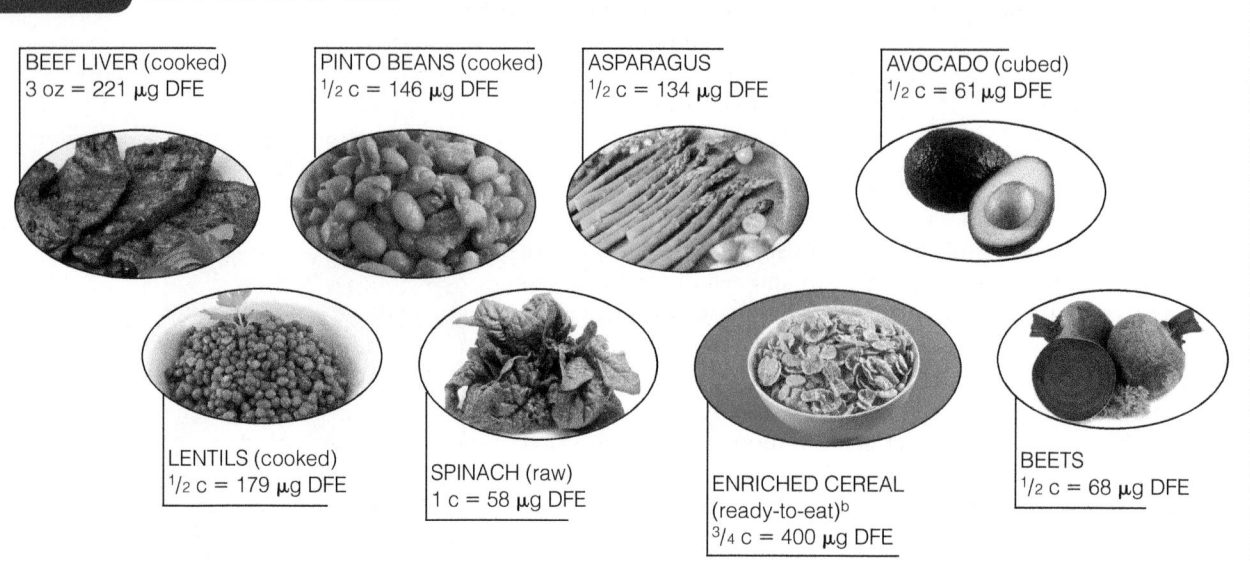

BEEF LIVER (cooked)
3 oz = 221 μg DFE

PINTO BEANS (cooked)
1/2 c = 146 μg DFE

ASPARAGUS
1/2 c = 134 μg DFE

AVOCADO (cubed)
1/2 c = 61 μg DFE

LENTILS (cooked)
1/2 c = 179 μg DFE

SPINACH (raw)
1 c = 58 μg DFE

ENRICHED CEREAL
(ready-to-eat)[b]
3/4 c = 400 μg DFE

BEETS
1/2 c = 68 μg DFE

[a]Folate recommendations are expressed in dietary folate equivalents (DFE). Note that for natural folate sources, 1 microgram equals 1 DFE; for enriched sources, 1 microgram equals 1.7 DFE. These foods provide 10 percent or more of the folate Daily Value in a serving. For a 2000-kcalorie diet, the DV is 400 micrograms DFE per day.

[b]Some highly enriched cereals may provide 400 or more micrograms DFE in a serving.

foliage). In the fruit group, oranges, orange juice, and cantaloupe are the best sources. With fortification, grain products are good sources of folate, too. Heat and oxidation during cooking and storage can destroy up to half of the folate in foods.

The difference in absorption between naturally occurring food folate and synthetic folate that enriches foods and is added to supplements must be considered when establishing folate recommendations. **Dietary folate equivalents (DFE)** convert all forms of folate into units that are equivalent to the folate in foods.

Vitamin B$_{12}$

Vitamin B$_{12}$ and folate share a special relationship: vitamin B$_{12}$ assists folate in cell division. Their roles intertwine, but each performs a specific task that the other cannot accomplish.

Vitamin B$_{12}$, Folate, and Cell Division Vitamin B$_{12}$ (in coenzyme form) stands by to accept carbon groups from folate as folate removes them from other compounds. The passing of these carbon groups from folate to vitamin B$_{12}$ regenerates the active form of folate so that it can continue its dismantling tasks. In the absence of vitamin B$_{12}$, folate is trapped in its inactive, metabolically useless form, unable to do its job. When folate is either trapped due to a vitamin B$_{12}$ deficiency or unavailable due to a deficiency of folate itself, cells that are growing most rapidly—notably, the blood cells—are the first to be affected. Thus, a deficiency of either nutrient—vitamin B$_{12}$ or folate—impairs maturation of the blood cells and produces **macrocytic anemia**. The anemia is identifiable by microscopic examination of the blood, which reveals many large, immature red blood cells. Either vitamin B$_{12}$ or folate will clear up the anemia.

Vitamin B$_{12}$ and the Nervous System Although either vitamin will reverse the anemia caused by vitamin B$_{12}$ deficiency, providing folate when vitamin B$_{12}$ is needed is disastrous to the nervous system. The reason: vitamin B$_{12}$ also helps maintain nerve fibers. A vitamin B$_{12}$ deficiency can ultimately result in devastating neurological symptoms, undetectable by a blood test. A deceptive folate "cure" of the anemia in vitamin B$_{12}$ deficiency allows the nerve deterioration to progress, leading to paralysis and permanent

dietary folate equivalents (DFE): the amount of folate available to the body from naturally occurring sources, fortified foods, and supplements, accounting for differences in bioavailability from each source.

macrocytic anemia: large-cell anemia; also known as *megaloblastic anemia.*

nerve damage. Even marginal vitamin B_{12} deficiency impairs memory and cognition.[33] This interaction between folate and vitamin B_{12} raises safety concerns about the use of folate supplements and fortification of foods. In an effort to prevent excessive folate intakes that could mask symptoms of a vitamin B_{12} deficiency, the FDA specifies the exact amounts of folic acid that can be added to enriched foods.

The way folate masks vitamin B_{12} deficiency underlines a point already made several times: It takes a skilled diagnostician to make a correct diagnosis. A person who self-diagnoses on the basis of a single observed symptom takes a serious risk.

Vitamin B_{12} Absorption Absorption of vitamin B_{12} requires **intrinsic factor**, a compound made by the stomach with instructions from the genes. With the help of the stomach's acid to liberate vitamin B_{12} from the food proteins that bind it, intrinsic factor attaches to the vitamin and the complex is absorbed into the bloodstream.

A few people have an inherited defect in the gene for intrinsic factor, which makes vitamin B_{12} absorption abnormal beginning in midadulthood. Many others lose the ability to produce enough stomach acid and intrinsic factor to allow efficient absorption of vitamin B_{12} in later life due to **atrophic gastritis**. In these cases, vitamin B_{12} must be supplied by injection to bypass the defective absorptive system. The anemia of the vitamin B_{12} deficiency caused by lack of intrinsic factor is known as **pernicious anemia**.

Vitamin B_{12} in Foods A unique characteristic of vitamin B_{12} is that it is found almost exclusively in foods derived from animals. People who eat meat are guaranteed an adequate intake, and lacto-ovo vegetarians (who consume milk, cheese, and eggs) are also protected from deficiency. It is a myth, however, that fermented soy products, such as miso (a soybean paste), or sea algae, such as spirulina, provide vitamin B_{12} in its active form. Extensive research shows that the amounts of vitamin B_{12} listed on the labels of these plant products are inaccurate and misleading because the vitamin B_{12} in these products occurs in an inactive, unavailable form. Vegans need a reliable source such as vitamin B_{12}–fortified soy milk or vitamin B_{12} supplements. Some loss of vitamin B_{12} occurs when foods are heated in microwave ovens.

Vitamin B_{12} Deficiency in Vegans Vegans are at special risk for undetected vitamin B_{12} deficiency for two reasons: First, they receive none in their diets, and second, they consume large amounts of folate in the vegetables they eat. Because the body can store many times the amount of vitamin B_{12} used each day, a deficiency may take years to develop in a new vegetarian. When a deficiency does develop, though, it may progress to a dangerous extreme because the deficiency of vitamin B_{12} may be masked by the high folate intake.

Worldwide, vitamin B_{12} deficiency among vegetarians is a growing problem.[34] A pregnant or lactating vegetarian woman who eats no foods of animal origin should be aware that her infant can develop a vitamin B_{12} deficiency, even if the mother appears healthy. Breastfed infants born to vegan mothers with low concentrations of vitamin B_{12} in their breast milk can develop severe neurological symptoms such as seizures and cognitive problems.

Choline Although not defined as a vitamin, choline is an essential nutrient that is commonly grouped with the B vitamins. The body uses choline to make the neurotransmitter acetylcholine and the phospholipid lecithin. During pregnancy, choline supports the neurological development of the fetus, and during adulthood, choline may improve cognition.[35]

Choline Recommendations The body can make choline from the amino acid methionine, but synthesis alone is insufficient to fully meet the body's needs; dietary choline is also needed. For this reason, the DRI Committee established an AI for choline.

Choline Deficiency and Toxicity Average choline intakes fall below the AI, but the impact of deficiencies are not fully understood. The UL for choline is based on its life-threatening effect in lowering blood pressure.

intrinsic factor: a substance secreted by the stomach cells that binds with vitamin B_{12} in the small intestine to aid in the absorption of vitamin B_{12}. Anemia that reflects a vitamin B_{12} deficiency caused by lack of intrinsic factor is known as *pernicious anemia*.

intrinsic = on the inside

atrophic gastritis (a-TROH-fik gas-TRY-tis): a chronic inflammation of the stomach accompanied by a diminished size and functioning of the stomach's mucous membrane and glands.

pernicious (per-NISH-us) **anemia:** a blood disorder that reflects a vitamin B_{12} deficiency caused by lack of intrinsic factor and characterized by large, immature red blood cells and damage to the nervous system (*pernicious* means "highly injurious or destructive").

Choline Food Sources Choline is found in a variety of common foods such as milk, eggs, and peanuts. Choline is also a part of lecithin, a food additive commonly used as emulsifying agent.

Non–B Vitamins

Other compounds are sometimes inappropriately called B vitamins because, like the true B vitamins, they serve as coenzymes in metabolism. Even if they were essential, however, supplements would be unnecessary because these compounds are abundant in foods.

Inositol and Carnitine Among the non–B vitamins are the compounds inositol and carnitine, which can be made by the body. Inositol is a part of cell membrane structures, and carnitine functions in cellular activities. Researchers are exploring the possibility that these substances may be essential.

Other Non–B Vitamins Other substances have also been mistaken for essential nutrients. They include para-aminobenzoic acid (PABA), bioflavonoids (vitamin P or hesperidin), and ubiquinone. Other names you may hear are "vitamin B_{15}" (a hoax) and "vitamin B_{17}" (laetrile, a fake cancer-curing drug and not a vitamin by any stretch of the imagination). There is, however, one other water-soluble vitamin of great interest and importance: vitamin C.

Vitamin C

More than 300 years ago, any man who joined the crew of a seagoing ship knew he had only half a chance of returning alive—not because he might be slain by pirates or die in a storm, but because he might contract the dread disease **scurvy**. Then, a physician with the British navy found that citrus fruit could cure the disease, and thereafter, all ships were required to carry lime juice for every sailor. (This is why British sailors are still called "limeys" today.) In the 1930s, the antiscurvy factor in citrus fruit was isolated from lemon juice and named **ascorbic acid**. Today, hundreds of millions of vitamin C pills are produced in pharmaceutical laboratories.

Metabolic Roles of Vitamin C Vitamin C's action defies a simple, tidy description. It plays many important roles in the body, and its modes of action differ in different situations.

Vitamin C's Role in Collagen Formation The best-understood action of vitamin C is its role in helping to form **collagen**, the single most important protein of connective tissue. Collagen serves as the matrix on which bone is formed, the material of scars, and an important part of the "glue" that attaches one cell to another. This latter function is especially important in the artery walls, which must expand and contract with each beat of the heart, and in the walls of the capillaries, which are thin and fragile.

Vitamin C as an Antioxidant Vitamin C is also an important antioxidant. Recall that the antioxidants beta-carotene and vitamin E protect fat-soluble substances from oxidizing agents; vitamin C protects water-soluble substances the same way. By being oxidized itself, vitamin C regenerates already-oxidized substances such as iron and copper to their original, active form. In the intestines, it protects iron from oxidation and so enhances iron absorption. In the cells and body fluids, it helps to protect other molecules, including the fat-soluble compounds vitamin A, vitamin E, and the polyunsaturated fatty acids.

Vitamin C in Amino Acid Metabolism Vitamin C is also involved in the metabolism of several amino acids. Some of these amino acids end up being used to make substances of great importance in body functioning, among them the neurotransmitter norepinephrine and the hormone thyroxine. Vitamin C also plays a role in the production of carnitine, important for transporting fatty acids within cells.

Role of Stress During stress, the adrenal glands release large quantities of vitamin C together with the stress hormones epinephrine and norepinephrine. The vitamin's

scurvy: the vitamin C–deficiency disease.

ascorbic acid: one of the two active forms of vitamin C. Many people refer to vitamin C by this name.

a = without
scorbic = having scurvy

collagen: the characteristic protein of connective tissue.

kolla = glue
gennan = produce

exact role in the stress reaction remains unclear, but physical stresses (described in a later section) raise vitamin C needs.

Vitamin C in the Prevention and Treatment of the Common Cold Vitamin C has been a popular option for the prevention and treatment of the common cold for decades, but research supporting such claims has been conflicting and controversial. Some studies find no relationship between vitamin C and the occurrence of the common cold, whereas others report modest benefits—fewer colds and shorter duration of severe symptoms, especially for those exposed to physical and environmental stresses. A review of the research on the treatment and prevention of the common cold reveals some reduction in the duration and severity of the common cold in those taking vitamin C supplements.[36] The question for consumers to consider is, " Is it enough to warrant routine supplementation?"

Vitamin C's Role in Cancer Prevention and Treatment The role of vitamin C in the prevention and treatment of cancer is still being studied.[37] Evidence to date indicates that foods containing vitamin C probably protect against cancer of the esophagus. The correlation may reflect not just an association with vitamin C but the broader benefits of a diet rich in fruit and vegetables and low in fat. It does not support the taking of vitamin C supplements to prevent or treat cancer.

Vitamin C Deficiency When intake of vitamin C is inadequate, the body's vitamin C pool dwindles, and the blood vessels show the first deficiency signs. The gums around the teeth begin to bleed easily, and capillaries under the skin break spontaneously, producing pinpoint hemorrhages. As vitamin C concentrations continue to fall, the symptoms of scurvy appear. Muscles, including the heart muscle, may degenerate. The skin becomes rough, brown, scaly, and dry. Wounds fail to heal because scar tissue will not form without collagen. Bone rebuilding falters; the ends of the long bones become softened, malformed, and painful; and fractures occur. The teeth may become loose in the jawbone and fall out. Anemia and infections are common. Sudden death is likely, perhaps because of massive bleeding into the joints and body cavities.

It takes only 10 or so milligrams of vitamin C a day to prevent scurvy, and not much more than that to cure it. Once diagnosed, scurvy is readily reversible with moderate doses, in the neighborhood of 100 milligrams per day. Such an intake is easily achieved by including vitamin C–rich foods in the diet.

Vitamin C Toxicity The easy availability of vitamin C in pill form and the publication of books recommending vitamin C to prevent everything from the common cold to life-threatening cancer have led thousands of people to take large doses of vitamin C. Not surprisingly, instances of vitamin C causing harm have surfaced. The Tolerable Upper Intake Level for vitamin C is 2000 milligrams per day.

Some of the suspected toxic effects of excess vitamin C have not been confirmed, but others have been seen often enough to warrant concern. Nausea, abdominal cramps, and diarrhea are often reported. Several instances of interference with medical regimens are known. Large amounts of vitamin C excreted in the urine obscure the results of tests used to detect diabetes. People taking anticoagulants may unwittingly counteract the effect of these medications if they also take massive doses of vitamin C. Large doses of vitamin C can also enhance iron absorption too much, resulting in iron overload (see Chapter 9).

People with sickle-cell anemia may be especially vulnerable to excessive intakes of vitamin C. Those who have a tendency toward **gout**, as well as those who have a genetic abnormality that alters the way they metabolize vitamin C, are more prone to forming kidney stones if they take large doses of vitamin C.

Recommended Intakes of Vitamin C The vitamin C RDA is 90 milligrams for men and 75 milligrams for women. These amounts are far higher than the 10 milligrams per day

gout (GOWT): a metabolic disease in which crystals of uric acid precipitate in the joints.

needed to prevent the symptoms of scurvy. In fact, they are close to the amount at which the body's pool of vitamin C is full to overflowing: about 100 milligrams per day.

Special Needs for Vitamin C As is true of all nutrients, unusual circumstances may raise vitamin C needs. Among the stresses known to do so are infections; burns; surgery; extremely high or low temperatures; toxic doses of heavy metals, such as lead, mercury, and cadmium; and the chronic use of certain medications, including aspirin, barbiturates, and oral contraceptives. Smoking, too, has adverse effects on vitamin C status. Cigarette smoke contains oxidants, which deplete this potent antioxidant. Accordingly, the vitamin C recommendation for smokers is set high, at 125 milligrams for men and 110 milligrams for women.

Safe Limits Few instances warrant the taking of more than 100 to 300 milligrams of vitamin C a day. The risks may not be great for adults who dose themselves with 1 to 2 grams a day, but those taking more than 2 grams, and especially those taking more than 3 grams per day, should be aware of the distinct possibility of harm.

Vitamin C in Foods The inclusion of intelligently selected fruit and vegetables in the daily diet guarantees a generous intake of vitamin C. Even those who wish to ingest amounts well above the RDA can easily meet their goals by eating certain foods (see Figure 8-14). Citrus fruit is rightly famous for its vitamin C contents. Certain other fruit and vegetables are also rich sources: cantaloupe, strawberries, broccoli, and brussels sprouts. No animal foods other than organ meats, such as chicken liver and kidneys, contain vitamin C. The humble potato is an important source of vitamin C in Western countries, where potatoes are eaten so frequently that they make substantial contributions overall: about 20 percent of the vitamin C in the average diet. Vitamin C in foods is easily oxidized, so store cut produce and juices in airtight containers.

Vitamin C and Iron Absorption Eating foods containing vitamin C at the same meal with foods containing iron can double or triple the absorption of iron from those foods.

FIGURE 8-14 Good Sources of Vitamin C[a]

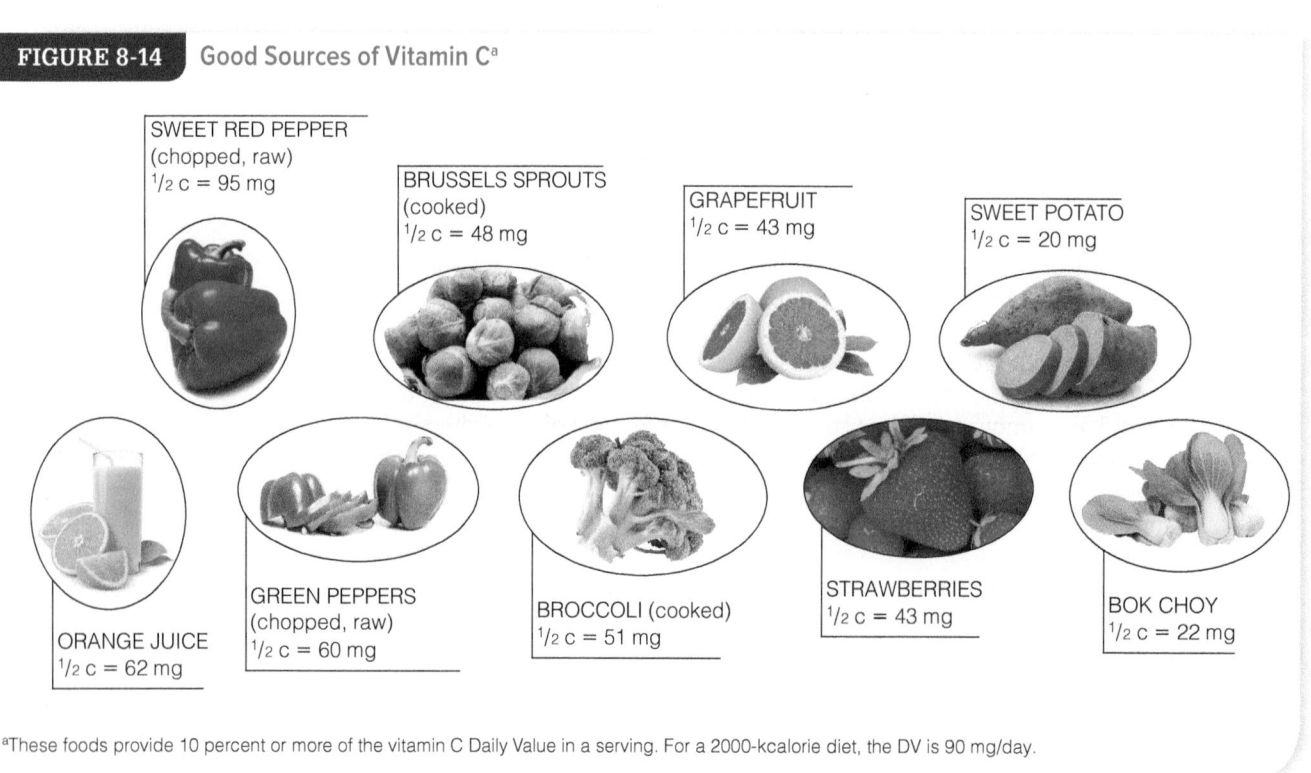

SWEET RED PEPPER (chopped, raw)
1/2 c = 95 mg

BRUSSELS SPROUTS (cooked)
1/2 c = 48 mg

GRAPEFRUIT
1/2 c = 43 mg

SWEET POTATO
1/2 c = 20 mg

ORANGE JUICE
1/2 c = 62 mg

GREEN PEPPERS (chopped, raw)
1/2 c = 60 mg

BROCCOLI (cooked)
1/2 c = 51 mg

STRAWBERRIES
1/2 c = 43 mg

BOK CHOY
1/2 c = 22 mg

[a]These foods provide 10 percent or more of the vitamin C Daily Value in a serving. For a 2000-kcalorie diet, the DV is 90 mg/day.

This strategy is highly recommended for women and children, whose energy intakes are not large enough to guarantee that they will get enough iron from the foods they eat. Iron is discussed in Chapter 9.

Table 8-5 summarizes functions, deficiency and toxicity symptoms, and food sources of the water-soluble vitamins.

TABLE 8-5 The Water-Soluble Vitamins: A Summary

VITAMIN NAME	CHIEF FUNCTIONS	DEFICIENCY SYMPTOMS	TOXICITY SYMPTOMS	SIGNIFICANT SOURCES
Thiamin (Vitamin B_1)	Part of a coenzyme used in energy metabolism	Beriberi (edema or muscle wasting), anorexia and weight loss, neurological disturbances, muscular weakness, heart enlargement and failure	None reported	Enriched, fortified, or whole-grain products; pork
Riboflavin (Vitamin B_2)	Part of coenzymes used in energy metabolism	Inflammation of the mouth, skin, and eyelids; sensitivity to light; sore throat	None reported	Milk products; enriched, fortified, or whole-grain products; liver
Niacin (Nicotinic acid, nicotinamide, niacinamide, vitamin B_3; precursor is dietary tryptophan, an amino acid)	Part of coenzymes used in energy metabolism	Pellagra (diarrhea, dermatitis, and dementia)	Niacin flush, liver damage, impaired glucose tolerance	Milk, eggs, meat, poultry, fish, whole-grain and enriched breads and cereals, nuts, and all protein-containing foods
Biotin	Part of a coenzyme used in energy metabolism	Skin rash, hair loss, neurological disturbances	None reported	Widespread in foods; GI bacteria synthesis
Pantothenic acid	Part of a coenzyme used in energy metabolism	Digestive and neurological disturbances	None reported	Widespread in foods
Vitamin B_6 (Pyridoxine, pyridoxal, pyridoxamine)	Part of coenzymes used in amino acid and fatty acid metabolism	Scaly dermatitis, depression, confusion, convulsions, anemia	Nerve degeneration, skin lesions	Meats, fish, poultry, potatoes, legumes, non-citrus fruit, fortified cereals, liver, soy products
Folate (Folic acid, folacin, pteroylglutamic acid)	Activates vitamin B_{12}; helps synthesize DNA for new cell growth	Anemia; smooth, red tongue; mental confusion; elevated homocysteine	Masks vitamin B_{12} deficiency	Fortified grains, leafy green vegetables, legumes, seeds, liver
Vitamin B_{12} (Cobalamin)	Activates folate; helps synthesize DNA for new cell growth; protects nerve cells	Anemia; nerve damage and paralysis	None reported	Foods derived from animals (meat, fish, poultry, shellfish, milk, cheese, eggs), fortified cereals
Vitamin C (Ascorbic acid)	Synthesis of collagen, carnitine, hormones, neurotransmitters; antioxidant	Scurvy (bleeding gums, pinpoint hemorrhages, abnormal bone growth, and joint pain)	Diarrhea, GI distress	Citrus fruit, cabbage-type vegetables, dark green vegetables (such as bell peppers and broccoli), cantaloupe, strawberries, lettuce, tomatoes, potatoes, papayas, mangoes

Review Notes

- The B vitamins and vitamin C are the water-soluble vitamins.
- Each B vitamin is part of an enzyme helper known as a coenzyme.
- As parts of coenzymes, the B vitamins assist in the release of energy from glucose, amino acids, and fats and help in many other body processes.
- Folate and vitamin B_{12} are important in cell division.
- Vitamin C's primary role is as an antioxidant.
- Historically, famous vitamin B–deficiency diseases are beriberi (thiamin) and pellagra (niacin). The vitamin C–deficiency disease is known as scurvy.

Self Check

1. Which of the following vitamins are fat soluble?
   a. Vitamins B, C, and E
   b. Vitamins B, C, D, and E
   c. Vitamins A, C, E, and K
   d. Vitamins A, D, E, and K

2. Which of the following describes fat-soluble vitamins?
   a. They include thiamin, vitamin A, and vitamin K.
   b. They cannot be stored to any great extent and so must be consumed daily.
   c. Toxic levels can be reached by consuming deep orange and dark green vegetables.
   d. They can be stored in the liver and fatty tissues and can reach toxic concentrations.

3. Night blindness and susceptibility to infection result from a deficiency of which vitamin?
   a. Niacin
   b. Vitamin C
   c. Vitamin A
   d. Vitamin B_{12}

4. Good sources of vitamin D include:
   a. eggs, fortified milk, and sunlight.
   b. citrus fruit, sweet potatoes, and spinach.
   c. leafy, green vegetables, cabbage, and liver.
   d. breast milk, polyunsaturated plant oils, and citrus fruit.

5. Which of the following describes water-soluble vitamins?
   a. They all play key roles in bone maintenance.
   b. They are frequently toxic.
   c. They are stored extensively in tissues.
   d. They are easily absorbed and excreted.

6. A coenzyme is:
   a. a fat-soluble vitamin.
   b. a molecule cells use to communicate.
   c. a connective tissue protein.
   d. a molecule that combines with an enzyme to make it active.

7. Good food sources of folate include:
   a. citrus fruit, dairy products, and eggs.
   b. liver, legumes, and leafy green vegetables.
   c. dark green vegetables, corn, and cabbage.
   d. potatoes, broccoli, and whole-wheat bread.

8. Which vitamin is present only in foods of animal origin?
   a. Riboflavin
   b. Pantothenic acid
   c. Vitamin B_{12}
   d. The inactive form of vitamin A

9. Which of the following nutrients is an antioxidant that protects water-soluble substances from oxidizing agents?
   a. Beta-carotene
   b. Thiamin
   c. Vitamin C
   d. Vitamin D

10. Eating foods containing vitamin C at the same meal can increase the absorption of which mineral?
    a. Iron
    b. Calcium
    c. Magnesium
    d. Folate

Answers: 1. d, 2. d, 3. c, 4. a, 5. d, 6. d, 7. b, 8. c, 9. c, 10. a

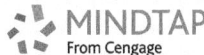

For more chapter resources visit **www.cengage.com** to access MindTap, a complete digital course.

Clinical Applications

1. How might a vitamin deficiency weaken a client's resistance to disease?

2. Pull together information from Chapter 1 about the different food groups and the significant sources of vitamins shown in the figures throughout this chapter. Consider which vitamins might be lacking in the diet of a client who reports the following:

- Dislikes leafy, green vegetables
- Never uses milk, milk products, or cheese
- Follows a very low-fat diet
- Eats a fruit or vegetable once a day

What additional information would help you pinpoint problems with vitamin intake?

Notes

1. O. Oyebode and coauthors, Fruit and vegetable consumption and all-cause, cancer, and CVD mortality: An analysis of Health Survey for England data, *Journal of Epidemiology and Community Health* 68 (2014): 856–862; C. K. Desai and coauthors, The role of vitamin supplementation in the prevention of cardiovascular disease events, *Clinical Cardiology* 37 (2014): 576–581.

2. E. Doldo and coauthors, Vitamin A, cancer treatment and prevention: The new role of cellular retinol binding proteins, *BioMed Research International* 2015, doi: 10.1155/2015/624627; C. C. Brown and R. J. Noelle, Seeing through the dark: New Insights into the immune regulatory functions of vitamin A, *European Journal of Immunology* 45 (2015): 1287–1295.

3. Doldo and coauthors, 2015; Z. Zhou and coauthors, TRIM14 is a mitochondrial adaptor that facilitates retinoic acid-inducible gene-l-like receptor-mediated innate immune response, *Proceedings of the National Academy of Sciences of the United States of America* 111 (2014): E245–E254.

4. T. A. Yorgan and coauthors, Immediate effects of retinoic acid on gene expression in primary murine osteoblasts, *Journal of Bone and Mineral Metabolism* 34 (2016): 161–170; Zhou and coauthors, 2014; D. M. Benbrook and coauthors, History of retinoic acid receptors, *Sub-cellular Biochemistry* 70 (2014): 1–20.

5. A. Janesick, S. C. Wu, and B. Blumberg, Retinoic acid signaling and neuronal differentiation, *Cellular and Molecular Life Sciences* 72 (2015): 1559–1576.

6. P. Ghezzi and coauthors, The oxidative stress theory of disease: Levels of evidence and epistemological aspects, *British Journal of Clinical Pharmacology* 174 (2017): 1784–1796; A. M. Pisoschi and A. Pop, The role of antioxidants in the chemistry of oxidative stress: A review, *European Journal of Medicinal Chemistry* 97 (2015): 55–74; F. Bonomini, L. F. Rodella, and R. Rezzani, Metabolic syndrome, aging and involvement of oxidative stress, *Aging and Disease* 6 (2015): 109–120.

7. Pisoschi and Pop, 2015; Bomomini, Rodella, Rezzani, 2015.

8. World Health Organization, Micronutrient deficiencies: Vitamin A deficiency, www.who.int/nutrition/topics/vad/en, 2017.

9. World Health Organization, Measles fact sheet, July 2017, www.who.int/mediacentre/factsheets/fs286/en/index.html.

10. E. D'Aniello and J. S. Waxman, Input overload: Contributions of retinoic acid signaling feedback mechanisms to heart development and teratogenesis, *Developmental Dynamics* 244 (2015): 513–523.

11. C. Annweiler and coauthors, Vitamin D and cognition in older adults: updated international recommendations, *Journal of Internal Medicine* 277 (2015): 45–57; L. Wang and coauthors, Vitamin D from different sources is inversely associated with Parkinson disease, *Movement Disorders* 30 (2015): 560–566; M. J. Berridge, Vitamin D: A custodian of cell signaling stability in health and disease, *Biochemical Society Transactions* 43 (2015): 349–358; L. Shen and H. F. Ji, Associations between vitamin D status, supplementation, outdoor work and risk of Parkinson's disease:

A meta-analysis assessment, *Nutrients* 7 (2015): 4817–4827; T. J. Littlejohns and coauthors, Vitamin D and the risk of dementia and Alzheimer disease, *Neurology* 83 (2014): 920–928.

12. E. K. McCarthy and M. Kiely, Vitamin D and muscle strength throughout the life course: A review of epidemiological and intervention studies, *Journal of Human Nutrition and Dietetics* 28 (2015): 636–645; M. Halfon, O. Phan, and D. Teta, Vitamin D: A review on its effects on muscle strength, the risk of fall, and frailty, *Biomed Research International,* 2015, doi: 10.1155/2015/953241; R. J. Moon and coauthors, Vitamin D and skeletal health in infancy and childhood, *Osteoporosis International* 25 (2014): 2673–2684.

13. J. C. Kroner, A. Sommer, and M. Fabri, Vitamin D every day to keep the infection away? *Nutrients* 7 (2015): 4170–4188; M. D. Kerns and coauthors, Impact of vitamin D on infectious disease: A systematic review of controlled trials, *American Journal of the Medical Sciences* 349 (2015): 245–262; H. Korf, B. Decallonne, and C. Mathieu, Vitamin D for infections, *Current Opinion in Endocrinology, Diabetes, and Obesity* 21 (2014): 431–436.

14. A. L. Slusher, M. J. McAllister, and C. J. Huang, A therapeutic role for vitamin D on obesity-associated inflammation and weight-loss intervention, *Inflammation Research* 64 (2015): 565–575; F. G. Cändido and J. Bressan, Vitamin D: Link between osteoporosis, obesity, and diabetes? *International Journal of Molecular Sciences* 15 (2014): 6569–6591.

15. S. R. Mallard, A. S. Howe, and L. A. Houghton, Vitamin D status and weight loss: A systematic review and meta-analysis of randomized and nonrandomized controlled weight-loss trials, *American Journal of Clinical Nutrition* 104 (2016): 1151–1159; A. Hannemann and coauthors, Adiposity measures and vitamin D concentrations in Northeast Germany and Denmark, *Nutrition and Metabolism* 12 (2015): 24; M. Pereira-Santos and coauthors, Obesity and vitamin D deficiency: A systematic review and meta-analysis, *Obesity Reviews* 16 (2015): 341–349; S. J. Mutt and coauthors, Vitamin D and adipose tissue—more than storage, *Frontiers in Physiology* 5 (2014): 228; Cändido and Bressan, 2014.

16. J. E. Heller and coauthors, Relation between vitamin D status and body composition in collegiate athletes, *International Journal of Sport Nutrition and Exercise Metabolism* 25 (2015): 128–135; L. K. Pourshahidi, Vitamin D and obesity: Current perspectives and future directions, *Proceedings of the Nutrition Society* 74 (2015): 115–124; Cändido and Bressan, 2014.

17. J. S. Walsh, S. Bowles, and A. L. Evans, Vitamin D in obesity, *Current Opinion in Endocrinology, Diabetes, and Obesity,* 2017, doi: 10.1097/MED.0000000000000371.

18. R. Zhang and coauthors, Serum 25-hydroxyvitamin D and the risk of cardiovascular disease: Dose-response meta-analysis of prospective studies, *American Journal of Clinical Nutrition* 105 (2017): 810–819; S. Chandrashekara and A. Patted, Role of vitamin D supplementation in improving disease activity in rheumatoid arthritis: An exploratory study,

International Journal of Rheumatic Diseases 20 (2017): 825–831; M. Song and coauthors, Plasma 25-hydroxyvitamin D and colorectal cancer risk according to tumour immunity status, *Gut* 65 (2016): 296–304; S. L. McDonnell and coauthors, Serum 25-hydroxyvitamin D concentrations ≥ 40 ng/ml are associated with >65% lower cancer risk: Pooled analysis of randomized trial and prospective cohort study, *PLoS One* 11 (2016): e0152441; C. Mathieu, Vitamin D and diabetes: Where do we stand? *Diabetes Research and Clinical Practice* 108 (2015): 201–209; L. Ke and coauthors, Vitamin D status and hypertension: A review, *Integrated Blood Pressure Control* 8 (2015): 13–35; A. E. Millen and coauthors, Association between vitamin D status and age-related macular degeneration by genetic risk, *JAMA Ophthalmology* 133 (2015): 1171–1179; I. Mozos and O. Marginean, Links between vitamin D deficiency and cardiovascular diseases, *Biomed Research International*, 2015, doi: 10.1155/2015/109275; Kroner, Sommer, and Fabri, 2015; Cändido and Bressan, 2014; C. F. Garland and coauthors, Meta-analysis of all-cause mortality according to serum 25-hydroxyvitamin D, *American Journal of Public Health* 104 (2014): e43–e50.

19. U. S. Preventive Services Task Force, September, 2017, *Draft Recommendation Statement: Vitamin D, Calcium, or Combined Supplementation for the Primary Prevention of Fractures in Adults:* www.uspreventiveservicestaskforce.org/Page/Document/draft-recommendation-statement/vitamin-d-calcium-or-combined-supplementation-for-the-primary-prevention-of-fractures-in-adults-preventive-medication; L. A. Beveridge and coauthors, Effect of vitamin D supplementation on blood pressure: A systematic review and meta-analysis incorporating individual patient data, *JAMA Internal Medicine* 175 (2015): 745–754; M. R. Hoffman, P. A. Senior, and D. R. Mager, Vitamin D supplementaion and health-related quality of life: A systematic review of the literature, *Journal of the Academy of Nutrition and Dietetics* 115 (2015): 406–418; K. Amrein and coauthors, Effect of high-dose vitamin D3 on hospital length of stay in critically ill patients with vitamin D deficiency: The VITdAL-ICU Randomized Clinical Trial, *Journal of the American Medical Association* 312 (2014): 1520–1530.

20. R.L. Schleicher and coauthors, The vitamin D status of the US population from 1988 to 2010 using standardized serum concentrations of 25-hydroxyvitamin D shows recent modest increases, *American Journal of Clinical Nutrition* 104 (2016): 454–461.

21. K. E. Hansen and coauthors, Treatment of vitamin D insufficiency in postmenopausal women, *JAMA Internal Medicine* 175 (2015): 1612–1621.

22. Q. Jiang, Natural forms of vitamin E: Metabolism, antioxidant, and anti-inflammatory activities and their role in disease prevention and therapy, *Free Radical Biology and Medicine* 72 (2014): 76–90.

23. H. N. Siti, Y. Kamisah, and J. Kamsiah, The role of oxidative stress, antioxidants and vascular inflammation in cardiovascular disease (a review), *Vascular Pharmacology* 71 (2015): 40–56.

24. R. H. Eckel and coauthors, 2013 AHA/ACC Guideline on Lifestyle management to reduce cardiovascular risk: A Report of the American College of Cardiology/American Heart Association Task Force on Practice Guidelines, *Circulation* 129 (2014): S76–S99.

25. M. Karpinski and coauthors, Roles of vitamins E and K, nutrition, and lifestyle in low-energy bone fractures in children and young adults, *Journal of the American College of Nutrition* 36 (2017): 399–412.

26. K. Shah, L. Gleason, and D. T. Villareal, Vitamin K and bone health in older adults, *Journal of Nutrition in Gerontology and Geriatrics* 33 (2014): 10–22; M. S. Hamidi and A. M. Cheung, Vitamin K and musculoskeletal

health in postmenopausal women, *Molecular Nutrition and Food Research* 58 (2014): 1647–1657.

27. M. Witt and coauthors, Prophylactic dosing of vitamin K to prevent bleeding, *Pediatrics* 137 (2016): e20154222; M. Weddle and coauthors, Are pediatricians complicit in vitamin K deficiency bleeding? *Pediatrics* 136 (2015): 753–757.

28. A. A. Badway, Pellagra and alcoholism: A biochemical perspective, *Alcohol and Alcoholism* 49 (2014): 238–250.

29. J. Zempleni and coauthors, Novel roles of holocarboxylase synthetase in gene regulation and intermediary metabolism, *Nutrition Reviews* 72 (2014): 369–376.

30. B. Gylling and coauthors, Vitamin B-6 and colorectal cancer risk: A prospective population-based study using 3 distinct plasma markers of vitamin B-6 status, *American Journal of Clinical Nutrition* 105 (2017): 897–904; B. Debreceni and L. Debreceni, The role of homocysteine-lowering B-vitamins in the primary prevention of cardiovascular disease, *Cardiovascular Therapeutics* 32 (2014): 130–138.

31. S. Mocellin, M. Briarava, and P. Pilati, Vitamin B6 and cancer risk: A field synopsis and meta-analysis, *Journal of the National Cancer Institute* 109 (2017): 1–9; Gylling and coauthors, 2017; Debreceni and Debreceni, 2014.

32. Centers for Disease Control and Prevention, Folic acid data and statistics, available at www.cdc.gov/ncbddd/folicacid/data.html, updated March 30, 2016; J. Williams and coauthors, Updated estimates of neural tube defects prevented by mandatory folic acid fortification—United States, 1995–2011, *Morbidity and Mortality Weekly Report* 64 (2015): 1–5.

33. T. Köbe and coauthors, Vitamin B-12 concentration, memory performance, and hippocampal structure in patients with mild cognitive impairment, *American Journal of Clinical Nutrition* 103 (2016): 1045–1054.

34. R. Pawlak, S. E. Lester, and T. Babatunde, The prevalence of cobalamin deficiency among vegetarians assessed by serum vitamin B12: A review of literature, *European Journal of Clinical Nutrition* 68 (2014): 541–548.

35. E. T. M. Leermakers and coauthors, Effects of choline on health across the life course: A systematic review, *Nutrition Reviews* 73 (2016): 500–522; S. P. Masih and coauthors, Pregnant Canadian women achieve recommended intakes of one-carbon nutrients through prenatal supplementation but the supplement composition, including choline, requires reconsideration, *Journal of Nutrition* 145 (2015): 1824–1834; X. Jiang, A. A. West, and M. A. Caudill, Maternal choline supplementation: A nutritional approach for improving offspring health? *Trends in Endocrinology and Metabolism* 25 (2014): 263–273.

36. H. Hemila, Vitamin C and infections, *Nutrients* 9 (2017): 339.

37. Q. Chen and coauthors, The unpaved journey of vitamin C in cancer treatment, *Canadian Journal of Physiology and Pharmacology* 93 (2015): 1055–1063; P. Kong and coauthors, Vitamin intake reduce the risk of gastric cancer: Meta-analysis and systematic review of randomized and observational studies, *PLoS One* 9 (2014): e116060; P. Li and coauthors, Association between dietary antioxidant vitamins intake/blood level and risk of gastric cancer, *International Journal of Cancer* 135 (2014): 1444–1453; C. Kuiper and M. C. Vissers, Ascorbate as a co-factor for fe- and 2-oxoglutarate dependent dioxygenases: Physiological activity in tumor growth and progression, *Frontiers in Oncology* 4 (2014): 349.

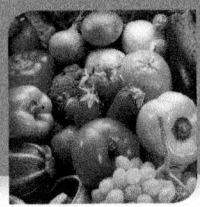

8.4 Nutrition in Practice

Phytochemicals and Functional Foods

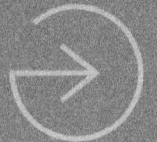

The wisdom of the familiar advice, "Eat your vegetables; they're good for you," stands on firmer scientific ground today than ever before as population studies around the world suggest that diets rich in vegetables and fruit protect against heart disease, cancer, and other chronic diseases.[1] We now know that the "goodness" of vegetables, fruit, and other whole foods such as legumes and grains comes not only from the nutrients they contain but also from the **phytochemicals** that they offer.[2] Phytochemicals often act as **bioactive food components**, food constituents with the ability to alter body processes. (Terms are defined in Table NP8-1.)

Vegetables, fruit, and other whole foods are the simplest examples of foods now known as **functional foods**. Functional foods provide health benefits beyond basic nutrition by altering one or more physiological processes. Foods that have been fortified, enriched, or enhanced with nutrients, phytochemicals, herbs, or other food components are also functional foods.[3] Functional foods that fit this description include orange juice fortified with calcium,

---

| **TABLE NP8-1** | Phytochemical and Functional Food Terms |

- **antioxidants** (anti-OX-ih-dants): compounds that protect other compounds from damaging reactions involving oxygen by themselves reacting with oxygen (*anti-* means "against"; *oxy-* means "oxygen"); oxidation is a potentially damaging effect of normal cell chemistry involving oxygen.
- **bioactive food components**: compounds in foods, either nutrients or phytochemicals, that alter physiological processes in the body.
- **carotenoids** (kah-ROT-eh-noyds): pigments commonly found in plants and animals, some of which have vitamin A activity. The carotenoid with the greatest vitamin A activity is beta-carotene.
- **edamame**: fresh green soybeans.
- **flavonoids** (FLAY-von-oyds): a common and widespread group of phytochemicals, with more than 6000 identified members; physiologic effects may include antioxidant, antiviral, anticancer, and other activities. Some flavonoids are yellow pigments in foods; *flavus* means "yellow."
- **flaxseed**: small brown seed of the flax plant; used in baking, cereals, and other foods. Valued in nutrition as a source of fiber, lignans, and the omega-3 fatty acid linolenic acid.
- **functional foods**: whole, fortified, enriched, or enhanced foods that have a potentially beneficial effect on health when consumed as part of a varied diet on a regular basis at effective levels.
- **genistein** (GEN-ih-steen): a phytoestrogen found primarily in soybeans that both mimics and blocks the action of estrogen in the body; a type of flavonoid.
- **lignans**: phytochemicals present mostly in seeds, particularly flaxseed, that are converted to phytoestrogens by intestinal bacteria and are under study as possible anticancer agents.
- **lutein** (LO-teen): a plant pigment of yellow hue; a phytochemical believed to play roles in eye functioning and health.
- **lycopene** (LYE-koh-peen): a pigment responsible for the red color of tomatoes and other red-hued vegetables; a phytochemical that may act as an antioxidant in the body.
- **miso**: fermented soybean paste used in Japanese cooking.
- **organosulfur compounds**: a large group of phytochemicals containing the mineral sulfur. Organosulfur phytochemicals are responsible for the pungent flavors and aromas of foods belonging to the onion, leek, chive, shallot, and garlic family and are thought to stimulate cancer defenses in the body.
- **phytochemicals** (FIGH-toe-CHEM-ih-cals): compounds in plants that confer color, taste, and other characteristics. Some phytochemicals are bioactive food components in functional foods.
- **phytoestrogens** (FIGHT-toe-ESS-troh-gens): phytochemicals structurally similar to human estrogen. Phytoestrogens weakly mimic or modulate estrogen in the body.
- **plant sterols**: phytochemicals that resemble cholesterol in structure but that lower blood cholesterol by interfering with cholesterol absorption in the intestine. Plant sterols include sterol esters and stanol esters. Formerly called *phytosterols*.
- **resveratrol** (rez-VER-ah-trol): a phytochemical of grapes under study for potential health benefits.
- **soy milk**: a milk-like beverage made from ground soybeans. Soy milk should be fortified with vitamin A, vitamin D, riboflavin, and calcium to approach the nutritional equivalency of milk.
- **tofu**: a white curd made of soybeans, popular in Asian cuisines, and considered to be a functional food.

folate-enriched cereal, beverages with herbal additives, and margarine enhanced with **plant sterols**. This Nutrition in Practice begins with a look at the evidence concerning the effectiveness and safety of a few selected phytochemicals in the simplest of functional foods—vegetables, fruit, and other whole foods. Then, the discussion turns to examine the most controversial of functional foods—novel foods to which phytochemicals have been added to promote health. How these foods fit into a healthy diet is still unclear.

What are phytochemicals, and what do they do?

Phytochemicals are bioactive compounds found in plants. In foods, phytochemicals impart tastes, aromas, colors, and other characteristics. They give hot peppers their burning sensation, garlic and onions their pungent flavor, chocolate its bitter tang, and tomatoes their dark red color. In the body, phytochemicals can have profound physiological effects—acting as antioxidants, mimicking hormones, stimulating or inhibiting enzymes, interfering with DNA replication, destroying bacteria, and binding physically to cell walls. Any of these actions may suppress the development of diseases, depending in part on how genetic factors interact with the phytochemicals.[4] Notably, cancer and heart disease are linked to processes involving oxygen compounds in the body, and **antioxidants** are thought to oppose these actions.[5]

Why are phytochemicals receiving so much attention these days, and what are some examples of those in the spotlight?

Diets rich in whole grains, legumes, vegetables, and fruit seem to be protective against heart disease and cancer, but identifying *the* specific foods or components of foods that are responsible is difficult. Scientists are conducting extensive research studies to discover phytochemical connections to disease prevention, but, so far, solid evidence is generally lacking. Some of the likeliest candidates include **flavonoids** and **carotenoids** (including **lycopene**).

What are flavonoids, and in which foods are they found?

Flavonoids, a large group of phytochemicals known for their health-promoting qualities, are found in whole grains, soy, vegetables, fruit, herbs, spices, teas, chocolate, nuts, olive oil, and red wine. Flavonoids are powerful antioxidants that may help to protect LDL against oxidation, minimize inflammation, and reduce blood platelet stickiness, thereby slowing the progression of atherosclerosis and making blood clots less likely.[6] Whereas an abundance of flavonoid-containing *foods* in the diet may lower the risks of chronic diseases, no claims can be made for flavonoids themselves as the protective factor, particularly when they are extracted from foods and sold as supplements. In fact, purified flavonoids may even be harmful.[7]

Flavonoids impart a bitter taste to foods, so manufacturers often refine away the natural flavonoids to please consumers, who usually prefer milder flavors. For example, for white grape juice or white wine, manufacturers remove the red, flavonoid-rich grape skins to lighten the flavor and color of the product, while greatly reducing its beneficial flavonoid content. One such flavonoid in purple grape juice and red wine, **resveratrol**, seems to hold promise as a disease fighter.[8] In laboratory studies, resveratrol demonstrates the potential to reduce harmful tissue inflammation that often accompanies cancer, diabetes, obesity, and heart disease and to oppose heart disease development in many other ways.[9] As tempting as it may be to conclude that grapes and red wine prevent human diseases, the controlled clinical human trials needed to confirm that people actually benefit from consuming grapes and red wine are still lacking.[10]

What about carotenoids?

In addition to flavonoids, fruit and vegetables are rich in carotenoids—the red and yellow pigments of plants. Some carotenoids, such as beta-carotene, are vitamin A precursors. Some research suggests that a diet rich in carotenoids is associated with a lower risk of hypertension and heart disease.[11] Among the carotenoids that may defend against heart disease as well as stroke is lycopene.[12] Lycopene possesses powerful antioxidant activity. Lycopene may also protect against certain types of cancer.[13] Theoretically, the potent antioxidant capability of lycopene may play a role in its action against cancer, but research suggests that several other mechanisms may underlie lycopene's possible anti-cancer activity.[14]

What is lycopene, and what foods contain it?

Lycopene is a red pigment found in guava, papaya, pink grapefruit, tomatoes (especially cooked tomatoes and tomato products), and watermelon. More than 80 percent of the lycopene consumed in the United States comes from tomato products such as tomato sauce, tomato juice, and catsup.

The Food and Drug Administration (FDA) concludes that no or very little solid evidence links lycopene or tomato consumption with reduced cancer risks. Tomatoes contain many other phytochemicals and nutrients that may contribute to the beneficial health effects of eating tomatoes and tomato products.

Do foods contain other phytochemicals that may help to protect people from cancer or other diseases?

Foods contain thousands of different phytochemicals, and so far only a few have been researched at all. There are still many questions about the phytochemicals that have been studied and only tentative answers about their roles in human health. For example, compared with people in the West, Asians living in Asia consume far more soybeans and soy products such as **edamame, miso, soy milk,** and **tofu**, and they suffer less frequently from heart disease and certain cancers.* When Asian populations adopt Western diets and habits, however, rates of obesity and chronic diseases increase.[15]

In research, evidence concerning soy and heart health seems promising.[16] Soy's cholesterol-like plant sterols may inhibit cholesterol absorption in the intestine, and thus lower blood cholesterol.[17] Soy protein may also speed up excretion of cholesterol from the body.[18]

Cancers of the breast, colon, and prostate can be estrogen-sensitive—meaning that they grow when exposed to estrogen. In addition to plant sterols, soy contains **phytoestrogens**, chemical relatives of human estrogen that may mimic or oppose its effects.[19] Phytoestrogens also have antioxidant activity that appears to slow the growth of some cancers. Soy foods appear to be most effective when consumed in moderation early and throughout life.[20] A study of women in China suggests a somewhat better outcome for breast cancer among soy consumers.[21] Soy intake may lower the risk of breast cancer for women in Asian countries, but for women in Western nations, evidence does not suggest a benefit.[22] Clearly, more research is needed before conclusions may be drawn about soy intake and cancer risk.

Low doses of one soy phytoestrogen, **genistein**, appear to speed up division of breast cancer cells in laboratory cultures and in mice. It seems unlikely, however, that moderate intakes of soy foods cause harm in people.

The opposing actions of phytoestrogens should raise a red flag against taking supplements, especially by people who have had cancer or have close relatives with cancer. The American Cancer Society recommends that breast cancer survivors and those under treatment for breast cancer should consume only moderate amounts of soy foods as part of a healthy plant-based diet and should not intentionally ingest very high levels of soy products.

Other foods under study for potential health benefits include **flaxseed**, found as a whole seed, ground meal, or flaxseed oil. Flaxseed is of interest for its possible benefits to heart health because it is a good source of soluble fiber, and it is the richest known source of both the omega-3 fatty acid linolenic acid and **lignans**. Lignans are converted into biologically active phytoestrogens by bacteria that normally reside in the human intestine.[23] Flaxseed oil, though rich in linolenic acid, does not contain fiber or lignans. Large quantities of flaxseed can cause digestive distress, and severe allergic reactions to flaxseed have been reported.

What about other phytochemical supplements?

Even when people don't make healthy food choices, taking supplements of purified phytochemicals is not the way to go. Phytochemicals can alter body functions, sometimes powerfully. Researchers are just beginning to understand how a handful of phytochemicals work, and what is current today may change tomorrow. Foods deliver thousands of bioactive food components, all within a food matrix that maximizes their availability and effectiveness.[24] The body is equipped to handle phytochemicals in diluted form, mixed with all of the other constituents of foods. The best way to reap the benefits of phytochemicals is by eating foods, not taking supplements (see Figure NP8-1).

How do whole foods compare with processed foods that have been enriched with phytochemicals?

Good question. The American food supply is being transformed by a proliferation of functional foods—foods claimed to provide health benefits beyond those of the traditional nutrients. Virtually all whole foods have some special value in supporting health and are therefore functional foods. Cranberries may protect against urinary tract infections because cranberries contain a phytochemical that dislodges bacteria from the tract. Cooked tomatoes, as mentioned, provide lycopene, along with **lutein** (an antioxidant associated with healthy eye function), vitamin C (an antioxidant vitamin), and many other healthful attributes. This has not stopped food manufacturers from trying to create functional foods as well. As consumer demand for healthful foods continues to grow, so will the development of functional foods.

What are some examples of manufactured functional foods?

Many processed foods become functional foods when they are fortified with nutrients (calcium-fortified orange juice to support bone health, for example). In other cases, processed foods are enhanced with bioactive food components (margarine blended with a plant sterol to lower cholesterol, for example). The creation of some novel manufactured functional foods raises the question—is it a food or a drug?

Isn't the distinction between a food and a drug pretty clear?

Not long ago, most of us could agree on what was a food and what was a drug. Today, functional foods blur the

---

*Among the cancers occurring less often in Asia are breast, colon, and prostate cancers.

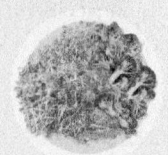

Broccoli and broccoli sprouts contain an abundance of the cancer-fighting phytochemical sulforaphane.

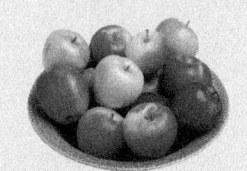

An apple a day—rich in flavonoids—may protect against lung cancer.

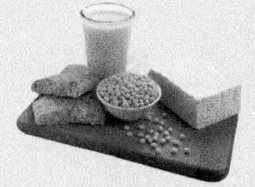

The phytoestrogens of soybeans seem to starve cancer cells and inhibit tumor growth; the phytosterols may lower blood cholesterol and protect cardiac arteries.

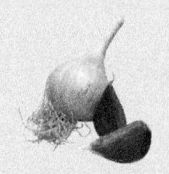

Garlic, with its abundant organosulfur compounds, may lower blood cholesterol and protect against stomach cancer.

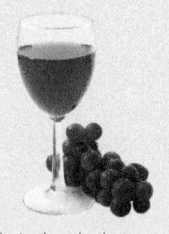

The phytochemical resveratrol found in grapes (and nuts) protects against cancer by inhibiting cell growth and against heart disease by limiting clot formation and inflammation.

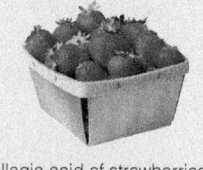

The ellagic acid of strawberries may inhibit certain types of cancer.

Tomatoes, with their abundant lycopene, may defend against cancer by protecting DNA from oxidative damage.

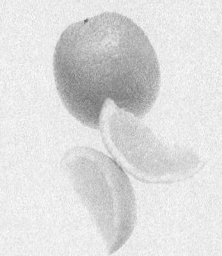

The monoterpenes of citrus fruit (and cherries) may inhibit cancer growth.

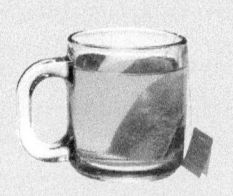

The flavonoids in black tea may protect against heart disease, whereas those in green tea may defend against cancer.

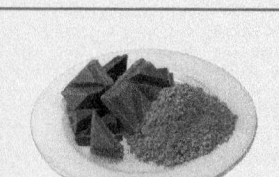

The flavonoids in cocoa and chocolate defend against oxidation and reduce the tendency of blood to clot.

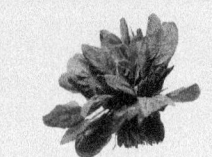

Spinach and other colorful vegetables contain the carotenoids lutein and zeaxanthin, which help protect the eyes against macular degeneration.

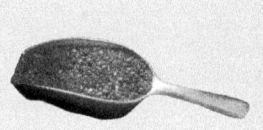

Flaxseed, the richest source of lignans, may prevent the spread of cancer.

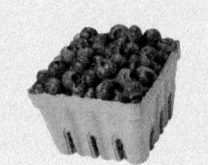

Blueberries, a rich source of flavonoids, improve memory in animals.

Garlic, Citrus fruits, © EyeWire, Inc.; Flaxseed, Courtesy of Flax Council of Canada; Broccoli, Courtesy of Brassica Protection Products; Apples, Strawberries, Blueberries, C Squared Studios/Photodisc/Getty Images; Grapes, Photodisc/Getty Images; Tomatoes, Photodisc, Inc/Getty Images; Black Tea, John A. Rizzo/Photodisc/Getty Images; Soybeans, Mitch Hrdlicka/PhotoDisc/Getty Images; Orange, Spinach, Cocoa by Matthew Farruggio

distinctions. They have characteristics similar to both foods and drugs but do not fit neatly into either category. Consider the margarine example above.

Eating nonhydrogenated margarine sparingly instead of butter generously may lower blood cholesterol slightly over several months and clearly falls into the food category. Taking a statin drug, on the other hand, lowers blood cholesterol significantly within weeks and clearly falls into the drug category. But margarine enhanced with a plant sterol that lowers blood cholesterol is in a gray area between the two.† The margarine looks and tastes like a food, but it acts like a drug.

What are the health advantages and disadvantages of eating manufactured functional foods?

To achieve a desired health effect, which is the better choice: to eat a food designed to affect some body function or simply to adjust the diet? Does it make more sense to use a margarine enhanced with a plant sterol that lowers blood cholesterol or simply to limit the amount of butter eaten? Is it smarter to eat eggs enriched with omega-3 fatty acids or to restrict egg consumption? Might functional foods offer a sensible solution for improving our nation's health—if done correctly?

---

†Margarine products that lower blood cholesterol contain either sterol esters—from vegetable oils, soybeans, and corn—or stanol esters from wood pulp.

Perhaps so, but there is a problem with functional foods: the food industry is moving too fast for either scientists or the FDA to keep up. Consumers were able to buy soup with St. John's wort that claimed to enhance mood and fruit juice with echinacea that was supposed to fight colds while scientists were still conducting their studies on these ingredients. Research to determine the safety and effectiveness of these substances is still in progress. Until this work is complete, consumers are on their own in finding the answers to the following questions:

- *Does it work?* Research is generally lacking, and findings are often inconclusive.
- *How much does it contain?* Food labels are not required to list the quantities of added phytochemicals. Even if they were, consumers have no standard for comparison and cannot deduce whether the amounts listed are a little or a lot. Most importantly, until research is complete, food manufacturers do not know what amounts (if any) are most effective—or most toxic.
- *Is it safe?* Functional foods can act like drugs. They contain ingredients that can alter body functions and cause allergies, drug interactions, drowsiness, and other side effects. Yet, unlike drug labels, food labels do not provide instructions for the dosage, frequency, or duration of treatment.
- *Has the FDA issued warnings about any of the ingredients?* Check the FDA's website (www.fda.gov) to find out.
- *Is it healthy?* Adding phytochemicals to a food does not magically make it a healthy choice. A candy bar may be fortified with phytochemicals, but it is still made mostly of sugar and fat.

Critics suggest that the designation "functional foods" may be nothing more than a marketing tool (see Photo NP8-1). After all, even the most experienced researchers cannot yet identify the perfect combination of nutrients and phytochemicals to support optimal health. Yet manufacturers are freely experimenting with various concoctions as if they possessed that knowledge. Is it okay for them to sprinkle phytochemicals on fried snack foods and label them "functional," thus implying health benefits?

What is the final word regarding phytochemicals and functional foods?

Nature has elegantly designed foods to provide us with a complex array of dozens

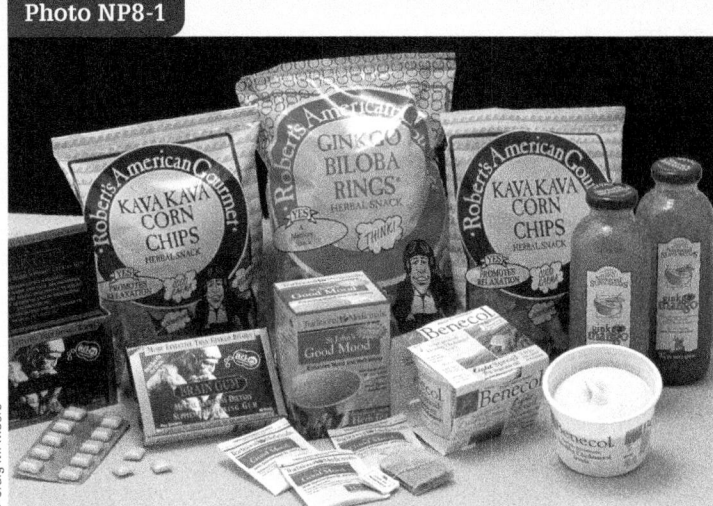

Photo NP8-1

Functional foods currently on the market promise to "enhance mood," "promote relaxation and good karma," "increase alertness," and "improve memory," among other claims.

© Craig M. Moore

of nutrients and thousands of additional compounds that may benefit health—most of which we have yet to identify or understand (see Photo NP8-2). Over the years, we have taken those foods and first deconstructed them and then reconstructed them in an effort to "improve" them. With new scientific understandings of how nutrients—and the myriad other compounds in foods—interact with genes, we may someday be able to design *specific* eating patterns to meet the *exact* health needs of *each* individual. Indeed, our knowledge of the human genome and of human nutrition may well merge to allow specific recommendations for individuals based on their predisposition to diet-related diseases.

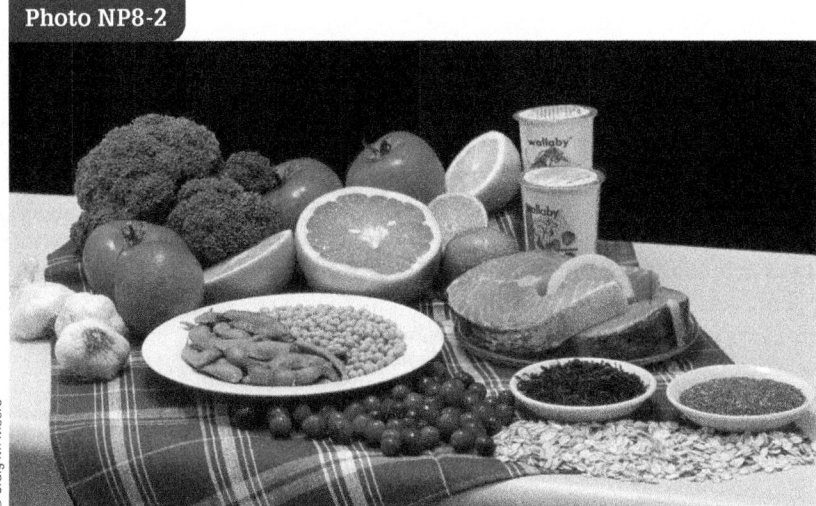

Photo NP8-2

Nature offers a variety of functional foods that provide us with many health benefits.

© Craig M. Moore

- *Eat more fruit.* The average U.S. diet provides little more than ½ cup fruit per day. Remember to choose juices and raw, dried, or cooked fruit and vegetables at mealtimes as well as for snacks. Choose dried fruit in place of candy.

- *Increase vegetable portions to meet recommendations.* Choose 1 cup of cut-up raw or cooked vegetables, or 2 cups of raw, leafy greens.

- *Use herbs and spices.* Cookbooks offer ways to include parsley, basil, garlic, hot peppers, oregano, and other beneficial seasonings.

- *Replace some meat with grains, legumes, and vegetables.* Oatmeal, soy meat replacer, or grated carrots mixed with ground meat and seasonings make a luscious, nutritious meatloaf, for example.

- *Add grated vegetables.* Carrots in chili or meatballs and celery, mushrooms, and squash in spaghetti sauce or other sauces add phytochemicals without greatly changing the taste of the food.

- *Try new foods.* Try a new fruit, vegetable, or whole grain each week. Walk through vegetable aisles and visit farmers' markets. Read recipes. Try tofu, fortified soy milk, or soybeans in cooking.

If the present trend continues, then someday physicians may be able to prescribe the perfect foods to enhance a person's health, and farmers will be able to grow them. In the meantime, however, it seems clear that a moderate approach to phytochemicals and functional foods is warranted. People who eat the recommended amounts of a variety of fruits and vegetables may cut their risk of many diseases by as much as half. Replacing some meat with soy foods and other legumes may also lower heart disease and cancer risks. Beneficial constituents are widespread among foods. Take a no-nonsense approach where your health is concerned: Choose a wide variety of whole grains, legumes, fruit, and vegetables in the context of an adequate, balanced, and varied diet, and receive all of the health benefits that these foods offer. Table NP8-2 offers some tips for consuming the whole foods known to provide phytochemicals.

Notes

1. L. Schwingshackl and coauthors, Food groups and risk of all-cause mortality: A systematic review and meta-analysis of prospective studies, *American Journal of Clinical Nutrition* 105 (2017): 1462–1473; J. Zhan and coauthors, Fruit and vegetable consumption and risk of cardiovascular disease: A meta-analysis of prospective cohort studies, *Critical Reviews in Food Science and Nutrition* 57 (2017): 1650–1663; A. Fardet and Y. Boirie, Associations between food and beverage groups and major diet-related chronic diseases: An exhaustive review of pooled/meta-analyses and systematic reviews, *Nutrition Reviews* 72 (2014): 741–762; O. Oyebode and coauthors, Fruit and vegetable consumption and all-cause, cancer and CVD mortality: Analysis of Health Survey for England data, *Journal of Epidemiology and Community Health* 68 (2014): 856–862; D. Hu and coauthors, Fruits and vegetables consumption and risk of stroke: A meta-analysis of prospective cohort studies, *Stroke* 45 (2014): 1613–1619.

2. D. Li and coauthors, Health benefits of anthocyanins and molecular mechanisms: Update from recent decade, *Critical Reviews in Food Science and Nutrition* 57 (2017): 1729–1741; A. Cassidy and coauthors, Habitual intake of anthocyanins and flavanones and risk of cardiovascular disease in men, *American Journal of Clinical Nutrition* 104 (2016): 587–594; Y. J. Zhang and coauthors, Antioxidant phytochemicals for the prevention and treatment of chronic diseases, *Molecules* 20 (2015): 21138–21156; S. Vendrame and D. Klimis-Zacas, Anti-inflammatory effect of anthocyanins via modulation of nuclear factor kB and mitogen-activated protein kinase signaling cascades, *Nutrition Reviews* 73 (2015): 348–358; M. J. Howes and M. S. Simmonds, The role of phytochemicals as micronutrients in health and disease, *Current Opinion in Clinical Nutrition and Metabolic Care* 17 (2014): 558–566.

3. Position of the Academy of Nutrition and Dietetics: *Functional foods, Journal of the Academy of Nutrition and Dietetics* 113 (2013): 1096–1103.

4. E. Shankar and coauthors, Dietary phytochemicals as epigenetic modifiers in cancer: Promise and challenges, *Seminars in Cancer Biology* 40 (2016):
82–99; Y. Guo, Z-Y Su, and A-N Kong, Current perspectives on epigenetic modifications by dietary chemopreventive and herbal phytochemicals, *Current Pharmacology Reports* 1 (2015): 245–257.

5. Zhang and coauthors, 2015.

6. Cassidy and coauthors, 2016; C. P. Bondonno and coauthors, Dietary flavonoids and nitrate: Effects on nitric oxide and vascular function, *Nutrition Reviews* 73 (2015): 216–235; K. L. Ivey and coauthors, Flavonoid intake and all-cause mortality, *American Journal of Clinical Nutrition* 101 (2015): 1012–1020; A. L. Macready and coauthors, Flavonoid-rich fruit and vegetables improve microvascular reactivity and inflammatory status in men at risk of cardiovascular disease—FLAVURS: A randomized controlled trial, *American Journal of Clinical Nutrition* 99 (2014): 479–489.

7. Bondonno and coauthors, 2015.

8. K. Liu and coauthors, Effect of resveratrol on glucose control and insulin sensitivity: A meta-analysis of 11 randomized controlled trials, *American Journal of Clinical Nutrition* 99 (2014): 1510–1519.

9. M. M. Poulsen and coauthors, Resveratrol and inflammation: Challenges in translating pre-clinical findings to improved patient outcomes, *Biochimica Biophysica Acta* 1852 (2015): 1124–1136; Y. Liu and coauthors, Effect of resveratrol on blood pressure: A meta-analysis of randomized controlled trials, *Clinical Nutrition* 34 (2015): 27–34.

10. Poulsen and coauthors, 2015; R. D. Semba and coauthors, Resveratrol levels and all- cause mortality in older community-dwelling adults, *JAMA: Internal Medicine* 174 (2014): 1077–1084; S. D. Anton and coauthors, Safety and metabolic outcomes of resveratrol supplementation in older adults: Results of a twelve-week, placebo-controlled pilot study, *Experimental Gerontology* 57 (2014): 181–187.

11. L. Müller and coauthors, Lycopene and its antioxidant role in the prevention of cardiovascular diseases—A critical review, *Critical Reviews in Food Science and Nutrition* 56 (2016): 1868–1879; T. Bohn and coauthors, Mind the gap-deficits in our knowledge of aspects impacting

the bioavailability of phytochemicals and their metabolites—A position paper focusing on carotenoids and polyphenols, *Molecular Nutrition and Food Research* 59 (2015): 1307–1323; M. A. Gammone, G. Riccioni, and N. D'Orazio, Carotenoids: Potential allies of cardiovascular health? *Food and Nutrition Research* 59 (2015): 26762.

12. Muller and coauthors, 2016; Gammone, Riccioni, and D'Orazio, 2015; X. Li and J. Xu, Dietary and circulating lycopene and stroke risk: A meta-analysis of prospective studies, *Scientific Reports* 4 (2014): 5031.

13. J. L. Rowles and coauthors, Increased dietary and circulating lycopene are associated with reduced prostate cancer risk: A systematic review and meta-analysis, *Prostate Cancer and Prostatic Diseases*, 2017, doi: 10.1038/pcan.2017.25; R. E. Graff and coauthors, Dietary lycopene intake and risk of prostate cancer defined by ERG protein expression, *American Journal of Clinical Nutrition* 103 (2016): 851–860; A. H. Eliassen and coauthors, Plasma carotenoids and risk of breast cancer over 20 y of follow-up, *American Journal of Clinical Nutrition* 101 (2015): 1197–1205.

14. J. Chen and coauthors, The effect of lycopene on the P13K/Akt signaling pathway in prostate cancer, *Anticancer Agents in Medicinal Chemistry* 14 (2014): 800–805.

15. Y. X. Zhang and coauthors, Trends in overweight and obesity among rural children and adolescents from 1985 to 2014 in Shandong, China, *European Journal of Preventive Cardiology* 23 (2016): 1314–1320.

16. Z. Yan and coauthors, Association between consumption of soy and riskof cardiovascular disease: A meta-analysis of observational studies, *European Journal of Preventive Cardiology* 24 (2017): 735–747.

17. T. Chalvon-Demersay and coauthors, A systematic review of the effects of plant compared with animal protein sources on features of metabolic syndrome, *Journal of Nutrition* 147 (2017): 281–292; H. Gylling and coauthors, Plant sterols and plant stanols in the management of dyslipidaemia and prevention of cardiovascular disease, *Atherosclerosis* 232 (2014): 346–360.

18. G. L. Arellano-Martinez and coauthors, Soya protein stimulates bile acid excretion by the liver and intestine through direct and indirect pathways influenced by the presence of dietary cholesterol, *British Journal of Nutrition* 111 (2014): 2059–2066.

19. G. Leclercq and Y. Jacquot, Interactions of isoflavones and other plant derived estrogens with estrogen receptors for prevention and treatment of breast cancer—Considerations concerning related efficacy and safety, *Journal of Steroid Biochemistry and Molecular Biology* 139 (2014): 237–244.

20. X. Guo and coauthors, Long-term soy consumption and tumor tissue MicroRNA and gene expression in triple-negative breast cancer, *Cancer* 122 (2016): 2544–2551; M. Messina, Soy foods, isoflavones, and the health of postmenopausal women, *American Journal of Clinical Nutrition* 100 (2014): 423S–430S.

21. X.O. Liu and coauthors, Association between dietary factors and breast cancer risk among Chinese females: Systematic review and meta-analysis, *Asian Pacific Journal of Cancer Prevention* 15 (2014): 1291–1298.

22. M. Chen and coauthors, Association between soy isoflavone intake and breast cancer risk for pre-and post-menopausal women: A meta-analysis of epidemioalogical studies, *PloS One* 9 (2014): e89288.

23. J. M. Landete and coauthors, Bioactivation of phytoestrogens: Intestinal bacteria and *Health, Critical Reviews in Food Science and Nutrition* 56 (2016): 1826–1843.

24. T. Bohn, Dietary factors affecting polyphenol bioavailability, *Nutrition Reviews* 72 (2014): 429–452.

chapter 9

Water and the Minerals

Chapter Sections and Learning Objectives (LOs)

9.1 Water and Body Fluids

LO 9.1 Explain how the body regulates fluid, electrolyte, and acid–base balance.

9.2 The Major Minerals

LO 9.2 Identify the main roles, deficiency and toxicity symptoms, and food sources for each of the major minerals (sodium, chloride, potassium, calcium, phosphorus, magnesium, sulfate).

9.3 The Trace Minerals

LO 9.3 Identify the main roles, deficiency and toxicity symptoms, and food sources for each of the trace minerals (iron, zinc, selenium, iodine, copper, manganese, fluoride, chromium, and molybdenum).

9.4 Nutrition in Practice: Vitamin and Mineral Supplements

LO 9.4 Present arguments for and against the use of dietary supplements.

Don Hammond/Design Pics/Corbis

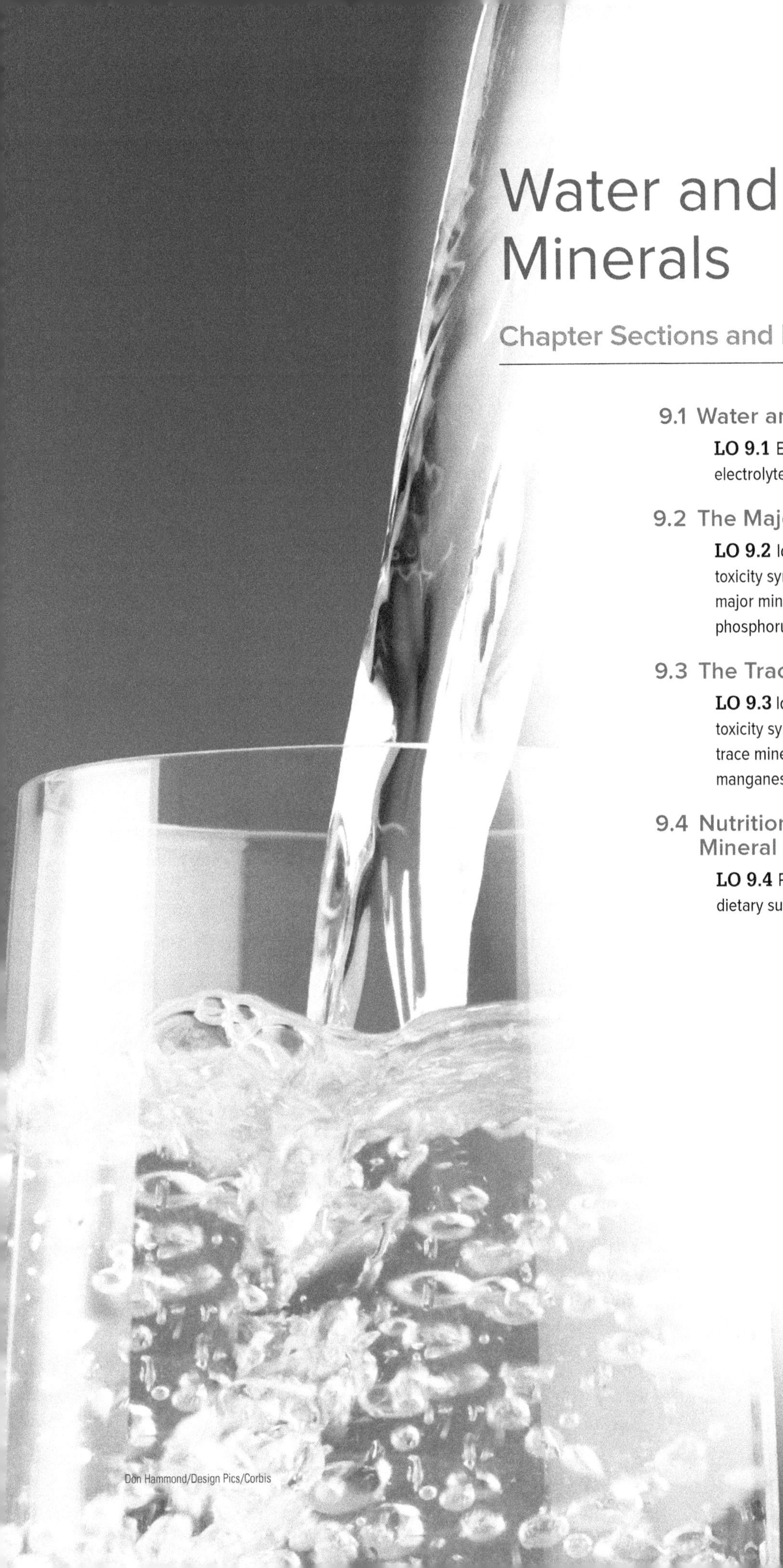

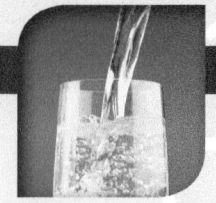

minerals dissolved in it. A person can drink pure water, but in the body, water mingles with minerals to become fluids in which all life processes take place. This chapter begins by discussing the body's fluids and their chief minerals. The focus then shifts to other functions of the minerals.

water balance: the balance between water intake and water excretion that keeps the body's water content constant.

dehydration: the loss of water from the body that occurs when water output exceeds water input. The symptoms progress rapidly from thirst, to weakness, to exhaustion and delirium, and end in death if not corrected.

water intoxication: the rare condition in which body water contents are too high. The symptoms may include confusion, convulsion, coma, and even death in extreme cases.

hypothalamus (high-poh-THAL-ah-mus): a brain center that controls activities such as maintenance of water balance, regulation of body temperature, and control of appetite.

9.1 Water and Body Fluids

Water constitutes about 60 percent of an adult's body weight and a higher percentage of a child's. Because water makes up about 75 percent of the weight of lean tissue and less than 25 percent of the weight of fat, a person's body composition influences how much of the body's weight is water. The proportion of water is generally smaller in females, obese people, and the elderly because of their smaller proportion of lean tissue.[1]

Every cell in the body is bathed in a fluid of the exact composition that is best for that cell. The body fluids bring to each cell the ingredients it requires and carry away the end products of the life-sustaining reactions that take place within the cell's boundaries. Without water, cells quickly die. The water in the body fluids:

- Carries nutrients and waste products throughout the body.
- Maintains the structure of large molecules such as proteins and glycogen.
- Participates in metabolic reactions.
- Serves as the solvent for minerals, vitamins, amino acids, glucose, and many other small molecules so that they can participate in metabolic activities.
- Maintains blood volume.
- Aids in the regulation of normal body temperature, as the evaporation of sweat from the skin removes excess heat from the body.
- Acts as a lubricant and cushion around joints and inside the eyes, spinal cord, and amniotic sac surrounding a fetus in the womb.

To support these and other vital functions, the body actively regulates its **water balance**.

Water Balance

The cells themselves regulate the composition and amounts of fluids within and surrounding them. The entire system of cells and fluids remains in a delicate but firmly maintained state of dynamic equilibrium. Imbalances such as **dehydration** (see Table 9-1) and **water intoxication** can occur, but the body quickly restores the balance to normal if it can. The body controls both water intake and water excretion to maintain water equilibrium.

Water Intake Regulation The body can survive for only a few days without water (see photo 9-1). In healthy people, thirst and satiety govern water intake. When the blood becomes too concentrated (having lost water but not salt and other dissolved substances), the mouth becomes dry, and the brain center known as the **hypothalamus** initiates drinking behavior.

Thirst lags behind the lack of water. A water deficiency that develops slowly can switch on drinking behavior in time to prevent serious dehydration, but a deficiency that develops quickly may not. Also, thirst itself does not remedy a water deficiency; a person must respond to the thirst signal by drinking. With aging, thirst sensations may diminish.[2] Dehydration can threaten older adults who do not develop the habit of drinking water regularly.

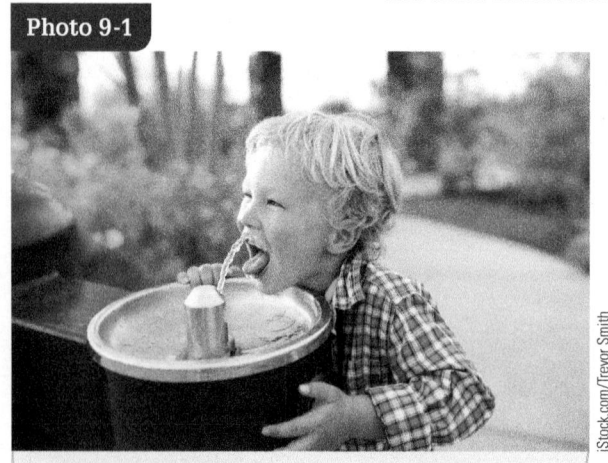

Photo 9-1

Water is the most indispensable nutrient of all.

iStock.com/Trevor Smith

TABLE 9-1	Signs of Mild and Severe Dehydration
MILD DEHYDRATION (LOSS OF < 5% BODY WEIGHT)	**SEVERE DEHYDRATION (LOSS OF > 5% BODY WEIGHT)**
• Thirst • Sudden weight loss • Rough, dry skin • Dry mouth, throat, body linings • Rapid pulse • Low blood pressure • Lack of energy; weakness • Impaired kidney function • Reduced quantity of urine; concentrated urine • Decreased mental functioning • Decreased muscular work and athletic performance • Fever or increased internal temperature • Fainting	• Pale skin • Bluish lips and fingertips • Confusion; disorientation • Rapid, shallow breathing • Weak, rapid, irregular pulse • Thickening of blood • Shock; seizures • Coma; death

Source: Based on Standing Committee on the Scientific Evaluation of Dietary Reference Intakes, Food and Nutrition Board, Institute of Medicine, *Dietary Reference Intakes: Water, Potassium, Sodium, Chloride, and Sulfate* (Washington, D.C.: National Academies Press, 2005), pp. 90–122.

Water intoxication, on the other hand, is rare but can occur with excessive water consumption and kidney disorders that reduce urine production. The symptoms may include severe headache, confusion, convulsions, and even death in extreme cases. Excessive water ingestion (several gallons) within a few hours dilutes the sodium concentration of the blood and contributes to a dangerous condition known as **hyponatremia**.

Water Excretion Regulation Water excretion is regulated by the brain and the kidneys. The cells of the brain's hypothalamus, which monitor blood salts, stimulate the **pituitary gland** to release **antidiuretic hormone (ADH)** whenever the salts are too concentrated, or the blood volume or blood pressure is too low. ADH stimulates the kidneys to reabsorb water rather than excrete it. Thus, the more water you need, the less you excrete.

If too much water is lost from the body, blood volume and blood pressure fall. Cells in the kidneys respond to the low blood pressure by releasing **renin**. Through a complex series of events involving the hormone **aldosterone**, this enzyme also causes the kidneys to retain more water. Again, the effect is that, when more water is needed, less is excreted.

Minimum Water Needed These mechanisms can maintain water balance only if a person drinks enough water. The body must excrete a minimum of about 500 milliliters (about ½ quart) each day as urine—enough to carry away the waste products generated by a day's metabolic activities. Above this amount, excretion adjusts to balance intake, so the more a person drinks, the more dilute the urine becomes. In addition to urine, some water is lost from the lungs as vapor, some is excreted in feces, and some evaporates from the skin. A person's water losses from all of these routes total about 2½ liters (about 2½ quarts) a day on the average. Table 9-2 (p. 240) shows how fluid intake and output naturally balance out.

Water Recommendations and Sources Water needs vary greatly depending on the foods a person eats, the environmental temperature and humidity, the person's activity level, and other factors. Accordingly, a general water requirement is difficult to establish. In the past, recommendations for adults were expressed in proportion to the amount of energy expended under normal environmental conditions. For the person who expends

hyponatremia (HIGH-po-na-TREE-me-ah): a decreased concentration of sodium in the blood.

pituitary (pit-TOO-ih-tary) **gland:** in the brain, the "king gland" that regulates the operation of many other glands.

antidiuretic hormone (ADH): a hormone released by the pituitary gland in response to high salt concentrations in the blood. The kidneys respond by reabsorbing water. ADH elevates blood pressure and so is also called *vasopressin* (VAS-oh-PRES-in).

vaso = vessel
press = press

renin (REN-in): an enzyme released by the kidneys in response to low blood pressure that helps them retain water through the renin-angiotensin mechanism.

aldosterone (al-DOS-ter-own): a hormone secreted by the adrenal glands that stimulates the reabsorption of sodium by the kidneys; also regulates chloride and potassium concentrations.

TABLE 9-2 Water Balance

WATER SOURCES	AMOUNT (mL)	WATER LOSSES	AMOUNT (mL)
Liquids	550 to 1500	Kidneys (urine)	500 to 1400
Foods	700 to 1000	Skin (sweat)	450 to 900
Metabolic water	200 to 300	Lungs (breath)	350
		GI tract (feces)	150
Total	1450 to 2800	Total	1450 to 2800

TABLE 9-3 Percentage of Water in Selected Foods

- 100%: Water, diet soft drinks, plain tea
- 90–99%: Fat-free milk, black coffee, Gatorade, strawberries, watermelon, grapefruit, tomato, lettuce, celery, spinach, broccoli
- 80–89%: Fruit juice, regular soft drinks, whole milk, yogurt, apples, grapes, oranges, carrots
- 70–79%: Shrimp, bananas, potatoes, avocados, ricotta cheese
- 60–69%: Pasta, cooked rice, legumes, salmon, chicken breast, ice cream
- 50–59%: Ground beef, pork chop, hot dogs, feta cheese
- 40–49%: Pizza, cheeseburger
- 30–39%: Cheddar cheese, bagels, bread
- 20–29%: Pepperoni sausage, cake, biscuits
- 10–19%: Butter, margarine, raisins
- 1–9%: Crackers, ready-to-eat cereals, peanut butter, nuts
- 0%: Oils, white sugar, meat fats, shortening

about 2000 kcalories a day, this works out to 2 to 3 liters, or about 8 to 12 cups. This recommendation is in line with the Adequate Intake (AI) for *total* water (3.7 liters for men and 2.7 liters for women) set by the DRI committee. Total water includes not only drinking water but also water in other beverages and in foods.

Because a wide range of water intakes will prevent dehydration and its harmful consequences, the AI is based on average intakes. Strenuous physical activity and heat stress can increase water needs considerably, however.[3] In general, you can tell from the color of the urine whether a person needs more water. Pale yellow urine reflects appropriate dilution.

The obvious dietary sources of water are water itself and other beverages, but nearly all foods also contain water. Water constitutes up to 95 percent of the volume of most fruit and vegetables and at least 50 percent of many meats and cheeses (see Table 9-3). The energy nutrients in foods also give up water during metabolism.

Which beverages are best? Any beverage can readily meet the body's fluid needs, but those with few or no kcalories do so without contributing to weight gain. Given that obesity is a major health problem and that beverages contribute more than 20 percent of the total energy intake in the United States, water is the best choice for most people. Other choices include tea, coffee, nonfat and low-fat milk and soy milk, artificially sweetened beverages, fruit and vegetable juices, sports drinks, and, lastly, sweetened nutrient-poor beverages. Carbonated soft drinks are chosen most often but this choice crowds more nutritious beverages out of the diet, and the regular sugar-sweetened varieties provide many empty kcalories from added sugars.

People often ask whether caffeine-containing beverages such as coffee, tea, or soda can help to meet water needs. People who drink caffeinated beverages lose a little more fluid than when they drink water because caffeine acts as a mild diuretic. The DRI committee considered such findings in making its recommendations for water intake and concluded that "caffeinated beverages contribute to the daily total water intake similar to that contributed by non-caffeinated beverages." In other words, it doesn't seem to matter whether people rely on caffeine-containing beverages or other beverages to meet their fluid needs.

In contrast, alcohol should probably not be used to meet fluid needs. As Nutrition in Practice 19 explains, alcohol acts as a diuretic, and it has many adverse effects on health and nutrition status.

Fluid and Electrolyte Balance

When mineral **salts** dissolve in water, they separate (dissociate) into charged particles known as ions, which can conduct electricity. For this reason, a salt that dissociates in water is known as an **electrolyte.*** The body fluids, which contain water and partly dissociated salts, are **electrolyte solutions.**

salts: compounds composed of charged particles (ions). An example of a salt is potassium chloride K^+Cl^-.

electrolyte: a salt that dissolves in water and dissociates into charged particles called ions.

electrolyte solutions: solutions that can conduct electricity.

---

*Exceptions: A compound in which the positive ions are hydrogen ions (H^+) is an acid (example: hydrochloric acid, or H^+Cl^-); a compound in which the negative ions are hydroxyl ions (OH^-) is a base (example: potassium hydroxide, or K^+OH^-).

The body's electrolytes are vital to the life of the cells and therefore must be closely regulated to help maintain the appropriate distribution of body fluids. The major minerals form salts that dissolve in the body fluids; the cells direct where these salts go; and the movement of the salts determines where the fluids flow because water follows salt (see Photo 9-2). Cells use this force, called *osmosis*, to move fluids back and forth across their membranes. Thanks to the electrolytes, water can be held in compartments where it is needed.

Proteins in the cell membranes move ions into or out of the cells. These protein pumps tend to concentrate sodium and chloride outside cells and potassium and other ions inside. By maintaining specific amounts of sodium outside and potassium inside, cells can regulate the exact amounts of water inside and outside their boundaries.

Healthy kidneys regulate the body's sodium, as well as its water, with remarkable precision. The intestinal tract absorbs sodium readily, and it travels freely in the blood, but the kidneys excrete unneeded amounts. The kidneys actually filter all of the sodium out of the blood; then they return to the bloodstream the exact amount the body needs to retain. Thus, the body's total electrolytes remain constant, while the urinary electrolytes fluctuate according to what is eaten.

In some cases, the body's mechanisms for maintaining fluid and electrolyte balances cannot compensate for a sudden loss of large amounts of fluid and electrolytes. Vomiting, diarrhea, heavy sweating, fever, burns, wounds, and the like may incur great fluid and electrolyte losses, precipitating an emergency that demands medical intervention. The body's responses to severe stress and trauma are discussed in Chapter 16.

Photo 9-2

© Craig M. Moore

Water follows salt. Notice the beads of "sweat," formed on the right-hand slices of eggplant, which were sprinkled with salt. Cellular water moves across each cell's membrane (water-permeable divider) toward the higher concentration of salt (dissolved particles) on the surface.

Acid–Base Balance

The body uses ions not only to help maintain water balance but also to regulate the acidity (pH) of its fluids. Like proteins, electrolyte mixtures in the body fluids protect the body against changes in acidity by acting as **buffers**—substances that can accommodate excess acids or bases.

The body's buffer systems serve as a first line of defense against changes in the fluids' acid–base balance. The lungs, skin, gastrointestinal (GI) tract, and kidneys provide other defenses. Of these organ systems, the kidneys play the primary role in maintaining acid–base balance. Thus, disorders of the kidneys impair the body's ability to regulate its acid–base balance, as well as its fluid and electrolyte balances.

Review Notes

- Water makes up about 60 percent of the body's weight.
- Water helps transport nutrients and waste products throughout the body, participates in metabolic reactions, acts as a solvent, assists in maintaining blood volume and body temperature, acts as a lubricant and cushion around joints, and serves as a shock absorber.
- To maintain water balance, intake from liquids, foods, and metabolism must equal losses from the kidneys, skin, lungs, and feces.
- Electrolytes help maintain the appropriate distribution of body fluids and acid–base balance.

buffers: compounds that can reversibly combine with hydrogen ions to help keep a solution's acidity or alkalinity constant.

TABLE 9-4	The Major and Trace Minerals	
MAJOR MINERALS	**TRACE MINERALS**	
Calcium	Chromium	
Chloride	Copper	
Magnesium	Fluoride	
Phosphorus	Iodine	
Potassium	Iron	
Sodium	Manganese	
Sulfur	Molybdenum	
	Selenium	
	Zinc	

9.2 The Major Minerals

Table 9-4 lists the major minerals and the nine essential trace minerals. Other trace minerals are recognized as essential nutrients for some animals but have not been proved to be required for human beings. Figure 9-1 shows the amounts of the major minerals found in the body, and for comparison, some of the trace minerals. As you can see, the most prevalent minerals are calcium and phosphorus, the chief minerals of bone. The distinction between the **major minerals** and the **trace minerals** does not mean that one group is more important than the other. A deficiency of the few micrograms of iodine needed daily is just as serious as a deficiency of the several hundred milligrams of calcium. The major minerals are so named because they are present, and needed, in larger amounts in the body than the trace minerals.

According to the Dietary Guidelines 2015 committee, intakes of the following minerals may fall below recommended intakes—they are shortfall nutrients:

- Calcium (for everyone).
- Magnesium (for everyone).
- Iron (for some people).
- Potassium (for everyone).

In addition, one mineral stands out as being overconsumed by most people:

- Sodium.[4]

Although all the major minerals influence the body's fluid balance, sodium, chloride, and potassium are most noted for that role. For this reason, these three minerals are discussed first. Each major mineral also plays other specific roles in the body. Sodium, potassium, calcium, and magnesium are critical to nerve transmission and muscle contractions. Phosphorus and magnesium are involved in energy metabolism.

FIGURE 9-1	Amounts of Minerals in a 60-Kilogram (132-Pound) Human Body

Not only are the major minerals present in the body in larger amounts than the trace minerals, but they are also needed by the body in large amounts. Recommended intakes for the major minerals are stated in hundreds of milligrams or grams, whereas those for the trace minerals are listed in tens of milligrams or even micrograms.

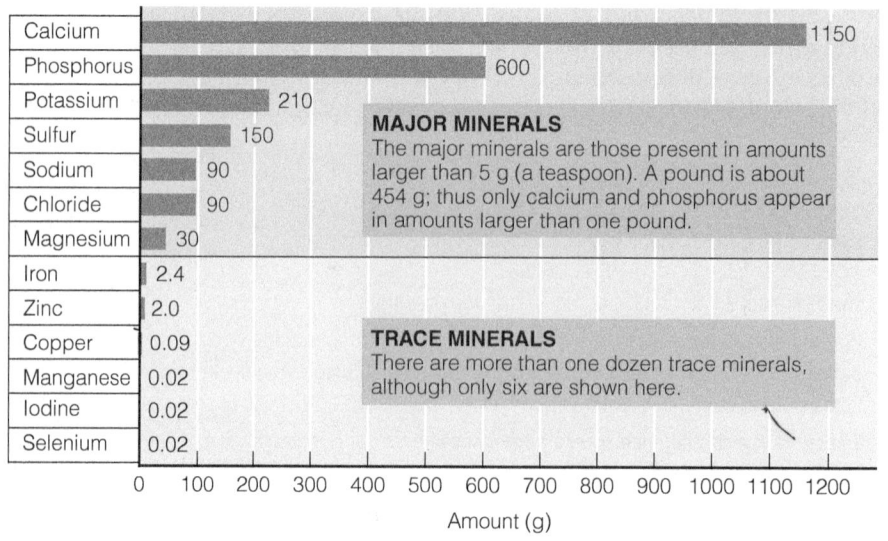

major minerals: essential mineral nutrients required in the adult diet in amounts greater than 100 milligrams per day.

trace minerals: essential mineral nutrients required in the adult diet in amounts less than 100 milligrams per day.

Calcium, phosphorus, and magnesium contribute to the structure of the bones. Sulfur helps determine the shape of proteins. Table 9-8, shown later in the chapter, provides a summary of information about the major minerals.

Sodium

Sodium is the principal electrolyte in the **extracellular fluid** (the fluid outside the cells) and the primary regulator of the extracellular fluid volume. When the blood concentration of sodium rises, as when a person eats salted foods, thirst prompts the person to drink water until the appropriate sodium-to-water ratio is restored. Sodium also helps maintain acid–base balance and is essential to muscle contraction and nerve transmission. Too much sodium, however, can contribute to high blood pressure (hypertension).

Sodium Recommendations and Food Sources Diets rarely lack sodium, and even when intakes are low, the body adapts by reducing sodium losses in urine and sweat, thus making deficiencies unlikely. Sodium recommendations (see the inside front cover) are set low enough to protect against high blood pressure but high enough to allow an adequate intake of other nutrients. Because high sodium intakes correlate with high blood pressure, the Tolerable Upper Intake Level (UL) for adults is set at 2300 milligrams per day—equivalent to about 1 teaspoon of salt (sodium chloride). Nearly 90 percent of the U.S. adult population meets or exceeds this amount daily.[5] The average U.S. sodium intake is more than 3400 milligrams per day.[6] People who need to reduce their blood pressure for the sake of their health are urged to cut their sodium intakes.[7] For example, people with hypertension or prehypertension are advised to take in no more than 1500 milligrams per day because this level of restriction often lowers blood pressure. Even without meeting the recommended levels, reducing sodium by at least 1000 milligrams per day reduces blood pressure. This is a worthy goal—hypertension is a leading cause of death and disability in this country.[8] Box 9-1 offers strategies for cutting salt (and, therefore, sodium) intake.

People who eat mostly processed and fast foods have the highest sodium intakes, whereas those who eat mostly whole, unprocessed foods, such as fresh fruit and vegetables, have the lowest intakes. In fact, about three-fourths of the sodium in people's diets comes from salt added to foods by manufacturers.

Many experts today are calling for reductions of sodium in the food supply to give consumers more low-salt options to choose from, yet manufacturers seem slow to comply.[9]

extracellular fluid: fluid residing outside the cells; includes the fluid between the cells (interstitial fluid), plasma, and the water of structures such as the skin and bones. Extracellular fluid accounts for about one-third of the body's water.

Box 9-1	***HOW TO* Cut Salt Intake**

Strategies to cut salt intake include:

- Select fresh, unprocessed foods.
- Cook with little or no added salt.
- Prepare foods with sodium-free spices such as basil, bay leaves, curry, garlic, ginger, mint, oregano, pepper, rosemary, and thyme; lemon juice; vinegar; or wine.
- Add little or no salt at the table; taste foods before adding salt.
- Read labels with an eye open for sodium. (See Table 1–11 on pp. 28–29 for terms used to describe the sodium contents of foods on labels.)
- Select low-salt or salt-free products when available.

Use these foods sparingly:

- Foods prepared in brine, such as pickles, olives, and sauerkraut.

- Salty or smoked meats, such as bologna, corned or chipped beef, bacon, frankfurters, ham, lunch meats, salt pork, sausage, and smoked tongue.
- Salty or smoked fish, such as anchovies, caviar, salted and dried cod, herring, sardines, and smoked salmon.
- Snack items such as potato chips, pretzels, salted popcorn, salted nuts, and crackers.
- Condiments such as bouillon cubes; seasoned salts; MSG; soy, teriyaki, Worcestershire, and barbeque sauces; prepared horseradish, catsup, and mustard.
- Cheeses, especially processed types.
- Canned and instant soups.

TABLE 9-5	Top Contributors of Sodium in the Diet

- Breads and rolls
- Cold cuts and cured meats
- Pizza
- Fresh and processed poultry
- Soups
- Sandwiches (including cheeseburgers)
- Cheese
- Pasta dishes
- Meat mixtures (including meatloaf)
- Salty snacks (including popcorn, chips, and pretzels)

Reducing the sodium content in processed foods could prevent an estimated 100,000 deaths and save billions in health care costs in the United States annually. Table 9-5 lists the top 10 sodium sources.[10]

Sodium and Blood Pressure High intakes of salt among the world's people correlate with high rates of **hypertension**, heart disease, and stroke.[11] Over time, a high-salt diet may damage the linings of blood vessels in ways that make hypertension likely to develop.[12] In many people, the relationship between salt intake and blood pressure is direct—as chronic sodium intakes increase, blood pressure rises with them in a stepwise fashion.[13] Once hypertension sets in, the risk of death from stroke and heart disease climbs steeply. More than one-third of U.S. adults have hypertension and the rate among African-American adults is one of the highest in the world at 45 percent.[14] An additional 30 percent of U.S. adults have **prehypertension**.

An eating pattern proven to help people to reduce sodium and increase potassium intakes, and thereby often reduce their blood pressure, is DASH (Dietary Approaches to Stop Hypertension).[15] The DASH approach emphasizes potassium-rich fruit and vegetables and fat-free or low-fat milk products; includes whole grains, nuts, poultry, and fish; and calls for reduced intakes of red and processed meats, sweets, and sugar-containing beverages. The DASH diet in combination with a reduced sodium intake is even more effective at lowering blood pressure than either strategy alone (see Chapter 21). Incorporating physical activity provides further benefits because regular moderate exercise reliably lowers blood pressure.

Chloride

The chloride ion is the major negative ion of the extracellular fluids, where it occurs primarily in association with sodium. Like sodium, chloride is critical to maintaining fluid, electrolyte, and acid–base balances in the body. In the stomach, the chloride ion is part of hydrochloric acid, which maintains the strong acidity of the gastric fluids.

Salt is a major food source of chloride, and, as with sodium, processed foods are a major contributor of this mineral to people's diets. Because salt contains a higher proportion of chloride (by weight) than sodium, chloride recommendations are slightly higher than, but still equivalent to, those of sodium. In other words, ¾ teaspoon of salt will deliver some sodium and more chloride, and still meet the AI for both.

Potassium

Outside the body's cells, sodium is the principal positively charged ion. *Inside* the cells, potassium takes the role of the principal positively charged ion. Potassium plays a major role in maintaining fluid and electrolyte balance and cell integrity. During nerve impulse transmission and muscle contraction, potassium and sodium trade places briefly across the cell membrane. The cell then quickly pumps them back into place. Controlling potassium distribution is a high priority for the body because it affects many aspects of homeostasis, including maintaining a steady heartbeat. The sudden deaths that occur with fasting, eating disorders, severe diarrhea, or severe malnutrition in children may be due to heart failure caused by potassium loss.

Potassium Deficiency and Toxicity Potassium deficiency is characterized by an increase in blood pressure, kidney stones, and bone turnover. As deficiency progresses, symptoms include irregular heartbeats, muscle weakness, and glucose intolerance. Potassium deficiency results more often from excessive losses than from deficient intakes. Deficiency arises in abnormal conditions such as diabetic acidosis, dehydration, or prolonged vomiting or diarrhea; potassium deficiency can also result from the regular use of certain medications, including **diuretics**, **steroids**, and **cathartics**.

hypertension: high blood pressure.

prehypertension: blood pressure values that predict hypertension.

diuretics (dye-yoo-RET-ics): medications that promote the excretion of water through the kidneys. Some diuretics increase the urinary loss of potassium; others, called potassium-sparing diuretics, are less likely to result in a potassium deficiency (see Chapter 21).

steroids (STARE-oids): medications used to reduce tissue inflammation, to suppress the immune response, or to replace certain steroid hormones in people who cannot synthesize them.

cathartics (ca-THART-ics): strong laxatives.

Potassium toxicity does not result from overeating foods high in potassium; therefore, a UL was not set. Toxicity can result from overconsumption of potassium salts or supplements and from certain diseases or medications. Given more potassium than the body needs, the kidneys accelerate their excretion. If the GI tract is bypassed, however, and potassium is injected directly into a vein, it can stop the heart.

Potassium Recommendations and Food Sources In healthy people, almost any reasonable diet provides enough potassium to prevent the dangerously low blood potassium that indicates a severe deficiency. Potassium is abundant inside all living cells, both plant and animal, and because cells remain intact until foods are processed, the richest sources of potassium are *fresh* foods of all kinds—especially fruit and vegetables (see Figure 9-2). A typical U.S. eating pattern, however, is low in fruit and vegetables and provides far less potassium than the recommended intake.[16] Although blood potassium may remain normal on such a diet, chronic diseases are more likely to occur.

Potassium and Hypertension Low potassium intakes, especially when combined with high sodium intakes, raise blood pressure and increase the risk of death from stroke.[17] Higher intakes of dietary potassium may or may not lower blood pressure, but diets with ample potassium are associated with a reduced risk of cardiovascular disease and stroke.[18] These effects, along with low U.S. consumption earn potassium its status as a Dietary Guidelines nutrient of public health concern.[19] Recall that the DASH eating pattern described earlier emphasizes potassium-rich foods such as fruit and vegetables.

Calcium

Calcium occupies more space in this chapter than any other major mineral. Other minerals with key roles in heart disease and kidney disease are revisited later in this book, but calcium deserves emphasis here because an adequate intake of calcium early in life helps grow a healthy skeleton and prevent bone disease in later life.

Calcium Roles in the Body Calcium is the most abundant mineral in the body. Ninety-nine percent of the body's calcium is stored in the bones (and teeth), where it plays two important roles. First, it is an integral part of bone structure. Second, it serves as a calcium bank available to the body fluids should a drop in blood calcium occur.

Calcium in Bone As bones begin to form, calcium salts form crystals on a matrix of the protein collagen. As the crystals become denser, they give strength and rigidity to the maturing bones. As a result, the long leg bones of children can support their weight by the time they have learned to walk. Figure 9-3 shows the lacy network of calcium-containing crystals in the bone.

Many people have the idea that bones are inert, like rocks. Not so. Bones continuously gain and lose minerals in an ongoing process of remodeling. Growing children gain more bone than they lose, and healthy

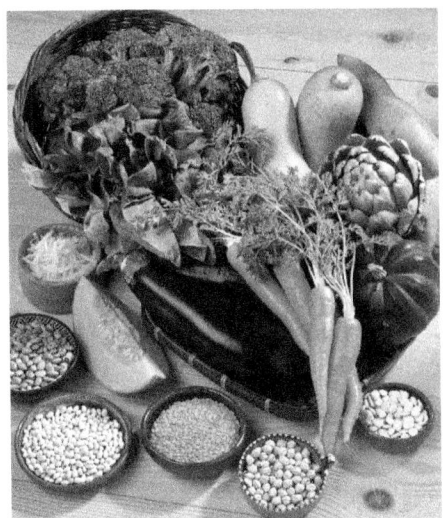
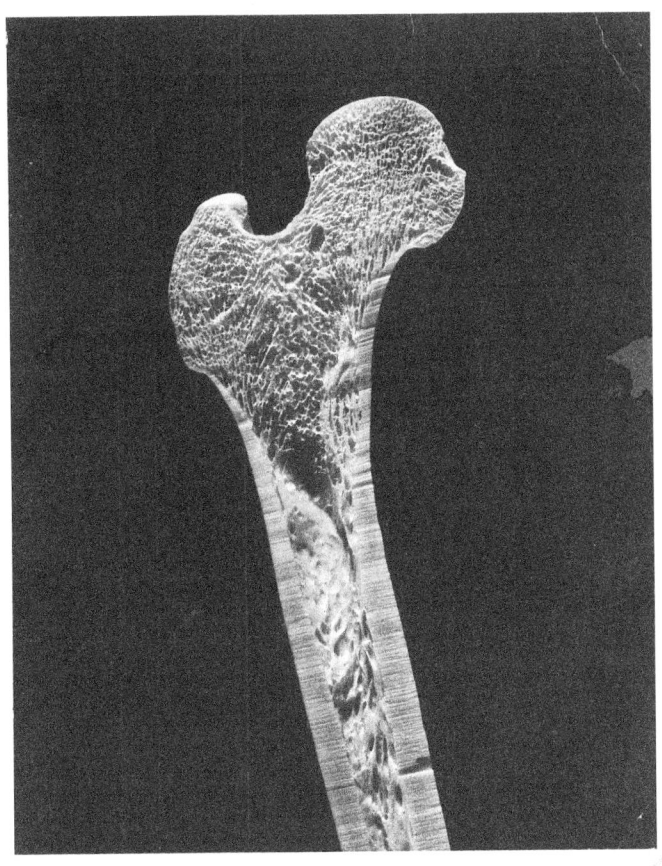

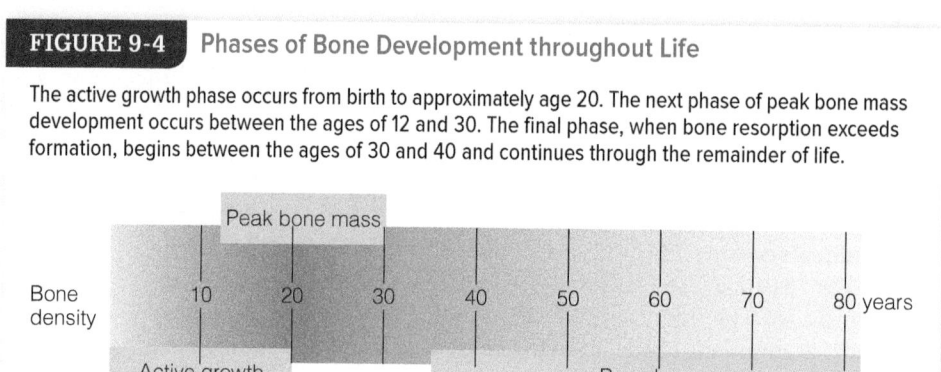

FIGURE 9-4 Phases of Bone Development throughout Life

The active growth phase occurs from birth to approximately age 20. The next phase of peak bone mass development occurs between the ages of 12 and 30. The final phase, when bone resorption exceeds formation, begins between the ages of 30 and 40 and continues through the remainder of life.

adults maintain a reasonable balance. When withdrawals substantially exceed deposits, however, problems such as osteoporosis develop.

From birth to approximately age 20, the bones are actively growing by modifying their length, width, and shape (see Figure 9-4). This rapid growth phase overlaps with the next period of peak bone mass development, which occurs between the ages of 12 and 30. During this period, skeletal mass increases. Bones grow thicker and denser by remodeling, a maintenance and repair process involving the loss of existing bone and the deposition of new bone. In the final phase, which begins between 30 and 40 years of age and continues throughout the remainder of life, bone loss exceeds new bone formation.

Calcium in Body Fluids The 1 percent of the body's calcium that circulates in the fluids as ionized calcium is vital to life. It plays these major roles:

- Regulates the transport of ions across cell membranes and is particularly important in nerve transmission.
- Helps maintain normal blood pressure.
- Plays an essential role in the clotting of blood.
- Is essential for muscle contraction and therefore for the heartbeat.
- Allows secretion of hormones, digestive enzymes, and neurotransmitters.
- Activates cellular enzymes that regulate many processes.

Because of its importance, blood calcium is tightly controlled.

Calcium Balance Whenever blood calcium rises too high, a system of hormones, including vitamin D, promotes its deposit into bone.* Whenever blood calcium falls too low, the regulatory system acts in three locations to raise it: (1) the small intestine absorbs more calcium; (2) the bones release more calcium into the blood; and (3) the kidneys excrete less calcium.[20] Thus, blood calcium rises to normal.

The calcium stored in bone provides a nearly inexhaustible source of calcium for the blood. Even in a calcium deficiency, blood calcium remains normal. Blood calcium changes only in response to abnormal regulatory control. Thus, a chronic deficiency of calcium due to a low dietary intake or poor absorption does not change blood calcium, but does deplete the calcium in the bones. To restate: it is the bones, not the blood, that are robbed by calcium deficiency.

Calcium and Osteoporosis As mentioned earlier, bone mass peaks at the time of skeletal maturity (about age 30), and a high peak bone mass is the best protection against later age-related bone loss and fracture. Adequate calcium nutrition during the growing years is essential to achieving optimal peak bone mass.[21] Following menopause, women may lose up to 20 percent of their bone mass, as may middle-aged and

*The regulators are hormones from the thyroid and parathyroid glands, as well as vitamin D. One hormone, parathormone, raises blood calcium. Another hormone, calcitonin, lowers blood calcium by inhibiting release of calcium from bone.

TABLE 9-6	Risk Factors for Osteoporosis	
NONMODIFIABLE	**MODIFIABLE**	
• Female gender	• Sedentary lifestyle	
• Older age	• Diet inadequate in calcium and vitamin D	
• Small frame	• Diet excessive in sodium, caffeine	
• Caucasian, Asian, or Hispanic/Latino heritage	• Cigarette smoking	
• Family history of osteoporosis or fractures	• Alcohol abuse	
• Personal history of fractures	• Low body weight	
• Estrogen deficiency in women (amenorrhea or menopause, especially early or surgically induced); testosterone deficiency in men	• Certain medications, such as glucocorticoids and anticonvulsants	

older men. When bone loss has reached such an extreme that bones fracture under even common, everyday stresses, the condition is known as **osteoporosis**. In the United States well over half of all adults 50 years of age and older—most of them women—have or are developing osteoporosis.[22] Men, however, are not immune to osteoporosis. Each year, 2 million people break a hip, leg, arm, hand, ankle, or other bone as a result of osteoporosis. Both men and women are urged to do whatever they can to prevent fractures related to osteoporosis.

Both genetic and environmental factors contribute to osteoporosis; Table 9-6 summarizes these risk factors. Osteoporosis is more prevalent in women than in men for several reasons. First, women consume less dietary calcium than men do. Second, at all ages, women's bone mass is lower than men's because women generally have smaller bodies. Finally, women often lose more bone, particularly in the 6 to 8 years following menopause when the hormone estrogen diminishes.[23]

In addition to calcium, many other minerals and vitamins, including phosphorus, magnesium, vitamin K, and vitamin D, help to form and stabilize the structure of bones. Any or all of these elements are needed to prevent bone loss. The first, most obvious lines of defense, however, are to maintain a lifelong adequate intake of calcium and to "exercise it into place." Physical activity supports bone growth during adolescence and may protect the bones later on.[24] Weight-bearing physical activity, such as walking, running, dancing, and weight training, prompts the bones to deposit minerals. It has long been known that, when people are confined to bed, both their muscles and their bones lose strength. Muscle strength and bone strength go together: when muscles work, they pull on the bones, and both are stimulated to grow stronger.

Calcium Recommendations As mentioned earlier, blood calcium concentration does not reflect calcium status. Calcium recommendations are therefore based on balance studies, which measure daily intake and excretion. An optimal calcium intake reflects the amount needed to retain the most calcium. The more calcium retained, the greater the bone density (within genetic limits) and, potentially, the lower the risk of osteoporosis. Calcium recommendations during adolescence are set high (1300 milligrams) to help ensure that the skeleton will be strong and dense. Between the ages of 19 and 50, recommendations are lowered slightly, and for women over age 50 and all adults over age 70, recommendations are raised again to minimize bone loss. Many people in the United States have calcium intakes well below current recommendations. The relationship between low calcium intakes and risks for osteoporosis led the Dietary Guidelines committee to designate calcium a nutrient of public health concern. Findings about the effectiveness of calcium supplements in reducing fractures in older women, however, are inconclusive or negative. Because adverse effects such as kidney stone formation are possible with high supplemental doses, a UL has been established (see inside front cover).

osteoporosis (os-tee-oh-pore-OH-sis): literally, porous bones; reduced density of the bones, also known as *adult bone loss*.

TABLE 9-7	Suggested Minimum Daily Fluid Milk Intakes	
Young children (4–8 years of age)		2½ cups
Older children and adolescents		3 cups
Adults		3 cups
Pregnant or lactating women		3 cups
Women past menopause		3 cups

Calcium in Foods Calcium is found most abundantly in a single food group—milk and milk products. For this reason, dietary recommendations advise daily consumption of low-fat or fat-free milk products. A cup of milk offers about 300 milligrams of calcium, so an adult who drinks 3 cups of milk a day (or eats the equivalent in yogurt) is well on the way to meeting daily calcium needs (see Table 9-7). The other dairy food that contains comparable amounts of calcium is cheese. One slice of cheese (1 ounce) contains about two-thirds as much calcium as a cup of milk. Cottage cheese, however, contains much less. Figure 9-5 shows foods that are rich in calcium, and Box 9-2 suggests ways of adding calcium to meals.

Some foods offer large amounts of calcium because of fortification. Calcium-fortified juice, high-calcium milk (milk with extra calcium added), and calcium-fortified cereals are examples. Some calcium-rich mineral waters may also be a useful source, providing calcium that may be as absorbable as that from milk but accompanied by zero kcalories.

Among the vegetables, beet greens, bok choy (a Chinese cabbage), broccoli, kale, mustard greens, rutabaga, and turnip greens provide some available calcium. So do collard greens, green cabbage, kohlrabi, parsley, and watercress. Some dark green, leafy vegetables—notably, spinach and Swiss chard—appear to be calcium rich but actually provide very little, if any, calcium to the body. These foods contain **binders** that prevent calcium absorption. Aided by vitamin D, the body is able to regulate its absorption of calcium by altering its production of the calcium-binding protein. More of this protein is made if more calcium is needed. Infants and children absorb up to 60 percent of the calcium they ingest, and pregnant women, about 50 percent. Other adults, who are not growing, absorb about 20 to 30 percent.[25]

People may think that taking a calcium supplement is preferable to getting calcium from food, but foods offer important fringe benefits. For example, drinking 3 cups of milk fortified with vitamins A and D will supply substantial amounts of other nutrients. Furthermore, the vitamin D and possibly other nutrients in the milk enhance calcium absorption. Some people absorb calcium better from milk and milk products than from even the most absorbable supplements. The National Institutes of Health concludes that foods are the best sources of calcium and recommends supplements only when intake from food is insufficient.

binders: chemical compounds in foods that combine with nutrients (especially minerals) to form complexes the body cannot absorb. Examples include *phytates* and *oxalates*.

FIGURE 9-5 Good Sources of Calcium[a]

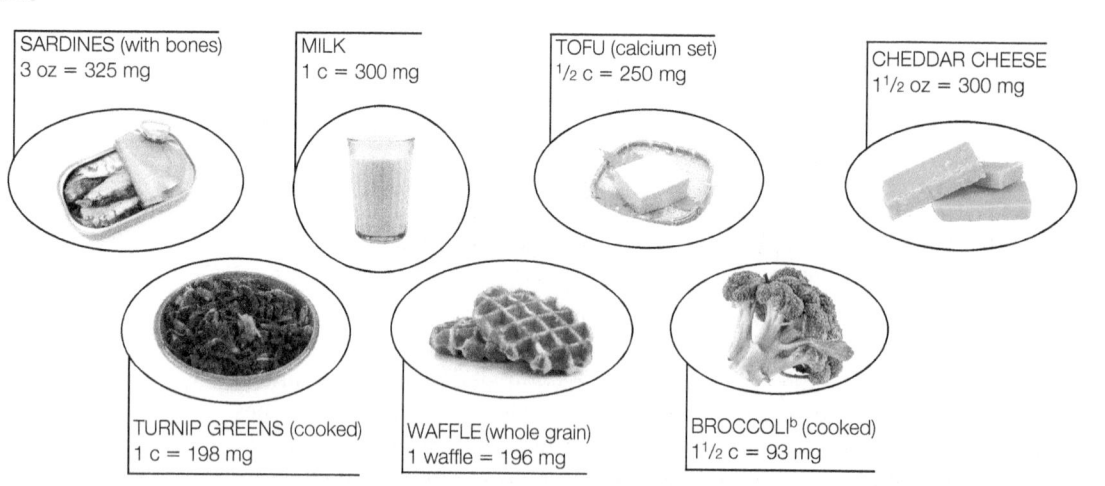

SARDINES (with bones)
3 oz = 325 mg

MILK
1 c = 300 mg

TOFU (calcium set)
½ c = 250 mg

CHEDDAR CHEESE
1½ oz = 300 mg

TURNIP GREENS (cooked)
1 c = 198 mg

WAFFLE (whole grain)
1 waffle = 196 mg

BROCCOLI[b] (cooked)
1½ c = 93 mg

[a]These foods provide 10 percent or more of the calcium Daily Value in a serving. For a 2000-kcalorie diet, the DV is 1300 mg/day.
[b]Broccoli, kale, and some other cooked green leafy vegetables are important sources of bioavailable calcium. Almonds also supply calcium.
Other greens, such as spinach and chard, contain calcium in an unabsorbable form. Some calcium-rich mineral waters may also be good sources.

Box 9-2 *HOW TO* Add Calcium to Daily Meals

For those who tolerate milk, many cooks slip extra calcium into meals by sprinkling a tablespoon or two of fat-free dry milk into almost everything. The added kcalorie value is small, and changes to the taste and texture of the dish are practically nil. Yet each 2 tablespoons adds about 100 extra milligrams of calcium and moves people closer to meeting the recommendation to obtain 3 cups of milk each day. Here are some more tips for including calcium-rich foods in your meals.

At Breakfast

- Choose calcium-fortified orange or vegetable juice.
- Serve tea or coffee, hot or iced, with milk.
- Choose cereals, hot or cold, with milk.
- Cook hot cereals with milk instead of water; then mix in 2 table-spoons of fat-free dry milk.
- Make muffins or quick breads with milk and extra fat-free powdered milk.
- Add milk to scrambled eggs.
- Moisten cereals with flavored yogurt.

At Lunch

- Add low-fat cheeses to sandwiches, burgers, or salads.
- Use a variety of green vegetables, such as watercress or kale, in salads and on sandwiches.
- Drink fat-free milk or calcium-fortified soy milk as a beverage or in a smoothie.

- Drink calcium-rich mineral water as a beverage (studies suggest significant calcium absorption).
- Marinate cabbage shreds or broccoli spears in low-fat Italian dressing for an interesting salad that provides calcium.
- Choose coleslaw over potato and macaroni salads.
- Mix the mashed bones of canned salmon into salmon salad or patties.
- Eat sardines with their bones.
- Stuff potatoes with broccoli and low-fat cheese.
- Try pasta such as ravioli stuffed with low-fat ricotta cheese instead of meat.
- Sprinkle Parmesan cheese on pasta salads.

At Dinner

- Toss a handful of thinly sliced green vegetables, such as kale or young turnip greens, with hot pasta; the greens wilt pleasingly in the steam of the freshly cooked pasta.
- Serve a green vegetable every night and try new ones—how about kohlrabi? It tastes delicious when cooked like broccoli.
- Learn to stir-fry Chinese cabbage and other Asian foods.
- Try tofu (the calcium-set kind); this versatile food has inspired whole cookbooks devoted to creative uses.
- Add fat-free powdered milk to almost anything—meatloaf, sauces, gravies, soups, stuffings, casseroles, blended beverages, puddings, quick breads, cookies, brownies. Be creative.
- Choose frozen yogurt, ice milk, or custards for dessert.

Phosphorus

Phosphorus is the second most abundant mineral in the body. About 85 percent of the body's phosphorus is found combined with calcium in the crystals of the bones and teeth. As part of one of the body's buffer systems (phosphoric acid), phosphorus is also found in all body tissues. Phosphorus is a part of DNA and RNA, the genetic material present in every cell. Thus, phosphorus is necessary for all growth. Phosphorus also plays many key roles in the transfer of energy that occurs during cellular metabolism. Phosphorus-containing lipids (phospholipids) help transport other lipids in the blood. Phospholipids are also principal components of cell membranes.

Animal protein is the best source of phosphorus because the mineral is so abundant in the cells of animals. Milk and cheese are also rich sources. Diets that provide adequate energy and protein also supply adequate phosphorus. Dietary deficiencies are rare. A summary of facts about phosphorus appears in Table 9-8 later in the chapter.

Magnesium

Magnesium barely qualifies as a major mineral. Only about 1 ounce of magnesium is present in the body of a 130-pound person, more than half of it in the bones. Most of the rest is in the muscles, heart, liver, and other soft tissues, with only 1 percent in the body fluids. Bone magnesium seems to be a reservoir to ensure that some will be on hand for vital reactions regardless of recent dietary intake.

Magnesium is critical to the operation of hundreds of enzymes and other cellular functions.[26] It acts in all the cells of the soft tissues, where it forms part of the protein-making machinery and is necessary for the release of energy. Magnesium and calcium work together for proper functioning of the muscles: calcium promotes contraction, and magnesium helps relax the muscles afterward. Magnesium is also critical to normal heart function.[27]

Magnesium Deficiency Average magnesium intakes typically fall below recommendations, and a chronically low intake may worsen inflammation and potentially contribute to heart failure, stroke, hypertension, and diabetes.[28] The Dietary Guidelines 2015 committee names magnesium among shortfall nutrients for the U.S. population.

An acute magnesium deficiency may occur with prolonged, vomiting, diarrhea, alcohol abuse, or severe malnutrition; in people who have been fed nutritionally incomplete fluids intravenously for too long after surgery; or in people using diuretics. Magnesium deficiency symptoms include a low blood calcium level, muscle cramps, and seizures. Magnesium deficiency is thought to cause the hallucinations commonly experienced during withdrawal from alcohol intoxication.

Magnesium Toxicity Magnesium toxicity is rare, but it can be fatal. Toxicity occurs only with high intakes from nonfood sources such as supplements or magnesium salts. Accidental poisonings may occur in children with access to medicine cabinets and in older adults who abuse magnesium-containing laxatives, antacids, and other medications. The consequences include diarrhea, abdominal cramps, and, in severe cases, acid–base imbalance and potassium depletion.

Magnesium Recommendations and Food Sources Magnesium recommendations vary only slightly among adult age groups; see the inside front cover. In some areas of the country, the water naturally contains both calcium and magnesium. This so-called "hard" water can contribute significantly to magnesium intakes.

Magnesium-rich food sources include dark green, leafy vegetables; nuts; legumes; whole-grain breads and cereals; seafood; chocolate; and cocoa (see Figure 9-6). Magnesium is easily lost from foods during processing, so unprocessed foods are the best choices.

FIGURE 9-6 Good Sources of Magnesium[a]

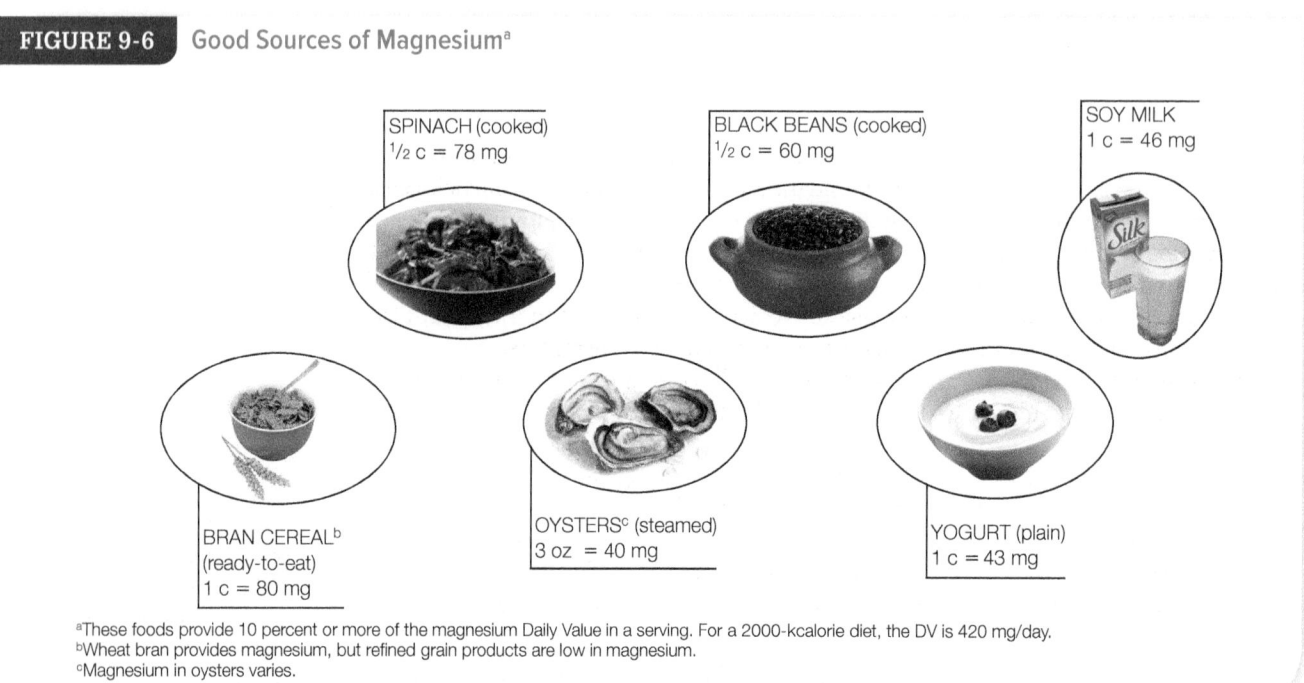

SPINACH (cooked)
½ c = 78 mg

BLACK BEANS (cooked)
½ c = 60 mg

SOY MILK
1 c = 46 mg

BRAN CEREAL[b]
(ready-to-eat)
1 c = 80 mg

OYSTERS[c] (steamed)
3 oz = 40 mg

YOGURT (plain)
1 c = 43 mg

[a]These foods provide 10 percent or more of the magnesium Daily Value in a serving. For a 2000-kcalorie diet, the DV is 420 mg/day.
[b]Wheat bran provides magnesium, but refined grain products are low in magnesium.
[c]Magnesium in oysters varies.

Sulfate

Sulfate is the oxidized form of sulfur as it exists in foods and water. The body requires sulfate for the synthesis of many important sulfur-containing compounds. Sulfur-containing amino acids play an important role in helping to shape strands of protein.* The particular shape of a protein enables it to do its specific job, such as enzyme work. Skin, hair, and nails contain some of the body's more rigid proteins, which have high sulfur contents.

There is no recommended intake for sulfur, and no deficiencies are known. Only a person who lacks protein to the point of severe deficiency will lack the sulfur-containing amino acids.

Review Notes

- All of the major minerals influence the body's fluid balance, but sodium, chloride, and potassium are most noted for this role.
- Excess sodium in the diet contributes to high blood pressure.
- Most of the body's calcium is in the bones, where it provides a rigid structure and a reservoir of calcium for the blood.
- Magnesium is critical to the operation of hundreds of enzymes and other cellular functions.

Table 9-8 offers a summary of the major minerals and their functions.

9.3 The Trace Minerals

Figure 9-1, earlier in this chapter, shows how tiny the quantities of trace minerals in the human body are. If you could remove all of them from your body, you would have only a bit of dust, hardly enough to fill a teaspoon. Yet each of the trace minerals performs some vital role for which no substitute will do. A deficiency of any of them can be fatal, and an excess of many can be equally deadly. Table 9-9, at the end of the chapter, provides a summary of the trace minerals.

Iron

Every living cell—both plant and animal—contains iron. Most of the iron in the body is a component of the proteins **hemoglobin** in red blood cells and **myoglobin** in muscle cells. The iron in both hemoglobin and myoglobin helps them carry and hold oxygen and then release it. Hemoglobin in the blood carries oxygen from the lungs to tissues throughout the body. Myoglobin holds oxygen for the muscles to use when they contract. As part of many enzymes, iron is vital to the processes by which cells generate energy. Iron is also needed to make new cells, amino acids, hormones, and neurotransmitters.

The special provisions the body makes for iron's handling show that it is a precious mineral to be tightly hoarded. For example, when a red blood cell dies, the liver saves the iron and returns it to the bone marrow, which uses it to build new red blood cells. The body does lose iron from the digestive tract, in nail and hair trimmings, and in shed skin cells, but only in tiny amounts. Bleeding, however, can cause significant iron loss from the body.

Special measures are needed to maintain an appropriate iron balance in the body. Iron is a powerful oxidant that generates free-radical reactions. Free radicals increase oxidative stress and inflammation associated with diseases such as diabetes, heart

hemoglobin: the oxygen-carrying protein of the red blood cells.

hemo = blood
globin = globular protein

myoglobin: the oxygen-carrying protein of the muscle cells.

myo = muscle

---

*The sulfur-containing amino acids are methionine and cysteine. Cysteine in one part of a protein chain can bind to cysteine in another part of the chain by way of a sulfur-sulfur bridge, thus helping to stabilize the protein structure.

TABLE 9-8 The Major Minerals: A Summary

MINERAL NAME	CHIEF FUNCTIONS IN THE BODY	DEFICIENCY SYMPTOMS	TOXICITY SYMPTOMS	SIGNIFICANT SOURCES
Sodium	With chloride and potassium (electrolytes), maintains cells' normal fluid balance and acid–base balance in the body. Also critical to nerve impulse transmission and muscle contraction.	Muscle cramps, mental apathy, loss of appetite	Hypertension	Salt, soy sauce, processed foods
Chloride	Part of the hydrochloric acid found in the stomach and necessary for proper digestion.	Does not occur under normal circumstances	Normally harmless (the gas chlorine is a poison but evaporates from water); can cause vomiting	Salt, soy sauce; moderate quantities in whole, unprocessed foods; large amounts in processed foods
Potassium	Facilitates reactions, including the making of protein; the maintenance of fluid and electrolyte balance; the support of cell integrity; the transmission of nerve impulses; and the contraction of muscles, including the heart.	Moderate deficiency: elevated blood pressure, increased salt sensitivity, increased risk of kidney stones, increased bone turnover. Severe deficiency: cardiac arrhythmias, muscle weakness, glucose intolerance.	Causes muscular weakness; triggers vomiting; if given into a vein, can stop the heart	All whole foods: meats, milk, fruit, vegetables, grains, legumes
Calcium	The principal mineral of bones and teeth. Also acts in normal muscle contraction and relaxation, nerve functioning, blood clotting, blood pressure, and immune defenses.	Stunted growth in children; adult bone loss (osteoporosis)	Constipation; increased risk of urinary stone formation and kidney dysfunction; interference with absorption of other minerals	Milk and milk products, oysters, small fish (with bones), tofu (bean curd), greens, legumes
Phosphorus	Involved in the mineralization of bones and teeth. Important in cells' genetic material, in cell membranes as phospholipids, in energy transfer, and in buffering systems.	Phosphorus deficiency unknown	Calcification of nonskeletal tissues, particularly the kidneys	Foods from animal sources (meat, fish, poultry, eggs, milk)
Magnesium	Another factor involved in bone mineralization, the building of protein, enzyme action, normal muscular contraction, and transmission of nerve impulses.	Low blood calcium; muscle cramps; confusion; if extreme, seizures, bizarre movements, hallucinations, and difficulty in swallowing; in children, growth failure.	From nonfood sources only; diarrhea, nausea, and abdominal cramps; acid–base imbalance; potassium depletion	Nuts, legumes, whole grains, dark green vegetables, seafoods, chocolate, cocoa
Sulfate	A component of certain amino acids; part of the vitamins biotin and thiamin and the hormone insulin; stabilizes protein shape by forming sulfur-sulfur bridges.	None known; protein deficiency would occur first	Would occur only if sulfur amino acids were eaten in excess; this (in animals) depresses growth	All protein-containing foods (meats, fish, poultry, eggs, milk, legumes, nuts)

disease, and cancer.[29] To ensure that enough iron is available to meet the body's needs and yet guard against excessive and damaging levels, special proteins transport and store the body's iron supply, and its absorption is tightly regulated.[30] Because the body has no active means of excreting excess iron, regulation of absorption plays a critical role in iron homeostasis.[31]

Normally, only about 10 to 15 percent of dietary iron is absorbed, but if the body's supply is diminished or if the need increases for any reason (such as pregnancy), absorption increases. The body makes several provisions for absorbing iron. A special protein in the intestinal cells captures iron and holds it in reserve for release into the body as needed; another protein transfers the iron to **transferrin**, an iron carrier in the blood. Transferrin carries the iron to tissues throughout the body. When more iron is needed, more of these proteins are produced so that more than the usual amount of iron can be absorbed and carried. If there is a surplus, iron storage proteins—ferritin and hemosiderin—in the liver, bone marrow, and other organs store it.

Researchers are discovering genes that participate in the regulation of the body's iron at an extraordinary pace. Along the way, new information about how the body controls the uptake, storage, and distribution of iron is emerging. The hormone **hepcidin**, produced by the liver, is central to the regulation of iron balance.[32] Hepcidin helps to maintain blood iron within the normal range by limiting absorption from the small intestine and controlling release from the liver, spleen, and bone marrow. Many details are known about this process, but simply described, hepcidin works in an elegant feedback system to control blood iron: Elevated levels of iron in the blood (and liver) trigger hepcidin secretion, which reduces iron absorption and inhibits the release of stored iron, thereby reducing the blood iron concentration. Low levels of iron in the blood suppress hepcidin secretion, which increases iron absorption and mobilizes storage iron, raising the blood iron concentrations. Thus, the body adjusts to changing iron needs and iron availability in the diet.[33]

Iron Deficiency Worldwide, **iron deficiency** is the most common nutrient deficiency, with **iron-deficiency anemia** affecting 2 billion people—mostly preschool children and pregnant women.[34] In the United States, iron deficiency is less prevalent, but it still affects about 10 percent of toddlers, adolescent girls, and women of childbearing age. Iron deficiency is also relatively common among those who are overweight.[35] The association between iron deficiency and obesity has yet to be explained, but researchers are currently examining the relationships between the inflammation that develops with excess body fat and reduced iron absorption.[36]

Some stages of life demand more iron but provide less, making deficiency likely. Women are especially prone to iron deficiency during their reproductive years because of blood losses during menstruation. Pregnancy places further iron demands on women: iron is needed to support the added blood volume, the growth of the fetus, and blood loss during childbirth. Infants (six months or older) and young children receive little iron from their high-milk diets, yet they need extra iron to support their rapid growth and brain development. The rapid growth of adolescence, especially for males, and the blood losses of menstruation for females also demand extra iron that a typical teen diet may not provide. To summarize, an adequate iron intake is especially important for women in their reproductive years, pregnant women, infants, toddlers, and adolescents.

Causes of Iron Deficiency The cause of iron deficiency is usually inadequate intake resulting from iron-poor food choices or a sheer lack of food altogether. In the Western world, high sugar and fat intakes are often associated with low iron intakes. Blood loss is the primary nonnutritional cause, especially in poor regions of the world where parasitic infections of the GI tract may lead to blood loss.

Assessment of Iron Deficiency Iron deficiency develops in three stages that can be identified using laboratory tests (Appendix E provides more details). In the first stage of iron deficiency both iron stores and ferritin levels diminish. Measures of serum ferritin (in the blood) reflect iron stores and are most valuable in assessing iron status at this earliest stage.

transferrin (trans-FERR-in): the body's iron-carrying protein.

hepcidin (HEP-sid-in): a hormone secreted by the liver in response to elevated blood iron. Hepcidin reduces iron's absorption from the intestine and its release from storage.

iron deficiency: the condition of having depleted iron stores.

iron-deficiency anemia: a blood iron deficiency characterized by small, pale red blood cells; also called *microcytic hypochromic anemia*.

> micro = small
> cytic = cells
> hypo = too little
> chrom = color

The second stage of iron deficiency is characterized by a decrease in transport iron: levels of serum iron fall, and levels of the iron-carrying protein transferrin *increase* (an adaptation that enhances iron absorption). Together, these two measures can determine the severity of the deficiency—the more transferrin and the less iron in the blood, the more advanced the deficiency is. Transferrin saturation—the percentage of transferrin that is saturated with iron—decreases as iron stores decline.

The third stage of iron deficiency occurs when the lack of iron limits hemoglobin production. Now the hemoglobin precursor, **erythrocyte protoporphyrin**, begins to accumulate as hemoglobin and **hematocrit** values decline.

Hemoglobin and hematocrit tests are easy, quick, and inexpensive, so they are the tests most commonly used in evaluating iron status. Their usefulness is limited, however, because they are late indicators of iron deficiency. Furthermore, other nutrient deficiencies and medical conditions can influence their values.

Iron Deficiency and Anemia Iron deficiency and iron-deficiency anemia are not the same: people may be iron deficient without being anemic. The term *iron deficiency* refers to depleted body iron stores without regard to the degree of depletion or to the presence of anemia. The term *iron-deficiency anemia* refers to the severe depletion of iron stores that results in a low hemoglobin concentration. In iron-deficiency anemia, red blood cells are pale and small (see Figure 9-7). They can't carry enough oxygen from the lungs to the tissues. Without adequate iron, energy metabolism in the cells falters. The result is fatigue, weakness, headaches, apathy, pallor, and poor resistance to cold temperatures. Because hemoglobin is the bright red pigment of the blood, the skin of a fair person who is anemic may become noticeably pale. In a dark-skinned person, the tongue and eye lining, normally pink, will be very pale.

The fatigue that accompanies iron-deficiency anemia differs from the tiredness a person experiences from a simple lack of sleep. People with anemia feel fatigue only when they exert themselves. Iron supplementation can, over time, relieve the fatigue and improve the body's response to physical activity.

Less severe iron deficiency produces symptoms, too. Long before the red blood cells are affected and anemia is diagnosed, a developing iron deficiency affects behavior.[37] Even at slightly lowered iron levels, energy metabolism is impaired and neurotransmitter synthesis is altered, reducing physical work capacity and mental productivity. Without the physical energy and mental alertness to work, plan, think, play, sing, or learn, people simply do these things less. They have no obvious deficiency signs; they just appear unmotivated, apathetic, and less physically fit. Children deprived of iron become irritable, restless, and unable to pay attention (see Chapter 11). These symptoms are among the first to appear when the body's iron begins to fall and among the first to disappear when iron status is restored.

FIGURE 9-7 Normal and Anemic Blood Cells

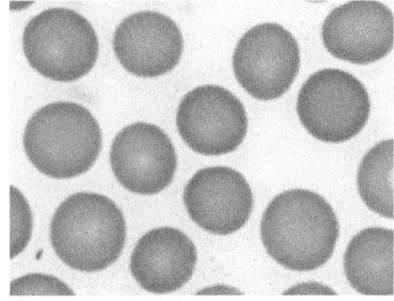

Well-nourished red blood cells. Both size and color are normal.

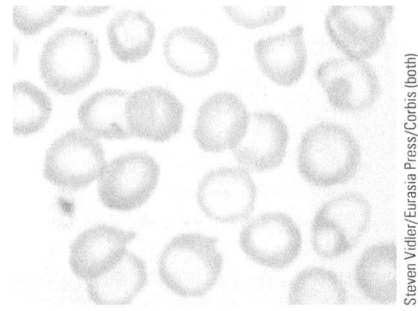

Blood cells in iron-deficiency anemia. These cells are small and pale because they contain less hemoglobin.

Steven Vidler/Eurasia Press/Corbis (both)

erythrocyte protoporphyrin (PRO-toh-PORE-fe-rin): a precursor to hemoglobin.

hematocrit (hee-MAT-oh-crit): measurement of the volume of the red blood cells packed by centrifuge in a given volume of blood.

Iron Deficiency and Pica A curious behavior seen in some iron-deficient (and sometimes zinc-deficient) people, especially in women and children of low-income groups, is **pica**—the craving for and consumption of ice, chalk, starch, and other nonfood substances. These substances contain no iron and cannot remedy a deficiency; in fact, clay actually inhibits iron absorption, which may explain the iron deficiency that accompanies such behavior. Pica is poorly understood. Its cause is unknown, but researchers hypothesize that it may be motivated by hunger, nutrient deficiencies, or an attempt to protect against toxins or microbes.

Caution on Self-Diagnosis Low hemoglobin may reflect an inadequate iron intake, and, if it does, the physician may prescribe iron supplements. Any nutrient deficiency, disease, or agent that interferes with hemoglobin synthesis, disrupts hemoglobin function, or causes a loss of red blood cells can precipitate anemia, however. Thus, feeling fatigued, weak, and apathetic is a sign that something is wrong and that a person should consult a physician, not an indication that he or she should take supplements. In fact, iron supplements can mask a serious medical condition, such as hidden bleeding from cancer or an ulcer. Furthermore, a person can waste precious time by not seeking treatment. Remember, don't self-diagnose.

Iron Overload As mentioned earlier, because too much iron can be toxic, its levels in the body are closely regulated and absorption normally decreases when iron stores are full. Even a diet that includes fortified foods usually poses no risk for most people, but some people are vulnerable to excess iron. Once considered rare, **iron overload** has emerged as an important disorder of iron metabolism and regulation.

Iron overload, known as **hemochromatosis**, is usually caused by a genetic failure to prevent unneeded iron in the diet from being absorbed. Research suggests that just as insulin supports normal glucose homeostasis, and its absence or ineffectiveness causes diabetes, the hormone hepcidin supports iron homeostasis and a deficiency causes hemochromatosis.[38] Other causes of iron overload include repeated blood transfusions, massive doses of supplementary iron, and other rare metabolic disorders.

Some of the signs and symptoms of iron overload are similar to those of iron deficiency: apathy, lethargy, and fatigue. Therefore, taking iron supplements before assessing iron status is clearly unwise; hemoglobin tests alone would fail to make the distinction because excess iron accumulates in storage. Iron overload assessment tests measure transferrin saturation and serum ferritin.

Iron overload is characterized by free-radical tissue damage, especially in iron-storing organs such as the liver.[39] Infections are likely because bacteria thrive on iron-rich blood. Symptoms are most severe in people who abuse alcohol because alcohol damages the intestine, further impairing its defenses against absorbing excess iron. Untreated hemochromatosis aggravates the risk of diabetes, liver cancer, heart disease, and arthritis.

Iron overload is much more common in men than in women and is twice as prevalent among men as iron deficiency. The widespread fortification of foods with iron makes it difficult for people with hemochromatosis to follow an iron-restricted diet.

Iron Poisoning The rapid ingestion of massive amounts of iron can cause sudden death. Iron-containing supplements can easily cause accidental poisonings in young children. As few as five iron tablets have caused death in a child. Keep iron-containing supplements out of children's reach. If you suspect iron poisoning, call the nearest poison center or a physician immediately.

Iron Recommendations The average eating pattern in the United States provides only about 6 to 7 milligrams of iron for every 1000 kcalories. Men need 8 milligrams of iron each day; most men easily take in more than 2000 kcalories, so a man can meet his iron needs without special effort. The recommendation for women during childbearing years, however, is 18 milligrams. Because women have higher iron needs and typically

pica (PIE-ka): a craving for nonfood substances; also known as *geophagia* (jee-oh-FAY-jee-uh) when referring to clay-eating behavior.

picus = woodpecker or magpie
geo = earth
phagein = to eat

iron overload: toxicity from excess iron.

hemochromatosis (heem-oh-crome-a-TOH-sis): iron overload characterized by deposits of iron-containing pigment in many tissues, with tissue damage. Hemochromatosis is usually caused by a hereditary defect in iron absorption.

FIGURE 9-8   Good Sources of Iron[a]

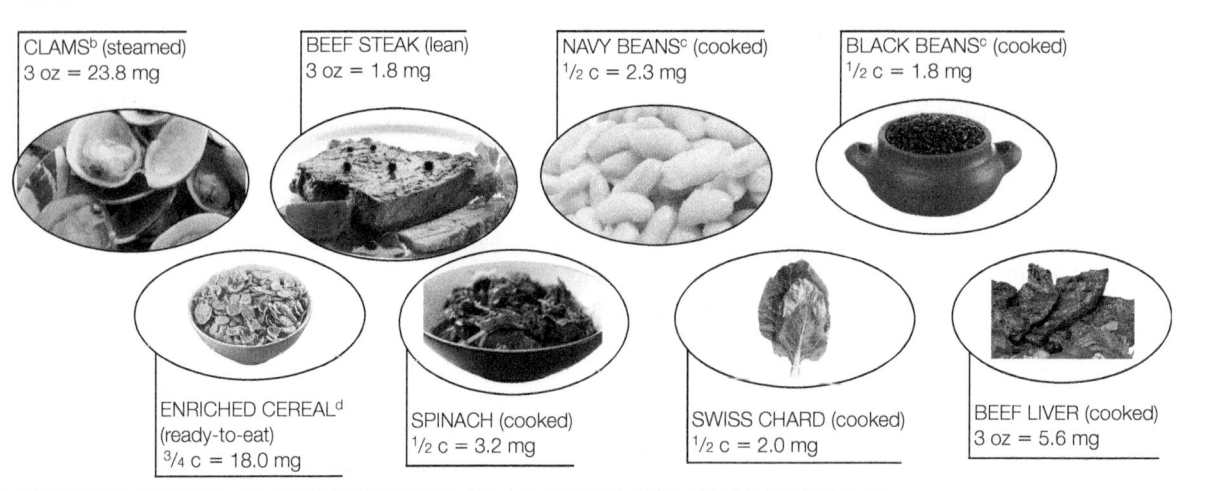

CLAMS[b] (steamed)
3 oz = 23.8 mg

BEEF STEAK (lean)
3 oz = 1.8 mg

NAVY BEANS[c] (cooked)
½ c = 2.3 mg

BLACK BEANS[c] (cooked)
½ c = 1.8 mg

ENRICHED CEREAL[d]
(ready-to-eat)
¾ c = 18.0 mg

SPINACH (cooked)
½ c = 3.2 mg

SWISS CHARD (cooked)
½ c = 2.0 mg

BEEF LIVER (cooked)
3 oz = 5.6 mg

[a]These foods provide 10 percent or more of the iron Daily Value in a serving. For a 2000-kcalorie diet, the DV is 18 mg/day.
[b]Some clams may contain less, but most types are iron-rich foods.
[c]Legumes contain phytates that reduce iron absorption.
[d]Enriched cereals vary widely in iron content.

Photo 9-3

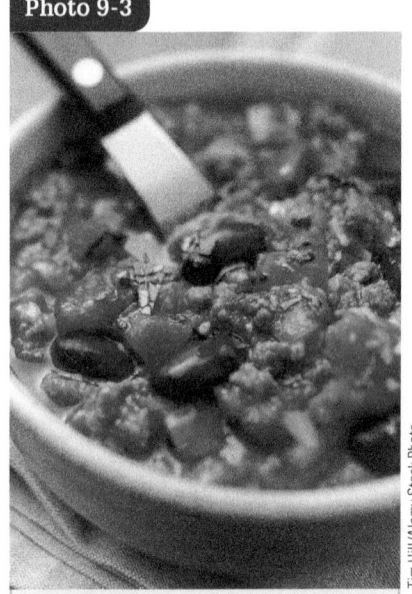

Tim Hill/Alamy Stock Photo

This chili dinner provides iron and MFP factor from meat, iron from legumes, and vitamin C from tomatoes. The combination of heme iron, nonheme iron, MFP factor, and vitamin C helps to achieve maximum iron absorption.

tannins: compounds in tea (especially black tea) and coffee that bind iron.

phytates: nonnutrient components of grains, legumes, and seeds. Phytates can bind minerals such as iron, zinc, calcium, and magnesium in insoluble complexes in the intestine, and the body excretes them unused.

consume fewer than 2000 kcalories per day, they have trouble achieving appropriate iron intakes. On average, women receive only 12 to 13 milligrams of iron per day, not enough until after menopause. To meet their iron needs from foods, premenopausal women need to select iron-rich foods at every meal. Vegetarians, because vegetable sources of iron are poorly absorbed, should aim for 1.8 times the normal requirement (see Nutrition in Practice 5).

Iron in Foods Iron occurs in two forms in foods: heme and nonheme. Heme iron, which is up to 10 times more absorbable than nonheme iron, is bound into the iron-carrying proteins hemoglobin and myoglobin in meat, poultry, and fish. Heme iron contributes a small portion of the iron consumed by most people, but it is absorbed at a fairly constant rate of about 23 percent. Nonheme iron is found in both meats and plant foods. People absorb nonheme iron at a lower rate (2 to 20 percent); its absorption depends on several dietary factors and iron stores. Most of the iron people consume is nonheme iron from vegetables, grains, eggs, meat, fish, and poultry. Figure 9-8 shows the iron contents of several different foods.

Iron absorption from foods can be maximized by two substances that enhance iron absorption: MFP factor and vitamin C (see Photo 9-3). Meat, fish, and poultry contain MFP factor, a factor other than heme that promotes the absorption of iron—even nonheme iron from other foods eaten at the same time. Vitamin C eaten in the same meal also doubles or triples nonheme iron absorption. Additionally, cooking with iron skillets can contribute iron to the diet. Some substances impair iron absorption; they include the **tannins** of tea and coffee, the calcium in milk, and the **phytates** that accompany fiber in legumes and whole-grain cereals. Box 9-3 offers suggestions for obtaining adequate iron.

Zinc

Zinc is a versatile trace mineral necessary for the activation of more than 300 different enzymes. These zinc-requiring enzymes perform tasks in the eyes, liver, kidneys, muscles, skin, bones, and male reproductive organs. Zinc works with the enzymes that make genetic material; manufacture heme; digest food; metabolize carbohydrate, protein, and fat; liberate vitamin A from storage in the liver; and dispose of damaging free radicals. Zinc also interacts with platelets in blood

Box 9-3   *HOW TO* Add Iron to Daily Meals

The following set of guidelines can be used for planning an iron-rich diet:

- *Grains.* Use only whole-grain, enriched, and fortified products (iron is one of the enrichment nutrients).

- *Vegetables.* The dark green, leafy vegetables are good sources of vitamin C and iron. Eat vitamin C–rich vegetables often to enhance absorption of the iron from foods eaten with them.

- *Fruit.* Dried fruit (raisins, apricots, peaches, and prunes) is high in iron. Eat vitamin C–rich fruit often with iron-containing foods.

- *Milk and milk products.* Do not overdo foods from the milk group; they are poor sources of iron. But do not omit them either because they are rich in calcium. Drink fat-free milk to free kcalories to be invested in iron-rich foods.

- *Protein foods.* Meat, seafood, and poultry are excellent iron sources. Include legumes frequently. One cup of peas or beans can supply up to 7 milligrams of iron.

clotting, affects thyroid hormone function, assists in immune function, and affects behavior and learning performance. Zinc is needed to produce the active form of vitamin A in visual pigments and is essential to wound healing, taste perception, the making of sperm, and fetal development. When zinc deficiency occurs, it impairs all these and other functions.

The body's handling of zinc differs from that of iron but with some interesting similarities. For example, like iron, extra zinc that enters the body is held within the intestinal cells, and only the amount needed is released into the bloodstream. As with iron, zinc status influences the percentage of zinc absorbed from the diet; if more is needed, more is absorbed.

Zinc's main transport vehicle in the blood is the protein albumin. This may account for observations that serum zinc concentrations decline in conditions that lower plasma albumin concentrations—for example, pregnancy and malnutrition.

Zinc Deficiency Zinc deficiency in human beings was first reported in the 1960s in studies of growing children and male adolescents in Egypt, Iran, and Turkey. Their diets were typically low in zinc and high in fiber and phytates (which impair zinc absorption). The zinc deficiency was marked by dwarfism, or severe growth retardation, and arrested sexual maturation—symptoms that were responsive to zinc supplementation.

Since that time, zinc deficiency has been recognized elsewhere and is known to affect more than growth. It drastically impairs immune function, causes loss of appetite, and, during pregnancy, may lead to growth and developmental disorders. In the developing world, more than 2 billion people are zinc deficient, and zinc deficiency is a substantial contributor to illness and death.[40] A detailed list of symptoms of zinc deficiency is presented later in Table 9-9.

Pronounced zinc deficiency is not widespread in developed countries, but deficiencies do occur in the most vulnerable groups of the U.S. population—pregnant women, young children, older adults, and the poor. Even mild zinc deficiency can result in metabolic changes such as impaired immune response, abnormal taste, and abnormal dark adaptation (zinc is required to produce the active form of vitamin A, retinal, in visual pigments).

Some people are at greater risk of zinc deficiency than others. Pregnant teenagers need zinc for their own growth as well as for the developing fetus. Vegetarians whose diets emphasize whole grains, legumes, and other plant foods may also be at risk. These foods, though rich in zinc, also contain phytate, a potent inhibitor of zinc absorption. Protein enhances zinc absorption, but most plant-protein foods also contain phytate. The DRI committee suggests that the dietary zinc requirement for vegetarians who exclude all animal-derived foods may be as much as 50 percent greater than the RDA, but so far evidence is insufficient to establish zinc recommendations based on the presence of other food components or nutrients. Vegetarians who include cheese, eggs, or other animal protein in their diet absorb more zinc than those who exclude these foods.

Zinc Toxicity Zinc can be toxic if consumed in large enough quantities. A high zinc intake is known to produce copper-deficiency anemia by inducing the intestinal cells to synthesize large amounts of a protein (metallothionein) that captures copper in a nonabsorbable form. Accidental consumption of high levels of zinc can cause vomiting, diarrhea, headaches, exhaustion, and other symptoms (see Table 9-9, later in the chapter). Large doses can even be fatal. The UL for zinc for adults is 40 milligrams per day.

Zinc Recommendations and Food Sources Most people in the United States have zinc intakes that approximate recommendations. Zinc is most abundant in foods high in protein, such as shellfish (especially oysters), meats, poultry, and milk products. In general, two 3-ounce servings a day of animal protein foods provide most of the zinc a healthy person needs. Legumes and whole-grain products are good sources of zinc if eaten in large quantities. For infants, breast milk is a good source of zinc, which is more efficiently absorbed from human milk than from cow's milk. Commercial infant formulas are fortified with zinc, of course. Figure 9-9 shows zinc-rich foods.

Zinc supplements are not recommended unless prescribed for an accurately diagnosed zinc deficiency or as a medication to displace other ions in unusual medical circumstances. Normally, it is possible to obtain enough zinc from the diet. Zinc lozenges to treat the common cold may sometimes shorten the duration of a cold, but they can upset the stomach and can contribute supplemental zinc to the body.[41]

Selenium

Selenium is an essential trace mineral that functions as an antioxidant nutrient, working primarily as a part of proteins—most notably, the glutathione peroxidase enzymes.[42] Glutathione peroxidase and vitamin E work in tandem. Glutathione peroxidase prevents free-radical formation, thus blocking the damaging chain reaction before it begins; if free radicals do form, and a chain reaction starts, vitamin E halts it. Selenium-containing enzymes are necessary for the proper functioning of the iodine-containing thyroid hormones that regulate metabolism.

Selenium and Cancer The question of whether selenium protects against the development of certain cancers, particularly prostate cancer, is under intense investigation.[43] Adequate *blood* selenium seems protective against cancers of the prostate,

---

FIGURE 9-9 Good Sources of Zinc[a]

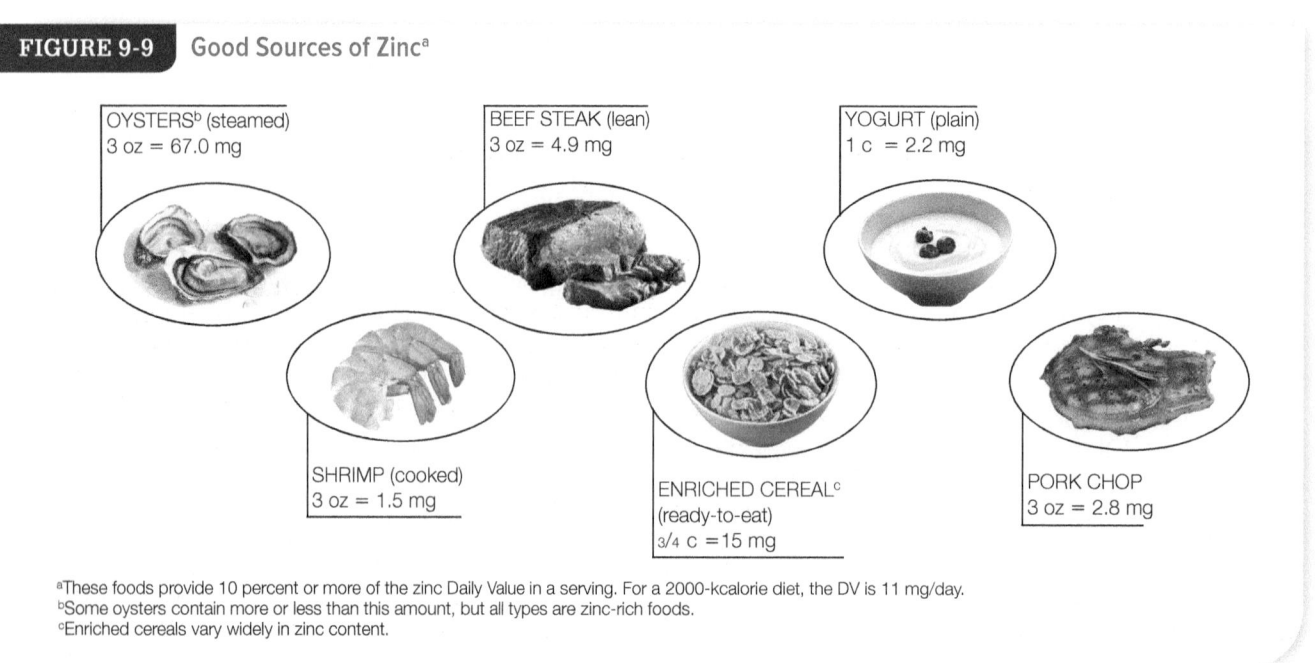

OYSTERS[b] (steamed)
3 oz = 67.0 mg

BEEF STEAK (lean)
3 oz = 4.9 mg

YOGURT (plain)
1 c = 2.2 mg

SHRIMP (cooked)
3 oz = 1.5 mg

ENRICHED CEREAL[c]
(ready-to-eat)
3/4 c = 15 mg

PORK CHOP
3 oz = 2.8 mg

[a]These foods provide 10 percent or more of the zinc Daily Value in a serving. For a 2000-kcalorie diet, the DV is 11 mg/day.
[b]Some oysters contain more or less than this amount, but all types are zinc-rich foods.
[c]Enriched cereals vary widely in zinc content.

breast, and other sites.[44] Many questions remain unanswered regarding selenium status, intake, and cancer, however. For example, the range of selenium status and the levels of intakes most beneficial to reducing cancer risk have not been established. Given the potential for harm from excess selenium and the lack of conclusive evidence, recommending selenium supplements to prevent cancer would be premature and possibly harmful.

Selenium Deficiency Selenium deficiency is associated with Keshan disease—a heart disease observed in children and young women living in regions of China where the soil and foods lack selenium. Keshan disease is named for one of the provinces where it was studied. Although the primary cause of Keshan disease is probably a virus, selenium deficiency appears to predispose people to it, and adequate selenium seems to prevent it.

Selenium Toxicity Because high doses of selenium are toxic, a UL has been set (see inside front cover). Selenium toxicity causes vomiting, diarrhea, loss of hair and nails, and lesions of the skin and nervous system.

Selenium Recommendations and Intakes Anyone who eats a normal diet composed mostly of unprocessed foods need not worry about meeting selenium recommendations. Selenium is widely distributed in foods such as meats and shellfish and in vegetables and grains grown on selenium-rich soil. Some regions in the United States and Canada produce crops on selenium-poor soil, but people are protected from deficiency because they eat selenium-rich meat and supermarket foods transported from other regions. Eating as few as two Brazil nuts a day effectively improves selenium status.

Iodine

Traces of the iodine ion (called iodide) are indispensible to life. In the GI tract, iodine from foods becomes iodide. This chapter uses the term *iodine* when referring to the nutrient in foods, and *iodide* when referring to it in the body. Iodide occurs in the body in minuscule amounts, but its principal role in human nutrition is well known, and the amount needed is well established. Iodide is an integral part of the thyroid hormones, which regulate body temperature, metabolic rate, reproduction, growth, the making of blood cells, nerve and muscle function, and more.

Iodine Deficiency and Toxicity When the iodide concentration in the blood is low, the cells of the thyroid gland enlarge in an attempt to trap as many particles of iodide as possible. If the gland enlarges until it is visible, the swelling is called a **goiter** (see Figure 9-10). People with iodine deficiency this severe become sluggish and may gain weight. In most cases of goiter, the cause is iodine deficiency, but some people have goiter because they overconsume foods of the cabbage family and others that contain an antithyroid substance (**goitrogen**) whose effect is not counteracted by dietary iodine. An estimated 2 billion people worldwide are at risk of iodine deficiency, including hundreds of millions of school-aged children.[45] This is a huge number, but one that reflects some improvement over past decades thanks to programs that provide iodized salt to people in iodine-poor areas.

Goiter may be the earliest and most obvious sign of iodine deficiency, but the most tragic and prevalent damage occurs in the brain. Iodine deficiency is the most common cause of *preventable* mental retardation and brain damage in the world.[46] Children with even a mild iodine deficiency typically have goiters and perform poorly in school. With sustained treatment, however, mental performance in the classroom as well as thyroid function improves.

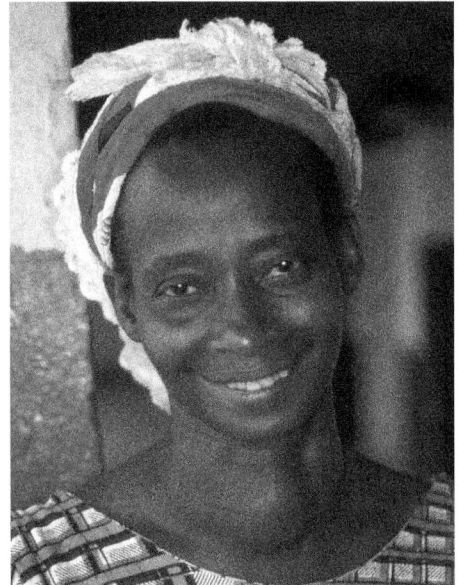

FIGURE 9-10 Iodine-Deficiency Symptom: The Enlarged Thyroid of Goiter

In iodine deficiency, the thyroid gland enlarges—a condition known as simple goiter.

Scott Camazine/Science Source

goiter (GOY-ter): an enlargement of the thyroid gland due to an iodine deficiency, malfunction of the gland, or overconsumption of a thyroid antagonist. Goiter caused by iodine deficiency is sometimes called *simple goiter*.

goitrogen (GOY-troh-jen): a substance that enlarges the thyroid gland and causes *toxic goiter*. Goitrogens occur naturally in such foods as cabbage, kale, brussels sprouts, cauliflower, broccoli, and kohlrabi.

A severe iodine deficiency during pregnancy causes the extreme and irreversible mental and physical retardation known as **cretinism**.[47] Much of the mental retardation can be averted if the pregnant woman's deficiency is detected and treated within the first six months of pregnancy, but if treatment comes too late or not at all, the child's IQ and other developmental indicators are likely to be substantially below normal.

Excessive intakes of iodine can enlarge the thyroid gland, just as deficiencies can. For this reason, a UL of 1100 micrograms per day for adults has been set.

Iodine Sources and Intakes The ocean is the world's major source of iodine. In coastal areas, seafood, water, and even iodine-containing sea mist are important iodine sources.* Further inland, the amount of iodine in the diet is variable and generally reflects the amount present in the soil in which plants are grown or on which animals graze. In the United States and Canada, the use of iodized salt has largely wiped out the iodine deficiency that once was widespread. In the United States, you have to read the label to find out whether salt is iodized; in Canada, all table salt is iodized. Average intakes in the United States are slightly above the recommended intake of 150 micrograms but still below the UL.

Copper

The body contains about 100 milligrams of copper. About one-fourth is in the muscles; one-fourth is in the liver, brain, and blood; and the rest is in the bones, kidneys, and other tissues. The primary function of copper in the body is to serve as a constituent of enzymes. The copper-containing enzymes have diverse metabolic roles: they catalyze the formation of hemoglobin, help manufacture the protein collagen, inactivate histamine, degrade serotonin, assist in the healing of wounds, and help maintain the sheaths around nerve fibers. One of copper's most vital roles is to help cells use iron.[48] Like iron, copper is needed in many reactions related to respiration and energy metabolism. The copper-dependent enzyme superoxide dismutase helps to control damage from free-radical activity in the tissues.

Copper Deficiency Copper deficiency is rare but not unknown. It has been seen in premature infants and malnourished infants. High intakes of zinc interfere with copper absorption and can lead to deficiency.

Copper Toxicity Some genetic disorders create a copper toxicity. Copper toxicity from foods, however, is unlikely. The UL for copper is set at 10,000 micrograms per day.

Copper Recommendations and Food Sources The RDA for copper is 900 micrograms per day, which is slightly below the average intake for adults in the United States. The best food sources of copper are organ meats, legumes, whole grains, seafood, nuts, and seeds.

Manganese

The human body contains a tiny 20 milligrams of manganese, mostly in the bones and metabolically active organs such as the liver, kidneys, and pancreas. Manganese is a cofactor for many enzymes, helping to facilitate dozens of different metabolic processes. Deficiencies of manganese have not been noted in people, but toxicity may be severe. Miners who inhale large quantities of manganese dust on the job over prolonged periods show many symptoms of a brain disease, along with abnormalities in appearance and behavior. The UL for manganese is 11 milligrams per day.

Manganese requirements are low, and plant foods such as nuts, whole grains, and leafy green vegetables contain significant amounts of this trace mineral. Deficiencies are therefore unlikely.

cretinism (CREE-tin-ism): an iodine-deficiency disease characterized by mental and physical retardation.

---

*Iodine in sea mist combines with particles in the air or with water. Iodine may then enter the soil or surface water or land on plants when these particles fall to the ground or when it rains.

Fluoride

Fluoride's primary role in health is the prevention of dental caries throughout life. Only a trace of fluoride occurs in the human body, but it is important to the mineralization of the bones and teeth. When bones and teeth become mineralized, first a crystal called hydroxyapatite forms from calcium and phosphorus. Then fluoride replaces the hydroxy portion of hydroxyapatite, forming **fluorapatite**. During development, fluorapatite enlarges crystals in bones and teeth, improving their resistance to demineralization and making the teeth more resistant to decay. Once the teeth have erupted, the topical application of fluoride by way of toothpaste or mouth rinse continues to exert a caries-reducing effect.

Fluoride Deficiency   Where fluoride is lacking in the water supply, the incidence of dental decay is high. Fluoridation of water is thus recommended as an important public health measure.[49] Those fortunate enough to have had sufficient fluoride during the tooth-forming years of infancy and childhood are protected throughout life from dental decay. Dental problems are of great concern because they can lead to a multitude of other health problems affecting the whole body. Based on the accumulated evidence of its beneficial effects, water fluoridation has been endorsed by nearly 100 national and international organizations including the National Institute of Dental Health, the Academy of Nutrition and Dietetics, the American Medical Association, the National Cancer Institute, and the Centers for Disease Control and Prevention (CDC). About 70 percent of the U.S. population served by public water systems receives optimal levels of fluoride (about 0.7 milligram per liter). Most bottled waters lack fluoride.

Fluoride Sources   All normal diets include some fluoride, but drinking water; processed soft drinks and fruit juice made with fluoridated water; and fluoride toothpastes, gels, and oral rinses are the most common fluoride sources in the United States. Fish and tea may supply substantial amounts as well.

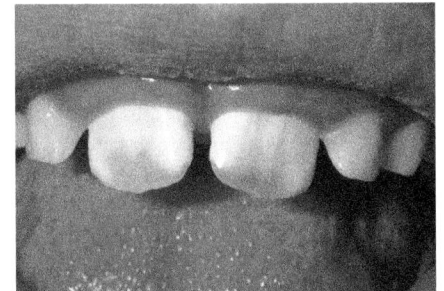

FIGURE 9-11   Fluoride Toxicity Symptom: The Mottled Teeth of Fluorosis

In some areas, the natural fluoride concentration in water is high, and too much fluoride can damage teeth, causing **fluorosis**. For this reason, a UL (10 mg per day for adults) has been established. In mild cases, the teeth develop small white specks; in severe cases, the enamel becomes pitted and permanently stained (see Figure 9-11). Fluorosis occurs only during tooth development and cannot be reversed, making its prevention during the first three years of life a high priority. To limit fluoride ingestion, take care not to swallow fluoride-containing dental products such as toothpaste and mouthwash and use fluoride supplements only as prescribed by a physician.

Chromium

Chromium is an essential mineral that participates in carbohydrate and lipid metabolism. Chromium enhances the activity of the hormone insulin.* When chromium is lacking, a diabetes-like condition with elevated blood glucose and impaired glucose tolerance, insulin response, and glucagon response may develop. Research suggests that chromium supplements provide little or no benefit to people with type 2 diabetes.[50]

Chromium deficiency is unlikely, given the small amount of chromium required and its presence in a variety of foods. The more refined foods people eat, however, the less chromium they obtain from their diets. Unrefined foods such as liver, brewer's yeast, whole grains, nuts, and cheeses are the best sources.

Other Trace Minerals

An RDA has been established for one other trace mineral, molybdenum. **Molybdenum** functions as a working part of several metal-containing enzymes, some of which are giant proteins. Deficiencies or toxicities of molybdenum are unknown.

---

*Small organic compounds that enhance insulin's activity are called glucose tolerance factors (GTF). Some glucose tolerance factors contain chromium.

fluorapatite (floor-APP-uh-tite): the stabilized form of bone and tooth crystal, in which fluoride has replaced the hydroxy portion of hydroxyapatite.

fluorosis (floor-OH-sis): mottling of the tooth enamel from ingestion of too much fluoride during tooth development.

molybdenum (mo-LIB-duh-num): a trace element.

Several other trace minerals are known or suspected to contribute to the health of the body. Nickel is recognized as important for the health of many body tissues. Nickel deficiencies harm the liver and other organs. Silicon is involved in the formation of bones and collagen. Cobalt is found in the large vitamin B_{12} molecule. Boron influences the activity of many enzymes and may play a key role in bone health, brain activities, and immune response. The future may reveal that other trace minerals also play key roles. Even arsenic—famous as the deadly poison in many murder mysteries and known to be a carcinogen—may turn out to be an essential nutrient in tiny quantities.

Review Notes

- The body requires trace minerals in tiny amounts, and they function in similar ways—assisting enzymes all over the body.
- Eating a diet that consists of a variety of foods is the best way to ensure an adequate intake of these important nutrients.
- Many dietary factors, including the trace minerals themselves, affect the absorption and availability of these nutrients.

Table 9-9 offers a summary of facts about trace minerals in the body.

TABLE 9-9	The Trace Minerals: A Summary			
MINERAL NAME	CHIEF FUNCTIONS IN THE BODY	DEFICIENCY SYMPTOMS	TOXICITY SYMPTOMS	SIGNIFICANT SOURCES
Iron	Part of the protein hemoglobin, which carries oxygen in the blood; part of the protein myoglobin in muscles, which makes oxygen available for muscle contraction; necessary for the utilization of energy	Anemia: weakness, pallor, headaches, reduced work productivity, inability to concentrate, impaired cognitive function (children), lowered cold tolerance	Iron overload: infections, liver injury, possible increased risk of heart attack, acidosis, bloody stools, shock	Red meats, fish, poultry, shellfish, eggs, legumes, dried fruit
Zinc	Part of the hormone insulin and many enzymes; involved in making genetic material and proteins, immune reactions, transport of vitamin A, taste perception, wound healing, the making of sperm, and normal fetal development	Growth retardation, delayed sexual maturation, impaired immune function, loss of taste, poor wound healing, eye and skin lesions	Loss of appetite, impaired immunity, low HDL, nausea, vomiting, diarrhea, headaches, copper and iron deficiencies	Protein-containing foods: meats, fish, shellfish, poultry, grains, vegetables
Selenium	Assists a group of enzymes that break down reactive chemicals that harm cells	Predisposition to heart disease characterized by cardiac tissue becoming fibrous (uncommon)	Nausea, abdominal pain, nail and hair changes, nerve damage	Seafoods, organ meats, other meats, whole grains and vegetables (depending on soil content)
Iodine	A component of two thyroid hormones, which help to regulate growth, development, and metabolic rate	Goiter, cretinism	Depressed thyroid activity; goiterlike thyroid enlargement	Iodized salt; seafood; bread; plants grown in most parts of the country and animals fed those plants

(Continued)

TABLE 9-9   The Trace Minerals: A Summary (continued)

MINERAL NAME	CHIEF FUNCTIONS IN THE BODY	DEFICIENCY SYMPTOMS	TOXICITY SYMPTOMS	SIGNIFICANT SOURCES
Copper	Necessary for the absorption and use of iron in the formation of hemoglobin; part of several enzymes	Anemia, bone abnormalities	Vomiting, diarrhea, liver damage	Organ meats, seafood, nuts, seeds, whole grains, drinking water
Manganese	Facilitator, with enzymes, of many cell processes; bone formation	Rare	Nervous system disorders	Nuts, whole grains, leafy vegetables, tea
Fluoride	An element involved in the formation of bones and teeth; helps to make teeth resistant to decay	Susceptibility to tooth decay	Fluorosis (pitting and discoloration of teeth); skeletal fluorosis (weak, malformed bones)	Drinking water (if fluoride containing or fluoridated), tea, seafood
Chromium	Enhances insulin action and may improve glucose tolerance	Diabetes-like condition marked by an inability to use glucose normally	None reported	Meats, whole grains

Self Check

1. Which of the following body structures helps to regulate thirst?
   a. Brainstem
   b. Cerebellum
   c. Optic nerve
   d. Hypothalamus

2. Which of the following is *not* a function of water in the body?
   a. Lubricant
   b. Source of energy
   c. Maintains protein structure
   d. Participant in chemical reactions

3. Two situations in which a person may experience fluid and electrolyte imbalances are:
   a. vomiting and burns.
   b. diarrhea and cuts.
   c. broken bones and fever.
   d. heavy sweating and excessive carbohydrate intake.

4. Three-fourths of the sodium in people's diets comes from:
   a. fresh meats.
   b. home-cooked foods.
   c. frozen vegetables and meats.
   d. salt added to food by manufacturers.

5. Which mineral is critical to keeping the heartbeat steady and plays a major role in maintaining fluid and electrolyte balance?
   a. Sodium
   b. Calcium
   c. Potassium
   d. Magnesium

6. The two best ways to prevent age-related bone loss and fracture are to:
   a. take calcium supplements and estrogen.
   b. participate in aerobic activity and drink eight glasses of milk daily.
   c. eat a diet low in fat and salt and refrain from smoking.
   d. maintain a lifelong adequate calcium intake and engage in weight-bearing physical activity.

7. Three good food sources of calcium are:
   a. milk, sardines, and broccoli.
   b. spinach, yogurt, and sardines.
   c. cottage cheese, spinach, and tofu.
   d. Swiss chard, mustard greens, and broccoli.

8. Foods high in iron that help prevent or treat anemia include:
   a. green peas and cheese.
   b. dairy foods and fresh fruit.
   c. homemade breads and most fresh vegetables.
   d. meat and dark green, leafy vegetables.

9. Two groups of people who are especially at risk for zinc deficiency are:
   a. Asians and children.
   b. infants and teenagers.
   c. smokers and athletes.
   d. pregnant adolescents and vegetarians.

10. A deficiency of _____ is one of the world's most common preventable causes of mental retardation.
   a. zinc
   b. iodine
   c. selenium
   d. magnesium

Answers: 1. d, 2. b, 3. a, 4. d, 5. c, 6. d, 7. a, 8. d, 9. d, 10. b

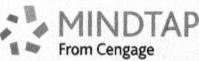

For more chapter resources visit **www.cengage.com** to access MindTap, a complete digital course.

Clinical Applications

1. Pull together information from Chapter 1 about the different food groups and the significant sources of minerals shown or discussed in this chapter. Consider which minerals might be lacking (or excessive) in the diet of a client who reports the following:

   • Relies on highly processed foods, snack foods, and fast foods as mainstays of the diet.
   • Never uses milk, milk products, or cheese.
   • Dislikes green, leafy vegetables.
   • Never eats meat, fish, poultry, or even other protein foods such as legumes.

   What additional information would help you pinpoint problems with mineral intake?

Notes

1. A. E. Stanhewicz and W. L. Kenney, Determinants of water and sodium intake and output, *Nutrition Reviews* 73 (2015): 73–82.
2. D. Benton and H. A. Young, Do small differences in hydration status affect mood and mental performance? *Nutrition Reviews* 73 (2015): 83–96.
3. R. J. Maughan, P. Watson, and S. M. Shirreffs, Implications of active lifestyles and environmental factors for water needs and consequences of failure to meet those needs, *Nutrition Reviews* 73 (2015): 130–140.
4. U.S. Department of Health and Human Services and U.S. Department of Agriculture, *2015–2020 Dietary Guidelines for Americans*, 8th ed. (2015), health.gov/dietaryguidelines/2015/guidelines/.
5. S. L. Jackson and coauthors, Prevalence of excess sodium intake in the United States—NHANES, 2009–2012, *Morbidity and Mortality Weekly Report* 64 (2016): 1393–1397.
6. U.S. Department of Health and Human Services and U.S. Department of Agriculture, *2015–2020 Dietary Guidelines for Americans*, 8th ed. (2015), health.gov/dietaryguidelines/2015/guidelines/; M. D. Ritchey and coauthors, Million hearts: Prevalence of leading cardiovascular disease risk factors—United States, 2005–2012, *Morbidity and Mortality Weekly Report* 63 (2014): 462–467.
7. U.S. Department of Health and Human Services and U.S. Department of Agriculture, *2015–2020 Dietary Guidelines for Americans*, 8th ed. (2015), health.gov/dietaryguidelines/2015/guidelines/; R. H. Eckel and coauthors, 2013 AHA/ ACC Guideline on Lifestyle Management to Reduce Cardiovascular Risk: A report of the American College of Cardiology/American Heart Association Task Force on Practice Guidelines, *Circulation* 129 (2014): S76–S99.
8. S. L. Lennon and coauthors, 2015 evidence analysis library evidence-based nutrition practice guideline for the management of hypertension in adults, *Journal of the Academy of Nutrition and Dietetics* 117 (2017): 1445–1458; B. M. Davy, T. M. Halliday, and K. P. Davy, Sodium intake and blood pressure: New controversies, new labels . . . new guidelines? *Journal of the Academy of Nutrition and Dietetics* 115 (2015): 200–203; Eckel and coauthors, 2014.
9. M. E. Cogswell and coauthors, Modeled changes in US sodium intake from reducing sodium concentrations of commercially processed and prepared foods to meet voluntary standards established in North America: NHANES, *American Journal of Clinical Nutrition* 106 (2017): 530–540; C. Gillespie and coauthors, Sodium content in major brands of US packaged foods, 2009, *American Journal of Clinical Nutrition* 101 (2015): 344–353.
10. R. S. Sebastian and coauthors, Sandwiches are major contributors of sodium in the diets of American adults: Results from What We Eat in America, National Health and Nutrition Examination Survey 2009–2010, *Journal of the Academy of Nutrition and Dietetics* 115 (2015): 272–277; U.S. Department of Health and Human Services and U.S. Department of Agriculture, *2015–2020 Dietary Guidelines for Americans*, 8th ed. (2015), health.gov/dietaryguidelines/2015/guidelines/.
11. V. Reddy and coauthors, High sodium causes hypertension: Evidence from clinical trials and animals experiments, *Journal of Integrative Medicine* 13 (2015): 1–8; D. Mozaffarian and coauthors, Global sodium consumption and death from cardiovascular causes, *New England Journal of Medicine* 371 (2014): 624–634.
12. W. B. Farquhar and coauthors, Dietary sodium and health: More than just blood pressure, *Journal of the American College of Cardiology* 65 (2015): 1042–1050.
13. V. Ponzo and coauthors, Blood pressure and sodium intake from snacks in adolescents, *European Journal of Clinical Nutrition* 69 (2015): 681–686; C. A. Anderson and coauthors, Commentary on making sense of the science of sodium, *Nutrition Today* 50 (2015): 66–71.
14. E. J. Benjamin and coauthors, Heart disease and stroke statistics—2017 update: A report from the American Heart Association, *Circulation* 135 (2017): e146–e603; Q. Chan, J. Stamler, and P. Elliott, Dietary factors and higher blood pressure in African-Americans, *Current Hypertension Reports* 17 (2015): 10.
15. Lennon and coauthors, 2017; U.S. Department of Health and Human Services and U.S. Department of Agriculture, *2015–2020 Dietary*

Guidelines for Americans, 8th ed. (2015), health.gov/dietaryguidelines/2015/guidelines/; M. Siervo and coauthors, Effects of the Dietary Approach to Stop Hypertension (DASH) diet on cardiovascular risk factors: A systematic review and meta-analysis, *British Journal of Nutrition* 113 (2015): 1–15; P. Saneei and coauthors, Influence of Dietary Approaches to Stop Hypertension (DASH) diet on blood pressure: A systematic review and meta-analysis on randomized controlled trials, *Nutrition, Metabolism, and Cardiovascular Diseases* 24 (2014): 1253–1261.

16. U.S. Department of Health and Human Services and U.S. Department of Agriculture, *2015–2020 Dietary Guidelines for Americans,* 8th ed. (2015), health.gov/dietaryguidelines/2015/guidelines/.

17. L. J. Ware and coauthors, Associations between dietary salt, potassium and blood pressure in South African adults: WHO SAGE Wave 2 Salt & Tobacco, *Nutrition Metabolism, and Cardiovascular Diseases* 27 (2017): 784–791; S. N. Adebamowo and coauthors, Association between intakes of magnesium, potassium, and calcium and risk of stroke: 2 cohorts of US women and updated meta-analysis, *American Journal of Clinical Nutrition* 101 (2015): 1269–1277; H. J. Adrogue and N. E. Madias, The impact of sodium and potassium on hypertension risk, *Seminars in Nephrology* 34 (2014): 257–272; L. D'Elia and coauthors, Potassium-rich diet and risk of stroke: Updated meta-analysis, *Nutrition, Metabolism, and Cardiovascular Diseases* 24 (2014): 585–587.

18. C. Ekmekcioglu and coauthors, The role of dietary potassium in hypertension and diabetes, *Journal of Physiology and Biochemistry* 72 (2016): 93–106; Adebamowo and coauthors, 2015; S. Sharma and coauthors, Dietary sodium and potassium is not associated with elevated blood pressure in US adults with no prior history of hypertension, *Journal of Clinical Hypertension* 16 (2014): 418–423; A. Seth and coauthors, Potassium intake and risk of stroke in women with hypertension and nonhypertension in the Women's Health Initiative, *Stroke* 45 (2014): 2874–2880; L. D'Elia and coauthors, Potassium-rich diet and risk of stroke: Updated meta-analysis, *Nutrition, Metabolism, and Cardiovascular Diseases* 24 (2014): 585–587.

19. U.S. Department of Health and Human Services and U.S. Department of Agriculture, *2015–2020 Dietary Guidelines for Americans,* 8th ed. (2015), health.gov/dietaryguidelines/2015/guidelines/.

20. D. Goltzman, Approach to Hypercalcemia, *Endotext* (2016), www.ncbi.nim.nih.gov/books/NBK279129.

21. C. Julián-Almárcegui and coauthors, Combined effects of interaction between physical activity and nutrition on bone health in children and adolescents: A systematic review, *Nutrition Reviews* 73 (2015): 127–139; N. H. Golden, S. A. Abrams and Committee on Nutrition, Optimizing bone health in children and adolescents, *Pediatrics* 134 (2014): e1229–e1243.

22. N. C. Wright and coauthors, The recent prevalence of osteoporosis and low bone mass in the United States based on bone mineral density at the femoral neck or lumbar spine, *Journal of Bone and Mineral Research* 29 (2014): 2520–2526.

23. P. Andreopoulou and R. S. Bockman, Management of postmenopausal osteoporosis, *Annual Review of Medicine* 66 (2015): 329–342; A. Giusti and G. Bianchi, Treatment of primary osteoporosis in men, *Clinical Interventions in Aging* 10 (2014): 105–115.

24. C. M. Weaver and coauthors, The National Osteoporosis Foundation's position statement on peak mass development and lifestyle factors: A systematic review and implementation recommendations, *Osteoporosis International* 27 (2016): 1281–1386; Julián-Almárcegui and coauthors, 2015; J. M. Lappe and coauthors, The longitudinal effects of physical activity and dietary calcium on bone mass accrual across stages of pubertal development, *Journal of Bone and Mineral Research* 30 (2015): 156–164; S. J. Warden and coauthors, Physical activity when young provides lifelong benefits to cortical bone size and strength in men, *Proceedings of the National Academy of Sciences of the United States of America* 111 (2014): 5337–5342.

25. Goltzman, 2016.

26. U. Gröber, J. Schmidt, and K. Kisters, Magnesium in prevention and therapy, *Nutrients* 7 (2015): 8199–8226.

27. Gröber, Schmidt, and Kisters, 2015; P. L. Lutsey and coauthors, Serum magnesium, phosphorus, and calcium are associated with risk of incident heart failure: The Atherosclerosis Risk in Communities (ARIC) study, *American Journal of Clinical Nutrition* 100 (2014): 756–764; D. Kolte and coauthors, Role of magnesium in cardiovascular diseases, *Cardiology in Review* 22 (2014): 182–192.

28. Lennon and coauthors, 2017; H. Han and coauthors, Dose-response relationship between dietary magnesium intake, serum magnesium concentration and risk of hypertension: A systematic review and meta-analysis of prospective cohort studies, *Nutrition Journal* 16 (2017): 26; X. Fang and coauthors, Dietary magnesium intake and the risk of cardiovascular disease, type 2 diabetes, and all-cause mortality: a dose-response meta-analysis of prospective cohort studies, *BMC Medicine* 14 (2016): 210; Adebamowo and coauthors, 2015.

29. H. Aljwaid and coauthors, Non-transferrin-bound iron is associated with biomarkers of oxidative stress, inflammation and endothelial dysfunction in type 2 diabetes, *Journal of Diabetes and Its Complications* 29 (2015): 943–949; P. J. Schmidt, Regulation of iron metabolism by hepcidin under conditions of inflammation, *Journal of Biological Chemistry,* 290 (2015): 18975–18983; E. Gammella and coauthors, Iron-induced damage in cardiomyopathy: Oxidative-dependent and independent mechanisms, *Oxidative Medicine and Cellular Longevity* 2015, doi:10.1155/2015/230182; H. Padmanabhan, M. J. Brookes, and T. Iqbal, Iron and colorectal cancer; Evidence from in vitro and animal studies, *Nutrition Reviews* 73 (2015): 308–317.

30. S. R. Hennigar and J. P. McClung, Homeostatic regulation of trace mineral transport by ubiquitination of membrane transporters, *Nutrition Reviews* 74 (2016): 59–67.

31. C. Camaschella, Iron-deficiency anemia, *New England Journal of Medicine* 372 (2015): 1832–1843.

32. S. R. Pasricha, K. McHugh, and H. Drakesmith, Regulation of hepcidin by erythropoiesis: The story so far, *Annual Review of Nutrition* 36 (2016): 417–434; Schmidt, 2015; D. M. Frazer and G. J. Anderson, The regulation of iron transport, *Biofactors* 40 (2014): 206–214.

33. Pasricha, McHugh, and Drakesmith, 2016; Camaschella, 2015.

34. Camaschella, 2015; World Health Organization, 2015, Micronutrient deficiencies, available at www.who.int/nutrition/topics/ida/en.

35. E. Aigner, A. Feldman, and C. Datz, Obesity as an emerging risk factor for iron deficiency, *Nutrients* 6 (2014): 3587–3600; Y. Manios and coauthors, The double burden of obesity and iron deficiency on children and adolescents in Greece: The Healthy Growth Study, *Journal of Human Nutrition and Dietetics* 26 (2014): 470–478.

36. C. Becker and coauthors, Iron metabolism in obesity: How interaction between homoeostatic mechanisms can interfere with their original purpose. Part 1: Underlying homoeostatic mechanisms of energy storage and iron metabolisms and their interaction, *Journal of Trace Elements in Medicine and Biology* 30 (2015): 195–201; A. A. Nikonorov and coauthors, Mutual interaction between iron homeostasis and obesity pathogenesis, *Journal of Trace Elements in Medicine and Biology* 30 (2015): 207–214; Aigner, Feldman, and Datz, 2014.

37. I. Jauregui-Lobera, Iron deficiency and cognitive functions, *Neuropsychiatric Disease and Treatment* 10 (2014): 2087–2095.

38. J. Liu and coauthors, Hepcidin: A promising therapeutic target for iron disorders: A systematic review, *Medicine* 95 (2016): e3150; R. J. Salgia and K. Brown, Diagnosis and management of hereditary hemochromatosis, *Clinics in Liver Disease* 19 (2015): 187–198.

39. P. C. Adams, Epidemiology and diagnostic testing for hemochromatosis and iron overload, *International Journal of Laboratory Hematology* 37 (2015): 25–30.

40. K. Jurowski and coauthors, Biological consequences of zinc deficiency in the pathomechanisms of selected diseases, *Journal of Biological Inorganic Chemistry* 19 (2014): 1069–1079.

41. H. Hemilä, Zinc lozenges and the common cold: A meta-analysis comparing zinc acetate and zinc gluconate, and the role of zinc dosage, *JRSM Open* 2017, doi: 10.1177/2054270417694291. eCollection 2017; R. R. Das and M. Singh, Oral zinc for the common cold, *Journal of the American Medical Association* 311 (2014): 1440–1441.

42. Z. Touat-Hamici and coauthors, Selective up-regulation of human selenoproteins in response to oxidative stress, *Journal of Biological Chemistry* 289 (2014): 14750–14761.

43. N. E. Allen and coauthors, Selenium and prostate cancer: Analysis of individual participant data from fifteen prospective studies, *Journal of the National Cancer Institute* 2016, doi: 10.1093/jnci/djw153; X. Cai and coauthors, Selenium exposure and cancer risk: An updated meta-analysis and meta-regression, *Scientific Reports* 6 (2016): 19213; C. Méplan, Selenium and chronic diseases: A nutritional genomics perspective, *Nutrients* 7 (2015): 3621–3651; M. Vinceti and coauthors, Selenium for

preventing cancer, *Cochrane Database of Systematic Reviews* 3 (2014): CD005195.

44. Cai and coauthors, 2016; Allen and coauthors, 2016; Vinceti and coauthors, 2014.

45. M. Kramer and coauthors, Association between household unavailability of iodized salt and child growth: Evidence from 89 demographic and health surveys, *American Journal of Clinical Nutrition* 104 (2016): 1093–1100.

46. K. Redman and coauthors, Iodine deficiency and the brain: Effects and mechanisms, *Critical Reviews in Food Science and Nutrition* 56 (2016): 269S–271S.

47. E. N. Pearce and coauthors, Consequences of iodine deficiency and excess in pregnant women: An overview of current knowns and unknowns, *American Journal of Clinical Nutrition* 104 (2016): 918S–923S.

48. S. Gulec and J. F. Collins, Molecular mediators governing iron-copper interactions, *Annual Review of Nutrition* 34 (2014): 95–116.

49. U.S. Public Health Service recommendation for fluoride concentration in drinking water for the prevention of dental caries, Public Health Reports 130 (2015): 318–331.

50. R. B. Costello, J. T. Dwyer, and R. L. Bailey, Chromium supplements for glycemic control in type 2 diabetes: Limited evidence of effectiveness, *Nutrition Reviews* 74 (2016): 455–468; C. H. Bailey, Improved meta-analytic methods show no effect of chromium supplements on fasting glucose, *Biological Trace Element Research* 157 (2014): 1–8.

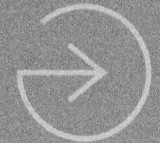

9.4 Nutrition in Practice
Vitamin and Mineral Supplements

More than half of U.S. adults collectively spend tens of *billions* of dollars a year on dietary supplements.[1] Most people take supplements as a part of their efforts to live a healthy life.[2] Yet most vitamin and mineral supplements do not prevent chronic diseases or delay death.[3] This Nutrition in Practice focuses on vitamin and mineral supplements. (Amino acid and protein supplements are discussed in Chapter 5; weight loss products in Chapter 7; and herbal supplements in Nutrition in Practice 14.)

An estimated 30 percent of U.S. adults take multivitamin-mineral supplements regularly.[4] Others take large doses of single nutrients, most commonly vitamin D and calcium. In many cases, taking supplements is a costly but harmless practice; sometimes, it is both costly and harmful to health. Every year, more than 7000 emergency department visits in the United States are attributed to adverse effects of vitamin and/or mineral supplements; an additional 16,000 visits are attributed to other herbal and nutritional products.[5] The truth is that most healthy people can get the nutrients they need from foods. Supplements cannot substitute for a healthy diet. For some people, however, certain nutrient supplements may be desirable, either to correct deficiencies or to reduce the risks of disease.

Do foods really contain enough vitamins and minerals to supply all that most people need?

Emphatically, yes, for both healthy adults and children who choose a variety of foods. The USDA Food Patterns described in Chapter 1 are the guide to follow to achieve adequate intakes. People who meet their nutrient needs from foods, rather than supplements, have little risk of deficiency or toxicity. When a health care professional finds a person's diet inadequate, the right corrective step is to improve the person's food choices and eating patterns, not to begin supplementation.

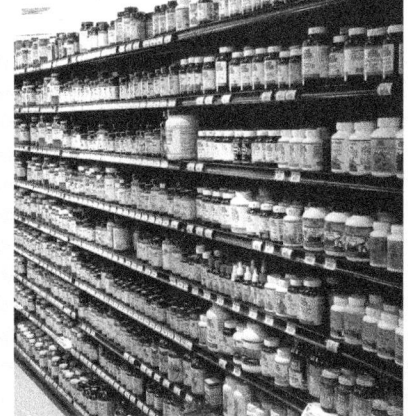

Tom Carter/PhotoEdit

Do some people need supplements?

Yes, some people may suffer marginal nutrient deficiencies due to illness, alcohol or drug addiction, or other conditions that limit food intake. People who may benefit from nutrient supplements in amounts consistent with the RDA include the following:

- People with specific nutrient deficiencies need specific nutrient supplements.
- People whose energy intakes are particularly low (fewer than 1600 kcalories per day) need multivitamin and mineral supplements.
- Vegetarians who eat all-plant diets (vegans) and older adults with atrophic gastritis need vitamin B_{12}.
- People who have lactose intolerance or milk allergies or who otherwise do not consume enough milk products to forestall extensive bone loss need calcium.
- People in certain stages of the life cycle who have increased nutrient requirements need specific nutrient supplements. For example, infants may need vitamin D, iron, and fluoride; women who are capable of becoming pregnant and pregnant women need folate and iron; and older adults may benefit from some of the vitamins and minerals in a balanced supplement (they may choose poor diets, have trouble chewing, or absorb or metabolize nutrients less efficiently; see Chapter 12).
- People who have inadequate intakes of milk or milk products, limited sun exposure, or heavily pigmented skin may need vitamin D.
- People who have diseases, infections, or injuries or who have undergone surgery that interferes with the intake, absorption, metabolism, or excretion of nutrients may need specific nutrient supplements (see Chapter 16).
- People taking medications that interfere with the body's use of specific nutrients may need specific nutrient supplements.

Why do so many people take supplements?

People frequently take supplements for mistaken reasons, such as "They give me energy" or "They make me strong."

Vitamin and Mineral Supplements   **267**

Other invalid reasons why people may take supplements include:

- Their feeling of insecurity about the nutrient content of the food supply.
- Their belief that extra vitamins and minerals will help them cope with stress.
- Their belief that supplements can enhance athletic performance or build lean body tissue without physical work.
- Their desire to prevent, treat, or cure symptoms or diseases ranging from the common cold to cancer.

Study after study has found that well-nourished people are the ones who take supplements, whereas people with low nutrient intakes from food generally do not. In addition, little relationship exists between the nutrients people need and the ones they take in supplements. In fact, an argument against supplements is that they may lull people into a false sense of security.

Are there other arguments against taking supplements?

Yes, there are several arguments against taking supplements. First, foods rarely cause nutrient imbalances or toxicities, but supplements can. The higher the dose, the greater the risk of harm. The Tolerable Upper Intake Levels (UL) of the DRI (see inside front cover) answer the question "How much is too much?" by defining the highest amount that appears safe for *most* healthy people. However, people's tolerances for high doses of nutrients vary, just as their risks of deficiencies do. Amounts that some can tolerate may produce toxicities in others, and no one knows who falls where along the spectrum.

Supplement users may have excessive intakes of certain nutrients. The extent and severity of supplement toxicity remain unclear. Only a few alert health care professionals can recognize toxicity, even when it is acute. When it is chronic, with the effects developing subtly and progressing slowly, it often goes unrecognized and unreported. In view of the potential hazards, some authorities believe supplements should bear warning labels, advising consumers that large doses may be toxic.

Toxic overdoses of vitamins and minerals in children are more readily recognized and, unfortunately, fairly common.[6] Fruit-flavored, chewable vitamins shaped like cartoon characters entice young children to eat them like candy in amounts that can cause poisoning. High-potency iron supplements (30 milligrams of iron or more per tablet) are especially toxic and are the leading cause of accidental ingestion fatalities among children.

Second, some dietary supplements sold on the U.S. market are contaminated. Toxic plant material, toxic heavy metals, bacteria, and other substances have shown up in a wide variety of dietary supplements. Even some children's chewable vitamins have contained appreciable lead, a destructive heavy metal. Even though hazardous products are quickly removed from the market upon discovery, many others remain on store shelves because current regulations make the supplement market difficult to monitor and control. Plain multivitamin and mineral supplements from reputable sources, without herbs or add-ons, often test free from contamination.

A third argument against taking supplements arises when people who are ill come to believe that high doses of vitamins or minerals can be therapeutic. Not only can high doses be toxic, but the person may take them instead of seeking medical help.

A final argument against taking supplements is that the body absorbs nutrients best from foods that dilute and disperse them among other substances to facilitate their absorption and use by the body. Taken in pure, concentrated form, nutrients are likely to interfere with one another's absorption or with the absorption of other nutrients from foods eaten at the same time. Such effects are particularly well known among the minerals. For example, zinc hinders copper and calcium absorption, iron hinders zinc absorption, and calcium hinders magnesium and iron absorption. Among vitamins, vitamin C supplements *enhance* iron absorption, making iron overload likely in susceptible people. These and other interactions represent drawbacks to supplement use.

Do antioxidant supplements prevent cancer?

Again, it is better advice to eat a nutrient-dense diet. Some evidence links high intakes of antioxidant-rich fruit and vegetables with good health and disease prevention.[7] More than 200 population studies have examined the effects of fruit and vegetables on cancer risk, and many show that people who eat more of these foods are less likely to develop certain cancers. Findings from other types of studies, such as intervention studies and clinical trials, however, show weaker associations between fruit and vegetable intake and reduced risk of cancer. Some researchers speculate that fruit and vegetable intake may play a smaller role in total cancer protection than previously thought.[8] However, some fruit and vegetables do contain protective factors for specific cancers. For example, research suggests dietary fiber protects against colorectal cancer.[9] When research combines many different fruit and vegetables, specific protective factors may not stand out. Many experts agree that the antioxidant vitamins in these foods are probably important protective factors, but they also note that other constituents of fruit and vegetables (see Figure NP8-1 on p. 232) certainly have not been ruled out as contributing factors.

The way to apply this information is to eat nutritious foods. Taking antioxidant supplements instead of making needed lifestyle changes may sound appealing, but evidence does not support a role for supplements against chronic diseases.[10] In some cases, supplements may even be harmful.

When a person needs a vitamin-mineral supplement, what kind should be used?

Ask your health care professional for advice. A single, balanced vitamin-mineral supplement with no added extras such as herbs should suffice. Choose the kind that provides all the nutrients in amounts less than, equal to, or very close to the RDA (remember, you get some nutrients from foods). For those who require a higher dose, such as young women who need supplemental folate in the childbearing years, choose a supplement with just the needed nutrient or in combination with a reasonable dose of others. Avoid any preparations that, in a daily dose, provide more than the recommended intake of vitamin A, vitamin D, or any mineral or more than the UL for any nutrient. In addition, avoid the following:

- High doses of iron (more than 10 milligrams per day), except for menstruating women.
- "Organic" or "natural" preparations with added substances. They are no better than standard types, but they cost more.
- "High-potency" or "therapeutic dose" supplements. More is not better.
- Substances not needed in human nutrition such as inositol and carnitine. These particular ingredients won't harm you, but they reveal a marketing strategy that makes the whole mix suspect.

As for price, be aware that local or store brands may be just as good as or better than nationally advertised brands. They may be less expensive because the price does not have to cover the cost of national advertising. Finally, be aware that if you see a USP symbol on the label (see Figure NP9-1), it means that the manufacturer has voluntarily paid an independent laboratory to test the product and affirm that it contains the ingredients listed and will dissolve or disintegrate in the digestive tract to make the ingredients available for absorption. The symbol does not imply that the supplement has been tested for safety or effectiveness with regard to health, however.

Can supplement labels help consumers make informed choices?

Yes, to some extent. To enable consumers to make more informed choices about nutrient supplements, the FDA, with the encouragement of the Academy of Nutrition and Dietetics, published labeling regulations for supplements. The Dietary Supplement Health and Education Act subjects supplements to the same general labeling requirements that apply to foods. Specifically:

- Nutrition labeling for dietary supplements is required. The nutrition panel on supplements is called "Supplement Facts" (see Figure NP9-2). The Supplement Facts panel lists the quantity and the percentage of the Daily Value for each nutrient in the supplement. Ingredients that have no Daily Value—for example, sugars and gelatin—appear in a list below the Supplement Facts panel.
- Labels may make nutrient claims (such as "high" or "low") according to specific criteria (for example, "an excellent source of vitamin C").
- Labels may make health claims that are supported by significant scientific agreement and are not brand specific (for example, "Folate protects against neural tube defects").
- Labels may claim that the lack of a nutrient can cause a deficiency disease, but if they do, they must also include the prevalence of that deficiency disease in the United States.
- Labels may claim to diagnose, treat, cure, or relieve common complaints such as menstrual cramps or memory loss, but they may *not* make claims about specific diseases (except as noted previously).
- Labels may make structure–function claims (see Chapter 1) about the role a nutrient plays in the body, explain how the nutrient performs its function, and indicate that consuming the nutrient is associated with general well-being. These claims must be accompanied by an FDA disclaimer statement: "This statement has not been evaluated by the Food and Drug Administration. This product is not intended to diagnose, treat, cure, or prevent any disease."

Note, however, that despite these requirements, in effect, the Dietary Supplement Health and Education Act resulted in the deregulation of the supplement industry. Under current law, the FDA is responsible only for taking action against unsafe dietary supplements already on the market. No advance registration or approval by the FDA is needed before a manufacturer can put a supplement on store shelves.[11] To act against unsafe supplements, the FDA must receive manufacturers' reports concerning serious adverse health effects reported to them by consumers. Manufacturers do list contact information on supplement labels for this

---

FIGURE NP9-1 USP Symbol

This symbol means that a supplement contains the nutrients stated and that it will dissolve in the digestive system—the symbol does not guarantee safety or health advantages.

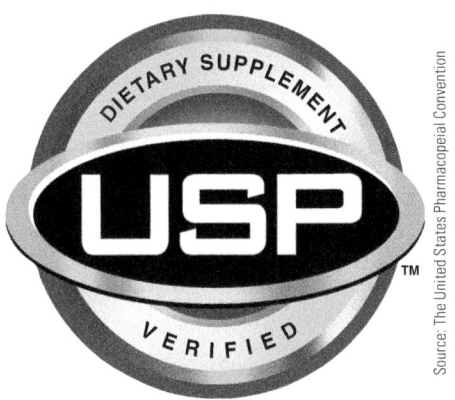

Source: The United States Pharmacopeial Convention

Check the Supplement Facts panel, left, for a list of included nutrients, quantity per serving, and "% Daily Value." Less-reliable structure–function claims, shown on the right, do not need FDA approval, but must be accompanied by a disclaimer

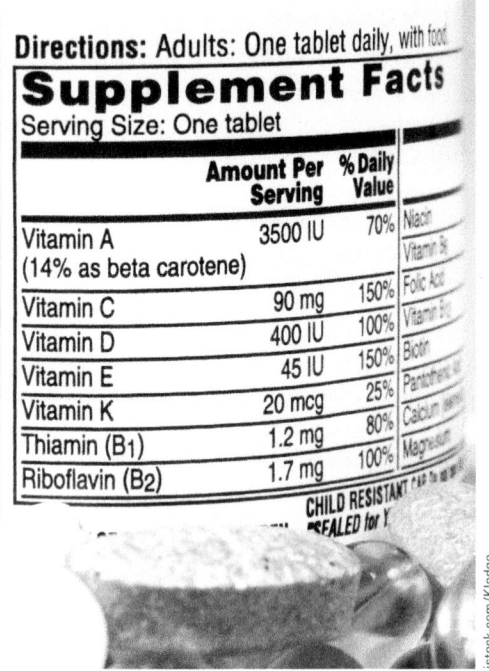

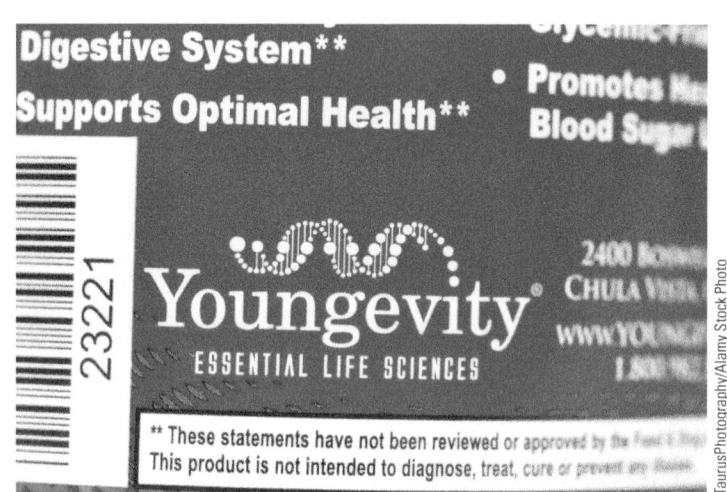

purpose, but many symptoms of adverse reactions are easily mistaken for something else—stomach flu or headache or fatigue. Consumers can also report adverse reactions from supplements directly to the FDA via its hotline or website, but most people are unaware of these options.*

People in developed nations are far more likely to suffer from *overnutrition* and poor lifestyle choices than from nutrient deficiencies. People wish that swallowing vitamin pills would boost their health. The truth—that they need to improve their eating and exercise habits—is harder to swallow.

Notes

1. E.D. Kantor and coauthors, Trends in dietary supplement use among US adults from 1999–2012, *Journal of the American Medical Association* 14 (2016): 1464–1474; M. L. Garcia-Cazarin and coauthors, Dietary supplement research portfolio at the NIH, 2009–2011, *Journal of Nutrition* 144 (2014): 414–418.
2. A. Dickinson and D. MacKay, Health habits and other characteristics of supplement users: A review, *Nutrition Journal* 13 (2014): 14.
3. S. Rautiainen and coauthors, Effect of baseline nutritional status on long-term multivitamin use and cardiovascular disease risk, *JAMA Cardiology*, 2017, doi: 10.1001/jamacardio.2017.017; P. Lance and coauthors, Colorectal adenomas in participants of the SELECT Randomized Trial of Selenium and Vitamin E for Prostate Cancer Prevention, *Cancer Prevention Research*, 2016, doi: 10.1158/1940-6207.CAPR-16-0104; G. Angelo, V. J. Drake, and B. Friel, Efficacy of multivitamin/mineral supplementation to reduce chronic disease risk: A critical review of the evidence from observational studies and randomized controlled trials, *Critical Reviews in Food Science and Nutrition* 55 (2015): 1968–1991.
4. Kantor and coauthors, 2016.
5. A. I. Geller and coauthors, Emergency department visits for adverse events related to dietary supplements, *New England Journal of Medicine* 373 (2015): 1531–1540.
6. FDA 101: Dietary supplements, www.fda.gov/forconsumers/consumerupdates/ucm050803.htm, updated July 15, 2015.
7. O. Oyebode and coauthors, Fruit and vegetable consumption and all-cause, cancer, and CVD mortality: Analysis of Health Survey for England data, *Journal of Epidemiology and Community Health* 68 (2014): 856–862.
8. T. Norat and coauthors, Fruits and vegetables: Updating the epidemiologic evidence for WCRF/AICR lifestyle recommendations for cancer prevention, *Cancer Treatment and Research* 159 (2014): 35–50.
9. Norat and coauthors, 2014; K. E. Bradbury, P. N. Appleby, and T. J. Key, Fruit, vegetable, and fiber intake in relation to cancer risk: Findings from the European Prospective Investigation into Cancer and Nutrition (EPIC), *American Journal of Clinical Nutrition* 100 (2014): 394S–398S.
10. V. A. Moyer, Vitamin, mineral, and multivitamin supplements for the primary prevention of cardiovascular disease and cancer: U.S. Preventive Services Task Force Recommendation Statement, Annals of Internal Medicine 160 (2014): 558–564.
11. U.S. Food and Drug Administration, Center for Food Safety and Applied Nutrition, Dietary Supplements, www.fda.gov/food/dietarysupplements/default.htm, updated September 5, 2017.

*Consumers should report suspected harm from dietary supplements to their health providers or to the FDA's MedWatch program at (800) FDA-1088 or on the Internet at www.fda.gov/medwatch/.

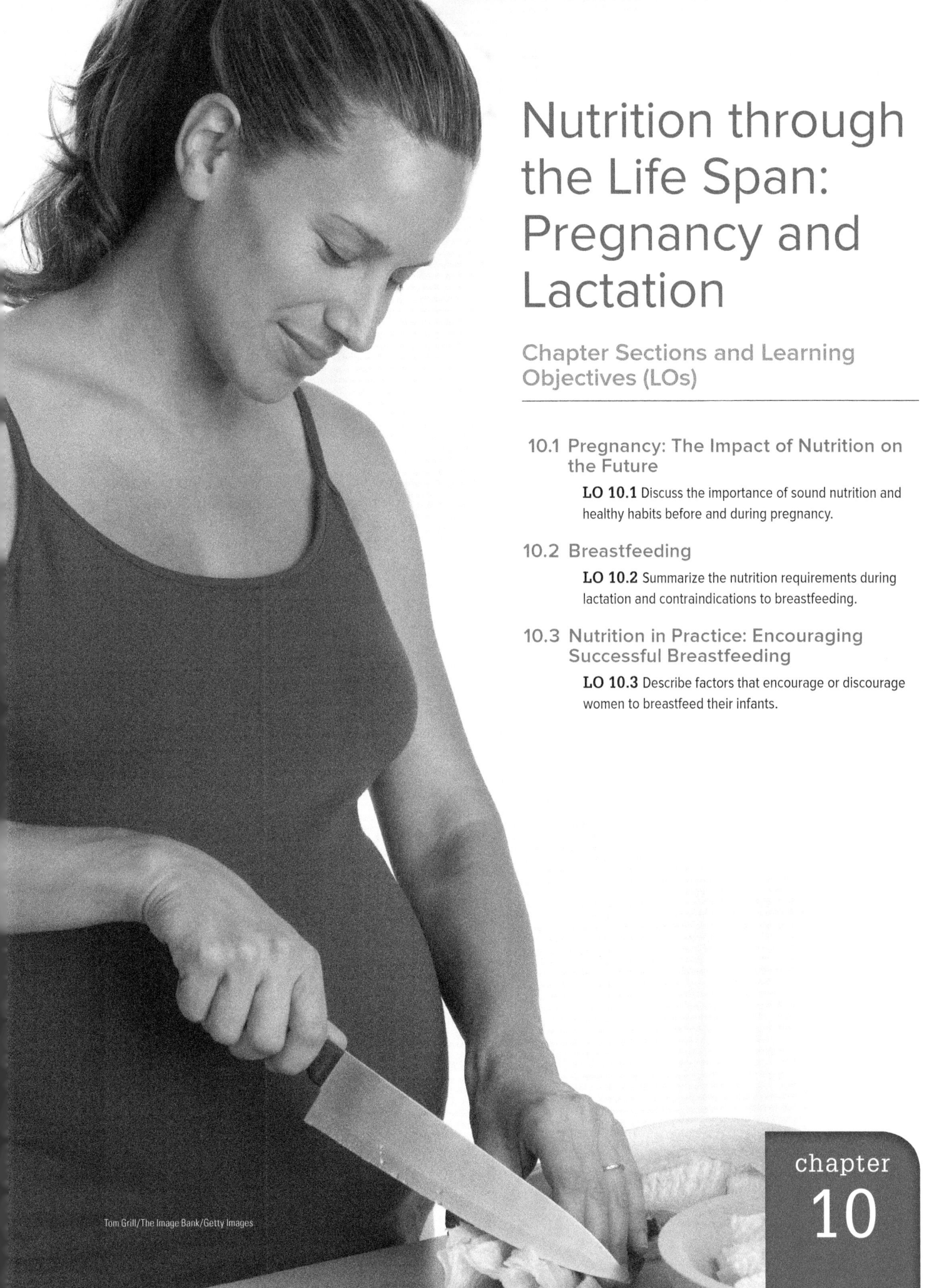

Nutrition through the Life Span: Pregnancy and Lactation

Chapter Sections and Learning Objectives (LOs)

10.1 Pregnancy: The Impact of Nutrition on the Future

LO 10.1 Discuss the importance of sound nutrition and healthy habits before and during pregnancy.

10.2 Breastfeeding

LO 10.2 Summarize the nutrition requirements during lactation and contraindications to breastfeeding.

10.3 Nutrition in Practice: Encouraging Successful Breastfeeding

LO 10.3 Describe factors that encourage or discourage women to breastfeed their infants.

Tom Grill/The Image Bank/Getty Images

chapter

10

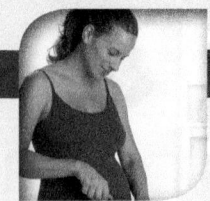

vary depending on their stage of life. This chapter focuses on nutrition in preparation for, and support of, pregnancy and lactation. The next two chapters address the needs of infants, children, adolescents, and older adults.

10.1 Pregnancy: The Impact of Nutrition on the Future

The woman who enters pregnancy with full nutrient stores, sound eating habits, and a healthy body weight has done much to ensure an optimal pregnancy. Then, if she eats a variety of nutrient-dense foods during pregnancy, her own and her infant's health will benefit further.

Nutrition Prior to Pregnancy

A discussion on nutrition prior to pregnancy must, by its nature, focus mainly on women. A man's nutrition may affect his **fertility** and possibly the genetic contributions he makes to his children, but nutrition exerts its primary influence through the woman.[1] Her body provides the environment for the growth and development of a new human being. Full nutrient stores *before* pregnancy are essential both to conception and to healthy infant development during pregnancy. In the early weeks of pregnancy, before many women are even aware that they are pregnant, significant developmental changes occur that depend on a woman's nutrient stores. In preparation for a healthy pregnancy, a woman can establish the following habits:

Both parents can prepare in advance for a healthy pregnancy.

- *Achieve and maintain a healthy body weight.* Both underweight and overweight women, and their newborns, face increased risks of complications.
- *Choose an adequate and balanced diet.* Malnutrition reduces fertility and impairs the early development of an infant should a woman become pregnant.
- *Be physically active.* A woman who wants to be physically active *when* she is pregnant needs to become physically active *beforehand.*
- *Receive regular medical care.* Regular health care visits can help ensure a healthy start to pregnancy.
- *Avoid harmful influences.* Both maternal and paternal ingestion of, or exposure to, harmful substances (such as cigarettes, alcohol, drugs, or environmental contaminants) can cause miscarriage or abnormalities, alter genes or their expression, and interfere with fertility.[2]

Young adults who nourish and protect their bodies do so not only for their own sakes but also for future generations (see Photo 10-1).

Prepregnancy Weight

Appropriate weight prior to pregnancy benefits pregnancy outcome. Being either underweight or overweight (see Table 10-4 on p. 282) presents medical risks during pregnancy and childbirth. Underweight women are therefore advised to gain weight before becoming pregnant and overweight women to lose excess weight.

Underweight Infant birthweight correlates with prepregnancy weight and weight gain during pregnancy and is the most potent single predictor of the infant's future health and survival. An underweight woman has a high risk of having a

fertility: the capacity of a woman to produce a normal ovum periodically and of a man to produce normal sperm; the ability to reproduce.

low-birthweight infant, especially if she is unable to gain sufficient weight during pregnancy.[3] Compared with normal-weight infants, low-birthweight infants are more likely to contract diseases and are nearly 40 times more likely to die in the first month of life. Impaired growth and development during pregnancy may have long-term health effects as well. Research suggests that, when nutrient supplies fail to meet demands, permanent adaptations take place that may make obesity or chronic diseases such as heart disease and hypertension more likely in later life.[4] Other potential problems of low birthweight may include low adult IQ and other brain impairments, short stature, and educational disadvantages.[5] Underweight women are therefore advised to gain weight before becoming pregnant and to strive to gain adequately during pregnancy.

Nutritional deficiency, coupled with low birthweight, is the underlying cause of more than half of all the deaths worldwide of children younger than five years of age. In the United States, the infant mortality rate in 2013 was slightly less than 6 deaths per 1000 live births.[6] This rate, though higher than that of some other developed countries, has seen a significant steady decline over the past several decades and stands as a tribute to public health efforts aimed at reducing infant deaths.

Not all cases of low birthweight reflect poor nutrition. Heredity, disease conditions, smoking, and drug use (including alcohol use) during pregnancy all contribute. Even with optimal nutrition and health during pregnancy, some women give birth to small infants for unknown reasons. But poor nutrition is a major factor in low birthweight—and an avoidable one, as later sections make clear.[7]

Overweight and Obesity Obese women are also urged to strive for healthy weights before pregnancy. Infants born to obese women are more likely to be large for gestational age, weighing more than 9 pounds.[8] Problems associated with a high birthweight include increased likelihood of a difficult labor and delivery, birth trauma, and **cesarean section**. Consequently, these infants have a greater risk of poor health and death than infants of normal weight. Infants of obese mothers also may be likely to be born with neural tube defects. Folate's role has been examined, but a more likely explanation may be poor glycemic control. Obese women themselves are likely to suffer from gestational diabetes, hypertension, and complications during and infections and hemorrhage after the birth.[9] In addition, both overweight and obese women have a greater risk of giving birth to infants with heart defects and other abnormalities.[10]

Obesity and overnutrition during pregnancy may also have long-term effects. Maternal obesity increases a child's risk of obesity, heart disease, type 2 diabetes, and asthma throughout life.[11] An obese woman who strives for a healthy body weight before her pregnancy will be helping to protect both herself and her child.

Healthy Support Tissues

A major reason that the mother's prepregnancy nutrition is so crucial is that it determines whether her **uterus** will be able to support the growth of a healthy **placenta** during the first month of **gestation**. The placenta is both a supply depot and a waste-removal system for the fetus. If the placenta works perfectly, the fetus wants for nothing; if it doesn't, no alternative source of sustenance is available, and the fetus will fail to thrive. Figure 10-1 shows that the placenta is a mass of tissue in which maternal and fetal blood vessels intertwine and exchange materials. The two bloods never mix, but the barrier between them is thin. Using the **umbilical cord** as a conduit, nutrients and oxygen easily move from the mother's blood into the fetus's blood, and wastes move out of the fetal blood to be excreted by the mother. Thus, by way of the placenta, the mother's digestive tract, respiratory system, and kidneys serve not only her own needs, but those of the fetus, whose organs are not yet functional. The **amniotic sac** surrounds and cradles the fetus, cushioning it with fluids.

low-birthweight (LBW): a birthweight less than 5½ lb (2500 g); indicates probable poor health in the newborn and poor nutrition status of the mother during pregnancy. Optimal birthweight for a full-term infant is 6.8 to 7.9 lb (about 3100 to 3600 g). Low-birthweight infants are of two different types. Some are **premature**; they are born early and are of a weight **appropriate for gestational age (AGA)**. Others have suffered growth failure in the uterus; they may or may not be born early, but they are **small for gestational age (SGA)**.

cesarean (si-ZAIR-ee-un) **section:** surgical childbirth, in which the infant is taken through an incision in the woman's abdomen.

uterus (YOO-ter-us): the womb, the muscular organ within which the infant develops before birth.

placenta (pla-SEN-tuh): an organ that develops inside the uterus early in pregnancy, in which maternal and fetal blood circulate in close proximity and exchange materials. The fetus receives nutrients and oxygen across the placenta; the mother's blood picks up carbon dioxide and other waste materials to be excreted via her lungs and kidneys.

gestation: the period of about 40 weeks (three trimesters) from conception to birth; the term of a pregnancy.

umbilical (um-BIL-ih-cul) **cord:** the ropelike structure through which the fetus's veins and arteries reach the placenta; the route of nourishment and oxygen into the fetus and the route of waste disposal from the fetus.

amniotic (am-nee-OTT-ic) **sac:** the "bag of waters" in the uterus in which the fetus floats.

FIGURE 10-1 The Placenta

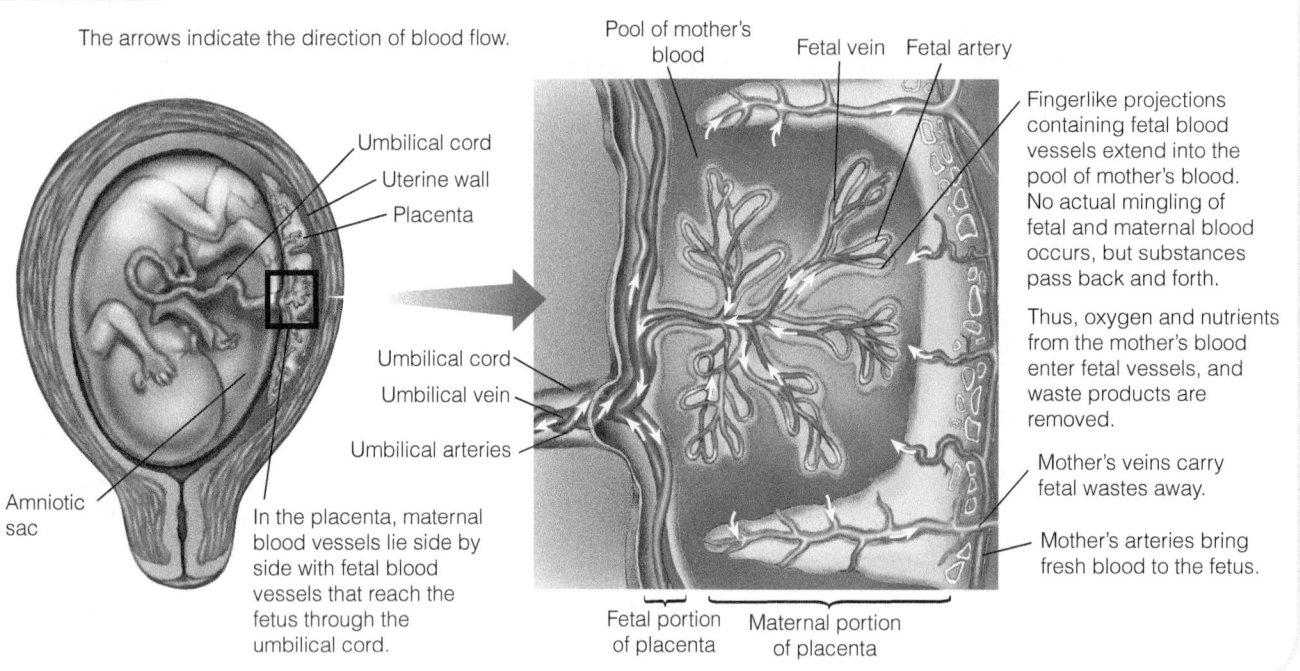

The arrows indicate the direction of blood flow.

Umbilical cord
Uterine wall
Placenta

Pool of mother's blood
Fetal vein   Fetal artery

Fingerlike projections containing fetal blood vessels extend into the pool of mother's blood. No actual mingling of fetal and maternal blood occurs, but substances pass back and forth.

Thus, oxygen and nutrients from the mother's blood enter fetal vessels, and waste products are removed.

Umbilical cord
Umbilical vein
Umbilical arteries

Mother's veins carry fetal wastes away.

Mother's arteries bring fresh blood to the fetus.

Amniotic sac

In the placenta, maternal blood vessels lie side by side with fetal blood vessels that reach the fetus through the umbilical cord.

Fetal portion of placenta   Maternal portion of placenta

The placenta is a highly metabolic organ that actively gathers up hormones, nutrients, and antibodies from the mother's blood and releases them into the fetal bloodstream. The placenta also produces numerous and diverse of hormones that act to maintain pregnancy and prepare the mother's breasts for **lactation**. A healthy placenta is essential for the developing fetus to attain its full potential.

Review Notes

- Adequate nutrition before pregnancy establishes physical readiness and nutrient stores to support fetal growth.
- Both underweight and overweight women should strive for appropriate body weights before pregnancy.
- Newborns who weigh less than 5½ pounds face greater health risks than normal-weight infants.
- The healthy development of the placenta depends on adequate nutrition before pregnancy.

lactation: production and secretion of breast milk for the purpose of nourishing an infant.

ovum (OH-vum): the female reproductive cell, capable of developing into a new organism upon fertilization; commonly referred to as an egg.

zygote (ZY-goat): the product of the union of ovum and sperm; a fertilized ovum.

blastocyst (BLASS-toe-sist): the developmental stage of the zygote when it is about 5 days old and ready for implantation.

implantation: the stage of development in which the blastocyst embeds itself in the wall of the uterus and begins to develop; occurs during the first two weeks after conception.

The Events of Pregnancy

The newly fertilized **ovum** is called a **zygote**. It begins as a single cell and rapidly divides to become a **blastocyst**. During the first week, the blastocyst floats down into the uterus, where it will embed itself in the inner uterine wall—a process known as **implantation**. Minimal growth in size takes place at this time, but it is a crucial period in development. Adverse influences such as smoking, drug abuse, and malnutrition at this time lead to failure to implant or to abnormalities such as neural tube defects that can cause the loss of the developing embryo, possibly before the woman knows she is pregnant.

FIGURE 10-2   Stages of Embryonic and Fetal Development

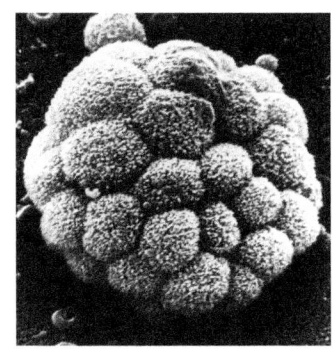

(1) A newly fertilized ovum is called a zygote and is about the size of the period at the end of this sentence. Less than one week after fertilization the zygote has rapidly divided multiple times and has become a blastocyst ready for implantation.

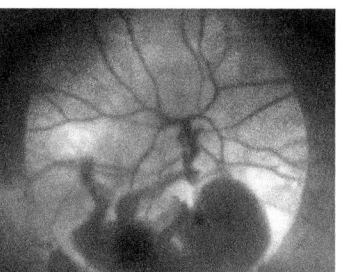

(3) A fetus after 11 weeks of development is just over an inch long. Notice the umbilical cord and blood vessels connecting the fetus with the placenta.

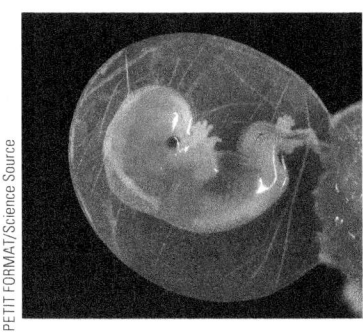

(2) After implantation, the placenta develops and begins to provide nourishment to the developing embryo. An embryo five weeks after fertilization is about 1/2 inch long.

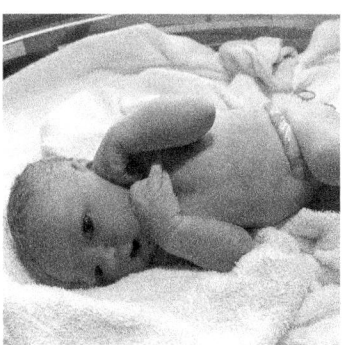

(4) A newborn infant after nine months of development measures close to 20 inches in length. The average birthweight is about 7¹/₂ pounds. From eight weeks to term, the infant has grown 20-fold in length and 50-fold in weight.

The Embryo and Fetus During the next six weeks of development, the **embryo** registers astonishing physical changes (see Figure 10-2). At eight weeks, the **fetus** has a complete central nervous system, a beating heart, a fully formed digestive system, well-defined fingers and toes, and the beginnings of facial features.

In the last seven months of pregnancy, the fetal period, the fetus grows prodigiously. Critical periods of cell division and development occur in organ after organ. Most successful pregnancies last 38 to 42 weeks and produce a healthy infant weighing between 6.8 and 7.9 pounds. The 40 or so weeks of pregnancy are divided into thirds, each of which is called a **trimester**.

A Note about Critical Periods Each organ and tissue type grows with its own characteristic pattern and timing. The development of each takes place only at a certain time—the **critical period**. Whatever nutrients and other environmental conditions are necessary during this period must be supplied on time if the organ is to reach its full potential. If the development of an organ is limited during a critical period, recovery is impossible. For example, the fetus's heart and brain are well developed at 14 weeks; the lungs, 10 weeks later. Therefore, early malnutrition impairs the heart and brain; later malnutrition impairs the lungs.

The effects of malnutrition during critical periods of pregnancy are seen in defects of the nervous system of the embryo (explained later), in the child's poor dental health, and in the adolescent's and adult's vulnerability to infections and possibly higher risks of diabetes, hypertension, stroke, or heart disease.[12] The effects of malnutrition during critical periods are irreversible: abundant and nourishing food consumed after the critical time cannot remedy harm already done.

Table 10-1 identifies characteristics of a **high-risk pregnancy**; the more factors that apply, the higher the risk. A woman with none of these factors is said to have a **low-risk pregnancy**. All pregnant women, especially those in high-risk categories, need prenatal medical care, including dietary advice.

embryo (EM-bree-oh): the developing infant from two to eight weeks after conception.

fetus (FEET-us): the developing infant from eight weeks after conception until its birth.

trimester: a period representing one-third of the term of gestation. A trimester is about 13 to 14 weeks.

critical period: a finite period during development in which certain events occur that will have irreversible effects on later developmental stages; usually a period of rapid cell division.

high-risk pregnancy: a pregnancy characterized by risk factors that make it likely the birth will be surrounded by problems such as premature delivery, difficult birth, retarded growth, birth defects, and early infant death.

low-risk pregnancy: a pregnancy characterized by factors that make it likely the birth will be normal and the infant healthy.

TABLE 10-1   High-Risk Pregnancy Factors

- Prepregnancy BMI either <18.5 or >25.0
- Insufficient or excessive pregnancy weight gain
- Nutrient deficiencies or toxicities; eating disorders
- Poverty, lack of family support, low level of education, limited food availability
- Smoking, alcohol, or other drug use
- Age, especially 15 years or younger or 35 years or older
- Many previous pregnancies (three or more to mothers younger than age 20; four or more to mothers age 20 or older)
- Short or long intervals between pregnancies (<18 months or >59 months)
- Previous history of problems
- Twins or triplets
- Low- or high-birthweight infants
- Development of gestational hypertension
- Development of gestational diabetes
- Diabetes; hypertension; heart, respiratory, and kidney disease; genetic disorders; special diets and medications

Review Notes

- Placental development, implantation, and early critical periods of embryonic and fetal development depend on maternal nutrition before and during pregnancy.
- The effects of malnutrition during critical periods are irreversible.

Nutrient Needs during Pregnancy

Nutrient needs during pregnancy increase more for certain nutrients than for others (see the inside front cover). Figure 10-3 shows the percentage increase in selected nutrient intakes recommended for pregnant women compared with nonpregnant women: notice how much longer the yellow and purple bars are than the green ones. To meet the high nutrient demands of pregnancy, a woman must make mindful food choices, but her body will also do its part by maximizing nutrient absorption and minimizing losses.

Energy, Carbohydrate, Protein, and Fat Energy needs change as pregnancy progresses. In the first trimester, the pregnant woman needs no additional energy, but as pregnancy progresses, her energy needs rise. She requires an additional 340 kcalories daily during the second trimester and an extra 450 kcalories each day during the third trimester.[13] Well-nourished pregnant women meet these demands for more energy in several ways: some eat more food, some reduce their activity, and some store less of their food energy as fat.[15] A woman can easily meet the need for extra kcalories by selecting more nutrient-dense foods from the five food groups. Table 1-6 on p. 19 provides suggested eating patterns for several kcalorie levels, and Table 10-2 offers sample menus for pregnant and lactating women.

If a woman chooses less nutritious options such as sugary soft drinks or fatty snack foods to meet her energy needs, she will undoubtedly come up short on nutrients (Box 10-1). The increase in the need for nutrients is even greater than that for energy, so the mother-to-be should choose nutrient-dense foods such as whole-grain breads and cereals, legumes, dark green vegetables, citrus fruit, low-fat milk and milk products, and lean meats, fish, poultry, and eggs.

Ample carbohydrate (ideally, 175 grams or more per day and certainly no less than 135 grams) is necessary to fuel the fetal brain and spare the protein needed for fetal growth. Fiber in carbohydrate-rich foods such as whole grains, vegetables, and fruit can help alleviate the constipation that many pregnant women experience.

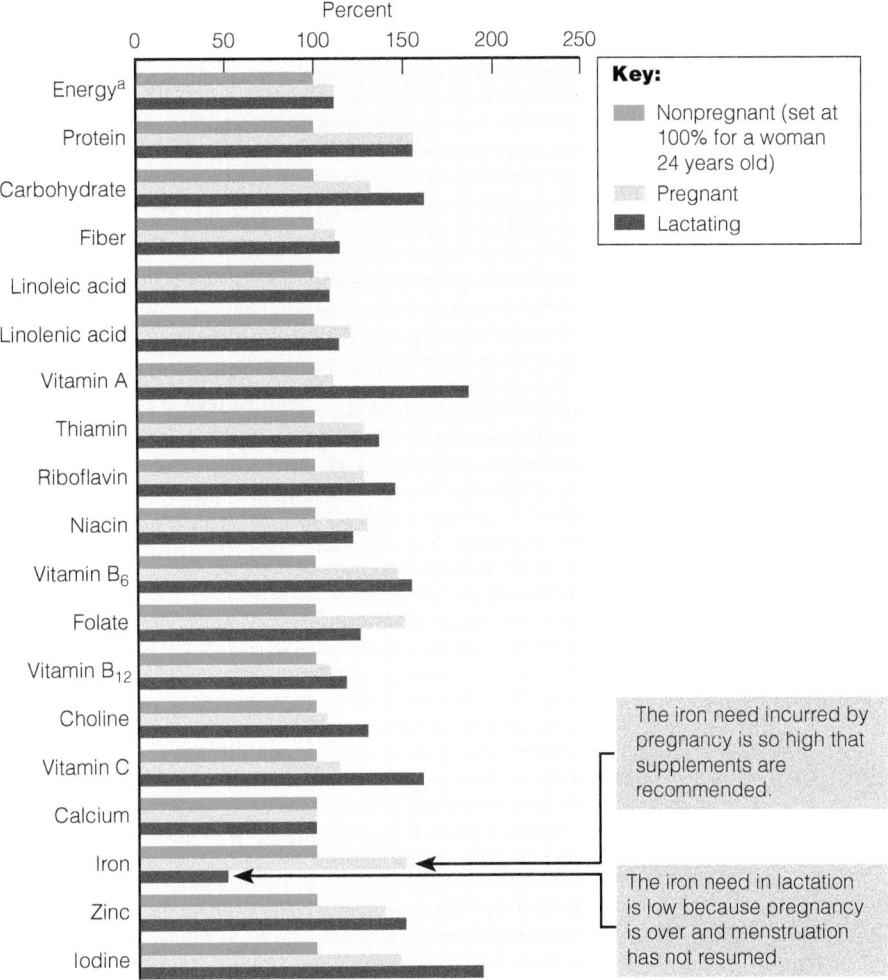

Key:
- Nonpregnant (set at 100% for a woman 24 years old)
- Pregnant
- Lactating

The iron need incurred by pregnancy is so high that supplements are recommended.

The iron need in lactation is low because pregnancy is over and menstruation has not resumed.

[Chart categories, top to bottom: Energy,ᵃ Protein, Carbohydrate, Fiber, Linoleic acid, Linolenic acid, Vitamin A, Thiamin, Riboflavin, Niacin, Vitamin B₆, Folate, Vitamin B₁₂, Choline, Vitamin C, Calcium, Iron, Zinc, Iodine. X-axis: Percent, 0 to 250.]

ᵃEnergy allowance during pregnancy is for the second trimester; energy allowance during the third trimester is slightly higher; no additional allowance is provided during the first trimester. Energy allowance during lactation is for the first six months; energy allowance during the second six months is slightly higher.

TABLE 10-2 Daily Food Choices for Pregnancy (Second and Third Trimesters) and Lactation

FOOD GROUP	AMOUNTS	SAMPLE MENU	
Fruit	2 c	**BREAKFAST** 1 whole-wheat English muffin 2 tbs peanut butter 1 c low-fat vanilla yogurt ½ c fresh strawberries 1 c orange juice	**DINNER** Chicken cacciatore 3 oz chicken ½ c stewed tomatoes 1 c rice
Vegetables	3 c		½ c summer squash
Grains	8 oz		1½ c salad (spinach, mushrooms, carrots)
Protein foods	6½ oz	**MIDMORNING SNACK** ½ c cranberry juice 1 oz pretzels	1 tbs salad dressing 1 slice Italian bread
Milk	3 c	**LUNCH** Sandwich (tuna salad on whole-wheat bread) ½ carrot (sticks) 1 c low-fat milk	2 tsp soft margarine 1 c low-fat milk

Note: This sample meal plan provides about 2500 kcalories (55 percent from carbohydrate, 20 percent from protein, and 25 percent from fat) and meets most of the vitamin and mineral needs of pregnant and lactating women.

TABLE 10-3	Rich Folate Sources

NATURAL FOLATE SOURCES

- Liver (3 oz): 221 μg DFE
- Lentils (½ c): 179 μg DFE
- Chickpeas or pinto beans (½ c): 145 μg DFE
- Asparagus (½ c): 134 μg DFE
- Spinach (1 c raw): 58 μg DFE
- Avocado (½ c): 61 μg DFE
- Orange juice (1 c): 74 μg DFE
- Beets (½ c): 68 μg DFE

FORTIFIED FOLATE SOURCES

- Highly enriched ready-to-eat cereals (¾ c): 680 μg DFE[a]
- Pasta, cooked (1 c): 154 μg DFE (average value)
- Rice, cooked (1 c): 153 μg DFE
- Bagel (1 small whole): 156 μg DFE
- Waffles, frozen (2): 78 μg DFE
- Bread, white (1 slice): 48 μg DFE

[a]Folate in cereals varies; read the Nutrition Facts panel of the label.

neural tube: the embryonic tissue that later forms the brain and spinal cord.

neural tube defect (NTD): a serious central nervous system birth defect that often results in lifelong disability or death.

anencephaly (AN-en-SEF-a-lee): an uncommon and always fatal type of neural tube defect; characterized by the absence of a brain.

an = not (without)
encephalus = brain

spina (SPY-nah) bifida (BIFF-ih-dah): one of the most common types of neural tube defects; characterized by the incomplete closure of the spinal cord's bony encasement, allowing the spinal cord to bulge through.

spina = spine
bifida = split

The protein RDA for pregnancy calls for 25 grams per day more than for nonpregnant women. Pregnant women can easily meet their protein needs by selecting meats, seafood, poultry, low-fat milk and milk products, and protein-containing plant foods such as legumes, tofu, whole grains, nuts, and seeds. Some vegetarian women limit or omit protein-rich meats, eggs, and milk products from their diets. For them, meeting the recommendation for food energy each day and including generous servings of protein-containing plant foods are imperative. Because use of high-protein supplements during pregnancy may be harmful to the infant's development, it is discouraged unless medically prescribed to treat fetal growth problems and carefully monitored.

The high nutrient requirements of pregnancy leave little room in the diet for excess fat, especially solid fats such as fatty meats and butter. The essential fatty acids, however, are particularly important to the growth and development of the fetus. The brain contains a substantial amount of lipid material and depends heavily on long-chain omega-3 and omega-6 fatty acids for its growth, function, and structure.[14] Fish consumption during pregnancy provides a rich source of omega-3 fatty acids and improves brain development and cognition in infants.[15] (See Table 4-4 on p. 104 for a list of good food sources of the essential fatty acids.)

Of Special Interest: Folate and Vitamin B$_{12}$ The vitamins famous for their roles in cell reproduction—folate and vitamin B$_{12}$—are needed in large amounts during pregnancy. New cells are laid down at a tremendous pace as the fetus grows and develops. At the same time, because the mother's blood volume increases, the number of her red blood cells must rise, requiring more cell division and therefore more vitamins. To accommodate these needs, the recommendation for folate during pregnancy increases from 400 to 600 micrograms a day.

As described in Chapter 8, folate plays an important role in preventing neural tube defects. To review, the early weeks of pregnancy are a critical period for the formation and closure of the **neural tube** that will later develop to form the brain and spinal cord. By the time a woman suspects she is pregnant, usually around the sixth week of pregnancy, the embryo's neural tube normally has closed. A **neural tube defect (NTD)** occurs when the tube fails to close properly. Each year in the United States, an estimated 3000 pregnancies are affected by an NTD.[16] The two most common types of NTD are anencephaly (no brain) and spina bifida (split spine).

In **anencephaly**, the upper end of the neural tube fails to close. Consequently, the brain is either missing or fails to develop. Pregnancies affected by anencephaly often end in miscarriage; infants born with anencephaly die shortly after birth.

Spina bifida is characterized by incomplete closure of the spinal cord and its bony encasement (see Figure 10-4). The membranes covering the spinal cord and sometimes the cord itself may protrude from the spine as a sac. Spina bifida often produces paralysis in varying degrees, depending on the extent of spinal cord damage. Mild cases may not be noticed. Moderate cases may involve curvature of the spine, muscle weakness, mental handicaps, and other ills, while severe cases can lead to death.

To reduce the risk of neural tube defects, women who are capable of becoming pregnant are advised to obtain 400 micrograms of folic acid daily from supplements, fortified foods, or both, *in addition* to eating folate-rich foods (see Table 10-3). The DRI committee recommends intake of synthetic folate, called folic acid, in supplements and fortified food because it is absorbed better than the folate naturally present in foods. Foods that naturally contain folate are still important, however, because they contribute to folate intakes while providing other needed vitamins, minerals, fiber, and phytochemicals.

The enrichment of grain products (cereal, grits, pasta, rice, bread, and the like) sold commercially in the United States with folic acid has improved folate status in women of childbearing age and lowered the number of neural tube defects that occur each year.[17] A safety concern arises, however. The pregnant woman also needs a greater amount of

FIGURE 10-4 Spina Bifida—A Neural Tube Defect

Spina bifida, a common neural tube defect, occurs when the vertebrae of the spine fail to close around the spinal cord, leaving it unprotected. The B vitamin folate—consumed prior to and during pregnancy—helps prevent spina bifida and other neural tube defects.

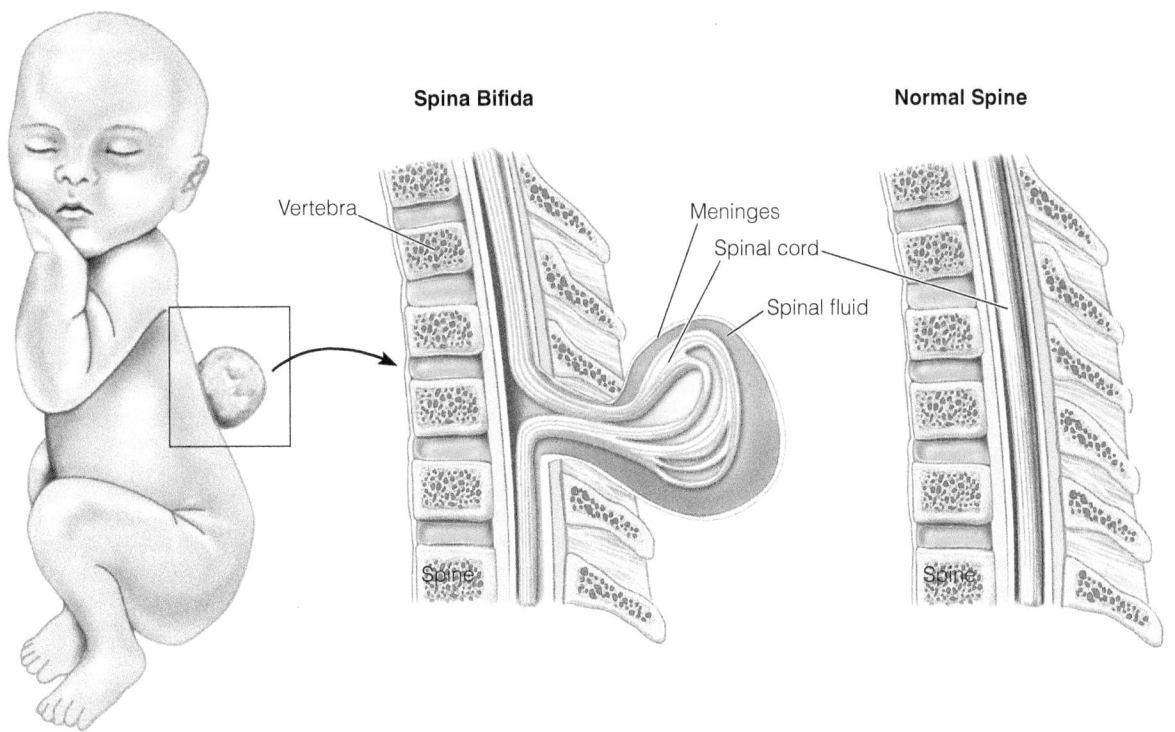

vitamin B_{12} to assist folate in the manufacture of new cells. Because high intakes of folate complicate the diagnosis of a vitamin B_{12} deficiency (see Chapter 8), quantities of 1 milligram or more require a prescription. Most over-the-counter multivitamin supplements contain 400 micrograms of folic acid; supplements for pregnant women usually contain at least 800 micrograms.

People who eat meat, eggs, or dairy products receive all the vitamin B_{12} they need, even for pregnancy. Those who exclude all animal-derived foods from the diet, however, need vitamin B_{12}–fortified foods or supplements.

Another Nutrient of Interest: Choline Choline is a dietary component that is vital for the structural integrity of cell membranes, the synthesis of an important neurotransmitter, and in lipid metabolism. During fetal development, choline is needed for the normal development of the brain and spinal cord.[18] During pregnancy, large amounts of choline are delivered to the fetus via the placenta. Transport of choline from mother to fetus depletes maternal stores.

Although an RDA for choline has not been established, the AI for pregnant women is set at 450 milligrams per day, which is slightly higher than the AI for nonpregnant women. Because **prenatal supplements** do not typically contain choline, pregnant women are advised to include choline-rich foods such as eggs, milk and milk products, legumes, and meats and seafood in their eating patterns.

Vitamin D and Calcium for Bones Vitamin D and the minerals involved in building the skeleton—calcium, phosphorus, magnesium, and fluoride—are in great demand during pregnancy. Insufficient intakes may produce abnormal fetal bone growth and tooth development.

prenatal supplements: nutrient supplements specifically designed to provide the nutrients needed during pregnancy, particularly folate, iron, and calcium, without excesses or unneeded constituents.

Vitamin D plays a vital role in calcium absorption and utilization. Consequently, severe maternal vitamin D deficiency interferes with normal calcium metabolism, which, in rare cases, may cause rickets in the infant.[19] Regular exposure to sunlight and consumption of vitamin D–fortified milk are usually sufficient to provide the recommended amount of vitamin D during pregnancy (15 μg/day), which is the same as for nonpregnant women. The vitamin D in prenatal supplements helps to protect many, but not all, pregnant women from inadequate intakes.[20]

Intestinal absorption of calcium doubles early in pregnancy, when the mother's bones store the mineral. Later, as the fetal bones begin to calcify, a dramatic shift of calcium across the placenta occurs. In the final weeks of pregnancy, more than 300 milligrams a day are transferred to the fetus. Recommendations to ensure an adequate calcium intake during pregnancy are aimed at conserving the mother's bone mass while supplying fetal needs.

Typically, young women in the United States take in too little calcium. Of particular importance, pregnant women under age 25, whose own bones are still actively depositing minerals, should strive to meet the recommendation for calcium by increasing their intakes of milk, cheese, yogurt, and other calcium-rich foods. The USDA Healthy U.S.-Style Eating Pattern suggests consuming 3 cups per day of fat-free or low-fat milk or the equivalent in milk products. Less preferred, but still acceptable, is a daily supplement of 600 milligrams of calcium. The RDA for calcium intake is the same for nonpregnant and pregnant women in the same age group. Women who exclude milk products need calcium-fortified foods such as soy milk, orange juice, and cereals. Read the labels: contents vary and products fortified with both calcium and vitamin D are recommended.

Iron The body conserves iron especially well during pregnancy: menstruation ceases, and absorption of iron increases up to threefold due to a rise in the blood's iron-absorbing and iron-carrying protein transferrin. Still, iron needs are so high that stores dwindle during pregnancy. To help improve the iron status of women before and during pregnancy, all women capable of becoming pregnant are advised to choose foods that supply heme iron (meat, seafood, and poultry), which is most readily absorbed; choose additional sources of iron such as eggs, vegetables, and legumes; and consume foods that enhance iron absorption, such as vitamin C–rich fruit and vegetables.

The developing fetus draws heavily on the mother's iron stores to create stores of its own to last through the first four to six months after birth. During the second and third trimesters of pregnancy, the hormone hepcidin, which regulates iron balance, is suppressed, and the mobilization of iron from maternal stores is enhanced.[21] The transfer of significant amounts of iron to the fetus is regulated by the placenta, which gives the iron needs of the fetus priority over those of the mother.[22] Even a woman with inadequate iron stores transfers a considerable amount of iron to the fetus. In addition, blood (and thus iron) losses are inevitable at birth, especially during a delivery by cesarean section.

Few women enter pregnancy with adequate iron stores, so a daily iron supplement is recommended early in pregnancy, if not before.[23] Women who enter pregnancy with iron-deficiency anemia are at increased risk of delivering low-birthweight or preterm infants. When a low hemoglobin or hematocrit level is confirmed by a repeat test, more than the standard iron dose of 30 milligrams may be prescribed. To enhance iron absorption, the supplement should be taken between meals and with liquids other than milk, coffee, or tea, which inhibit iron absorption.

Zinc Zinc is required for protein synthesis and cell development during pregnancy. Typical zinc intakes of pregnant women are lower than recommendations but, fortunately, zinc absorption increases when intakes are low. Large doses of iron can interfere with zinc absorption and metabolism, but most prenatal supplements supply the right balance of these minerals for pregnancy. Zinc is abundant in protein-rich foods such as shellfish, meat, and nuts.

Nutrient Supplements A healthy pregnancy and optimal infant development depend on the mother's diet.[24] Pregnant women can meet their nutrient needs—except for iron—by making wise food choices. Even so, physicians often recommend daily multi-vitamin-mineral supplements for pregnant women. These prenatal supplements typically provide more folic acid, iron, and calcium than regular supplements. Prenatal supplements are especially beneficial for women who do not eat adequately and for those in high-risk groups: women carrying twins or triplets, cigarette smokers, and alcohol or drug abusers. For these women, prenatal supplements may be of some help in reducing the risks of preterm delivery, low infant birthweights, and birth defects. Be aware, however, that supplements cannot prevent the vast majority of fetal harm from tobacco, alcohol, and drugs, which continues unopposed, as later sections explain.

Review Notes

- The pregnant woman needs no additional energy intake during the first trimester, an increase of 340 kcalories per day during the second trimester, and an increase of 450 kcalories per day during the third trimester as compared with her nonpregnant needs.

- An additional 25 grams per day of protein are needed during pregnancy, but pregnant women can easily meet this need by choosing meats, poultry, seafood, eggs, low-fat milk and milk products, and plant-protein foods such as legumes, whole grains, nuts, and seeds.

- Due to their key roles in cell reproduction, folate and vitamin B$_{12}$ are needed in large amounts during pregnancy.

- Folate plays an important role in preventing neural tube defects.

- Choline is needed for the normal development of the brain and spinal cord.

- Maternal vitamin D deficiency interferes with calcium metabolism in the infant.

- All pregnant women, but especially those who are younger than 25 years of age, need to pay special attention to calcium to ensure adequate intakes.

- Iron supplements are recommended for pregnant women.

- Large doses of iron can interfere with zinc absorption and metabolism, but most prenatal supplements supply the right balance of these minerals.

- Physicians often recommend daily multivitamin-mineral supplements for pregnant women.

- Women most likely to benefit from prenatal supplements during pregnancy include those who do not eat adequately, those carrying twins or triplets, and those who smoke cigarettes or abuse alcohol or drugs.

Food Assistance Programs

Women of limited financial means may eat diets too low in calcium, iron, vitamins A and C, and protein. Often, they and their children need help in obtaining food and benefit from nutrition counseling. At the federal level, the **Special Supplemental Nutrition Program for Women, Infants, and Children (WIC)** provides vouchers redeemable for nutritious foods, nutrition education, and referrals to health and social services to low-income pregnant and lactating women and their children.[25] WIC offers vouchers for the following nutritious foods: baby foods; eggs; dried and canned beans and peas; tuna fish; peanut butter; fruit, vegetables, and their juices; iron-fortified cereals; milk and cheese; soy-based beverages and tofu; and whole-wheat and other whole-grain products. For infants given infant formula, WIC also provides iron-fortified formula. WIC encourages mothers to breastfeed their infants, however, and offers incentives to those who do.

More than 9 million people—most of them infants and young children—receive WIC benefits each month. Participation in the WIC program benefits both the nutrient status and the growth and development of infants and children. WIC participation

Special Supplemental Nutrition Program for Women, Infants, and Children (WIC): a high-quality, cost-effective health care and nutrition services program administered by the U.S. Department of Agriculture for low-income women, infants, and children who are nutritionally at risk. WIC provides supplemental foods, nutrition education, and referrals to health care and other social services.

during pregnancy can effectively reduce iron deficiency, infant mortality, low birth-weight, and maternal and newborn medical costs.

The Supplemental Nutrition Assistance Program (SNAP) provides a debit card that can also help to stretch the low-income pregnant woman's grocery dollars. In addition, many communities and organizations such as the Academy of Nutrition and Dietetics (AND) provide educational services and materials, including nutrition, food budgeting, and shopping information.

Review Notes

- Food assistance programs such as WIC can provide nutritious food for pregnant women of limited financial means.
- Participation in WIC during pregnancy can reduce iron deficiency, infant mortality, low birth-weight, and maternal and newborn medical costs.

Weight Gain

Women must gain weight during pregnancy—fetal and maternal well-being depend on it. Ideally, a woman will have begun her pregnancy at a healthy weight, but even more importantly, she will gain within the recommended weight range based on her prepregnancy body mass index (BMI) as shown in Table 10-4. Pregnancy weight gains within the recommended ranges are associated with fewer surgical births, a greater number of healthy birthweights, and other positive outcomes for both mothers and infants, but many women do not gain within these ranges.[26] Among women in the United States, excessive weight gain during pregnancy is more prevalent than inadequate weight gain. To improve pregnancy outcomes, researchers and health care providers are placing greater emphasis on preventing excessive weight gains during pregnancy than in the recent past.[27]

Weight loss during pregnancy is not recommended.[28] Obese women are advised to gain between 11 and 20 pounds for the best chance of delivering a healthy infant. Ideally, overweight and obese women will achieve a healthy body weight before becoming pregnant, avoid excessive weight gain during pregnancy, and postpone weight loss until after childbirth.

According to current recommendations, pregnant adolescents who are still growing should strive for gains at the upper end of the target range. Current concerns about obesity raise questions as to whether such recommendations are always appropriate. Compared with older mothers, for example, the risk of lifetime weight retention after pregnancy may be far greater for young adolescents.

TABLE 10-4 Recommended Pregnancy Weight Gains Based on Prepregnancy Weight

PREPREGNANCY WEIGHT	RECOMMENDED WEIGHT GAIN	
	FOR SINGLE BIRTH	FOR TWIN BIRTH
Underweight (BMI <18.5)	28–40 lb (12.5–18.0 kg)	Insufficient data to make recommendation
Healthy weight (BMI 18.5–24.9)	25–35 lb (11.5–16.0 kg)	37–54 lb (17–25 kg)
Overweight (BMI 25.0–29.9)	15–25 lb (7.0–11.5 kg)	31–50 lb (14–23 kg)
Obese (BMI ≥30)	11–20 lb (5–9 kg)	25–42 lb (11–19 kg)

Source: Institute of Medicine, *Weight Gain During Pregnancy: Reexamining the Guidelines.* Reprinted with permission from The National Academies Press, Copyright © 2009, National Academy of Sciences.

FIGURE 10-5 Components of Weight Gain during Pregnancy

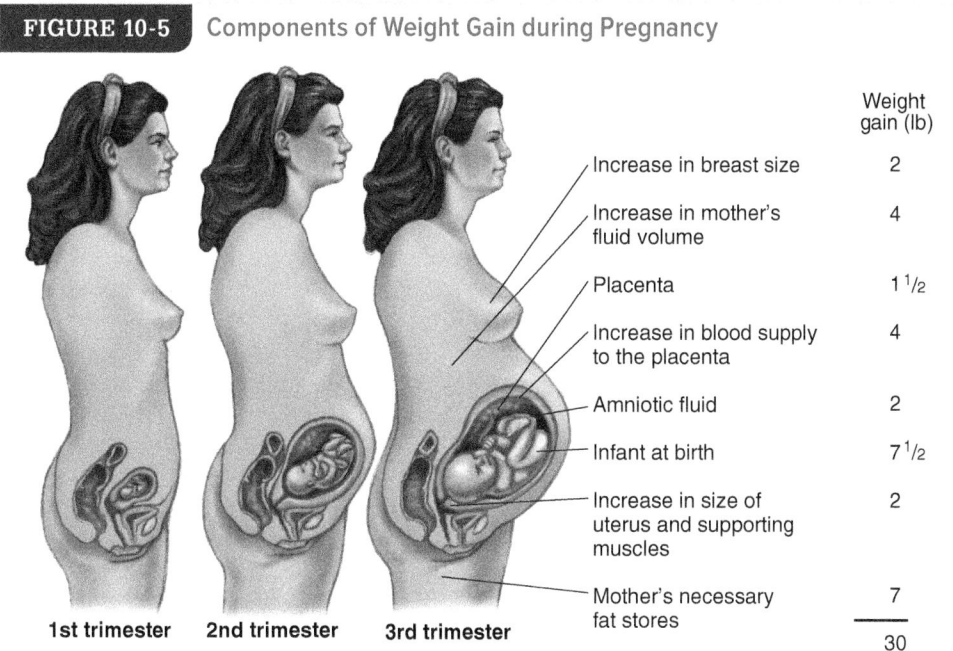

	Weight gain (lb)
Increase in breast size	2
Increase in mother's fluid volume	4
Placenta	1 ½
Increase in blood supply to the placenta	4
Amniotic fluid	2
Infant at birth	7 ½
Increase in size of uterus and supporting muscles	2
Mother's necessary fat stores	7
	30

1st trimester   2nd trimester   3rd trimester

The ideal weight gain pattern for a woman who begins pregnancy at a healthy weight is 3½ pounds during the first trimester and 1 pound per week thereafter (see the prenatal weight-gain grid in Appendix E). If a woman gains more than is recommended early in pregnancy, she should not restrict her energy intake later on in order to lose weight. A sudden, large weight gain is a danger signal, however, because it may indicate the onset of preeclampsia (discussed later in the chapter).

The weight the pregnant woman gains is nearly all lean tissue: placenta, uterus, blood, milk-producing glands, and the fetus itself (see Figure 10-5). The fat she gains is needed later for lactation. Physical activity can help a pregnant woman cope with the extra weight, as a later section explains.

Weight Loss after Pregnancy

The pregnant woman loses some weight at delivery. In the following weeks, she loses more as her blood volume returns to normal and she loses accumulated fluids. The typical woman does not, however, return to her prepregnancy weight. In general, the more weight a woman gains beyond the needs of pregnancy, the more she retains and the more likely she will continue to gain over the next several years. Even with an average weight gain during pregnancy, most women tend to retain a few pounds with each pregnancy. When the weight gain has added up to seven or more pounds and the BMI has increased by a unit or more, complications such as diabetes and hypertension in future pregnancies as well as chronic diseases later in life can increase—even for women who are not overweight. Women who achieve a healthy weight prior to the first pregnancy and maintain it between pregnancies best avoid the cumulative weight gain that threatens health later on.

Review Notes

- Appropriate (adequate but not excessive) weight gain is essential for a healthy pregnancy.
- A woman's prepregnancy BMI, her own nutrient needs, and the number of fetuses she is carrying help to determine appropriate weight gain.
- Most women tend to retain a few pounds with each pregnancy.

Physical Activity

An active, physically fit woman experiencing a normal pregnancy can and should continue to exercise throughout pregnancy, adjusting the intensity and duration as the pregnancy progresses. Staying active during the course of a normal, healthy pregnancy improves the fitness of the mother-to-be, facilitates labor, helps to prevent or manage gestational diabetes and gestational hypertension, and reduces psychological stress.[29] Women who remain active report fewer discomforts throughout their pregnancies, are more likely to meet weight gain recommendations, and retain habits that help in losing excess weight and regaining fitness after the birth.[30]

Pregnant women should choose "low-impact" activities and avoid sports in which they might fall or be hit by other people or objects. Swimming and water aerobics are particularly beneficial because they allow the body to remain cool and move freely with the water's support, thus reducing back pain.

As is true for everyone, the frequency, duration, and intensity of the activity affect the likelihood of the benefits or risks. A few guidelines are offered in Figure 10-6. Several of the guidelines are aimed at preventing excessively high internal body temperatures and dehydration, both of which can harm fetal development. To this end, a pregnant woman should also stay out of saunas, steam rooms, and hot whirlpools. A pregnant woman with a medical condition or pregnancy complication should undergo a thorough evaluation by her health care provider before engaging in physical activity.

Review Notes

- Physically fit women can continue physical activity throughout pregnancy but should choose activities wisely.
- Pregnant women should avoid sports in which they might fall or be hit by other people or objects and should take care not to become dehydrated or overheated.

FIGURE 10-6 Guidelines for Physical Activity during Pregnancy

DO

Do exercise regularly (most, if not all, days of the week).

Do warm up with 5 to 10 minutes of light activity.

Do 30 minutes or more of moderate physical activity.

Do cool down with 5 to 10 minutes of slow activity and gentle stretching.

Do drink water before, during, and after exercise.

Do eat enough to support the additional needs of pregnancy plus exercise.

Do rest adequately.

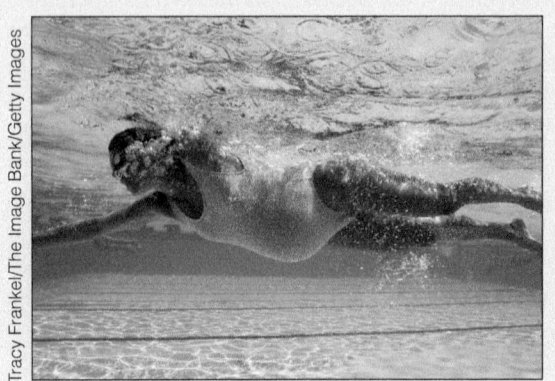

Tracy Frankel/The Image Bank/Getty Images

Pregnant women can enjoy the benefits of physical activity.

DON'T

Don't exercise vigorously after long periods of inactivity.

Don't exercise in hot, humid weather.

Don't exercise when sick with fever.

Don't exercise while lying on your back after the first trimester of pregnancy or stand motionless for prolonged periods.

Don't exercise if you experience any pain or discomfort.

Don't participate in activities that may harm the abdomen or involve jerky, bouncy movements.

Don't scuba dive.

Common Nutrition-Related Concerns of Pregnancy

Food sensitivities, nausea, heartburn, and constipation are common during pregnancy. A few simple strategies can help alleviate maternal discomforts (see Table 10-5).

Food Cravings and Aversions Some women develop cravings for, or aversions to, certain foods and beverages during pregnancy. Individual **food cravings** during pregnancy do not seem to reflect real physiological needs. In other words, a woman who craves pickles does not necessarily need salt. Similarly, cravings for ice cream are common during pregnancy but do not signify a calcium deficiency. **Food aversions** and cravings that arise during pregnancy are probably due to hormone-induced changes in taste and sensitivities to smells, and they quickly disappear after the birth.

Nonfood Cravings Some pregnant women develop cravings for and ingest nonfood items such as laundry starch, clay, soil, or ice—a practice known as pica.[31] Pica may be practiced for cultural reasons that reflect a society's folklore. Pica is often associated with iron deficiency, but whether iron deficiency leads to pica or pica leads to iron deficiency is unclear. Eating clay or soil may interfere with iron absorption and displace iron-rich foods from the diet. Furthermore, if the soil or clay contains environmental contaminants such as lead or parasites, health and nutrition suffer.

Morning Sickness Not all women have queasy stomachs in the early months of pregnancy, but many do. The nausea of "morning sickness" may actually occur anytime and may even be a welcome sign of a healthy pregnancy because it arises from the hormonal changes of early pregnancy (Box 10-2).[32] The problem typically peaks at nine weeks' gestation and resolves within a month or two. Many women complain that odors, especially cooking smells, make them sick. Thus, minimizing odors may

---

TABLE 10-5 Strategies to Alleviate Maternal Discomforts

To alleviate the nausea of pregnancy:

- On waking, arise slowly.
- Eat dry toast or crackers.
- Chew gum or suck hard candies.
- Eat small, frequent meals whenever hunger strikes.
- Avoid foods with offensive odors.
- When nauseated, do not drink citrus juice, water, milk, coffee, or tea.

To prevent or alleviate constipation:

- Eat foods high in fiber.
- Exercise daily.
- Drink at least eight glasses of liquids a day.
- Respond promptly to the urge to defecate.
- Use laxatives only as prescribed by a physician; avoid mineral oil—it carries needed fat-soluble vitamins out of the body.

To prevent or relieve heartburn:

- Relax and eat slowly.
- Chew food thoroughly.
- Eat small, frequent meals.
- Drink liquids between meals.
- Avoid spicy or greasy foods.
- Sit up while eating.
- Wait an hour after eating before lying down.
- Wait two hours after eating before exercising.

food cravings: deep longings for particular foods.

food aversions: strong desires to avoid particular foods.

alleviate morning sickness for some women. Traditional strategies for quelling nausea are listed in Table 10-5, but little evidence exists to support such advice.[33] Some women do best by simply eating what they desire whenever they feel hungry. Morning sickness can be persistent, however. If morning sickness interferes with normal eating for more than a week or two, the woman should seek medical advice to prevent nutrient deficiencies.

Heartburn Heartburn, a burning sensation in the lower esophagus near the heart, is common during pregnancy and is also benign. As the growing fetus puts increasing pressure on the woman's stomach, acid may back up and create a burning sensation in her throat. Tips to relieve heartburn are listed in Table 10-5.

Constipation As the hormones of pregnancy alter muscle tone and the thriving infant crowds intestinal organs, an expectant mother may complain of constipation, another harmless but annoying condition (Box 10-3). A high-fiber diet, physical activity, and plentiful fluids will help relieve this condition. Also, responding promptly to the urge to defecate can help. Laxatives should be used only as prescribed by a physician.

BOX 10-3 *Nursing Diagnosis*

The nursing diagnosis *risk for constipation* applies to clients who are pregnant.

Review Notes

- Food cravings typically do not reflect physiological needs.
- Pica is the ingestion of nonfood items such as laundry starch, clay, soil, or ice. In some cases, pica can be harmful to health and nutrition.
- The nausea, heartburn, and constipation that sometimes accompany pregnancy can usually be alleviated with a few simple strategies.

Problems in Pregnancy

Just as adequate nutrition and normal weight gain support the health of the mother and growth of the fetus, maternal diseases can have an adverse effect. If discovered early, many diseases can be controlled—another reason why early prenatal care is recommended. Some nutrition measures can help alleviate the most common problems encountered during pregnancy.

Preexisting Diabetes Pregnancy presents special challenges for the management of diabetes. Insulin-induced hypoglycemia has a more rapid onset during pregnancy and is a danger to the mother, especially in those with type 1 diabetes. Women with type 2 diabetes often start pregnancy with insulin resistance and obesity, making optimal glycemic control difficult.[34] The risks of diabetes during pregnancy depend on how well it is managed before, during, and after. Excellent glycemic control in the first trimester and throughout the pregnancy is associated with the lowest frequency of maternal, fetal, and newborn complications. Without proper management, women face high infertility rates, and those who do conceive may experience episodes of severe hypoglycemia or hyperglycemia, preterm labor, and pregnancy-related hypertension. Infants may be large, suffer physical and mental abnormalities, and experience other complications such as severe hypoglycemia or respiratory distress, both of which can be fatal. Signs of fetal health problems are apparent even when maternal glucose is above normal but still below the level diagnostic for diabetes. Ideally, a woman will receive the prenatal care needed to achieve glucose control before conception and continued glucose control throughout pregnancy. For optimal long-term outcomes, continuation of intensified diabetes management after pregnancy is in the best interest of the mother's health.

Gestational Diabetes Some women are prone to developing a pregnancy-related form of diabetes, **gestational diabetes**. Gestational diabetes usually resolves after the infant is born, but some women go on to develop type 2 diabetes later in life, especially if they are overweight.[35] For this reason, health care professionals strongly advise against excessive weight gain during and after pregnancy. Weight gains after pregnancy increase the risk of gestational diabetes in the next pregnancy. Gestational diabetes can lead to fetal or infant sickness or death, though the risk of these outcomes falls dramatically when it is identified early and managed properly. More commonly, gestational diabetes leads to surgical birth and high infant birthweight. To ensure prompt diagnosis and treatment, physicians screen all women who are overweight (BMI ≥25) and have one or more additional risk factors for type 2 diabetes (for example, high blood pressure, family history of diabetes or heart disease, previous gestational diabetes, family background that is Latinx American, African American, Native American, Asian American, or Pacific Islander) at the first prenatal visit. In addition, all pregnant women not previously diagnosed with diabetes are tested for glucose intolerance at 24 to 28 weeks' gestation.[36] Chapter 20 provides information about medical nutrition therapy for gestational diabetes.

Hypertension Hypertension complicates pregnancy and affects its outcome in different ways, depending on how severe it becomes. Hypertension during pregnancy may be **chronic hypertension** or **gestational hypertension**.[37] Chronic hypertension can be a preexisting condition that develops before a woman becomes pregnant. In women whose prepregnancy blood pressure is unknown, diagnosis of chronic hypertension is based on the presence of sustained hypertension before 20 weeks of gestation. In contrast, gestational hypertension develops after the 20th week of gestation. In women with gestational hypertension, blood pressure usually returns to normal during the first few weeks after childbirth.

Both types of hypertension pose risks to the mother and fetus. In addition to the health risks normally imposed by hypertension (heart attack and stroke), high blood pressure increases the risks of growth restriction, preterm birth, and separation of the placenta from the wall of the uterus before the birth.[38] Both chronic hypertension and gestational hypertension also increase the risk of preeclampsia.

Preeclampsia **Preeclampsia** is a condition characterized not only by high blood pressure but also by protein in the urine.[39] Table 10-6 presents the signs and symptoms of preeclampsia. Preeclampsia usually occurs with first pregnancies and almost always appears after 20 weeks' gestation. Symptoms typically regress within 48 hours of delivery. Because delivery is the only known cure, preeclampsia is a leading cause of indicated preterm delivery and accounts for about 15 percent of infants who are growth restricted.

Preeclampsia affects almost all of the woman's organs—the circulatory system, liver, kidneys, and brain. If it progresses, she may experience seizures; when this occurs, the condition is called **eclampsia**. Maternal deaths during pregnancy are rare in developed countries, but among those that do occur, eclampsia is a common cause. Preeclampsia demands prompt medical attention. Treatment focuses on regulating blood pressure and preventing seizures.

TABLE 10-6	Signs and Symptoms of Preeclampsia

- Hypertension
- Protein in the urine
- Upper abdominal pain
- Severe headaches
- Swelling of hands, feet, and face
- Vomiting
- Blurred vision
- Sudden weight gain (1 lb/day)

gestational diabetes: glucose intolerance with first onset or first recognition during pregnancy.

chronic hypertension: in pregnant women, hypertension that is present and documented before pregnancy; in women whose prepregnancy blood pressure is unknown, the presence of sustained hypertension before 20 weeks of gestation.

gestational hypertension: high blood pressure that develops in the second half of pregnancy and usually resolves after childbirth.

preeclampsia (PRE-ee-KLAMP-see-ah): a condition characterized by hypertension and protein in the urine during pregnancy.

eclampsia (eh-KLAMP-see-ah): a severe complication during pregnancy in which seizures occur.

Review Notes

- Conditions such as gestational diabetes, hypertension, and preeclampsia can threaten the health and life of both mother and infant.
- Maternal diseases require medical and nutrition treatment.

BOX 10-4 *Nursing Diagnosis*

The nursing diagnosis *ineffective health maintenance* applies to clients who lack knowledge regarding basic health practices.

Practices to Avoid

A general guideline for the pregnant woman is to eat a normal, healthy diet and practice moderation. A woman's daily choices during pregnancy take on enormous importance. Forewarned, pregnant women can choose to abstain from or avoid potentially harmful practices (Box 10-4).

Cigarette Smoking One practice to be avoided during pregnancy is cigarette smoking, which is associated with many complications (see Table 10-7). Parental smoking can kill an otherwise healthy fetus or newborn. Unfortunately, an estimated 10 percent of pregnant women in the United States smoke.[40]

Constituents of cigarette smoke, such as nicotine, carbon monoxide, arsenic, and cyanide, are toxic to a fetus. Smoking during pregnancy can cause damage to fetal chromosomes, which can lead to developmental defects or diseases such as cancer. Smoking also restricts the blood supply to the growing fetus and so limits the delivery of oxygen and nutrients and the removal of wastes. It slows fetal growth, can reduce brain size, and may impair the intellectual and behavioral development of the child later in life. Smoking during pregnancy damages fetal blood vessels, an effect that is still apparent at the age of five years. It interferes with fetal lung development and increases the risks of respiratory infections and childhood and adolescent asthma.[41]

A mother who smokes is more likely to have a complicated birth and a low-birthweight infant.[42] The more a mother smokes, the smaller her infant will be. Of all preventable causes of low birthweight in the United States, smoking has the greatest impact. Sudden infant death syndrome (SIDS), the unexplained death that sometimes occurs in an otherwise healthy infant, has also been linked to the mother's cigarette smoking during pregnancy.[43] Even in women who do not smoke, exposure to **environmental tobacco smoke (ETS)**, or secondhand smoke, during pregnancy increases the risk of low birthweight and the likelihood of SIDS.

Alternatives to smoking—such as e-cigarettes, using snuff, chewing tobacco, or nicotine-replacement therapy—are not safe during pregnancy.[44] Any woman who uses nicotine in any form and is considering pregnancy or who is already pregnant needs to quit.

Medicinal Drugs and Herbal Supplements Medicinal drugs taken during pregnancy can cause serious birth defects. Pregnant women should not take over-the-counter drugs or any other medications without consulting their physicians, who must weigh the benefits against the risks.

Some pregnant women mistakenly consider herbal supplements to be safe alternatives to medicinal drugs and take them to relieve nausea, promote water loss, alleviate depression, help them sleep, or for other reasons. Some herbal products may be safe, but very few have been tested for safety or effectiveness during pregnancy. Pregnant women are advised to stay away from herbal supplements, teas, or other products unless their safety during pregnancy has been ascertained. Nutrition in Practice 14 offer more information about herbal supplements and other alternative therapies.

Drugs of Abuse Drugs of abuse such as methamphetamine and cocaine easily cross the placenta and impair fetal growth and development. Furthermore, they can cause preterm births, low infant birthweight, and sudden infant deaths. If these newborns survive, central nervous system damage is evident: Their cries, sleep, and behaviors early in life are abnormal, and their cognitive development later in life is impaired.[45] They may be hypersensitive or underaroused; many suffer the symptoms of withdrawal. Delays in their growth and development persist throughout childhood and adolescence.

Environmental Contaminants Infants and young children of pregnant women exposed to environmental contaminants such as lead and mercury show signs of impaired mental and psychomotor development. During pregnancy, lead readily

---

TABLE 10-7 Complications Associated with Smoking during Pregnancy

- Fetal growth restriction
- Low birthweight
- Preterm birth
- Premature separation of the placenta
- Miscarriage
- Stillbirth
- Sudden infant death syndrome
- Congenital malformations

---

environmental tobacco smoke (ETS): the combination of exhaled smoke (mainstream smoke) and smoke from lighted cigarettes, pipes, or cigars (sidestream smoke) that enters the air around smokers and may be inhaled by other people.

TABLE 10-8	Advice for Pregnant (and Lactating) Women Eating Fish
Best choices Eat 2–3 servings/week	Anchovy, Atlantic croaker, Atlantic mackerel, black sea bass, butterfish, catfish, clam, cod, crab, crawfish, flounder, haddock, hake, herring, lobster, mullet, oyster, Pacific chub mackerel, perch, pickerel, plaice, pollock, salmon, sardine, scallop, shad, shrimp, skate, smelt, sole, squid, tilapia, trout, tuna (canned light), whitefish, whiting
Good choices Eat 1 serving/week	Atlantic tilefish, bluefish, buffalo fish, carp, Chilean sea bass, grouper, halibut, mahi mahi, monkfish, Pacific croaker, rockfish, sablefish, sea trout, sheepshead, snapper, Spanish mackerel, striped bass, tuna (yellowfin and albacore, white tuna, canned and fresh/frozen), white croaker
Poor choices Avoid eating	King mackerel, marlin, orange roughy, shark, swordfish, Gulf of Mexico tilefish, tuna (bigeye)

listeriosis: a serious foodborne infection that can cause severe brain infection or death in a fetus or newborn; caused by the bacterium *Listeria monocytogenes*, which is found in soil and water.

moves across the placenta, inflicting severe damage on the developing fetal nervous system. In addition, infants exposed to even low levels of lead during gestation weigh less at birth and consequently struggle to survive. For these reasons, it is particularly important that pregnant women consume foods and beverages free of contamination. Dietary calcium can help to defend against lead toxicity by reducing its absorption.

Mercury is a contaminant of concern as well. As discussed in Chapter 4, fatty fish are a good source of omega-3 fatty acids, but some fish contain large amounts of the pollutant mercury, which can impair fetal growth and harm the developing brain and nervous system. Because the benefits of moderate seafood consumption outweigh the risks, pregnant (and lactating) women need reliable information on which fish are safe to eat. Because many pregnant women do not consume any fish or shellfish, however, the FDA and EPA encourage pregnant and lactating women to eat *at least 8* ounces and up to 12 ounces (cooked or canned) of seafood weekly (see Table 10-8).[46] However, the FDA and EPA continue to recommend that no more than 6 ounces (cooked or canned) of white (albacore) tuna be consumed weekly. Supplements of fish oil are not recommended because they may contain concentrated toxins and because their effects on pregnancy remain unknown.

Foodborne Illness The vomiting and diarrhea caused by many foodborne illnesses can leave a pregnant woman exhausted and dangerously dehydrated. Particularly threatening, however, is **listeriosis**, which can cause miscarriage, stillbirth, or severe brain or other infections to fetuses and newborns.[47] Pregnant women are 11 times more likely than other healthy adults to get listeriosis. A woman with listeriosis may develop symptoms such as fever, vomiting, and diarrhea within about 12 hours after eating a contaminated food, and serious symptoms may develop one to six weeks later. A blood test can reliably detect listeriosis, and antibiotics given promptly to the pregnant sufferer can often prevent infection of the fetus or newborn. Table 10-9 presents tips to prevent listeriosis. Nutrition in Practice 2 includes precautions to minimize the risks of other common foodborne illnesses.

Large Doses of Vitamin-Mineral Supplements Pregnant women who are trying eat well may mistakenly assume that more is better when it comes to multivitamin-mineral supplements. This is simply not true; excess vitamin and mineral supplementation during pregnancy can be harmful.[48] Excess vitamin A is particularly infamous for its role in fetal malformations of the cranial nervous system. Intakes before the

TABLE 10-9 Tips to Prevent Listeriosis

- Use only pasteurized juices and dairy products; do not eat soft cheeses such as feta, brie, Camembert, Panela, "queso blanco," "queso fresco," and blue-veined cheeses such as Roquefort; do not drink raw (unpasteurized) milk or eat foods that contain it.
- Do not eat hot dogs or luncheon or deli meats unless heated until steaming hot.
- Thoroughly cook meat, poultry, eggs, and seafood.
- Wash all fruit and vegetables.
- Do not eat refrigerated patés or meat spreads.
- Do not eat ham salad, chicken salad, or seafood salad made in a store. Make these salads at home following the basic food safety guidelines: clean, separate, cook, and chill.
- Do not eat smoked seafood, or any fish labeled "nova-style," "lox," or "kippered."

FIGURE 10-7 Typical Facial Characteristics of FAS

These facial traits are typical of fetal alcohol syndrome, caused by drinking alcohol during pregnancy—low nasal bridge, short eyelid opening, underdeveloped groove in the center of the upper lip, thin upper lip, short nose, and small head circumference.

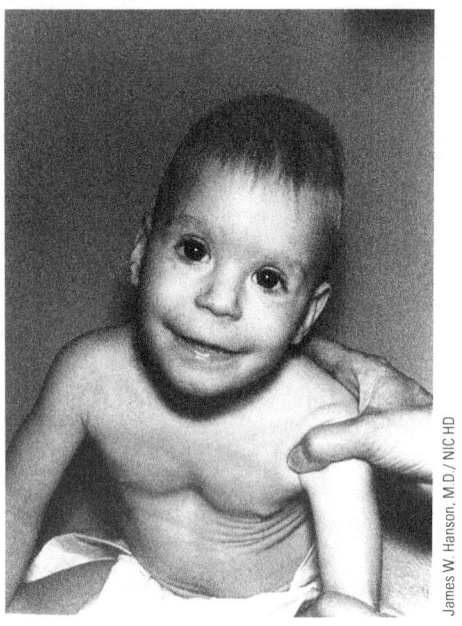

James W. Hanson, M.D. / NIC HD

seventh week of pregnancy appear to be the most damaging. For this reason, vitamin A supplements are not given during pregnancy unless there is specific evidence of deficiency, which is rare.

Restrictive Dieting Restrictive dieting, even for short periods, can be hazardous during pregnancy. Low-carbohydrate diets or fasts that cause ketosis deprive the growing fetal brain of needed glucose and may impair cognitive development. Such diets are also likely to be deficient in other nutrients vital to fetal growth. Regardless of prepregnancy weight, pregnant women need adequate diets to support healthy fetal development.

Sugar Substitutes Artificial sweeteners have been studied extensively and found to be acceptable during pregnancy if used within the FDA's guidelines (see Chapter 3). Advice to pregnant women includes a caution to use sweeteners in moderation and within an otherwise nutritious and well-balanced diet. Women with phenylketonuria should not use aspartame, as Chapter 3 explains.

Caffeine Caffeine crosses the placenta, and the fetus has only a limited ability to metabolize it. Even so, women can safely consume less than 200 milligrams per day without apparent ill effects on their pregnancy duration or outcome.[49] Limited evidence suggests that heavy use—intake equaling more than 3 cups of coffee a day—increases the risk of miscarriage and low birthweight.[50] All things considered, it seems most sensible to limit caffeine consumption to the equivalent of one or two cups of coffee a day.

Alcohol Drinking alcohol during pregnancy threatens the fetus with irreversible brain damage, growth retardation, mental retardation, facial abnormalities, vision abnormalities, and many more health problems—a spectrum of symptoms known as **fetal alcohol spectrum disorders (FASD)**. Children at the most severe end of the spectrum (those with all of the symptoms) are defined as having **fetal alcohol syndrome (FAS)**, which results in the facial abnormalities shown in Figure 10-7.[51] Less obvious is the internal harm: The fetal brain is extremely vulnerable to a glucose or oxygen deficit, and alcohol causes both by disrupting placental functioning. The lifelong mental retardation and other tragedies of FAS can be prevented by abstaining from drinking alcohol during pregnancy. Once the damage is done, however, the child remains impaired. FASDs are the leading known preventable cause of developmental delays and intellectual disabilities in the world.[52]

Despite alcohol's injurious potential, 1 out of every 10 pregnant women drinks alcohol sometime during her pregnancy, and 1 out of 33 reports binge drinking (four or more drinks on one occasion).[53] Almost half of all pregnancies are unintended, and many are conceived during a binge-drinking episode.

Women who know they are pregnant and desire to drink may wonder: How much alcohol is too much? Even one drink a day threatens neurological development and behaviors. Low birthweight is reported among infants born to women who drink 1 ounce (two drinks) of alcohol per day during pregnancy, and FAS is also known to occur with as few as two drinks a day. Birth defects have been reliably observed among the children of women who drink 2 ounces (four drinks) of alcohol daily during pregnancy. The most severe impact is likely to occur in the first two months, possibly before the woman is aware that she is pregnant.

fetal alcohol spectrum disorders (FASD): a spectrum of physical, behavioral, and cognitive disabilities caused by prenatal alcohol exposure.

fetal alcohol syndrome (FAS): the cluster of symptoms seen in an infant or child whose mother consumed excessive alcohol during her pregnancy. FAS includes, but is not limited to, brain damage, growth retardation, mental retardation, and facial abnormalities.

Even when a child does not develop full FAS, prenatal exposure to alcohol can lead to less severe, but nonetheless serious, mental and physical problems. The cluster of mental problems is known as **alcohol-related neurodevelopmental disorder (ARND)**, and the physical malformations are referred to as **alcohol-related birth defects (ARBD)**. Some of these children show no outward sign of impairment, but others are short in stature or display subtle facial abnormalities. Many perform poorly in school and in social interactions and suffer a subtle form of brain damage.[54] Mood disorders and problem behaviors, such as aggression, are common.

For every child diagnosed with full-blown FAS, many more with FASD go undiagnosed until problems develop in the preschool years. Upon reaching adulthood, such children are ill equipped for employment, relationships, and the other facets of life most adults take for granted. Anyone exposed to alcohol before birth may always respond differently to it, and also to certain drugs, than if no exposure had occurred, making addictions likely.

The American Academy of Pediatrics (AAP) takes the position that women should stop drinking as soon as they *plan* to become pregnant. Researchers have looked for a "safe" alcohol intake limit during pregnancy and have found none. Their conclusion: abstinence from alcohol is the best policy for pregnant women.

For pregnant women who have already drunk alcohol, the advice is "stop now." A woman who has drunk heavily during the first two-thirds of her pregnancy can still prevent some organ damage by stopping heavy drinking during the third trimester.

alcohol-related neurodevelopmental disorder (ARND): a condition caused by prenatal alcohol exposure that is diagnosed when there is a confirmed history of substantial, regular maternal alcohol intake or heavy episodic drinking and behavioral, cognitive, or central nervous system abnormalities known to be associated with alcohol exposure.

alcohol-related birth defects (ARBD): a condition caused by prenatal alcohol exposure that is diagnosed when there is a history of substantial, regular maternal alcohol intake or heavy episodic drinking and birth defects known to be associated with alcohol exposure.

Review Notes

- Smoking during pregnancy delivers toxins to the fetus, damages DNA, restricts fetal growth, and limits delivery of oxygen and nutrients and the removal of wastes.

- Abstaining from smoking and other drugs, including alcohol, limiting intake of foods known to contain unsafe levels of contaminants such as mercury, taking precautions against foodborne illness, avoiding large doses of nutrients, refraining from restrictive dieting, using artificial sweeteners in moderation, and limiting caffeine use are recommended during pregnancy.

- Drinking alcohol during pregnancy threatens the fetus with irreversible brain damage, growth retardation, mental retardation, facial abnormalities, vision abnormalities, and many more health problems—a spectrum of symptoms known as fetal alcohol spectrum disorders, or FASD.

Adolescent Pregnancy

The number of infants born to teenage mothers has steadily declined during the last 50 years. Despite the long-term decline, however, the U.S. teen birth rate is still one of the highest among industrialized nations. More than 209,000 adolescent girls give birth each year in the United States; almost 20 percent of them already have at least one child.[55]

A pregnant adolescent presents a special case of intense nutrient needs. Young teenage girls have a hard enough time meeting nutrient needs for their own rapid growth and development, let alone those of pregnancy. Many teens enter pregnancy with deficiencies of vitamins B$_{12}$ and D, folate, calcium, and iron that can impair fetal growth (Box 10-5).[56] Pregnant adolescents are less likely to receive early prenatal care and are more likely to smoke during pregnancy—two factors that predict low birthweight and infant death (Box 10-6).[57]

BOX 10-5 *Nursing Diagnosis*

The nursing diagnosis *imbalanced nutrition: less than body requirements* applies to clients with reported food intakes less than the RDA and those who lack nutrition knowledge.

BOX 10-6 *Nursing Diagnosis*

The nursing diagnosis *risk for delayed development* applies to clients who are young, are pregnant, and lack prenatal care.

The rates of stillbirths, preterm births, and low-birthweight infants are high for teenagers—both for teen moms and for teen dads. Their greatest risk, though, is death of the infant: Mothers younger than 16 years of age bear more infants who die within the first year than do women in any other age group. These factors combine to make adolescent pregnancy a major public health problem.

Adequate nutrition is an indispensable component of prenatal care for adolescents and can substantially improve the outlook for both mother and infant. To support the needs of both mother and fetus, a pregnant teenager with a BMI in the normal range is encouraged to gain about 35 pounds to reduce the likelihood of a low-birthweight infant. As mentioned earlier, however, compared with older mothers, the lifetime risk of postpartum weight retention in young adolescents may be far greater. Researchers agree that optimal weight gain recommendations for pregnant adolescents need focused attention. Meanwhile, pregnant and lactating adolescents would do well to follow the eating pattern presented in Table 1-6 (on p. 19) for a kcalorie level that will support adequate, but not excessive, weight gain.

Review Notes

- Pregnant adolescents have extraordinarily high nutrient needs and an increased likelihood of problem pregnancies.
- Proper nutrition and adequate weight gain are especially important in reducing the risk of poor pregnancy outcome in adolescents.

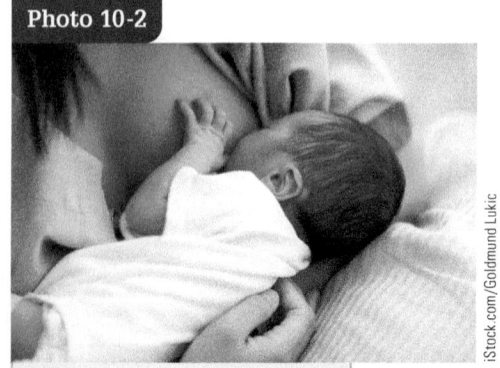

Photo 10-2

A woman who decides to breastfeed provides her infant with a full array of nutrients and protective factors to support optimal health and development.

iStock.com/Goldmund Lukic

exclusive breastfeeding: an infant's consumption of human milk with no supplementation of any type (no water, no juice, no nonhuman milk, and no foods) except for vitamins, minerals, and medications.

10.2 Breastfeeding

The AAP recommends that infants receive breast milk for at least the first 12 months of life and beyond for as long as mutually desired by mother and child.[58] The Academy of Nutrition and Dietetics (AND) advocates breastfeeding for the nutritional health it confers on the infant as well as for the physiological, social, economic, and other benefits it offers the mother (see Table 10-10).[59] The AAP and the AND recognize **exclusive breastfeeding** for 6 months and breastfeeding with complementary foods for at least 12 months as an optimal feeding pattern for infants. Breast milk's unique nutrient composition and protective factors promote optimal infant health and development (see Photo 10-2).

The only acceptable alternative to breast milk is iron-fortified formula. Adequate nutrition of the mother supports successful lactation, and without it, lactation is likely to falter or fail. Health care professionals play an important role in providing encouragement and accurate information on breastfeeding.

Nutrition during Lactation

By continuing to eat nutrient-dense foods, not restricting weight gain unduly, and enjoying ample food and fluids at frequent intervals throughout lactation, the mother who chooses to breastfeed her infant will be nutritionally prepared to do so. An inadequate diet does not support the stamina, patience, and self-confidence that nursing an infant demands. Figure 10-3 (on p. 277) shows how a lactating woman's nutrient needs differ from those of a nonpregnant woman, and Table 10-2 (on p. 277) presents sample menus that meet those needs.

TABLE 10-10	Benefits of Breastfeeding

FOR INFANTS
- Provides the appropriate composition and balance of nutrients with high bioavailability
- Provides hormones that promote physiological development
- Improves cognitive development
- Protects against a variety of infections and illnesses
- May protect against some chronic diseases—such as diabetes (both types), obesity, atherosclerosis, asthma, and hypertension—later in life
- Protects against food allergies
- Supports healthy weight
- Reduces the risk of sudden infant death syndrome (SIDS)

FOR MOTHERS
- Contracts the uterus
- Delays the return of regular ovulation, thus lengthening birth intervals (this is not, however, a dependable method of contraception)
- Conserves iron stores (by prolonging amenorrhea)
- May protect against breast and ovarian cancer and reduce the risk of diabetes (type 2)

OTHER
- Cost and time savings from not needing medical treatment for childhood illnesses or leaving work to care for sick infants
- Cost and time savings from not needing to purchase and prepare formula (even after adjusting for added foods in the diet of a lactating mother)
- Environmental savings for society from not needing to manufacture, package, and ship formula and dispose of the packaging

Energy A nursing woman produces about 25 ounces of milk a day, with considerable variation from woman to woman and in the same woman from time to time, depending primarily on the infant's demand for milk. Producing this milk costs a woman almost 500 kcalories per day above her regular need during the first six months of lactation. To meet this energy need, the woman is advised to eat foods providing an extra 330 kcalories each day. The other 170 kcalories can be drawn from the fat stores she accumulated during pregnancy. During the second 6 months of lactation, an additional 400 kcalories each day are recommended. The food energy consumed by the nursing mother should carry with it abundant nutrients. Severe energy restriction hinders milk production and can compromise the mother's health.

Weight Loss After the birth of the infant, many women actively try to lose the extra weight and body fat they accumulated during pregnancy. How much weight a woman retains after pregnancy depends on her gestational weight gain and the duration and intensity of breastfeeding.[60] Many women who follow recommendations for gestational weight gain and breastfeeding can readily return to prepregnancy weight by 6 months. Neither the quality nor the quantity of breast milk is adversely affected by moderate weight loss, and infants grow normally.

Women often choose to be physically active to lose weight and improve fitness, and this is compatible with breastfeeding and infant growth.[61] A gradual weight loss (1 pound per week) is safe and does not reduce milk output. Too large an energy deficit, however, especially soon after birth, will inhibit lactation.

Vitamins and Minerals   A question often raised is whether a mother's milk may lack a nutrient if she fails to get enough in her diet. The answer differs from one nutrient to the next, but, in general, nutritional deprivation of the mother reduces the *quantity*, not the *quality*, of her milk. Women can produce milk with adequate protein, carbohydrate, fat, folate, and most minerals, even when their own supplies are limited. For these nutrients, milk quality is maintained at the expense of maternal stores. This is most evident in the case of calcium: Dietary calcium has no effect on the calcium concentration of breast milk, but maternal bones lose some of their density during lactation if calcium intakes are inadequate. Such losses are generally made up quickly when lactation ends, and breastfeeding has no long-term harmful effects on women's bones. The nutrients in breast milk that are most likely to decline in response to prolonged inadequate intakes are the vitamins—especially vitamins B_6, B_{12}, A, and D. Vitamin supplementation of undernourished women appears to help normalize the vitamin concentrations in their milk and may be beneficial.

Water   The volume of breast milk produced depends on how much milk the infant demands, not on how much fluid the mother drinks. The nursing mother is nevertheless advised to drink plenty of liquids each day (about 13 cups) to protect herself from dehydration. To help themselves remember to drink enough liquid, many women make a habit of drinking a glass of milk, juice, or water each time the infant nurses as well as at mealtimes.

Particular Foods   Foods with strong or spicy flavors (such as onions or garlic) may alter the flavor of breast milk. A sudden change in the taste of the milk may annoy some infants, whereas familiar flavors may enhance enjoyment. Flavors imparted to breast milk by the mother's diet can influence the infant's later food preferences.[62] A mother who is breastfeeding her infant is advised to eat whatever nutritious foods she chooses. Then, if a particular food seems to cause the infant discomfort, she can try eliminating that food from her diet for a few days and see if the problem goes away.

Current evidence does not support a major role for maternal dietary restrictions during lactation to prevent or delay the onset of food allergy in infants.[63] Generally, infants with a strong family history of food allergies benefit from breastfeeding.

The case study in Box 10-7 presents a woman who is 4 months pregnant. Answering the questions offers practice in thinking through some of the issues related to pregnancy and breastfeeding.

Contraindications to Breastfeeding

Some substances impair maternal milk production or enter the breast milk and interfere with infant development. Some medical conditions prohibit breastfeeding (Box 10-8).

Alcohol Alcohol easily enters breast milk and can adversely affect the production, volume, composition, and ejection of breast milk as well as overwhelm an infant's immature alcohol-degrading system. Alcohol concentration in breast milk peaks within one hour after ingestion of even moderate amounts (equivalent to a can of beer). It may alter the taste of the milk unfavorably such that the nursing infant may, in protest, drink less milk than normal.

Tobacco and Caffeine Many women who quit smoking during pregnancy resume after delivery. Lactating women who smoke produce less milk, and milk with a lower fat content, than do nonsmokers. Consequently, infants of smokers gain less weight than infants of nonsmokers.

A lactating woman who smokes not only transfers nicotine and other chemicals to her infant via her breast milk but may also expose the infant to secondhand smoke. Infants who are "smoked over" experience a wide array of health problems—poor growth, hearing impairment, vomiting, breathing difficulties, and even unexplained death.[64] Health care professionals should actively discourage smoking by lactating women.

Excessive caffeine can make an infant jittery and wakeful. As during pregnancy, caffeine consumption during lactation should be moderate.

Medications and Illicit Drugs Many prescription medications do not reach nursing infants in sufficient quantities to affect them adversely and so have no impact on breastfeeding. Other drugs are incompatible with breastfeeding, either because they are secreted into the milk and can harm the infant or because they suppress lactation. A nursing mother should consult with the prescribing physician before taking medicines or even herbal supplements—herbs may have unpredictable effects on breastfeeding infants. If a nursing mother must take medication that is secreted in breast milk and is known to affect the infant, then breastfeeding must be put off for the duration of treatment. Meanwhile, the flow of milk can be sustained by pumping the breasts and discarding the milk. Breastfeeding is also contraindicated if the mother uses illicit drugs. Breast milk can deliver such high doses of illicit drugs as to cause irritability, tremors, hallucinations, and even death in infants.

Many women wonder about using oral contraceptives during lactation. Those that combine the hormones estrogen and progestin seem to suppress milk output, lower the nitrogen content of the milk, and shorten the duration of breastfeeding. In contrast, progestin-only pills have no effect on breast milk or breastfeeding and are considered appropriate for lactating women.

Maternal Illness If a woman has an ordinary cold, she can go on nursing without worry. If susceptible, the infant will catch it from her anyway, and, thanks to immunological protection, a breastfed baby may be less susceptible than a formula-fed infant would be. A woman who has tuberculosis should not breastfeed, but she can resume or begin once she has been treated and it is documented that she is no longer infectious.

The human immunodeficiency virus (HIV), responsible for causing AIDS, can be passed from an infected mother to her infant during pregnancy, at birth, or through breast milk, especially during the early months of breastfeeding. In developed countries such as the United States, where safe alternatives are available, HIV-positive women should not breastfeed their infants.

Throughout the world, breastfeeding prevents millions of infant deaths each year. In developing countries, where the feeding of inappropriate or contaminated formulas causes more than 1 million infant deaths annually, breastfeeding can be critical to infant survival. Thus, the question of whether HIV-infected women in developing countries should breastfeed comes down to a delicate balance between risks and benefits. For these women, the most appropriate infant-feeding option depends on individual circumstances, including the health status of the mother and the local situation, as well as the health services, counseling, and support available. The World Health Organization

(WHO) recommends exclusive breastfeeding for infants of HIV-infected women for the first six months of life unless replacement feeding is acceptable, feasible, affordable, sustainable, and safe for mothers and their infants before that time. Alternatively, HIV-exposed infants may be protected by receiving antiretroviral treatment while being breastfed.

Review Notes

- The lactating woman needs enough energy and nutrients to produce about 25 ounces of milk a day. She also needs extra fluids.
- Alcohol, smoking, caffeine, and drugs may reduce milk production or enter breast milk and impair infant development.
- Some maternal illnesses are incompatible with breastfeeding.

Nutrition Assessment Checklist for Pregnant and Lactating Women

MEDICAL HISTORY
Check the medical record for:

- Alcohol or illicit drug abuse
- Chronic diseases
- Gestational diabetes
- History of previous pregnancies (number, intervals, outcomes, multiple births, gestational age, and birth weights)
- Hypertension
- Neural tube defect in an infant born previously
- Preeclampsia

Note risk factors for complications during pregnancy, including:

- Cigarette smoking
- Food faddism
- Lactose intolerance
- Low socioeconomic status
- Significant or prolonged vomiting
- Very young or old age
- Weight-loss dieting

Note any complaints of:

- Constipation
- Heartburn
- Morning sickness

MEDICATIONS
For pregnant women who are using drug therapy for medical conditions, note:

- Potential for contraindication to breastfeeding
- GI-tract side effects that might reduce food intake or change nutrient needs

DIETARY INTAKE
For all pregnant and lactating women, especially those considered at risk nutritionally, assess the diet for:

- Total energy
- Protein
- Calcium, phosphorus, magnesium, iron, and zinc
- Folate and vitamin B_{12}
- Vitamin D

ANTHROPOMETRIC DATA
Measure baseline height and weight:

- Prepregnancy weight

Reassess weight at each medical check-up and determine whether gains are appropriate. Note:

- Weight gain during pregnancy
- Gestational age

LABORATORY TESTS
Monitor the following laboratory tests for pregnant women:

- Hemoglobin, hematocrit, or other tests of iron status
- Blood glucose

PHYSICAL SIGNS
Blood pressure measurement is routine in physical exams but is especially important for pregnant women. Look for physical signs of:

- Iron deficiency
- Edema
- Protein-energy malnutrition
- Folate deficiency

1. The most important single predictor of an infant's future health and survival is:
   a. the infant's birthweight.
   b. the infant's iron status at birth.
   c. the mother's weight at delivery.
   d. the mother's prepregnancy weight.

2. A mother's prepregnancy nutrition is important to a healthy pregnancy because it determines the development of:
   a. the largest baby possible.
   b. adequate maternal iron stores.
   c. an adequate fat supply for the mother.
   d. healthy support tissues—the placenta, amniotic sac, umbilical cord, and uterus.

3. A pregnant woman needs an extra 450 calories above the allowance for nonpregnant women during which trimester(s)?
   a. First
   b. Second
   c. Third
   d. First, second, and third

4. Two nutrients needed in large amounts during pregnancy for rapid cell proliferation are:
   a. vitamin B_{12} and vitamin C.
   b. calcium and vitamin B_6.
   c. folate and vitamin B_{12}.
   d. copper and zinc.

5. For a woman who is at the appropriate weight for height and is carrying a single fetus, the recommended weight gain during pregnancy is:
   a. 40 to 60 pounds.
   b. 25 to 35 pounds.
   c. 10 to 20 pounds.
   d. 20 to 40 pounds.

6. Rewards of physical activity during pregnancy may include:
   a. weight loss.
   b. decreased incidence of pica.
   c. relief from morning sickness.
   d. reduced stress and easier labor.

7. During pregnancy, the combination of high blood pressure and protein in the urine signals:
   a. jaundice.
   b. preeclampsia.
   c. gestational diabetes.
   d. gestational hypertension.

8. Which of the following preventative measures should pregnant women take to avoid contracting listeriosis?
   a. Choose soft rather than aged cheeses.
   b. Avoid pasteurized milk.
   c. Thoroughly heat hot dogs.
   d. Avoid raw fruit and vegetables.

9. To facilitate lactation, a mother needs:
   a. about 5000 kcalories a day.
   b. adequate nutrition and fluid intake.
   c. vitamin and mineral supplements.
   d. a glass of wine or beer before each feeding.

10. A woman who breastfeeds her infant should drink plenty of water to:
    a. produce more milk.
    b. suppress lactation.
    c. prevent dehydration.
    d. dilute nutrient concentrations.

Answers: 1. a, 2. d, 3. c, 4. c, 5. b, 6. d, 7. b, 8. c, 9. b, 10. c

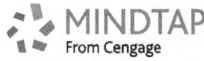 **MINDTAP** From Cengage   For more chapter resources visit **www.cengage.com** to access MindTap, a complete digital course.

Clinical Applications

1. Consider the different factors in a pregnant woman's history that can affect her nutrition status and the outcome of her pregnancy. Describe what steps you would take to remedy potential problems for the following clients:
   a. A 15-year-old adolescent of low socioeconomic status is in her first trimester of pregnancy. She began the pregnancy at a normal, healthy weight, but her weight gain during pregnancy so far has been less than expected. Her favorite beverages are soft drinks; her favorite foods are French fries and boxed macaroni and cheese.

b. A lactose-intolerant, 22-year-old pregnant woman has been eating a vegan diet for the past year or so. She began the pregnancy slightly underweight (BMI = 18.4), but her weight gain has been adequate and consistent during the 4 months of her pregnancy. She complains of feeling tired all the time.

2. What information would you give to a pregnant woman who is considering breastfeeding her infant, but isn't quite sure why she should?

Notes

1. L. Giahi and coauthors, Nutritional modifications in male infertility: A systematic review covering 2 decades, *Nutrition Reviews* 74 (2016): 118–130.

2. J. Abbasi, The paternal epigenome makes its mark, *Journal of the American Medical Association* 317 (2017): 2049–2051; T. K. Jensen and coauthors, Habitual alcohol consumption associated with reduced semen quality and changes in reproductive hormones; a cross sectional study among 1221 young Danish men, *British Medical Journal Open* 4 (2014): e005462R.

3. R. F. Goldstein and coauthors, Association of gestational weight gain with maternal and infant outcomes, *Journal of the American Medical Association* 317 (2017): 2207–2225; E. Gresham and coauthors, Effects of dietary interventions on neonatal and infant outcomes: A systematic review and meta-analysis, *American Journal of Clinical Nutrition* 100 (2014): 1298–1321.

4. C. Berti and coauthors, Early-life nutritional exposures and lifelong health: Immediate and long-lasting impacts of probiotics, vitamin D, and breastfeeding, *Nutrition Reviews* 75 (2017): 83–97; D. Ley and coauthors, Early-life origin of intestinal inflammatory disorders, *Nutrition Reviews* 75 (2017): 175–187; J. G. O. Avila and coauthors, Impact of oxidative stress during pregnancy on fetal epigenetic patterns and early origin of vascular diseases, *Nutrition Reviews* 73 (2015): 12–21; T. L. Crume and coauthors, The long-term impact of intrauterine growth restriction in a diverse U.S. cohort of children; The EPOCH study, *Obesity (Silver Springs)* 22 (2014): 608–615.

5. A. M. W. Laerum and coauthors, Psychiatric disorders and general functioning in low birth weight adults: A longitudinal study, *Pediatrics* 139 (2017): e20162135; C. Xie and coauthors, Stunting at 5 years among SGA newborns, *Pediatrics* 137 (2016): e20152636; E. E. Ziegler, Nutrient needs for catch-up growth in low-birthweight infants, *Nestle Nutrition Institute Workshop Series* 81 (2015): 135–143; A. Lahat and coauthors, ADHD among young adults born at extremely low birth weight: The role of fluid intelligence in childhood, *Frontiers in Psychology* 19 (2014): 446.

6. S. L. Murphy and coauthors, Annual summary of vital statistics: 2013–2014, *Pediatrics* 139 (2017): e20163239.

7. Position of the Academy of Nutrition and Dietetics: Nutrition and lifestyle for a healthy pregnancy outcome, *Journal of the Academy of Nutrition and Dietetics* 114 (2014): 1099–1103.

8. Goldstein and coauthors, 2017; Position of the Academy of Nutrition and Dietetics: Obesity, reproduction, and pregnancy outcomes, *Journal of the Academy of Nutrition and Dietetics* 116 (2016): 677–691.

9. Position of the Academy of Nutrition and Dietetics, Obesity, reproduction, and pregnancy outcomes, 2016; R. C. Ma and coauthors, Clinical management of pregnancy in the obese mother: Before conception, during pregnancy and post partum, *Lancet Diabetes and Endocrinology* 4 (2016): 1037–1049.

10. Position of the Academy of Nutrition and Dietetics, Obesity, reproduction, and pregnancy outcomes, 2016; J. Marchi and coauthors, Risks associated with obesity in pregnancy, for the mother and the baby: A systematic review of reviews, *Obesity Reviews* 16 (2015): 621–638.

11. K. M. Godfrey and coauthors, Influence of maternal obesity on the long-term health of offspring, *Lancet Diabetes and Endocrinology* 5 (2017): 53–64; S. A. Leonard and coauthors, Trajectories of maternal weight from before pregnancy through postpartum and associations with childhood obesity, *American Journal of Clinical Nutrition* 106 (2017): 1295–1301.

12. Berti and coauthors, 2017; Ley and coauthors, 2017; Avila and coauthors, 2015; J. Zheng and coauthors, DNA methylation: The pivotal interaction between early-life nutrition and glucose metabolism in later life, *British Journal of Nutrition* 112 (2014): 1850–1857.

13. C. G. Campbell and L. L. Kaiser, Practice Paper of the Academy of Nutrition and Dietetics: Nutrition and lifestyle for a healthy pregnancy outcome, 2014, www.eatright.org/members/practicepapers/.

14. V. Leventakou and coauthors, Fish intake during pregnancy, fetal growth, and gestational length in 19 European cohort studies, *American Journal*

of Clinical Nutrition 99 (2014): 506–516; K. A. Mulder, D. J. King, and S. M. Innis, Omega-3 fatty acid deficiency in infants before birth identified using a randomized trial of maternal DHA supplementation in pregnancy, *PLoS One* 9 (2014): e83764.

15. P. M. Emmett, L. R. Jones, and J. Golding, Pregnancy diet and associated outcomes in the Avone Longitudinal Study of Parents and Children, Nutrition Reviews 73 (Suppl 3) (2015): 154–174.

16. Centers for Disease Control and Prevention, Birth defects COUNT, www.cdc.gov/ncbddd/birthdefectscount/data.html, updated March 31, 2016.

17. Centers for Disease Control and Prevention, Birth defects COUNT, www.cdc.gov/ncbddd/birthdefectscount/data.html, updated March 31, 2016.

18. E. T. M. Leermakers and coauthors, Effects of choline on health across the life course: A systematic review, *Nutrition Reviews* 73 (2015): 500–522. mothers, *Clinical Nutrition* 34 (2015): 793–798.

19. C. R. Peterson and D. Ayoub, Congenital rickets due to vitamin D deficiency in the mothers, *Clinical Nutrition* 34 (2015): 793–798.

20. M. K. Ozias and coauthors, Typical prenatal vitamin D supplement intake does not prevent decrease of plasma 25-hydroxyvitamin D at birth, *Journal of the American College of Nutrition* 33 (2014): 394–399.

21. A. L. Fisher and E. Nemeth, Iron homeostasis during pregnancy, *American Journal of Clinical Nutrition* 106 (2017): 1567S–1574S.

22. C. Cao and M. D. Fleming, The placenta: The forgotten essential organ of iron transport, *Nutrition Reviews* 74 (2016): 421–431.

23. C. G. Campbell and L. L. Kaiser, Practice paper of the Academy of Nutrition and Dietetics: Nutrition and lifestyle for a healthy pregnancy outcome, 2014, www.eatright.org/members/practicepapers/.

24. D. G. Weismiller and K. M. Kolasa, Special concerns through an early pregnancy journey, *Nutrition Today* 51 (2016): 175–185; L. Englund-Ogge and coauthors, Maternal dietary patterns and Preterm delivery: Results from large prospective cohort study, *British Medical Journal* 348 (2014): g1446; J. A. Grieger, L. E. Grzeskowiak, and V. L. Clifton, Preconception dietary patterns in human pregnancies are associated with preterm delivery, *Journal of Nutrition* 144 (2014): 1075–1080.

25. Women, Infants, and Children, WIC, Frequently asked questions about www.fns.usda.gov/wic/frequently-asked-questions-about-wic, May 4, 2017.

26. Goldstein and coauthors, 2017; N. P. Deputy, A. J. Sharma, and S. Y. Kim, Gestational weight gain—United States, 2012 and 2013, *Morbidity and Mortality Weekly Report* 64 (2015): 1215–1220; Position of the Academy of Nutrition and Dietetics: Nutrition and lifestyle for a healthy pregnancy outcome, 2014.

27. Position of the Academy of Nutrition and Dietetics: Obesity, reproduction, and pregnancy outcomes, 2016; Ma and coauthors, 2016; A. B. Berenson and coauthors, Obesity risk knowledge, weight misperception, and diet and health-related attitudes among women intending to become pregnant, *Journal of the Academy of Nutrition and Dietetics* 116 (2016): 69–75; A. C. Flynn coauthors, Dietary interventions in overweight and obese pregnant women: A systematic review of the content, delivery, and outcomes of randomized controlled trials, *Nutrition Reviews* 74 (2016): 312–328.

28. M. Z. Kapadia and coauthors, Weight loss instead of weight gain within the guidelines in obese women during pregnancy: A systematic review and meta-analyses of maternal and infant outcomes, *PLoS One* 10 (2015): e0132650.

29. M. Perales, R. Artal, and A. Lucia, Exercise during pregnancy, *Journal of the American Medical Association* 317 (2017): 1113–1114; M. Perales and coauthors, Maternal cardiac adaptations to a physical exercise program during pregnancy, *Medicine and Science in Sports and Exercise* 48 (2016): 896–906; S. E. Badon and coauthors, Leisure time physical activity and gestational diabetes mellitus in the Omega Study, *Medicine and Science in Sports and Exercise* 48 (2016): 1044–1052; Position of the Academy of Nutrition and Dietetics: Nutrition and Lifestyle for a healthy pregnancy outcome, 2014.

30. S. T. Harris and coauthors, Exercise during pregnancy and its association with gestational weight gain, *Maternal and Child Health Journal* 19 (2015): 528–537; R. Barakat and coauthors, A program of exercise throughout pregnancy: Is it safe to mother and newborn? *American Journal of Health Promotion* 29 (2014): 2–8. (2014): 101–108.

31. R. W. Corbett and K. M. Kolasa, Pica and weight gain in pregnancy, Nutrition today 49 (2014): 101–108.

32. G. Koren, S. Madjunkova, and C. Maltepe, The protective effects of nausea and vomiting of pregnancy against adverse fetal outcome—A systematic review, *Reproductive Toxicology* 47 (2014): 77–80.

33. A. Matthews and coauthors, Interventions for nausea and vomiting in early pregnancy, *Cochrane Database of Systemic Reviews* 3 (2014): CD007575.

34. S. K. Abell and coauthors, Type 1 and type 2 diabetes preconception and in pregnancy: Health impacts, influence of obesity and lifestyle, and principles of management, *Seminars in Reproductive Medicine* 34 (2016): 110–120; G. H. Visser and H. W. de Valk, Management of diabetes in pregnancy: Antenatal follow-up and decisions concerning timing and mode of delivery, *Best Practice and Research. Clinical Obstetrics and Gynaecology* 29 (2015): 237–243.

35. Position of the Academy of Nutrition and Dietetics, Obesity, reproduction, and pregnancy outcomes, 2016; A. Allalou and coauthors, A predictive metabolic signature for the transition from gestational diabetes to type 2 diabetes, *Diabetes* 65 (2016): 2529–2539; W. Bao and coauthors, Long-term risk of type 2 diabetes mellitus in relation to BMI and weight change among women with a history of gestational diabetes mellitus: A prospective cohort study, *Diabetologia* 58 (2015): 1212–1219.

36. American Diabetes Association, Classification and diagnosis of diabetes, *Diabetes Care* 40 (2017): S11–S24.

37. H. N. Moussa, S. E. Arian, and B. M. Sibai, Management of hypertension disorders in pregnancy, *Women's Health* 10 (2014): 385–404.

38. Moussa, Arian, and Sibai, 2014.

39. Moussa, Arian, and Sibai, 2014.

40. Centers for Disease Control and Prevention, Reproductive Health: Tobacco use and pregnancy, www.cdc.gov/reproductivehealth /maternalinfanthealth/tobaccousepregnancy/index.htm, updated September 29, 2017.

41. E. M. Hollams and coauthors, Persistent effects of maternal smoking during pregnancy on lung function and asthma in adolescents, *American Journal of Respiratory and Critical Care Medicine* 189 (2014): 401–407.

42. Centers for Disease Control and Prevention, Reproductive Health: Tobacco use and pregnancy, www.cdc.gov/reproductivehealth /maternalinfanthealth/tobaccousepregnancy/index.htm, updated September 29, 2017; S. Phelan, Smoking Cessation in Pregnancy, *Obstetrics and Gynecology Clinics of North America* 41 (2014): 255–266.

43. American Academy of Pediatrics, Task Force on Sudden Infant Death Syndrome, SIDS and other sleep-related infant deaths: Updated 2016 Recommendations for a Safe Infant Sleeping Environment, *Pediatrics* 138 (2016): e20162938.

44. Centers for Disease Control and Prevention, Reproductive Health: Tobacco use and pregnancy, www.cdc.gov/reproductivehealth /maternalinfanthealth/tobaccousepregnancy/index.htm, updated September 29, 2017.

45. M. Neri and coauthors, Drugs of abuse in pregnancy, poor neonatal development, and future neurodegeneration. Is oxidative stress the culprit? *Current Pharmaceutical Design* 21 (2015): 1358–1368; A. M. Cressman and coauthors, Cocaine abuse during pregnancy, *Journal of Obstetrics and Gynaecology Canada* 36 (2014): 628–631.

46. Unites States Food and Drug Administration, Eating fish: What pregnant women and parents should know, www.fda.gov/Food/ResourcesForYou /Consumers/ucm393070.htm, updated October 19, 2017.

47. Centers for Disease Control and Prevention, People at risk—Pregnant women and newborns, www.cdc.gov/listeria/risk-groups/pregnant-women.html, updated June 29, 2017.

48. E. Pannia and coauthors, Role of maternal vitamins in programming health and chronic disease, *Nutrition Reviews* 74 (2016): 166–180.

49. The American College of Obstetricians and Gynecologists, Committee Opinion, Moderate caffeine consumption during pregnancy, www.acog .org/Resources-And-Publications/Committee-Opinions/Committee-on -Obstetric-Practice/Moderate-Caffeine-Consumption-During-Pregnancy, reaffirmed 2016.

50. L. W. Chen and coauthors, Maternal caffeine intake during pregnancy and risk of pregnancy loss: A categorical and dose-response meta-analysis of prospective studies, *Public Health Nutrition* 19 (2016): 1233–1244; J. Li and coauthors, A meta-analysis of risk of pregnancy loss and caffeine and coffee consumption during pregnancy, *International Journal of Gynaecology and Obstetrics* 130 (2015): 116–122; J. Rhee and coauthors, Maternal caffeine consumption during pregnancy and risk of low birth weight: A dose-response meta-analysis of observational studies, *PLoS One* 10 (2015): e0132334; D. C. Greenwood and coauthors, Caffeine intake during pregnancy and adverse birth outcomes: A systematic review and dose-response meta-analysis, *European Journal of Epidemiology* 29 (2014): 725–734; A. T. Hoyt and coauthors, Maternal caffeine consumption and small for gestational age births: Results from a population-based case - control study, *Maternal and Child Health Journal* 18 (2014): 1540–1551.

51. Centers for Disease Control, *Fetal Alcohol Spectrum Disorders*, www.cdc .gov/ncbddd/fasd/facts.html, updated June 6, 2017.

52. H. E. Hoyme and coauthors, Updated clinical guidelines for diagnosing fetal alcohol spectrum disorders, *Pediatrics* 138 (2016): e20154256.

53. Centers for Disease Control, *Fetal Alcohol Spectrum Disorders*, www.cdc .gov/ncbddd/fasd/facts.html, updated June 6, 2017.

54. P. Gautam and coauthors, Developmental trajectories for visuo-spatial attention are altered by prenatal alcohol exposure: A longitudinal FMRI study, *Cerebral Cortex* 25 (2015): 4761–4771.

55. U.S. Department of Health and Human Services, Office of Adolescent Health, Teen pregnancy and childbearing, 2016, www.hhs.gov/ash/oah /adolescent-development/reproductive-health-and-teen-pregnancy/teen -pregnancy-and-childbearing/index.html.

56. S. V. Dean and coauthors, Preconception care: Nutritional risks and interventions, *Reproductive Health* 11 (2014): S3.

57. J. L. Bottorff and coauthors, Tobacco and alcohol use in the context of adolescent pregnancy and postpartum: A scoping review of the literature, *Health and Social Care in the Community* 22 (2014): 561–574.

58. Breastfeeding, in Committee on Nutrition, American Academy of Pediatrics, *Pediatric Nutrition*, 7th ed., ed. R. E. Kleinman (Elk Grove Village, Ill.: American Academy of Pediatrics, 2014), pp. 41–59; American Academy of Pediatrics, Policy statement: Breastfeeding and the use of human milk, *Pediatrics* 129 (2012): e827–e841, available at www. pediatrics. org/content/129/3/e827.full.

59. Position of the Academy of Nutrition and Dietetics: Promoting and supporting breastfeeding, *Journal of the Academy of Nutrition and Dietetics* 115 (2015): 444–449.

60. C. G. Perrine and coauthors, Lactation and maternal cardio-metabolic health, *Annual Review of Nutrition* 36 (2016): 627–645; Position of the Academy of Nutrition and Dietetics, Obesity, reproduction, and pregnancy outcomes, 2016; N. López-Olmedo and coauthors, The associations of maternal weight change with breastfeeding, diet and physical activity during the postpartum period, *Maternal and Child Health Journal* 20 (2016): 270–280; M. P. Jarlenski and coauthors, Effects of breastfeeding on postpartum weight loss among U.S. women, *Preventive Medicine* 69 (2014): 146–150.

61. A. Zourladani and coauthors, The effect of physical exercise on postpartum fitness, hormone and lipid levels: A randomized controlled trial in primiparous, lactating women, *Archives of Gynecology and Obstetrics* 291 (2015): 525–530; K. R. Evenson and coauthors, Summary of international guidelines for physical activity after pregnancy, *Obstetrical and Gynecological Survey* 69 (2014): 407–414.

62. J. A. Mennella, L. M. Daniels, and A. R. Reiter, Learning to like vegetables during breastfeeding: A randomized clinical trial of lactating mothers and infants, *American Journal of Clinical Nutrition* 106 (2017): 67–76; S. Nicklaus, The role of dietary *and Metabolism* 70 (2017): 67–76; S. Nicklaus, The role of dietary reference_Prev.pdf experience in the development of eating behavior during the first years of life, *Nutrition and Metabolism* 70 (2017): 241–245.

63. Committee on Food Allergies: Global burden, causes, treatment, prevention, and public policy, in V. A. Stallings and M. P. Oria, eds., Food and Nutrition Board, Health and Medicine Division, National Academies of Sciences, Engineering, and Medicine, *Finding a Path to Safety in Food Allergy: Assessment of the Global Burden, Causes, Prevention, Management, and Public Policy* (Washington, D.C.: National Academies Press, 2016), www.nnap.edu/23658.

64. Centers for Disease Control and Prevention, Health effects of Secondhand smoke, www.cdc.gov/tobacco/data_statistics/ fact_sheets/secondhand _smoke/health_effects, updated January 11, 2017; J. D. Thacher and coauthors, Pre- and postnatal exposure to parental Smoking and allergic disease through adolescence, *Pediatrics* 134 (2014): 428–434.

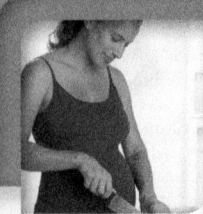

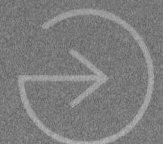

10.3 Nutrition in Practice

Encouraging Successful Breastfeeding

As discussed in Chapter 10, breastfeeding offers benefits to both mother and infant. The American Academy of Pediatrics (AAP) and the Academy of Nutrition and Dietetics, and advocate breastfeeding as the preferred means of infant feeding.[1] Promotion of breastfeeding is an integral part of the WIC program's nutrition education component. National efforts to promote breastfeeding seem to be working, at least to some extent: The percentage of infants who were breastfed at least for a while rose from 60 percent among those born in 1994 to 81 percent among infants born in 2013.[2] Despite this encouraging trend, by 6 months, breastfeeding rates fall to 52 percent. The AAP and many other health organizations recommend exclusive breastfeeding for the first six months of life.[3] Exclusive breastfeeding is defined as an infant's consumption of human milk with no supplementation of any kind (no water, no other type of milk, no juice, and no other foods) except for vitamins, minerals, and medications. The AAP recommends that breastfeeding continue for at least a year and thereafter for as long as mutually desired. In the United States, the prevalence of exclusive breastfeeding at six months is low (about 22 percent) and only about one in three infants is still breastfeeding at one year of age.[4] Increasing the rates of breastfeeding initiation and duration is one of the goals of *Healthy People 2020*:

> Increase the proportion of infants who are breastfed ever, at 6 months, and at 1 year. Increase the proportion of infants who are breastfed exclusively through 3 months, and through 6 months.[5]

Despite the trend toward increasing breastfeeding, the percentage of mothers choosing to breastfeed their infants and continuing to do so still falls short of goals.

Why don't more women choose to breastfeed their infants?

Many experts cite two major deterrents: infant formula manufacturers' public advertising and promotion of their products and the medical community's failure to encourage breastfeeding. Infant formula manufacturers spend millions of dollars each year marketing their products, often claiming that formula "is like breast milk." Infant formula is an appropriate substitute for breast milk when breastfeeding is specifically contraindicated, but for most infants, the benefits of breast milk outweigh those of formula. Despite medical evidence of the benefits of breast milk, medical practice is not always supportive.[6]

As an example of the medical lack of encouragement, some hospitals routinely separate mother and infant soon after birth.[7] The child's first feeding then comes from the bottle rather than the breast. Furthermore, many hospitals send new mothers home with free samples of infant formula. According to a recent survey, however, this practice is on the decline. Between 2007 and 2013, the percentage of U.S. hospitals distributing infant formula discharge samples to mothers breastfeeding their infants decreased markedly from 73 percent to 32 percent.[8] Such findings may reflect increased participation in the Baby-Friendly Hospital Initiative, a global effort to promote and support breastfeeding.

The World Health Organization opposes the distribution of infant formula discharge samples because it sends a misleading message that medical authorities favor infant formula over breast milk for infants. Even in hospitals where women are encouraged to breastfeed and are supported in doing so, little, if any, assistance is available after hospital discharge when many breastfeeding women still need assistance. More than half of mothers who initially breastfeed their infants stop within six months—seemingly due to lack of knowledge and support.

Women who receive early and repeated breastfeeding information and support breastfeed their infants longer than other women do. Information and instruction are especially important during the *prenatal* period when most women decide whether to breastfeed or to feed formula.[9] Nurses and other health care professionals can play a crucial role in encouraging successful breastfeeding by offering women adequate, accurate information about breastfeeding that permits them to make informed choices. Table NP10-1 lists tips for successful breastfeeding.

TABLE NP10-1	Tips for Successful Breastfeeding

- Learn about the benefits of breastfeeding.
- Initiate breastfeeding within 1 hour of birth.
- Ask a health care professional to explain how to breastfeed and how to maintain lactation.
- Give newborn infants no food or drink other than breast milk, unless medically indicated.
- Breastfeed on demand.
- Give no artificial nipples or pacifiers to breastfeeding infants.[a]
- Find breastfeeding support groups, books, or websites to help troubleshoot breastfeeding problems.

[a]Compared with nonusers, infants who use pacifiers breastfeed less frequently and stop breastfeeding at a younger age.

If breastfeeding is a natural process, what do mothers need to learn?

Although lactation is an automatic physiological process, breastfeeding requires some learning. This learning is most successful in a supportive environment. It begins with preparatory steps taken before the infant is born.

What are these preparatory steps?

Toward the end of pregnancy and throughout lactation, a woman who intends to breastfeed should stop using soap and lotions on her breasts. The natural secretions of the breasts themselves lubricate the nipple area best. A woman who plans to breastfeed should also acquire at least two nursing bras before her infant is born. The bras should provide good support and have drop-flaps so that either breast can be freed for nursing.

How soon after birth should breastfeeding start?

As soon as possible. Immediately after the delivery, for a short period, the infant is intensely alert and intent on suckling. This is the ideal time for the first breastfeeding and facilitates successful lactation.

What does the new mother need to know to continue breastfeeding her infant successfully?

She needs to learn how to relax and position herself so that she and the infant will be comfortable and the infant can breathe freely while nursing (Box NP10-1). She also needs to understand that infants have a **rooting reflex** that makes them turn toward any touch on the face (see the glossary in Box NP10-2). Consequently, she should touch the infant's cheek to her nipple so that the infant will turn the right way to nurse. The mother can then place four fingers under the breast and her thumb on top to support the breast and present the nipple

Box NP10-2 Glossary

engorgement: overfilling of the breasts with milk.
letdown reflex: the reflex that forces milk to the front of the breast when the infant begins to nurse.
mastitis: infection of a breast.
rooting reflex: a reflex that causes an infant to turn toward whichever cheek is touched, in search of a nipple.

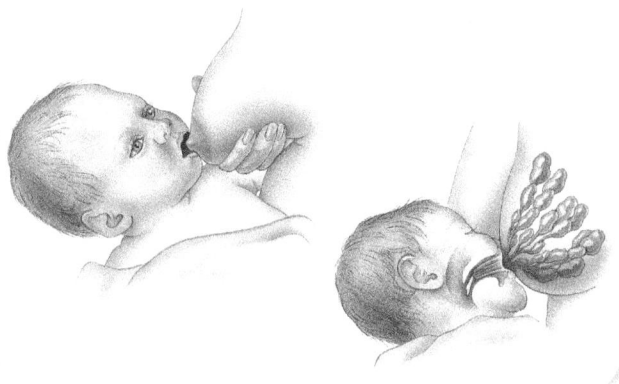

FIGURE NP10-1 Infant's Grasp on Mother's Breast

The mother supports the breast with her fingers and thumb behind the areola to present the nipple to the infant. Once the infant latches onto the breast, the infant's lips and gums pump the areola, releasing milk from the mammary glands into the milk ducts that lie beneath the areola.

to the infant. The mother's fingers and thumb should be behind the areola, the colored ring around the nipple, so as not to interfere with the infant latching onto the breast (see Figure NP10-1). With the breast supported, the mother tickles the infant's lips with the breast until the infant's mouth opens wide. The mother can then gently bring the infant forward onto the breast. The nipple must rest well back on the infant's tongue so that the infant's gums will squeeze on the glands that release the milk and swallowing will be effortless. To break the suction, if necessary, the mother can slip a finger between the infant's mouth and her breast.

Does it hurt to have the infant sucking so hard on the breast?

Breastfeeding should not be painful if the infant is positioned correctly. The mother has a **letdown reflex** that forces milk to the front of her breast when the infant begins to nurse, virtually propelling the milk into the infant's mouth. Letdown is necessary for the infant to obtain milk easily, and the mother needs to relax for letdown to occur. The mother who assumes a comfortable position in an environment without interruptions will find it easiest to relax.

How long should the infant be allowed to nurse at each feeding?

Even though the infant obtains about half the milk from the breast during the first two or three minutes of suckling, and 80 to 90 percent of it within four minutes, the infant should be encouraged to breastfeed on the first breast for as long as he or she wishes before being offered the second breast. The suckling itself, as well as the complete removal of milk from the breast, stimulates the mammary glands to produce milk for the next nursing session. Successive sessions should start on alternate breasts to ensure that each breast is emptied regularly. This pattern maintains the same supply and demand for each breast and thus prevents either breast from overfilling.

Infants should be fed "on demand" and not be held to a rigid schedule. The breastfed infant may average 8 to 12 feedings per 24-hour period during the first month or so. Once the mother's milk supply is well established and the infant's capacity has increased, the intervals between feedings will become longer.

What if a mother wants to skip one or two feedings daily—for example, because she works outside the home?

The mother can express breast milk into a bottle ahead of time, properly store the breast milk, and, when needed, substitute the expressed breast milk for a nursing session. Breast milk can be kept refrigerated for 48 hours or frozen. Freeze bottles of expressed milk in the back of the freezer where the temperature is coldest, not in the door. Milk can be frozen for up to nine months.[10]

The mother can hand-express her breast milk or use one of several different breast pumps available. The bicycle-horn type of manual breast pump is difficult to keep clean and is not recommended. Cylinder-type manual pumps or electric breast pumps are safer and are also more efficient. Alternatively, a mother can substitute formula for those missed feedings and continue to breastfeed at other times.

What about problems associated with breastfeeding such as sore nipples or infection of the breast?

Most problems associated with breastfeeding can be resolved. Many mothers experience sore nipples during the initial days of breastfeeding. Sore nipples need to be treated kindly, but nursing can continue. Improper feeding position is a frequent cause of sore nipples: the mother should make sure the infant is taking the entire nipple and part of the areola onto the tongue. She should nurse on the less sore breast first to get letdown going while the infant is suckling hardest; then she can switch to the sore breast. Between times, she should expose her nipples to light and air to heal them.

Before lactation is well established, when the schedule changes, or when a feeding is missed, the breasts may become full and hard—an uncomfortable condition known as **engorgement**. The infant cannot grasp an engorged nipple and so cannot provide relief by nursing. A gentle massage or warming the breasts with a cloth soaked in warm water or in a shower helps to initiate letdown and to release some of the accumulated milk; then the mother can pump out some of her milk and allow the infant to nurse.

Infection of the breast, known as **mastitis,** is best managed by continuing to breastfeed. By drawing off the milk, the infant helps to relieve pressure in the infected area. The infant is safe because the infection is between the milk-producing glands, not inside them.

Even if everything is going smoothly, the nursing mother should ideally have enough help and support so that she can rest in bed a few hours each day for the first week or so. Successful breastfeeding requires the support of all those who care. This, plus adequate nutrition, ample fluids, fresh air, and physical activity, will do much to enhance the well-being of mother and infant.

Notes

1. Position of the Academy of Nutrition and Dietetics: Promoting and Supporting breastfeeding, *Journal of the Academy of Nutrition and Dietetics* 115 (2015): 444–449; Breastfeeding, in *Pediatric Nutrition*, 7th ed., ed. R. E. Kleinman (Elk Grove Village, Ill.: American Academy of Pediatrics, 2014), pp. 41–59.

2. Centers for Disease Control and Prevention, *Breastfeeding Report Card United States, 2016,* available at www.cdc.gov/breastfeeding/data /reportcard.htm.

3. Position of the Academy of Nutrition and Dietetics: Promoting and Supporting breastfeeding, 2015; American Academy of Pediatrics, Breastfeeding, 2014.

4. Centers for Disease Control and Prevention, *Breastfeeding Report Card United States, 2016,* available at www.cdc.gov/breastfeeding/data /reportcard.htm.

5. Centers for Disease Control and Prevention, *Breastfeeding Report Card United States, 2016,* available at www.cdc.gov/breastfeeding/data /reportcard.htm.

6. L. P. Ward, Widespread hospital variation in supplementation of breastfed newborns, *Pediatrics* 140 (2017): e20170946; J. M. Nelson, R. Li, and

C. G. Perrine, Trends of US hospitals distributing infant formula packs to breastfeeding mothers, 2007 to 3013, *Pediatrics* 135 (2015): 1051–1056; C. J. Chantry and coauthors, In-hospital formula use increases early breastfeeding cessation among first-time mothers intending to exclusively breastfeed, *Journal of Pediatrics* 164 (2014): 1339–1345.

7. L. P. Ward and coauthors, Improving exclusive breastfeeding in an urban academic hospital, *Pediatrics* 139 (2017): e20160344.

8. J. M. Nelson, R. Li, and C. G. Perrine, Trends of US hospitals distributing infant formula packs to breastfeeding mothers, 2007 to 2013, *Pediatrics* 135 (2015): 1051–1056.

9. R. L. Dunn and coauthors, Engaging field-based professionals in a qualitative assessment of barriers and positive contributors to breastfeeding using the social ecological model, *Maternal and Child Health Journal* 19 (2015): 6–16; A. M. Stuebe, Enabling women to achieve their breastfeeding goals, *Obstetrics and Gynecology* 123 (2014): 643–652.

10. Breastfeeding beyond infancy, in *American Academy of Pediatrics, New Mother's Guide to Breastfeeding*, ed. J. Y. Meek (New York: Bantam Books, 2017), pp. 180–206.

Nutrition through the Life Span: Infancy, Childhood, and Adolescence

Chapter Sections and Learning Objectives (LOs)

11.1 Nutrition of the Infant

LO 11.1 Describe the nutritional needs of infants, the beneficial components of breast milk, and the appropriate foods and feeding practices for infants.

11.2 Nutrition during Childhood

LO 11.2 Explain how children's appetites and nutrient needs reflect their stage of growth; why hunger, iron deficiency, lead poisoning, food allergies, hyperactivity, and obesity are often concerns during childhood; and how parents and other caregivers can foster healthful eating habits and food choices in children.

11.3 Nutrition during Adolescence

LO 11.3 Describe the nutrient needs of adolescents and some of the challenges in meeting these needs.

11.4 Nutrition in Practice: Childhood Obesity and the Early Development of Chronic Diseases

LO 11.4 Describe the lifestyle factors that can help prevent childhood obesity and the development of type 2 diabetes and heart disease.

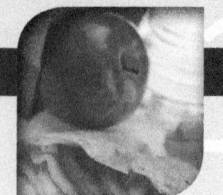

development. After the first year, a child continues to grow and change, but more slowly. Sound nutrition throughout infancy and childhood promotes normal growth and development; facilitates academic and physical performance; and helps prevent obesity, diabetes, heart disease, cancer, and other degenerative diseases in adulthood. As children enter their teens, a foundation built by years of eating nutritious foods best prepares them to meet the upcoming demands of rapid growth. This chapter examines the special nutrient needs of infants, children, and adolescents.

11.1 Nutrition of the Infant

Early nutrition affects later development, and early feeding sets the stage for eating habits that will influence nutrition status for a lifetime. Trends change, and experts argue about the fine points, but properly nourishing an infant is relatively simple, overall. The infant initially drinks only breast milk or formula but later begins to eat some foods, as appropriate. Common sense in the selection of infant foods and a nurturing, relaxed environment go far to promote an infant's health and well-being. The remainder of this discussion is devoted to feeding the infant and identifying the nutrients most often deficient in infant diets.

Nutrient Needs during Infancy

An infant grows faster during the first year than ever again, as Figure 11-1 shows. The growth of infants and children directly reflects their nutritional well-being and is an important parameter in assessing their nutrition status. Health care professionals use growth charts to evaluate the growth and development of children from birth to 20 years of age (see Appendix E).

Nutrients to Support Growth An infant's birthweight doubles by about five months of age and triples by the age of one year, typically reaching 20 to 25 pounds. (Consider that if an adult, starting at 120 pounds, were to do this, the person's weight would increase to 360 pounds in a single year.) The infant's length changes more slowly than weight, increasing about 10 inches from birth to one year. By the end of the first year, the growth rate slows considerably. An infant typically gains less than 10 pounds during the second year and grows about 5 inches in height. At the age of two, healthy children have attained approximately half of their adult height.

Not only do infants grow rapidly, but, in proportion to body weight, their basal metabolic rate is remarkably high—about twice that of an adult. The rapid growth and metabolism of the infant demand an ample supply of all the nutrients. Of special importance during infancy are the energy nutrients and the vitamins and minerals critical to the growth process, such as vitamin A, vitamin D, and calcium.

Because they are small, infants need smaller *total* amounts of these nutrients than adults do, but as a percentage of body weight, infants need more than twice as much of most nutrients. Infants require about 100 kcalories per kilogram of body weight per day; most adults require fewer than 40 (see Table 11-1). Figure 11-2 compares a five-month-old infant's needs (per unit of body weight) with those of an adult man. You can see that differences in vitamin D and iodine, for instance, are extraordinary. Around 6 months of age, energy needs begin to increase less rapidly as the

FIGURE 11-1 Weight Gain of Human Infants in Their First Five Years of Life

In the first year, an infant's birthweight may triple, but over the following several years, the rate of weight gain gradually diminishes.

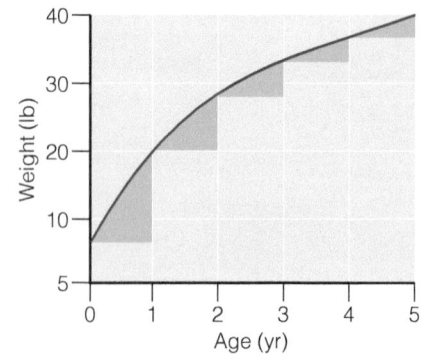

	INFANTS	ADULTS
TABLE 11-1		

TABLE 11-1 Infant and Adult Heart Rate, Respiration Rate, and Energy Needs Compared

	INFANTS	ADULTS
Heart rate (beats/minute)	120 to 140	70 to 80
Respiration rate (breaths/minute)	20 to 40	15 to 20
Energy needs (kcal/body weight)	45/lb (100/kg)	<18/lb (<40/kg)

growth rate begins to slow, but some of the energy saved by slower growth is spent on increased activity (see Photo 11-1). When their growth slows, infants spontaneously reduce their energy intakes. Parents can expect their infants to adjust their own food intakes to their changing needs; there is no need to force or coax them to eat more than they need.

FIGURE 11-2 Nutrient Recommendations for a Five-Month-Old Infant and an Adult Male Compared on the Basis of Body Weight

Infants may be relatively small and inactive, but they use large amounts of energy and nutrients in proportion to their body size to keep all their metabolic processes going.

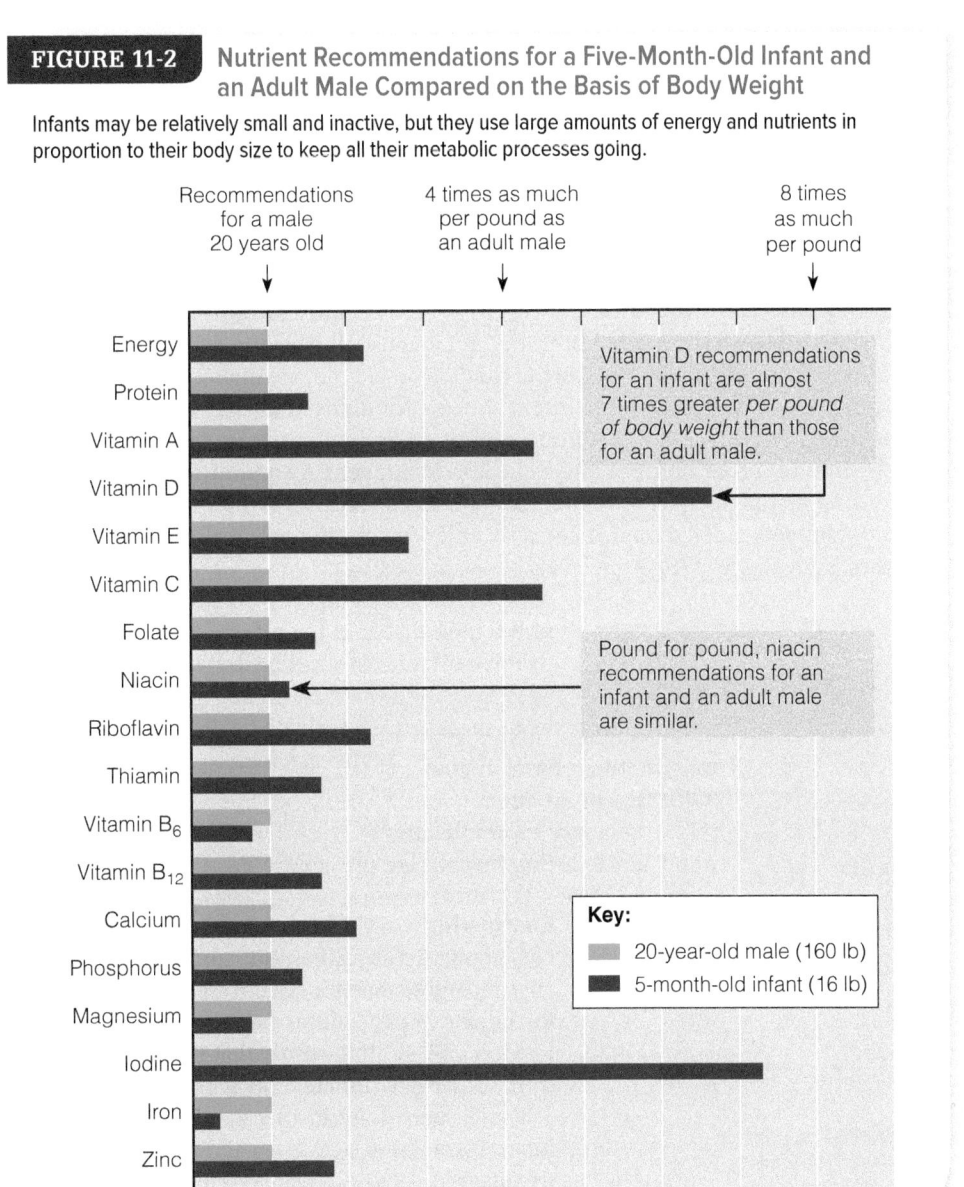

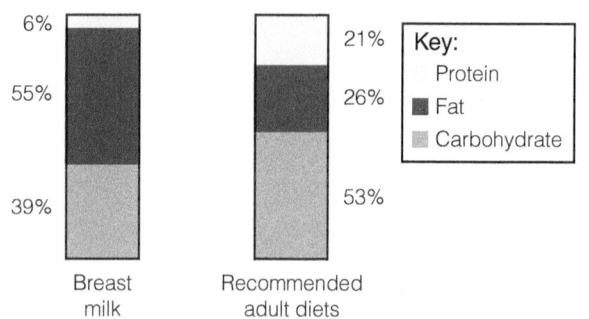

Photo 11-1

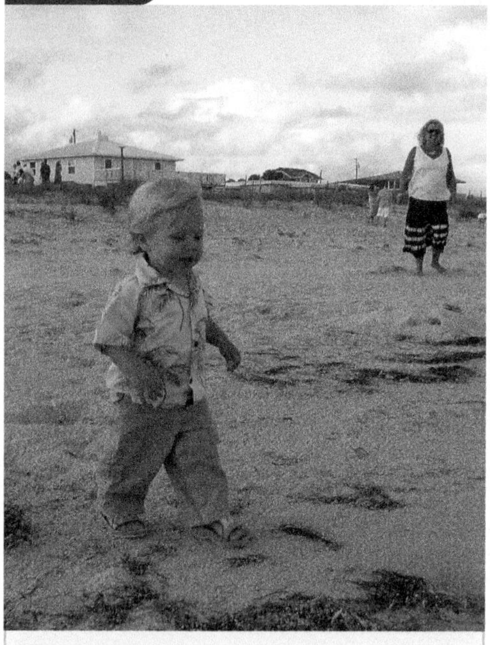

After six months of age, energy saved by slower growth is spent on increased activity.

Linda DeBruyne

Water One of the most important nutrients for infants, as for everyone, is water. The younger a child is, the more of the child's body weight is water. Breast milk or infant formula normally provides enough water to replace fluid losses in a healthy infant. If the environmental temperature is extremely high, however, infants need supplemental water.[1] Because proportionately more of an infant's body water than an adult's is between the cells and in the vascular space, this water is easy to lose. In the event of rapid fluid loss due to vomiting or diarrhea, an electrolyte solution designed for infants (available in drug stores) is needed.

Review Notes

- An infant's birthweight doubles by about five months of age and triples by one year.
- Infants' rapid growth and development depend on adequate nutrient supplies, including water from breast milk and formula.

Breast Milk

Breast milk excels as a source of nutrients for the young infant. With the possible exception of vitamin D (discussed later), breast milk meets all of a healthy infant's needs for the first six months of life. It provides many other health benefits as well.

BOX 11-1 *Nursing Diagnosis*

The nursing diagnosis *effective breastfeeding* applies to clients with effective mother/infant communication patterns and an infant who is content after feeding.

Frequency and Duration of Breastfeeding Breast milk is more easily and completely digested than formula, so breastfed infants usually need to eat more frequently than formula-fed infants do. During the first few weeks, approximately 8 to 12 feedings a day—on demand, as soon as the infant shows early signs of hunger such as increased alertness, activity, or suckling motions—promote optimal milk production and infant growth (Box 11-1). Crying is a late indicator of hunger.[2] An infant who nurses every two to three hours and sleeps contentedly between feedings is adequately nourished. As the infant gets older, stomach capacity enlarges and the mother's milk production increases, allowing for longer intervals between feedings.

When breastfeeding, the infant draws about half of the milk that is in the breast within the first two or three minutes of suckling, but should be encouraged to continue to nurse on that breast for as long as he or she is actively suckling before being offered the second breast. Begin each feeding on the breast that was offered second, the last time. The infant's suckling, as well as the complete removal of milk from the breast, stimulates lactation.

Energy Nutrients The distribution of energy nutrients in breast milk differs dramatically from the balance recommended for adults (see Figure 11-3). Yet, for infants, breast milk is nature's most nearly perfect food, illustrating clearly that people at different stages of life have different nutrient needs.

The carbohydrate in breast milk (and standard infant formula) is lactose. In addition to being easily digested, lactose enhances calcium absorption. The carbohydrate component of breast milk also

FIGURE 11-3 Percentages of Energy-Yielding Nutrients in Breast Milk and in Recommended Adult Diets

The proportions of energy-yielding nutrients in human breast milk differ from those recommended for adults.

Breast milk: 6%, 55%, 39%
Recommended adult diets: 21%, 26%, 53%

Key:
Protein
Fat
Carbohydrate

Note: The values listed for adults represent approximate midpoints of the acceptable ranges for protein (10 to 35 percent), fat (20 to 35 percent), and carbohydrate (45 to 65 percent).

contains abundant oligosaccharides, which are present only in trace amounts in cow's milk and infant formula made from cow's milk. Human milk oligosaccharides help protect the infant from infection by preventing the binding of pathogens to the infant's intestinal cells.[3]

Human breast milk contains less protein than cow's milk, but this is actually beneficial because less protein places less stress on the infant's immature kidneys to excrete the major end product of protein metabolism, urea. The protein in breast milk is largely **alpha-lactalbumin**, which is efficiently digested and absorbed.

The lipids in breast milk (and infant formula) provide the infant's main source of energy. Breast milk contains a generous proportion of the essential fatty acids linoleic acid and linolenic acid, as well as their longer-chain derivatives arachidonic acid and docosahexaenoic acid (DHA). Most formulas today also contain added arachidonic acid and DHA (read the label). Infants can produce some arachidonic acid and DHA from linoleic and linolenic acid, respectively, but some infants may need more than they can make.

As Chapter 4 mentioned, DHA is the most abundant fatty acid in the brain and is also present in the retina of the eye. DHA accumulation in the brain is greatest during fetal development and early infancy.[4] Research has focused on the visual and mental development of breastfed infants and infants fed standard formula with and without DHA added.[5] Results of studies for visual acuity development in term infants have been inconsistent. Factors such as the amount of DHA provided, its sources, and the sensitivity of different measures for visual acuity may have contributed to the inconsistent outcomes. Some of the evidence from studies that have examined the effects of DHA status on cognitive function suggests that DHA supplementation during development can influence certain measures of cognitive function.[6] Studies that follow children beyond infancy, when more detailed tests of cognitive function can be employed, are needed to confirm the importance of DHA for optimal infant and child development.

Vitamins and Minerals With the exception of vitamin D, the vitamin content of the breast milk of a well-nourished mother is ample. Even vitamin C, for which cow's milk is a poor source, is supplied generously. The concentration of vitamin D in breast milk is low, however, and vitamin D deficiency impairs bone mineralization.[7] Vitamin D deficiency is most likely in infants who are not exposed to sunlight daily, have darkly pigmented skin, and receive breast milk without vitamin D supplementation. Reports of infants in the United States developing the vitamin D–deficiency disease rickets and recommendations by the American Academy of Pediatrics (AAP) to keep infants under six months of age out of direct sunlight prompted revisions in vitamin D guidelines. The AAP recommends a vitamin D supplement for all infants who are breastfed exclusively and for any infants who do not receive at least 1 liter (1000 milliliters) or 1 quart (32 ounces) of vitamin D–fortified formula daily.[8] Despite these recommendations, many infants in the United States are consuming inadequate amounts of vitamin D.

As for minerals, the calcium content of breast milk is ideal for infant bone growth, and the calcium is well absorbed. Breast milk is also appropriately low in sodium. The limited amount of iron in breast milk is highly absorbable. Zinc is absorbed well, too, thanks to the presence of a zinc-binding protein.

Supplements for Infants Pediatricians may prescribe supplements containing vitamin D, iron, and fluoride (after six months of age). Table 11-2 offers a schedule of supplements during infancy. Vitamin K nutrition for newborns presents a unique case: the AAP recommends giving a single dose of vitamin K to infants at birth to prevent uncontrolled bleeding. (See Chapter 8 for a description of vitamin K's role in blood clotting.)

Immunological Protection In addition to its nutritional benefits, breast milk offers unsurpassed immunological protection.[9] Not only is breast milk sterile, but it also actively fights disease and protects infants from illnesses. Protective factors include antiviral agents, anti-inflammatory agents, antibacterial agents, and infection inhibitors.

During the first two or three days after delivery, the breasts produce **colostrum**, a premilk substance containing mostly serum with antibodies and white blood cells.

alpha-lactalbumin (lact-AL-byoo-min): a major protein in human breast milk, as opposed to *casein* (CAY-seen), a major protein in cow's milk.

colostrum (co-LAHS-trum): a milklike secretion from the breasts, present during the first few days after delivery before milk appears; rich in protective factors.

TABLE 11-2   Supplement Recommendations for Full-Term Infants

Recommendations for all supplements should be based on the health care provider's assessment of the infant.

SUPPLEMENTS	BIRTH	4 MONTHS	6 MONTHS
Vitamin D	All infants who are: • Exclusively breastfed. • Receiving less than 1 qt (32 oz) of vitamin D–fortified formula per day.	As recommended at birth.	As recommended at birth.
Iron (1 mg per kg of body weight per day)		All infants who are: • Exclusively breastfed. • Receiving more than one-half of their daily feedings as breast milk and no iron-containing comple-mentary foods.	May not be needed once iron containing foods are introduced.
Fluoride			All infants who are: • Exclusively breastfed. • Receiving ready-to-use formulas (which are made with water low in fluoride). • Receiving formula mixed with water that contains little or no fluoride (less than 0.3 ppm).

Source: Adapted from the American Academy of Pediatrics, *Pediatric Nutrition*, 7th ed., ed. R. E. Kleinman (Elk Grove Village, IL: American Academy of Pediatrics, 2014).

Colostrum (like breast milk) helps protect the newborn from infections against which the mother has developed immunity—precisely those that the infant is most likely to be exposed to. The maternal antibodies in colostrum and breast milk inactivate disease-causing bacteria within the infant's digestive tract before they can start infections.[10] This explains, in part, why breastfed infants have fewer intestinal infections than formula-fed infants. In addition to antibodies, colostrum and breast milk provide other powerful agents that help to fight against bacterial infection (see Table 11-3).

Breastfeeding also protects against other common illnesses of infancy such as middle ear infection and respiratory illness.[11] Breast milk offers protection against the development of allergies as well. Compared with formula-fed infants, breastfed infants have a lower incidence of allergic reactions such as asthma, wheezing, and skin rash.[12] This protection is especially noticeable among infants with a family history of allergies. Breastfeeding also reduces the risk of sudden infant death syndrome (SIDS).[13] This protective effect is stronger when breastfeeding is exclusive, but any amount of breast milk for any duration is protective against SIDS.

Clearly, breast milk is a very special substance. Nutrition in Practice 10 offers suggestions for successful breastfeeding.

TABLE 11-3 Protective Factors in Breast Milk

- **Antibodies:** Offer protection in the upper respiratory tract and gastrointestinal tract, preventing adherence of pathogens to the mucosa, protecting against invasive infections; may stimulate the infant's own immune system

- **Bifidus factors:** Favor the growth of the "friendly" bacterium *Lactobacillus bifidus* in the infant's digestive tract so that other, harmful bacteria cannot become established

- **Growth factors:**
  - Epidermal growth factor: Regulates cell growth, proliferation, and differentiation
  - Transforming growth factor-beta (TGF-β): Anti-inflammatory; epithelial barrier function

- **Lactadherin:** Inhibits binding of pathogens to the intestinal mucosa

- **Lactoferrin:** Prevents bacteria from getting the iron they need to grow; helps absorb iron into the infant's bloodstream; kills some bacteria directly; antiviral effects

- **Lysozyme:** Together with lactoferrin, kills bacteria

- **Oligosaccharides:** Help to establish and maintain growth of desired bacteria in gastrointestinal tract; prevent binding of pathogens in gastrointestinal tract

Sources: Adapted from J. T. Smilowitz and coauthors, Breast milk oligosaccharides: Structure-function relationships in the neonate, *Annual Review of Nutrition* 34 (2014): 143–169; B. Lonnerdal, Bioactive proteins in breast milk, *Journal of Paediatrics and Child Health* (Supplement S1) 49 (2013): 1–7; D. E. W. Chatterton and coauthors, Anti-inflammatory mechanisms of bioactive milk proteins in the intestine of newborns, *International Journal of Biochemistry and Cell Biology* 45 (2013): 1730–1747; P. V. Jeurink and coauthors, Mechanisms underlying immune effects of dietary oligosaccharides, *American Journal of Clinical Nutrition* 98 (2013): 572S–577S.

Other Potential Benefits Breast milk may offer protection against the development of cardiovascular disease, but more well-conducted research, using consistent and precise definitions of breastfeeding, is needed to confirm this effect.[14] Breastfeeding may also offer some protection against excessive weight gain later, although findings are inconsistent.[15] Researchers note that many other factors—socioeconomic status, other infant and child feeding practices, and especially the mother's weight—strongly predict a child's body weight.[16]

Many studies suggest a beneficial effect of breastfeeding on later intelligence, but when subjected to strict standards of methodology (for example, large sample sizes and appropriate intelligence testing), the evidence is less convincing.[17] Nevertheless, the possibility that breastfeeding may positively affect later intelligence is intriguing. It may be that some specific component of breast milk, such as DHA, contributes to brain development or that certain factors associated with the feeding process itself promote the intellect. Most likely, several factors are more large, well-controlled studies are needed to confirm the effects, if any, of breastfeeding on later intelligence.

Infant Formula

Breastfeeding offers many benefits to both mother and infant, and it should be encouraged whenever possible. The mother who has decided to use formula, however, should be supported in her choice just as the breastfeeding mother should be. She can offer the same closeness, warmth, and stimulation during feedings as the breastfeeding mother can. An advantage of feeding formula is that other family members can participate in feeding the infant, giving them a chance to develop the special closeness that feeding fosters.

Many mothers choose to breastfeed at first but **wean** their children within the first 1 to 12 months. If infants are less than a year old, mothers must wean them onto *infant formula*, not onto plain cow's milk of any kind—whole, reduced-fat, low-fat, or fat-free.

wean: to gradually replace breast milk with infant formula or other foods.

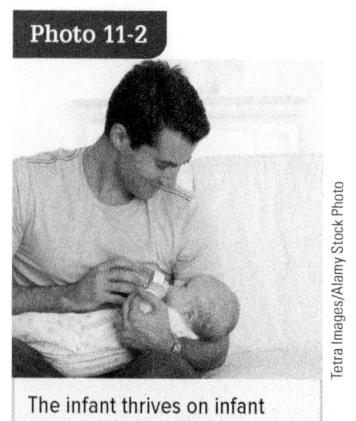

The infant thrives on infant formula offered with affection.

Infant formula is available as a powdered or liquid concentrate that must be mixed with water according to label directions, and as a ready-to-feed liquid. The powdered form is the least expensive.

Infant Formula Composition Manufacturers can prepare formulas from cow's milk in such a way that they do not differ significantly from human milk in nutrient content. All currently available infant formulas meet all of the energy and nutrient requirements for healthy, full-term infants during the first four to six months of life (see Photo 11-2). After the infant is six months of age, formulas, along with a variety of complementary foods, continue to supply a significant part of the infant's nutrient needs.

Figure 11-4 illustrates the energy nutrient distributions of breast milk, infant formula, and cow's milk. Notice the higher protein concentration of cow's milk, which stresses an infant's kidneys. The AAP recommends that all formula-fed infants receive iron-fortified infant formulas.[18] Use of iron-fortified formulas has risen in recent decades and is credited with the decline of iron-deficiency anemia in U.S. infants.

Infant Formula Standards National and international standards have been set for the nutrient contents of infant formulas. U.S. standards are based on AAP recommendations, and the Food and Drug Administration (FDA) mandates quality control procedures to ensure that these standards are met. All standard formulas are therefore nutritionally similar. Small differences in nutrient content are sometimes confusing but usually unimportant. Recently, the FDA issued new quality control procedures to further ensure that infant formulas are safe and support healthy growth.[19] These specify how and when manufacturers must inform the FDA about new formulas and changes to formulas, and require testing for contamination with harmful bacteria such as *Salmonella*.

Special Formulas Standard cow's milk–based formulas are inappropriate for some infants. Special formulas have been designed to meet the dietary needs of infants with specific conditions such as prematurity or inherited diseases. Most infants allergic to milk protein can drink formulas based on soy protein.[20] Soy formulas contain cornstarch and sucrose instead of lactose and so are recommended for infants with lactose intolerance as well. They are also useful as an alternative to milk-based formulas for vegan families. Infants who are allergic to both cow's milk protein and soy protein can be given special formulas based on hydrolyzed protein.

Risks of Formula Feeding Infant formulas contain no protective antibodies for infants, but, in general, vaccinations, purified water, and clean environments in developed

FIGURE 11-4 Percentages of Energy-Yielding Nutrients in Breast Milk, Infant Formula, and Cow's Milk

The average proportions of energy-yielding nutrients in human breast milk and formula differ slightly. In contrast, cow's milk provides too much protein and too little carbohydrate.

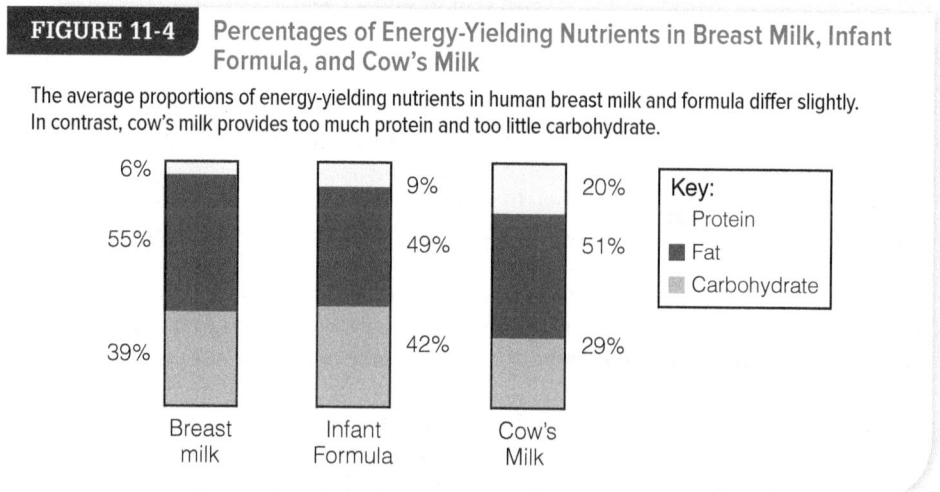

Key:
Protein
Fat
Carbohydrate

countries help protect infants from infections. Formulas can be prepared safely by following the rules of proper food handling and by using water that is free of contamination. Of particular concern is lead-contaminated water, a major source of lead poisoning in infants. Because the first water drawn from the tap each day is highest in lead, a person living in a house with old, lead-soldered plumbing should let the water run a few minutes before drinking or using it to prepare formula or food.

In developing countries and in poor areas of the United States, formula may be unavailable, overdiluted in an attempt to save money, or prepared with contaminated water. Overdilution of formula can cause malnutrition and growth failure. Contaminated formula often causes infections leading to diarrhea, dehydration, and malabsorption. Wherever sanitation is poor, breastfeeding should be encouraged over feeding formula. Breast milk is sterile, and its antibodies enhance an infant's resistance to disease.

FIGURE 11-5 Nursing Bottle Tooth Decay— An Extreme Example

The teeth have decayed all the way to the gum line.

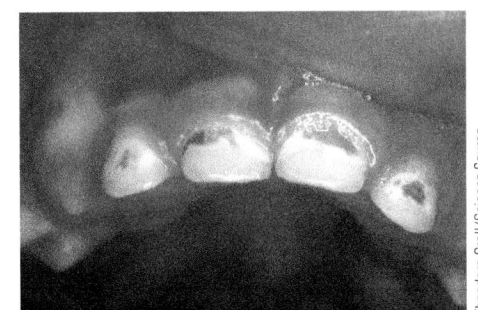

Theodore Croll/Science Source

Nursing Bottle Tooth Decay Dentists advise against putting an infant to bed with a bottle. Salivary flow, which normally cleanses the mouth, diminishes as the infant falls asleep. Prolonged sucking on a bottle of formula, milk, or juice bathes the upper teeth in a carbohydrate-rich fluid that nourishes decay-producing bacteria. (The tongue covers and protects most of the lower teeth, but they, too, may be affected.) The result is extensive and rapid tooth decay (see Figure 11-5). To prevent **nursing bottle tooth decay**, no child should be put to bed with a bottle as a pacifier.

The Transition to Cow's Milk

The AAP advises that cow's milk is not appropriate during the first year.[21] In some infants, particularly those younger than six months of age, cow's milk causes intestinal bleeding, which can lead to or aggravate iron deficiency. Cow's milk is also a poor source of iron. Consequently, it both causes iron loss and fails to replace iron. Furthermore, the bioavailability of iron from infant cereal and other foods is reduced when cow's milk replaces breast milk or iron-fortified formula during the first year. Compared with breast milk or iron-fortified formula, cow's milk is higher in calcium and lower in vitamin C, characteristics that reduce iron absorption. To repeat, then, cow's milk is a poor choice during the first year of life; infants need breast milk or iron-fortified infant formula.

Once an infant has reached a year of age and is receiving at least two-thirds of total daily food energy from a balanced mixture of cereals, vegetables, fruit, and other foods, reduced-fat or low-fat cow's milk is an acceptable and recommended accompanying beverage.[22] After the age of two, a transition to fat-free milk can take place, but care should be taken to avoid excessive restriction of dietary fat.

Introducing First Foods

Changes in the body organs during the first year affect the infant's readiness to accept solid foods. Until the child is several months old, the immature stomach and intestines can digest milk sugar (lactose) but not starch. This is one of the many reasons why breast milk and formula are such good foods for an infant; they provide simple, easily digested carbohydrate that supplies energy for the infant's growth and activity.

When to Introduce Solid Food The AAP supports exclusive breastfeeding for approximately six months but recognizes that infants are often developmentally ready to accept **complementary foods** between four and six months of age.[23] The main purpose of introducing solid foods is to provide needed nutrients that are no longer supplied adequately by breast milk or formula alone. The foods chosen must be those that the infant is capable of handling both physically and metabolically. The exact timing depends on the individual infant's needs and developmental readiness

nursing bottle tooth decay: extensive tooth decay due to prolonged tooth contact with formula, milk, fruit juice, or other carbohydrate-rich liquid offered to an infant in a bottle.

complementary foods: nutrient- and energy-containing solid or semisolid foods (or liquids) fed to infants in addition to breast milk or infant formula.

(see Table 11-4), which vary from infant to infant because of differences in growth rates, activities, and environmental conditions. The addition of foods to an infant's diet should be governed by three considerations: the infant's nutrient needs, the infant's physical readiness to handle different forms of foods, and the need to detect and control allergic reactions.

How to Introduce First Foods   It bears repeating that early feeding strategies are critical in establishing healthy food preferences and habits that last throughout life. Infants (and toddlers) learn solely from their caregivers what, when, and how to eat. Caregivers

TABLE 11-4   Infant Development and Recommended Foods

AGE (MO)	PHYSICAL AND DEVELOPMENTAL MILESTONES	HUNGER SIGNALS	SATIETY SIGNALS	FOODS INTRODUCED INTO THE DIET
0 to 4	Turns head toward any object that brushes cheek. Initially swallows using back of tongue; gradually begins to swallow using front of tongue as well. Strong reflex (extrusion) to push food out during first two to three months.	Wakes and moves around. Sucks on fist. Cries or fusses. Opens mouth while feeding to indicate wanting more.	Seals lips together. Turns head away. Stops sucking. Falls asleep when full.	Feed breast milk or infant formula.
4 to 6	Extrusion reflex diminishes, and the ability to swallow nonliquid foods develops. Sits erect with support at six months. Begins chewing action. Brings hand to mouth. Grasps objects with palm of hand.	Cries or fusses. Indicates desire for food by smiling or cooing during feeding. Indicates desire for food by opening mouth and leaning forward.	Slows rate of sucking or stops sucking. Turns head away and leans back.	Begin iron-fortified cereal mixed with breast milk, formula, or water. Begin pureed meats, legumes, vegetables, and fruit.
6 to 8	Able to self-feed finger foods. Develops pincher (finger to thumb) grasp. Begins to drink from cup.	Reaches for spoon or food. Points to food.	Slows eating. Pushes food away.	Begin textured vegetables and fruit.
8 to 10	Begins to hold own bottle. Sits unsupported.	Reaches for and grabs spoon and food. Shows excitement when food is presented.	Shuts mouth tightly or pushes food away.	Begin breads and cereals from table. Begin yogurt. Begin pieces of soft, cooked vegetables and fruit from table. Gradually begin finely cut meats, fish, casseroles, cheese, eggs, and mashed legumes.
10 to 12	Begins to master spoon but still spills some.	Indicates desire for specific food with words or sounds.	Uses words such as *no, all done,* or *get down.* Plays with or throws food when done.	Add variety. Gradually increase portion sizes.[a]

[a]Portion sizes for infants and young children are smaller than those for an adult. For example, a grain serving might be ½ slice of bread instead of 1 slice, or ¼ cup rice instead of ½ cup.

Note: Because each stage of development builds on the previous stage, the foods from an earlier stage continue to be included in all later stages.

Source: Adapted in part from Committee on Nutrition, American Academy of Pediatrics, *Pediatric Nutrition,* 7th ed., ed. R. E. Kleinman (Elk Grove Village, Ill.: American Academy of Pediatrics, 2014), pp. 123–139.

must therefore understand how infants signal hunger and satiety (see Table 11-4) and how to respond to these signals appropriately—a process known as **responsive feeding**.[24] By clearly and consistently responding to a child's needs at mealtimes, the child learns to identify internal hunger, thirst, and satiety signals; to ask for food or beverages when hungry or thirsty; and to stop eating when full.

Foods to Provide Iron, Zinc, and Vitamin C Rapid growth demands iron. At about four to six months, an infant begins to need more iron than body stores plus breast milk or iron-fortified formula can provide. In addition to breast milk or iron-fortified formula, infants can receive iron from iron-fortified cereals and, once they readily accept solid foods, from meat or meat alternates such as legumes (see Figure 11-6). Iron-fortified cereals contribute a significant amount of iron to an infant's diet, but the iron's bioavailability is poor.[25] Caregivers can enhance iron absorption from iron-fortified cereals by serving vitamin C–rich foods with meals.

The concentration of zinc in breast milk is initially high, but decreases sharply over the first few months of lactation. The high efficiency of zinc absorption from breast milk does not compensate for this low concentration over time. Infant formulas are fortified with zinc concentrations higher than those found in breast milk. Thus, breastfed infants depend more on complementary foods to provide adequate zinc intakes than do formula-fed infants. Infant cereals are not routinely fortified with zinc, so the best sources are protein foods such as meats, poultry, seafood, eggs, and legumes. Zinc is less well absorbed from legumes than from the other protein foods.

The best sources of vitamin C are fruit and vegetables (see Figure 8-14 on p. 224 in Chapter 8). Fruit juice is a source of vitamin C, too much juice can cause diarrhea in young children.[26] Furthermore, too much fruit juice contributes excess kcalories and displaces other nutrient-rich foods. The AAP recommends no fruit juice for infants before one year of age and limiting juice for toddlers (1 to 3 years of age) to 4 ounces per day. For young children (4 to 6 years of age), limiting juice to 6 ounces per day is recommended.[27] Fruit juices should be diluted and served in a cup, not a bottle.

Physical Readiness for Solid Foods The ability to swallow solid food develops at around four to six months, and food offered by spoon helps to develop swallowing ability. At eight months to one year, an infant can sit up, can handle finger foods, and begins to teethe. At that time, hard crackers and other hard finger foods may be introduced to promote the development of manual dexterity and control of the jaw muscles. These feedings must take place under the watchful eye of an adult because infants cannot safely chew and swallow some foods without choking.

Some parents want to feed solids at an earlier age, on the theory that "stuffing the baby" at bedtime promotes sleeping through the night. There is no proof for this theory. On average, infants start to sleep through the night at about the same age (three to four months) regardless of when solid foods are introduced.

Food Allergies To prevent allergies or identify them promptly, experts recommend introducing each new food singly in a small portion and waiting three to five days before introducing the next new food.[28] For example, rice cereal is usually the first cereal introduced because it is the least allergenic. When it is clear that rice cereal is not causing an allergy, another grain, perhaps barley or oats, is introduced. Wheat cereal is offered last because it is the most common offender. If a cereal causes an allergic reaction such as a skin rash, digestive upset, or respiratory discomfort, it should

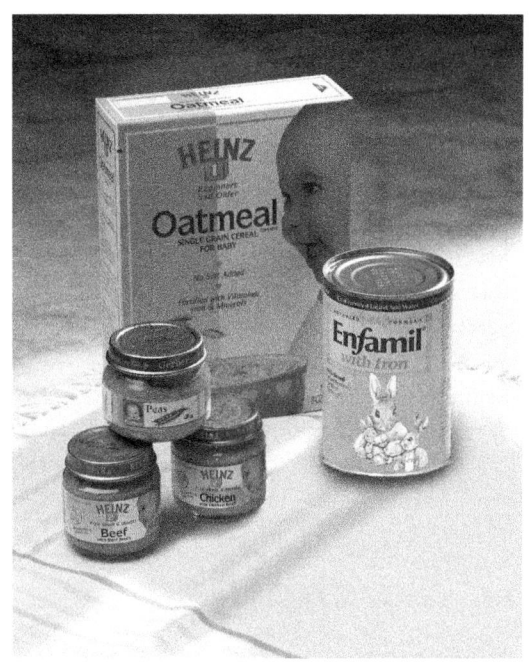

FIGURE 11-6 Iron Sources for Infants

Foods such as iron-fortified cereals and formulas, mashed legumes, and strained meats provide iron.

Polara Studios, Inc.

responsive feeding: an interactive feeding process in which a young child signals hunger and satiety vocally, through facial expressions, and through motor actions; the caregiver recognizes these cues and responds promptly in an emotionally supportive and developmentally appropriate manner. In this way, the child experiences a predictable response to hunger and satiety signals that supports healthy eating behaviors.

TABLE 11-5 Examples of Foods and Nonfood Items Children Can Choke On

To prevent choking, do not give infants or young children:

- Gum
- Hard or gel-type candies
- Hot dog slices
- Large raw apple slices
- Marshmallows
- Nuts
- Peanut butter
- Popcorn, chips, and pretzel nuggets
- Raw carrots
- Raw celery
- Sausage sticks or slices
- Whole beans
- Whole cherries
- Whole grapes

Keep these nonfood items out of their reach:

- Balloons
- Coins
- Pen tops
- Small balls and marbles
- Other items of similar size

be discontinued before introducing the next food. Food allergies in the United States have increased over the last few decades, especially allergy to peanuts. New guidelines recommend introducing peanut-based foods early (between 4 and 11 months), rather than later (between 12 and 36 months) to prevent peanut allergy. Infants at high risk—those with severe skin rash or egg allergies—need medical approval and oversight, but for most other infants, parents may start adding peanut-containing foods such as watered down peanut butter or peanut puffs to the diet in the same way oatmeal and mashed vegetables are introduced.[29]

Choice of Infant Foods Infant foods should be selected to provide variety, balance, and moderation. Commercial baby foods offer a wide variety of palatable, nutritious foods in a safe and convenient form. Parents or caregivers should not feed directly from the jar—remove the infant's portion and place it in a dish so as not to contaminate the leftovers that will be stored in the jar. Homemade infant foods can be as nutritious as commercially prepared ones, as long as the cook minimizes nutrient losses during preparation. Ingredients for homemade foods should be fresh, whole foods without added salt, sugar, or seasonings. Pureed food can be frozen in ice cube trays, providing convenient-sized blocks of food that can be thawed, warmed, and fed to the infant. Infants and young children are vulnerable to foodborne illnesses. An infant's caregiver must be on guard against food poisoning and take precautions against it as described in Nutrition in Practice 2. For example, hands and equipment must be kept clean.

Foods to Omit Sweets of any kind (including baby food "desserts") have no place in an infant's diet. The added food energy conveys few, if any, nutrients to support growth and contributes to obesity. Canned vegetables are also inappropriate for infants; they often contain too much sodium. Honey and corn syrup should never be fed to infants because of the risk of botulism.

Infants and even young children cannot safely chew and swallow any of the foods listed in Table 11-5; they can easily choke on these foods, a risk not worth taking. Nonfood items of small size should always be kept out of the infant's reach to prevent choking.

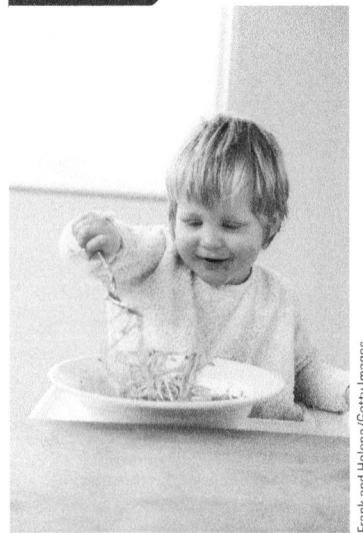

Photo 11-3

Ideally, a one-year-old eats many of the same healthy foods as the rest of the family.

Frank and Helena/Getty Images

Foods at One Year At one year of age, reduced-fat or low-fat cow's milk can become a primary source of most of the nutrients an infant needs; 2 to 3 cups a day meet those needs sufficiently. More milk than this displaces iron-rich foods and can lead to the iron-deficiency anemia known as milk anemia. Other foods—meat and meat alternates, iron-fortified cereals, whole-grain or enriched bread, fruit, and vegetables—should be supplied in variety and in amounts sufficient to round out total energy needs. Ideally, a one-year-old will sit at the table, eat many of the same foods everyone else eats, and drink liquids from a cup—not a bottle (see Photo 11-3). Table 11-6 shows a sample menu that meets a one-year-old's requirements.

Looking Ahead

Probably the most important single measure to undertake during the first year is to encourage eating habits that will support continued normal weight as the child grows. This means introducing a variety of nutritious foods in an inviting way, not forcing the infant to finish the bottle or the baby food jar, avoiding concentrated sweets and empty-kcalorie foods, and encouraging physical activity. Parents should avoid teaching infants to seek food as a reward, to expect food as comfort for unhappiness, or to associate food deprivation with punishment. Normal dental development is also promoted by supplying nutritious foods, avoiding sweets, and discouraging the association of food with reward or comfort. Oral health is the subject of Nutrition in Practice 17.

Mealtimes

The nurturing of a young child involves more than just nutrition. Those who care for young children are responsible for providing not only food, milk, and water but also a safe, loving environment in which a child can grow and develop physical and emotional health and security. The person feeding a one-year-old should be aware that exploring and experimenting are normal and desirable behaviors at this time in a child's life. The child is developing a sense of autonomy that, if allowed to develop, will lay the foundation for later assertiveness in choosing when and how much to eat and when to stop eating. In light of the developmental and nutrient needs of one-year-olds, and in the face of their often contrary and willful behavior, a few feeding guidelines may be helpful:

- *Discourage unacceptable behavior (such as standing at the table or throwing food) by removing the child from the table to wait until later to eat.* Be consistent and firm, not punitive. For example, instead of saying "You make me mad when you don't sit down," say "The fruit salad tastes good—please sit down and eat some with me." The child will soon learn to sit and eat.
- *Let young children explore and enjoy food.* This may mean eating with fingers for a while. Learning to use a spoon will come in time. Children who are allowed to touch, mash, and smell their food while exploring it are more likely to accept it.
- *Don't force food on children.* Rejecting new foods is normal, and acceptance is more likely as children become familiar with new foods through repeated opportunities to taste them. Instead of saying "You cannot go outside to play until you taste your carrots," say "You can try the carrots again another time."
- *Provide nutritious foods, and let children choose which ones, and how much, they will eat.* Gradually, they will acquire a taste for different foods.
- *Limit sweets.* Infants and young children have little room for empty-kcalorie foods in their daily energy allowance. Do not use sweets as a reward for eating meals.
- *Don't turn the dining table into a battleground.* Make mealtimes enjoyable. Teach healthy food choices and eating habits in a pleasant atmosphere. Mealtimes are not the time to fight, argue, or scold.

These recommendations reflect a spirit of tolerance that best serves the emotional and physical interests of the infant. This attitude, carried throughout childhood, helps the child to develop a healthy relationship with food.

TABLE 11-6 Sample Menu for a One-Year-Old

BREAKFAST
1 scrambled egg
1 slice whole-wheat toast
½ c reduced-fat milk

MORNING SNACK
½ c yogurt
¼ c fruit[a]

LUNCH
½ grilled cheese sandwich: 1 slice whole-wheat bread with 1 slice cheese
½ c vegetables[b] (steamed carrots)
¼ c 100% fruit juice

AFTERNOON SNACK
½ c fruit[a]
½ c toasted oat cereal

DINNER
1 oz chopped meat or ¼ c well-cooked mashed legumes
½ c rice or pasta
½ c vegetables[b] (chopped broccoli)
½ c reduced-fat milk

[a]Include citrus fruit, melons, and berries.
[b]Include dark green, leafy, and deep yellow vegetables.

Note: This sample menu provides about 1000 kcalories.

Review Notes

- The primary food for infants during the first 12 months is either breast milk or iron-fortified formula.
- In addition to nutrients, breast milk also offers immunological protection.
- At about four to six months, infants should gradually begin eating solid foods.
- The addition of foods to an infant's diet should be governed by three considerations: the infant's nutrient needs, the infant's physical readiness to handle different forms of foods, and the need to detect and control allergic reactions.
- By the time infants are one year old, they are drinking from a cup and eating many of the same foods as the rest of the family.

11.2 Nutrition during Childhood

After the age of one, growth rate slows, but the body continues to change dramatically (see Figure 11-7). At age one, infants have just learned to stand and toddle; by age two, they walk confidently and are learning to run, jump, and climb. Nutrition and physical activity have helped them prepare for these new accomplishments by adding to the mass and density of their bone and muscle tissue. Thereafter, their bones continue to grow longer and their muscles to gain size and strength, though unevenly and more slowly, until adolescence.

Energy and Nutrient Needs

Children's appetites begin to diminish around the first birthday, consistent with the slowed growth rate. Thereafter, the appetite fluctuates. At times children seem to be insatiable, and at other times they seem to live on air and water. Parents and other caregivers need not worry: given an ample selection of nutritious foods at regular intervals, internal appetite regulation in healthy, normal-weight children guarantees that their food energy intakes will be right for each stage of growth.

Ideally, children accumulate stores of nutrients before adolescence. Then, when they take off on the adolescent growth spurt and their nutrient intakes cannot keep pace with the demands of rapid growth, they can draw on the nutrient stores accumulated earlier. This is especially true of calcium; the denser the bones are in childhood, the better prepared they will be to support teen growth and still withstand the inevitable bone losses of later life.[30] Consequently, the way children eat influences their nutritional health during childhood, during their teen years, and for the rest of their lives.

Children's Appetites Many people mistakenly believe that they must "make" their children eat the right amounts of food, and children's erratic appetites often reinforce this belief. Although children's food energy intakes vary widely from meal to meal, total daily energy intake remains remarkably constant. If children eat less at one meal, they typically eat more at the next, and vice versa.

Parents do, however, need to help children choose the right foods, and, with overweight children, they may need to help more, as described later. Overweight children may not adjust their energy intakes appropriately and may disregard appetite-regulation signals and eat in response to external cues, such as television commercials.[31]

FIGURE 11-7 Body Shape of a One-Year-Old and a Two-Year-Old Compared

The body shape of a one-year-old (left) changes dramatically by age two (right). The two-year-old has lost much of the baby fat; the muscles (especially in the back, buttocks, and legs) have firmed and strengthened; and the leg bones have lengthened.

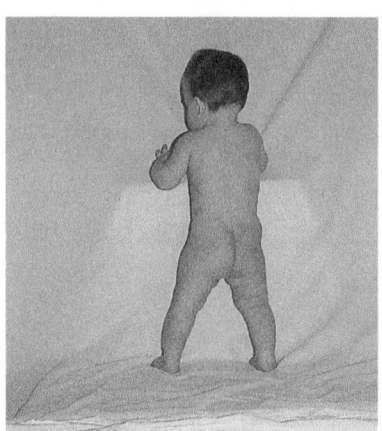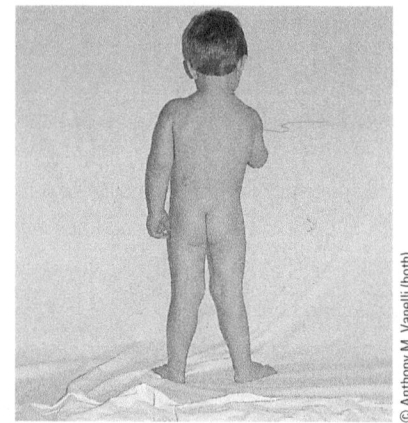

© Anthony M. Vanelli (both)

Energy Individual children's energy needs vary widely, depending on their growth and physical activity. A one-year-old child needs approximately 800 kcalories a day; an active six-year-old needs twice as many. By age 10, an active child needs about 2000 kcalories a day. Total energy needs increase gradually with age, but energy needs per kilogram of body weight actually decline. Physically active children of any age need more energy because they expend more, and inactive children can become obese even when they eat less food than the average. Unfortunately, our nation's children are becoming less and less active; childcare programs and schools would serve our children well by offering more activities to promote physical fitness.[32]

Some children, notably those adhering to a vegan diet, may have difficulty meeting their energy needs. Grains, vegetables, and fruit provide plenty of fiber, adding bulk, but may provide too few kcalories to support growth (Box 11-2). Soy products, other legumes, and nut or seed butters offer more concentrated sources of energy to support optimal growth and development.[33]

Carbohydrate and Fiber Carbohydrate recommendations are based on glucose use by the brain. After one year of age, brain glucose use remains fairly constant and is within the adult range. Carbohydrate recommendations for children after one year are therefore the same as for adults (see inside front cover).

Fiber recommendations (see inside front cover) derive from adult intakes shown to reduce the risk of coronary heart disease and are based on energy intakes. Consequently, fiber recommendations are lower for younger children with low energy intakes than for older ones with high energy intakes.

Fat and Fatty Acids No RDA for total fat has been established, but the DRI committee recommends a fat intake of 30 to 40 percent of energy for children 1 to 3 years of age and 25 to 35 percent for children 4 to 18 years of age. However, as long as children's energy intakes are adequate, fat intakes below 30 percent of total energy do not impair growth. Children who eat low-fat diets, however, tend to have low intakes of some vitamins and minerals. Recommended intakes of the essential fatty acids are based on average intakes (see inside front cover).

Protein Like energy needs, total protein needs increase slightly with age but actually decline slightly per unit of body weight (see inside front cover). Protein recommendations must address the requirements for maintaining nitrogen balance, the quality of protein consumed, and the added needs of growth.

Vitamins and Minerals The vitamin and mineral needs of children increase with age (see inside front cover). A balanced diet of nutritious foods can meet children's needs for these nutrients, with the notable exception of iron and possibly vitamin D. Iron-deficiency anemia, a major problem worldwide, is prevalent among U.S. and Canadian children, especially toddlers one to three years of age.[34] During the second year of life, toddlers progress from a diet of iron-rich infant foods such as breast milk, iron-fortified formula, and iron-fortified infant cereal to a diet of adult foods and iron-poor cow's milk. In addition, their appetites often fluctuate—some become finicky about the foods they eat, and others prefer milk and juice to solid foods. These situations can interfere with children eating iron-rich foods at a critical time for brain growth and development.

To prevent iron deficiency, children's foods must deliver 7 to 10 milligrams of iron per day. To achieve this goal, snacks and meals should include iron-rich foods (see Table 11-7), and milk intake should be reasonable so that it will not displace lean meats, fish, poultry, eggs, legumes, and whole-grain or enriched products. That means 2½ cups of milk per day up to age eight, increasing to 3 cups per day from age nine on. After age one, as long as the overall diet supplies 30 percent of total kcalories from fat, reduced-fat or low-fat milk can be used instead of whole milk.[35] The saved kcalories can be invested in iron-rich

TABLE 11-7 Iron-Rich Foods Children Like[a]

BREADS, CEREALS, AND GRAINS

Cream of wheat (½ c)

Fortified dry cereals (1 oz)[b]

Noodles, rice, or barley (½ c)

Tortillas (1 flour or whole-wheat, 2 corn)

Whole-wheat, enriched, or fortified bread (1 slice)

VEGETABLES

Cooked snow peas (½ c)

Cooked mushrooms (½ c)

Green peas (½ c)

Mixed vegetable juice (1 c)

FRUIT

Canned plums (3 plums)

Cooked dried apricots (¼ c)

Dried peaches (4 halves)

Raisins (1 tbs)

MEATS AND LEGUMES

Bean dip (¼ c)

Lean chopped roast beef or cooked ground beef (1 oz)

Liverwurst on crackers (½ oz)

Meat casseroles (½ c)

Mild chili or other bean/meat dishes (¼ c)

Peanut butter and jelly sandwich (½ sandwich)

Sloppy joes (½ sandwich)

[a]Each serving provides at least 1 milligram of iron. Vitamin C–rich foods included with these snacks increase iron absorption.
[b]Some fortified breakfast cereals contain more than 10 milligrams of iron per half-cup serving (read the labels).

TABLE 11-8 USDA Food Patterns: Recommended Daily Amounts for Each Food Group (1000 to 1800 kCalories)

FOOD GROUP	1000 kcal	1200 kcal	1400 kcal	1600 kcal	1800 kcal
Fruit	1 c	1 c	1½ c	1½ c	1½ c
Vegetables	1 c	1½ c	1½ c	2 c	2½ c
Grains	3 oz	4 oz	5 oz	5 oz	6 oz
Protein Foods	2 oz	3 oz	4 oz	5 oz	5 oz
Milk	2 c	2½ c	2½ c	3 c	3 c

TABLE 11-9 Estimated Daily kCalorie Needs for Children

AGE (YEARS)	SEDENTARY[a]	ACTIVE[b]
2	1000	1000
3	1000	1400
FEMALES		
4	1200	1400
5 to 6	1200	1600
7	1200	1800
8 to 9	1400	1800
10	1400	2000
11	1600	2000
12 to 13	1600	2200
MALES		
4 to 5	1200	1600
6 to 7	1400	1800
8	1400	2000
9	1600	2000
10	1600	2200
11	1800	2200
12	1800	2400
13	2000	2600

[a]Sedentary describes a lifestyle that includes only the activities typical of day-to-day life.
[b]Active describes a lifestyle that includes at least 60 minutes per day of moderate physical activity (equivalent to walking more than 3 miles per day at 3 to 4 miles per hour) in addition to the activities of day-to-day life.

Source: U.S. Department of Health and Human Services and U.S. Department of Agriculture, *2015–2020 Dietary Guidelines for Americans*, 8th ed. (2015), health.gov /dietaryguidelines/2015/guidelines/.

foods such as lean meats, fish, poultry, eggs, and legumes. Whole-grain or enriched breads and cereals also contribute iron.

Children typically obtain most of their vitamin D from fortified milk (2.5 micrograms per cup) and dry cereals (1 microgram per ½ cup). Children who do not meet their RDA (15 micrograms) from these sources should receive a vitamin D supplement.[36] Remember that sunlight is also a source of vitamin D, especially in warm climates and warm seasons.

Supplements With the exception of specific recommendations for fluoride, iron, and vitamin D during infancy and childhood, the AAP and other professional groups agree that well-nourished children do not need vitamin and mineral supplements—yet many children and adolescents take them. Researchers are still studying the safety of supplement use by children. The Federal Trade Commission has warned parents about giving children supplements advertised to prevent or cure childhood illnesses such as colds, ear infections, or asthma. Dietary supplements on the market today include many herbal products that have not been tested for safety and effectiveness in children.

Food Patterns for Children To provide all the needed nutrients, a child's meals and snacks should include a variety of foods from each food group—in amounts suited to the child's appetite and needs. Table 11-8 provides USDA Food Patterns for several kcalorie levels. (For kcalorie levels over 1800, see Table 1-6 on p. 19.) Estimated daily kcalorie needs for active and sedentary children of various ages are shown in Table 11-9. MyPlate online resources for preschoolers (two to five years) translate the eating patterns into messages that can help parents ensure that the foods they provide meet their child's needs. For children 6 to 11 years, the site provides interactive nutrition games, videos, and other resources for teachers, parents, and children themselves (Figure 11-8). These guidelines and resources also stress the importance of balancing kcalorie intake with kcalorie expenditure through adequate physical activity to promote growth without excessive weight gain (as discussed later in this chapter).

Children whose diets follow the pattern presented in Table 11-8 meet their nutrient needs fully, but few children eat according to these recommendations. Many children in the United States do not eat the types and amounts of foods consistent with recommendations to promote normal growth and development and reduce the risk of future disease.[37] For example, while children's intakes of solid fats and added sugars exceed recommendations, intakes of fruit, vegetables, whole grains, and milk and milk products fall short.[38] In other words, many children's eating patterns are energy-dense and nutrient-poor. Of great concern is the finding that during a 20-year period, preschoolers'

FIGURE 11-8   MyPlate Resources for Children

Abundant MyPlate resources for preschool children and older children can be found at *www.choosemyplate.gov*.

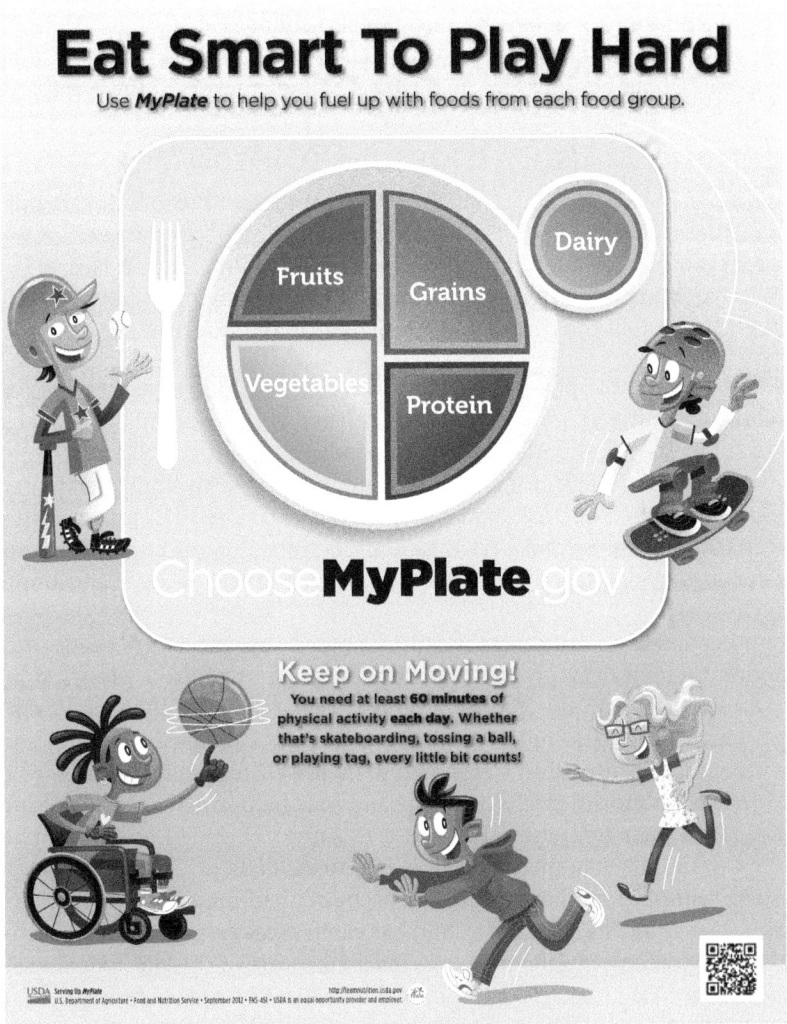

consumption of foods high in added sugars (candy, sweet snacks), solid fats (pizza, mixed Mexican dishes), and sodium (salty snacks) increased sharply; on a positive note, their intake of fruit also increased slightly. Parents and caregivers of infants and toddlers thus need to offer a much greater variety of nutrient-dense meals and snacks to help ensure adequate nutrition. Importantly, reading food labels can help parents identify appropriate foods for young children. Some commercial foods marketed to infants and toddlers—infant and toddler dinners, cereal bars, crackers, and ready-to-serve mixed cereals and fruits—may have added sugars or high sodium levels.[39]

Children's Food Choices The childhood years are the parents' best chance to influence their child's food choices. Appropriate eating habits and attitudes toward food, developed in childhood, can help future adults emerge with healthy habits that reduce risks of chronic diseases in later life. The challenge is to deliver nutrients in the form of meals and snacks that are both nutritious and appealing so that children will learn to enjoy a variety of health-promoting foods.

Permitting large quantities of candy, cola, and other concentrated sweets in children's diets will result in nutrient deficiencies, obesity, or both. Children can't be trusted to choose nutritious foods on the basis of taste; the preference for sweets is innate, and children naturally gravitate to them. Overweight children, especially, need help in selecting nutrient-dense foods that will meet their nutrient needs within their energy allowances. Underweight children or active, healthy-weight children can enjoy higher-kcalorie foods, but these should still be nutritious. Examples are ice cream and pudding in the milk group and whole-grain or enriched pancakes and crackers in the bread group.

Hunger and Malnutrition in Children

Most children in the United States and Canada have access to regular meals, but hunger and malnutrition do appear in certain circumstances. Children in very low-income families, for example, are more likely to be hungry and malnourished. Nearly 16 million U.S. children are hungry at least some of the time and are living in poverty.[40] Nutrition in Practice 12 examines the causes and consequences of hunger in the United States.

Hunger and Behavior Both short-term and long-term hunger exert negative effects on behavior and health. Short-term hunger, such as when a child misses a meal, impairs the child's ability to pay attention and to be productive. Hungry children are irritable, apathetic, and uninterested in their environment. Long-term hunger impairs growth and immune defenses. Food assistance programs such as the WIC program (discussed in Chapter 10) and the School Breakfast and National School Lunch Programs (discussed later in this chapter) are designed to protect against hunger and improve the health of children.[41]

A nutritious breakfast is a central feature of a diet that meets the needs of children and supports their healthy growth and development.[42] Children who skip breakfast typically do not make up the deficits at later meals—they simply have lower intakes of energy, vitamins, and minerals than those who eat breakfast. Malnourished children are particularly vulnerable. Compared to their well-fed peers, children who eat no breakfast may have shorter attention spans and may be more likely to perform poorly in tasks requiring concentration, but more research is needed to substantiate these findings.[43] Common sense dictates that it is unreasonable to expect anyone to learn and perform without fuel. For the child who hasn't had breakfast, the morning's lessons may be lost altogether. Even if a child has eaten breakfast, discomfort from hunger may become distracting by late morning. Teachers aware of the late-morning slump in their classrooms wisely request that midmorning snacks be provided; snacks improve classroom performance all the way to lunchtime.

Iron Deficiency and Behavior Iron deficiency has well-known and widespread effects on children's behavior and intellectual performance.[44] In addition to carrying oxygen in the blood, iron transports oxygen within cells, which use it for energy metabolism. Iron is also used to make neurotransmitters—most notably, those that regulate the ability to pay attention, which is crucial to learning. Consequently, iron deficiency not only causes an energy crisis but also directly impairs attention span and learning ability.

Iron deficiency is often diagnosed by a quick, easy, inexpensive hemoglobin or hematocrit test that detects a deficit of iron in the *blood*. A child's *brain*, however, is sensitive to low iron concentrations long before the blood effects appear. Iron deficiency lowers the motivation to persist in intellectually challenging tasks and impairs overall intellectual performance. Anemic children perform poorly on tests and are disruptive in the classroom; iron supplementation improves learning and memory. When combined with other nutrient deficiencies, iron-deficiency anemia has synergistic effects that are especially detrimental to learning. Furthermore, children who had iron-deficiency anemia *as infants* continue to perform poorly as they grow older, even if their iron status improves.[45] The long-term damaging effects on mental development make prevention and treatment of iron deficiency during infancy and early childhood a high priority.

Other Nutrient Deficiencies A child with any of several nutrient deficiencies may be irritable, aggressive, and disagreeable, or sad and withdrawn. Such a child may be labeled "hyperactive," "depressed," or "unlikable," when in fact these traits may be due to simple, even marginal, malnutrition. Though parents and medical practitioners often overlook this possibility, any departure from normal, healthy appearance and behavior is a sign of possible poor nutrition (see Photo 11-4). In any such case, inspection of the child's diet by a registered dietitian nutritionist or other qualified health care professional is in order. Any suspicion of dietary inadequacies, *no matter what other causes may be implicated*, should prompt steps to correct those inadequacies immediately.

Lead Poisoning in Children

Children who are malnourished are vulnerable to lead poisoning. They absorb more lead if their stomachs are empty; if they have low intakes of calcium, zinc, vitamin C, or vitamin D; and, of greatest concern because it is so common, if they have an iron deficiency. Iron deficiency weakens the body's defenses against lead absorption, and lead poisoning can cause iron deficiency.[46] Circumstances associated with both iron deficiency and lead poisoning are a low socioeconomic status and a lack of immunizations against infectious diseases. Another common factor is pica—a craving for nonfood items. Many children with lead poisoning eat dirt or chips of old paint, two common sources of lead (see Photo 11-5).

The anemia brought on by lead poisoning may be mistaken for a simple iron deficiency and therefore may be incorrectly treated. Like iron deficiency, mild lead toxicity has nonspecific symptoms, including diarrhea, irritability, and fatigue. Adding iron to the diet does not reverse the symptoms; exposure to lead must stop and treatment for lead poisoning must begin. With further exposure, the symptoms become more pronounced, and children develop learning disabilities and behavior problems (Box 11-3). Still more severe lead toxicity can cause irreversible nerve damage, paralysis, mental retardation, and death.

Approximately half a million children between the ages of one and five in the United States have blood lead levels above 5 micrograms per deciliter, the level at which the Centers for Disease Control and Prevention recommend public health actions be initiated.[47] Lead toxicity in young children results from their own behaviors and activities—putting their hands in their mouths, playing in dirt and dust, and chewing on nonfood items. Unfortunately, the body readily absorbs lead during times of rapid growth and hoards it possessively thereafter. Lead is not easily excreted and accumulates mainly in the bones but also in the brain, teeth, and kidneys. Because a child's neuromuscular system is maturing during these first few years of life, children with elevated lead levels experience impairment of balance, motor development, and the relaying of nerve messages to and from the brain. Deficits in intellectual development are only partially reversed when lead levels decline.

Federal laws mandating reductions in leaded gasolines, lead-based solder, and other products over the past four decades have helped to reduce the amounts of lead in food and in the environment in the United States. As a consequence, the prevalence of lead toxicity in children has declined dramatically for most of the nation.

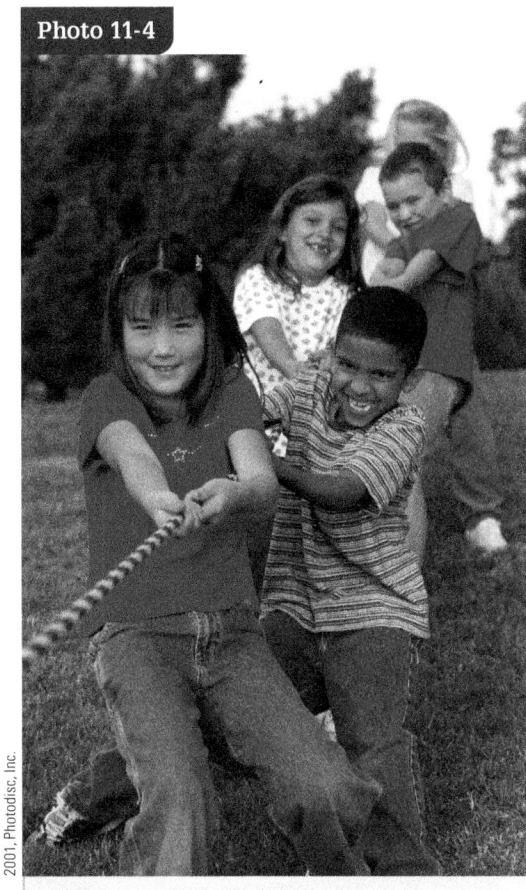

Photo 11-4

2001. Photodisc, Inc.

Healthy, well-nourished children are alert in the classroom and energetic at play.

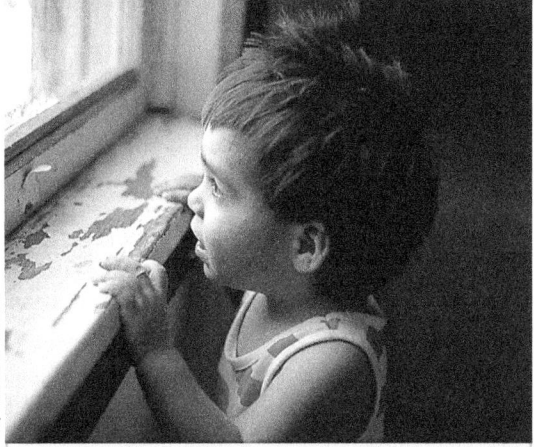

Photo 11-5

Tony Freeman/PhotoEdit

Old lead-based paint can threaten the health of an exploring child.

BOX 11-3 *Nursing Diagnosis*

The nursing diagnosis *risk for poisoning* applies to children who have dangerous products placed within their reach.

Box 11-4 | *HOW TO* Protect against Lead Toxicity

- Ask a pediatrician whether your child should be tested for lead poisoning.

- Clean floors, window frames, window sills, and other surfaces regularly. Use a mop or sponge with warm water and a general all-purpose cleaner.

- Prevent children from putting dirty or old painted objects in their mouths, and make sure children wash their hands before eating.

- Feed children balanced, timely meals with ample iron and calcium.

- Wash children's bottles, pacifiers, and toys often.

- Do not use lead-contaminated water to make infant formula.

- Have your water tested for lead. If the cold water hasn't been used for more than a few hours, let it run for 15 to 30 seconds before drinking it.

- Be aware that other countries do not have the same regulations protecting consumers against lead. Children have been poisoned by eating crayons made in China, putting toys from China in their mouths, and drinking fruit juice canned in Mexico.

Nevertheless, lead exposure is still a threat in certain communities. Box 11-4 presents strategies for defending children against lead toxicity. Unfortunately, regulations and precautions to protect people from lead contamination sometimes fail. In Flint, Michigan, dangerous levels of lead and other toxins in the water supply occurred when the city switched water sources to cut costs. Residents of Flint, including many children, were exposed to the contamination and the health risks posed by high concentrations of lead in the water.

Food Allergy

Food allergy is frequently blamed for physical and behavioral abnormalities in children, but only 4 to 8 percent of children younger than four years of age are diagnosed with true food allergies.[48] Food allergies diminish with age, until in adulthood they affect less than 4 percent of the population. The prevalence of food allergy, especially peanut allergy, is on the rise, however.[49] Reasons for an increase in peanut allergy are not yet clear, but possible contributing factors include genetics, composition and diversity of GI microbiota during infancy, food preparation methods (roasting peanuts at very high temperatures makes them more allergenic), and exposure to medicinal skin creams containing peanut oil.[50]

A true food allergy occurs when fractions of a food protein or other large molecule are absorbed into the blood and elicit an immunologic response. (Recall that proteins are normally dismantled in the digestive tract to amino acids that are absorbed without such a reaction.) The body's immune system reacts to these large food molecules as it does to other **antigens**—by producing antibodies or other defensive agents.

Detecting Allergy Allergies may have one or two components. They always involve antibodies; they may or may not involve symptoms. Moreover, symptoms exactly like those of an allergy may have other causes. Therefore, allergies cannot be diagnosed from symptoms alone. Physicians use clinical guidelines to diagnose and manage food allergy. Food allergy should be considered when an individual—especially a young child—experiences symptoms such as skin rash, respiratory difficulties, vomiting, diarrhea, or anaphylactic shock (described later) within minutes to hours of eating.

Diagnosis of food allergy requires medical testing and food challenges. Once a food allergy has been diagnosed, the required treatment is strict elimination of the offending food. Children with allergies, like all children, need all their nutrients, so it is important to include other foods that offer the same nutrients as the omitted foods. Nutritional counseling and growth monitoring are recommended for all children with food allergies.[51]

Immediate and Delayed Reactions Allergic reactions to food may be immediate or delayed. In either case, the antigen interacts immediately with the immune system, but

food allergy: an adverse reaction to food that involves an immune response; also called *food-hypersensitivity reactions*.

antigens: substances that elicit the formation of antibodies or an inflammation reaction from the immune system. A bacterium, a virus, a toxin, and a protein in food that causes allergy are all examples of antigens.

symptoms may appear within minutes or after several (up to 24) hours. Identifying the food that causes an immediate allergic reaction is easy because symptoms correlate closely with the time the food is eaten. Identifying the food that causes a delayed reaction is more difficult because the symptoms may not appear until much later. By this time, many other foods may have been eaten, complicating the picture.

Anaphylactic Shock The life-threatening food allergy reaction known as **anaphylactic shock** is most often caused by peanuts, tree nuts, milk, eggs, wheat, soybeans, fish, or shellfish (see Figure 11-9). Among these foods, eggs, milk, soy, and peanuts most often cause problems in children. Children are more likely to outgrow allergies to eggs, milk, wheat, and soy than allergies to peanuts, tree nuts, fish, and shellfish. Peanut allergies cause more life-threatening reactions than do all other food allergies combined. Research is currently under way to help those with peanut allergies tolerate small doses, thus saving lives and minimizing reactions.[52] Families of children with a life-threatening food allergy and school personnel who supervise those children must guard them against any exposure to the allergen. The child must learn to identify which foods pose a problem and then to use refusal skills for all foods that may contain the allergen.

Parents of allergic children can pack safe foods for lunches and snacks and ask school officials to strictly enforce a "no swapping" policy in the lunchroom. The child must be able to recognize the symptoms of impending anaphylactic shock (see Table 11-10). Any person with food allergies severe enough to cause anaphylactic shock should wear a medical alert bracelet or necklace. Finally, the responsible child and the school staff should be prepared to administer injections of **epinephrine**, which prevents anaphylaxis after exposure to the allergen. Many preventable deaths occur each year when people with food allergies accidentally ingest the allergen but have no epinephrine available.

Technology may soon offer new solutions. New drugs that may interfere with the immune response that causes allergic reactions are being developed. Also, through genetic engineering, scientists may one day banish allergens from peanuts, soybeans, and other foods to make them safer.

Food Labeling Food labels must identify any common allergens present in plain language, using the names of the eight most common allergy-causing foods. For example, a food containing "textured vegetable protein" must say "soy" on its label, and "casein" must be identified as "milk." Food producers must also prevent cross-contamination during production and clearly label the foods in which it is likely to occur. For example, equipment used for making peanut butter must be scrupulously clean before being used to pulverize cashew nuts for cashew butter to protect unsuspecting cashew butter consumers from peanut allergens.

Other Adverse Reactions to Foods Not all **adverse reactions** to foods are food allergies, although even physicians may describe them as such. Signs of adverse reactions to foods include stomachaches, headaches, rapid pulse rate, nausea, wheezing, hives, bronchial irritation, coughs, and other such discomforts. Among the causes may be reactions to chemicals in foods, such as the flavor enhancer monosodium glutamate

FIGURE 11-9 Common Food Allergens

These eight normally wholesome foods—milk, shellfish, fish, peanuts, tree nuts, eggs, wheat, and soybeans (and soy products)—may cause life-threatening symptoms in people with allergies.

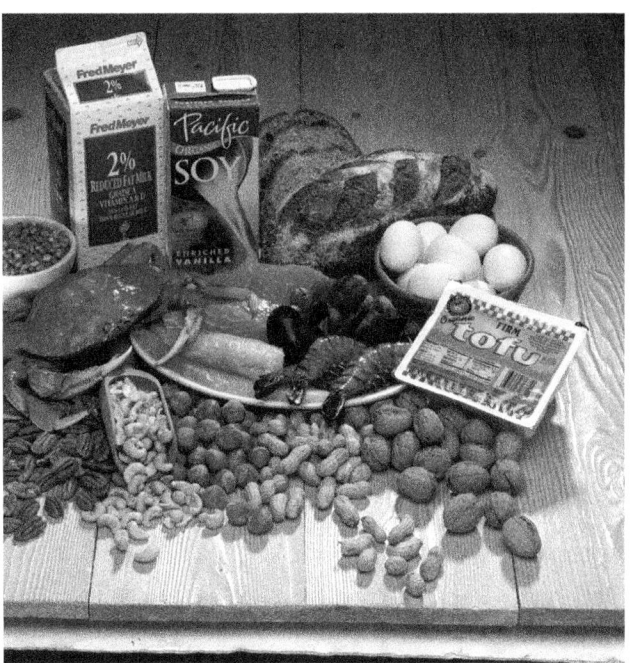

Polara Studios, Inc.

TABLE 11-10 Symptoms of Impending Anaphylactic Shock

- Tingling sensation in mouth
- Swelling of the tongue and throat
- Irritated, reddened eyes
- Difficulty breathing, asthma
- Hives, swelling, rashes
- Vomiting, abdominal cramps, diarrhea
- Drop in blood pressure
- Loss of consciousness

anaphylactic (AN-ah-feh-LAC-tic) **shock:** a life-threatening whole-body allergic reaction to an offending substance.

epinephrine: one of the stress hormones secreted whenever emergency action is needed; prescribed therapeutically to relax the bronchioles during allergy or asthma attacks.

adverse reactions: unusual responses to food (including intolerances and allergies).

(MSG), the natural laxative in prunes, or the mineral sulfur; digestive diseases, obstructions, or injuries; enzyme deficiencies, such as lactose intolerance; and even psychological aversions. These reactions involve symptoms but no antibody production. Therefore, they are **food intolerances**, not allergies.

Pesticides applied to produce in fields may linger on foods and cause adverse reactions. Health risks from pesticide exposure may be low for healthy adults, but children are vulnerable. Therefore, government agencies have set a **tolerance level** for each pesticide by first identifying foods that children commonly eat in large amounts and then considering the effects of pesticide exposure during each developmental stage.

Food Dislikes Parents are advised to watch for signs of food dislikes and take them seriously. Children's food aversions may be the result of nature's efforts to protect them from allergic or other adverse reactions. Test for allergies, and then apply nutrition knowledge conscientiously in deciding how to alter the diet.

Hyperactivity

Hyperactivity affects behavior and learning in about 11 percent of young school-aged children.[53] Left untreated, it can interfere with a child's social development and ability to learn. Treatment focuses on relieving the symptoms and controlling the associated problems. Physicians often manage hyperactivity through behavior modification, special educational techniques, and psychological counseling. In many cases, they prescribe medication.

Research on hyperactivity has focused on several nutritional factors as possible causes or treatments.[54] Parents of hyperactive children often blame sugar. They hopefully believe that simply eliminating candy and other sweet treats will solve the problem. Studies have found no convincing evidence that sugar causes hyperactivity or worsens behavior but dietary changes may still be helpful. Sugar-sweetened foods and beverages displace more nutritious choices from the diet, and, as stated previously, nutrient deficiencies are known to cause behavioral problems.

Food additives have also been blamed for hyperactivity and other behavior problems in children, but scientific evidence to substantiate the connection has been elusive.[55] Limited research suggests that food additives such as artificial colors or sodium benzoate preservative (or both) may exacerbate hyperactive symptoms such as inattention and impulsivity. Additional studies are needed to confirm the findings and to determine which additives studied might be responsible for negative behaviors.

Children can become excitable, rambunctious, and unruly as a result of a desire for attention, lack of sleep, overstimulation, watching too much television or playing too many computer games, too much caffeine from colas or chocolate, or a lack of physical activity. Such behaviors may suggest that more consistent care is needed. It helps to insist on regular hours of sleep, regular mealtimes, and regular outdoor activity. Box 11-5 offers an opportunity to think about these issues in relation to a specific child.

| Box 11-5 | **Case Study: Boy with Disruptive Behavior** |

Freddie Willis is a 6-year-old boy who seldom sits still, often misbehaves, and is frequently sick. Freddie's eating habits are erratic and poor, as is his appetite. He often misses breakfast because he is too tired to get up in time to eat before school. By midmorning, Freddie is irritable and disruptive in the classroom. At lunchtime, he trades the peanut butter and banana sandwich his mother packed in his lunchbox for a piece of cake. After school, he hurries home to watch television while he eats his favorite snack: cola and potato chips. At dinnertime, Freddie picks at his food because he isn't very hungry.

Later on, when it's time for bed, Freddie complains that he's hungry. His parents let him stay up to have a bowl of cereal (the kind with marshmallows) before he finally falls asleep.

1. What factors in Freddie's daily routine might be contributing to his restless behavior?

2. Discuss some changes in diet that might improve Freddie's health and disposition.

Childhood Obesity

The number of overweight children has increased dramatically over the past three decades. Like their parents, children in the United States are becoming fatter. An estimated 32 percent of U.S. children and adolescents 2 to 19 years of age are overweight or obese and 17 percent are obese.[56] Based on data from the BMI-for-age growth charts (see Figure E-5 in Appendix E), children and adolescents are categorized as *overweight* above the 85th percentile and as *obese* at the 95th percentile and above. One exception: for older adolescents, BMI at the 95th percentile is higher than 30, the adult obesity cutoff point. Therefore, obesity in young people is defined as BMI at the 95th percentile or BMI of 30 or greater, whichever is lower. For children younger than two years of age, BMI values are not available. For this age group, weight-for-height values above the 95th percentile are classified as overweight.

A third cutoff point (BMI greater than 120 percent of the 95th percentile or a BMI of 35 or greater, whichever is lower) defines severe obesity in childhood.[57] Unfortunately, severe obesity in children is becoming more prevalent. Many of these children have multiple risk factors for cardiovascular disease and a high risk of severe obesity in adulthood.[58] The special risks and treatment needs of severely obese children need to be recognized.

Obesity in children is especially troubling because overweight children may become obese adults with all the social, economic, and medical ramifications that often accompany obesity. They have additional problems, too, arising from differences in their growth, physical health, and psychological development. In trying to explain the rise in childhood obesity, researchers point to both genetic and environmental factors.

Genetic and Environmental Factors Parental obesity predicts an early increase in a young child's BMI, and it more than doubles the chances that a young child will become an obese adult.[59] Children with neither parent obese have a less than 10 percent chance of becoming obese in adulthood, whereas overweight teens with at least one obese parent have a greater than 80 percent chance of being obese adults. An obese child's risk of becoming an obese adult increases as the child grows older.[60] The link between parental and child obesity reflects both genetic and environmental factors (as described in Chapter 7).

Diet and physical inactivity are the two strongest environmental factors explaining why children are heavier today than they were 40 or so years ago. As the prevalence of childhood obesity throughout the United States has more than doubled for young children and more than tripled for children 6 to 11 years of age and adolescents, the society our children live in has changed considerably. In many families today, both parents work long hours outside the home; more emphasis is placed on convenience foods and foods eaten away from home; meal choices at school are more diverse and often less nutritious; sedentary activities such as watching television and playing computer games occupy much of children's free time; and opportunities for physical activity and outdoor play both during and after school have declined.[61] All of these factors—and many others—influence children's eating and activity patterns.

Children learn food behaviors from their families, and research confirms the significant roles parents play in teaching their children about healthy food choices, providing nutrient-dense foods, and serving as role models.[62] When parents eat fruit and vegetables frequently, their children do, too. The more fruit and vegetables children eat, the more vitamins, minerals, and fiber, and the less saturated fat, in their diets.

In children 2 to 18 years of age, about one third of total energy intake comes from solid fats and added sugars—in other words, empty kcalories.[63] About half of these empty kcalories are contributed by six specific foods: soda, fruit drinks, dairy desserts (ice cream, frozen yogurt, sorbet, sherbet, pudding, and custard), grain desserts (cakes, cookies, pies, cobblers, donuts, and granola bars), pizza, and whole milk. Not surprisingly, researchers have found that children's food choices today provide more kcalories than those of 40 years ago.

As Chapter 3 discussed, as the prevalence of obesity has surged over the past four decades, so has the consumption of added sugars, especially high-fructose corn syrup—the easily consumed, energy-dense liquid sugar added to soft drinks.[64] Each 12-ounce can of soft drink provides the equivalent of about 10 teaspoons of sugar and 150 kcalories. More than half of school-age children consume at least one soft drink each day at school; adolescent males consume the most—two or more cans daily. Research shows that consumption of sugar-sweetened beverages such as soft drinks is associated with increased energy intake and body weight.[65]

No doubt, the tremendous increase in soft drink consumption plays a role, but much of the obesity epidemic can be explained by lack of physical activity. Children have become more sedentary, and sedentary children are more often overweight.[66] Television watching may contribute most to physical inactivity. Children 8 to 18 years of age spend an average of 4.5 hours per day watching television. Longer television time is linked with overweight in children.[67] Television fosters overweight and obesity because it:

- Requires no energy beyond basal metabolism.
- Replaces vigorous activities.
- Encourages snacking.
- Promotes a sedentary lifestyle.

A child who spends more than an hour or two each day in front of a television, computer monitor, or other media can become overweight even while eating fewer kcalories than a more active child. Too much screen time and not enough activity time also contributes to a child's psychological distress.

Children who have television sets in their bedrooms spend more time watching TV, less time being physically active, less time sleeping, and are more likely to be overweight than children who do not have televisions in their rooms.[68] Children who watch a great deal of television are most likely to be overweight and least likely to eat family meals or fruit and vegetables.[69] They often snack on the nutrient-poor, energy-dense foods that are advertised.[70] Child-targeted food ads on television peddle foods high in sugar, saturated fat, and salt such as sugar-coated breakfast cereals, candy bars, chips, fast foods, and carbonated beverages.[71] More than half of all food advertisements are aimed specifically at children and market their products as fun and exciting. Not surprisingly, the more time children spend watching television, the more they request these advertised foods and beverages—and they get them about half of the time. The most popular foods and beverages are marketed to children and adolescents on the Internet as well, using "advergaming" (advertised product as part of a game), cartoon characters or "spokes-characters," and designated children's areas. Food marketing to children, including TV and Internet ads, as well as marketing in local communities by way of store giveaways, restaurant promotions, school activities, and sporting events, has a profound effect on children's nutrition and health.[72] Despite initiatives by the food industry to answer public health concerns about child-targeted advertising, much remains to be done to reduce the marketing of unhealthy foods to children.[73]

The physically inactive time spent watching television (and playing video and computer games) is second only to time spent sleeping. Compared to sedentary screen-time activities, playing active video games does expend a little more energy, but more research is needed to ascertain whether playing active video games increases habitual physical activity or decreases sedentary behaviors.[74] Simply reducing the amount of time spent watching television (and playing video games) can improve a child's BMI. The AAP recommends no television viewing before two years of age and thereafter limiting television and video time to two hours per day as a strategy to help prevent childhood obesity.[75]

Growth Overweight children develop a characteristic set of physical traits. They typically begin puberty earlier and so grow taller than their peers at first, but then they stop growing at a shorter height. They develop greater bone and muscle mass in response to the demand of having to carry more weight—both fat and lean weight. Consequently, they appear "stocky" even when they lose their excess fat.

Physical Health Like overweight adults, overweight children display a blood lipid profile indicating that atherosclerosis is beginning to develop—high levels of total cholesterol, triglycerides, and LDL cholesterol. Overweight children also tend to have high blood pressure; in fact, obesity is a leading cause of pediatric hypertension.[76] Their risks for developing type 2 diabetes and respiratory diseases (such as asthma) are also exceptionally high.[77] These relationships between childhood obesity and chronic diseases are discussed fully in Nutrition in Practice 11.

Psychological Development In addition to the physical consequences, childhood obesity brings a host of emotional and social problems.[78] Because people frequently judge others on appearance more than on character, overweight and obese children are often victims of prejudice and bullying. Many suffer discrimination by adults and rejection by their peers. They may have poor self-images, a sense of failure, and a passive approach to life. Television shows, which are a major influence in children's lives, often portray the fat person as the bumbling misfit. Overweight children may come to accept this negative stereotype in themselves and in others, which can lead to additional emotional and social problems. Researchers investigating children's reactions to various body types find that both normal-weight and underweight children respond unfavorably to overweight bodies.

Prevention and Treatment of Obesity Medical science has worked wonders in preventing or curing many of even the most serious childhood diseases, but obesity remains a challenge. Parents are encouraged to make major efforts to prevent childhood obesity, starting at birth, or to begin treatment early. Unopposed, obesity often advances through childhood into adulthood, steadily worsening with age. Importantly, not every overweight child grows to become an obese adult. Those who avoid adult obesity and its health risks often reduce their rates of gain early in childhood, before age 5 or so.[79] Their rate of gain begins to slow or hold steady as they grow. The same thing shows up again in many adolescents—the rate of gain slows, allowing them to grow into healthy weight adults. Therefore, parents of overweight children, particularly those with obese children, should not delay in taking action during early childhood and adolescence. These ages seem to offer critical windows of opportunity for changing a child's weight gain trajectory and helping them to launch into adulthood with a healthy BMI. Table 11-11 presents specific eating and physical activity behaviors to prevent obesity, for all children.

Treatment of obesity must consider the many aspects of the problem and possible solutions. The main goal of obesity treatment is to improve long-term physical health through permanent healthy lifestyle habits. The most successful approach integrates diet, physical activity, psychological support, and behavioral changes.[80] As a first step, overweight and obese children and their families are advised to adopt the same healthy eating and activity behaviors presented in Table 11-11 for obesity prevention. The goal for overweight and obese children is to improve BMI. If the child's BMI does not improve after several months, the intensity of the treatment is increased. The level of intensity depends on treatment response, age, degree of obesity, health risks, and the family's readiness to change.[81] Advanced treatment involves close follow-up monitoring by a health care provider and greater support and structure for the child.

Diet The initial goal for overweight children is to reduce the rate of weight gain, that is, to maintain weight as the child grows taller. Continued growth will then accomplish the desired change in BMI. Weight loss is usually not recommended because diet restriction can interfere with growth and development. Intervention for some overweight children with accompanying medical conditions may warrant weight loss, but this treatment requires an individualized approach based on the degree of overweight and severity of the medical conditions. Dietary strategies begin with those listed in Table 11-11 and progress to more structured family meal plans when necessary. For example, the child or the parent may be instructed to keep detailed logs of dietary intake.

Physical Activity The many benefits of physical activity are well known but often are not enough to motivate overweight people, especially children. Yet regular vigorous

---

TABLE 11-11 Recommended Eating and Physical Activity Behaviors to Prevent Obesity

The following healthy habits are recommended for children 2 to 18 years of age to help prevent childhood obesity:

- Limit or avoid consumption of sugar-sweetened beverages, such as soft drinks and fruit-flavored punches.
- Eat the recommended amounts of fruit and vegetables every day (2 to 4.5 cups per day based on age).
- Learn to eat age-appropriate portions of foods.
- Eat foods low in energy density such as those high in fiber and/or water and modest in fat.
- Eat a nutritious breakfast every day.
- Eat foods rich in calcium every day.
- Choose a dietary pattern balanced in recommended proportions for carbohydrate, fat, and protein.
- Eat foods high in fiber every day.
- Eat together as a family as often as possible.
- Limit the frequency of restaurant meals.
- Limit television watching or other screen time to no more than two hours per day, and do not have televisions or computers in sleeping areas.
- Engage in at least 60 minutes of moderate to vigorous physical activity every day.

activity can improve a child's weight, body composition, and physical fitness.[82] Ideally, parents will limit sedentary activities and encourage at least one hour of daily physical activity to promote strong skeletal, muscular, and cardiovascular development and instill in their children the desire to be physically active throughout life. Opportunities to be physically active can include team, individual, and recreational activities (see Table 11-12). Most importantly, parents need to set a good example. Physical activity is a natural and lifelong behavior of healthy living. It can be as simple as riding a bike, playing tag, jumping rope, or doing chores. The AAP supports the efforts of schools to include more physical activity in the curriculum and encourages parents to support their children's participation.

Behavioral Changes In contrast to traditional weight-loss programs that focus on *what* to eat, behavioral programs focus on *how* to eat. These techniques involve changing learned habits that lead a child to eat excessively. Weight-loss programs that involve parents and other caregivers in treatment report greater success than those without parental involvement. Because obesity in parents and their children tends to be positively correlated, both benefit when parents participate in a weight-loss program. Parental attitudes about food greatly influence children's eating behavior, so it is important that the influence be positive. Otherwise, eating problems may become exacerbated.

TABLE 11-12 Examples of Aerobic, Muscle-Strengthening, and Bone-Strengthening Physical Activities for Children and Adolescents

MODERATE-TO-VIGOROUS AEROBIC ACTIVITIES	MUSCLE-STRENGTHENING ACTIVITIES	BONE-STRENGTHENING ACTIVITIES
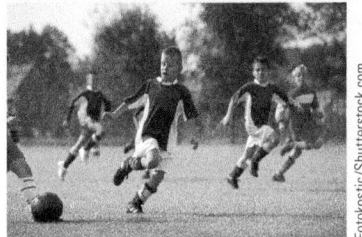	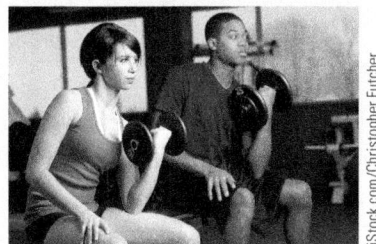	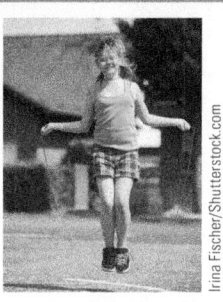
MODERATE • Active recreation such as hiking, skateboarding, rollerblading • Bicycle riding[a] • Brisk walking **VIGOROUS** • Active games involving running and chasing, such as tag • Bicycle riding[a] • Cross-country skiing • Jumping rope • Martial arts • Running • Sports such as soccer, ice or field hockey, basketball, swimming, tennis	• Games such as tug of war • Modified push-ups (with knees on the floor) • Resistance exercises using body weight, free weights, or resistance bands • Rope or tree climbing • Sit-ups (curl-ups or crunches) • Swinging on playground equipment/bars	• Games such as hopscotch • Hopping, skipping, jumping • Jumping rope • Running • Sports such as gymnastics, basketball, volleyball, tennis

[a]Some activities, such as bicycling, can be moderate or vigorous, depending on level of effort.

TABLE 11-13	Selection Criteria for Obesity Surgery in Adolescents

- Physically mature
- BMI ≥40, or BMI >35 with significant weight-related health problems
- History of failure in a formal, six-month weight-loss program
- Capable of adhering to the long-term lifestyle changes required after surgery

Drugs The use of weight-loss drugs to treat obesity in children merits special concern because the long-term effects of these drugs on growth and development have not been studied. The drugs may be used in addition to structured lifestyle changes for carefully selected children or adolescents who are at high risk for severe obesity in adulthood. Orlistat (see Chapter 7) is the only prescription weight-loss medication that has been approved for use in adolescents 12 years of age and older. Alli, the over-the-counter version of orlistat, should not be given to anyone younger than age 18.

Surgery The efficacy of surgery as a treatment for severe obesity in adults (see Chapter 7) has created interest in its use for adolescents. Limited research shows that, after surgery, extremely obese adolescents lose significant weight and experience improvements in type 2 diabetes and cardiovascular risk factors.[83] The selection criteria for surgery to treat obesity in adolescents listed in Table 11-13 are based on recommendations of a panel of pediatricians and surgeons.

Obesity is prevalent in our society. Because treatment of obesity is frequently unsuccessful, it is most important to prevent its onset. Above all, be sensible in teaching children how to maintain appropriate body weight. Children can easily get the impression that their worth is tied to their body weight. Parents and the media are most influential in shaping self-concept, weight concerns, and dieting practices.[84] Some parents fail to realize that society's ideal of slimness can be perilously close to starvation and that a child encouraged to "diet" cannot obtain the energy and nutrients required for normal growth and development. Even healthy children without diagnosable eating disorders have been observed to limit their growth through "dieting." Weight loss in truly overweight children can be managed without compromising growth, but it should be overseen by a health care professional.

Review Notes

- Childhood obesity has become a major health problem.
- Genetics, energy-dense diets, and physical inactivity play roles in childhood obesity.
- Childhood obesity can impair physical and psychological health.
- The main goal of obesity treatment in children is to improve long-term physical health through permanent healthy lifestyle habits.

Mealtimes at Home

The childhood years are the parents' last chance to influence their children's food choices. Parents who want to promote nutritious choices and healthful habits provide access to nutrient-dense, delicious foods and opportunities for active play at home.

In today's consumer-oriented society, children have greater influence over family decisions concerning food—the fast-food restaurant the family chooses when eating out, the snacks the family eats at home, and the specific brands the family purchases at the grocery store. Parental guidance in food choices is still necessary, but teaching children consumer skills to help them make informed choices is equally important.

Feeding children requires not only providing a variety of nutritious foods but also nurturing the children's self-esteem and well-being. Parents face a number of challenges in preparing meals that both appeal to their children's tastes and provide needed nutrients. Because the interactions between parents and children can set the stage for lifelong attitudes and habits, a child's preferences should be treated with respect, even when nutrient needs must take precedence (Box 11-6).

BOX 11-6 *Nursing Diagnosis*

The nursing diagnosis *readiness for enhanced parenting* applies to clients who have children whose needs (physical and emotional) are met.

Honoring Children's Preferences Researchers attempting to explain children's food preferences encounter many contradictions. Children say they like colorful foods yet most often reject green and yellow vegetables while favoring brown peanut butter and white potatoes, apple wedges, and bread. They do like raw vegetables better than cooked ones, though, so it is wise to offer vegetables that are raw or slightly undercooked, crunchy, and bright in color. They should be warm, not hot, because a child's mouth is much more sensitive than an adult's. The flavor should be mild (a child has more taste buds), and smooth foods such as mashed potatoes or pea soup should have no lumps (a child wonders, with some disgust, what the lumps might be).

Make mealtimes fun for children. Young children like to eat at little tables and to be served little portions of food. They also love to eat with other children and have been observed to stay at the table longer and eat more food when in the company of their friends (see Photo 11-6). Children are also more likely to give up their prejudices against foods when they see their peers eating them. Parents who serve food in a relaxed and casual manner, without anxiety, provide an environment in which a child's negative emotions will be minimized.

Photo 11-6

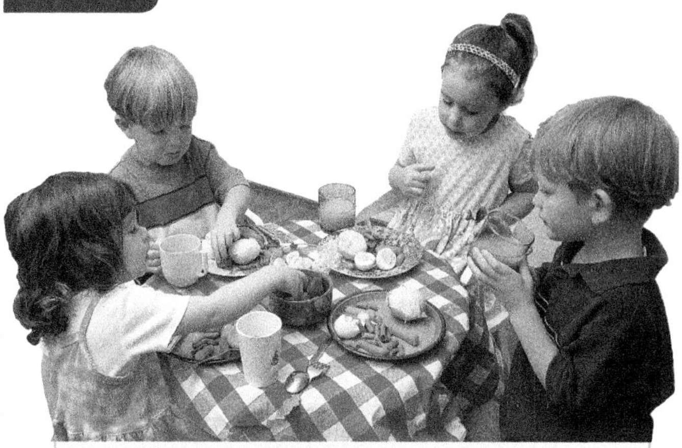

Eating is more fun when friends are there.

Avoiding Power Struggles Problems over food often arise during the second or third year, when children begin asserting their independence. Many of these problems stem from the conflict between children's developmental stages and capabilities and parents who, in attempting to do what they think is best for their children, try to control every aspect of eating. Such conflicts can disrupt children's abilities to regulate their own food intakes or to determine their own likes and dislikes.[85] For example, many people share the misconception that children must be persuaded or coerced to try new foods. In fact, the opposite is true. When children are forced to try new foods, especially when offered rewards for eating a particular food, they are less likely to try those foods again than are children who are left to decide for themselves. Similarly, when children are restricted from eating their favorite foods, they are more likely to want those foods. Wise parents provide nutritious foods and allow their child to determine *how much* and even *whether* to eat.

When introducing new foods at the table, parents are advised to offer them one at a time and only in small amounts at first. The more often a food is presented to a young child, the more likely the child will accept that food.[86] Between 5 and 10 exposures to a new food are necessary before a toddler shows an enhanced preference for the food. Offer the new food at the beginning of the meal, when the child is hungry, and allow the child to make the decision to accept or reject it. Parents have their own inclinations and dislikes; so do children. Never make an issue of food acceptance. Table 11-14 on p. 332 offers tips for feeding picky eaters.

Choking Prevention Parents must always be alert to the dangers of choking. A choking child is silent, so an adult should be present whenever a child is eating. Make sure the child sits when eating; choking is more likely when a child is running or falling. (See Table 11-5 on p. 314 for a list of foods and nonfood items most likely to cause choking.)

Play First Ideally, each meal is preceded, not followed, by the activity the child looks forward to the most. A number of schools have discovered that children eat a much better lunch if it is served after, rather than before, recess. Otherwise, children "hurry up and eat" so that they can go play.

Child Participation Allowing children to help plan and prepare the family's meals provides enjoyable learning experiences and encourages children to eat the foods they have prepared. Vegetables are pretty, especially when fresh, and provide opportunities

TABLE 11-14 **Tips for Feeding Picky Eaters**

GET THEM INVOLVED

Children are more likely to feel a sense of ownership and may be more interested in trying foods when they participate in meal planning, grocery shopping, cooking, gardening, and harvesting the foods they eat.

BE CREATIVE

- Try serving veggies as finger foods with dips or spreads.
- Use cookie cutters to cut fruit and veggies into fun shapes.
- Put healthy snacks in ice cube trays or muffin pans where children can easily reach them and graze on them as they play.
- Serve traditional meals out of order (for example, breakfast for dinner).
- Use healthy foods such as veggies and whole grains in craft projects to help kids become familiar with them and encourage their interest and enthusiasm for these foods.

ENHANCE FAVORITE RECIPES

- Include sliced or shredded veggies in sauces, casseroles, pancakes, and muffins.
- Serve fruit over cereal, yogurt, or ice cream.
- Bake brownies with black beans or cookies with lentils as an ingredient.

MODEL AND SHARE

- Be a role model to children by eating healthy foods with them. Offer to share your healthy snack with them, too.
- Sometimes children need to be exposed to a new food multiple times before they develop a taste for the food, so make sure healthy options are always available and don't give up on repeatedly offering foods your child might not seem interested in.
- Encourage your child to taste at least one bite of each food served at a meal.

RESPECT AND RELAX

- Remember that it is not uncommon for children to eat sporadically. They have smaller stomachs and therefore are likely to feel full faster and become hungry again not long after a snack or meal.
- Focus on your child's overall weekly intake of food and nutrients rather than daily consumption.
- If you suspect that your child might not be eating enough to support healthy growth and development, discuss your concerns with your child's doctor. It might be helpful to maintain a food log of everything your child eats over a period of three days to bring along to the doctor appointment.

Source: Based on Mayo Clinic Staff, Children's nutrition: 10 tips for picky eaters, 2011, available at www.mayoclinic.com/health/childrens-health/HQ01107.

for children to learn about color, growing things and their seeds, and shapes and textures—all of which are fascinating to young children. Measuring, stirring, decorating, and arranging foods are skills that even a very young child can practice with enjoyment and pride (see Table 11-15).

Snacks Parents may find that their children often snack so much that they aren't hungry at mealtimes. Instead of teaching children *not* to snack, teach them *how* to snack. Provide snacks that are as nutritious as the foods served at mealtime. Snacks can even be mealtime foods that are served individually over time, instead of all at once on one plate. When providing snacks to children, think of the food groups and offer such snacks as pieces of cheese, sliced strawberries, cooked baby carrots, and egg salad on whole-wheat crackers (see Table 11-16). Replacing nutrient-poor, high-kcalorie snacks such as potato chips with nutrient-rich, low-kcalorie snacks such as vegetables not only reduces children's energy intakes but improves their nutrient intakes as well. Snacks that are easy to prepare should be readily available to children, especially if the children arrive home after school before their parents.

Preventing Dental Caries Children frequently snack on sticky, sugary foods that stay on the teeth and provide an ideal environment for the growth of bacteria that cause dental caries. Teach children to brush and floss after meals, to brush or rinse after eating snacks, to avoid sticky foods, and to select crisp or fibrous foods frequently.

TABLE 11-15 Food Skills and Developmental Milestones of Preschool Children[a]

AGE (YEARS)	FOOD SKILLS	DEVELOPMENTAL MILESTONES
1 to 2	• Uses a spoon • Lifts and drinks from a cup • Helps scrub fruit and vegetables, tear lettuce or greens, snap green beans, or dip foods • Can be messy; can be easily distracted	• Large muscles develop • Experiences slowed growth and decreased appetite • Develops likes and dislikes • May suddenly refuse certain foods
3	• Spears food with a fork • Feeds self independently • Helps wrap, pour, mix, shake, stir, or spread foods • Follows simple instructions	• Medium hand muscles develop • May suddenly refuse certain foods • Begins to request favorite foods • Makes simple either/or food choices
4	• Uses all utensils and napkin • Helps measure dry ingredients • Learns table manners	• Small finger muscles develop • Influenced by TV, media, and peers • May dislike many mixed dishes
5	• Measures liquids • Helps grind, grate, and cut (soft foods with dull knife) • Uses hand mixer with supervision	• Fine coordination of fingers and hands develops • Usually accepts food that is available • Eats with minor supervision

[a]These ages are approximate. Healthy, normal children develop at their own pace.

Source: Adapted from MyPlate for Preschoolers, Behavioral Milestones, available at www.choosemyplate.gov/preschoolers/healthy-habits/Milestones.pdf.

TABLE 11-16 Healthful Snack Ideas—Think Food Groups, Alone and in Combination

Selecting two or more foods from different food groups adds variety and nutrient balance to snacks. The combinations are endless, so be creative.

Grains: Grain products are filling snacks, especially when combined with other foods:
• Cereal with fruit and milk
• Crackers and cheese
• Whole-grain toast with melted cheese
• Oatmeal raisin cookies with milk

Vegetables: Lightly steamed, cut-up fresh vegetables make great snacks alone or in combination with foods from other food groups:
• Lightly steamed broccoli, cauliflower, and carrot sticks with a flavored cottage cheese dip or hummus

Fruit: Fruit is a delicious snack and can be eaten alone—fresh, dried, or juiced—or combined with other foods:
• Peeled apple slices and cheese
• Bananas and peanut butter
• Peaches with yogurt
• Raisins and crunchy cereal mix

Protein Foods: Meat, poultry, seafood, legumes, soy products, nuts, and seeds add protein to snacks:
• Refried beans and cheese on a flour tortilla
• Peanut butter, hummus, or tuna on crackers
• Luncheon meat or tuna salad on whole-grain bread

Milk and Milk Products: Milk can be used as a beverage with any snack, and many other milk products, such as yogurt and cheese, can be eaten alone or with other foods as listed above.

Serving as Role Models In an effort to practice these many tips, parents may overlook perhaps the single most important influence on their children's food habits—themselves. Parents who do not eat oranges should not be surprised when their children refuse to eat oranges. Likewise, parents who dislike the smell of brussels sprouts may not be able to persuade children to try them. Children learn much through imitation. Parents, older siblings, and other caregivers set an irresistible example by sitting with younger children, eating the same foods, and having pleasant conversations during mealtime.

While serving and enjoying food, caregivers can promote both physical and emotional health at every stage of a child's life. They can help their children to develop both a positive self-concept and a positive attitude toward food. If the beginnings are right, children will grow without the conflicts and confusions over foods that lead to nutrition and health problems.

Nutrition at School

While parents are doing what they can to establish good eating habits in their children at home, others are preparing and serving foods to their children at daycare centers and schools. In addition, children begin learning about food and nutrition in the classroom. Meeting the nutrition and education needs of children is critical to supporting their healthy growth and development.

The U.S. government funds programs to provide nutritious, high-quality meals for children at school. Both the School Breakfast Program and the National School Lunch Program provide meals at a reasonable cost to children from families with the financial means to pay. Meals are available free or at reduced cost to children from low-income families.

The National School Lunch and Breakfast Programs

More than 30 million children receive lunches through the National School Lunch Program—more than half of them free or at a reduced price. School lunches are designed to provide at least a third of the recommendation for energy, protein, vitamin A, vitamin C, iron, and calcium. They must also include specified numbers of servings from each food group. In an effort to help reduce disease risk, all government-funded meals served at schools must follow the Dietary Guidelines for Americans. Table 11-17 shows school lunch patterns for children of different ages.

Current school meal patterns and nutrition standards ensure the greater availability of fruit, vegetables, whole grains, and fat-free and low-fat milk, and decreased levels of sodium, saturated fat, and *trans* fat in meals served to school children. Guidelines also specify that nutrient needs must be met within specified kcalorie ranges based on age/grade groups for children.

Parents often rely on school lunches to meet a significant part of their children's nutrient needs on school days. Indeed, students who regularly eat school lunches have higher intakes of many nutrients and fiber than students who do not. Interestingly, research shows

TABLE 11-17 School Lunch Patterns

| FOOD GROUP | GRADES | | |
	K–5	6–8	9–12
	Amount per week (minimum per day)		
Fruit[a] (cups)	2½ (½)	2½ (½)	5 (1)
Vegetables[a] (cups)	3¾ (¾)	3¾ (¾)	5 (1)
Dark green	≥½	≥½	≥½
Red and orange	≥¾	≥¾	≥1¾
Legumes	≥½	≥½	≥½
Starchy	≥½	≥½	≥½
Other	≥½	≥½	≥¾
Any additional vegetables to meet total requirement	1	1	1½
Grains (oz equivalents)	8–9 (1)	8–10 (1)	10–12 (2)
Protein foods (oz equivalents)	8–10 (1)	9–10 (1)	10–12 (2)
Fluid milk[b] (cups)	5 (1)	5 (1)	5 (1)
OTHER			
kCalories	550–650	600–700	750–850
Saturated fat (% of total kcalories)	<10	<10	<10
Sodium (mg)	≤640	≤710	≤740
Trans fat (g per serving)	0	0	0

[a]No more than half of the fruit or vegetable servings may be in the form of juice. All juice must be 100 percent full strength.

[b]Fluid milk must be low-fat (unflavored) or fat-free (flavored or unflavored).

Source: U.S. Department of Agriculture, Nutrition Standards in the National School Lunch and School Breakfast Programs, January 25, 2012.

many more students will self-serve fruit and vegetables from a salad bar located inside the serving line compared with one located outside the line.[87]

The School Breakfast Program is available in most of the nation's schools that offer school lunch, and more than 14 million children participate in it. Nevertheless, many children who need the School Breakfast Program either do not have access to the program or do not participate in it.

Competing Influences at School Serving nutritious lunches is only half the battle; students need to eat them, too. Short lunch periods and long lines prevent some students from eating a school lunch and leave others with too little time to complete their meals.[88] Nutrition efforts at schools are also undermined when students can buy what the USDA labels "competitive foods"—meals from fast-food restaurants or à la carte foods such as pizza or snack foods and carbonated beverages from snack bars, school stores, and vending machines. These foods and beverages compete with nutritious school lunches. When students have access to competitive foods, participation in the school lunch program decreases, nutrient intake from lunch declines, and more food is discarded.[89]

Nation-wide, USDA's Smart Snacks in School regulations now require that competitive foods and beverages, including those sold in vending machines, offer students healthier options with more fruit, vegetables, dairy products, and whole grains.[90] The foods and beverages must also meet standards for kcalories, sodium, fat, saturated fat, *trans* fat, and added sugars (see Table 11-18).

| **TABLE 11-18** | USDA Nutrition Standards for Foods Sold in Schools |

Any food sold in schools must:
- be a "whole grain–rich" grain product; or
- have a fruit, vegetable, dairy product, or protein food as the first ingredient; or
- be a combination food that contains at least ¼ cup of fruit, vegetable, or both
- Limit kcalories, sodium, fat, *trans* fat, and sugar

All schools may sell the following beverages:
- Plain or carbonated water
- Unflavored low-fat milk
- Unflavored or flavored fat-free milk/milk alternatives
- 100% fruit or vegetable juice with no added sugars

Source: U.S. Department of Agriculture, Food and Nutrition Service, School meals, Tools for schools: Focusing on smart snacks, November 28, 2017, www.fns.usda.gov/school-meals/tools-school-focusing-smart-snacks.

Review Notes

- Adults at home and at school need to provide children with nutrient-dense foods and teach them how to make healthful choices. Adults also need to provide ample opportunity for children to be physically active.

- School meals are designed to provide at least a third of certain nutrients that children need daily while emphasizing increased availability of fruit, vegetables, whole grains, and low-fat and fat-free fluid milk. Standards for reduced sodium, and reduced levels of saturated and *trans* fats must also be met.

11.3 Nutrition during Adolescence

As children pass through **adolescence** on their way to becoming adults, they change in many ways. Their physical changes make their nutrient needs high, and their emotional, intellectual, and social changes make meeting those needs a challenge.

Teenagers make many more choices for themselves than they did as children. They are not fed; they eat. Food choices made during the teen years profoundly affect present and future health. At the same time, social pressures thrust choices at them: whether to drink alcoholic beverages and whether to develop their bodies to meet extreme ideals of slimness or athletic prowess. Their interest in nutrition—both valid information and misinformation—derives from personal, immediate experiences. They are concerned with how diet can improve their lives now—they try the latest fad diet to fit into a new bathing suit, avoid greasy foods in an effort to clear acne, or eat a plate of pasta to prepare for a big sporting event. In presenting information on the nutrition and health of adolescents, this chapter includes topics of interest to teens.

adolescence: the period of growth from the beginning of puberty until full maturity. Timing of adolescence varies from person to person.

Growth and Development during Adolescence

With the onset of adolescence, the steady growth of childhood speeds up abruptly and dramatically, and the growth patterns of females and males become distinct. Hormones direct the intensity and duration of the adolescent growth spurt, profoundly affecting every organ of the body, including the brain. After two to three years of intense growth and a few more at a slower pace, physically mature adults emerge.

In general, the adolescent growth spurt begins at age 10 or 11 for females and at age 12 or 13 for males. It lasts about 2.5 years. Before **puberty**, male and female body compositions differ only slightly, but during the adolescent spurt, differences between the genders become apparent in the skeletal system, lean body mass, and fat stores. In females, fat assumes a larger percentage of total body weight, and in males, the lean body mass—principally muscle and bone—increases much more than in females. On average, males grow 8 inches taller, and females, 6 inches taller. Males gain approximately 45 pounds, and females, about 35 pounds.

Energy and Nutrient Needs

The energy needs of adolescents vary greatly, depending on the current rate of growth, gender, body composition, and physical activity. Boys' energy needs may be especially high; they typically grow faster than girls and, as mentioned, develop a greater proportion of lean body mass. An exceptionally active boy of 15 may need 3500 kcalories or more a day just to maintain his weight. Girls start growing earlier than boys and attain shorter heights and lower weights, so their energy needs peak sooner and decline earlier than those of their male peers. An inactive girl of 15 whose growth is nearly at a standstill may need fewer than 1800 kcalories a day if she is to avoid excessive weight gain. Thus, teenage girls need to pay special attention to being physically active and selecting foods of high nutrient density so that they will meet their nutrient needs without exceeding their energy needs.

Obesity The insidious problem of obesity becomes ever more apparent in adolescence and often continues into adulthood. Without intervention, overweight teens will face numerous physical and socioeconomic consequences for years to come. The consequences of obesity are so dramatic and our society's attitude toward obese people is so negative that even healthy-weight or underweight teens may perceive a need to lose weight. When taken to extremes, restrictive diets bring dramatic physical consequences of their own, as Nutrition in Practice 6 explains.

Vitamin D Recommendations for most vitamins increase during the teen years (see the tables on the inside front cover). Several of the vitamin recommendations for adolescents are similar to those for adults, including recommendations for vitamin D. Vitamin D is essential for bone growth and development. Recent studies of vitamin D status in adolescents show that many are vitamin D deficient; blacks, females, and overweight adolescents are most at risk.[91] Adolescents who do not receive enough vitamin D from fortified foods such as milk and cereals, or from sun exposure each day, may need a supplement.

Iron The need for iron increases during adolescence for both females and males but for different reasons. Iron needs increase for females as they start to menstruate and for males as their lean body mass develops. Hence, the RDA increases at age 14 for both males and females. Because menstruation continues throughout a woman's childbearing years, the RDA for iron remains high for women into late adulthood. For males, the RDA returns to preadolescent values in early adulthood.

In addition, iron needs increase when the adolescent growth spurt begins, whether that occurs before or after age 14. Therefore, boys in a growth spurt need an additional 2.9 milligrams of iron per day above the RDA for their age; girls need an additional 1.1 milligrams per day. Furthermore, iron recommendations for girls before age 14

puberty: the period in life in which a person becomes physically capable of reproduction.

do not reflect the iron losses of menstruation, even though the average age of menarche (first menstruation) in the United States is 12.5 years. Therefore, for girls younger than age 14 who have started to menstruate, an additional 2.5 milligrams of iron per day is recommended. Thus, the RDA for iron depends not only on age and gender but also on whether the individual is in a growth spurt or has begun to menstruate, as listed in Table 11-19.

Iron intakes often fail to keep pace with increasing needs, especially for females, who typically consume fewer iron-rich foods such as meat and fewer total kcalories than males. Not surprisingly, iron deficiency is most prevalent among adolescent girls. Iron-deficient children and teens score lower on standardized tests than those who are not iron deficient.

Calcium Adolescence is a crucial time for bone development, and the requirement for calcium reaches its peak during these years.[92] Unfortunately, many adolescents, especially females, have calcium intakes below recommendations.[93] Low calcium intakes during times of active growth, especially if paired with physical inactivity, can compromise the development of peak bone mass, which is considered the best protection against adolescent fractures and adult osteoporosis. Increasing milk products in the diet to meet calcium recommendations greatly increases bone density.[94] Once again, however, teenage girls are most vulnerable, for their milk—and therefore their calcium—intakes begin to decline at the time when their calcium needs are greatest. Furthermore, women have much greater bone losses than men in later life. In addition to dietary calcium, physical activity makes bones grow stronger. However, because some high schools do not require students to attend physical activity classes, many adolescents must make a point to be physically active during leisure time.

Food Choices and Health Habits

Teenagers like the freedom to come and go as they choose. They eat what they want if it is convenient and if they have the time. With a multitude of afterschool, social, and job activities, they almost inevitably fall into irregular eating habits. At any given time on any given day, a teenager may be skipping a meal, eating a snack, preparing a meal, or consuming food prepared by a parent or restaurant. Adolescents who frequently help prepare and eat meals with their families, however, eat more fruit, vegetables, grains, and calcium-rich foods and drink fewer soft drinks than those who seldom eat with their families.[95] Many adolescents begin to skip breakfast on a regular basis, missing out on important nutrients that are not made up at later meals during the day. Compared with those who skip breakfast, teenagers who do eat breakfast have higher intakes of vitamins A, D, and folate, as well as calcium, iron, and zinc.[96] Teenagers who eat breakfast are therefore more likely to meet their nutrient recommendations.

Breakfast skipping may also lead to weight gain in adolescents. Eating breakfast each day, especially a breakfast rich in fiber and protein, improves satiety and reduces hunger and the desire to eat throughout the day. As adolescents make the transition to adulthood, not only do they skip breakfast more often, but they also eat fast food more often. Both skipping breakfast and eating fast foods lead to weight gain.[97]

Ideally, in light of adolescents' busy schedules and desire for freedom, the adult becomes a **gatekeeper**, controlling the type and availability of food in the teenager's environment. Teenage sons and daughters and their friends should find plenty of nutritious, easy-to-grab food in the refrigerator (meats for sandwiches; low-fat cheeses; fresh, raw vegetables and fruit; fruit juices; and milk) and more in the cabinets (whole-grain breads, peanut butter, nuts, popcorn, and cereal). In many

TABLE 11-19 Iron Recommendations for Adolescents

Iron RDA for males:
- 9–13 yr: 8 mg/day
- 9–13 yr in growth spurt: 10.9 mg/day
- 14–18 yr: 11 mg/day
- 14–18 yr in growth spurt: 13.9 mg/day

Iron RDA for females:
- 9–13 yr: 8 mg/day
- 9–13 yr in menarche: 10.5 mg/day
- 9–13 yr in menarche and growth spurt: 11.6 mg/day
- 14–18 yr: 15 mg/day
- 14–18 yr in growth spurt: 16.1 mg/day

gatekeeper: with respect to nutrition, a key person who controls other people's access to foods and thereby exerts a profound impact on their nutrition. Examples are the spouse who buys and cooks the food, the parent who feeds the children, and the caregiver in a daycare center.

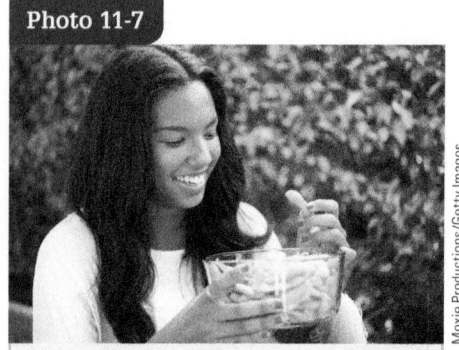
Photo 11-7

Nutritious snacks contribute valuable nutrients to an active teen's diet.

Moxie Productions/Getty Images

households today, all the adults work outside the home, and teenagers perform some of the gatekeeper's roles, such as shopping for groceries or choosing fast or prepared foods.

Snacks On average, about a fourth of an adolescent's total daily energy intake comes from snacks, which, if chosen carefully, can contribute some of the needed nutrients (see Table 11-16 on p. 333 and Photo 11-7). Energy-dense, nutrient-poor snack foods are readily available in settings where teens spend their time, however, and frequent snacking on these foods can contribute to higher total energy intakes as well as higher energy intakes from added sugars.[98]

Beverages Most frequently, adolescents drink soft drinks instead of fruit juice or milk with lunch, supper, and snacks. About the only time they select fruit juices is at breakfast. When teens drink milk, they are more likely to consume it with a meal (especially breakfast) than as a snack. Because of their greater food intakes, boys are more likely than girls to drink enough milk to meet their calcium needs.[99]

Soft drinks, when chosen as the primary beverage, may affect bone density, partly because they displace milk from the diet. Over the past three decades, teens (especially girls) have been drinking more soft drinks and less milk. Adolescents who drink soft drinks regularly have a higher energy intake and a lower calcium intake than those who do not.[100]

Soft drinks and energy drinks containing caffeine present a different problem if caffeine intake becomes excessive. Many adolescents consume energy drinks on a regular basis and these beverages contain much more caffeine than soft drinks.* Caffeine seems to be relatively harmless, however, when used in moderate doses (less than 100 milligrams per day, roughly equivalent to fewer than three 12-ounce cola beverages a day). In greater amounts, it can cause the symptoms associated with anxiety—sweating, tenseness, and inability to concentrate.

Eating Away from Home Adolescents eat about one-third of their meals away from home, and their nutritional welfare is enhanced or hindered by the choices they make.[101] A lunch consisting of a hamburger, a chocolate shake, and french fries supplies substantial quantities of many nutrients at a kcalorie cost of about 800, an energy intake some adolescents can afford. When they eat this sort of lunch, teens can adjust their breakfast and dinner choices to include fruit and vegetables for vitamin A, vitamin C, folate, and fiber, and lean meats and legumes for iron and zinc. Fortunately, many fast-food restaurants are offering more nutritious choices than the standard hamburger meal.

Peer Influence Physical maturity and growing independence present adolescents with new choices whose consequences influence their health and nutrition status both today and throughout life. Many of the food and health choices adolescents make reflect the opinions and actions of their peers. When others perceive milk as "babyish," a teen may choose soft drinks instead; when others skip lunch and hang out in the parking lot, a teen may join in for the camaraderie, regardless of hunger. Some teenagers begin using drugs, alcohol, and tobacco; others wisely refrain. Adults can set up the environment so that nutritious foods are available and can stand by with reliable information and advice about health and nutrition, but the rest is up to the adolescents. Ultimately, they make the choices.

---

*Caffeine-containing soft drinks typically deliver about 30 milligrams of caffeine per 12-ounce can; energy drinks typically deliver about 100 milligrams of caffeine for equivalent amounts. A pharmacologically active dose of caffeine is defined as 200 milligrams.

- Nutrient needs rise dramatically as children enter the rapid growth phase of the teen years.
- The busy lifestyles of teenagers add to the challenge of meeting their nutrient needs, especially for iron and calcium.

Assessment of nutrition status in healthy infants, children, and adolescents can confirm that development is normal or can catch potential problems early. (Chapter 13 offers details about nutrition assessment.) The Nutrition Assessment Checklist highlights problems to look for when working with infants, children, and adolescents.

Nutrition Assessment Checklist for Infants, Children, and Adolescents

MEDICAL HISTORY

Check the medical record for:

- ○ Alcohol, tobacco, or illicit drug abuse
- ○ Attention deficit/hyperactivity disorder (ADHD)
- ○ Diabetes or other chronic disorders
- ○ Eating disorders
- ○ Food allergies
- ○ Lactose intolerance
- ○ Obesity
- ○ Pregnancy

MEDICATIONS

For children or adolescents being treated with drug therapy for medical conditions, note:

- ○ Side effects that might reduce food intake or change nutrient needs
- ○ Proper administration of medication with respect to food intake

DIETARY INTAKE

For infants, note:

- ○ Method of feeding (breastfeeding, formula, or both)
- ○ Frequency and duration of breastfeeding
- ○ Amount of infant formula
- ○ Practice of putting infant to bed with bottle
- ○ Solid foods the infant is fed, if any
- ○ Amount of food the infant is fed

For all children and adolescents, especially those considered at risk nutritionally, assess the diet for:

- ○ Total energy
- ○ Protein
- ○ Calcium and iron
- ○ Vitamin A, vitamin C, vitamin D, and folate
- ○ Fiber

Note the following:

- ○ Number of days each week a nutritious breakfast is eaten
- ○ Number of hours the child or teen sleeps each day

- ○ Number of soft drinks the child or teen drinks each day
- ○ Number of fast-food meals eaten each day
- ○ Number and type of snacks eaten each day
- ○ Type and amount of physical activity
- ○ Amount of caffeine consumed

ANTHROPOMETRIC DATA

Measure baseline height and weight.

- ○ Note infant birth weight.
- ○ Reassess height, weight, and growth patterns at each medical checkup.
- ○ Note weight, length, and head circumference of infants.
- ○ Note significant obesity or underweight and any intervention strategies employed.

LABORATORY TESTS

Monitor the following laboratory tests for infants:

- ○ Blood glucose of infants born to mothers with gestational diabetes
- ○ Results of tests for inborn errors of metabolism (see Nutrition in Practice 15)

Monitor the following laboratory tests for children and adolescents:

- ○ Hemoglobin, hematocrit, or other tests of iron status
- ○ Blood glucose for children or adolescents with diabetes
- ○ Blood lead concentrations

PHYSICAL SIGNS

Look for physical signs of:

- ○ Protein-energy malnutrition
- ○ Iron deficiency
- ○ Vitamin A deficiency
- ○ Vitamin C deficiency
- ○ Folate deficiency

1. Which of the following is a characteristic of iron deficiency in children?
   a. It rarely develops in those with high intakes of milk.
   b. It affects brain function before anemia sets in.
   c. It is a primary factor in hyperactivity.
   d. It is difficult to detect using standard blood tests.

2. Three symptoms of lead toxicity are:
   a. diarrhea, irritability, and fatigue.
   b. low blood sugar, hair loss, and skin rash.
   c. increased heart rate, hyperactivity, and dry skin.
   d. bleeding gums, brittle fingernails, and swollen glands.

3. Allergic reactions to foods are most often caused by:
   a. corn, rice, or meats.
   b. eggs, peanuts, or milk.
   c. sulfur, milk, or MSG.
   d. wheat, dark greens, or lactose.

4. When introducing new foods to children:
   a. reward children as they try new foods.
   b. offer many choices to encourage variety.
   c. offer one new food at the end of the meal.
   d. offer one new food at the beginning of the meal.

5. Which of the following is *not* true? Children who watch a lot of television are likely to:
   a. become obese.
   b. spend less time being physically active.
   c. learn healthy eating tips from programs.
   d. eat the foods most often advertised on television.

6. Which of the following strategies is *not* effective?
   a. Play first, eat later.
   b. Provide small portions.
   c. Encourage children to help prepare meals.
   d. Use dessert as a reward for eating vegetables.

7. During the growth spurt of adolescence:
   a. females gain more weight than males.
   b. males gain more fat, proportionately, than females.
   c. differences in body composition between males and females become apparent.
   d. similarities in body composition between males and females become apparent.

8. Two nutrients that are usually lacking in adolescents' diets are:
   a. zinc and fat.
   b. iron and calcium.
   c. protein and thiamin.
   d. vitamin A and riboflavin.

9. To help teenagers consume a balanced diet, parents can:
   a. monitor the teens' food intake.
   b. give up—parents can't influence teenagers.
   c. keep the cabinets and refrigerator well stocked.
   d. forbid snacking and insist on regular, well-balanced meals.

10. To balance the day's intake, an adolescent who eats a hamburger, fries, and chocolate shake at lunch might benefit most from a dinner of:
    a. fried chicken, rice, and banana.
    b. ribeye steak, baked potato, and salad.
    c. pork chop, mashed potatoes, and apple juice.
    d. spaghetti with tomato-vegetable sauce, broccoli, and milk.

Answers: 1. b, 2. a, 3. b, 4. d, 5. c, 6. d, 7. c, 8. b, 9. c, 10. a

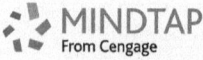 **MINDTAP** From Cengage

For more chapter resources visit **www.cengage.com** to access MindTap, a complete digital course.

Clinical Applications

1. At two and a half years old, Travis is healthy, though slightly underweight, and headstrong. Travis's mother hovers over him at every meal and insists that he take several bites of every food on his plate, even if he dislikes the food or is not familiar with it. Even though Travis is hungry when he sits down to a meal, his mother's constant urging to get him to eat quickly quells any interest he had in eating. Travis simply folds his arms across his chest, closes his mouth tightly, and refuses to eat any more food. After more begging, pleading, and nagging, Travis's mother becomes angry and sends him away from the table. Travis is not allowed to snack between meals because his mother is concerned that snacks will ruin his appetite.
   - What factors might be contributing to Travis's refusal to eat?
   - Travis's mother is concerned about her son's underweight. What strategies would you suggest to help Travis gain weight?
   - What advice would you offer Travis's mother to help her improve mealtimes with her son?

2. Loni is a physically inactive, overweight 15-year-old girl who enjoys watching television and playing computer games in her spare time. She typically buys a cola and a bag of chips from the vending machine for lunch and then stops by a fast-food restaurant after school for chicken nuggets or a hamburger with french fries. She has noticed that she has gained weight and lacks energy.

- What nutrients might be excessive or lacking in her current diet plan?
- What dietary advice would you offer to help Loni look and feel healthier?
- What would you tell Loni to motivate her to become physically active?

Notes

1. Formula feeding of term infants, in *Pediatric Nutrition,* 7th ed., ed. R. E. Kleinman (Elk Grove Village, Ill.: American Academy of Pediatrics, 2014), pp. 61–81.
2. American Academy of Pediatrics, *New Mother's Guide to Breastfeeding,* 3rd. ed., ed. J. Y. Meek (New York, Bantam Books, 2017), pp. 64–94.
3. T. Jost and coauthors, Impact of human milk bacteria and oligosaccharides on neonatal gut microbiota establishment and gut health, *Nutrition Reviews* 73 (2015): 426–437; J. T. Smilowitz and coauthors, Breast milk oligosaccharides: Structure-function relationships in the neonate, *Annual Review of Nutrition* 34 (2014): 143–169.
4. J. T. Brenna and S. E. Carlson, Docosahexaenoic acid and human brain development: Evidence that a dietary supply is needed for optimal development, *Journal of Human Evolution* 77 (2014): 99–106.
5. S. M. Innis, Impact of maternal diet on human milk composition and neurological development of infants, *American Journal of Clinical Nutrition* 99 (2014): 734S–741S; Brenna and Carlson, 2014.
6. U. Ramakrishnan and coauthors, Prenatal supplementation with DHA improves attention at 5 y or age: A randomized controlled trial, *American Journal of Clinical Nutrition* 104 (2016): 1075–1082; J. J. Qingqing and coauthors, Effect of n-3 PUFA supplementation on cognitive function throughout the life span from infancy to old age: A systematic review and meta-analysis of randomized controlled trials, *American Journal of Clinical Nutrition* 100 (2014): 1422–1436.
7. Fat-soluble vitamins, in American Academy of Pediatrics, *Pediatric Nutrition,* 7th ed., ed. R. E. Kleinman (Elk Grove Village, Ill.: American Academy of Pediatrics, 2014), pp. 495–515.
8. Breastfeeding, in *Pediatric Nutrition,* 7th ed., ed. R. E. Kleinman (Elk Grove Village, Ill.: American Academy of Pediatrics, 2014), pp. 41–59.
9. B. Lönnerdal, Human Milk: Bioactive proteins /peptides and functional properties, *Nestle Nutrition Institute Workshop Series* 86 (2016): 97–107; M. A. Koch and coauthors, Maternal IgG and IgA antibodies dampen mucosal T helper cell responses in early life, *Cell* 165 (2016): 827–841; Jost and coauthors, 2015; Position of the Academy of Nutrition and Dietetics: Promoting and supporting breastfeeding, *Journal of the Academy of Nutrition and Dietetics* 115 (2015): 444–449; Smilowitz and coauthors, 2014.
10. Jost and coauthors, 2015; B. M. Jakaitis and P. W. Denning, Human breast milk and the gastrointestinal innate immune system, *Clinics in Perinatology* 41 (2014): 423–435.
11. I. Tromp and coauthors, Breastfeeding and the risk of respiratory tract infections after infancy: The Gerneration R Study, *PLoS One* 12 (2017): e0172763; G. Bowatte and coauthors, Breastfeeding and childhood acute otitis media: A systematic review and meta-analysis, *Acta Paediatrica* 104 (2015): 85–95.
12. K. Grimshaw and coauthors, Modifying the infant's diet to prevent food allergy, *Archives of Disease in Childhood* 102 (2017): 179–186; V. Bion and coauthors, Evaluating the efficacy of breastfeeding guidelines on long-term outcomes for allergic disease, *Allergy* 71 (2016): 661–670; C. J. Lodge and coauthors, Breastfeeding and asthma and allergies: A systematic review and meta-analysis, *Acta Paediatrica* 104 (2015): 38–53.
13. J. M. D. Thompson and coauthors, Duration of breastfeeding and risk of SIDS: An individual participant data meta-analysis, *Pediatrics* 140 (2017): e20171324; R. A. Danall and coauthors, American Academy of Pediatrics' Task Force on SIDS fully supports breastfeeding, *Breastfeeding Medicine* 9 (2014): 486–487.
14. I. Ramirez-Silva and coauthors, Breastfeeding status at age 3 months is associated with adiposity and cardiometabolic markers at age 4 years in Mexican children, *Journal of Nutrition* 145 (2015): 1295–1302;

T. W. McDade and coauthors, Long-term effects of birth weight and breastfeeding duration on inflammation in early adulthood, *Proceedings. Biological Sciences* 281 (2014): 20133116; S. Pirilä and coauthors, Breast-fed infants and their later cardiovascular health: A prospective study from birth to age 32 years, *British Journal of Nutrition* 111 (2014): 1069–1076.
15. P. Rzehak and coauthors, Infant feeding and growth trajectory patterns in childhood and body composition in young adulthood, *American Journal of Clinical Nutrition* 106 (2017): 568–580; W. Liang and coauthors, Breastfeeding reduces childhood obesity risks, *Childhood Obesity* 13 (2017): 197–204; A. Zamora-Kapoor and coauthors, Breastfeeding in infancy is associated with body mass index in adolescence: A retrospective cohort study comparing American Indians/Alaska Natives and Non-Hispanic whites, *Journal of the Academy of Nutrition and Dietetics* 117 (2017): 1049–1056; R. J. Hancox and coauthors, Association between breastfeeding and body mass index at age 6–7 years in an international survey, *Pediatric Obesity* 10 (2015): 283–287; C. M. Lefebvre and R. M. John, The effect of breastfeeding on childhood overweight and obesity: A systematic review of the literature, *Journal of the American Association of Nurse Practitioners* 26 (2014): 386–401.
16. Lefebvre and John, 2014.
17. S. Bar, R. Milanaik, and A. Adesman, Long-term neurodevelopmental benefits of breastfeeding, *Current Opinion in Pediatrics* 28 (2016): 559–566; S. Cai and coauthors, Infant feeding effects on early neurocognitive development in Asian children, *American Journal of Clinical Nutrition* 101 (2015): 326–336.
18. American Academy of Pediatrics, Formula feeding of term infants, 2014.
19. U. S. Food and Drug Administration, FDA takes final step on infant formula protections, www.fda.gov/ForConsumers/ConsumerUpdates/ucm048694.htm, updated November 8, 2017.
20. American Academy of Pediatrics, Formula feeding of term infants, 2014.
21. American Academy of Pediatrics, Formula feeding of term infants, 2014.
22. Complementary feeding, in *Pediatric Nutrition,* 7th ed., ed. R. E. Kleinman (Elk Grove Village, Ill.: American Academy of Pediatrics, 2014), pp. 123–139.
23. American Academy of Pediatrics, Complementary feeding, 2014.
24. R. Pérez-Escamilla, S. Segura-Pérez, and M. Lott, Feeding guidelines for infants and young toddlers, *Nutrition Today* 52 (2017): 223–231.
25. American Academy of Pediatrics, Complementary feeding, 2014.
26. M. B. Heyman and S. A. Abrams, Fruit juice in infants, children, and adolescents: Current recommendations, *Pediatrics* 139 (2017): e20170967.
27. Heyman and Abrams, 2017.
28. American Academy of Pediatrics, Complementary feeding, 2014.
29. P. J. Turner and D. E. Campbell, Implementing primary prevention for peanut allergy at a population level, *Journal of the American Medical Association* 317 (2017): 1111–1112; A. Togias and coauthors, Addendum guidelines for the prevention of peanut allergy in the United States: Report of the National Institute of Allergy and Infectious Diseases—Sponsored expert panel, *Annals of Allergy, Asthma, and Immunology,* doi: dx.doi.org/10.1016/j.anai.2016.10.004; G. Du Toit and coauthors, Randomized trial of peanut consumption in infants at risk for peanut allergy, *New England Journal of Medicine* 372 (2015): 803–813; D. M. Fleischer and coauthors, Consensus communication on early peanut introduction and the prevention of peanut allergy in high-risk infants, *Pediatrics* 136 (2015): 600–604.
30. C. M. Weaver and coauthors, The National Osteoporosis Foundation's position statement on peak bone mass development and lifestyle factors: A systematic review and implementation recommendations, *Osteoporosis International* 27 (2016): 1281–1386; N. H. Golden, S. A. Abrams, and

Committee on Nutrition, Optimizing bone health in children and adolescents, *Pediatrics* 134 (2014): e1229–e1243; R. Rizzoli, Dairy products, yogurt, and bone health, *American Journal of Clinical Nutrition* 99 (2014): 1256S–1262S.

31. Position of the Academy of Nutrition and Dietetics: Nutrition guidance for healthy children ages 2 to 11 years, *Journal of the Academy of Nutrition and Dietetics* 114 (2014): 1257–1276; D. M. Hoelscher and coauthors, Position of the Academy of Nutrition and Dietetics: Interventions for the prevention and treatment of pediatric overweight and obesity, *Journal of the Academy of Nutrition and Dietetics* 113 (2013): 1375–1394, reaffirmed, 2017.

32. Position of the Academy of Nutrition and Dietetics, Nutrition guidance for healthy children ages 2 to 11 years, 2014.

33. Nutritional aspects of vegetarian diets, in *Pediatric Nutrition*, 7th ed., ed. R. E. Kleinman (Elk Grove Village, Ill.: American Academy of Pediatrics, 2014), pp. 241–264.

34. P. M. Gupta and coauthors, Iron, anemia, and iron deficiency anemia among young children in the United States, *Nutrients* 2016, doi: 10.3390/nu8060330; M. Domellöf and coauthors, Iron requirements of infants and toddlers, *Journal of Pediatric Gastroenterology* 58 (2014): 119–129; G. Paoletti, D. L. Bogen, and A. K. Ritchey, Severe iron-deficiency anemia still an issue in toddlers, *Clinical Pediatrics* 53 (2014): 1352–1358.

35. American Academy of Pediatrics, Complementary feeding, 2014.

36. Golden, Abrams, and Committee on Nutrition, 2014.

37. U. S. Department of Health and Human Services and U.S. Department of Agriculture, *2015–2020 Dietary Guidelines for Americans,* 8th ed. (2015), health.gov/dietaryguidelines/2015/guidelines/.

38. Position of the Academy of Nutrition and Dietetics, Nutrition guidance for health children ages 2 to 11 years, 2014.

39. M. E. Cogswell and coauthors, Sodium and sugar in complementary infant and toddler foods sold in the United States, *Pediatrics* 135 (2015): 416–423.

40. Bread for the World, About hunger, www.breadorg//where-does-hunger-exist, accessed January 18, 2018.

41. Position of the Academy of Nutrition and Dietetics, Nutrition guidance for health children ages 2–11 years, 2014.

42. J. D. Coulthard, L. Palla, and G. K. Pot, Breakfast consumption and nutrient intakes in 4-18-year-olds: UK National Diet and Nutrition Survey Rolling Programme (2008–2012), *British Journal of Nutrition* 17 (2017): 1–11; S. S. Pineda Vargas and coauthors, Eating ready-to-eat cereal for breakfast is positively associated with daily nutrient intake, but not weight, in Mexican-American children and adolescents, *Nutrition Today* 51 (2016): 206–215; S. I. Barr, L. DiFrancesco, and V. L. Fulgoni, Breakfast consumption is positively associated with nutrient adequacy in Canadian children and adolescents, *British Journal of Nutrition* 112 (2014): 1373–1383.

43. I. Iovino and coauthors, Breakfast consumption has no effect on neuropsychological functioning in children: A repeated-measures clinical trial, *American Journal of Clinical Nutrition* 104 (2016): 715–721; V. Edefonti and coauthors, The effect of breakfast composition and energy contribution on cognitive and academic performance: A systematic review, *American Journal of Clinical Nutrition* 100 (2014): 626–656.

44. Gupta and coauthors, 2016; J. R. Doom and M. K. Georgieff, Striking while the iron is hot: Understanding the biological and neurodevelopmental effects of iron deficiency to optimize intervention in early childhood, *Current Pediatric Reports* 2 (2014): 291–298.

45. Doom and Georgieff, 2014.

46. B. P. Lanphear and Council on Environmental Health, American Academy of Pediatrics Policy Statement, Prevention of childhood lead toxicity, *Pediatrics* 138 (2016): 146–160; C. S. Sim and coauthors, Iron deficiency increases blood lead levels in boys and pre-menarche girls surveyed in KNHANES 2010–2011, *Environmental Research* 130 (2014): 1–6.

47. Centers for Disease Control and Prevention, Lead, www.cdc.gov/nceh/lead, updated December 4, 2017.

48. Food and Drug Administration, Food allergies: Reducing the risks, www.fda.gov/forconsumers/consumerupdates/ucm089307.htm; updated December 18, 2017.

49. S. M. Jones and A. W. Burks, Food allergy, *New England Journal of Medicine* 377 (2017): 1168–1176; S. Benedė and coauthors, The rise of food allergy: Environmental factors and emerging treatments, *EBioMedicine* 7 (2016): 27–34; D. M. Fleischer and coauthors, Consensus communication on early peanut introduction and the prevention of peanut allergy in high-risk infants, *Pediatrics* 136 (2015): 600–604; Food

and Drug Administration, Food allergies: Reducing the risks, www.fda.gov/forconsumers/consumerupdates/ucm089307.htm; updated December 18, 2017.

50. Benedė and coauthors, 2016.

51. S. C. Collins, Practice paper of the Academy of Nutrition and Dietetics: Role of the registered dietitian nutritionist in the diagnosis and management of food allergies, *Journal of the Academy of Nutrition and Dietetics* 116 (2016): 1621–1631; R. B. Canani and coauthors, The effects of dietary counseling on children with food allergy: A prospective, multicenter intervention study, *Journal of the Academy of Nutrition and Dietetics* 114 (2014): 1432–1439.

52. B. P. Vickery and coauthors, Early oral immunotherapy in peanut-allergic preschool children is safe and highly effective, *Journal of Allergy and Clinical Immunology,* 2016, doi: 10.1016/jaci.2016.05027; K. Anagnostou and coauthors, Assessing the efficacy of oral immunotherapy for the desensitization of peanut allergy in children (STOPII): A phase 2 randomised controlled trial, *Lancet* 383 (2014): 1297–1304.

53. Centers for Disease Control and Prevention, Attention-Deficit/Hyperactivity Disorder, Data and Statistics, www.cdc.gov/ncbddd/ adhd/data.html, updated November 13, 2017.

54. S. Cruchet, Y. Lucero, and V. Cornejo, Truths, myths, and needs of special diets: Attention-deficit/hyperactivity disorder, autism, non-celiac gluten sensitivity, and vegetarianism, *Annals of Nutrition and Metabolism* 68 (2016): 43–50.

55. J. Stevenson and coauthors, Research review: The role of diet in the treatment of attention-deficit/hyperactivity disorder—An appraisal of the evidence on efficacy and recommendations on the design of future studies, *Journal of Child Psychology and Psychiatry* 55 (2014): 416–427.

56. U.S. Preventive Services Task Force, Screening for obesity in children and adolescents; U.S. Preventive Services Task Force Recommendation Statement, *Journal of the American Medical Association* 317 (2017): 2417–2426; C. L. Ogden and coauthors, Trends in obesity prevalence among children and adolescents in the United State, 1988–1994 through 2013–2014, *Journal of the American Medical Association* 315 (2016): 2292–2299.

57. A. C. Skinner and J. A. Skelton, Prevalence and trends in obesity and severe obesity among children in the United States, 1999–2012, *JAMA Pediatrics* 168 (2014): 561–566.

58. A. C. Skinner and coauthors, Cardiometabolic risks and severity of obesity in children and young adults, *New England Journal of Medicine* 373 (2015): 1307–1317.

59. P. Dolton and M. Xiao, The intergenerational transmission of body mass index across countries, *Economics and Human Biology* 24 (2017): 140–152; K. Silventoinen and coauthors, Genetic and environmental effects on body mass index from infancy to the onset of adulthood: An individual-based pooled analysis of 45 twin cohorts participating in the Collaborative project of Development of Anthropometrical measures in Twins (CODATwins) study, *American Journal of Clinical Nutrition* 104 (2016): 371–379; M. G. Hohenadel and coauthors, The impact of genetic variants on BMI increase during childhood versus adulthood, *International Journal of Obesity* 40 (2014): 1301–1309.

60. Skinner and Skelton, 2014.

61. Centers for Disease Control and Prevention, Childhood obesity: Causes and consequences, www.cdc.gov/obesity/childhood/causes.html, updated December 15, 2016.

62. S. M. Robson and coauthors, Parent diet quality and energy intake are related to child diet quality and energy intake, *Journal of the Academy of Nutrition and Dietetics* 116 (2016): 984–990; J. K. Larsen and coauthors, How parental dietary behavior and food parenting practices affect children's dietary behavior: Interacting forces of influence? *Appetite* 89 (2015): 246–257; J. Martin-Biggers and coauthors, Translating it into real life: A qualitative study of the cognitions, barriers and supports for key obesogenic behaviors of parents of preschoolers, *BMC Public Health* 15 (2015): 189; S. C. couch and coauthors, Home food environment in relation to children's diet quality and weight status, *Journal of the Academy of Nutrition and Dietetics* 114 (2014): 1569–1579; A. W. Watts and coauthors, Parent-child associations in selected food group and nutrient intakes among overweight and obese adolescents, *Journal of the Academy of Nutrition and Dietetics* 114 (2014): 1580–1586.

63. J. M. Poti, M. M. Slining, and B. M. Popkin, Where are kids getting their empty calories? Stores, schools, and fast-food restaurants each played an important role in empty calorie intake among US children during

2009–2010, *Journal of the Academy of Nutrition and Dietetics* 114 (2014): 908–917.

64. C. W. Leung and coauthors, Sugar-sweetened beverage and water intake in relation to diet quality in U.S. children, *American Journal of Preventive Medicine* 2018, doi: 10.1016/jamepre.2017.11.005; M. B. Vos and coauthors, Added sugars and cardiovascular disease risk in children: A Scientific Statement from the American Heart Association, *Circulation* 135 (2017): e1017–e1034; L. Tappy and K. A. Lê, Health effects of fructose and fructose-containing caloric sweeteners: Where do we stand 10 years after the initial whistle blowings? *Current Diabetes Reports* 15 (2015): 54; G. A. Brady and B. M. Popkin, Dietary sugar and body weight: Have we reached a crisis in the epidemic of obesity and diabetes? *Diabetes Care* 37 (2014): 950–956; S. C. Bundrick and coauthors, Soda consumption during ad libitum food intake predicts weight change, *Journal of the Academy of Nutrition and Dietetics* 114 (2014): 444–449.

65. Leung and coauthors, 2018; M. Luger and coauthors, Sugar-sweetened beverages and weight gain in children and adults: A systematic review from 2013 to 2015 and a comparison with previous studies, *Obesity Facts* 14 (2017): 674–693; S. D. Poppitt, Beverage consumption: Are alcoholic and sugary drinks tipping the balance towards overweight and obesity? *Nutrients* 7 (2015): 6700–6718; The Obesity Society, Position statement: Reduced Consumption of sugar-sweetened beverages can reduce total caloric intake, 2014, www.obesity.org/publications/reduced-consumption-of-sugar-sweetened-beverages-can-reduce-total-caloric-intake.htm; Bray and Popkin, 2014; Bundrick and coauthors, 2014.

66. A. Marques and coauthors, Association between physical activity, sedentary time, and healthy fitness in youth, *Medicine* and *Science in Sports and Exercise* 47 (2015): 575–580; T. Remmers and coauthors, Relationship between physical activity and the development of body mass index in children, *Medicine and Science in Sports and Exercise* 46 (2014): 177–184.

67. V. Carson and coauthors, Systematic review of sedentary behavior and health indicators in school-aged children and youth: An update, *Applied Physiology, Nutrition, and Metabolism* 41 (2016): S240–265; A. G. LeBlanc and coauthors, Correlates of total sedentary time and screen time in 9–11 year-old children around the world: The International Study of Childhood Obesity, Lifestyle and the Environment, *PLoS One* 10 (2015): e0129622.

68. M. M. Borghese and coauthors, Mediating role of television time, diet patterns, physical activity and sleep duration in the association between television in the bedroom and adiposity in 10 year-old children, *International Journal of Behavioral Nutrition and Physical Activity* 13 (2015): 60; E. M. Cespedes and coauthors, Television viewing, bedroom television, and sleep duration from infancy to mid-childhood, *Pediatrics* 133 (2014): e1163–1171; J. Owens, Insufficient sleep in adolescents and young adults: An update on causes and consequences, *Pediatrics* 134 (2014): e921–e932.

69. Carson and coauthors, 2016; Borghese and coauthors, 2015; M. M. Borghese and coauthors, Independent and combined associations of total sedentary time and television viewing time with food patterns of 9- to 11-year-old Canadian children, *Applied Physiology, Nutrition, and Metabolism* 39 (2014): 937–943; J. Falbe and coauthors, Longitudinal relations of television, electronic games, and digital versatile discs with changes in diet in adolescents, *American Journal of Clinical Nutrition* 100 (2014): 1173–1181.

70. Carson and coauthors, 2014; Borghese and coauthors, 2014.

71. M. R. Longacre and coauthors, Child-targeted TV advertising and preschoolers' consumption of high-sugar breakfast cereals, *Appetite* 108 (2016): 295–302; E. J. Boyland and R. Whalen, Food advertising to children and its effects on diet: Review of recent prevalence and impact data, *Pediatric Diabetes* 16 (2015): 331–337.

72. M. Nestle, WHO Europe takes on food marketing to children, November 7, 2016, www.foodpolitics.com/2016/11/who-europe-takes-on-food-marketing-to-children; Boyland and Whalen, 2015.

73. D. L. Kunkel, J. S. Castonguay, and C. R. Filer, Evaluating industry self-regulation of food marketing to children, *American Journal of Preventive Medicine* 49 (2015): 181–187; M. D. Hingle and coauthors, Alignment of children's food advertising with proposed Federal Guidelines, *American Journal of Preventive Medicine* 48 (2015): 707–713; A. M. Bernhardt and coauthors, Children's recall of fast food television advertising—Testing the adequacy of food marketing regulation, *PLoS One* 10 (2015): e0119300.

74. K. L. R. Canabrava and coauthors, Energy expenditure and intensity of active video games in children and adolescents, *Research Quarterly for Exercise and Sport* 15 (2018): 1–10; M. Simmons and coauthors,

Associations between active video gaming and other energy-balance related behaviours in adolescents: A 24-hour recall diary study, *International Journal of Behavioral Nutrition and Physical Activity* 12 (2015): 32; A. Gribbon and coauthors, Active video games and energy balance in male adolescents: A randomized crossover trial, *American Journal of Clinical Nutrition* 101 (2015): 1126–1134.

75. American Academy of Pediatrics, Policy statement, Council on Communications and media, Media and young minds, *Pediatrics* 138 (2016): e20162592; American Academy of Pediatrics, Policy statement, Council on Communications and media, Media use in school-aged children and adolescents, *Pediatrics* 138 (2016): e20162592.

76. A. C. Skinner and coauthors, Cardiometabolic risks and severity of obesity in children and young adults, *New England Journal of Medicine* 373 (2015): 1307–1317; K. R. Armstrong and coauthors, Childhood obesity, arterial stiffness, and prevalence and treatment of hypertension, *Current Treatment Options in Cardiovascular Medicine* 16 (2014): 339.

77. G. Twig and coauthors, Body mass index at age 17 and diabetes mortality in midlife: A nationwide cohort of 2.3 million adolescents, *Diabetes Care* 39 (2016): 1996–2003; B. Tobisch, L. Blatniczky, and L. Barkai, Cardiometabolic risk factors and insulin resistance in obese children and adolescents: Relation to puberty, *Pediatric Obesity* 10 (2015): 37–44.

78. R. M. Puhl and coauthors, Experiences of weight teasing in adolescence and weight-related outcomes in adulthood: A 15-year longitudinal study, *Preventive Medicine* 100 (2017): 173–179; A. W. Harrist and coauthors, The social and emotional lives of overweight, obese, and severely obese children, *Child Development* 87 (2016): 1564–1580.

79. M. J. Buscot and coauthors, BMI trajectories associated with resolution of elevated youth BMI and incident adult obesity, *Pediatrics* 141 (2018): e20172003.

80. U.S. Preventive Services Task Force, Screening for obesity in children and adolescents, *Journal of the American Medical Association* 317 (2017): 2417–2426; D. M. Styne and coauthors, Pediatric obesity—assessment, treatment, and prevention: An Endocrine Society Clinical Practice Guideline, *Journal of Clinical Endocrinology and Metabolism* (2017): jc2016–2573; P. T. Katzmarzyk and coauthors, An evolving scientific basis for the prevention and treatment of pediatric obesity, *International Journal of Obesity* 38 (2014): 887–905.

81. Katzmarzyk and coauthors, 2014.

82. J. Bangsbo and coauthors, The Copenhagen Consensus Conference 2016: Children, youth, and physical activity in schools and during leisure time, *British Journal of Sports Medicine* 50 (2016): 1177–1178; P. T. Katzmarzyk and coauthors, Physical activity, sedentary time, and obesity in an international sample of children, *Medicine and Science in Sports and Exercise* 47 (2015): 2062–2069; A. Marques and coauthors, Association between physical activity, sedentary time, and healthy fitness in youth, *Medicine and Science in Sports and Exercise* 47 (2015): 575–580.

83. T. H. Inge and coauthors, Weight loss and health status 3 years after bariatric surgery in adolescents, *New England Journal of Medicine* 374 (2016): 113–123; Katzmarzyk and coauthors, 2014.

84. A. Ek and coauthors, Associations between parental concerns about preschoolers' weight and eating and parental feeding practices: Results from analyses of the Child Eating Behavior Questionnaire, the Child Feeding Questionnaire, and the Lifestyle Behavior Checklist, *PLoS One* 11 (2016): e0147257; S. R. Damiano, L. M. Hart, and S. J. Paxton, Correlates of parental feeding practices with pre-schoolers: Parental body image and eating knowledge, attitudes, and behaviours, *Appetite* 101 (2016): 192–198.

85. N. C. Cole and coauthors, Correlates of picky eating and food neophobia in young children: A systematic review and meta-analysis, *Nutrition Reviews* 75 (2017): 515–532; H. Bergmeier, H. Skouteris, and M. Hetherington, Systematic research review of observational approaches used to evaluate mother-child mealtime interactions during preschool years, *American Journal of Clinical Nutrition* 101 (2015): 7–15.

86. Position of the Academy of Nutrition and Dietetics, Nutrition guidance for health children ages 2–11 years, 2014.

87. M. A. Adams and coauthors, Location of school lunch salad bars and fruit and vegetable consumption in middle schools: A cross-sectional plate waste study, *Journal of the Academy of Nutrition and Dietetics* 116 (2016): 407–416.

88. J. F. W. Cohen and coauthors, Amount of time to eat lunch is associated with children's selection and consumption of school meal entrée, fruits, vegetables, and milk, *Journal of the Academy of Nutrition and Dietetics* 116 (2016): 123–128.

89. Position of the Academy of Nutrition and Dietetics, Nutrition guidance for health children ages 2–11 years, 2014.

90. U.S. Department of Agriculture, Food and Nutrition Service, School meals, Tools for schools: Focusing on smart snacks, November 28, 2017, www.fns.usda.gov/school-meals/tools-school-focusing-smart -snacks.

91. T. J. Smith and coauthors, Vitamin D in adolescence: Evidence-based dietary requirements and implications for public health policy, *Proceedings of the Nutrition Society*, 2017, doi: 10.1017/S0029665117004104.

92. C. M. Weaver and coauthors, The National Osteoporosis Foundation's position statement on peak bone mass development and lifestyle factors: A systematic review and implementation recommendations, *Osteoporosis International* 27 (2016): 1281–1386.

93. D. K. Dror and L. H. Allen, Dairy product intake in children and adolescents in developed countries: Trends, nutritional contribution, and a review of association with health outcomes, *Nutrition Reviews* 72 (2014): 68–81.

94. Dror and Allen, 2014.

95. L. M. Lipsky and coauthors, Diet quality of US adolescents during the transition to adulthood: Changes and predictors, *American Journal of Clinical Nutrition* 105 (2017): 1424–1432; J. M. Berge and coauthors, Family food preparation and its effects on adolescent dietary quality and eating patterns, *Journal of Adolescent Health* 59 (2016): 530–536.

96. J. D. Coulthard, L. Palla, and G. K. Pot, Breakfast consumption and nutrient intakes in 4-18-year-olds: UK National Diet and Nutrition Survey rolling Programme (2008–2012), *British Journal of Nutrition* 17 (2017): 1–11; S. I. Barr, L. DiFrancesco, and V. L. Fulgone, Breakfast consumption is positively associated with nutrient adequacy in Canadian children and adolescents, *British Journal of Nutrition* 112 (2014): 1373–1383.

97. J. M. Poti, K. J. Duffey, and B. M. Popkin, The association of fast food consumption with poor dietary outcomes and obesity among children: Is it the fast food or the remainder of the diet? *American Journal of Clinical Nutrition* 99 (2014): 162–171.

98. E. W. Evans and coauthors, The role of eating frequency on total energy intake and diet quality in a low-income, racially diverse sample of schoolchildren, *Public Health Nutrition* 18 (2015): 474–481; F. Bellisle, Meals and snacking, diet quality and energy balance, *Physiology and Behavior* 134 (2014): 38–43.

99. Dror and Allen, 2014.

100. S. D. Poppitt, Beverage consumption: Are alcoholic and sugary drinks tipping the balance towards overweight and obesity? *Nutrients* 7 (2015): 6700–6715; Obesity Society, Position statement: Reduced consumption of sugar-sweetened beverages can reduce total caloric intake, April, 2014, www.obesity.org/publications/position-and-policies/sugar-sweetened; Dror and Allen, 2014.

101. Poti, Duffey, and Popkin, 2014.

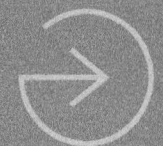

11.4 Nutrition in Practice

Childhood Obesity and the Early Development of Chronic Diseases

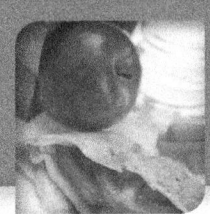

When people think about the health problems of children and adolescents, they typically think of ear infections, colds, and acne—not heart disease, diabetes, or hypertension. Today, however, unprecedented numbers of U.S. children are being diagnosed with obesity and the serious "adult diseases," such as type 2 diabetes, that accompany overweight.[1] When type 2 diabetes develops before the age of 20, the incidence of diabetic kidney disease and death in middle age increases dramatically, largely because of the long duration of the disease. For children born in the United States in the year 2000, the risk of developing type 2 diabetes sometime in their lives is estimated to be 30 percent for boys and 40 percent for girls. U.S. children are not alone—rapidly rising rates of obesity threaten the health of an alarming number of children around the globe.[2] Without immediate intervention, millions of children are destined to develop type 2 diabetes and hypertension in childhood followed by **cardiovascular disease (CVD)** in early adulthood.[3]

Over the past three decades, researchers have been observing how changes in body weight, blood lipids, blood pressure, and individual behaviors correlate with the development of CVD over time—from infancy to childhood through adolescence and into young adulthood. Some major findings have emerged from this research:

- Changes inside the arteries—changes predictive of CVD—are evident in childhood.
- Obesity in children affects these changes.
- Behaviors that influence the development of obesity and of CVD are learned and begin early in life. These behaviors include overeating, physical inactivity, and cigarette smoking.

This Nutrition in Practice focuses on efforts to prevent childhood obesity, type 2 diabetes, and CVD (see Box NP11-1 for definitions of the relevant terms), but the benefits extend to other obesity-related diseases as well. The years of childhood (ages 2 to 18) are emphasized here, for the earlier in life health-promoting habits become established, the better they will stick.

What about genetics? Do some people inherit the tendency to become obese or develop diabetes or CVD regardless of the lifestyle habits they adopt?

For obesity, as well as for CVD, hypertension, and type 2 diabetes, genetics does not appear to play a *determining* role; that is, a person is not simply destined at birth to develop them. Instead, genetics appears to play a *permissive* role—the potential is inherited and will then develop, if given a push by factors in the environment such as poor diet, sedentary lifestyle, and cigarette smoking.[4] Researchers note that the relationship between genes and the environment is a synergistic one—their combined effects are greater than the sum of their individual effects.

Many experts agree that preventing or treating obesity in childhood will reduce the rate of chronic diseases in adulthood. Without intervention, most overweight children become overweight adolescents who become overweight adults, and being overweight exacerbates every chronic disease that adults face.[5] Fatty liver, a condition that correlates directly with BMI, was not even recognized in pediatric research until recently. Today, fatty liver disease affects about one in three obese children.[6]

Box NP11-1 Glossary

atherosclerosis (ATH-er-oh-scler-OH-sis): a type of artery disease characterized by plaques (accumulations of lipid-containing material) on the inner walls of the arteries (see Chapter 21).

- *athero = porridge or soft*
- *scleros = hard*
- *osis = condition*

cardiovascular disease (CVD): a general term for all diseases of the heart and blood vessels. Atherosclerosis is the main cause of CVD. When the arteries that carry blood to the heart muscle become blocked, the heart suffers damage, known as coronary heart disease (CHD).

- *cardio = heart*
- *vascular = blood vessels*

fatty streaks: accumulation of cholesterol and other lipids along the walls of the arteries.

plaque (PLACK): an accumulation of fatty deposits, smooth muscle cells, and fibrous connective tissue that develops in the artery walls. Plaque associated with atherosclerosis is known as **atheromatous** (ATH-er-OH-ma-tus) **plaque**.

What about events that take place during fetal development—malnutrition, for example? Can they affect a person's tendency to develop diseases later in life?

A theory called *fetal programming*, or *developmental origins of health and disease*, states that maternal malnutrition or other harmful conditions at a critical period of fetal development may have lifelong effects on an individual's pattern of genetic expression and therefore on the tendency to develop obesity and certain diseases.[7] Poor maternal diet or health during pregnancy may alter the infant's bodily functions that influence disease development, such as blood pressure, cholesterol metabolism, glucose metabolism, and immune functions.[8] For example, malnutrition during fetal development may encourage metabolic programming that promotes nutrient storage and thus provides a survival advantage in an environment of poor postnatal nutrition. In a postnatal environment of adequate nutrition or overnutrition, however, such adaptations can lead to the development of glucose intolerance, type 2 diabetes, cardiovascular disease, and hypertension.

Why has type 2 diabetes become so prevalent?

In recent years, type 2 diabetes, a chronic disease closely linked with obesity, has been on the rise among children and adolescents as the prevalence of obesity in U.S. youth has increased.[9] Type 2 diabetes is most likely to occur in those who are obese and sedentary and have a family history of diabetes. Obesity is the most important risk factor—most of the children diagnosed with type 2 diabetes are obese. Most are diagnosed during puberty, but as children become more obese and less active, the disease is appearing in younger and younger children.

How does type 2 diabetes develop?

In type 2 diabetes, the body's cells become insulin resistant—that is, the cells become less sensitive to insulin, reducing the amount of glucose entering the cells from the blood. The combination of obesity and insulin resistance produces a cluster of symptoms, including high blood pressure and high blood lipids, which in turn promotes the development of atherosclerosis and the early development of CVD.[10] Other common problems evident by early adulthood include kidney disease, blindness, and miscarriages. The complications of diabetes, especially when encountered at a young age, can shorten life expectancy. Chapter 20 offers a detailed discussion of diabetes.

Prevention and treatment of type 2 diabetes depend on weight management, which can be particularly difficult in a young person's world of food advertising, video games, and pocket money for candy bars. The activity and dietary suggestions to help defend against heart disease later in this discussion apply to type 2 diabetes as well.

How does CVD develop, and when does its development begin?

Most CVD involves **atherosclerosis**. Atherosclerosis develops when regions of an artery's walls become progressively thickened with **plaque**—an accumulation of fatty deposits, smooth muscle cells, and fibrous connective tissue. Frequently, atherosclerosis and its complications interfere with the flow of blood to the heart and can lead to coronary heart disease (CHD), which, in turn, raises the likelihood of a heart attack. When atherosclerosis interferes with blood flow to the brain, a stroke can result. Infants are born with healthy, smooth, clear arteries, but within the first decade of life, **fatty streaks** may begin to appear. During adolescence, these fatty streaks may begin to turn into plaques (Figure 21-2 in Chapter 21 on p. 599 shows the formation of plaques in atherosclerosis). By early adulthood, the fibrous plaques may begin to calcify and become raised lesions, especially in boys and young men. As the lesions grow more numerous and thicken, the heart disease rate begins to rise, and the rise becomes dramatic at about age 45 in men and 55 in women. From this point on, arterial damage and blockage progress rapidly, and heart attacks and strokes threaten life. In short, the consequences of atherosclerosis, which become apparent only in adulthood, have their beginnings in the first decades of life.[11]

Children with the highest risks of developing heart disease are sedentary and obese; they may also have diabetes, high blood pressure, and high blood cholesterol. In contrast, children with the lowest risks of heart disease are physically active and of normal weight, with low blood pressure and favorable lipid profiles.

Parents do not need to worry about their children's blood cholesterol, do they?

Atherosclerotic lesion formation reflects blood cholesterol: as blood cholesterol rises, lesion coverage increases. Cholesterol values at birth are similar in all populations; differences emerge in early childhood. Standard values for cholesterol screening in children and adolescents are listed in Table NP11-1. Cholesterol concentrations change with age in children and adolescents, however, and are especially variable during puberty. Thus, using a single cut point for all pediatric age groups has limitations.

In general, blood cholesterol tends to rise as dietary saturated fat intakes increase. Blood cholesterol also correlates with childhood obesity, especially abdominal obesity. LDL cholesterol rises with obesity, and HDL declines.

TABLE NP11-1	Cholesterol Values for Children and Adolescents	
DISEASE RISK	TOTAL CHOLESTEROL (mg/dL)	LDL CHOLESTEROL (mg/dL)
Acceptable	<170	<110
Borderline	170–199	110–129
High	≥200	≥130

Note: Adult values appear in Table 21-2 on p. 599.

These relationships are apparent throughout childhood, and their magnitude increases with age.

Children who are both overweight and have high blood cholesterol are likely to have parents who develop heart disease early. For this reason, selective screening is recommended for children and adolescents of any age who are overweight or obese; those whose parents (or grandparents) have premature (≤55 years of age for men and ≤65 years of age for women) heart disease; those whose parents have elevated blood cholesterol; those who have other risk factors for heart disease such as hypertension, cigarette smoking, or diabetes; and those whose family history is unavailable. Because blood cholesterol in children is a good predictor of adult values, some experts recommend universal screening for all children aged 9 to 11.[12] The U.S. Preventive Services Task Force, however, concludes there is insufficient evidence of the benefits and harms of lipid screening in children and adolescents to make a recommendation.[13] Early—but not advanced—atherosclerotic lesions are reversible, making screening and education a high priority. Both those with family histories of heart disease and those with multiple risk factors need intervention.

Is hypertension a concern for children and adolescents?

Pediatricians routinely monitor blood pressure in children and adolescents. High blood pressure may signal an underlying disease or the early onset of hypertension. Childhood hypertension, left untreated, can accelerate the development of atherosclerosis.[14] Diagnosing hypertension in children and adolescents requires consideration of age, gender, and height, and blood pressure cannot be assessed using the simple tables applied to adults.

Like atherosclerosis and high blood cholesterol, hypertension may develop in the first decades of life, especially among obese children, and worsen with time. Children can control their hypertension by participating in regular aerobic activity and by losing weight or maintaining their weight as they grow taller. Restricting dietary sodium also causes an immediate drop in most children's and adolescents' blood pressure.[15]

Regular physical activity lowers risks for heart disease and hypertension in adults; does it do so in children as well?

Yes. Research has confirmed an association between blood lipids and physical activity in children, similar to that seen in adults. Physically active children have a better lipid profile and lower blood pressure than physically inactive children, and these positive findings often persist into adulthood.[16] Table 11-12 on p. 329 offers examples of aerobic, muscle-strengthening, and bone-strengthening physical activities for children and adolescents.

Just as blood cholesterol and obesity track over the years, so does a child's level of physical activity.[17] Those who are inactive now are likely to still be inactive years later. Similarly, those who are physically active now tend to remain so. Compared with inactive teens, those who are physically active weigh less, smoke less, eat a diet lower in saturated fats, and have better blood lipid profiles. Both obesity and blood cholesterol correlate with the inactive pastime of watching television. The message is clear: Physical activity offers numerous health benefits, and children who are active today are most likely to be active for years to come.

Are adult dietary recommendations appropriate for children?

Regardless of family history, all children older than age two should eat a variety of foods and maintain a desirable weight (see Table NP11-2 on p. 348). For heart health, children older than two years of age benefit from the same dietary pattern recommended for older individuals—that is, a diet limited in saturated fat, *trans* fat, sodium, and added sugars, while rich in nutrients and age-appropriate in kcalories. Such a diet benefits blood lipids without compromising nutrient adequacy, physical growth, or neurological development.

Healthy children older than age two can begin the transition to these recommendations by selecting more fruit and vegetables and fewer foods high in saturated fat, sodium, and added sugars. Like saturated fat and sodium, excess intakes of added sugars may increase the risk of obesity, heart disease, and hypertension.[18] Healthy meals can occasionally include moderate amounts of a child's favorite food, such as ice cream, even if it is high in saturated fat. A steady diet from the children's menus in some restaurants—which feature chicken nuggets, hot dogs, french fries, and sugar-sweetened beverages—easily exceeds a prudent intake of saturated fat, *trans* fat, and kcalories, however, and invites both nutrient shortages and weight gains.[19] Fortunately, most restaurant chains are

TABLE NP11-2 American Heart Association Dietary Guidelines and Strategies for Children[a]

- Balance dietary kcalories with physical activity to maintain normal growth.
- Every day, engage in 60 minutes of moderate to vigorous play or physical activity.
- Eat a variety of vegetables and fruit daily while limiting juice intake. Serve fresh, frozen, or canned vegetables and fruit at every meal; limit those with added fats, salt, and sugar.
- Eat foods low in saturated fat, trans fat, sodium, and added sugars.
- Use vegetable oils (canola, soybean, olive, safflower, or other unsaturated oils) and soft margarines low in saturated fat and trans-fatty acids instead of butter or most other animal fats in the diet.
- Choose whole-grain breads and cereals rather than refined products; read labels and make sure that "whole grain" is the first ingredient.
- Limit or avoid the intake of sugar-sweetened beverages; encourage water.
- Consume low-fat and nonfat milk and milk products daily.
- Include two servings of fish per week, especially fatty fish such as broiled or baked salmon.
- Choose legumes and tofu in place of meat for some meals.
- Choose only lean cuts of meat and reduced-fat meat products; remove the skin from poultry.
- Serve age-appropriate portion sizes on/in appropriately sized plates and bowls.

[a]These guidelines are for children two years of age and older.

www.heart.org/HEARTORG/HealthyLiving/HealthyKids/HowtoMakeaHealthyHome/Dietary-Recommendations-for-Healthy-Children_UCM_303886_Article.jsp#.WhNLCUqnGzc, September, 2014.

changing children's menus to include steamed vegetables, fruit cups, and broiled or grilled chicken—additions welcomed by busy parents who often dine out or purchase take-out foods.

Other fatty foods—such as nuts, vegetable oils, and some varieties of fish such as tuna or salmon—contribute essential fatty acids. Low-fat milk and milk products also deserve special attention in a child's diet for the needed calcium and other nutrients they supply.

Parents and caregivers play a key role in helping children establish healthy eating habits. Balanced meals need to provide lean meat, poultry, fish, and legumes; fruit and vegetables; whole grains; and low-fat milk products. Such meals can provide enough energy and nutrients to support growth and maintain blood cholesterol within a healthy range.

Pediatricians warn parents to avoid extremes. Although intentions may be good, excessive food restriction may create nutrient deficiencies and impair growth. Furthermore, parental control over eating may instigate battles and foster attitudes about foods that can lead to inappropriate eating behaviors.

Do pediatricians ever prescribe drugs to lower blood cholesterol in children?

Experts agree that children with high blood cholesterol should first be treated with diet. If high blood cholesterol persists despite dietary intervention in children 10 years of age and older, then drugs may be necessary to lower blood cholesterol. Drugs can effectively lower blood cholesterol without interfering with adolescent growth or development.

Can parents or caregivers do anything else to help children reduce their risks of CVD?

Even though the focus of this text is nutrition, another risk factor for heart disease that starts in childhood and carries over into adulthood—cigarette smoking—must also be addressed. Each day more than 3000 young people between the ages of 12 and 17 light up for the first time, and an estimated 2000 become daily cigarette smokers.[20] Among high school students, about 20 percent use some type of tobacco product (electronic cigarettes, cigars, smokeless tobacco, pipes). Approximately 90 percent of all adult smokers began smoking before the age of 18.

Of those teenagers who continue smoking, half will eventually die of smoking-related causes. Efforts to teach children about the dangers of smoking need to be aggressive. Children are not likely to consider the long-term health consequences of tobacco use. They are more likely to be struck by the immediate health consequences, such as shortness of breath when playing sports, or social consequences, such as having bad breath. Whatever the context, the message to all children and teens should be clear: Don't start smoking. If you've already started, quit.

In conclusion, *adult* heart disease is a major *pediatric* problem. Without intervention, some 60 million children are destined to suffer its consequences within the next 30 years. Optimal prevention efforts focus on children, especially on those who are overweight. Just as young children receive vaccinations against infectious diseases, they need screening for, and education about, chronic diseases. Many health education programs have been implemented in schools around the country. These programs are most effective when they include education in the classroom, heart-healthy meals in the lunchroom, fitness activities on the playground, and parental involvement at home.

Notes

1. C. M. Hales and coauthors, Prevalence of obesity among adults and youth: United States, 2015–2016, *NCHS Data Brief*, no. 288 (Hyattsville, MD: National Center for Health Statistics, 2017); C.L. Ogden and coauthors, Trends in obesity prevalence among children and adolescents in the United States, 1988–1994 through 2013–2014, *Journal of the American Medical Association* 315 (2016): 2292–2299; D. Dabelea and coauthors, Prevalence of type 1 and type 2 diabetes among children and adolescents from 2001 to 2009, *Journal of the American Medical Association* 311 (2014): 1778–1786; N. K. Güngör, Overweight and obesity in children and adolescents, *Journal of Clinical Research in Pediatric Endocrinology* 6 (2014): 129–143.

2. M. Ezzati and coauthors, Worldwide trends in body-mass index, underweight, overweight, and obesity from 1975 to 2016: A pooled analysis of 2416 population-based measurement studies in 128.9 million children, adolescents, and adults, Lancet, 2017, DOI: dx.doi.org/10.1016/S0140-6736(17)32129-3; World Health Organization, Global strategy on diet, physical activity and health, Childhood overweight and obesity, www.who.int/dietphysicalactivity/childhood/en/, 2017.

3. T. Lobstein and R. Jackson-Leach, Planning for the worst: Estimates of obesity and comorbidities in school-age children in 2025, *Pediatric Obesity* 11 (2016): 321–325; G. Twig and coauthors, Body mass index at age 17 and diabetes mortality in midlife: A nationwide cohort of 2.3 million adolescents, *Diabetes* Care 39 (2016): 1996–2003; E. D. Parker and coauthors, Change in weight status and development of hypertension, *Pediatrics* 137 (2016): e20151662; A. C. Skinner and coauthors, Cardiometabolic risks and severity of obesity in children and young adults, *New England Journal of Medicine* 373 (2015): 1307–1317; N. Mangner and coauthors, Childhood obesity: Impact on cardiac geometry and function, *Journal of the American College of Cardiology*, 2014, doi: 10.101016/j.jcmg.2014.08.006; K. R. Armstrong and coauthors, Childhood obesity, arterial stiffness, and prevalence and treatment of hypertension, *Current Treatment Options in Cardiovascular Medicine* 16 (2014): 339.

4. W. H. Dietz, C. E. Douglas, and R. C. Brownson, Chronic disease prevention: Tobacco avoidance, physical activity, and nutrition for a healthy start, *Journal of the American Medical Association* 316 (2016): 1645–1646; R. D. Telford and coauthors, Sensitivity of blood lipids to changes in adiposity, exercise, and diet in children, *Medicine and Science in Sports and Exercise* 47 (2015): 974–982; Skinner and coauthors, 2015.

5. Dietz, Douglas, and Brownson, 2016; A. Llewellyn and coauthors, Childhood obesity as a predictor of morbidity in adulthood: A systematic review and meta-analysis, *Obesity Reviews* 17 (2016): 56–67; C. Y. Lee and coauthors, Association of parental overweight and cardiometabolic diseases and pediatric adiposity and lifestyle factors with cardiovascular risk factor clustering adolescents, *Nutrients* 8 (2016): 567; Mangner and coauthors, 2014; Güngor, 2014.

6. M. G. Clemente and coauthors, Pediatric non-alcoholic fatty liver disease: Recent solutions, unresolved issues, and future research directions, *World Journal of Gastroenterology* 22 (2016): 8078–8093.

7. C. Berti and coauthors, Early-life nutritional exposures and lifelong health: Immediate and long-lasting impacts of probiotics, vitamin D, and breastfeeding, *Nutrition Reviews* 75 (2017): 83–97; D. Ley and coauthors, Early-life origin of intestinal inflammatory disorders, *Nutrition Reviews* 75 (2017): 175–187; J. G. O. Avila and coauthors, Impact of oxidative stress during pregnancy on fetal epigenetic patterns and early origin of vascular diseases, *Nutrition Reviews* 73 (2015): 12–21; J. Zheng and coauthors, DNA methylation: The pivotal interaction between early-life nutrition and glucose metabolism in later life, *British Journal of Nutrition* 112 (2014): 1850–1857; T. L. Crume and coauthors, The long-term impact of intrauterine growth restriction in a diverse U.S. cohort of children; The EPOCH study, *Obesity* (Silver Springs) 22 (2014): 608–615.

8. B. T. Alexander, J. H. Dasinger, and S. Intapad, Fetal programming and cardiovascular pathology, *Comprehensive Physiology* 5 (2015): 997–1025.

9. Llewellyn and coauthors, 2016; B. Tobisch, L. Blatniczky, and L. Barkai, Cardiometabolic risk factors and insulin resistance in obese children and adolescents: Relation to puberty, *Pediatric Obesity* 10 (2015): 37–44.

10. Tobisch, Blatniczky, and Barkai, 2015; N. F. Butte and coauthors, Global metabolomics profiling targeting childhood obesity in the Hispanic population, *American Journal of Clinical Nutrition* 102 (2015): 256–267.

11. Lobstein and Jackson-Leach, 2016; Llewellyn and coauthors, 2016; K. A. LaBresh and coauthors, Adoption of cardiovascular risk reduction guidelines: A cluster-randomized trial, *Pediatrics* 134 (2014): e732–e738.

12. S. S. Gidding and coauthors, American Heart Association Atherosclerosis, Hypertension, and Obesity in Young Committee of Council on Cardiovascular Disease in Young, Council on Cardiovascular and Stroke Nursing, Council on Functional Genomics and Translational Biology, and Council on Lifestyle and Cardiometabolic Health, The agenda for familial hypercholesterolemia: A Scientific Statement from the American Heart Association, *Circulation* 132 (2015): 2167–2192.

13. U.S. Preventive Services Task Force, Screening for lipid disorders in children and adolescents, US Preventive Services Task Force Recommendation Statement, *Journal of the American Medical Association* 316 (2016): 625–633.

14. J. T. Flynn and coauthors, Clinical practice guideline for screening and management of high blood pressure in children and adolescents, *Pediatrics* 140 (2017): e20171904.

15. L. J. Appel and coauthors, Reducing sodium intake in children: A public health investment, *Journal of Clinical Hypertension* 17 (2015): 657–662.

16. B. Gopinath and coauthors, Activity behaviors in schoolchildren and subsequent 5-yr change in blood pressure, *Medicine and Science in Sports and Exercise* 46 (2014): 724–729.

17. R. Telama and coauthors, Tracking of physical activity from early childhood through youth into adulthood, *Medicine and Science in Sports and Exercise* 46 (2014): 955–962.

18. M. B. Vos and coauthors, Added sugars and cardiovascular disease risk in children, A Scientific Statement from the American Heart Association, *Circulation* 135 (2017): e1017–e1034; K. P. Kell and coauthors, Added sugars in the diet are positively associated with diastolic blood pressure and triglycerides in children, *American Journal of Clinical Nutrition* 100 (2014): 46–52.

19. M. Altman and coauthors, Reduction in food away from home is associated with improved child relative weight and body composition outcomes and this relation is mediated by changes in diet quality, *Journal of the Academy of Nutrition and Dietetics* 115 (2015): 1400–1407.

20. Centers for Disease Control and Prevention, Youth and tobacco use, www.cdc.gov/tobacco/data_statistics/fact_sheets/youth_data/tobacco_use/index.htm, updated September 20, 2017.

Nutrition through the Life Span: Later Adulthood

Chapter Sections and Learning Objectives (LOs)

Ulrich Kerth/StockFood Creative/Getty Images

chapter

12

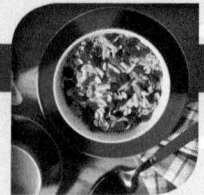

that require special nutrition attention: pregnancy, lactation, infancy, childhood, and adolescence. Much of the text before that focused on nutrition to support wellness during adulthood. This chapter describes the special nutrition needs of the later adult years.

The most urgent nutrition need of older people, however, is to have made good food choices in the past! All of life's nutrition choices incur health consequences for the better or for the worse. A single day's intake of nutrients may exert only a minute effect on body organs and their functions, but, over years and decades, the repeated effects accumulate to have major impacts. This being the case, it is of great importance for everyone, of every age, to pay close attention today to nutrition.

The "graying" of America is a continuing trend. The majority of citizens are now middle aged, and the ratio of old people to young is increasing, as Figure 12-1 shows. Our society uses the arbitrary age of 65 to define the transition point between middle age and old age, but growing "old" happens day by day, with changes occurring gradually over time. Commonly used age groups include young old (65–74 years), old (75–84 years), and oldest old (≥85 years).

Since 1950 the population older than age 65 has almost tripled. Remarkably, the fastest-growing age group has been people older than age 85; since 1950 their numbers have increased sevenfold. The U.S. Bureau of the Census projects that by the year 2040 more than a million Americans will be 100 years old or older.

Life expectancy in the United States is 79 years, up from about 47 years in 1900.[1] Advances in medical science—antibiotics and other treatments—are largely responsible for almost doubling the life expectancy in the 20th century. Improved nutrition and an abundant food supply have also contributed to lengthening life expectancy. Ironically, this abundant food supply has also jeopardized the chances of further lengthening life expectancy as obesity rates increase.[2]

The human **life span**, currently estimated at 125 years, is the upper limit of human **longevity**, even given optimal nutrition. With work progressing in medical and genetic technologies, however, the human life span may be extended significantly.

Research in the field of aging is active—and difficult. Researchers are challenged by the diversity of older adults. When older adults experience health problems, it is hard to know whether to attribute these problems to genetics, aging, or other environmental factors such as nutrition. The idea that nutrition can influence the way the human body ages is particularly appealing because diet is a factor that people can control and change.

12.1 Nutrition and Longevity

What has been learned so far about the effects of nutrition and environment on longevity provides incentive for researchers to keep asking questions about how and why human beings age. Among their questions are:

- To what extent is aging inevitable, and can it be slowed through changes in lifestyle and environment?
- What role does nutrition play in the aging process, and what role can it play in slowing aging?

With respect to the first question, it seems that aging is an inevitable, natural process, programmed into the genes at conception. People can, however, slow the process within

---

FIGURE 12-1 The Aging of the U.S. Population

In 1940, 6.8 percent of the population was age 65 or older. In 1990, 12.7 percent of us had reached age 65; by 2040, 21.7 percent will have reached age 65; and by 2090, nearly one out of four Americans will be age 65 or older.

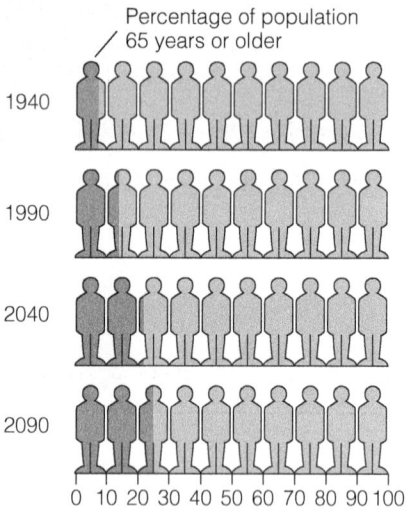

Percentage of population 65 years or older

1940

1990

2040

2090

0 10 20 30 40 50 60 70 80 90 100
Percentage of total population

life expectancy: the average number of years lived by people in a given society.

life span: the maximum number of years of life attainable by a member of a species.

longevity: long duration of life.

the natural limits set by heredity by adopting healthy lifestyle habits such as following a dietary pattern that emphasizes plant-based foods and engaging in physical activity. In fact, a person's life expectancy depends on both individual health-related behaviors and genes.[3]

With respect to the second question, good nutrition helps to maintain a healthy body and can therefore ease the aging process in many significant ways.[4] Clearly, nutrition can improve the **quality of life** in the later years.[5]

Slowing the Aging Process

One approach researchers use to search out the secret of long life is to study older people. Some people are young for their ages, whereas others are old for their ages. What makes the difference?

Healthy Habits Some lifestyle habits seem to have a profound influence on people's health and therefore on their **physiological age**:[6]

- Following a healthy, plant-based eating pattern such as the Mediterranean diet (rich in fruit, vegetables, whole grains, legumes, poultry, fish, and low-fat milk products)[7]
- Maintaining a healthy body weight
- Engaging in regular physical activity daily
- Not smoking
- Not using alcohol, or using it in moderation
- Sleeping regularly and adequately
- Having a sense of purpose
- Relieving stress (through meditation, prayer, naps, or other calming activity)
- Belonging to a community of loving family and friends (home, church, or other social network)

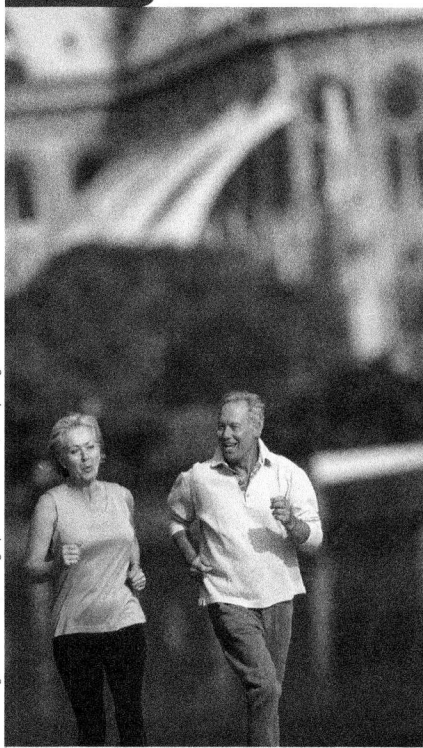

Photo 12-1

Regular physical activity promotes a healthy, independent lifestyle.

Over the years, the effects of these lifestyle choices accumulate—that is, those who follow all of these practices live longer and have fewer disabilities as they age. They are in better health, even if older in **chronological age**, than people who do not adopt these behaviors. Even though people cannot alter their birth dates, they may be able to add years to, and enhance the quality of, their lives. Physical activity seems to be most influential in preventing or slowing the many changes that many people seem to accept as an inevitable consequence of old age (see Photo 12-1). In other words, physical activity and long life seem to go together.[8]

Physical Activity The many and remarkable benefits of regular physical activity are not limited to the young. Compared with those who are inactive, older adults who are active weigh less; have greater flexibility, more endurance, better balance, and better health; and live longer.[9] They reap additional benefits from various types of activities as well: Aerobic activities improve cardiorespiratory endurance, blood pressure, and blood lipid concentrations; moderate endurance activities improve the quality of sleep; and resistance training significantly improves posture and mobility.[10] In fact, regular physical activity is a powerful predictor of a person's mobility in the later years (Box 12-1).[11] Mobility, in turn, is closely associated with longevity. Physical activity also increases blood flow to the brain, thereby preserving mental ability, alleviating depression, and supporting independence.[12]

Muscle mass and muscle strength tend to decline with aging, making older people vulnerable to falls and immobility (Box 12-2). Falls are a major cause of fear, injury, disability, dependence, and even death among older adults. Regular physical activity tones, firms, and strengthens muscles, helping to improve confidence, reduce the risk of falling, and minimize the risk of injury should a fall occur.[13]

Even without a fall, older adults may become so weak that they can no longer perform life's daily tasks, such as climbing stairs, carrying packages, and opening jars. Resistance training helps older adults to maintain independence by strengthening the muscles needed to perform these tasks.[14] Even in frail, elderly people older than

quality of life: a person's perceived physical and mental well-being.

physiological age: a person's age as estimated from her or his body's health and probable life expectancy.

chronological age: a person's age in years from his or her date of birth.

BOX 12-1 *Nursing Diagnosis*

The nursing diagnosis *impaired physical mobility* applies to clients with slowed movement, decreased muscle mass, and decreased muscle strength.

BOX 12-2 *Nursing Diagnosis*

The nursing diagnosis *risk for falls* applies to clients who are 65 years of age or older, those who have a history of falls, those who live alone, and those who use assistive devices such as a walker or a cane.

85 years of age, resistance training has been shown not only to improve balance, muscle strength, and mobility but also to increase energy expenditure and energy intake. This finding highlights another reason to be physically active: A person spending energy on physical activity can afford to eat more food and, with it, more nutrients. People who are committed to an ongoing fitness program can benefit from higher energy and nutrient intakes and still maintain healthy body weights.

Ideally, physical activity should be part of each day's schedule and should be intense enough to prevent muscle loss and to speed up the heartbeat and respiration rate. Although aging affects both speed and endurance to some degree, older adults can still train and achieve exceptional performances. Healthy older adults who have not been active can ease into a suitable routine. They can start by walking short distances until they are walking at least 10 minutes continuously and then gradually increase the distance to a 30- to 60-minute walk at least five days a week. With persistence, people can achieve great improvements at any age. Table 12-1 provides exercise goals and guidelines for older adults. Relatively few older adults meet these goals. People with medical conditions should check with a physician before beginning an exercise routine, as should sedentary men older than 40 and sedentary women older than 50 who want to participate in a vigorous program.

TABLE 12-1 Exercise Guidelines for Older Adults

	AEROBIC	STRENGTH	BALANCE	FLEXIBILITY
Examples	Geoff Manasse/PhotoDisc/PictureQuest/Jupiter Images	IT Stock Free/PictureQuest/Jupiter Images	IT Stock Free/PictureQuest/Jupiter Images	Ron Chapple/Thinkstock/PictureQuest/Jupiter Images
Start easy and progress gradually	Be active five minutes on most or all days	Using 0- to 2-pound weights, do one set of 8–12 repetitions twice a week	Hold onto table or chair with one hand, then with one finger	Hold stretch for 10 seconds; do each stretch three times
Frequency	At least five days per week of moderate activity or at least four days per week of vigorous activity	At least two (nonconsecutive) days per week	Two to three days each week	At least two days per week, preferably on all days that aerobic or strength activities are performed
Intensity[a]	Moderate, vigorous, or combination	Moderate to high; 10 to 15 repetitions per exercise	—	Moderate
Duration	At least 30 minutes of moderate activity in bouts of at least 10 minutes each or at least 20 minutes of continuous vigorous activity	Eight to 10 exercises involving the major muscle groups	—	Stretch major muscle groups for 10–30 seconds, repeating each stretch three to four times
Cautions and comments	Stop if you are breathing so hard you can't talk or if you feel dizziness or chest pain	Breathe out as you contract and in as you relax (do not hold your breath); use smooth, steady movements	Incorporate balance techniques with strength exercises as you progress	Stretch after strength and endurance exercises for 20 minutes, three times a week; use slow, steady movements; bend joints slightly

[a]On a 10-point scale, where 0 = sitting; 5–6 = moderate intensity; 7–8 = vigorous intensity; and 10 = maximum effort.

Note: Activity recommendations are in addition to routine activities of daily living (such as getting dressed, cooking, and grocery shopping) and moderate activities lasting less than 10 minutes.

Sources: C. E. Garber and coauthors, Quantity and quality of exercise for developing and maintaining cardiorespiratory, musculoskeletal, and neuromotor fitness in apparently healthy adults: Guidance for prescribing exercise, *Medicine and Science in Sports and Exercise* 43 (2011): 1334–1359; W. J. Chodzko-Zajko and coauthors, Position Stand of the American College of Sports Medicine: Exercise and physical activity for older adults, *Medicine and Science in Sports and Exercise* 41 (2009): 1510–1530.

Restriction of kCalories In their efforts to understand longevity, researchers have not only observed people but have also manipulated influencing factors, such as diet, in animals. This research has produced some interesting and suggestive findings. For example, animals live longer and have fewer age-related diseases when their energy intakes are restricted.[15] These life-prolonging benefits become evident when the diet provides enough food to prevent malnutrition and an energy intake of about 70 percent of normal; benefits decline as the age at which energy restriction begins is delayed.

Exactly how energy restriction prolongs life remains unexplained, although gene activity appears to play a key role. Energy restriction in animals prevents alterations in gene expression that are associated with aging.[16] Food restriction may also extend the life span by preventing damaging lipid oxidation, thereby delaying the onset of age-related diseases such as cancer and atherosclerosis.

Moderate energy restriction (80 to 90 percent of usual intake) in human beings may be valuable. When people restrict energy intake moderately, body weight, body fat, and blood pressure drop, and blood lipids and insulin response improve—favorable changes for preventing chronic diseases. The reduction in oxidative damage that occurs with energy restriction in animals also occurs in people whose diets include antioxidant nutrients and phytochemicals. Diets such as the Mediterranean diet that include an abundance of fruit, vegetables, olive oil, whole grains, and legumes—with their array of antioxidants and phytochemicals—support good health and long life.[17]

Nutrition and Disease Prevention

Nutrition alone, even if ideal, cannot ensure a long and robust life. Nevertheless, nutrition clearly affects aging and longevity in human beings by way of its role in disease prevention. Among the better-known relationships between nutrition and disease are the following:

- Appropriate energy intake helps prevent *obesity, diabetes,* and related *cardiovascular diseases* such as atherosclerosis and hypertension (Chapters 7, 20, and 21) and may influence the development of some forms of *cancer* (Chapter 23).
- Adequate intakes of essential nutrients prevent *deficiency diseases* such as scurvy, goiter, and anemia (Chapters 8 and 9).
- Variety in food intake, as well as ample intakes of certain fruit and vegetables, may be protective against certain types of *cancer* (Chapter 23).
- Moderation in sugar intake helps prevent *dental caries* (Nutrition in Practice 17).
- Appropriate fiber intakes may help prevent disorders of the digestive tract such as *constipation, diverticulosis,* and possibly *colon cancer* (Chapters 3, 18, and 23).
- Moderate sodium intake and adequate intakes of potassium, calcium, and other minerals help prevent *hypertension* (Chapters 9 and 21).
- An adequate calcium intake throughout life helps protect against *osteoporosis* (Chapter 9).

Other, less well-established links between nutrition and disease are being discovered each day. Research that focuses on how life factors affect aging and disease processes is vital to ensuring that more and more people can look forward to long, healthy lives.

Review Notes

- Life expectancy in the United States increased dramatically in the 20th century.
- Factors that enhance longevity include limited or no alcohol use, a plant-based eating pattern, weight management, adequate sleep, abstinence from smoking, and regular physical activity.
- Nutrition alone, even if ideal, cannot guarantee a long and robust life. At the very least, however, nutrition—especially when combined with regular physical activity—can influence aging and longevity in human beings by supporting good health and preventing disease.

12.2 Nutrition-Related Concerns during Late Adulthood

Nutrition through the prime years may play a greater role than has been realized in preventing many changes once thought to be inevitable consequences of growing older. The following discussions of cataracts and macular degeneration, arthritis, and the aging brain show that nutrition may provide at least some protection against some of the conditions commonly associated with aging.

Cataracts and Macular Degeneration

Cataracts are age-related thickenings in the lenses of the eye that impair vision. If not surgically removed, they ultimately lead to blindness. Oxidative stress appears to play a significant role in the development of cataracts but supplements of the antioxidant nutrients (vitamin C, vitamin E, and carotenoids) do not seem to prevent or slow the progression.[18] By comparison, a healthy diet that includes plenty of fruit and vegetables rich in these antioxidants does seem to slow the progression or reduce the risk of developing cataracts.[19]

Cataracts may develop as a result of ultraviolet lights exposure, oxidative damage, viral infections, toxic substances, genetic disorders, injury, or other trauma. Most cataracts are vaguely called "senile" cataracts, meaning "caused by aging." In the United States, half of all adults have a cataract by age 75.

One other diet-related factor may play a role in cataract development: obesity.[20] How obesity may influence the development of cataracts is not known. Risk factors that typically accompany overweight, such as inactivity, diabetes, or hypertension, do not explain the association.

The leading cause of visual loss among older people is **macular degeneration**, a deterioration of the macular region of the eye. As with cataracts, risk factors for age-related macular degeneration include oxidative stress from sunlight. A supplement containing the antioxidant vitamins C and E, and the minerals copper and zinc has been shown to reduce the risk of progression of macular degeneration in those who already have the disease.[21] Limited research suggests that folate, vitamin B_6, vitamin B_{12}, and the carotenoids lutein and zeaxanthin may help prevent macular degeneration or slow its progression, but more research is needed to confirm these possible relationships.

Arthritis

More than 54 million people in the United States have some form of **arthritis**.[22] As the population ages, it is expected that the prevalence will increase to 72 million by 2030. The most common type of arthritis that disables older people is **osteoarthritis**, a painful swelling of the joints. During movement, the ends of bones are normally protected from wear by cartilage and by small sacs of fluid that lubricate the joint. With age, the cartilage sometimes disintegrates, and the joints become malformed and painful to move.

Obesity is common among adults with arthritis.[23] Weight loss can help overweight people with osteoarthritis, partly because the joints affected are often weight-bearing joints that are stressed and irritated by having to carry excess poundage. Interestingly, though, weight loss often relieves the worst pain of osteoarthritis in the hands as well, even though they are not weight-bearing joints. Importantly, walking and other weight-bearing activities do not worsen osteoarthritis. In fact, low-impact aerobic activity and resistance training offer modest improvements in physical performance and pain relief, especially when accompanied by even modest weight loss.[24]

Traditional medical intervention for arthritis includes medication and surgery. Two popular supplements for treating osteoarthritis—glucosamine and chondroitin—may alleviate pain and improve mobility, but mixed reports from studies emphasize the

cataracts: clouding of the eye lenses that impairs vision and can lead to blindness.

macular (MACK-you-lar) degeneration: deterioration of the macular area of the eye that can lead to loss of central vision and eventual blindness. The **macula** is a small, oval, yellowish region in the center of the retina that provides the sharp, straight-ahead vision so critical to reading and driving.

arthritis: inflammation of a joint, usually accompanied by pain, swelling, and structural changes.

osteoarthritis: a painful, chronic disease of the joints that occurs when the cushioning cartilage in a joint breaks down; joint structure is usually altered, with loss of function; also called *degenerative arthritis*.

need for additional research.[25] Drugs and supplements used to relieve arthritis can impose nutrition risks; some affect appetite and alter the body's use of nutrients, as Chapter 14 explains.

Another type of arthritis, known as **rheumatoid arthritis**, has a possible link to diet through the immune system. In rheumatoid arthritis, the immune system mistakenly attacks the bone coverings as if they were made of foreign tissue. In some individuals, certain foods, notably a Mediterranean-type diet of fish, vegetables, and olive oil, may moderate the inflammatory responses and provide some relief.

The omega-3 fatty acids commonly found in fish oil may help prevent rheumatoid arthritis as well as reduce joint tenderness and improve mobility in some people with the condition.[26] The same diet recommended for heart health—one low in saturated fat from meats and milk products and high in omega-3 fats from fish—helps prevent or reduce the inflammation in the joints that makes arthritis so painful.

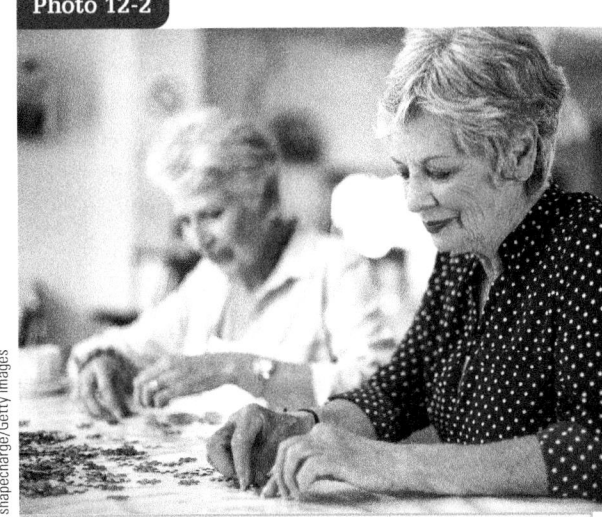

Photo 12-2

shapecharge/Getty Images

Both foods and mental challenges nourish the brain.

The Aging Brain

Dementia affects an estimated 15 percent of adults older than 70 years of age in the United States and represents a financial burden of hundreds of billions of dollars. The brain, like all of the body's organs, ages in response to both genetic and environmental factors—such as physical activities, intellectual challenges, social interactions, and nutritious diets—that enhance or diminish its amazing capacities (see Photo 12-2).[27] One of the challenges researchers face when studying the aging of the human brain is to distinguish among changes caused by normal, age-related, physiological processes; changes caused by diseases; and changes caused by cumulative, environmental factors such as diet.

The brain normally changes in some characteristic ways as it ages. For one thing, its blood supply decreases. For another, the number of **neurons**, the brain cells that specialize in transmitting information, diminishes as people age. Losses of neurons affect different functions depending on their location in the brain. For example, declines in the number of nerve cells in one part of the **cerebral cortex** affect hearing and speech, while losses in other parts of the cortex can impair memory and cognitive function. When the number of neurons in the hindbrain diminishes, balance and posture are affected.

Nutrient Deficiencies and Brain Function   Clinicians now recognize that much of the cognitive loss and forgetfulness generally attributed to aging is due in part to environmental, and therefore controllable, factors such as nutrient deficiencies. The ability of neurons to synthesize specific neurotransmitters depends in part on the availability of precursor nutrients that are obtained from the diet. The neurotransmitter serotonin, for example, derives from the amino acid tryptophan. In addition, the enzymes involved in neurotransmitter synthesis require vitamins and minerals to function properly. The B vitamins folate, vitamin B_6, and vitamin B_{12} slow brain atrophy and improve cognition and memory.[28] Some, but not all, research suggests that the essential fatty acid DHA may help to counteract the cognitive decline commonly seen in older adults.[29] Thus, nutrient deficiencies may contribute to the loss of memory and cognition that some older adults experience.[30] Such losses may be preventable or at least diminished or delayed through diet and physical activity. Healthy eating patterns such as the Mediterranean diet, seem to slow cognitive decline and lower the risk of dementia.[31]

In some instances, the degree of cognitive loss is extensive. Such **senile dementia** may be attributable to a specific disorder such as a brain tumor or Alzheimer's disease.

Alzheimer's Disease   In **Alzheimer's disease**, the most prevalent form of dementia, brain cell death occurs in the areas of the brain that coordinate memory and cognition.

rheumatoid arthritis: a disease of the immune system involving painful inflammation of the joints and related structures.

neurons: nerve cells; the structural and functional units of the nervous system. Neurons initiate and conduct nerve transmissions.

cerebral cortex: the outer surface of the cerebrum, which is the largest part of the brain.

senile dementia: the loss of brain function beyond the normal loss of physical adeptness and memory that occurs with aging.

Alzheimer's disease: a progressive, degenerative disease that attacks the brain and impairs thinking, behavior, and memory.

TABLE 12-2 Signs of Alzheimer's and Typical Age-Related Changes Compared

SIGNS OF ALZHEIMER'S	TYPICAL AGE-RELATED CHANGES
Memory loss that disrupts daily life such as asking for the same information repeatedly or asking others to handle tasks of daily living	Forgetting a name or missing an appointment
Challenges in planning or solving problems such as following a recipe or paying monthly bills	Missing a monthly payment or making an error when balancing the checkbook
Difficulty completing familiar tasks at home such as using the microwave, at work such as preparing a report, or at leisure such as playing a game	Needing help recording a television program
Confusion with time or place including current season and location	Not knowing today's date
Trouble understanding visual images and spatial relationships such as judging distances and recognizing self in a mirror	Experiencing visual changes due to cataracts
New problems with words in speaking or writing such as not knowing the name of a common object	Being unable to find the right word to use
Misplacing things and losing the ability to retrace steps such as putting the milk in the closet and having no idea when or where the milk was last seen	Misplacing a pair of glasses or the car keys
Decreased or poor judgment such as giving large sums of money to strangers	Making a bad decision on occasion
Withdrawal from work projects or social activities	Feeling too tired to participate in work, family, or social activities
Changes in mood and personality such as confusion, suspicion, depression, and anxiety, especially when in unfamiliar places or with unfamiliar people	Becoming irritable when routines are disrupted

Source: Adapted from Alzheimer's Association, www.alz.org/alzheimers_disease_10_signs_of_alzheimers.asp.

BOX 12-3 *Nursing Diagnosis*

The nursing diagnosis *chronic confusion* applies to clients with Alzheimer's disease.

Alzheimer's disease afflicts more than five million people in the United States, and that number is expected to triple by the year 2050.[32] Diagnosis of Alzheimer's depends on its characteristic symptoms: The victim gradually loses memory, reasoning ability, the ability to communicate, physical capabilities, and, eventually, life itself (Box 12-3). Table 12-2 compares the signs of Alzheimer's disease with typical age-related changes.

The primary risk factor for Alzheimer's disease is age, but the exact cause remains unknown. Clearly, genetic factors are involved. Free radicals and oxidative stress also seem to be involved. Nerve cells in the brains of people with Alzheimer's disease show evidence of free-radical attack—damage to DNA, cell membranes, and proteins—and of the minerals that trigger these attacks—iron, copper, zinc, and aluminum. Some research suggests that the antioxidant nutrients can limit free-radical damage and delay or prevent Alzheimer's disease, but more research is needed to confirm this possibility.[33]

Increasing evidence also suggests that overweight and obesity in middle age are associated with dementia in general, and with Alzheimer's disease in particular.[34] The possible relationship between obesity and Alzheimer's disease is disturbing given the current obesity epidemic. Efforts to prevent and treat obesity, however, may also help prevent Alzheimer's disease.

In Alzheimer's disease, the brain develops **senile plaques** and **neurofibrillary tangles**. Senile plaques are clumps of a protein fragment called beta-amyloid, whereas neurofibrillary tangles are snarls of the fibers that extend from the nerve cells. Both seem to occur in response to oxidative stress. The accumulation of beta-amyloid seems to be a consequence of both excessive production and impaired clearance.[35] Treatment research focuses on lowering beta-amyloid levels.

Cardiovascular disease risk factors such as high blood pressure, diabetes, obesity, smoking, and physical inactivity are associated with the development of Alzheimer's disease.[36] Diets designed to support a healthy heart, which include the omega-3 fatty acids of oily fish, may benefit brain health as well.[37] Similarly, physical activity supports heart health and slows the cognitive decline of Alzheimer's disease.[38]

Treatment for Alzheimer's disease involves providing care to clients and support to their families. Drugs are used to improve or at least to slow the loss of short-term memory and cognition, but they do not cure the disease. Other drugs may be used to control depression, anxiety, and behavior problems.

Maintaining appropriate body weight may be the most important nutrition concern for the person with Alzheimer's disease. Depression and forgetfulness can lead to changes in eating behaviors and poor food intake. Furthermore, changes in the body's weight-regulation system may contribute to weight loss. Perhaps the best that a caregiver can do nutritionally for a person with Alzheimer's disease is to supervise food planning and mealtimes. Providing well-liked and well-balanced meals and snacks in a cheerful atmosphere encourages food consumption. To minimize confusion, offer a few ready-to-eat foods, in bite-size pieces, with seasonings and sauces. To avoid mealtime disruptions, control distractions such as music, television, children, and the telephone.

senile plaques: clumps of the protein fragment beta-amyloid on the nerve cells, commonly found in the brains of people with Alzheimer's dementia.

neurofibrillary tangles: snarls of the threadlike strands that extend from the nerve cells, commonly found in the brains of people with Alzheimer's dementia.

Review Notes

- Cataracts, age-related macular degeneration, and arthritis afflict millions of older adults, while others face senile dementia and other losses of brain function.
- Oxidative stress plays a significant role in the development of cataracts, and the antioxidant nutrients and phytochemicals in fruit and vegetables may help minimize the damage.
- Weight loss can help overweight people with osteoarthritis. For some people with rheumatoid arthritis, a Mediterranean-type diet of fish, vegetables, and olive oil may moderate the inflammatory responses and provide some relief.
- Nutrient deficiencies may contribute to the loss of memory and cognition that some older adults experience. Such losses may be preventable or at least diminished or delayed through diet.
- The primary risk factor for Alzheimer's disease is age, but the exact cause remains unknown.

12.3 Energy and Nutrient Needs during Late Adulthood

Knowledge about the nutrient needs and nutrition status of older adults has grown considerably in recent years. The Dietary Reference Intakes (DRI) cluster people older than age 50 into two categories: 51 to 70 years old and 71 years and older. Research is showing that the nutrition needs of people 50 to 70 years old may be very different from those of people older than 70—a pattern that makes sense considering the wide age span involved.

Setting standards for older people is difficult, though, because individual differences become more pronounced as people grow older. People start out with different

TABLE 12-3	Examples of Physical Changes of Aging That Affect Nutrition
Mouth	Tooth loss, gum disease, and reduced salivary output impede chewing and swallowing. Swallowing disorders and choking may become likely. Discomfort and pain associated with eating may reduce food intake.
Digestive tract	Intestines lose muscle strength, resulting in sluggish motility that leads to constipation (see Chapter 18). Stomach inflammation, abnormal bacterial growth, and greatly reduced acid output impair digestion and absorption. Pain may cause food avoidance or reduced intake.
Hormones	For example, the pancreas secretes less insulin and cells become less responsive, causing abnormal glucose metabolism.
Sensory organs	Diminished senses of smell and taste can reduce appetite; diminished sight can make food shopping and preparation difficult.
Body composition	Weight loss and decline in lean body mass lead to lowered energy requirements. May be preventable or reversible through physical activity.
Urinary tract	Increased frequency of urination may limit fluid intake.

genetic predispositions and ways of handling nutrients, and the effects of these differences become magnified with years of unique dietary habits. For example, one person may tend to omit fruit and vegetables from his diet, and by the time he is old, he may have a set of nutrition problems associated with a lack of fiber and antioxidants. Another person who omitted milk and milk products all her life may have nutrition problems related to a lack of calcium. Also, as people age, they may suffer different chronic diseases and take different medications—both have impacts on nutrient needs. Table 12-3 lists some changes of aging that can affect nutrition. For all these reasons, researchers have difficulty even defining "healthy aging," a prerequisite to developing recommendations that are designed to meet the "needs of practically all healthy persons." Still, some generalizations are valid. The next sections give special attention to a few nutrients of concern.

FIGURE 12-2 Sarcopenia

These cross-sections of two women's thighs may appear to be about the same size from the outside, but the 20-year-old woman's thigh (left) is dense with muscle tissue. The 64-year-old woman's thigh (right) has lost muscle and gained fat, changes that may be largely preventable with strength-building physical activities.

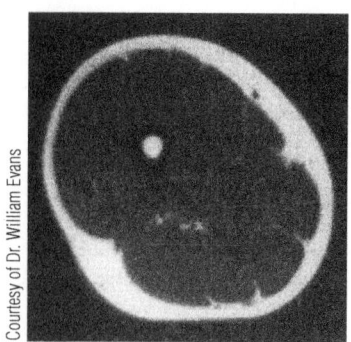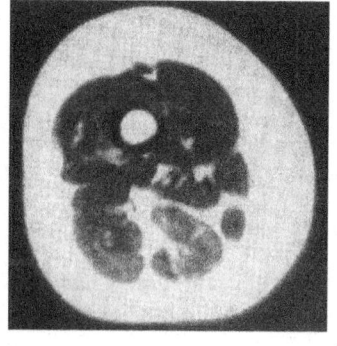

Courtesy of Dr. William Evans

sarcopenia (SAR-koh-PEE-nee-ah): age-related loss of skeletal muscle mass, muscle strength, and muscle function.

Energy and Energy Nutrients

Energy needs decline with advancing age. As a general rule, adult energy needs decline an estimated 5 percent per decade. One reason is that people usually reduce their physical activity as they age, although they need not do so. Another reason is that basal metabolic rate declines 1 to 2 percent per decade, in part because lean body mass and thyroid hormones diminish. Loss of muscle mass, known as **sarcopenia**, can be significant in the later years (its prevalence is more than 50 percent among those older than age 80) and its consequences, dramatic (see Figure 12-2).[39]

Sarcopenia is often accompanied by a gain in body fat. Research is underway to determine whether excess body fat in those with sarcopenia is detrimental to, or protective of, physical function.[40] As skeletal muscle mass diminishes, people lose their ability to move and to maintain balance, making falls likely. The limitations that accompany the loss of muscle mass and strength play a key role in the diminishing health that often accompanies aging. To some extent, however, declines in lean body mass and energy needs may not be entirely inevitable. Optimal nutrition with sufficient protein and regular physical activity, especially resistance training, can help maintain muscle mass and strength and minimize the changes in body composition associated with aging.[41] Physical activity not only increases energy expenditure but, along with sound nutrition, enhances bone density and supports many body functions as well.

The lower energy expenditures of many older adults require that they eat less food to maintain their weights. Accordingly, the estimated energy requirements for adults decrease steadily after age 19. Energy intakes typically decline in parallel with needs. Still, many older adults are overweight, indicating that their food intakes do not decline enough to compensate for their reduced energy expenditures. Chapter 6 presents the many health problems that accompany obesity and the BMI guidelines for a healthy body weight (18.5–24.9). These guidelines apply to all adults, regardless of age, but they may be too restrictive for older adults. The importance of body weight in defending against chronic diseases differs for older adults.[42] Being *moderately overweight* may not be harmful. Older adults who are *obese*, especially those with central obesity, however, face serious medical complications and can improve their quality of life with weight loss.[43]

On limited energy allowances, people must select mostly nutrient-dense foods. There is little leeway for added sugars, solid fats, or alcohol. Older adults can follow the USDA Food Groups and Subgroups (see pp. 20–21), making sure to choose the recommended daily amounts of food from each food group that are appropriate to their energy needs (see Table 1-6 on p. 19).

Protein Currently, the protein RDA for older adults is the same as that for younger adults (0.8 g/kg body weight). Emerging evidence suggests that the protein needs of older adults may be slightly higher (1.0 to 1.2 g/kg body weight) than those of younger people, however.[44] Older adults (> 65 years), especially those with sarcopenia, may need more protein to help limit age-related loss of muscle mass, muscle strength, and muscle function.[45] With advancing age, people take in fewer total kcalories from food and so may need a greater percentage of kcalories from protein at each meal in order to support a healthy immune system and prevent losing muscle tissue, bone tissue, and other lean body mass.[46]

As energy needs decrease, lower-kcalorie protein sources such as lean tender meats, poultry, fish, boiled eggs, fat-free milk products, and legumes can help hold weight to a healthy level. Underweight or malnourished older adults need the opposite—energy-dense protein sources such as eggs scrambled with margarine, tuna salad with mayonnaise, peanut butter on wheat toast, hearty soups, and milkshakes. Nutrient-fortified supplements in liquid, pudding, cookie, or other forms between meals can also boost energy and nutrient intakes.[47]

Carbohydrate and Fiber As always, abundant carbohydrate is needed to protect protein from being used as an energy source. Carbohydrate-rich foods such as legumes, vegetables, whole grains, and fruit are also rich in fiber and essential vitamins and minerals. High-fiber eating patterns support good physical, mental, and social health.[48] With age, fiber takes on extra importance for its role in alleviating constipation, a common complaint among older adults and among residents of **health care communities** in particular.

Fruit and vegetables supply soluble fibers and phytochemicals to help ward off chronic diseases, but factors such as transportation problems, limited cooking facilities, and chewing problems limit some elderly people's intakes of fresh fruit and vegetables. Even without such problems, many older adults fail to obtain the recommended daily 25 or more grams of fiber (14 grams per 1000 kcalories). When low fiber intakes are combined with low fluid intakes, inadequate physical activity, and constipating medications, constipation becomes inevitable.

Fat As is true for people of all ages, dietary fat intake needs to be moderate for most older adults—enough to enhance flavors and provide valuable essential fatty acids and other nutrients, but not so much as to raise risks of cancer, atherosclerosis, and other degenerative diseases. The recommendation should not be taken too far; limiting fat

health care communities: living environments for people with chronic conditions, functional limitations, or need for supervision or assistance; include assisted living facilities, group homes, short-term rehabilitation facilities, skilled nursing facilities, and hospice facilities.

BOX 12-4 *Nursing Diagnosis*

too severely may lead to nutrient deficiencies and weight loss—two problems that carry greater health risks in the elderly than overweight.

Water Dehydration is a risk for older adults, who may not notice or pay attention to their thirst or who find it difficult and bothersome to get a drink or to get to a bathroom (Box 12-4).[49] Older adults who have lost bladder control may be afraid to drink too much water. Despite real fluid needs, older people do not seem to feel as thirsty or notice mouth dryness as readily as younger people. Many employees of health care communities such as assisted living facilities say it is hard to persuade their older clients to drink enough water and fruit juices.

Total body water decreases as people age, so even mild stresses such as fever or hot weather can precipitate rapid dehydration in older adults. Dehydrated older adults seem to be more susceptible to urinary tract infections, pneumonia, pressure ulcers, confusion, and disorientation. An intake of 9 cups a day of total beverages, including water, is recommended for women; for men, the recommendation is 13 cups a day of total beverages, including water.

Vitamins and Minerals

As research reveals more about how specific vitamins and minerals influence disease prevention and how age-related physiological changes affect nutrient metabolism, optimal intakes of vitamins and minerals for different groups of older adults are being defined. This section highlights the vitamins and minerals of greatest concern to older adults.

Vitamin D Older adults face a greater risk of vitamin D deficiency than younger people do. Vitamin D–fortified milk is the most reliable source of vitamin D, but many older adults drink little or no milk. Further compromising the vitamin D status of many older people, especially those in assisted living facilities or group homes, is their limited exposure to sunlight. Finally, aging reduces the skin's capacity to make vitamin D and the kidneys' ability to convert it to its active form. Not only are older adults not getting enough vitamin D, but they may actually need more to improve both muscle and bone strength. To prevent bone loss and to maintain vitamin D status, especially in those who engage in minimal outdoor activity, adults 51 to 70 years old need 15 micrograms daily and those 71 and older need 20 micrograms. Supplements may be needed to achieve adequate levels of vitamin D.

Vitamin B_{12} The DRI committee recommends that adults aged 51 years and older obtain 2.4 micrograms of vitamin B_{12} daily *and* that vitamin B_{12}–fortified foods (such as fortified cereals) or supplements be used to meet much of the DRI recommended intake. The committee's recommendation reflects the finding that many older adults lose the ability to produce enough stomach acid to make the protein-bound form of vitamin B_{12} available for absorption. Synthetic vitamin B_{12} is reliably absorbed, however. Given the poor cognition, anemia, and other devastating neurological effects associated with a vitamin B_{12} deficiency, an adequate intake is imperative.

One cause of the malabsorption of protein-bound vitamin B_{12} is a condition known as **atrophic gastritis**. An estimated 10 to 30 percent of adults older than age 50 have atrophic gastritis.

Folate As is true of vitamin B_{12}, folate intakes of older adults typically fall short of recommendations. Older adults are also more likely to have medical conditions or to take medications that can compromise folate status.

atrophic gastritis (a-TRO-fik gas-TRI-tis): a condition characterized by chronic inflammation of the stomach accompanied by a diminished size and functioning of the mucosa and glands.

Iron Among the minerals, iron deserves first mention. Iron-deficiency anemia is less common in older adults than in younger people, but it still occurs in some, especially in those with low food energy intakes. Aside from diet, other factors in many older people's lives make iron deficiency likely: chronic blood loss from disease conditions and medicines and poor iron absorption due to reduced secretion of stomach acid and antacid use. Anyone concerned with older adults' nutrition should keep these possibilities in mind.

Zinc Zinc intake is commonly low in older people. Zinc deficiency can depress the appetite and blunt the sense of taste, thereby leading to low food intakes and worsening of zinc status. Zinc deficiency may also increase the likelihood of infectious diseases such as pneumonia. Many medications that older adults commonly use can impair zinc absorption or enhance its excretion and thus lead to deficiency.

Calcium The importance of abundant dietary calcium throughout life to protect against osteoporosis has been emphasized throughout this book. The calcium intakes of many people, especially women, in the United States are well below the recommendations. If milk causes stomach discomfort, as many older adults report, then lactose-modified milk or other calcium-rich foods should take its place.

Nutrient Supplements for Older Adults

People judge for themselves how to manage their nutrition, and many older adults turn to dietary supplements. Advertisers target older people with appeals to take supplements and eat "health" foods, claiming that these products prevent disease and promote longevity. Quite often those who take supplements are not deficient in the nutrients being supplemented.

Elderly people often benefit from a balanced low-dose vitamin and mineral supplement, however. Such supplements supply many of the needed minerals along with the vitamins often lacking in older adults' diets without providing too much of any one nutrient.

Nonetheless, food is still the best source of nutrients for everybody. Supplements are just that—supplements to foods, not substitutes for them. For anyone who is motivated to obtain the best possible health, it is never too late to learn to eat well, become physically active, and adopt other lifestyle changes such as quitting smoking and moderating alcohol use. Table 12-4 summarizes the nutrient concerns of aging. Table 12-5 offers strategies for growing old healthfully.

TABLE 12-4	Summary of Nutrient Concerns of Aging	
NUTRIENT	**EFFECT OF AGING**	**COMMENTS**
Water	Lack of thirst and decreased total body water make dehydration likely.	Mild dehydration is a common cause of confusion. Difficulty obtaining water or getting to the bathroom may compound the problem.
Energy	Need decreases as muscle mass decreases (sarcopenia).	Physical activity moderates the decline.
Fiber	Likelihood of constipation increases with low intakes and changes in the GI tract.	Inadequate water intakes and lack of physical activity, along with some medications, compound the problem.
Protein	Needs may stay the same or increase slightly.	Low-fat milk and other high-quality protein foods are appropriate. Low-fat, high-fiber legumes and grains meet both protein and other nutrient needs.
Vitamin B$_{12}$	Atrophic gastritis is common.	Deficiency causes neurological damage; supplements may be needed.
Vitamin D	Increased likelihood of inadequate intake; skin synthesis declines.	Daily sunlight exposure in moderation or supplements may be beneficial.
Calcium	Intakes may be low; osteoporosis is common.	Stomach discomfort commonly limits milk intake; calcium substitutes or supplements may be needed.
Iron	In women, status improves after menopause; deficiencies are linked to chronic blood losses and low stomach acid output.	Adequate stomach acid is required for absorption; antacid or other medicine use may aggravate iron deficiency; vitamin C and meat increase absorption.
Zinc	Intakes are often inadequate and absorption may be poor, but needs may also increase.	Medications interfere with absorption; deficiency may depress appetite and sense of taste.

| TABLE 12-5 | Strategies for Growing Old Healthfully |

- Choose nutrient-dense foods.
- Be physically active. Walk, run, dance, swim, bike, or row for aerobic activity. Lift weights, do calisthenics, or pursue some other activity to tone, firm, and strengthen muscles. Practice balancing on one foot or doing simple movements with your eyes closed. Modify activities to suit changing abilities and preferences.
- Maintain appropriate body weight.
- Reduce stress—cultivate self-esteem, maintain a positive attitude, manage time wisely, know your limits, practice assertiveness, release tension, and take action.
- For women, discuss with a physician the risks and benefits of estrogen replacement therapy.
- For people who smoke, discuss with a physician strategies and programs to help you quit.
- Expect to enjoy sex, and learn new ways of enhancing it.
- Use alcohol only moderately, if at all; use drugs only as prescribed.
- Take care to prevent accidents.
- Expect good vision and hearing throughout life; obtain glasses and hearing aids if necessary.
- Take care of your teeth; obtain dentures if necessary.

- Be alert to confusion as a disease symptom, and seek diagnosis.
- Take medications as prescribed; see a physician before self-prescribing medicines or herbal remedies and a registered dietitian nutritionist before self-prescribing supplements.
- Control depression through activities and friendships; seek professional help if necessary.
- Drink six to eight glasses of water every day.
- Practice mental skills. Keep solving math problems and crossword puzzles, playing cards or other games, reading, writing, imagining, and creating.
- Make financial plans early to ensure security.
- Accept change. Work at recovering from losses; make new friends.
- Cultivate spiritual health. Cherish personal values. Make life meaningful.
- Go outside for sunshine and fresh air as often as possible.
- Be socially active—play bridge, join an exercise or dance group, take a class, teach a class, eat with friends, or volunteer time to help others.
- Stay interested in life—pursue a hobby, spend time with grandchildren, take a trip, read, grow a garden, or go to the movies.
- Enjoy life.

The Effects of Drugs on Nutrients

As people grow older, the use of medicines—from over-the-counter drugs such as aspirin and laxatives to prescription medications of all kinds—becomes commonplace. Most drugs interact with one or more nutrients in several ways, usually resulting in greater-than-normal needs for these nutrients. Chapter 14 offers a discussion of diet-drug interactions and describes the many reasons why elderly people are vulnerable to such interactions.

The most common drug that can affect nutrition in older people is alcohol. The effects of alcohol on people of all ages are explained in Nutrition in Practice 19.

Review Notes

- Aging significantly affects nutrient needs and intakes, as summarized in Table 12-4.
- Older adults often benefit from a balanced low-dose vitamin and mineral supplement. Food is still the best source of nutrients, however.

12.4 Food Choices and Eating Habits of Older Adults

To provide any benefit, strategies and interventions to improve a person's nutrition status must be based on knowledge of food preferences and eating patterns. Menus and feeding programs for older adults must take into consideration not only food likes and dislikes but also the living conditions, economic status, and medical conditions of this diverse group of people. If nutrition intervention is to be successful, it is essential to know what foods people will eat, in what settings they like to eat these foods, and whether they can buy and prepare meals.

Older adults are, for the most part, independent, socially sophisticated, mentally lucid, fully participating members of society who report themselves to be happy and healthy. In fact, chronic disabilities among the elderly have declined dramatically in recent years. Older people spend more money per person on foods to eat at home than other age groups and less money on foods eaten away from home. Manufacturers would be wise to cater to the preferences of older adults by providing good-tasting, nutritious foods in easy-to-open, single-serving packages with labels that are easy to read. Such products enable older adults to maintain their independence; most of them want to take care of themselves and need to feel a sense of control and involvement in their own lives. As discussed earlier, another way older adults can take care of themselves is by remaining or becoming physically active. Physical activity helps preserve one's ability to perform daily tasks and so promotes independence.

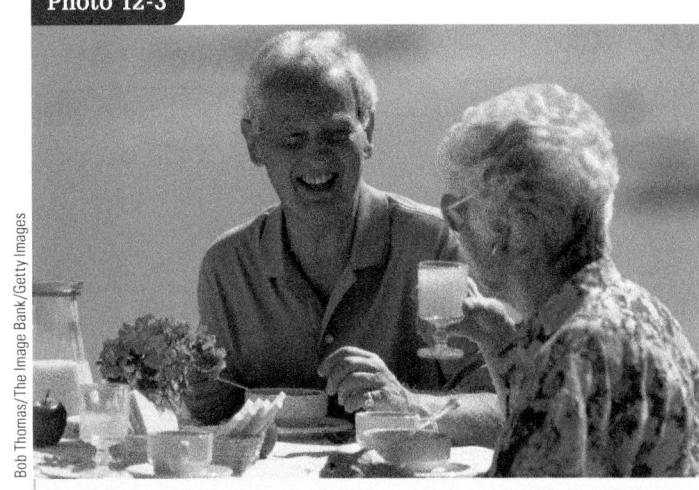

Photo 12-3

Shared meals can brighten the day and enhance the appetite.

Individual Preferences

Familiarity, taste, and health beliefs are most influential on older people's food choices. Eating foods that are familiar, especially ethnic foods that recall family meals and pleasant times, can be comforting. Older adults are choosing poultry and fish, low-fat milk and milk products, and high-fiber breads and grains, indicating that they recognize the importance of diet in supporting good health. Few older adults, however, consume the recommended amounts of milk products.

Meal Setting

The food choices and eating habits of older adults are also affected by the changes in lifestyle that often accompany aging in this society. Whether people live alone, with others, or in institutions affects the way they eat. For example, men living alone are most likely to be poorly nourished. Older adults who live alone do not make poorer food choices than those who live with companions; rather, they consume too little food. Loneliness is directly related to inadequacies, especially of energy intakes.

Depression

Another factor affecting food intake and appetite in older people is depression. Loss of appetite and motivation to cook or even to eat frequently accompanies depression. An overwhelming feeling of grief and sadness at the death of a spouse, friend, or family member may leave many people, particularly older adults, with a feeling of powerlessness to overcome the depression. The support and companionship of family and friends, especially at mealtimes, can help overcome depression and enhance appetite (see Photo 12-3). The case study in Box 12-5 on p. 366 presents a man who has several of these problems. Use the suggestions here, and in the last section of this chapter, to help develop solutions. The Nutrition Assessment Checklist for Older Adults at the end of this chapter helps to pinpoint nutrition-related factors to look for when working with older adults. To *determine* the risk of malnutrition in older clients, health care providers can keep in mind the characteristics listed in Table 12-6.

Food Assistance Programs

Federally funded programs can provide food and nutrition services for older adults. The Older Americans Act (OAA) provides many different support services to help older adults remain healthy and independent.

TABLE 12-6 Risk Factors for Malnutrition in Older Adults

These questions help *determine* the risk of malnutrition in older adults:

- *Disease:* Do you have an illness or condition that changes the types or amounts of foods you eat?
- *Eating poorly:* Do you eat fewer than two meals a day? Do you eat fruit, vegetables, and milk products daily?
- *Tooth loss or mouth pain:* Is it difficult or painful to eat?
- *Economic hardship:* Do you have enough money to buy the food you need?
- *Reduced social contact:* Do you eat alone most of the time?
- *Multiple medications:* Do you take three or more different prescribed or over-the-counter medications daily?
- *Involuntary weight loss or gain:* Have you lost or gained 10 pounds or more in the last six months?
- *Needs assistance:* Are you physically able to shop, cook, and feed yourself?
- *Elderly person:* Are you older than 80?

Mr. Brezenoff is 75 years old and lives alone. He has slowly been losing weight since his wife died a year ago. At 5 feet 8 inches tall, he currently weighs 124 pounds. His previous weight was 150 pounds. In talking with Mr. Brezenoff, you realize that he doesn't even like to talk about food, let alone eat it. "My wife always did the cooking before, and I ate well. Now I just don't feel like eating." You manage to find out that he skips breakfast, has soup and bread for lunch, and sometimes eats a cold-cut sandwich or a frozen dinner for supper. He seldom sees friends or relatives. Mr. Brezenoff has also lost several teeth and doesn't eat any raw fruit or vegetables because he finds them hard to chew. He lives on a meager but adequate income.

1. Consult the BMI table (inside back cover), and judge whether Mr. Brezenoff is at a healthy weight. What other assessments might you use to back up your judgment? Is his weight loss significant?

2. What factors are contributing to Mr. Brezenoff's poor food intake? What nutrients are probably deficient in his diet?

3. Look at Mr. Brezenoff as an individual and suggest ways he can improve his diet and his lifestyle.

4. What other aspects of Mr. Brezenoff's physical and mental health should you consider in helping him to improve his food intake?

| TABLE 12-7 | Food Assistance Programs for Older Adults |

OAA Nutrition Program

Services: Provides congregate and home-delivered meals to improve older people's nutrition status. Includes transportation to congregate meal sites; shopping assistance; information and referral; and, to some extent, nutrition counseling and education.

Impact: Improves the nutrient content of high-risk older adults' diets and offers socialization and recreation. Many of the nutrition programs around the country go above and beyond federal requirements of congregate and home meals by offering lunch clubs, ethnic meals, and meals for older homeless people.

Supplemental Nutrition Assistance Program (SNAP)

Services: Supplements income for low-income households by means of a card similar to a debit card that can be used to purchase food.

Impact: Serves more as an income supplement for some elderly participants than as a device to improve nutrition status. For other elderly participants, nutrient intakes are higher than those of nonparticipants with similar incomes.

Meals on Wheels

Services: Delivers meals directly to the homebound elderly; integrated into the meal delivery services provided by the OAA Nutrition Program.

Impact: Focuses on filling the need for weekend and holiday meals for homebound elderly people, a service that is limited in the OAA Nutrition Program.

Senior Farmers' Market Nutrition Program

Services: Provides low-income older adults with coupons that can be exchanged for fresh fruit, vegetables, and herbs at community-supported farmers' markets and roadside stands; administered by the USDA. State agencies may limit sales to specific foods that are locally grown to encourage recipients to support farmers in their own states.

Impact: Increases fresh fruit and vegetable consumption, provides nutrition information, and even reaches the homebound elderly, a group of people who normally do not have access to farmers' markets.

An integral component of the OAA is the OAA Nutrition Program. Table 12-7 summarizes this and other food assistance programs available to the elderly.

Meals for Singles

Many older adults live alone, and singles of all ages face challenges in purchasing, storing, and preparing food. Large packages of meat and vegetables are often intended for families of four or more, and even a head of lettuce can spoil before one person can use it all. Many singles live in small dwellings and have little storage space for foods. A limited income presents additional obstacles. This section offers suggestions that can help to solve some of the problems singles face.

Avoid Foodborne Illness The risk of foodborne illness is greater for older adults than for other adults. The consequences of an upset stomach, diarrhea, fever, vomiting, abdominal cramps, and dehydration are oftentimes more severe, sometimes leading to paralysis, meningitis, or even death. For these reasons, older adults need to carefully follow the food safety suggestions presented in Nutrition in Practice 2.

Spend Wisely People who have the means to shop and cook for themselves can cut their food bills just by being wise shoppers. Large supermarkets are usually less expensive than convenience stores. A grocery list helps reduce impulse buying, and specials and coupons can save money when the items featured are those that the shopper needs and uses.

Buying the right amount so as not to waste any food is a challenge for people eating alone. Fresh milk should be purchased in the size best suited for personal needs. Pint-size and even cup-size boxes of milk that can be stored unopened on a shelf for up to three months without refrigeration are available.*

Many foods that offer a variety of nutrients for practically pennies have a long shelf-life; staples such as rice, pastas, dry powdered milk, and dried legumes can be purchased in bulk and stored for months at room temperature. Other foods that are usually a good buy include whole pieces of cheese rather than sliced or shredded cheese, fresh produce in season, variety meats such as chicken livers, and cereals that require cooking instead of ready-to-serve cereals.

A person who has ample freezing space can buy large packages of meat, such as pork chops, ground beef, or chicken, when they are on sale. Then the meat can be immediately wrapped in individual servings for the freezer. All the individual servings can be put in a bag marked appropriately with the contents and the date. Alternatively, grocers will break open a package of wrapped meat and rewrap the portion needed. Similarly, eggs can be purchased by the half-dozen. Eggs do keep for long periods, though, if stored properly in the refrigerator.

Frozen vegetables are more economical in large bags than in small boxes. The amount needed can be taken out, and the bag closed tightly with a twist tie or rubber band. If the package is returned quickly to the freezer each time, the vegetables will stay fresh for a long time. Fresh fruit and vegetables can be purchased individually. A person can buy fresh fruit at various stages of ripeness: a ripe one to eat right away, a semiripe one to eat soon after, and a green one to ripen on the windowsill. If vegetables are packaged in large quantities, the grocer can break open the package so that a smaller amount can be purchased. Small cans of fruit and vegetables, even though they are more expensive per unit, are a reasonable alternative, considering that it is expensive to buy a regular-size can and let the unused portion spoil.

Finally, breads and cereals usually must be purchased in larger quantities. Again the amount needed for a few days can be taken out and the rest stored in the freezer.

Be Creative Creative chefs think of various ways to use foods when only large amounts are available. For example, a head of cauliflower can be divided into thirds. Then one-third is cooked and eaten hot, another third is put into a vinegar-and-oil marinade for use in a salad, and the last third can be used in a casserole or stew.

A variety of vegetables and meats can be enjoyed stir-fried; inexpensive vegetables such as cabbage, celery, and onion are delicious when crisp-cooked in a little oil with herbs or lemon added. Interesting frozen vegetable mixtures are available in larger grocery stores. Cooked, leftover vegetables can be dropped in at the last minute. A bonus of a stir-fried meal is that there is only one pan to wash. Similarly, a microwave oven allows a home chef to use fewer pots and pans. Meals and leftovers can also be frozen or refrigerated in microwavable containers to reheat as needed.

Many frozen dinners or grocery store take-out foods offer nutritious options. Adding a fresh salad, a whole-wheat roll, and a glass of milk can make a nutritionally balanced meal. Box 12-6 offers time-saving tips to turn convenience foods into nutritious meals.

Also, single people shouldn't hesitate to invite someone to share meals with them whenever there is enough food. It's likely that the person will return the invitation, and both parties will get to enjoy companionship and a meal prepared by others.

---

*Boxes of milk that can be stored at room temperature have been exposed to temperatures above those of pasteurization just long enough to sterilize the milk—a process called *ultrahigh temperature (UHT)*.

Box 12-6 **HOW TO Turn Convenience Foods into Nutritious Meals**

These time-saving tips can turn convenience foods into nutritious meals:

- Add extra nutrients and a fresh flavor to canned stews and soups by tossing in some frozen ready-to-use mixed vegetables. Choose vegetables frozen without salty, fatty sauces—prepared foods generally contain enough salt to season the whole dish, including added vegetables.

- Buy frozen vegetables in a bag, toss in a variety of herbs, and use as needed.

- When grilling burgers or chicken, wrap a mixture of frozen broccoli, onions, and carrots in a foil packet with a tablespoon of Italian dressing and grill alongside the meat for seasoned grilled vegetables.

- Use canned fruits in their own juices as desserts. Toss in some frozen berries or peach slices and top with flavored yogurt for an instant fruit salad.

- Prepared rice or noodle dishes are convenient, but those claiming to contain broccoli, spinach, or other vegetables seldom contain enough to qualify as a serving of vegetables. Pump up the nutrient value by adding a half-cup of frozen vegetables per serving of pasta or rice just before cooking.

- Purchase frozen onion, mushroom, and pepper mixtures to embellish jarred spaghetti sauce or small frozen pizzas. Top with parmesan cheese.

- Use frozen shredded potatoes, sold for hash browns, in soups or stews or mix with a handful of shredded reduced-fat cheese or a can of fat-free "cream of anything" soup and bake for a quick and hearty casserole.

- Purchase a bag of triple-washed, ready-to-eat salad and add any or all of the following to make a hearty, healthy salad: a small can of garbanzo beans or a package of frozen edamame (soybeans); a handful of shredded reduced-fat cheese; a hardboiled egg; a handful of toasted almonds or other nuts.

- Open a can of pinto beans or black beans, heat a tablespoon of olive oil, and sauté a little bit of frozen onion and pepper mixture. Add the beans and mash them in the oil and vegetables. Serve the bean mixture in a soft taco shell with shredded reduced-fat cheese, lettuce, and salsa for a tasty, nutritious bean taco.

Review Notes

- Food choices of older adults are affected by health status and changed life circumstances.
- Older people can benefit from both the nutrients provided and the social interaction available at congregate meals. Other government programs deliver meals to those who are homebound.
- With creativity and careful shopping, those living alone can prepare nutritious, inexpensive meals.

Nutrition Assessment Checklist for Older Adults

MEDICAL HISTORY

Check the medical record for:

- ○ Alcohol abuse
- ○ Alzheimer's disease or other dementia or confusion
- ○ Arthritis
- ○ Cataracts or macular degeneration
- ○ Chronic diseases (cancer, heart disease, hypertension, diabetes)
- ○ Cigarette, cigar, or pipe smoking; use of other tobacco products
- ○ Constipation
- ○ Dehydration
- ○ Dental disease or tooth loss
- ○ Depression
- ○ Inflammation of the stomach (gastritis)
- ○ Swallowing disorders

MEDICATIONS

For older adults being treated with drug therapy for medical conditions, note:

- ○ Use of multiple medications—prescription and/or over-the-counter medications such as laxatives and pain relievers
- ○ Side effects that might reduce food intake or change nutrient needs
- ○ Proper administration of medication with respect to food intake
- ○ Malnutrition—is the person's nutrition status questionable even before considering side effects of medications that worsen nutrition status?
- ○ Diminished mental capacity that might interfere with taking correct medications and doses
- ○ Dehydration (can alter effects of medications)

DIETARY INTAKE

For all older adults, especially those at risk nutritionally, assess the diet for:

- ○ Total energy
- ○ Protein
- ○ Calcium, iron, and zinc
- ○ Vitamin B_6, vitamin B_{12}, folate, and vitamin D

Note the following:

- ○ Number of meals eaten each day
- ○ Number and ages of people in household
- ○ Amount of milk consumed each day
- ○ Type and frequency of outdoor activity
- ○ Type and frequency of physical activity
- ○ Financial resources
- ○ Transportation resources
- ○ Physical disabilities
- ○ Mental alertness

ANTHROPOMETRIC DATA

Measure baseline height and weight.

- ○ Reassess height and weight at each medical checkup.
- ○ Note significant overweight or underweight, which warrants intervention.
- ○ Use skinfold measures to reveal altered body composition that may indicate malnutrition and loss of lean tissue.

LABORATORY TESTS

- ○ Hemoglobin, hematocrit, or other tests of iron status
- ○ Serum albumin or other measures of protein status
- ○ Serum folate
- ○ Serum B_{12}

PHYSICAL SIGNS

Look for physical signs of:

- ○ Protein-energy malnutrition
- ○ Iron and zinc deficiency
- ○ Folate deficiency

Self Check

1. The fastest-growing age group in the United States is:
   a. under 21 years of age.
   b. 30 to 45 years of age.
   c. 50 to 70 years of age.
   d. over 85 years of age.

2. Which of the following lifestyle habits can enhance the length and quality of people's lives?
   a. Moderate smoking
   b. Six hours of sleep daily
   c. Regular physical activity
   d. Skipping breakfast

3. Which of the following is among the better-known relationships between nutrition and disease prevention?
   a. Appropriate fiber intake helps prevent goiter.
   b. Moderate sodium intake helps prevent obesity.
   c. Moderate sugar intake helps prevent hypertension.
   d. Appropriate energy intake helps prevent diabetes and cardiovascular disease.

4. A disease of the immune system that involves painful inflammation of the joints is:
   a. sarcopenia.
   b. osteoarthritis.
   c. senile dementia.
   d. rheumatoid arthritis.

5. Examples of low-kcalorie, high-quality protein foods include:
   a. cottage cheese, sour cream, and eggs.
   b. green and yellow vegetables and citrus fruit.
   c. potatoes, rice, pasta, and whole-grain breads.
   d. lean meats, poultry, fish, legumes, fat-free milk, and eggs.

6. For malnourished and underweight people, protein- and energy-dense snacks include:
   a. fresh fruit and vegetables.
   b. yogurt and cottage cheese.
   c. whole grains and high-fiber legumes.
   d. scrambled eggs and peanut butter on wheat toast.

7. Which of the following does not contribute to dehydration risk in older adults?
   a. They do not seem to feel thirsty.
   b. Total body water increases with age.
   c. They may find it difficult to get a drink.
   d. They may have difficulty getting to the bathroom.

8. Inadequate milk intake and limited exposure to sunlight contribute to older adults' risk of:
   a. vitamin A deficiency.
   b. vitamin D deficiency.
   c. riboflavin deficiency.
   d. vitamin B_{12} deficiency.

9. Two risk factors for malnutrition in older adults are:
   a. loneliness and multiple medication use.
   b. increased energy needs and lack of fiber.
   c. decreased mineral absorption and antioxidant intake.
   d. high carbohydrate intake and lack of physical activity.

10. Strategies to improve nutrition status when growing old include:
    a. increasing vitamin A intake and exercising 30 minutes daily.
    b. choosing nutrient-dense foods and maintaining appropriate weight.

   c. avoiding high-fiber foods and taking a daily vitamin-mineral supplement.
   d. eating at least one big meal per day and drinking at least 10 glasses of water daily.

Answers: 1. d, 2. c, 3. d, 4. d, 5. d, 6. d, 7. b, 8. b, 9. a, 10. b

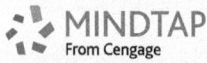 **MINDTAP** From Cengage   For more chapter resources visit **www.cengage.com** to access MindTap, a complete digital course.

Clinical Applications

1. Ms. Hamilton, an 80-year-old woman in excellent health, lives alone, eats a well-balanced diet, enjoys an active social life, and walks every day. Consider the way Ms. Hamilton's health and nutrition status might be affected by the following situations:

   • Many of Ms. Hamilton's friends pass away or move into extended care facilities.
   • Ms. Hamilton falls and breaks her hip.
   • Ms. Hamilton begins to feel isolated and depressed.

   Describe interventions the health care professional can take to help Ms. Hamilton deal with each situation to prevent her from falling into a downward spiral.

Notes

1. K. D. Kochanek and coauthors, Deaths: Final data for 2014, *National Vital Statistics Reports*, June 30, 2016, pp. 1–122.
2. S. H. Preston, Y. C. Vierboom, and A. Stokes, The role of obesity in exceptionally slow US mortality improvement, *Proceedings of the National Academy of Sciences of the United States of America* 115 (2018): 957–961.
3. G. Passarino, F. De Rango, and A. Montesanto, Human longevity: Genetics or lifestyle? It takes two to tango, *Immunity and Ageing*, 2016, doi: 10.1186/s12979-016-0066-z; A. M. May and coauthors, The impact of a healthy lifestyle on disability-adjusted life years: A prospective cohort study, *BMC Medicine* 13 (2015): 287; O. Oyebode and coauthors, Fruit and vegetable consumption and all cause, cancer and CVD mortality: Analysis of Health Survey for England data, *Journal of Epidemiology and Community Health* 68 (2014): 856–862.
4. M. Sotos-Prieto and coauthors, Association of changes in diet quality with total and cause-specific mortality, *New England Journal of Medicine* 377 (2017): 143–153; K. A. Hagan and coauthors, Greater adherence to the Alternative Healthy Eating Index is associated with lower incidence of physical function impairment in the Nurses' Health Study, *Journal of Nutrition* 146 (2017): 1341–1347.
5. J. C. Mathers, Impact of nutrition on the ageing process, *British Journal of Nutrition* 113 (2015): S18–S22; J. C. Kiefte-de Jong, J. C. Mathers, and O. H. Franco, Nutrition and healthy ageing: The key ingredients, *Proceedings of the Nutrition Society* 73 (2014): 249–259.
6. R. D. Pollock and coauthors, An investigation into the relationship between age and physiological function in highly active older adults, *Journal of Physiology* 593 (2015): 657–680; May and coauthors, 2015.
7. G. Kojuma and coauthors, Adherence to Mediterranean diet reduces incident frailty risk: Systematic review and meta-analysis, *Journal of the American Geriatric Society*, 2018, doi: 10.1111/jgs.15251; D. F. Romagnolo and O. I. Selmin, Mediterranean diet and prevention of chronic diseases, *Nutrition Today* 52 (2017): 208–222; S. Vasto and coauthors, Mediterranean diet and healthy ageing: A Sicilian perspective, *Gerontology* 60 (2014): 508–518.
8. R. A. Fielding and coauthors, Dose of physical activity, physical functioning and disability risk in mobility-limited older adults: Results from the LIFE study randomized trial, *PLoS One* 12 (2017): e0182155; May and coauthors, 2015; W. J. Brown, T. Pavey, and A. E. Bauman, Comparing population attributable risks for heart disease across the adult lifespan in women, *British Journal of Sports Medicine* 49 (2015): 1069–1076; L. Soares-Miranda and coauthors, Physical activity and heart rate variability in older adults: The Cardiovascular Health Study, *Circulation* 129 (2014): 2100–2110.
9. M. M. Robinson and coauthors, Enhanced protein translation underlies improved metabolic and physical adaptations to different exercise training modes in young and old humans, *Cell Metabolism* 25 (2017): 581–592; Pollock and coauthors, 2015; L. Soares-Miranda and coauthors, Physical activity and risk of coronary heart disease and stroke in older adults: The Cardiovascular Health Study, *Circulation* 133 (2015): 147–155.
10. S. A. Motalebi and coauthors, Effect of low-cost resistance training on lower-limb strength and balance in institutionalized seniors, *Experimental Aging Research* 44 (2018): 48–61; Ø. Støren and coauthors, The effect of age on the VO$_{2max}$ response to high-intensity interval training, *Medicine and Science in Sports and Exercise* 49 (2017): 78–85.
11. S. B. Kritchevsky and coauthors, Exercise's effect on mobility disability in older adults with and without obesity: The LIFE study randomized clinical trial, *Obesity* 25 (2017): 1199–1205; M. Bellumori, M. Uygur, and C. A. Knight, High-speed cycling intervention improves rate-dependent mobility in older adults, *Medicine and Science in Sports and Exercise* 49 (2017): 106–114; M. Pahor and coauthors, Effect of structured physical activity on Prevention of major mobility disability in older adults: The LIFE Study randomized Clinical Trial, *Journal of the American Medical Association* 311 (2014): 2387–2396.
12. W. Zhu and coauthors, Objectively measured physical activity and cognitive function in older adults, *Medicine and Science in Sports and Exercise* 49 (2017): 47–53; D. P. Gill and coauthors, The Healthy Mind, Healthy Mobility Trial: A novel exercise program for older adults,

Medicine and Science in Sports and Exercise 48 (2016): 297–306; G. Cooney, K. Dwan, and G. Mead, Exercise for depression, *Journal of the American Medical Association* 311 (2014): 2432–2433; P. Pereira, M. C. Geoffroy, and C. Power, Depressive symptoms and physical activity during 3 decades in adult life: Bidirectional associations in a prospective cohort study, *JAMA Psychiatry* 71 (2014): 1373–1380.

13. Y. H. Cho and coauthors, The effects of a multicomponent intervention program on clinical outcomes associated with falls in healthy older adults, *Aging Clinical and Experimental Research*, 2018, doi: 10.1007/s40520-018-0895-z; A. C. Tricco and coauthors, Comparisons of interventions for preventing falls in older adults: A systematic review and meta-analysis, *Journal of the American Medical Association* 318 (2017): 1687–1699; K. Uusi-Rasi and coauthors, Exercise and vitamin D in fall prevention among older women, *JAMA Internal Medicine* 175 (2015): 703–711.

14. J. A. Conlon and coauthors, Periodization strategies in older adults: Impacts on physical function and health, *Medicine and Science in Sports and Exercise* 48 (2016): 2426–2436.

15. S. Brandhorst and coauthors, A periodic diet that mimics fasting promotes multi-system regeneration, enhanced cognitive performance, and healthspan, *Cell Metabolism* 22 (2015): 86–99.

16. L. Fontana and L. Partridge, Promoting health and longevity through diet: From model organisms to humans, *Cell* 161 (2015): 106–118.

17. D. F. Romagnolo and O. I. Selmin, Mediterranean diet and prevention of chronic diseases, *Nutrition Today* 52 (2017): 208–222; Vasto and coauthors, 2014; Oyebode and coauthors, 2014.

18. W. G. Christen and coauthors, Age-related cataract in men in the Selenium and Vitamin E Cancer Prevention Trial Eye Endpoints Study: a randomized clinical trial, *JAMA Ophthalmology* 133 (2015): 17–24.

19. J. Mares, Food antioxidants to prevent cataract, *Journal of the American Medical Association* 313 (2015): 1048–1049; S. Rautiainen and coauthors, Total antioxidant capacity of the diet and risk of age-related cataract: A population-based prospective cohort of women, *JAMA Ophthalmology* 132 (2014): 247–252; K. A. Weikel and coauthors, Nutritional modulation of cataract, *Nutrition Reviews* 72 (2014): 30–47.

20. D. S. Lee and coauthors, The gender-dependent association between obesity and age-related cataracts in middle-aged Korean adults, *PLoS One* 10 (2015): e0124262; C. W. Pan and Y. Lin, Overweight, obesity, and age-related cataract: A meta-analysis, *Optometry and Vison Science* 91 (2014): 478–483; J. Ye and coauthors, Body mass index and risk of age-related cataract: A meta-analysis of prospective cohort studies, *PLoS One* 9 (2014): e89923.

21. G. K. Broadhead and coauthors, Dietary modification and supplementation for the treatment of age-related macular degeneration, *Nutrition Reviews* 73 (2015): 448–462; J. R. Evans and J. G. Lawrenson, A review of the evidence for dietary Interventions in preventing or slowing the progression of age-related macular degeneration, *Ophthalmic and Physiological Optics* 34 (2014): 390–396.

22. Centers for Disease Control and Prevention, Arthritis, www.cdc.gov/arthritis/data_statistics/national-statistics.html, updated October 25, 2017.

23. C. Reyes and coauthors, Association between overweight and obesity and risk of clinically diagnosed knee, hip, and hand osteoarthritis: A population-based cohort study, *Arthritis and Rheumatology* 68 (2016): 1869–1875; G. Musumeci and coauthors, Osteoarthritis in the 21st century: Risk factors and behaviours that influence disease onset and progression, *International Journal of Molecular Sciences* 16 (2015): 6093–6112; E. Thijssen, A. van Caam, and P. M. van der Kraan, Obesity and osteoarthritis, more than just wear and tear: Pivotal roles for inflamed adipose tissue and dyslipidaemia in obesity-induced osteoarthritis, *Rheumatology* 54 (2015): 588–600.

24. M. Taglietti and coauthors, Effectiveness of aquatic exercises compared to patient-education on health status in individuals with knee osteoarthritis: A randomized controlled trial, *Clinical Rehabilitation*, doi: 10.1177/0269215517754240; M. Fransen and coauthors, Exercise for osteoarthritis of the knee, *Cochrane Database of Systematic Reviews*, doi: 10.1002/14651858.CD004376.pub3.

25. M. Fransen and coauthors, Glucosamine and chondroitin for knee osteoarthritis: A double-blind randomized placebo-controlled clinical trial evaluating single and combination regimens, *Annals of the Rheumatic Diseases*, 74 (2015): 851–858.

26. D. Di Giuseppe and coauthors, Long-term intake of dietary long-chain n-3 polyunsaturated fatty acids and risk of rheumatoid arthritis: A prospective cohort study of women, *Annals of the Rheumatic Diseases* 73 (2014): 1949–1953.

27. P. B. Gorelick and coauthors, Defining optimal brain health in adults: A Presidential Advisory from the American Heart Association/American Stroke Association, *Stroke*, 2017, doi: 10.1161/STR.0000000000000148; D. G. Blazer, K. Yaffe, and J. Karlawish, Cognitive aging: A report from the Institute of Medicine, *Journal of the American Medical Association* 313 (2015): 2121–2122; M. P. Mattson, Lifelong brain health is a lifelong challenge: From evolutionary principles to empirical evidence, *Ageing Research Reviews* 20C (2015): 37–45.

28. T. Köbe and coauthors, Vitamin B-12 concentration, memory performance, and hippocampal structure in patients with mild cognitive impairment, *American Journal of Clinical Nutrition* 103 (2016): 1045–1054; A. D. Smith and H. Refsum, Homocysteine, B vitamins, and cognitive impairment, *Annual Review of Nutrition* 36 (2016): 211–239; J. C. Agnew-Blais and coauthors, Folate, vitamin B-6, and vitamin B-12 intake and mild cognitive impairment and probable dementia in the Women's Health Initiative Memory Study, *Journal of the Academy Nutrition and Dietetics* 115 (2015): 231–241; C. McGarel and coauthors, Emerging roles for folate and related B-vitamins in brain health across the lifecycle, *Proceedings of the Nutrition Society*, 74 (2015): 46–55; C. A. de Jager, Critical levels of brain Atrophy associated with homocysteine and cognitive decline, *Neurobiology of Aging* 35 (2014): S35–S39; M. Gallucci and coauthors, Serum folate, homocysteine, brain atrophy, and auto-CM system: The Treviso Dementia (TREDEM) study, *Journal of Alzheimers Disease* 38 (2014): 581–587.

29. Y. Zhang and coauthors, Intakes of fish and polyunsaturated fatty acids and milk-to-severe cognitive impairment risks: A dose-response meta-analysis of 21 cohort studies, *American Journal of Clinical Nutrition* 103 (2016): 330–340; M. C. Morris and coauthors, Association of seafood consumption, brain mercury level, and APOE ε4 status with brain neuropathology in older adults, *Journal of the American Medical Association* 315 (2016): 489–497; K. Yurko-Mauro, D. D. Alexander, and M. E. Van Elswyk, Docosahexaenoic acid and adult memory: A systematic review and meta-analysis, *PLoS One* 10 (2015): e0120391; W. Stonehouse, Does consumption of LC omega-3 PUFA enhance cognitive performance in healthy school-aged children and throughout adulthood?: Evidence from clinical trials, *Nutrients* 6 (2014): 27302758; J. Jiao and coauthors, Effect of n-3 PUFA supplementation on cognitive function throughout the life span from infancy to old age: A systematic review and meta-analysis of randomized controlled trials, *American Journal of Clinical Nutrition* 100 (2014): 1422–1436.

30. McGarel and coauthors, 2015; Yurko-Mauro, Alexander, and Van Elswyk, 2015; de Jager, 2014.

31. C. Valls-Padret and coauthors, Mediterranean diet and age-related cognitive decline: A randomized clinical trial, *JAMA Internal Medicine* 175 (2015): 1094–1103; A. Smyth and coauthors, Healthy eating and reduced risk of cognitive decline, *Neurology* 84 (2015): 2258–2265.

32. Centers for Disease Control and Prevention, Alzheimer's disease, www.cdc.gov/aging/aginginfo/alzheimers.htm, updated October 13, 2017.

33. E. Ahmed and A. Moneim, Oxidant/antioxidant imbalance and the risk of Alzheimer's disease, *Current Alzheimer Research* 12 (2015): 335–349.

34. L. Ronan and coauthors, Obesity associated with increased brain-age from mid-life, *Neurobiology of Aging* 47 (2016): 63–70; J. C. D. Nguyen, A. S. Killcross, and T. A. Jenkins, Obesity and cognitive decline: Role of inflammation and vascular changes, *Frontiers in Neuroscience* 8 (2014): 375.

35. Ahmed and Moneim, 2015.

36. Gorelick and coauthors, 2017.

37. Gorelick and coauthors, 2017; H. N. Yassine and coauthors, Association of serum docosahexaenoic acid with cerebral amyloidosis, *JAMA Neurology* 73 (2016): 1208–1216.

38. G. A. Panza and coauthors, Can exercise improve cognitive symptoms of Alzheimer's disease? A meta-analysis, *Journal of the American Geriatric Society*, 2018, doi: 10.1111/jgs.15241; W. Zhu and coauthors, Objectively measured physical activity and cognitive function in older adults, *Medicine and Science in Sports and Exercise* 49 (2017): 47–53; S. McNally and coauthors, Focus on physical activity can help avoid unnecessary social care, *BMJ* 359 (2017): j4609; T. Paillard, Y. Rolland, and P. de Souto Barreto, Protective effects of physical exercise in Alzheimer's disease and Parkinson's disease: A narrative review, *Journal of Clinical Neurology* 11 (2015): 212–219; C. P. Boyle and coauthors, Physical activity, body mass index, and brain atrophy in Alzheimer's disease, *Neurobiology of Aging* 36 (2015): S194–S202.

39. J. Morley, S. D. Anker, and S. von Haehling, Prevalence, incidence, and clinical impact of sarcopenia: Facts, numbers, and epidemiology—update 2014, *Journal of Cachexia, Sarcopenia and Muscle* 5 (2014): 253–259.
40. M. Hammer and F. O'Donovan, Sarcopenic obesity, weight loss, and mortality: The English Longitudinal Study of Aging, *American Journal of Clinical Nutrition* 106 (2017): 125–129.
41. L. Holm and N. B. Nordsborg, Supplementing a normal diet with protein yields a moderate improvement in the robust gains in muscle mass and strength induced by resistance training in older individuals, *American Journal of Clinical Nutrition* 106 (2017): 971–972; M. Steffl and coauthors, Relationship between sarcopenia and physical activity in older people: A systematic review and meta-analysis, *Clinical Interventions in Aging* 12 (2017): 835–845; A. Shao and coauthors, The emerging global phenomenon of sarcopenic obesity: Role of functional foods; a conference report, *Journal of Functional Foods* 33 (2017): 244–250; A. M. Martone and coauthors, Treating sarcopenia in older and oldest old, *Current Pharmaceutical Design* 21 (2015): 1715–1722; N. E. Deutz and coauthors, Protein intake and exercise for optimal muscle function with aging: Recommendations from the ESPEN Expert Group, *Clinical Nutrition* 33 (2014): 929–936; R. M. Daly and coauthors, Protein enriched diet, with the use of lean red meat, combined with progressive resistance training enhances lean tissue mass and muscle strength and reduces circulating IL-6 concentrations in elderly women: A cluster randomized controlled trial, *American Journal of Clinical Nutrition* 99 (2014): 899–910.
42. I. Holme and S. Tonstad, Survival in elderly men in relation to midlife and current BMI, *Age and Ageing* 44 (2015): 434–439.
43. B. Y. Cho and coauthors, BMI and central obesity with falls among community-dwelling older adults, *American Journal of Preventive Medicine*, 2018, doi: 10.1016/j.amepre.2017.12.020; K. Bowman and coauthors, Central adiposity and the overweight risk paradox in aging: Follow-up of 130473 UK Biobank participants, *American Journal of Clinical Nutrition* 106 (2017): 130–135; K. N. Porter Starr and C. W. Bates, Excessive body weight in older adults, *Clinics in Geriatric Medicine* 31 (2015): 311–326; N. Napoli and coauthors, Effect of weight loss, exercise, or both on cognition and quality of life in obese older adults, *American Journal of Clinical Nutrition* 100 (2014): 189–198.
44. J. I. Baum, I. Y. Kim, and R. R. Wolfe, Protein consumption and the elderly: What is the optimal level of intake? *Nutrients* 8 (2016): E359; R. R. Deer and E. Volpi, Protein intake and muscle function in older adults, *Current Opinion in Clinical Nutrition and Metabolic Care* 18 (2015): 248–253; Deutz and coauthors, 2014.
45. Deer and Volpi, 2015; Deutz and coauthors, 2014.
46. S. Farsijani and coauthors, Relation between mealtime distribution of protein intake and lean mass loss in free-living older adults of the NUAge study, *American Journal of Clinical Nutrition* 104 (2016): 694–703.
47. C. Giezenaar and coauthors, Effects of randomized whey-protein loads on energy intake, appetite, gastric emptying, and plasma gut-hormone concentrations in older men and women, *American Journal of Clinical Nutrition* 106 (2017): 865–877.
48. B. Gopinath and coauthors, Association between carbohydrate nutrition and successful aging over 10 years, *Journal of Gerontology* 71 (2016): 1335–1340.
49. L. Hooper, Why, oh why, are so many older adults not drinking enough fluid? *Journal of the Academy of Nutrition and Dietetics* 116 (2016): 774–777; M. V. Marra and coauthors, Elevated serum osmolality and total water deficit indicate impaired hydration status in residents of long-term care facilities regardless of low or high body mass index, *Journal of the Academy of Nutrition and Dietetics* 116 (2016): 828–836.

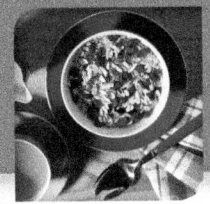

12.5 Nutrition in Practice
Hunger and Community Nutrition

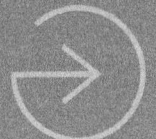

Worldwide, more than 800 million people (about 1 in 9) experience persistent hunger—not the healthy appetite triggered by anticipation of a hearty meal but the painful sensation caused by a lack of food.[1] Hunger deprives a person of the physical and mental energy needed to enjoy a full life and often leads to severe malnutrition and death. In 2016, nearly three million children younger than the age of five died as a result of hunger and malnutrition.[2]

Ideally, all people at all times would have access to enough food to support an active, healthy lifestyle. In other words, they would experience **food security**. Unfortunately, in the United States, where most people enjoy a life of relative abundance, 6.1 million households live with **very low food security**—one or more members of these households, many of them children, repeatedly had little or nothing to eat because of a lack of money (Box NP12-1).[3] Another 9.5 million households experience **low food security** or **marginal food security**, somewhat less dire conditions. Given the agricultural bounty and

enormous wealth in this country, do these numbers surprise you? The limited or uncertain availability of nutritionally adequate and safe foods is known as **food insecurity** and is a major social problem in our nation today.[4] Table NP12-1 presents questions used in national surveys to identify food insecurity in the United States, and Figure NP12-1 presents the most recent findings. Surveys like these provide crude,

FIGURE NP12-1 Prevalence of Food Security in U.S. Households

Most U.S. households are food secure.

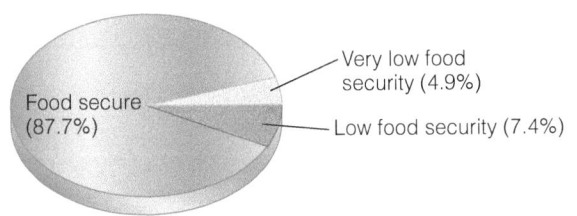

Source: A. Coleman-Jensen and coauthors, *Economic Research Service Report*, September 2017, Household food security in the United States in 2016.

TABLE NP12-1 Food Security Questions for U.S. Households

The USDA's Economic Research Service asks questions such as these to identify conditions that make it difficult for households to meet their basic food needs. Households reporting two or fewer of these conditions are classified as *food secure*; those with more than two are *food insecure* (for scoring details, visit the website below). For a household with children, additional questions determine their degree of food insecurity as well.

1. "We worried whether our food would run out before we got money to buy more." Was that often, sometimes, or never true for you in the last 12 months?

2. "The food that we bought just didn't last and we didn't have money to get more." Was that often, sometimes, or never true for you in the last 12 months?

3. "We couldn't afford to eat balanced meals." Was that often, sometimes, or never true for you in the last 12 months?

4. In the last 12 months, did you or other adults in the household ever cut the size of your meals or skip meals because there wasn't enough money for food? (Yes/No)

5. (If yes to question 4) How often did this happen—almost every month, some months but not every month, or in only one or two months?

6. In the last 12 months, did you ever eat less than you felt you should because there wasn't enough money for food? (Yes/No)

7. In the last 12 months, were you ever hungry, but didn't eat because there wasn't enough money for food? (Yes/No)

8. In the last 12 months, did you lose weight because there wasn't enough money for food? (Yes/No)

9. In the last 12 months, did you or other adults in your household ever not eat for a whole day because there wasn't enough money for food? (Yes/No)

10. (If yes to question 9) How often did this happen—almost every month, some months but not every month, or in only one or two months?

Source: A. Coleman-Jensen and coauthors, *Economic Research Service Report*, September 2017, Household food security in the United States in 2016. *www.ers.usda.gov/media/8271/hh2012.pdf*

emergency kitchens: programs that provide meals to be eaten on-site; often called soup kitchens.

food banks: facilities that collect and distribute food donations to authorized organizations feeding the hungry.

food deserts: urban and rural low-income areas with limited access to affordable and nutritious foods (also defined in Chapter 7).

food insecurity: limited or uncertain availability of nutritionally adequate and safe foods or limited or uncertain ability to acquire acceptable foods in socially acceptable ways. Food insecurity categories include:

- *low food security:* reduced dietary quality, variety, or desirability but with little or no indication of reduced food intake.

- *very low food security:* multiple indications of disrupted eating patterns and reduced food intake.

food pantries: community food collection programs that provide groceries to be prepared and eaten at home.

food poverty: hunger occurring when enough food exists in an area but some of the people cannot obtain it because they lack money, are being deprived for political reasons, live in a country at war, or suffer from other problems such as lack of transportation.

food recovery: the collection of wholesome food for distribution to low-income people who are hungry. Four common methods of food recovery are:

- *field gleaning:* collecting crops from fields that either have already been harvested or are not profitable to harvest.

- *perishable food rescue or salvage:* collection of perishable produce from wholesalers and markets.

- *prepared food rescue:* collection of prepared foods from commercial kitchens.

- *nonperishable food collection:* collection of processed foods from wholesalers and markets.

food security: access to enough food to sustain a healthy and active life. Food security categories include:

- *high food security:* no indications of food-access problems or limitations.

- *marginal food security:* one or two indications of food-access problems but with little or no change in food intake.

---

but necessary, data to estimate the degree of hunger in this country. Box NP12-2 defines related terms.

Why is hunger a problem in developed countries such as the United States where food is abundant?

Hunger has many causes, but in developed countries, the primary cause is **food poverty**. People are hungry not because there is no food available nearby, but because they lack sufficient money with which to buy nutritious food and pay for other necessities, such as housing, clothing, medicines, and utilities. More than 12 percent of the population of the United States lives in poverty.[5] Even those above the poverty line may not have food security. Physical and mental illnesses and disabilities, sudden job losses, and high living expenses threaten their financial stability. Further contributing to food poverty are other problems such as abuse of alcohol and other drugs; lack of awareness of food assistance programs; and the reluctance of people, particularly older adults, to accept what they perceive as "welfare" or "charity." Lack of financial resources remains the major cause of food poverty in developed countries, and solving this problem would do a lot to relieve hunger.

In the United States, poverty and hunger reach across various segments of society, touching some more than others—notably, single parents living in households with their children, Hispanics, African Americans, and those living in the inner cities or rural areas.[6] People living in poverty are simply unable to buy sufficient amounts of nourishing foods, even if they are skilled in food shopping. Consequently, their diets tend to be inadequate. For many of the children in these families, school lunch (and breakfast, where available) may be the only nourishment for the day. Otherwise, they go hungry, waiting for an adult to find money for food. Not surprisingly, these children are more likely to have health problems and iron-deficiency anemia than those who eat regularly. They also tend to perform poorly in school and in social situations. For adults, the risk of developing chronic diseases increases.[7]

Is it true that hunger and obesity often exist side by side—sometimes within the same household or even the same person?

Research findings on the relationship between food insecurity and obesity are inconsistent, but food insufficiency and obesity often exist side by side.[8] Low-income urban and rural communities that offer little or no access to affordable nutritious foods—**food deserts** (first mentioned in Chapter 7)—lack markets that sell fresh produce, dairy products, and other nutritious fresh foods. Not surprisingly, people living in food deserts often lack fruit and vegetables in their diets. High-fat, high-sugar, refined, energy-dense foods that are readily available in food deserts infamously lack other needed nutrients.

Economic uncertainty and stress greatly influence the prevalence of obesity.[9] People who are unsure about their next meal may overeat when food or money become available.

What U.S. food programs are directed at relieving hunger in the United States?

The Academy of Nutrition and Dietetics calls for aggressive action to bring an end to domestic hunger and to achieve food and nutrition security for all residents of the United States.[10] Many federal and local programs aim to prevent or relieve malnutrition and hunger.

An extensive network of federal assistance programs provides life-giving food daily to millions of U.S. citizens. Even so, the programs are not fully successful in preventing hunger, though they do seem to improve the nutrient intakes of those who participate. Programs described in the life cycle chapters include the WIC program for low-income pregnant women, breastfeeding mothers, and their young children (Chapter 10); the school lunch and breakfast programs for children (Chapter 11); and the food assistance programs for older adults such as congregate meals and Meals on Wheels (Chapter 12).

The centerpiece of food programs for low-income people in the United States is the Supplemental Nutrition Assistance Program (SNAP), administered by the U.S. Department of Agriculture (USDA). The USDA issues debit cards through state agencies to households—people who buy and prepare food together. The amount a household receives depends on its size, resources, and income. Recipients may use the cards to purchase food and food-bearing plants and seeds but not to buy tobacco, cleaning items, alcohol, or other nonfood items. Box NP12-3 offers tips for both saving money and preventing food waste.

SNAP is the largest of the federal food assistance programs, both in amount of money spent and in number of people participating. It provides assistance to more than 44 million people at a cost of 70 billion per year; about half of the recipients are children.

Box NP12-3 | *HOW TO* Stretch Food Dollars and Reduce Waste

Eating well on a limited budget can pose a challenge, but these tips ease the task. The Healthy Eating on a Budget section of the MyPlate website (www.choosemyplate.gov/budget) offers additional tips for planning meals and purchasing foods as well as menu ideas.

Plan Ahead
- Plan your menus, write grocery lists, and shop only for foods on your list to avoid expensive "impulse" buying.
- Center meals on whole grains, legumes, and vegetables; use smaller quantities of meat, poultry, fish, or eggs.
- Use cooked cereals such as oatmeal instead of ready-to-eat breakfast cereals.
- Cook large quantities when time and money allow; freeze portions for convenient later meals.
- Check for sales and use coupons for products you need; plan meals to take advantage of sale items.

Shop Smart
- Do not shop when hungry.
- Select whole foods instead of convenience foods (raw whole potatoes instead of refrigerated prepared mashed potatoes, for example).
- Try store brands.
- Buy fresh produce in season; buy canned or frozen items at other times.
- Buy large bags of frozen items or dry goods; use as needed and store the remainder.

- Buy fat-free dry milk; mix and refrigerate quantities needed for a day or two. Buy fresh milk by the gallon or half-gallon only if you can use it up before it spoils.
- Buy less expensive cuts of meat, such as beef chuck and pork shoulder roasts; cook with liquid long enough to make the meat tender.
- Buy whole chickens instead of pieces; ask a butcher to show you how to cut them up.
- Frequent discount stores instead of grocery stores for nonfood items such as toilet paper and detergent.

Reduce Waste
- Change your thinking from "what do I want to eat" to "what do I have available to eat." Consumers can search websites for recipes using ingredients they have on hand.
- Use leftovers to save time and money as well as to reduce waste.
- Buy only the amount of fresh foods that you will eat before it spoils.
- Peel away the tough outer layers from stems of asparagus and broccoli; slice and cook the tender stems or add raw to salads.
- Scrub, but don't peel, potatoes before cooking—the skins add color, texture, and nutrients to the dish.
- Before buying food in bulk, plan how to store it properly. If it spoils before use, you'll throw away your savings.
- If your "bargain" bulk food is more than you can use but is still fresh, donate it to your local food bank or homeless shelter. (It won't save you money, but it will provide a wealth of satisfaction.)
- If space permits, compost fruit and vegetable scraps to feed shrubs and other outdoor plants.

Why do health care professionals need to know about food assistance programs?

Health care professionals who work in public health are generally well acquainted with food assistance programs, and often many of their clients receive such assistance. Regardless of the setting in which health care professionals see clients, however, it is important to encourage those who may be having financial problems to talk with a social worker who can assess their eligibility for food assistance programs. The subject of food assistance must be approached in a nonjudgmental and tactful manner—the client may feel uncomfortable about seeking assistance.

Are there other programs aimed at reducing hunger in the United States?

Efforts to resolve the problem of hunger in the United States do not depend solely on federal assistance programs. National **food recovery** programs such as Feeding America coordinate the efforts of **food banks**, **food pantries**, **emergency kitchens**, and homeless shelters that provide food to tens of millions of people a year (see Photo NP12-1). Table NP12-2 lists websites for Feeding America and other hunger relief organizations.

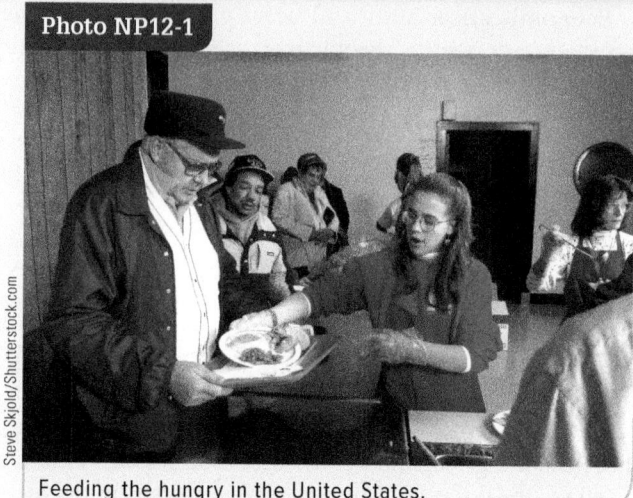

Photo NP12-1

Feeding the hungry in the United States.

Each year, a tremendous amount of our food supply is wasted in fields, commercial kitchens, grocery stores, and restaurants—enough food to feed millions of people. Food recovery programs collect and distribute good food that

TABLE NP12-2 Hunger-Relief Organizations

ORGANIZATION	MISSION STATEMENT
Bread for the World *www.bread.org*	Nonpartisan, Christian citizens' movement seeking to influence reform in policies, programs, and conditions that allow hunger and poverty to persist globally.
Catholic Relief Services *www.crs.org*	Humanitarian service agency assisting the impoverished and disadvantaged through community-based, sustainable development initiatives.
Congressional Hunger Center *www.hungercenter.org*	Bipartisan organization training and inspiring leaders with the intent to end hunger and advocating public policies to create a food-secure world.
Feeding America *www.feedingamerica.org*	Domestic charity organization providing food assistance through a nationwide network of member food banks and facilitating education to end hunger nationally.
Food and Agriculture Organization (FAO) of the United Nations *www.fao.org*	International organization leading efforts to achieve food security for all by helping to develop and modernize countries' agriculture, forestry, and fishery practices.
Food First *www.foodfirst.org*	North American coalition working to catalyze food systems that are healthy, sustainable, just, and democratic by building community voice and capacity for change.
Idealist *www.idealist.org*	International organization seeking to connect people, organizations, and resources to help build a world where all people can live free and dignified lives.
Oxfam America *www.oxfamamerica.org*	International relief and development organization aiming to create lasting solutions to poverty, hunger, and injustice.
Pan American Health Organization *new.paho.org*	International public health agency aiming to strengthen national and local health systems with the purpose of improving the quality of, and lengthening, the lives of the peoples in the Americas.
Society of St. Andrew *www.endhunger.org*	Ecumenical Christian ministry salvaging and redirecting large amounts of fresh produce to hunger agencies for distribution to the poor.

(continued)

ORGANIZATION	MISSION STATEMENT
The Hunger Project *www.thp.org*	International relief organization attempting to end hunger and poverty by pioneering sustainable, grassroots, women-centered strategies and advocating for their widespread adoption in countries throughout the world.
United Nations Children's Fund (UNICEF) *www.unicef.org*	International organization advocating for the protection of children's rights, to help meet their basic needs and to expand their opportunities to reach their full potentials.
WhyHunger *www.whyhunger.org*	Domestic organization supporting and funding community-based organizations intent on empowering individuals and building self-reliance to provide long-term solutions to end hunger and poverty.
World Food Programme *www.wfp.org*	Food aid branch of the United Nations aiming to prepare for, protect during, and provide assistance after emergencies, as well as reduce hunger and undernutrition.
World Health Organization (WHO) *www.who.int*	United Nations agency acting as the authority on international public health by influencing policy, setting research agendas, establishing standards, and providing technical support to monitor and assess health trends.

Photo NP12-2

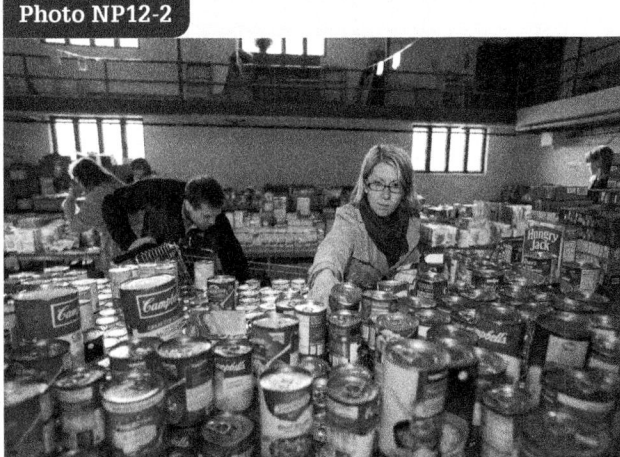

Community-based efforts to feed citizens include food pantries that provide groceries.

Jim West/AGE Fotostock

would otherwise go to waste. Volunteers might pick corn left in an already harvested field, a grocer might deliver ripe bananas to a local food bank, and a caterer might take leftover chicken salad to a community shelter, for example. All of these efforts help to feed the hungry in the United States.

What about local efforts and community nutrition programs?

Food recovery programs depend on volunteers. Concerned citizens work through local agencies and churches to feed the hungry. Community-based food pantries provide groceries, and soup kitchens serve prepared meals (see Photo NP12-2). Meals often deliver adequate nourishment, but most homeless people receive fewer than one and a half meals a day, so many are still inadequately nourished. Health care professionals can serve as valuable members of community groups seeking to provide food assistance.

Notes

1. *The State of Food Security and Nutrition in the World, 2017,* Food and Agriculture Organization, www.fao.org/state-of-food-security-nutrition/en.
2. World Health Organization, *Children: Reducing mortality,* Fact sheet, October, 2017, www.who.int/mediacentre/factsheets/fs178/en/index.html.
3. A. Coleman-Jensen and coauthors, *Economic Research Service Report,* September 2017, Household food security in the United States in 2016. www.ers.usda.gov/webdocs/publications/84973/err-237.pdf?v=42979.
4. Position of the Academy of Nutrition and Dietetics, Food insecurity in the United States, *Journal of the Academy of Nutrition and Dietetics* 117 (2017): 1991–2002.
5. J. L. Semega, K. R. Fontenot, and M. A. Kollar, *Income and Poverty in the United States: 2016,* September 12, 2017, www.census.gov/library/publications/2017/demo/p60-259.html.
6. Position of the Academy of Nutrition and Dietetics, Food insecurity in the United States, 2017.
7. S. M. Irving, R. S. Njai, and P. Z. Siegel, Food insecurity and self-reported hypertension among Hispanic, black, and white adults in 12 states, Behavioral Risk Factor Surveillance System, 2009, *Preventing Chronic Disease* 18 (2014): E161.
8. B. T. Nguyen and coauthors, Food security and weight status in children: Interactions with food assistance programs, *American Journal of Preventive Medicine* 52 (2017): S138–S144; K. R. Flórez and coauthors, Associations between depressive symptomatology, diet, and body mass index among participants in the Supplemental Nutrition Assistance Program, *Journal of the Academy of Nutrition and Dietetics,* 115 (2015): 1102–1108; J. Kaur, M. M. Lamb, and C. L. Ogden, The association between food insecurity and obesity in children—The National Health and Nutrition Examination Survey, *Journal of the Academy of Nutrition and Dietetics* 115 (2015): 751–758.
9. Flórez and coauthors, 2015.
10. Position of the Academy of Nutrition and Dietetics, Food insecurity in the United States, 2017.

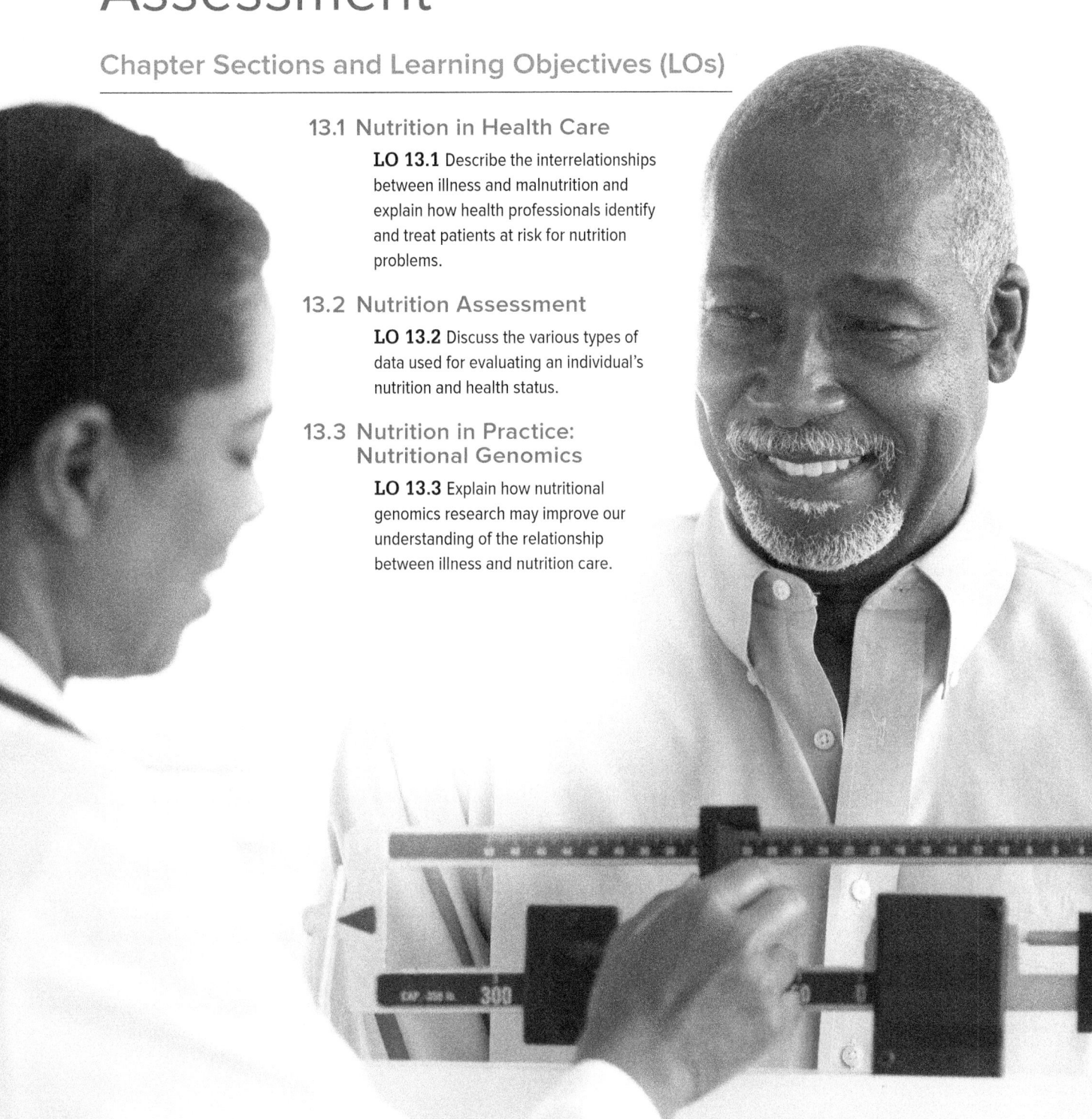

Nutrition Care and Assessment

chapter
13

Chapter Sections and Learning Objectives (LOs)

13.1 Nutrition in Health Care

LO 13.1 Describe the interrelationships between illness and malnutrition and explain how health professionals identify and treat patients at risk for nutrition problems.

13.2 Nutrition Assessment

LO 13.2 Discuss the various types of data used for evaluating an individual's nutrition and health status.

13.3 Nutrition in Practice: Nutritional Genomics

LO 13.3 Explain how nutritional genomics research may improve our understanding of the relationship between illness and nutrition care.

JGI/Tom Grill/Getty Images

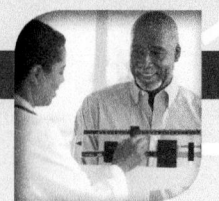
described how appropriate dietary choices can support good health. Turning now to clinical nutrition, the remaining chapters explain how various illnesses influence nutrition status and how nutrition therapy contributes to medical care. Nurses and other health care providers who consider nutrition care in their treatment decisions are best prepared to help patients* recover from illness and maintain an optimal quality of life. This chapter introduces the process used for providing nutrition care and the strategies used for assessing nutrition status.

13.1 Nutrition in Health Care

The busy nurse with many responsibilities may be tempted to put a patient's nutritional needs on the back burner; after all, the benefits of nutrition therapy are not always as obvious or immediate as those of other medical treatments. Correcting nutrition problems, however, may improve both short- and long-term outcomes of medical treatments and help to prevent complications. Moreover, patients are often concerned about the diet they should adopt to improve their health.

Malnutrition is frequently reported in patients hospitalized with an acute illness. Depending on the patient population, estimates of malnutrition in hospital patients range from 15 to 60 percent.[1] Poor nutrition status weakens immune function and compromises a person's healing ability, influencing both the course of illness and the body's response to treatment. Complications of malnutrition often lengthen hospital stays and increase the overall cost of patient care.[2]

How Illness Affects Nutrition Status

Illnesses and their treatments may lead to malnutrition by causing a reduction in food intake, interfering with digestion and absorption, or altering nutrient metabolism and excretion (see Figure 13-1). For example, the nausea caused by some illnesses or treatments can diminish appetite and reduce food intake; similarly, inflammation in the mouth or esophagus may cause discomfort when the patient consumes food. Some medications can cause **anorexia** (loss of appetite) or gastrointestinal (GI) discomfort or interfere with nutrient function and metabolism. Prolonged bedrest often results in **pressure sores**, which increase metabolic stress and raise protein and energy needs.

The dietary changes required during an acute illness are usually temporary and can be tailored to accommodate an individual's preferences and lifestyle. Conversely, chronic illnesses (those lasting three months or longer) may require long-term dietary adjustments. For example, diabetes treatment requires lifelong changes in diet and lifestyle that some people may find difficult to adhere to. The challenge for nurses and other health professionals is to help their patients understand the potential benefits of nutrition therapy and accept the dietary changes that can improve their health.

An illness may have indirect effects that influence nutrition status. For example, an individual may lack the strength and energy required for meal preparation while recovering from illness. Emotional health may suffer as a result of chronic disease or terminal illness, causing a lack of appetite and disinterest in food preparation. In some cases, the costs of health care can drain financial resources and limit the ability to make the appropriate food choices.

anorexia: loss of appetite.

pressure sores: regions of skin and tissue that are damaged due to prolonged pressure on the affected area by an external object, such as a bed, wheelchair, or cast; vulnerable areas of the body include buttocks, hips, and heels. Also called *decubitus* (deh-KYU-bih-tus) *ulcers*.

*Nurses may use the term *client* or *patient* when referring to an individual under their care. The clinical chapters emphasize the care of those with serious illnesses; thus, the term *patient* is used throughout these chapters.

FIGURE 13-1 Ways in Which Illness Can Affect Nutrition Status

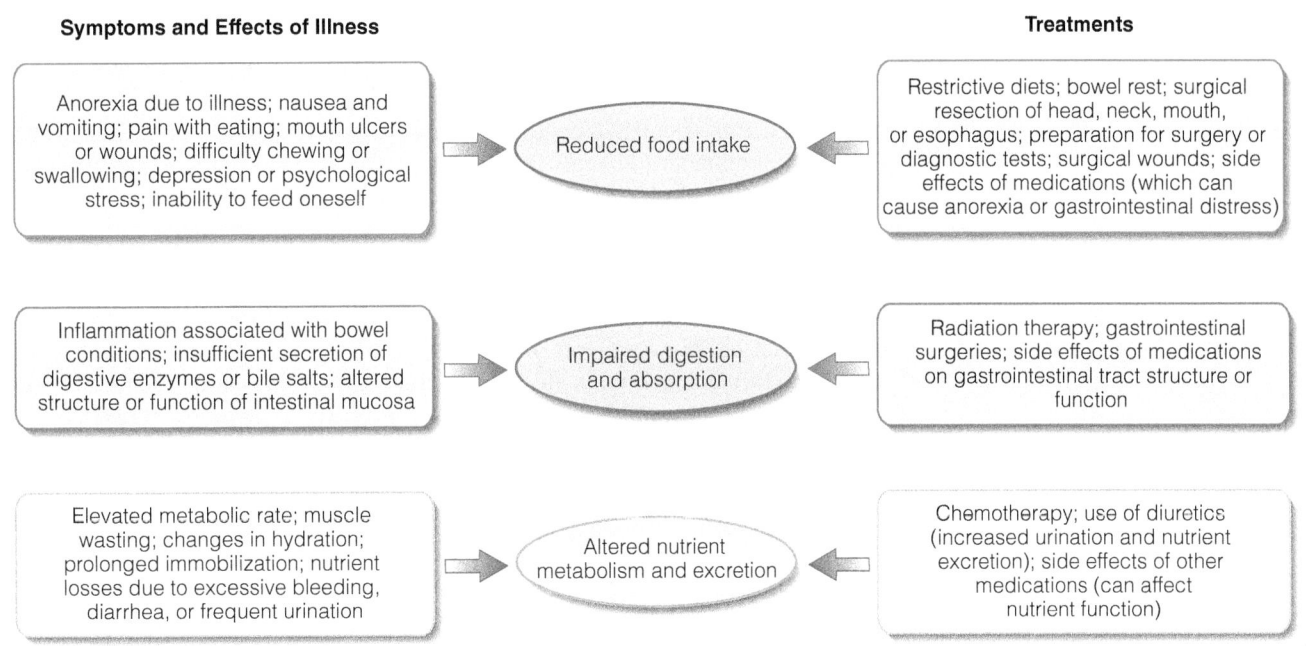

Symptoms and Effects of Illness   Treatments

Anorexia due to illness; nausea and vomiting; pain with eating; mouth ulcers or wounds; difficulty chewing or swallowing; depression or psychological stress; inability to feed oneself → Reduced food intake ← Restrictive diets; bowel rest; surgical resection of head, neck, mouth, or esophagus; preparation for surgery or diagnostic tests; surgical wounds; side effects of medications (which can cause anorexia or gastrointestinal distress)

Inflammation associated with bowel conditions; insufficient secretion of digestive enzymes or bile salts; altered structure or function of intestinal mucosa → Impaired digestion and absorption ← Radiation therapy; gastrointestinal surgeries; side effects of medications on gastrointestinal tract structure or function

Elevated metabolic rate; muscle wasting; changes in hydration; prolonged immobilization; nutrient losses due to excessive bleeding, diarrhea, or frequent urination → Altered nutrient metabolism and excretion ← Chemotherapy; use of diuretics (increased urination and nutrient excretion); side effects of other medications (can affect nutrient function)

Responsibility for Nutrition Care

Members of the health care team work together to ensure that the nutritional needs of patients are met during illness. The roles of health professionals vary among different institutions, and their responsibilities can sometimes overlap. In some cases, the patient's nutrition care is incorporated into the medical care plan developed by the entire health care team. Such plans, called **clinical pathways**, outline coordinated plans of care for specific medical diagnoses, procedures, or treatments.

Physicians Physicians are responsible for meeting all of a patient's medical needs, including nutrition. They prescribe **diet orders** and other instructions related to nutrition care, including referrals for nutrition assessment and dietary counseling. Physicians rely on nurses, registered dietitians, and other health professionals to alert them to nutrition problems, suggest strategies for handling nutrition care, and provide nutrition services.

Nurses Nurses interact closely with patients and thus are in an ideal position to identify people who would benefit from nutrition services. Nurses often screen patients for nutrition problems and may participate in nutrition and dietary assessments. Nurses also provide direct nutrition care, such as encouraging patients to eat, finding practical solutions to food-related problems, recording a patient's food intake, and answering questions about special diets. As members of **nutrition support teams**, nurses are responsible for administering tube and intravenous feedings. In facilities that do not employ registered dietitians, nurses often assume responsibility for much of the nutrition care.

Registered Dietitians A **registered dietitian** (or **registered dietitian nutritionist**) is a food and nutrition expert who is qualified to provide **medical nutrition therapy**. Registered dietitians may conduct nutrition and dietary assessments; diagnose nutrition problems; develop, implement, and evaluate **nutrition care plans** (described later); order patient diets; plan and approve menus; and provide dietary counseling and nutrition

clinical pathways: coordinated programs of treatment that merge the care plans of different health practitioners; also called *care pathways, care maps,* or *critical pathways.*

diet orders: specific instructions about dietary management; also called *diet prescriptions* or *nutrition prescriptions.*

nutrition support teams: health care professionals responsible for providing nutrients by tube feeding or intravenous infusion.

registered dietitian or **registered dietitian nutritionist:** a food and nutrition expert who has completed the education and training specified by the Academy of Nutrition and Dietetics (or Dietitians of Canada), including a bachelor's degree in nutrition or dietetics, a supervised internship, and a national registration examination.

medical nutrition therapy: nutrition care provided by a registered dietitian; includes assessing nutrition status, diagnosing nutrition problems, and providing nutrition care.

nutrition care plans: strategies for meeting an individual's nutritional needs.

education services. Registered dietitians may also manage foodservice operations in health care institutions.

Registered Dietetic Technicians Registered dietetic technicians often work in partnership with registered dietitians and assist in the implementation and monitoring of nutrition services. Depending on their background and experience, they may screen patients for nutrition problems, develop menus and recipes, ensure appropriate meal delivery, monitor patients' food choices and intakes, and provide patient education and counseling. Dietetic technicians sometimes supervise foodservice operations and may have roles in purchasing, inventory, quality control, sanitation, or safety.

Other Health Care Professionals Other health care professionals who may assist with nutrition care include pharmacists, physical therapists, occupational therapists, speech therapists, nursing assistants, home health care aides, and social workers. These individuals can be instrumental in alerting dietitians or nurses to nutrition problems or may share relevant information about a patient's health status or personal needs.

Identifying Risk for Malnutrition

To identify patients who are malnourished or at risk for malnutrition, a **nutrition screening** is conducted within 24 hours of a patient's admission to a hospital or other extended-care facility. A screening may also be included in certain types of outpatient services and community health programs. A nutrition screening involves collecting health-related data that can indicate the presence of **protein-energy malnutrition (PEM)** or other nutrition problems. The screening should be sensitive enough to identify patients who require nutrition care but simple enough to be completed within 10 to 15 minutes. Usually a nurse, nursing assistant, registered dietitian, or dietetic technician performs and documents the screening.

The information collected in a nutrition screening varies according to the patient population, the type of care offered by the health care facility, and the patient's medical problem. Often included are the admitting diagnosis, physical measurements and laboratory test results obtained during the admission process, relevant symptoms, and information about diet and health status provided by the patient or caregiver (see Table 13-1 for examples). Several screening tools that use different combinations of

nutrition screening: an assessment procedure that helps to identify patients who are malnourished or at risk for malnutrition.

protein-energy malnutrition (PEM): a state of malnutrition characterized by depletion of tissue proteins and energy stores, usually accompanied by micronutrient deficiencies.

nursing diagnoses: clinical judgments about actual or potential health problems that provide the basis for selecting appropriate nursing interventions.

nutrition care process: a systematic approach used by dietetics professionals to evaluate and treat nutrition-related problems.

TABLE 13-1	Criteria for Identifying Malnutrition Risk
CATEGORY	**SPECIFIC EXAMPLES**
Admission data	Age, medical diagnosis, severity of illness or injury
Anthropometric data	Height and weight, body mass index (BMI), unintentional weight changes, loss of muscle or subcutaneous fat
Functional assessment data	Low handgrip strength, general weakness, impaired mobility
Historical information	History of diabetes, renal disease, or other chronic illness; use of medications that can impair nutrition status; extensive dietary restrictions; food allergies or intolerances; requirement for nutrition support; difficulties with meal preparation or ingestion; depression, social isolation, or dementia
Laboratory test results	Blood test results that suggest the presence of inflammation (such as low serum protein levels) or anemia
Signs and symptoms	Reduced appetite or food intake, problems that interfere with food intake (such as chewing or swallowing difficulties or nausea and vomiting), localized or general edema, presence of pressure sores

TABLE 13-2 **Subjective Global Assessment**

The Subjective Global Assessment evaluates a person's risk of malnutrition by ranking key variables of the medical history and physical examination. These variables are each given an A, B, or C rating: A for well nourished, B for potential or mild malnutrition, and C for severe malnutrition. Patients are classified according to the final numbers of A, B, and C ratings.

MEDICAL HISTORY

- Body weight changes: percentage weight loss in past six months; weight loss or gain in past two weeks
- Dietary changes: suboptimal, low calorie, liquid diet, or starvation
- GI symptoms: nausea, diarrhea, vomiting, or anorexia for more than two weeks
- Functional ability: full capacity versus suboptimal, walking versus bedridden
- Degree of disease-related metabolic stress: low, medium, or high

PHYSICAL EXAMINATION

- Subcutaneous fat loss (triceps or chest)
- Muscle loss (quadriceps or deltoids)
- Ankle edema
- Sacral (lower spine) edema
- Ascites (abdominal edema)

CLASSIFICATION

A: Well nourished: if no significant loss of weight, fat, or muscle tissue and no dietary difficulties, functional impairments, or GI symptoms; also applies to patients with recent weight gain and improved appetite, functioning, or medical prognosis

B: Moderate malnutrition: if 5 to 10 percent weight loss, mild loss of muscle or fat tissue, decreased food intake, and digestive or functional difficulties that impair food intake; the B classification usually applies to patients with an even mix of A, B, and C ratings

C: Severe malnutrition: if more than 10 percent weight loss, severe loss of muscle or fat tissue, edema, multiple GI symptoms, and functional impairments

Sources: P. Charney and M. Marian, Nutrition screening and nutrition assessment, in P. Charney and A. M. Malone, eds., *ADA Pocket Guide to Nutrition Assessment* (Chicago: American Dietetic Association, 2009), pp. 1–19; A. S. Detsky and coauthors, What is subjective global assessment of nutritional status? *Journal of Parenteral and Enteral Nutrition* 11 (1987): 8–13.

these variables have become popular in recent years; one example is the Subjective Global Assessment, which ranks nutrition-related elements of the medical history and physical examination to assess malnutrition risk (see Table 13-2). Briefer screening methods use just two or three variables; for example, some tools screen for malnutrition risk by evaluating health status, unintentional weight changes, and reduced appetite or food intake.[3]

Nursing care plans often include **nursing diagnoses** that suggest the need for nutrition interventions (see Table 13-3). For example, a nursing diagnosis of "impaired swallowing" alerts the nurse to potential problems with food consumption and suggests the need for a modified diet. Such a diagnosis can accompany various medical disorders, including developmental disabilities, diseases involving the esophagus, and neurological conditions. Examples of relevant nursing diagnoses are provided throughout the clinical nutrition chapters.

A nutrition screening may lead to a referral for nutrition care. The following section describes the next stage of the process: the method used by dietitians to address nutritional concerns.

The Nutrition Care Process

Registered dietitians use a systematic approach to medical nutrition therapy called the **nutrition care process**.[4] The four steps of this process—nutrition assessment, nutrition diagnosis, nutrition intervention, and nutrition monitoring and evaluation—are shown in

TABLE 13-3 **Nursing Diagnoses with Nutritional Implications**

- Chronic confusion
- Chronic pain
- Constipation
- Diarrhea
- Disturbed body image
- Feeding self-care deficit
- Imbalanced nutrition: less than body requirements
- Impaired dentition
- Impaired oral mucous membrane integrity
- Impaired physical mobility
- Impaired swallowing
- Insufficient breast milk production
- Nausea
- Obesity
- Readiness for enhanced nutrition
- Risk for aspiration
- Risk for deficient fluid volume
- Risk for overweight
- Risk for unstable blood glucose level

Source: T. H. Herdman and S. Kamitsuru, eds., *NANDA International Nursing Diagnoses: Definitions and Classification 2018–2020* (New York: Thieme Publishers, 2017).

FIGURE 13-2   The Nutrition Care Process

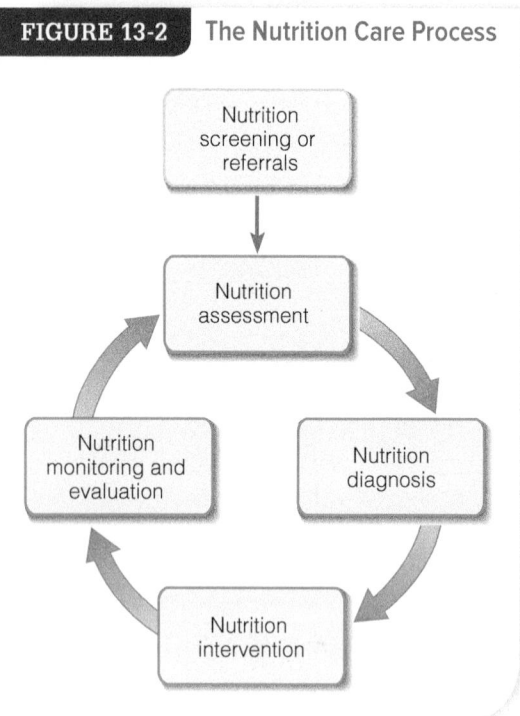

Figure 13-2. Although the nutrition care process is easiest to visualize as a series of steps, the steps are frequently revisited in order to reassess and revise diagnoses and intervention strategies. Each step must be documented in the medical record, providing a record for future reference and facilitating communication among members of the health care team. Note that the provision of nursing care involves a similar process, as shown in Box 13-1.

Nutrition Assessment A nutrition assessment involves the collection and analysis of health-related data in order to identify specific nutrition problems and their underlying causes. The information may be obtained from the medical record, physical examination, laboratory analyses, medical procedures, an interview with the patient or caregiver, and consultation with other health professionals. The assessment data are used to develop a plan of action to prevent or correct energy or nutrient imbalances, or to determine whether a care plan is working. The second half of this chapter describes the components of nutrition assessment in detail.

Nutrition Diagnosis Each nutrition problem identified by the nutrition assessment receives a separate diagnosis, which is formatted as a **PES statement**, a statement that includes the specific problem (P), etiology or cause (E), and signs and symptoms that provide evidence of the problem (S).[5] For example, a potential nutrition diagnosis might be, "Unintended weight gain *(the problem)* related to long-term use of corticosteroids *(the etiology or cause)* as evidenced by an involuntary weight gain of 10 percent of body weight over the past six months *(the sign or symptom)*." Like nursing diagnoses, a nutrition diagnosis can change during the course of an illness.

Nutrition Intervention After nutrition problems are identified, the appropriate nutrition care can be planned and implemented. A nutrition intervention may include counseling or education about appropriate dietary and lifestyle practices, a change in medication or other treatment, or adjustments in the meals or services offered to a hospital patient. To be successful, the intervention should consider the individual's food habits, lifestyle, and other personal factors. Goals are stated in terms of measurable outcomes; for example, goals for an overweight person with diabetes might include improvements in blood glucose levels and body weight. Other goals may be positive changes in dietary behaviors and lifestyle; for example, a diabetes patient may learn how to control carbohydrate intake or begin a regular exercise program. Chapter 14 provides additional information about nutrition intervention.

Nutrition Monitoring and Evaluation The effectiveness of the nutrition care plan must be evaluated periodically: the patient's progress should be monitored closely, and updated assessment data or diagnoses may require adjustments in goals or outcome measures. Sometimes a new situation alters nutritional needs; for example, a change in the medical treatment or a new medication may alter a person's tolerance to certain foods. The nutrition care plan must be flexible enough to adapt to the new situation.

If progress is slow or a patient is unable or unwilling to make the suggested changes, the care plan should be redesigned and take into account the reasons why the earlier plan was not successful. The new plan may need to include motivational techniques or additional patient education. If the patient remains unwilling to modify behaviors despite the expected benefits, the health practitioner can try again at a later time when the patient may be more receptive (see Box 13-2).

BOX 13-1

The nursing process, which is the approach used for providing nursing care, consists of these steps:

1. Assessment
2. Nursing diagnosis
3. Planning
4. Implementation
5. Evaluation

BOX 13-2 *Nursing Diagnosis*

The nursing diagnosis *readiness for enhanced nutrition* is appropriate for a person who is willing to improve dietary practices.

PES statement: a statement that describes a nutrition problem in a format that includes the problem (P), the etiology or cause (E), and the signs and symptoms (S).

13.2 Nutrition Assessment

As described earlier, a nutrition assessment provides the information needed for diagnosing nutrition problems and designing a nutrition care plan; follow-up assessments can determine whether the care plan has been effective. Ideally, the assessment should be sensitive enough to detect subtle nutrition problems and specific enough to identify problem nutrients. For most nutrient imbalances, a variety of tests are necessary to identify nutrition problems.

Historical Information

Historical information provides valuable clues about the patient's nutrition status and nutrient requirements; it also reveals personal preferences that should be considered when developing a nutrition care plan. Table 13-4 summarizes the various types of historical data that contribute to a nutrition assessment. This information can be obtained from the medical record or by interviewing the patient or caregiver.

Medical History The medical history helps the clinician identify health problems or medical treatments that may interfere with food intake or require dietary changes;

TABLE 13-4 Historical Information Used in Nutrition Assessment[a]

MEDICAL HISTORY	MEDICATION AND SUPPLEMENT HISTORY	PERSONAL AND SOCIAL HISTORY	FOOD AND NUTRITION HISTORY
Age	Prescription drugs	Cognitive abilities	Food intake
Current complaint(s)	Over-the-counter drugs	Cultural/ethnic identity	Food availability
Past medical problems	Dietary and herbal supplements	Educational level	Recent weight changes
Ongoing medical treatments		Employment status	Dietary restrictions
Surgical history		Home/family situation	Food allergies or intolerances
Family medical history		Religious beliefs	Nutrition and health knowledge
Chronic disease risk		Socioeconomic status	Physical activity level and exercise habits
Mental/emotional health status		Use of tobacco, alcohol, or illegal drugs	

[a]Historical information is classified in different ways among medical institutions.

TABLE 13-5 **Medical Problems Often Associated with Malnutrition**

- Acquired immunodeficiency syndrome (AIDS)
- Alcoholism
- Anorexia nervosa or bulimia nervosa
- Burns (extensive or severe)
- Cancer and cancer treatments
- Cardiovascular diseases
- Celiac disease
- Chewing or swallowing difficulties
- Chronic kidney disease
- Dementia or other mental illness
- Diabetes mellitus
- Feeding disabilities
- Infections
- Inflammatory bowel diseases
- Liver disease
- Malabsorption
- Pressure sores
- Surgery (major)
- Vomiting (prolonged or severe)

Table 13-5 lists examples. The medical history generally includes the family medical history as well; this information may reveal genetic susceptibilities for diseases that can potentially be prevented with dietary and lifestyle changes.

Medication and Supplement History A number of medications can have detrimental effects on nutrition status, and various components of foods and dietary supplements can alter the absorption and metabolism of drugs. Chapter 14 provides examples of diet-drug interactions that may need consideration when planning nutrition care.

Personal and Social History Personal and social factors can influence both food choices and the ability to manage health and nutrition problems. For example, cultural background or religious beliefs can affect food preferences, whereas financial concerns may restrict access to health care and nutritious foods. Some individuals may depend on others to prepare or procure food. A person who lives alone or is depressed may eat poorly or be unable to follow complex dietary instructions. Use of alcohol, tobacco, or street drugs may alter food intake or have disruptive effects on health and nutrition status.

Food and Nutrition History A food and nutrition history (often called a *diet history*) is a detailed account of a person's dietary practices. It includes information about food intake, lifestyle habits, and other factors that may affect food choices, such as food allergies or beliefs about nutrition and health. The procedure often includes an interview about recent food intake (for example, a *24-hour dietary recall*) and a survey about usual food choices (such as a *food frequency questionnaire*). In the hospital setting, direct observation of patients' food intakes is helpful. The following section describes the most common methods of gathering food intake information.

Dietary Assessment

Obtaining accurate food intake data is challenging, as the results may vary depending on an individual's memory and honesty and the assessor's skill and training. Each method has its own strengths and weaknesses, so the best results are obtained by using a combination of approaches. Table 13-6 summarizes the methods commonly used as well as each method's advantages and disadvantages.

24-Hour Dietary Recall The **24-hour dietary recall** is a guided interview in which an individual recounts all of the foods and beverages consumed in the past 24 hours or during the previous day. The interview includes questions about the times when meals or snacks were eaten, amounts consumed, and ways in which foods were prepared (see Photo 13-1).

The *multiple-pass method* is considered the most effective approach for conducting a 24-hour dietary recall.[6] In this procedure, the interview includes four or five separate passes through the 24-hour period of interest. In the first pass, the respondent provides a "quick list" of foods consumed without prompts by the interviewer. The second pass is conducted to help the respondent remember foods that are often forgotten, such as beverages, bread, additions to foods (such as butter on toast), savory snacks, and sweets. The third and fourth passes elicit additional details about the foods consumed, such as the amounts eaten, preparation methods, and places where foods were obtained or consumed. A fifth pass may be conducted to provide a final opportunity to recall foods and to probe for more details. The entire multiple-pass interview can be conducted in about 30 to 45 minutes.

24-hour dietary recall: a record of foods consumed during the previous day or in the past 24 hours; sometimes modified to include foods consumed in a typical day.

TABLE 13-6	Methods for Obtaining Food Intake Data		
METHOD	**DESCRIPTION**	**ADVANTAGES**	**DISADVANTAGES**
24-hour dietary recall	Guided interview in which the foods and beverages consumed in a 24-hour period are described in detail.	• Results are not dependent on literacy or educational level of respondent. • Interview occurs after food is consumed, so method does not influence dietary choices. • Results are obtained quickly; method is relatively easy to conduct. • Method does not require reading or writing ability.	• Process relies on memory. • Underestimation and overestimation of food intakes are common. • Food items that cause embarrassment (alcohol, desserts) may be omitted. • Data from a single day cannot accurately represent the respondent's usual intake. • Seasonal variations may not be addressed. • Skill of interviewer affects outcome.
Food frequency questionnaire	Written survey of food consumption during a specific period of time, often a 1-year period.	• Process examines long-term food intake, so day-to-day and seasonal variability should not affect results. • Questionnaire is completed after food is consumed, so method does not influence food choices. • Method is inexpensive to administer.	• Process relies on memory. • Food lists often include common foods only. • Serving sizes are often difficult for respondents to evaluate without assistance. • Calculated nutrient intakes may not be accurate. • Food lists for the general population are of limited value in special populations. • Method is not effective for monitoring short-term changes in food intake.
Food record	Written account of food consumed during a specified period, usually several consecutive days. Accuracy is improved by including weights or measures of foods.	• Process does not rely on memory. • Recording foods as they are consumed may improve accuracy of food intake data. • Process is useful for controlling intake because keeping records increases awareness of food choices.	• Recording process itself influences food intake. • Underreporting and portion size errors are common. • Process is time-consuming and burdensome for respondent; requires a high degree of motivation. • Method requires literacy and the physical ability to write. • Seasonal changes in diet are not taken into account.
Direct observation	Observation of meal trays or shelf inventories before and after eating; possible only in residential facilities.	• Process does not rely on memory. • Method does not influence food intake. • Method can be used to evaluate the acceptability of a prescribed diet.	• Process is possible only in residential situations. • Method is labor intensive.

After the day's intake is recounted, the interviewer can ask whether the intake that day was fairly typical and, if not, how it varied from the person's usual intake. Recall interviews may be conducted on several nonconsecutive days to get a better representation of a person's usual diet. A disadvantage of the 24-hour dietary recall is that it does not take into account fluctuations in food intake or seasonal variations. Moreover, food intakes are often underestimated because the process relies on an individual's memory and reporting accuracy.

Photo 13-1 Collecting Food Intake Data

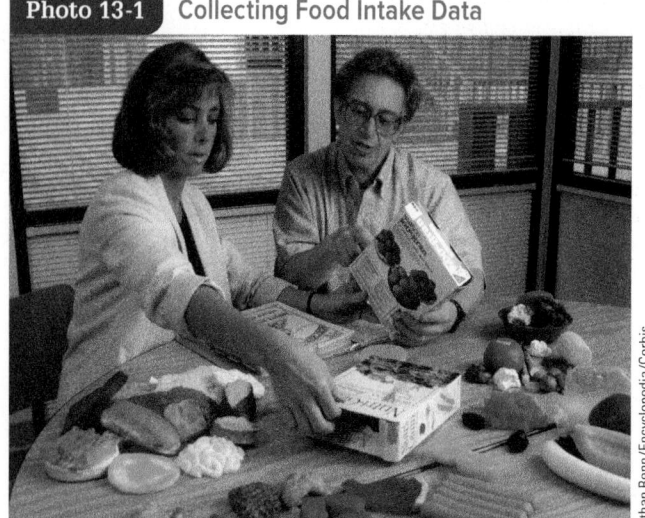

Nathan Benn/Encyclopedia/Corbis

The use of food models and measuring utensils can help an individual visualize portion sizes, improving the accuracy of food intake data.

food frequency questionnaire: a survey of foods routinely consumed. Some questionnaires ask about the types of food eaten and yield only qualitative information; others include questions about portions consumed and yield semiquantitative data as well.

Food Frequency Questionnaire A **food frequency questionnaire** surveys the foods and beverages regularly consumed during a specific time period. Some questionnaires are qualitative only: food lists contain common foods, organized by food group, with check boxes to indicate frequency of consumption. Other types of questionnaires can collect semiquantitative information by including portion sizes as well. Figure 13-3 shows a sample section of a semiquantitative questionnaire that surveys fruit intake over the previous year. Because the respondent is often asked to estimate food intakes over a one-year period, the results should not be affected by seasonal changes in diet. Conversely, a disadvantage of this method is its inability to determine recent changes in food intake. Another limitation is that the questionnaires typically list only common food items, so the accuracy of food intake data is reduced if an individual consumes atypical foods.

Some brief versions of food frequency questionnaires focus on food categories relevant to a person's medical condition. For example, a questionnaire designed to evaluate calcium intake may include only milk products, fortified foods, certain fruits and vegetables, and dietary supplements that contain calcium. A computer analysis can then quickly estimate the individual's calcium intake and compare it to recommendations.

Food Record A **food record** is a written account of foods and beverages consumed during a specified time period, usually several consecutive days. Foods are recorded as they are consumed in order to obtain the most complete and accurate record possible; thus, the process does not rely on memory. A detailed food record includes the types

FIGURE 13-3 Sample Section of a Food Frequency Questionnaire

FRUIT	Never or less than once per month	1 per mon.	2–3 per mon.	1 per week	2 per week	3–4 per week	5–6 per week	Every day	MEDIUM SERVING	YOUR SERVING SIZE S	M	L
EXAMPLE: Bananas	○	○	○	●	○	○	○	○	1 medium	○ 1/2	● 1	○ 2
Bananas	○	○	○	○	○	○	○	○	1 medium	○ 1/2	○ 1	○ 2
Apples, applesauce	○	○	○	○	○	○	○	○	1 medium or 1/2 cup	○ 1/2	○ 1	○ 2
Oranges (not including juice)	○	○	○	○	○	○	○	○	1 medium	○ 1/2	○ 1	○ 2
Grapefruit (not including juice)	○	○	○	○	○	○	○	○	1/2 medium	○ 1/4	○ 1/2	○ 1
Cantaloupe	○	○	○	○	○	○	○	○	1/4 medium	○ 1/8	○ 1/4	○ 1/2
Peaches, apricots (fresh, in season)	○	○	○	○	○	○	○	○	1 medium	○ 1/2	○ 1	○ 2
Peaches, apricots (canned or dried)	○	○	○	○	○	○	○	○	1 medium or 1/2 cup	○ 1/2	○ 1	○ 2
Prunes, or prune juice	○	○	○	○	○	○	○	○	1/2 cup	○ 1/4	○ 1/2	○ 1
Watermelon (in season)	○	○	○	○	○	○	○	○	1 slice	○ 1/2	○ 1	○ 2
Strawberries, other berries (in season)	○	○	○	○	○	○	○	○	1/2 cup	○ 1/4	○ 1/2	○ 1
Any other fruit, including kiwi, fruit cocktail, grapes, raisins, mangoes	○	○	○	○	○	○	○	○	1/2 cup	○ 1/4	○ 1/2	○ 1

CHAPTER 13 Nutrition Care and Assessment

and amounts of foods and beverages consumed, times of consumption, and methods of preparation. It may also include information about medication use, disease symptoms, physical activity, or other items of interest.

The food record provides valuable information about food intake as well as a person's response to and compliance with nutrition therapy. Unfortunately, food records require a great deal of time to complete, and people need to be highly motivated to keep accurate records. Another drawback is that the recording process itself may influence food intake. Furthermore, it is difficult to obtain accurate estimates of nutrient intakes in just a few days or even a week because of day-to-day and seasonal variations in food intake.

Direct Observation In facilities that serve meals, food intakes can be directly observed and analyzed. This method can also reveal a person's food preferences, changes in appetite, and any problems with a prescribed diet. Nurses use direct observation to conduct patients' **calorie counts**, which are estimates of the food energy (and often, protein) consumed by patients during a single day or several consecutive days. To perform a calorie count, the nurse records the dietary items that a patient is given at meals and subtracts the amounts remaining after meals are completed; this procedure allows an estimate of the caloric content of foods and beverages that are actually consumed. Although a useful means of discerning patients' intakes, direct observation requires regular and careful documentation and can be labor intensive and costly.

Anthropometric Data

Measures of body size, known as **anthropometric** measurements, can reveal problems related to both PEM and overnutrition. Height (or **length**) and weight are the most common anthropometric measurements and are used to evaluate growth in children and nutrition status in adults. Other helpful values include the results of body composition tests (see Appendix E) and circumferences of the head, waist, and limbs.

Height (or Length) Poor growth in children can be a sign of malnutrition. In adults, height measurements alone do not reflect current nutrition status but can be used for estimating a person's appropriate body weight or energy needs. Length is measured in infants and children younger than 24 months of age, and height is usually measured in older children and adults. Length can also be measured in adults and children who cannot stand unassisted due to physical or medical reasons. Box 13-3 describes some standard techniques for measuring length and height.

In adults who are bedridden or unable to stand, height can be estimated from equations that include either the knee height or the full arm span, both of which correlate well with height.[7] Knee height, which extends from the heel to the top of the knee when the leg is bent at a 90-degree angle, can be measured in either a sitting or supine position with a knee-height caliper; specific formulas are available for different ages, sexes, and ethnic groups. The full arm span is the distance from the tip of one middle finger to the other while the arms are extended horizontally. In children with disabilities that affect stature, alternative measures of linear growth include the full arm span, lower-leg lengths (knee to heel, similar to the knee-height measure), and upper-arm lengths (shoulder to elbow), all of which can be compared with reference percentiles.

Body Weight During clinical care, health care providers monitor body weights closely: weight changes may reflect changes in body water due to illness, and an involuntary weight loss can be a sign of PEM. Body weights can be compared with healthy ranges on height-weight tables and growth charts or used to calculate the **body mass index (BMI)**. A healthy body weight typically falls within a BMI range of 18.5 to 25; thus, an appropriate body weight can usually be estimated by using a BMI table or graph (see the inside back cover of this book). Box 13-4 includes suggestions for improving the accuracy of weight measurements.

food record: a detailed log of food eaten during a specified time period, usually several days; also called a *food diary*. A food record may also include information about medications, disease symptoms, and physical activity.

calorie counts: estimates of food energy (and often, protein) consumed by patients for one or more days.

anthropometric (AN-throw-poe-MEH-trik)**:** related to physical measurements of the human body, such as height, weight, body circumferences, and percentage of body fat.

length: the distance from the top of the head to the soles of the feet while a person is recumbent (lying down). In contrast, *height* is measured while a person is standing upright.

body mass index (BMI): a person's weight in relation to height; determined by dividing one's weight (in kilograms) by the square of the height (in meters).

Box 13-3 | *HOW TO* Measure Length and Height

To improve the accuracy of length and height measurements, keep the following in mind:

- Always measure—never ask. Self-reported heights are less accurate than measured heights. If height is not measured, document that the height is self-reported.

- Measure the length of infants and young children by using a measuring board with a fixed headboard and a movable footboard. It generally takes two people to measure length: one person gently holds the infant's head against the headboard; the other straightens the infant's legs and moves the footboard to the bottom of the infant's feet.

- Measure height next to a wall on which a nonstretchable measuring tape or board has been fixed. Ask the person to stand erect without shoes and with heels together. The person's eyes and head should be facing forward, with heels, buttocks, and shoulder blades touching the wall. Place a ruler or other flat, stiff object on the top of the head at a right angle to the wall and carefully note the height measurement. Immediately record length and height measurements to the nearest ⅛ inch or 0.1 centimeter.

- For evaluating the growth rate of young children, use the appropriate growth chart (Appendix E) when plotting results. If length is measured, use the growth chart for children between 0 and 36 months; if height is measured, use the chart for individuals between 2 and 20 years.

- Higher values are obtained from supine measurements than from vertical height measurements due to gravity.

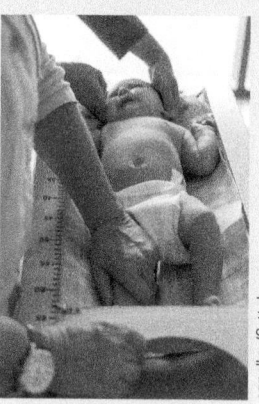

It generally takes two people to measure the length of an infant.

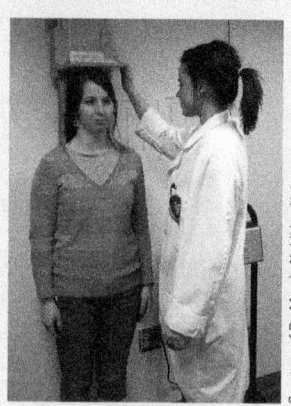

Standing erect allows for an accurate height measurement.

Head Circumference A measurement of head circumference helps to assess brain growth and malnutrition in children up to three years of age, although the measure is not necessarily reduced in a malnourished child. Head circumference values can also track brain development in premature and small-for-gestational-age infants. To measure head circumference, the assessor encircles the largest circumference mea-

Box 13-4 | *HOW TO* Measure Weight

Tips for measuring weight include:

- Always measure—never ask. Self-reported weights are often inaccurate. If weight is not measured, document that the weight is self-reported.

- Valid weight measurements require scales that have been carefully maintained, calibrated, and checked for accuracy at regular intervals. Beam balance and electronic scales are the most accurate. Bathroom scales are inaccurate and inappropriate for clinical use.

- Measure an infant's weight with a scale that allows the infant to sit or lie down. The tray should be large enough to support an infant or young child up to 40 pounds, and weight graduations should be in ½-ounce or 10-gram increments. For accurate results, weigh infants without clothes or diapers. Excessive movement by the infant can reduce accuracy.

- Children who can stand are weighed in the same way as adults, using beam balance or electronic scales with platforms large enough for standing comfortably.

- If repeated weight measurements are needed, each weighing should take place at the same time of day (preferably before breakfast), in the same amount of clothing, after the person has voided, and using the same scale. Record weights to the nearest ¼ pound or 0.1 kilogram.

- Special scales and hospital beds with built-in scales are available for weighing people who are bedridden.

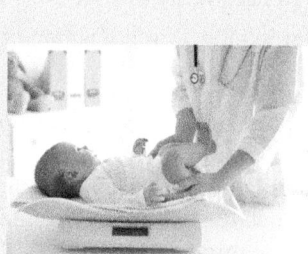

Infants are weighed on scales that allow them to sit or lie down.

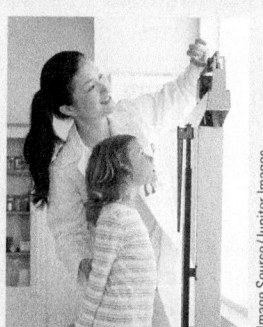

Beam balance scales allow accurate weight measurements for older children and adults.

sure of a child's head with a nonstretchable measuring tape: the tape is placed just above the eyebrows and ears and around the occipital prominence at the back of the head (see Photo 13-2). The measurement is read to the nearest ⅛ inch or 0.1 centimeter.

Circumferences of Waist and Limbs Circumferences of the waist and limbs are useful for evaluating body fat and muscle mass, respectively. The waist circumference correlates with intra-abdominal fat and can help in assessing overnutrition. Circumferences of the mid-upper arm, mid-thigh, and mid-calf regions can help in evaluating the effects of illness, aging, and PEM on skeletal muscle tissue. For improved accuracy, circumference measurements are often used together with skinfold measurements to correct for the subcutaneous fat in limbs.

Anthropometric Assessment in Infants and Children To evaluate growth patterns, the nurse takes periodic measurements of height (or length), weight, and head circumference and plots them on growth charts, such as those provided in Appendix E. The most commonly used growth charts compare height (or length) to age, weight to age, head circumference to age, weight to length, and BMI to age. Although individual growth patterns vary, a child's growth will generally stay at about the same percentile throughout childhood; a sharp drop in a previously steady growth pattern suggests malnutrition. Growth patterns that fall below the 5th percentile may also be cause for concern, although genetic influences must be considered when interpreting low values. Growth charts with BMI-for-age percentiles can be used to assess risk of underweight and overweight in children over two years of age: the 5th and 85th percentiles are used as cutoffs to identify children who may be malnourished or overweight, respectively.[8]

Anthropometric Assessment in Adults To evaluate the nutritional risks associated with illness, clinicians monitor both the total reduction in body weight and the rate of weight loss over time. As Table 13-7 shows, an unintended weight loss of more than 2 percent within one week or more than 5 percent within one month suggests the development of malnutrition.[9] Weight changes need to be evaluated carefully, however: although unintentional weight loss can indicate malnutrition, weight gain may result from fluid retention rather than recovery of muscle tissue or overnutrition. Fluid retention often accompanies worsening disease in patients with heart failure, liver cirrhosis, and kidney failure and it can mask the weight loss associated with PEM. Some medications can also contribute to weight changes.

Weight data are often expressed as a percentage of usual body weight (%UBW) or ideal body weight (%IBW). The %UBW is more effective than %IBW for interpreting weight changes that occur in underweight, overweight, or obese individuals. In overweight persons, the %IBW may fail to identify significant weight loss. Conversely, in underweight individuals, the %IBW can overstate the degree of weight loss due to illness. Box 13-5 describes how to estimate %UBW and %IBW, and Table 13-8 shows how to interpret these values.

Some illnesses discussed in later chapters are associated with losses in muscle tissue that resist nutritional intervention. In older adults, losses in both muscle tissue and height are common even though body weights may remain stable. Thus, clinicians may include skinfold and limb circumference measurements in a nutrition assessment to help them identify changes in body composition that need to be addressed in the treatment plan.

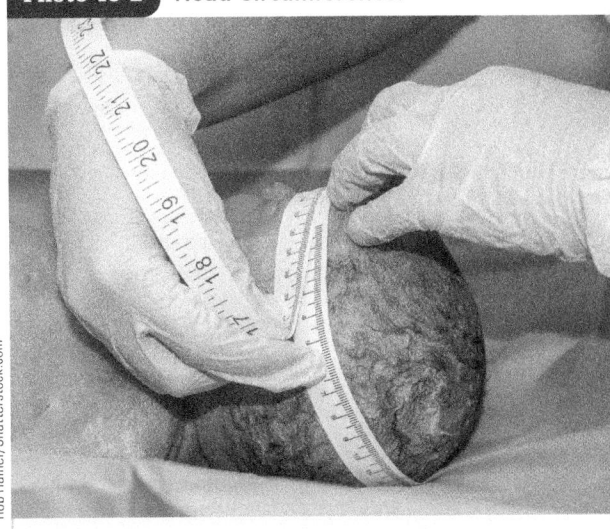

Photo 13-2 Head Circumference.

Head circumference measurements can help to assess brain growth.

Rob Hainer/Shutterstock.com

TABLE 13-7 Rate of Involuntary Weight Loss Associated with Nutritional Risk

% WEIGHT LOSS[a]	TIME PERIOD
>2%	1 week
>5%	1 month
>7.5%	3 months
>10%	6 months

[a] % weight loss = $\dfrac{\text{amount of weight loss}}{\text{usual weight}} \times 100$

Box 13-5 *HOW TO* Estimate and Evaluate Changes in Body Weight

%UBW: To estimate %UBW, compare an individual's current weight with the usual body weight:

$$\%UBW = \frac{\text{current weight}}{\text{usual weight}} \times 100$$

For example, if a man loses 32 pounds during illness and his usual weight is 180 pounds, his current weight would be 148 pounds. These values can be incorporated into the previous equation:

$$\%UBW = \frac{148}{180} \times 100 = 82.2\%$$

The man in this example weighs 82.2 percent of his usual weight. A look at Table 13-8 shows that a person who is at 82 percent of UBW may be moderately malnourished.

%IBW: To estimate %IBW, compare an individual's current weight with a reasonable (ideal) weight from a BMI table or other appropriate reference:

$$\%IBW = \frac{\text{current weight}}{\text{ideal weight}} \times 100$$

For example, suppose you wish to calculate the %IBW for a woman who is 5 feet 8 inches tall and weighs 116 pounds. The midpoint of the healthy BMI range is approximately 22, so using a BMI table (as shown on the inside back cover of this book), you estimate that a reasonable weight for this woman would be about 144 pounds:

$$\%IBW = \frac{116}{144} \times 100 = 80.6\%$$

The woman in this example weighs about 80.6 percent of her ideal body weight. A look at Table 13-8 suggests that, at 80.6 percent of IBW, she may be mildly malnourished. Keep in mind that the calculation of "ideal body weight" is somewhat arbitrary because the BMI table and various other references provide a range of weights for individuals of a given height.

TABLE 13-8	Body Weight and Nutritional Risk	
%UBW	**%IBW**	**NUTRITIONAL RISK**
85–95	80–90	Risk of mild malnutrition
75–84	70–79	Risk of moderate malnutrition
<75	<70	Risk of severe malnutrition

Biochemical Analyses

Biochemical data can help in the evaluation of PEM, vitamin and mineral status, fluid and electrolyte balances, and organ function. Most values are obtained by analyzing blood and urine samples, which contain proteins, nutrients, and metabolites that reflect various aspects of health and nutrition status. Repeated measures are more helpful than single values, as serial data can indicate whether a condition is improving or worsening. Table 13-9 lists and describes common blood tests that may be helpful in a nutrition assessment. Laboratory tests relevant to specific diseases are discussed in the chapters that follow.

Interpreting laboratory values can be challenging because a number of factors may influence test results. For example, fluid imbalances may alter test values: fluid retention dilutes substances and therefore lowers lab values, whereas dehydration can cause an increase in lab values. Serum protein levels may be influenced by fluid status, infections, inflammation, pregnancy, and other factors. Similarly, serum levels of vitamins and minerals are often poor indicators of nutrient deficiency because of the effects of other physiological factors. Taken together with other assessment data, however, laboratory test results help to present a clearer picture than is possible to obtain otherwise.

Serum Proteins Serum protein levels can aid in the assessment of protein-energy status, but, as mentioned earlier, the levels may fluctuate for other reasons as well.[10] Because serum proteins are synthesized in the liver, blood levels of these proteins can reflect liver function. Metabolic stress (often due to illness, injury, or infection) alters serum proteins because the liver responds to stress by increasing its synthesis of some proteins and reducing the synthesis of others. Serum protein values may also be influenced by hydration status, pregnancy, kidney function, zinc status, blood loss, and some medications. Because serum proteins are affected by so many factors, their values must be considered along with other data to evaluate health and nutrition status.

Albumin Albumin is the most abundant serum protein and is easily measured, so its levels are routinely monitored in hospital patients to help gauge the severity of

TABLE 13-9 Routine Laboratory Tests with Nutritional Implications

This table lists some commonly performed blood tests that have implications for nutritional problems. Unless whole blood is used, results are generally reported in terms of either *plasma* or *serum* levels. *Plasma* is the yellow fluid that remains after cells are removed and still contains clotting factors. *Serum* is the fluid remaining after both cells and clotting factors are removed.

LABORATORY TEST	ACCEPTABLE RANGE	DESCRIPTION
HEMATOLOGY (WHOLE BLOOD SAMPLES)		
Red blood cell (RBC) count	Male: 4.3–5.7 million/μL Female: 3.8–5.1 million/μL	RBC number; helps with anemia diagnosis.
Hemoglobin (Hb)	Male: 13.5–17.5 g/dL Female: 12.0–16.0 g/dL	RBC hemoglobin content; helps with anemia diagnosis.
Hematocrit (Hct)	Male: 39–49% Female: 35–45%	Percent RBC volume in blood; helps with anemia diagnosis.
Mean corpuscular volume (MCV)	80–100 fL	RBC size; helps to distinguish microcytic and macrocytic anemia.
Mean corpuscular hemoglobin concentration (MCHC)	31–37% Hb/cell	RBC Hb concentration; helps with diagnosis of iron-deficiency anemia.
White blood cell (WBC) count	4,500–11,000 cells/μL	WBC number; may indicate immune status, infection, or inflammation.
SERUM PROTEINS		
Total protein	6.4–8.3 g/dL	Levels are not highly sensitive or specific to disease; may reflect body protein content, illness, infection, inflammation, changes in hydration or metabolism, pregnancy, or use of certain medications.
Albumin	3.4–4.8 g/dL	Levels may reflect illness or PEM; slow to respond to improvement or worsening of disease.
Transferrin	200–360 mg/dL >60 yr: 160–340 mg/dL	Levels may reflect illness, PEM, or iron deficiency; slightly more sensitive to changes in health status than albumin.
Transthyretin (prealbumin)	20–40 mg/dL	Levels may reflect illness or PEM; more responsive to changes in health status than albumin or transferrin.
C-reactive protein	<0.5 mg/dL	Elevated levels may indicate inflammation or infection.
SERUM ENZYMES		
Creatine kinase (CK)	Male: 46–171 U/L Female: 34–145 U/L	Different forms are found in the muscle, brain, and heart. Elevated blood levels may indicate a heart attack, brain tissue damage, or skeletal muscle injury.
Lactate dehydrogenase (LDH)	125–220 U/L	Found in many tissues; specific types may be elevated after a heart attack, lung damage, or liver disease.
Alkaline phosphatase	Male: 53–128 U/L Female: 42–98 U/L	Found in many tissues; often measured to evaluate liver function.
Aspartate aminotransferase (AST; formerly SGOT)	Male: <35 U/L Female: <31 U/L	Elevated levels may indicate liver disease or liver damage; somewhat increased after muscle injury.
Alanine aminotransferase (ALT; formerly SGPT)	Male: <45 U/L Female: <34 U/L	Elevated levels may indicate liver disease or liver damage; somewhat increased after muscle injury.
SERUM ELECTROLYTES		
Sodium	136–145 mEq/L	Helps with assessment of hydration status or neuromuscular, kidney, and adrenal functions.
Potassium	3.5–5.1 mEq/L	Helps with assessment of acid–base balance or kidney function; can also detect potassium imbalances.

(Continued)

LABORATORY TEST	ACCEPTABLE RANGE	DESCRIPTION
Chloride	98–107 mEq/L	Helps with assessment of hydration status or detection of acid–base and electrolyte imbalances.
OTHER		
Glucose, fasting (serum)	Adult: 74–100 mg/dL > 60 yr: 82–115 mg/dL	Helps with diagnosis of glucose intolerance, diabetes mellitus, and hypoglycemia; also used for monitoring diabetes treatment.
Glycated hemoglobin (HbA$_{1c}$), whole blood	<6.5% of total Hb	Used for monitoring long-term blood glucose control (approximately 1 to 3 months prior).
Blood urea nitrogen (BUN), serum or plasma	6–20 mg/dL	Primarily used for monitoring kidney function; value altered by liver failure, dehydration, or shock.
Uric acid, serum	Male: 3.5–7.2 mg/dL Female: 2.6–6.0 mg/dL	Used for detection of gout or changes in kidney function; levels affected by age and diet and vary among different ethnic groups.
Creatinine, serum	Male: 0.62–1.10 mg/dL Female: 0.45–0.75 mg/dL	Used for monitoring renal function.

Note: μL = microliter; dL = deciliter; fL = femtoliter; U/L = units per liter; mEq = milliequivalents.

Source: L. Goldman and A. I. Schafer, eds., *Goldman-Cecil Medicine* (Philadelphia: Saunders, 2016).

BOX 13-6

Half-lives of blood proteins:

- Albumin: 14–20 days
- Transferrin: 8–10 days
- Transthyretin: 2–3 days
- Retinol-binding protein: 12 hours

half-life: in blood tests, refers to the length of time that a substance remains in plasma. The albumin in plasma has a half-life of 14 to 20 days, meaning that half of the amount circulating in plasma is degraded in this time period.

illness. Although many medical conditions influence albumin, it is slow to reflect changes in nutrition status because of its large body pool and slow rate of degradation. (Box 13-6 lists the **half-life** for albumin and other proteins discussed in this section.) In people with chronic PEM, albumin levels remain normal for a long period despite significant protein depletion, and levels fall only after prolonged malnutrition. Likewise, albumin levels increase slowly when malnutrition is treated, so albumin is not a sensitive indicator of effective treatment.

Transferrin Transferrin is an iron-transport protein, and its blood concentrations respond to iron status, PEM, and various illnesses. Transferrin levels rise as iron status worsens and fall as iron status improves, so using transferrin values to evaluate protein-energy status is difficult if an iron deficiency is also present. Transferrin degrades more rapidly than albumin, but its levels change relatively slowly in response to nutrition therapy.

Transthyretin and Retinol-Binding Protein Blood concentrations of transthyretin (also called *prealbumin*) and retinol-binding protein decrease rapidly during PEM and respond quickly to improved protein intakes. Thus, these proteins are more sensitive than albumin to short-term changes in protein status. Although sometimes used to evaluate malnutrition risk or improvement in nutrition status, they are more expensive to measure than albumin so they are not routinely included during a nutrition assessment. Like other serum proteins, their usefulness is somewhat limited because they are affected by a number of different factors, including metabolic stress, zinc deficiency, and various medical conditions.

C-Reactive Protein C-reactive protein (CRP) levels rise rapidly in response to inflammation or infection and are often elevated in individuals with critical illness, heart disease, and certain cancers. Elevated CRP values may help to identify individuals at risk for malnutrition, as well as aid in the interpretation of other serum protein tests.[11]

TABLE 13-10 Clinical Signs of Nutrient Deficiencies

PART OF BODY	ACCEPTABLE APPEARANCE	SIGNS OF MALNUTRITION	OTHER CAUSES OF ABNORMALITIES
Hair	Shiny, firm in scalp	Dull, brittle, dry, loose; falls out (PEM); corkscrew hair (vitamin C)	Excessive hair bleaching; hair loss from aging, chemotherapy, or radiation therapy
Eyes	Bright; clear; shiny; pink, moist membranes; adjust easily to light	Pale membranes (iron); spots, dryness, night blindness (vitamin A); redness at corners of eyes (B vitamins)	Anemia that is unrelated to nutrition, eye disorders, allergies, aging
Lips	Smooth	Dry, cracked, or with sores in the corners of the lips (B vitamins)	Sunburn, windburn, excessive salivation from ill-fitting dentures or various disorders
Mouth and gums	Oral tissues without lesions, swelling, or bleeding; red tongue; normal sense of taste; teeth without caries; ability to chew and swallow	Bleeding gums (vitamin C); smooth or magenta tongue (B vitamins); poor taste sensation (zinc)	Medications, periodontal disease (poor oral hygiene)
Skin	Smooth, firm, good color	Poor wound healing (PEM, vitamin C, zinc); dry, rough, lack of fat under skin (essential fatty acids, PEM, vitamin A, B vitamins); bruising or bleeding under skin (vitamins C and K); pale (iron)	Poor skin care, diabetes mellitus, aging, medications
Nails	Smooth, firm, uniform, pink	Ridged (PEM); spoon shaped, pale (iron)	—
Other	—	Dementia, peripheral neuropathy (B vitamins); swollen glands at front of neck (PEM, iodine); bowed legs (vitamin D)	Disorders of aging (dementia), diabetes mellitus (peripheral neuropathy)

Physical Examination

As with other assessment methods, interpreting physical signs of malnutrition requires skill and clinical judgment. Most physical signs are nonspecific; they can reflect any of several nutrient deficiencies, as well as conditions unrelated to nutrition. For example, cracked lips may be caused by several B vitamin deficiencies but may also result from sunburn, windburn, or dehydration. Dietary and laboratory data are usually needed as additional evidence to confirm suspected nutrient deficiencies.

Clinical Signs of Malnutrition Signs of malnutrition tend to appear most often in parts of the body where cell replacement occurs at a rapid rate, such as the hair, skin, and digestive tract (including the mouth and tongue). Table 13-10 lists some clinical signs of nutrient deficiencies, and Photo 13-3 illustrates some signs of malnutrition in a child with kwashiorkor. Note that many signs of nutrient deficiency appear only in the advanced stages. Chapters 8 and 9 provide additional examples of clinical signs that develop during nutrient imbalances.

Hydration Status As mentioned, fluid imbalances may accompany some illnesses and can also result from the use of certain medications. Recognizing the signs of fluid retention or dehydration is necessary for the correct interpretation of blood test results and body weight measurements.

Fluid retention (also called *edema*) may be caused by PEM, severe infection or injury, and some medications. It can also result from heart failure, disorders of the liver or kidneys, and obstructions in the veins or lymphatic system.

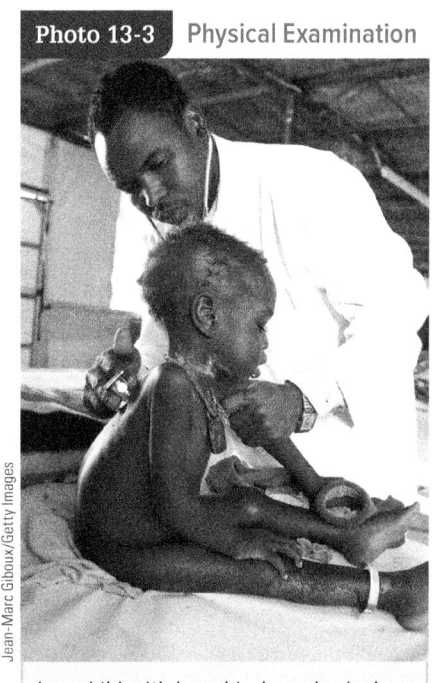

Photo 13-3 Physical Examination

Jean-Marc Giboux/Getty Images

In a child with kwashiorkor, physical signs of malnutrition may include sparse, brittle hair; loss of hair color; a swollen abdomen; and dermatitis.

Box 13-7   Case Study: Nutrition Screening and Assessment

Lisa Sawrey is an 80-year-old retired businesswoman who has been a widow for 10 years. She uses a walker and has poorly fitting dentures. She was recently admitted to the hospital with pneumonia and also has heart failure and diabetes. She routinely takes several medications to control her blood glucose levels, hypertension, and heart function. In addition to these medications, the physician has recently ordered antibiotics to treat the pneumonia. During an initial nutrition screening, Mrs. Sawrey stated that she had been eating very poorly over the past two weeks. She said that she usually weighs about 125 pounds—a fact that was documented in her medical chart from a previous visit. Although she felt she was losing weight, she didn't know how much weight she may have lost or when she started losing weight. Upon admission to the hospital, Mrs. Sawrey weighed 110 pounds and was 5 feet 3 inches tall. Her serum albumin level was 3.0 grams per deciliter. A physical exam revealed edema, and several other laboratory tests confirmed that she was retaining fluid. As a result of the nutrition screening, Mrs. Sawrey was referred to a nurse for a nutrition assessment.

1. From the brief description provided, which items in Mrs. Sawrey's medical history, personal and social history, and food and nutrition history might alert the nurse that this patient is at risk of malnutrition?

2. Identify a healthy body weight for Mrs. Sawrey, and calculate her %UBW and %IBW. What do the results reveal? How does the presence of edema influence your evaluation of Mrs. Sawrey's weight loss?

3. How might fluid retention alter Mrs. Sawrey's serum protein levels? What physical symptoms may have indicated that she was retaining excess fluid?

4. What tools can be used to estimate Mrs. Sawrey's usual food intake? What medical, physical, and personal factors are likely to influence her diet?

5. Describe other types of assessment information that may help the nurse determine whether Mrs. Sawrey should be referred to a registered dietitian.

Physical signs of fluid retention include weight gain, facial puffiness, tissue swelling, abdominal distention, and tight-fitting shoes.

Dehydration may be caused by vomiting, diarrhea, fever, excessive urination, blood loss, and wounds or burns (due to fluid loss through skin lesions). The risk of dehydration is especially high in older adults, who have a reduced thirst response and various other impairments in fluid regulation. Signs or symptoms include thirst, weight loss, dry skin or mouth, reduced skin tension, dark-colored urine, and low urine volume.

Functional Assessment Nutrient deficiencies sometimes impair physiological functions, so clinicians may conduct tests or procedures to evaluate some aspects of malnutrition. For example, both PEM and zinc deficiency can depress immunity, which can be evaluated by testing the skin's response to antigens that cause redness and swelling when immune function is adequate. Muscle weakness due to **wasting** (loss of muscle tissue) can be assessed by testing handgrip strength. Exercise tolerance, which is reduced in heart and lung disorders, may be evaluated using a treadmill or cycle ergometer.

The Case Study in Box 13-7 can help you review the different components of a nutrition assessment.

Review Notes

- Nutrition status can be assessed using historical information, anthropometric data, biochemical analyses, and a physical examination. Health care providers can collect food intake data using 24-hour dietary recall interviews, food frequency questionnaires, food records, and direct observation.

- Anthropometric measurements, such as height, weight, and body circumferences, help clinicians evaluate growth patterns, overnutrition and undernutrition, and body composition.

- Biochemical analyses may indicate nutrient imbalances but are also influenced by various other medical problems.

- Physical examinations can reveal signs of nutrient deficiencies, fluid imbalances, and functional impairments related to nutritional problems.

wasting: the gradual atrophy (loss) of body tissues; associated with protein-energy malnutrition or chronic illness.

1. Alex experiences loss of appetite, difficulty swallowing, and mouth pain as a consequence of illness. Alex is at risk of malnutrition due to:
   a. altered metabolism.
   b. reduced food intake.
   c. altered excretion of nutrients.
   d. altered digestion and absorption.

2. Because of their central role in health care, nurses are well positioned for:
   a. calculating patients' nutrient needs.
   b. providing medical nutrition therapy.
   c. conducting complete nutrition assessments.
   d. identifying patients at risk for malnutrition.

3. Of the following data collected during a nutrition screening, which item does *not* place the person at risk for malnutrition?
   a. Having a health problem that is frequently associated with PEM
   b. Using prescription medications that affect nutrient needs
   c. Residing with a spouse in a middle-income neighborhood
   d. Significantly reducing food intake over the past week

4. The nutrition care process is a systematic approach for:
   a. identifying the nutrient content of foods.
   b. ordering special diets.
   c. conducting a nutrition screening.
   d. identifying and meeting the nutrition needs of patients.

5. To conduct complete nutrition assessments, clinicians rely on several sources of information, which include all of the following *except*:
   a. nutrition care plans.
   b. body measurements.
   c. medical, medication, and social histories.
   d. biochemical analyses.

6. Which dietary assessment method does a nurse use to conduct a calorie count?
   a. 24-hour dietary recall interview
   b. Food frequency questionnaire
   c. Food record
   d. Direct observation

7. The %UBW of a person who weighs 135 pounds and has a usual body weight of 150 pounds is:
   a. 111 percent.
   b. 90 percent.
   c. 86 percent.
   d. 74 percent.

8. A malnourished, acutely ill patient has just begun to eat after days without significant amounts of food. Which of the following blood test results would change most quickly as the patient's nutrition and health status improves?
   a. Albumin
   b. Transferrin
   c. Serum electrolytes
   d. Retinol-binding protein

9. Which sign of PEM would be unlikely to show up in a physical examination?
   a. Low serum protein levels
   b. Dull, brittle hair
   c. Poor wound healing
   d. Wasting

10. Fluid retention may cause all of the following effects *except*:
    a. swelling of limbs.
    b. facial puffiness.
    c. weight loss.
    d. tight-fitting shoes.

Answers: 1. b, 2. d, 3. c, 4. d, 5. a, 6. d, 7. b, 8. d, 9. a, 10. c

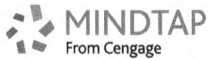 **MINDTAP** From Cengage   For more chapter resources visit **www.cengage.com** to access MindTap, a complete digital course.

Clinical Applications

1. Describe the potential nutritional implications of these findings from a patient's medical, personal, and social histories: age 78, lives alone, recently lost spouse, uses a walker, has no natural teeth or dentures, has a history of hypertension and diabetes, uses medications that cause frequent urination, sleeps poorly, often feels depressed.

2. Calculate the %UBW and %IBW for a man who is 5 feet 11 inches tall with a current weight of 150 pounds and a usual body weight of 180 pounds. What additional information do you need to interpret the implications of his weight loss?

3. Nurses and nurses' aides frequently shoulder much of the responsibility for collecting food intake data for calorie counts because they typically deliver food trays and snacks and later retrieve them. Why is it important to verify and record both what the patient receives (foods and amounts) and the foods that remain uneaten? When might patients be enlisted in the collection of food intake data, and when might such a course be unwise?

Notes

1. J. V. White and coauthors, Consensus statement of the Academy of Nutrition and Dietetics/American Society for Parenteral and Enteral Nutrition: Characteristics recommended for the identification and documentation of adult malnutrition (undernutrition), *Journal of the Academy of Nutrition and Dietetics* 112 (2012): 730–738.

2. M. I. Correia and coauthors, Evidence-based recommendations for addressing malnutrition in health care: An updated strategy from the feedM.E. Global Study Group, *Journal of the American Medical Directors Association* 15 (2014): 544–550.

3. A. Skipper, Nutrition screening, *Pocket Guide to Nutrition Assessment* (Chicago: Academy of Nutrition and Dietetics, 2016), pp. 15–33.

4. The Academy Quality Management Committee and Scope of Practice Subcommittee of the Quality Management Committee, Academy of Nutrition and Dietetics: Revised 2012 standards of practice in nutrition care and standards of professional performance for registered dietitians, *Journal of the Academy of Nutrition and Dietetics* 113 (2013): S29–S45.

5. The Academy Quality Management Committee and Scope of Practice Subcommittee of the Quality Management Committee, 2013.

6. F. E. Thompson and A. F. Subar, Dietary assessment methodology, in A. M. Coulston, C. J. Boushey, and M. G. Ferruzzi, eds., *Nutrition in the*

Prevention and Treatment of Disease (London: Academic Press/Elsevier, 2013), pp. 5–46; K. S. Stote and coauthors, The number of 24 h dietary recalls using the U.S. Department of Agriculture's automated multiple-pass method required to estimate nutrient intake in overweight and obese adults, *Public Health Nutrition* 14 (2011): 1736–1742.

7. E. Saltzman and K. M. Mogensen, Physical and clinical assessment of nutrition status, in A. M. Coulston, C. J. Boushey, and M. G. Ferruzzi, eds., *Nutrition in the Prevention and Treatment of Disease* (London: Academic Press/Elsevier, 2013), pp. 65–79.

8. S. Going, M. Hingle, and J. Farr, Body composition, in A. C. Ross and coeditors, eds., *Modern Nutrition in Health and Disease* (Baltimore: Lippincott Williams & Wilkins, 2014), pp. 635–648.

9. A. Malone and C. Hamilton, Academy of Nutrition and Dietetics/ American Society for Parenteral and Enteral Nutrition consensus malnutrition characteristics: Application in practice, *Nutrition in Clinical Practice* 28 (2013): 639–650.

10. C. W. Thompson, Biochemical tests, medical data, and procedures, in P. Charney and A. Malone, eds., *Pocket Guide to Nutrition Assessment* (Chicago: Academy of Nutrition and Dietetics, 2016), pp. 108–195.

11. Malone and Hamilton, 2013.

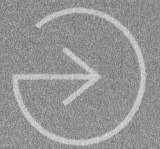

13.3 Nutrition in Practice

Nutritional Genomics

Consider this situation: A physician scrapes a sample of cells from inside your cheek and submits the sample to a **genomics** lab. In a short time, you receive a report that reveals your disease susceptibilities and suggests dietary and lifestyle changes that can improve your health. You may even be given a prescription for food choices or a dietary supplement that will best meet your personal nutrient requirements. Unlikely? Perhaps, but these possibilities are being explored by scientists working in the field of **nutritional genomics**, the study of dietary effects on **gene expression**. Recent research suggests that some dietary factors may be more helpful (or more harmful) in people who have particular genetic variations. The promise of nutritional genomics is a custom-designed dietary prescription that fits each person's specific needs. Box NP13-1 defines genomics and related terms.

What is a genome?

Genetic information is encoded in DNA molecules within the nuclei of almost all of the cells in our bodies. Figure NP13-1 shows how the genetic material is organized within the **genome**, the complete set of genetic information within our cells. The DNA molecules are tightly packed along with associated proteins within the 46 **chromosomes**. Segments of a DNA strand that can eventually be translated into proteins are called **genes**. The sequence of **nucleotides** within each gene encodes the amino acid sequence of a particular protein. Scientists estimate that there are about 23,000 genes in the human genome.[1] However, only a small percentage (about 1 to 2 percent) of the genome codes for proteins: most DNA consists of **noncoding sequences**, which may help to regulate gene expression or have other functions.

FIGURE NP13-1 The Human Genome

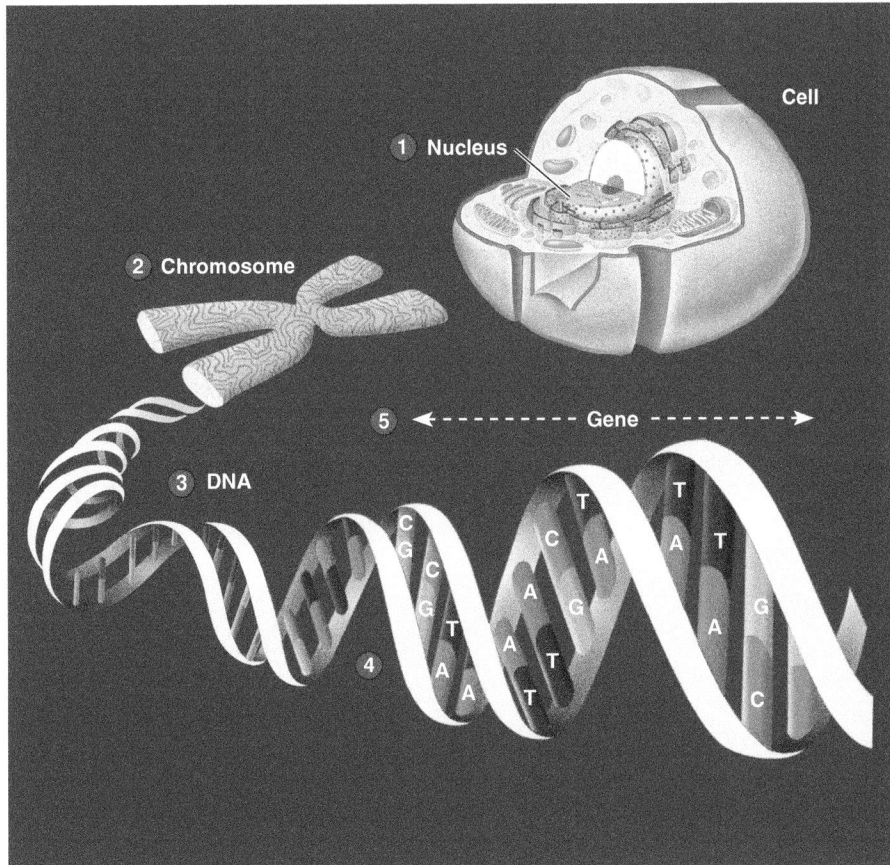

1. The human genome is a complete set of genetic material organized into 46 chromosomes, located within the nucleus of a cell.

2. A chromosome is made of DNA and associated proteins.

3. The double helical structure of a DNA molecule is made up of two long chains of nucleotides. Each nucleotide is composed of a phosphate group, a 5-carbon sugar, and a base.

4. The sequence of nucleotide bases (C, G, A, T) determines the amino acid sequence of proteins. These bases are connected by hydrogen bonding to form base pairs: adenine (A) with thymine (T) and guanine (G) with cytosine (C).

5. A gene is a segment of DNA that includes the information needed to synthesize one or more proteins.

Source: Office of Biological and Environmental Research of the U.S. Department of Energy Office of Science: science.energy.gov/ber/

chromosomes: structures within the nucleus of a cell that contain the cell's DNA and associated proteins.

epigenetics: processes that cause heritable changes in gene expression that are separate from the DNA nucleotide sequence.

gene expression: the process by which a cell converts the genetic code into RNA and protein.

genes: segments of DNA that contain the information needed to make proteins.

genome (JEE-nome): the full complement of genetic material in the chromosomes of a cell.

genomics (jee-NO-miks): the study of genomes.

inherited disorders: medical conditions resulting from genetic defects.

methylation: the addition of methyl ($-CH_3$) groups.

microarray technology: research technology that monitors the expression of thousands of genes simultaneously.

multigene or polygenic: involving a number of genes, rather than a single gene.

noncoding sequences: regions of DNA that do not code for proteins. Some noncoding sequences may have regulatory or structural properties, but most have no known function.

nucleotides: the subunits of DNA and RNA molecules. These compounds—cytosine (C), thymine (T), uracil (U), guanine (G), and adenine (A)—are each composed of a phosphate group, a five-carbon sugar (ribose), and a nitrogen-containing base. A DNA molecule is made up of two long chains of nucleotides held together by hydrogen bonding between nucleotide bases on opposing strands; each hydrogen-bonded nucleotide couple is called a *base pair*.

nutritional genomics: the study of dietary effects on genetic expression; also known as *nutrigenomics*.

polymorphisms: variations in DNA sequences of a particular gene. A *single-nucleotide polymorphism*, the most common type of polymorphism, involves the insertion, deletion, or substitution of a single nucleotide in the DNA strand.

- *poly* = many
- *morph* = form
- *ism* = condition

promoter: a region of DNA involved with gene activation.

transcription factors: proteins that bind DNA at specific sequences to regulate gene expression.

When proteins are made, the information in the DNA sequence is first transcribed (copied) to messenger RNA molecules, which carry the genetic information from the nucleus to the cytoplasm. Gene expression can be measured by determining the amounts of messenger RNA in a tissue sample. The expression of thousands of genes can be measured simultaneously using **microarray technology** (see Photo NP13-1).

Photo NP13-1

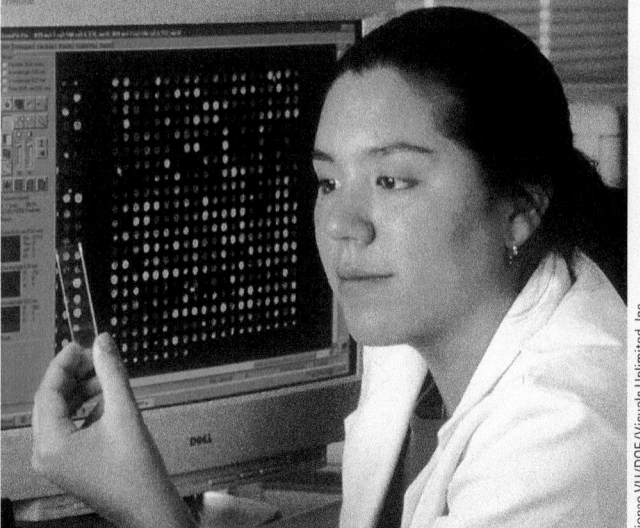

Science VU/DOE/Visuals Unlimited, Inc.

A DNA microarray allows researchers to monitor the expression of thousands of genes simultaneously.

How did research in nutritional genomics begin?

The current surge in genomics research grew from the Human Genome Project, an international effort by industry and government scientists to determine the complete nucleotide sequence of human DNA. Completed in 2003, the project led to enormous advances in the research technologies needed to study genes and genetic variation. Scientists are now working to identify the individual genes in the genome, the roles of their protein products, the genes and proteins associated with diseases, and the dietary and lifestyle choices that influence the expression of genes involved in disease. In addition, researchers are studying how variations in the noncoding regions of DNA molecules—which regulate gene expression—influence disease risk.

Genetic differences among individuals have been studied for years, as have the specialized dietary therapies used to treat various **inherited disorders**. For example, an individual may inherit a genetic defect that inhibits the normal metabolism of an essential nutrient and may therefore need to consume a diet that contains either more or less of this nutrient. (An example of this type of condition is phenylketonuria [PKU], discussed in Nutrition in Practice 15.) Genomic research takes this concept a bit further: Instead of focusing on alterations in just one or two genes, researchers have been able to study the expression of *multiple* genes.

How do nutrients alter gene expression?

Various nutrients can switch gene expression on or off.[2] The **promoter** region of a gene (a DNA sequence involved with gene activation) acts as the master switch. A large variety of proteins known as **transcription factors** can bind to areas on the promoter and either enhance or inhibit gene expression. A combination of dietary factors and hormones influences the types of transcription factors that reach the nucleus and their tendency to bind to DNA. Specific examples of how nutrients can influence transcription factors include:

- The transcription factor that enhances the gene expression of enzymes required for cholesterol synthesis enters the nucleus only when the cellular cholesterol content is low.
- The transcription factor that inhibits the expression of ferritin, an iron-storage protein, changes its affinity for DNA based on the iron content of the cell.

Gene expression is also influenced by modifications in the structure of DNA and its packaging in chromosomes. For example, **methylation** of DNA (the addition of methyl groups) can alter the expression of genes and depends on both inherited factors and the availability of certain nutrients. In individuals who are susceptible to a disease that is influenced by DNA methylation, an altered diet or nutrient supplementation can potentially reduce the risk of disease.[3] The field of **epigenetics** investigates processes that cause heritable changes in gene expression that are separate from the underlying DNA nucleotide sequence.

How much genetic variation is there among people?

Except for identical twins, no two individuals are genetically identical. However, the variation in the genomes of any two persons is only about 1 to 3 percent,[4] a difference of approximately one base in every few hundred. Genetic differences, known as **polymorphisms**, are variations in the DNA sequence of a particular gene. The most common type of polymorphism is a *single-nucleotide polymorphism*, characterized by a nucleotide insertion, deletion, or substitution in the DNA molecule. Genetic variations are significant only if they affect a protein's amino acid sequence in a way that alters the protein's function, or if the change in the DNA molecule changes how a particular gene is regulated.

Genetic variation gives rise to the diversity among human beings—it explains most of the differences in our physical appearances and metabolic characteristics. Along with environmental factors, it also determines our susceptibilities to disease. Diseases affected by a single gene tend to be relatively rare and usually exert their effects early in life. In contrast, common diseases such as heart disease and cancer are influenced by many genes and typically develop over several decades or even longer. In these more complex **multigene**, or **polygenic**, disorders, many genes can contribute to disease risk, but no single gene may be sufficient to cause the disease on its own. In addition, the specific genes that influence a person's susceptibility to disease may vary substantially among different individuals.

What are some examples of single-gene disorders?

Examples of single-gene disorders include phenylketonuria, cystic fibrosis (discussed in Chapter 18), sickle-cell anemia, and the iron-overload disease hemochromatosis. Single-gene disorders may seriously disrupt metabolism and often require significant dietary or medical intervention. However, not all single-gene disorders have life-threatening ramifications. For example, lactose intolerance is related to an alteration in the promoter of the lactase gene; the condition may cause gastrointestinal discomfort but is readily managed by simple dietary changes.

How are multigene disorders different from single-gene disorders?

Multigene disorders are usually sensitive to a number of environmental influences, including diet and lifestyle; these environmental factors can directly influence the expression of the genes involved. Multigene disorders tend to develop over many years, so determining genetic susceptibility may allow a person to modify diet and lifestyle appropriately and reduce his or her disease risk before signs and symptoms appear.

Heart disease is an example of a disease with multiple gene influences.[5] Its many risk factors represent the involvement of an assortment of genes, which affect disparate aspects of physiology and metabolism. Consider that the major risk factors for heart disease include elevated blood cholesterol levels, hypertension, type 2 diabetes, and obesity. The underlying cause of any of these risk factors is rarely known; currently, clinicians screen for the presence of risk factors but not for the reasons why they occur. Should genomic research prove successful, a future assessment might be to identify specific genetic variations that can lead to the development of individual risk factors. For example, tests may determine whether a person's high blood cholesterol levels are due to excessive cholesterol absorption, excessive cholesterol production in the liver, or reduced cholesterol degradation. This information could then guide health care providers to the most appropriate intervention, allowing a better match between treatment recommendations and a person's genetic profile.

Can genomic research be used to explore the differences in nutrient needs among people?

Even though most people apparently can meet their nutrient needs by consuming nutrients at recommended levels, it would be useful to learn more about genetic variations within healthy populations. The techniques that have emerged from genomic research may provide a means for fine-tuning nutrient recommendations for different individuals. Moreover, ideal indicators of nutrient status are still lacking for several of the minerals, such as zinc, magnesium, and chromium. Scientists hope to eventually produce genomic maps that will indicate how various nutrient deficiencies and combinations of deficiencies affect gene expression. These maps may eventually provide data that can help diagnose nutrient deficiencies.

Will knowledge about the human genome substantially change the manner in which health care is provided?

The enthusiasm surrounding genomic research should be put into perspective in terms of both the status of clinical medicine at present and people's willingness to make difficult lifestyle choices. Critics have questioned whether genetic markers for disease are more useful than simple and inexpensive clinical measurements, which reflect both genetic *and* environmental influences.[6] In other words, knowing that a person is genetically predisposed toward high cholesterol levels is not necessarily more useful than knowing the person's actual blood cholesterol level. Furthermore, a person's family history is already a simple genomic tool that indicates a higher genetic risk for certain illnesses. Understanding the family's medical history allows the clinician to use risk-reduction strategies that are appropriate to the culture and literacy of the patient, rather than focusing on genetic risk alone.[7]

Obtaining additional knowledge about disease risk is not necessarily useful unless people are motivated to make serious lifestyle changes. For example, despite the abundance of disease prevention recommendations, many people seem unwilling or unable to make the changes known to improve health.[8] Researchers have estimated that heart disease and type 2 diabetes are nearly 80 percent and 90 percent preventable, respectively, by changing one's lifestyle to include an appropriate diet, a healthy body weight, and regular exercise, among other factors.[9] Given the difficulty that people have with current recommendations, it is unlikely that they will enthusiastically adopt an even more detailed list of dietary and lifestyle modifications.

What ethical concerns are raised by having extensive knowledge about an individual's genome?

A primary concern with our newfound ability to obtain detailed genetic information is confidentiality: should information about a person's susceptibility to disease be released to others (including other family members at risk) without that person's consent? Concern about privacy issues has led to federal and state legislation that prevents discrimination by group health plans, health insurers, and employers on the basis of an individual's genetic predisposition to disease.[10]

Another consideration is whether genetic testing is always in the best interest of children. Although early knowledge of a child's predisposition to illnesses may be useful for parents who want to provide optimal care, awareness of disease risk could possibly cause stigma, alter family dynamics, and increase the potential for discrimination in the future.[11] In addition, children at high risk of developing a serious illness may grow up believing that their future choices are limited and may alter their life course to accommodate a disease that may never develop.[12]

Although genomic research has the potential to improve our ability to diagnose and treat disease, it is still unclear how knowledge of the genome will be translated into useful medical treatments. Health care professionals will need to keep informed of the ethical, legal, and social implications of nutritional and medical genomics as this remarkable research continues.

Notes

1. S. C. S. Nagamani, P. Stankiewicz, and J. R. Lupski, Gene, genomic, and chromosomal disorders, in L. Goldman and A. I. Schafer, eds., *Goldman-Cecil Medicine* (Philadelphia: Saunders, 2016), pp. 189–195.
2. R. J. Cousins and L. A. Lichten, Nutritional regulation of gene expression and nutritional genomics, in A. C. Ross and coeditors, eds., *Modern Nutrition in Health and Disease* (Baltimore: Lippincott Williams & Wilkins, 2014), pp. 515–522.
3. A. Arpón and coauthors, Adherence to Mediterranean diet is associated with methylation changes in inflammation-related genes in peripheral blood cells, *Journal of Physiology and Biochemistry* Feb 8 2017 (2017): doi: 10.1007/s13105-017-0552-6; A. Perfilyev and coauthors, Impact of polyunsaturated and saturated fat overfeeding on the DNA-methylation pattern in human adipose tissue: A randomized controlled trial, *American Journal of Clinical Nutrition* 105 (2017): 991–1000.
4. P. J. Stover and Z. Gu, Genetic variation: Effect on nutrient utilization and metabolism, in A. C. Ross and coeditors, eds., *Modern Nutrition in Health and Disease* (Baltimore: Lippincott Williams & Wilkins, 2014), pp. 523–533.
5. R. Roberts, Genomics in cardiovascular disease, *Journal of the American College of Cardiology* 61 (2013): 2029–2037.
6. R. San-Cristobal, F. I. Milagro, and J. A. Martinez, Future challenges and present ethical considerations in the use of personalized nutrition based on genetic advice, *Journal of the Academy of Nutrition and Dietetics* 113

(2013): 1447–1454; W. C. Willett, Balancing life-style and genomics research for disease prevention, *Science* 296 (2002): 695–698.
7. M. J. Khoury and coauthors, Do we need genomic research for the prevention of common diseases with environmental causes? *American Journal of Epidemiology* 161 (2005): 799–805.
8. R. W. Grant and coauthors, Personalized genetic risk counseling to motivate diabetes prevention, *Diabetes Care* 36 (2013): 13–19; T. H. G. Webster, S. J. Beal, and K. B. Brothers, Motivation in the age of genomics: Why knowing disease susceptibility might not motivate behavior change, *Life Sciences, Society and Policy* 9 (2013): doi: 10.1186/2195-7819-9-8; J. P. Evans and coauthors, Deflating the genomic bubble, *Science* 331 (2011): 861–862.
9. A. Akesson and coauthors, Low-risk diet and lifestyle habits in the primary prevention of myocardial infarction in men, *Journal of the American College of Cardiology* 64 (2014): 1299–1306; Khoury and coauthors, 2005.
10. P. R. Reilly and R. M. DeBusk, Ethical and legal issues in nutritional genomics, *Journal of the American Dietetic Association* 108 (2008): 36–40.
11. I. R. Yurkiewicz, B. R. Korf, and L. S. Lehmann, Prenatal whole-genome sequencing—Is the quest to know a fetus' future ethical? *New England Journal of Medicine* 370 (2014): 195–197.
12. B. R. Korf, Principles of genetics, in L. Goldman and A. I. Schafer, eds., *Goldman-Cecil Medicine* (Philadelphia: Saunders, 2016), pp. 186–189.

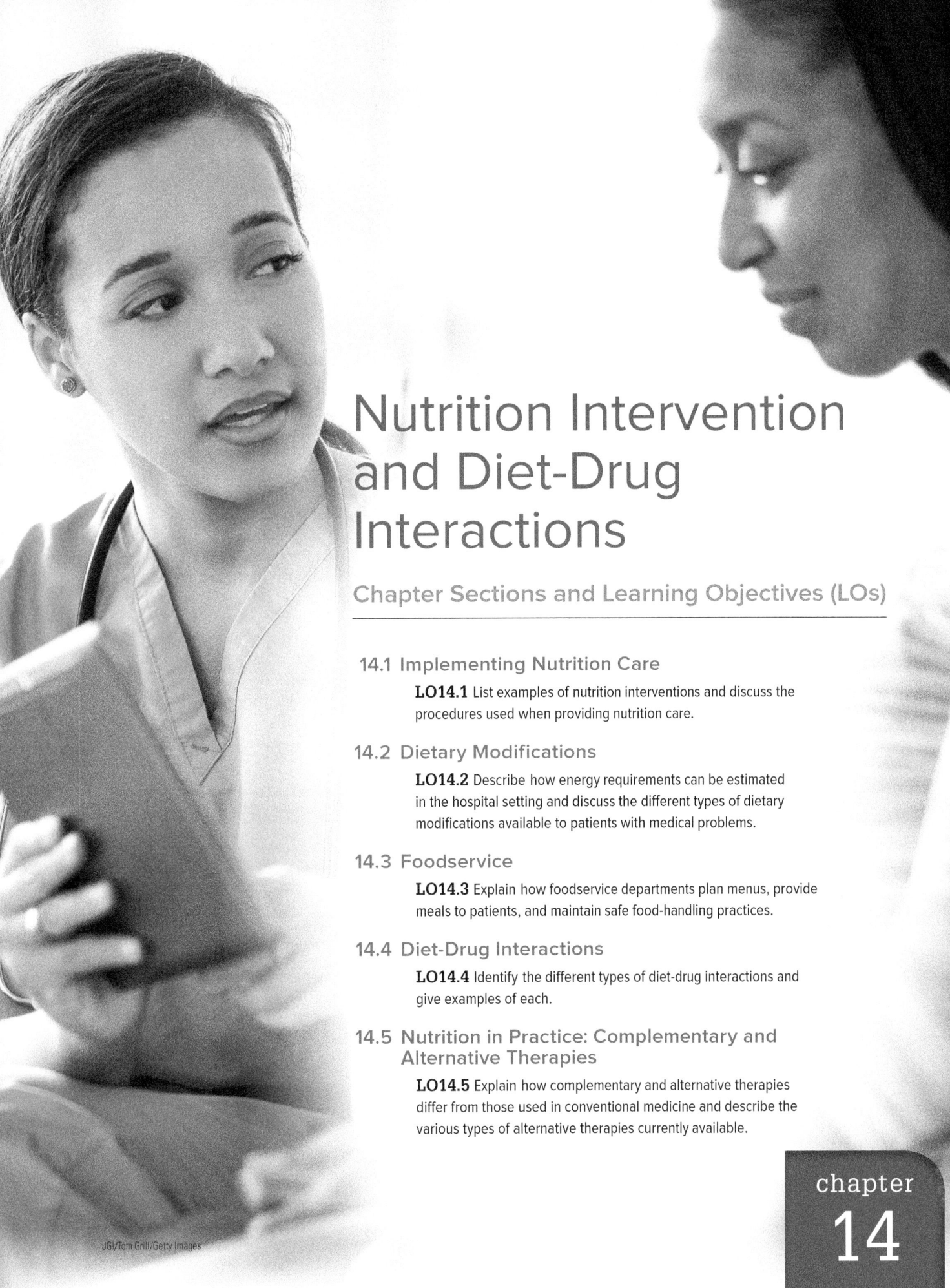

Nutrition Intervention and Diet-Drug Interactions

Chapter Sections and Learning Objectives (LOs)

14.1 Implementing Nutrition Care

LO14.1 List examples of nutrition interventions and discuss the procedures used when providing nutrition care.

14.2 Dietary Modifications

LO14.2 Describe how energy requirements can be estimated in the hospital setting and discuss the different types of dietary modifications available to patients with medical problems.

14.3 Foodservice

LO14.3 Explain how foodservice departments plan menus, provide meals to patients, and maintain safe food-handling practices.

14.4 Diet-Drug Interactions

LO14.4 Identify the different types of diet-drug interactions and give examples of each.

14.5 Nutrition in Practice: Complementary and Alternative Therapies

LO14.5 Explain how complementary and alternative therapies differ from those used in conventional medicine and describe the various types of alternative therapies currently available.

JGI/Tom Grill/Getty Images

chapter

14

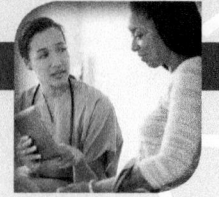

nutrition problems and provide nutrition care. A critical part of this process is ensuring that nutritional needs are met, so the chapter also introduces some common dietary modifications and reviews the procedures and challenges involved in foodservice delivery. The final section discusses diet-drug interactions that need consideration when health practitioners provide nutrition care.

14.1 Implementing Nutrition Care

As Chapter 13 explains, nurses are well positioned to identify patients with nutrition problems. In addition, nursing care plans may include nursing diagnoses that suggest the need for nutrition intervention. This section provides examples of typical nutrition interventions and describes how the nurse can incorporate nutrition care into a care plan.

Care Planning

Once the dietitian or nurse has collected and analyzed assessment information, the next steps of nutrition care can be carried out. Table 14-1 lists examples of nutrition interventions that may be appropriate in either the hospital or outpatient setting; note that some interventions may fall within the scope of nursing practice whereas others require the assistance of other health professionals. Many interventions include a diet order (prescribed by a physician or, in some cases, a registered dietitian), which provides specific recommendations regarding food, nutrient, or energy intake or feeding method. The care plan may also involve nutrition education or counseling (typically administered by a registered dietitian) to provide the knowledge, skills, and motivation that enable the patient to make dietary and lifestyle changes.

Table 14-2 shows an example of how nutrition care might be incorporated into a nursing care plan. The example describes a patient at risk for protein-energy malnutrition and wasting due to his swallowing difficulty and intolerance to physical activity. After diagnosing his nutrition-related problems, the nurse identifies **expected outcomes**

> **expected outcomes:** patient-oriented goals that are derived from nursing diagnoses.

TABLE 14-1	Examples of Nutrition Interventions
INTERVENTION	**EXAMPLES**
Food and/or nutrient delivery	Providing appropriate meals, snacks, and dietary supplements
	Providing specialized nutrition support (tube feedings or parenteral nutrition)
	Determining the need for feeding assistance or adjustment in feeding environment
	Managing nutrition-related medication problems
Nutrition education	Providing basic nutrition-related instruction
	Providing in-depth training to increase dietary knowledge or skills
	Providing information about a modified diet or change in formula
Nutrition counseling	Helping the individual set priorities and establish diet-related goals
	Motivating the individual to change behaviors to achieve goals
	Solving problems that interfere with the nutrition care plan
Coordination of nutrition care	Providing referrals or consulting other health professionals or agencies that can assist with treatment
	Organizing treatments that involve other health professionals or health care facilities
	Arranging transfer of nutrition care to another professional or location

TABLE 14-2 Incorporating Nutrition Care into the Nursing Care Plan

The following example illustrates how the nurse can address nutrition problems while working through the different phases of the nursing process.

NURSING PROCESS	NUTRITION-RELATED FEATURES
Assessment. The nurse includes nutrition assessment data in the overall assessment database.	The assessment data related to nutrition care are categorized and documented. *Subjective data:* • 74-year-old man with emphysema and dysphagia (difficulty swallowing); lives with wife. • Uses oxygen therapy at home but mostly while sleeping; frequently feels "out of breath" during the day. • Reports coughing while eating; senses that food gets "stuck" in his throat. • Believes he has lost weight recently because his clothes seem looser than usual. Says usual weight is 160 pounds, which is documented in the medical record. • Physically inactive; mostly watches TV during the day. *Objective data:* Height: 5′ 9″; weight: 145 lb; BMI: 21.5; %UBW: 90.6%; albumin: 3.6 g/dL; continually needs to clear throat; exhibits dyspnea (labored breathing) with walking.
Nursing diagnosis. The nurse develops diagnoses that indicate the need for nutrition intervention.	Nursing diagnoses with nutritional implications include: • *Impaired swallowing:* related to neuromuscular impairment. • *Risk for aspiration:* related to ineffective swallowing reflex. • *Imbalanced nutrition: less than body requirements* related to inability to ingest foods. • *Activity intolerance:* related to imbalance between oxygen supply and demand.
Planning: outcome identification. The nurse identifies outcomes associated with improved nutrition status.	Appropriate outcomes include the patient's ability to: • Identify foods and beverages that can be consumed without difficulty. • Consume meals without coughing or aspiration. • Consume adequate amounts of food and beverages to meet nutritional needs. • Avoid further weight loss. • Use oxygen therapy as needed to permit a steady increase in activity.
Planning: development of nursing strategies. The nurse determines the interventions that would allow the patient to reach goals.	To help the patient achieve the expected outcomes, the nurse plans to: • Educate the patient about body positioning and feeding techniques that can improve his ability to eat without coughing or discomfort. • Provide the patient with information about high-kcalorie and high-protein foods to minimize further weight and lean tissue losses. • Explain the need for daily physical activity, including suggestions that may improve the patient's ability to tolerate additional activity. • Teach the patient to conserve energy while performing activities of daily living. • Provide information about lightweight, portable, supplemental oxygen that can assist the patient during the day. Examples of interventions that would require the involvement of other health professionals include: • The attending physician may need to prescribe dysphagia testing to help determine the most appropriate food plan for the patient. • A dysphagia specialist may need to provide specific feeding recommendations related to the patient's type of dysphagia. • A registered dietitian may need to review and modify the patient's food plan so that he can improve his energy intake and make more appropriate food and beverage selections.

Implementation. The nurse performs the appropriate interventions and refers patient to other health practitioners, as necessary.

Evaluation: The nurse continually monitors and evaluates the patient's progress in achieving each outcome. The nursing care plan is revised as needed.

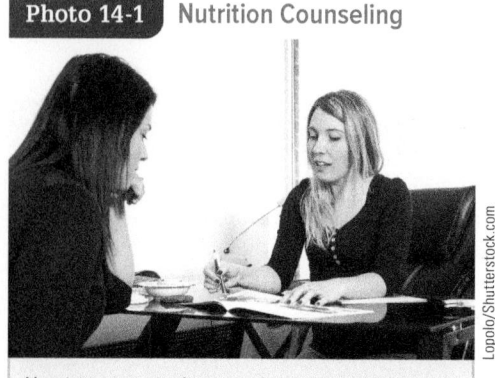

Photo 14-1 Nutrition Counseling

Nutrition counseling requires sensitivity to cultural orientation, educational background, and motivation for change.

and plans strategies that can correct the problems. This example includes interventions that require referrals to other health practitioners.

Approaches to Nutrition Care

A nutrition care plan often involves significant dietary modifications. To ensure better compliance, the plan must be compatible with the desires and abilities of the person it is designed to help. The challenge is greater if dietary changes are required for extended periods.

Long-Term Dietary Intervention When long-term changes are necessary, a care plan must take into account a person's current food practices, lifestyle, and degree of motivation (see Photo 14-1). Behavior change is a process that occurs in stages; therefore, more than one consultation is usually necessary. The following approaches may be helpful in implementing long-term dietary changes:[1]

- *Determine the individual's readiness for change.* Some people have little desire to change their food practices, and even those who are willing may not be fully prepared to take the necessary steps. The health practitioner needs to consider a patient's readiness to adopt new dietary behaviors before attempting to implement an ambitious care plan.
- *Emphasize what to eat, rather than what* not *to eat.* Emphasizing foods to include in the diet, rather than those to restrict, can make dietary changes more appealing. For example, encouraging additional fruits and vegetables is a more attractive message than advising the patient to restrict butter, cream sauces, and ice cream.
- *Suggest only one or two changes at a time.* People are more likely to adopt a nutrition care plan that does not deviate too much from their usual diet. If they succeed in adopting one or two changes, they are more likely to stick to the plan and be open to additional suggestions. Stricter plans may yield quicker results but are useful only for highly motivated people.

Nutrition Education Nutrition education allows patients to learn about the dietary factors that affect their particular medical condition. Ideally, this knowledge can motivate them to change their diet and lifestyle in order to improve their health status.

A nutrition education program should be tailored to a person's age, level of literacy, and cultural background. Learning style should also be considered: some people learn best by discussion supplemented with written materials, whereas others prefer visual examples, such as food models and measuring devices.[2] Information can be provided in one-on-one sessions or group discussions. The initial meeting should include an assessment of the person's understanding of the material and commitment to making changes. Follow-up sessions can reveal whether the person has successfully adopted the new dietary plan. For example, a nurse who counsels a woman who is lactose intolerant and hesitant to use milk products might proceed as follows:

- The nurse provides sample menus of a nutritionally adequate diet that limits milk and milk products. Together, the nurse and the woman design menus that consider the woman's food preferences.
- The nurse describes the types and amounts of milk products that would likely be tolerated without causing symptoms and explains how to gradually incorporate these foods into the diet.
- Using diet analysis software, the nurse demonstrates how altering intakes of calcium- and vitamin D–containing foods changes a meal's nutrient content.
- The nurse explains how to use the Daily Values on food labels to estimate the calcium content of packaged foods.
- The nurse provides information about the advantages and disadvantages of different calcium and vitamin D supplements.

Box 14-1   Case Study: Implementing Nutrition Care

Max is an 11-year-old boy who was admitted to the hospital after he passed out while playing with friends. Tests confirm a diagnosis of type 1 diabetes mellitus. Max remains in the hospital for several days until his blood glucose and ketone levels are under control. During this time, he and his family learn about diabetes, the diet Max needs to follow, the use of insulin, the monitoring of blood glucose levels, and the required coordination of food intake, insulin, and physical activity. The details of diabetes mellitus are reserved for Chapter 20, but for now you can consider the steps that are necessary for implementing Max's nutrition care.

1. The nurse handling Max's case must identify expected outcomes when writing the care plan. What expected outcomes are appropriate for Max's situation?

2. Given the chronic nature of Max's illness and his age, what approaches should the nurse use when discussing the required meal plan and insulin treatment with Max and his family?

3. What factors should be considered when designing a nutrition education program for Max and his parents?

4. Max will need additional care to learn more about diabetes and to make the adjustments that will allow him to cope with his condition. Why is it important to address follow-up care before Max leaves the hospital?

- The nurse assesses the woman's understanding by having her identify nonmilk products that are high in calcium or vitamin D.

Ideally, the nurse would be able to monitor the woman's progress in a subsequent counseling session.

Follow-Up Care For optimal results, the health care professional should monitor the patient's progress and periodically evaluate the effectiveness of the nutrition care plan. Doing so usually involves comparing relevant outcome measures (such as the results of blood tests) with initial values and meeting with the patient to learn whether the plan has been satisfactory from the patient's point of view. Such follow-up efforts can reveal whether the care plan needs to be revised or updated, as is often the case when a person's medical condition changes.

The Case Study in Box 14-1 provides an opportunity for you to review the implementation of nutrition care.

Review Notes

- Nutrition interventions are designed to correct the nutrition problems associated with illness. The intervention may involve food and/or nutrient delivery, nutrition education, nutrition counseling, and the coordination of nutrition care with other health professionals.
- Using the steps of the nursing process, a nurse can incorporate nutrition care into a nursing care plan.
- A nutrition intervention should take into account a person's food practices, lifestyle, and degree of motivation. Nutrition education should be individualized to accommodate a patient's needs and learning style.
- Nutrition care can be evaluated by reviewing relevant outcome measures of health status and determining the patient's understanding and acceptance of the intervention.

14.2 Dietary Modifications

During illness, many patients can meet their energy and nutrient needs by following a **regular diet**. Others may require a **modified diet**, which is altered by changing food consistency or texture, nutrient content, or the foods included in the diet. This section describes how energy needs may be estimated and introduces several types of dietary modifications.

regular diet: a diet that includes all foods and meets the nutrient needs of healthy people; may also be called a *standard diet, general diet, normal diet,* or *house diet.*

modified diet: a diet that contains foods altered in texture, consistency, or nutrient content or that includes or omits specific foods; may also be called a *therapeutic diet.*

TABLE 14-3 Selected Equations for Estimating Resting Metabolic Rate (RMR)

Harris–Benedict[a]

Women: RMR = 655.1 + [9.563 × weight (kg)] + [1.85 × height (cm)] − [4.676 × age (years)]

Men: RMR = 66.5 + [13.75 × weight (kg)] + [5.003 × height (cm)] − [6.755 × age (years)]

Mifflin–St. Jeor[b]

Women: RMR = [9.99 × weight (kg)] + [6.25 × height (cm)] − [4.92 × age (years)] − 161

Men: RMR = [9.99 × weight (kg)] + [6.25 × height (cm)] − [4.92 × age (years)] + 5

[a]Although the Harris–Benedict equations are sometimes used for estimating basal metabolic rate (BMR), they were derived from data measured during resting conditions in most cases.

[b]In overweight and obese individuals who are not critically ill, the Mifflin–St. Jeor equation may provide a more accurate estimate of RMR than other predictive equations.

Energy Intakes in Hospital Patients

To estimate the energy needs of hospital patients, the clinician may measure or calculate the resting metabolic rate (RMR) and then adjust the RMR value with a "stress factor" that accounts for the medical problem.[3] In ambulatory patients, a factor for activity level may also be applied. Table 14-3 lists examples of RMR equations in common use, and Box 14-2 presents an example of this method. To obtain more accurate RMR values, clinicians sometimes use **indirect calorimetry**, a procedure that estimates energy expenditure by measuring oxygen consumption and carbon dioxide production during a period of rest. In many bedridden, hospitalized individuals, the value obtained from indirect calorimetry may be an accurate indicator of total energy needs without need for further adjustment because the measured value includes the metabolic changes caused by illness.[4]

A quick method for estimating energy needs is to multiply a person's body weight by a factor considered appropriate for the medical condition. For example, the recommended energy intake for optimal wound healing is approximately 30 to 35 kilocalories per kilogram body weight per day[5]; a patient weighing 132 pounds (60 kilograms) may therefore require between 1800 and 2100 kcalories per day. The energy intake can be

indirect calorimetry: a procedure that estimates energy expenditure by measuring oxygen consumption and carbon dioxide production.

Box 14-2 | *HOW TO* Estimate Appropriate Energy Intakes for Hospital Patients

To estimate an appropriate energy intake for a hospital patient, the health practitioner may calculate the patient's resting metabolic rate (RMR) and then apply a "stress factor" to accommodate the additional energy needs imposed by illness. The stress factor 1.25 has been shown to be reasonably accurate for many hospitalized patients; other examples are listed in Box 16-6 on p. 475.

The following example uses the Mifflin–St. Jeor equation (shown in Table 14-3) and the stress factor 1.25 to determine the energy needs of a 57-year-old female patient who is 5 feet 3 inches tall, weighs 115 pounds, and is confined to bed.

Step 1: The patient's weight and height are converted to the units used in the equation:

Weight in kilograms = 115 lb ÷ 2.20 lb/kg = 52.3 kg
Height in centimeters = 63.0 in × 2.54 cm/in = 160 cm

Step 2: Using the Mifflin–St. Jeor equation for estimating RMR in women:

RMR = [9.99 × weight (kg)] + [6.25 × height (cm)] − [4.92 × age (years)] − 161

= (9.99 × 52.3) + (6.25 × 160) − (4.92 × 57) − 161
= 522 + 1000 − 280 − 161 = 1081 kcal

Step 3: The RMR value is multiplied by the appropriate stress factor:

RMR × stress factor = 1081 × 1.25 = 1351 kcal

Thus, an appropriate energy intake for this patient would be approximately 1350 kcal. Her weight should be monitored to determine if her actual needs are higher or lower.

For a patient who is not confined to bed, an additional activity factor may be applied to accommodate the extra energy needs. For example, if the patient in the example begins limited activity while in the hospital, an activity factor of 1.2 can be multiplied by the results obtained in Step 3:

1351 × activity factor = 1351 × 1.2 = 1621 kcal

The activity factor for a hospitalized patient often falls between 1.1 and 1.4, and it is likely to change as the patient's condition improves.

started within this range and then adjusted as the patient's body weight or other determinants of nutrition status change.

In patients who are critically ill, energy needs may be higher than normal because of fever, mechanical ventilation, restlessness, or the presence of open wounds. Patients who are critically ill are usually bedridden and inactive, however, so the energy needed for physical activity is minimal. Energy requirements for critical-care patients are described in Chapter 16.

Modified Diets

Diets that contain foods with altered texture and consistency may be advised for individuals with chewing or swallowing difficulties. Diets with modified nutrient or food content may be prescribed to correct malnutrition, relieve disease symptoms, or reduce the risk of developing complications. Patients who have several medical problems may require a number of dietary modifications. Keep in mind that modified diets should be adjusted to satisfy individual preferences and tolerances and may also need to be altered as a patient's condition changes. Table 14-4 lists examples of modified diets that are often prescribed during illness.[6] Later chapters discuss other types of dietary strategies that may be helpful for treating nutritional problems.

TABLE 14-4	Examples of Modified Diets	
TYPE OF DIET[a]	**DESCRIPTION OF DIET**	**APPROPRIATE USES**
Modified Texture and Consistency		
Mechanically altered diets	Contain foods that are modified in texture. Pureed food diets include only pureed foods; mechanically altered and soft food diets may include solid foods that are mashed, minced, ground, or soft.	Pureed food diets are used for people with swallowing difficulty, poor lip and tongue control, or oral hypersensitivity. Mechanically altered and soft food diets are appropriate for people with limited chewing ability or certain swallowing impairments.
Blenderized liquid diet	Contains fluids and foods that are blenderized to liquid form.	For people who cannot chew, swallow easily, or tolerate solid foods.
Clear liquid diet	Contains clear fluids or foods that are liquid at room temperature and leave minimal residue in the colon.	For preparation for bowel surgery or colonoscopy, for acute GI disturbances (such as after GI surgeries), or as a transition diet after intravenous feeding. For short-term use only.
Modified Nutrient or Food Content		
Fat-restricted diet	Limits dietary fat to low ($<$50 g/day) or very low ($<$25 g/day) intakes.	For people who have certain malabsorptive disorders or symptoms of diarrhea, flatulence, or steatorrhea (fecal fat) resulting from dietary fat intolerance.
Low-fiber diet	Limits dietary fiber; degree of restriction depends on the patient's condition and reason for restriction.	For acute phases of intestinal disorders or to reduce fecal output before surgery. Not recommended for long-term use.
Low-sodium diet	Limits dietary sodium; degree of restriction depends on symptoms and disease severity.	To help lower blood pressure or prevent fluid retention; used in hypertension, heart failure, renal disease, and liver disease.
High-kcalorie, high-protein diet	Contains foods that are kcalorie- and protein-dense.	Used for patients with high kcalorie and protein requirements (due to cancer, AIDS, burns, trauma, and other conditions); also used to reverse malnutrition, improve nutritional status, or promote weight gain.

[a]Registered dietitians may use the term *nutrition therapy* in place of *diet* when they provide nutrition care; for example, the *low-fiber diet* may be called *low-fiber nutrition therapy*.

Source: Academy of Nutrition and Dietetics, *Nutrition Care Manual* (Chicago: Academy of Nutrition and Dietetics, 2018).

TABLE 14-5 | Foods Included in Mechanically Altered Diets

Depending on the feeding problem, a pureed food, mechanically altered, or soft food diet may include foods that are pureed, mashed, ground, minced, or soft textured. Foods used in the different diets may overlap. Individual tolerances ultimately determine whether foods are included or excluded.

PUREED FOODS	MECHANICALLY ALTERED OR SOFT FOODS
Milk products: Milk, smooth yogurt, pudding, custard	**Milk products:** Milk, yogurt with soft fruit, pudding, cottage cheese
Fruit: Pureed fruit and fruit juice without pulp, seeds, skin, or chunks; well-mashed fresh bananas; applesauce	**Fruit:** Canned or cooked fruit without seeds or skin, fruit juice with small amounts of pulp, ripe bananas
Vegetables: Pureed cooked vegetables without seeds, skin, or chunks; mashed potatoes, pureed potatoes with gravy	**Vegetables:** Soft, well-cooked vegetables that are not rubbery or fibrous; well-cooked, moist potatoes
Meat and meat substitutes: Pureed meat; smooth, homogeneous soufflés; hummus or other pureed legume spreads	**Meat and meat substitutes:** Ground, minced, or tender meat, poultry, or fish with gravy or sauce; tofu; well-cooked, moist legumes; scrambled or soft-cooked eggs
Breads and cereals: Smooth cooked cereals such as Cream of Wheat, slurried bread or pancakes,ª pureed rice or pasta	**Breads and cereals:** Cooked cereals or moistened dry cereals with minimal texture, soft bread or pancakes, well-cooked noodles or dumplings in sauce or gravy

ªSlurried foods are foods that have been mixed with liquid to achieve an appropriate consistency; they may be gelled and shaped to improve their appearance.

Mechanically Altered Diets Individuals who have difficulty chewing or swallowing may benefit from mechanically altered diets. Chewing difficulties usually result from dental problems. Impaired swallowing, or **dysphagia**, may result from neurological disorders, surgical procedures involving the head and neck, and physiological or anatomical abnormalities that restrict the movement of food within the throat or esophagus. Dysphagia diets are highly individualized because swallowing problems vary in severity and swallowing ability can fluctuate over time. Chapter 17 provides details about the specific diets used for treating dysphagia.

Table 14-5 provides examples of foods that are usually included in mechanically altered diets. Although the names for these diets vary, a more restrictive diet may contain mostly pureed foods (*pureed food diet*), whereas a less restrictive diet may include ground or minced foods (*ground/minced food diet* or *mechanically altered diet*) or moist, soft-textured foods that easily form a bolus (*soft food diet*). Note that the foods used in these diets can overlap, and individual tolerances ultimately determine whether foods are included or excluded.

Blenderized Liquid Diet A *blenderized diet* is most often recommended following oral or facial surgeries (for example, jaw wiring). Foods that can be blenderized (often with added liquid) are available from all food groups: they include breads and cereals; boiled rice and pasta; cooked vegetables; fresh or cooked fruit without skins or seeds; and cooked, tender meats and fish. Foods that do not blend well should be excluded; examples include hard or rubbery foods such as nuts and seeds, coconut, dried fruit, hard cheese, sausages and frankfurters, and some raw vegetables.

Clear Liquid Diet Clear liquids, which require minimal digestion and are easily tolerated by the gastrointestinal (GI) tract, are often recommended before some GI procedures (such as GI examinations, X-rays, or surgeries), after GI surgery, or after fasting or intravenous feeding. The **clear liquid diet** consists of clear fluids and foods that are liquid at room temperature and leave little undigested material (called **residue**) in the colon. Permitted foods include clear or pulp-free fruit juices, carbonated beverages, clear meat and vegetable broths (such as consommé and bouillon), fruit-flavored

dysphagia: difficulty swallowing.

clear liquid diet: a diet that consists of foods that are liquid at room temperature, require minimal digestion, and leave little residue (undigested material) in the colon.

residue: material left in the intestine after digestion; includes mostly dietary fiber, undigested starches and proteins, GI secretions, and cellular debris.

gelatin, fruit ices made from clear juices, frozen juice bars, and plain hard candy. Although the clear liquid diet provides fluid and electrolytes, its nutrient and energy contents are extremely limited. If used for longer than a day or two, this diet should be supplemented with commercially prepared low-residue formulas that provide required nutrients. Figure 14-1 gives an example of a one-day clear liquid menu.

Fat-Restricted Diet Fat restriction may be necessary for reducing the symptoms of fat malabsorption, which often accompanies diseases of the liver, gallbladder, pancreas, and intestines. Fat restriction may also alleviate the symptoms of heartburn. Although the fat intake is occasionally limited to as little as 25 grams daily, it should not be restricted more than necessary because fat is an important source of energy.

Most foods included in a fat-restricted diet provide less than 1 gram of fat per serving. The diet includes fat-free milk products, most breads and cooked grains, fat-free broths and soups, vegetables prepared without fat, most fruits, and fat-free candies and sweets. Restricted foods include low-fat and full-fat milk products, baked products with added fat (such as muffins), and most prepared desserts. Lean meat and meat substitutes are permitted but may be restricted to 4 to 6 ounces per day, depending on the degree of restriction. Some patients with malabsorptive disorders cannot tolerate large amounts of lactose or dietary fiber, so foods that include these substances may also need to be excluded from the diet. Chapter 18 provides additional information about fat-restricted diets.

Low-Fiber Diet Fiber restriction is recommended during acute phases of intestinal disorders, when the presence of fiber may exacerbate intestinal discomfort or cause diarrhea or blockages. Low-fiber diets are sometimes used before surgery to minimize fecal volume and after surgery during transition to a regular diet. Long-term fiber restriction is discouraged, however, because it is associated with constipation and other problems.

Low-fiber diets often restrict whole-grain breads and cereals, nuts and nut butters, most fresh fruit (except peeled apples, ripe bananas, and melons), dried fruit, dried beans and peas, and many vegetables (including broccoli, cabbage, corn, onions, peppers, spinach, and winter squash); Chapter 3 provides additional information about the fiber content of foods. If necessary, even greater reductions in colonic residue can be achieved by excluding foods high in resistant starch (see p. 71), milk products that contain significant lactose, and foods that contain fructose or sugar alcohols (such as sorbitol); these foods contribute to colonic residue because some of their nutrients may be poorly digested (such as the lactose in milk) or poorly absorbed (such as sorbitol and fructose).

Low-Sodium Diet A low-sodium diet can help to prevent or correct fluid retention and may be prescribed for treatment of hypertension, heart failure, kidney disease, and liver disease. The sodium intake recommended depends on the illness, the severity of symptoms, and the specific drug treatment prescribed. In most cases, sodium is restricted to 2000 or 3000 milligrams daily, although more severe restrictions may be used in the hospital setting. Many patients find it difficult to significantly reduce their sodium intake, so while the low-sodium diet is prescribed in an attempt to improve the patient's medical problem, the recommended sodium intake may sometimes exceed the Tolerable Upper Intake Level (UL) for sodium of 2300 milligrams.*

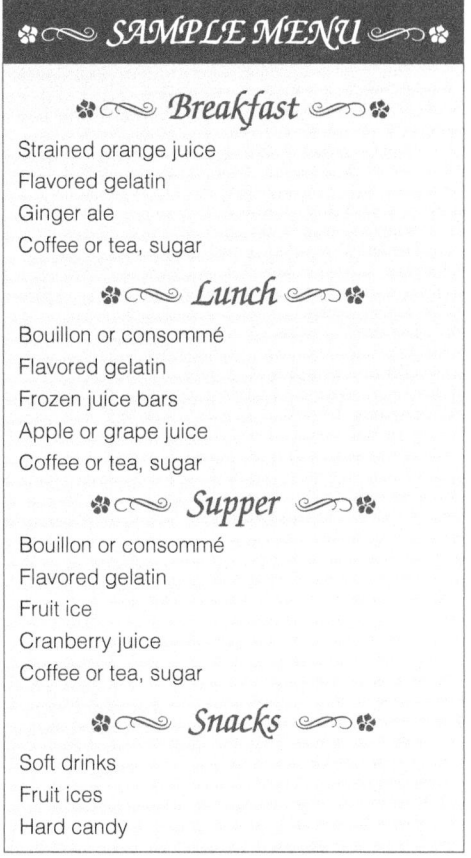

FIGURE 14-1 Menu for a Clear Liquid Diet

❧⌒ *SAMPLE MENU* ⌒❧

❧⌒ *Breakfast* ⌒❧
Strained orange juice
Flavored gelatin
Ginger ale
Coffee or tea, sugar

❧⌒ *Lunch* ⌒❧
Bouillon or consommé
Flavored gelatin
Frozen juice bars
Apple or grape juice
Coffee or tea, sugar

❧⌒ *Supper* ⌒❧
Bouillon or consommé
Flavored gelatin
Fruit ice
Cranberry juice
Coffee or tea, sugar

❧⌒ *Snacks* ⌒❧
Soft drinks
Fruit ices
Hard candy

---

*The average sodium intake in the United States is approximately 3400 mg per day. The sodium UL was set at 2300 mg to help prevent hypertension.

Low-sodium diets limit the use of salt when cooking and at the table, eliminate most prepared foods and condiments, and limit consumption of milk and milk products (if excessive). Because processed foods are often high in sodium, people following a low-sodium diet should check food labels and consume only low-sodium products. Sodium restrictions are difficult to implement on a long-term basis because many people find low-sodium foods unpalatable. Additional information about controlling dietary sodium is provided in Chapters 21 and 22.

High-kCalorie, High-Protein Diet The high-kcalorie, high-protein diet is used to increase kcalorie and protein intakes in patients who have unusually high requirements or in those who are eating poorly. High-fat foods are added to increase energy intakes; consequently, the diet may exceed 35 percent kcalories from fat (current guidelines recommend a total fat intake between 20 and 35 percent of kcalories). Consuming small, frequent meals and commercial liquid supplements (such as Ensure or Boost) can also help a patient meet increased energy, protein, and other nutrient needs.

Examples of foods included in high-kcalorie, high-protein diets are listed in Table 14-6. Some of these foods are high in saturated fat, which is limited in heart-healthy diets. These foods are used liberally in diets for malnourished patients to help correct their immediate nutrition problems—weight loss and muscle wasting. Chapter 23 offers additional suggestions for increasing the kcalorie and protein contents of meals.

TABLE 14-6 Foods Included in High-kCalorie, High-Protein Diets

Milk products	Whole milk, half-and-half, cream
	Milkshakes, eggnog
	Cheese
	Ice cream, whipped cream
Meat and other high-protein foods	All types of meat, fish, and poultry, including bacon, frankfurters, and luncheon meat; eggs; beans; tofu
	Meat prepared by frying or served with cream sauce or gravy
	Protein bars
	Nuts and seeds, peanut and other nut butters, coconut
Breads and cereals	Granola and other dry cereals prepared with whole milk or cream and dried fruit
	Hot cereal with whole milk or cream, or added fat
	Pasta, rice, and biscuits with added fat
	Pancakes, waffles, French toast
Vegetables	High-kcalorie vegetables such as potatoes, corn, and peas
	Vegetables prepared with butter, margarine, sour cream, cheese sauce, mayonnaise, or salad dressing
	Cream of vegetable soups
Fruit	Dried fruit
	Canned fruit in heavy syrup
	Avocado
Beverages	Fruit juices, fruit smoothies, sweetened beverages
	Meal replacement drinks
	Beverages with added protein powder

Variations in the Diet Order

In most cases, the physician is responsible for prescribing an appropriate diet for a patient in a medical facility. Diet orders must be precise to avoid confusion; for example, a "low-sodium diet" should specify the amount of sodium permitted, as "low sodium" could be interpreted to mean any amount between 500 and 3000 milligrams. The physician often relies on the dietitian or nurse to recommend changes in the diet order when warranted. If a diet order seems inappropriate or outdated, the nurse should alert the physician that a mistake may have been made.

Diet Progression A change in diet as a patient's food tolerance improves is called **diet progression**. For example, the diet order may read, "progress diet from clear liquids to a regular diet as tolerated." In practice, this means that the patient would be given clear beverages initially, and then gradually be provided with other beverages or solid foods that are unlikely to cause discomfort. As another example, the diet may progress from small, frequent feedings to larger meals as tolerance improves. Symptoms such as nausea, vomiting, diarrhea, and gastrointestinal pain suggest intolerance.

Nothing by Mouth (NPO) An order to not give a patient anything at all—food, beverages, or medications—is indicated by NPO, an abbreviation for *non per os*, meaning "nothing by mouth." For example, an order may read "NPO for 24 hours" or "NPO until after X-ray." The NPO order is commonly used during certain acute illnesses or diagnostic tests involving the GI tract.

Alternative Feeding Routes Most patients can meet their nutrient needs by consuming regular foods. If their nutrient needs are high or their appetites poor, oral supplements can be added to their diets to improve their intakes. Sometimes, however, a person's medical condition makes it difficult to meet nutrient needs orally. In such cases, the physician may order **tube feedings** or **parenteral nutrition**, which are described more fully in Chapter 15.

- *Tube feedings.* Nutritionally complete formulas can be delivered through a tube placed directly into the stomach or intestine. Tube feedings are preferred to parenteral nutrition if the GI tract is functioning normally.
- *Parenteral nutrition.* A person's medical condition sometimes prohibits the use of the GI tract to deliver nutrients. If the person is malnourished and the GI tract cannot be used for a significant period of time, parenteral nutrition, in which nutrients are supplied intravenously, can meet nutritional needs.

diet progression: a change in diet as a patient's tolerances permit.

tube feedings: liquid formulas delivered through a tube placed in the stomach or intestine.

parenteral nutrition: the provision of nutrients by vein, bypassing the intestine.

Review Notes

- Dietary modifications prescribed during illness may include changes in food texture or consistency, modified energy or nutrient content, or the inclusion or exclusion of certain foods.
- The energy needs of hospital patients can be estimated by multiplying a person's resting metabolic rate (RMR) or body weight by factors that account for the medical condition.
- Mechanically altered diets may be prescribed for people with chewing or swallowing difficulties. Diets with modified nutrient or food content are usually prescribed to correct malnutrition, relieve disease symptoms, or reduce the risk of developing complications.
- The diet order must include specific instructions about dietary modifications to avoid confusion. The diet prescribed may change during the course of illness.

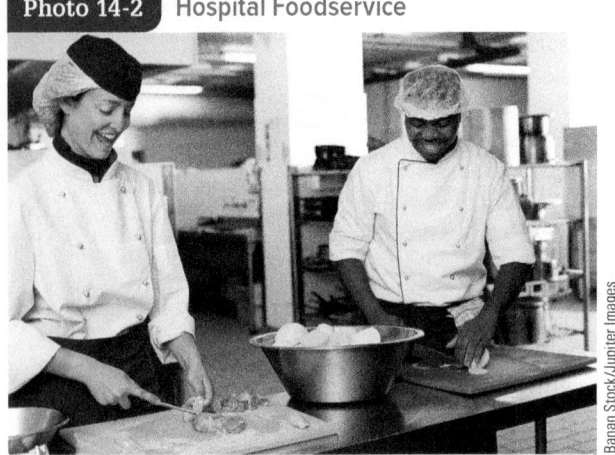

Photo 14-2 Hospital Foodservice

Foodservice departments strive to prepare appetizing and nutritious meals and may accommodate dozens of special diets.

FIGURE 14-2 Sample Selective Menu

SODIUM-CONTROLLED	SUNDAY
❀ ᎒ Lunch ᎒ ❀	
LF = Low Fat LSLF = Low Sodium, Low Fat	
Meats	
LSLF Baked chicken LSLF Baked fish (cod)	
Starchy Vegetables	
LSLF Rice	LSLF Boiled potatoes
Vegetables	
LSLF Baby carrots	LSLF Green beans
Soup/Salad/Juice	**Dressings**
LSLF Coleslaw	Diet French
LS Chicken broth	Diet Thousand Island
Apple juice	Diet Italian
Tossed salad	
Desserts	
Pears	Fresh fruit
Breads	
Dinner roll	Bran bread
White bread	LS Crackers
Whole wheat bread	
Beverages & Condiments	
Coffee	Sugar
Decaf. coffee	Sugar substitute
Hot tea	Creamer
Decaf. hot tea	Lemon
Iced tea	Herb seasoning
Whole milk	Margarine
2% milk	Diet mustard
Fat-free milk	Diet mayonnaise
No salt	Diet catsup
Name _____	Room ____

14.3 Foodservice

Foodservice departments face a daily challenge in planning, producing, and delivering hundreds of nutritious meals and accommodating dozens of special diets and food preferences (see Photo 14-2). When designing menus, the dietary and foodservice personnel refer to a **diet manual**, which details the specific foods or preparation methods to include in or exclude from modified diets. The diet manual may also outline the rationale and indications for use of the diets and include sample menus.

Food Selection

Most hospitals provide **selective menus** from which patients can select their meals (see Figure 14-2). If a patient is following a modified diet, the menu includes only foods that are permitted on that diet. To improve patient satisfaction, many hospitals are moving toward a room-service, cook-to-order system similar to what an individual might experience in a hotel. In these facilities, the menus list more food choices than usual and include more fresh foods, seasonal ingredients, and local specialties. Entrees are prepared as they are ordered, and food delivery hours are expanded to better accommodate the patients' varied schedules.

Food Safety

The protocols used by healthcare facilities for handling food products are based on a recognition of the potential hazards and critical control points in food preparation, usually referred to as **Hazard Analysis and Critical Control Points (HACCP)**. A HACCP program typically addresses food handling, cooking, and storage procedures; cleaning and disinfecting of utensils, surfaces, and equipment; and staff sanitation issues. The personnel involved with preparing or delivering meals need to be aware of the specific HACCP systems at their facility.

Improving Food Intake

People in medical facilities often lose their appetites as a result of their medical condition, treatment, or emotional distress. Moreover, some medications and other treatments can dramatically alter taste perceptions. Patients may receive meals at specified times, whether they are hungry or not, and often must eat in bed without companionship. Meals may also be unwelcome if the person is in pain or has been sedated.

To improve food intakes, health professionals should ensure that the patient's room remains calm and quiet during mealtime. Excessive activity, like room maintenance or ward rounds, can distract patients and reduce appetite. If the patient's appetite or sense of taste is affected by illness, the patient can be asked to identify foods that are the most enjoyable. Box 14-3 includes additional suggestions that may help to improve food intake at mealtimes.

Box 14-3 **HOW TO** Help Hospital Patients Improve Their Food Intakes

1. Empathize with the patient. Show that you understand how difficult eating may be when a person feels too sick to move or too tired to sit up. Help to motivate the patient by explaining how important good nutrition is to recovery.

2. Help patients select the foods they like and mark menus appropriately. When appropriate and permissible, let friends or family members bring favorite foods from outside the hospital.

3. For patients who are weak, suggest foods that require little effort to eat. Eating a roast beef sandwich, for example, requires less effort than cutting and eating a steak. Drinking soup from a cup may be easier than eating it with a spoon.

4. During mealtimes, make sure the patient's room is quiet and has sufficient lighting for viewing the food. See that the room is free of odors that may interfere with the appetite.

5. Help patients prepare for meals. Help them wash their hands and get comfortable, either in bed or in a chair. Adjust the extension

table to a comfortable distance and height and make sure it is clean. Take these steps before the food tray arrives so that the meal can be served promptly and at the right temperature.

6. When the food cart arrives, check the patient's tray. Confirm that the patient is receiving the right diet, the foods on the tray are those selected from the menu, and the foods look appealing. Order a new tray if the foods are not appropriate.

7. Help with eating, if necessary. Help patients open containers or cut foods, and assist with feeding if patients cannot feed themselves. Encourage patients with little appetite to eat the most nutritious foods first and to drink liquids between meals.

8. Take a positive attitude toward the hospital's food. Let patients know that the foodservice department tries to make foods appetizing. Placing an occasional "surprise" on the tray—a decoration or funny card, for example—may help patients look forward to meals or perk up sagging spirits.

Review Notes

- Foodservice personnel rely on diet manuals when preparing menus for modified diets.
- Many hospitals provide selective menus from which patients can choose meals; some facilities may use a room service model that allows patients more food choices.
- Foodservice departments must follow the specific HACCP protocols adopted by their institutions to ensure food safety.
- Hospital patients who lack appetite at mealtime may need encouragement to consume adequate amounts of food.

diet manual: a resource that specifies the foods or preparation methods to include in or exclude from modified diets and provides sample menus.

selective menus: menus that provide choices in some or all menu categories.

Hazard Analysis and Critical Control Points (HACCP): systems of food or formula preparation that identify food safety hazards and critical control points during foodservice procedures; pronounced *HAH-sip*.

14.4 Diet-Drug Interactions

When working with patients, medical personnel should be alert to possible interactions between drugs and dietary substances. These interactions can raise health care costs and result in serious, and sometimes fatal, complications. Accordingly, health professionals must learn to take steps to prevent or lessen their adverse consequences (see Photo 14-3). Diet-drug interactions (also called *food-drug interactions* or *drug-nutrient interactions*) generally fall into the following categories:

- Drugs may alter food intake by reducing the appetite or by causing complications that make food consumption difficult or unpleasant. Other drugs may increase the appetite and cause weight gain.
- Drugs may alter the absorption, metabolism, or excretion of nutrients. Conversely, nutrients and other food components may alter the absorption, metabolism, or excretion of drugs.
- Some interactions between dietary components and drugs can cause drug toxicity.

Examples of these types of diet-drug interactions are shown in Table 14-7.[7]

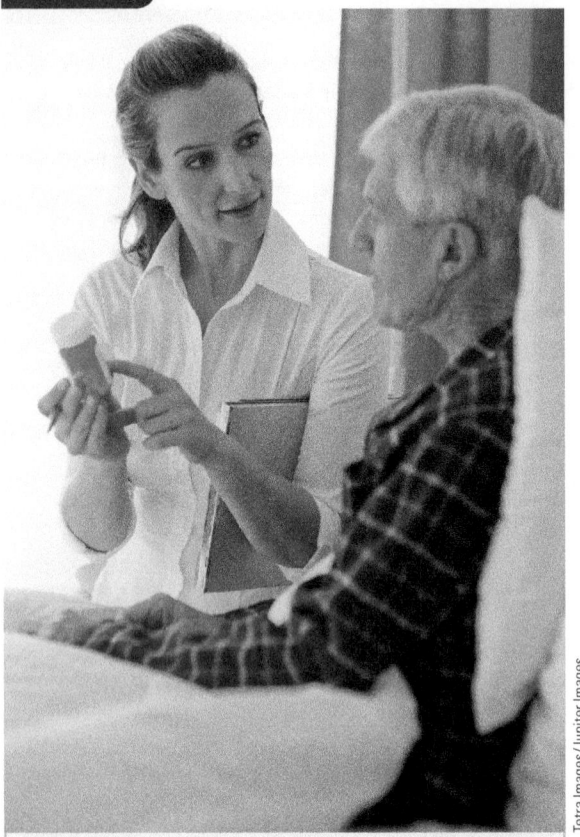

Photo 14-3

Because nurses interact closely with patients, they are often responsible for educating patients about potential diet-drug interactions.

Drug Effects on Food Intake

Some drugs can make food intake difficult or unpleasant: they may suppress the appetite, cause mouth dryness, alter the sense of taste, lead to inflammation or lesions in the mouth or GI tract, or induce nausea and vomiting. Certain side effects of drugs, including abdominal discomfort, constipation, and diarrhea, may be worsened by food consumption. Medications that cause drowsiness, such as sedatives and some painkillers, can make a person too tired to eat.

Drug complications that reduce food intake are significant only when they continue for a long period. Although many drugs can cause nausea in certain individuals, the nausea often subsides after the first few doses of the drug and therefore has little effect on nutrition status. If side effects persist, other medications may be prescribed to treat them; for example, antinauseants and **antiemetics** can help to reduce nausea and vomiting and thereby improve food intake.

Some medications stimulate the appetite and encourage weight gain. Unintentional weight gain may result from the use of some antidepressants, antipsychotics, antidiabetic drugs, and corticosteroids (such as prednisone).[8] For some conditions, however, weight gain is desirable. Patients with diseases that cause wasting, such as cancer or the acquired immunodeficiency syndrome (AIDS), are sometimes prescribed appetite enhancers such as megestrol acetate (Megace), a progesterone analog, or dronabinol (Marinol), which is derived from the active ingredient in marijuana.

Drug Effects on Nutrient Absorption

The medications that most often cause nutrient malabsorption are those that either upset GI function or damage the intestinal mucosa. **Antineoplastic drugs** and **antiretroviral drugs** are especially detrimental, whereas nonsteroidal anti-inflammatory drugs (NSAIDs) and some antibiotics can have similar, though milder, effects. This section describes additional ways in which medications may alter nutrient absorption.

Drug-Nutrient Binding Some medications bind to nutrients in the GI tract, preventing their absorption. For example, bile acid binders (such as cholestyramine, or Questran), which are used to reduce blood cholesterol levels, may bind to fat-soluble vitamins. Some antibiotics, notably tetracycline and ciprofloxacin (Cipro), bind to the calcium in foods and supplements, reducing the absorption of both the calcium and the antibiotic. Other minerals that may bind to these antibiotics include iron, magnesium, and zinc. Consumers are advised to use dairy products and all mineral supplements at least 2 hours before or after taking these medications.

Altered Stomach Acidity Medications that reduce stomach acidity can impair the absorption of vitamin B_{12}, folate, and iron. Examples include antacids, which neutralize stomach acid by acting as weak bases, and antiulcer drugs (such as proton pump inhibitors and H2 blockers), which interfere with acid secretion.

Direct Inhibition Several drugs impede nutrient absorption by interfering with their transport into mucosal cells. For example, the antibiotics trimethoprim (Proloprim) and pyrimethamine (Daraprim) compete with folate for absorption into intestinal cells. The anti-inflammatory medication colchicine, a treatment for gout, interferes with vitamin B_{12} absorption.

antiemetics: drugs that prevent vomiting.

antineoplastic drugs: drugs that control or kill cancer cells.

antiretroviral drugs: drugs that treat retroviral infections, such as infection with human immunodeficiency virus (HIV).

Tetra Images/Jupiter Images

TABLE 14-7   Examples of Diet-Drug Interactions

Drugs may alter food intake by:

- Altering the appetite (amphetamines suppress appetite; corticosteroids increase appetite).
- Interfering with taste or smell (amphetamines change taste perception).
- Inducing nausea or vomiting (digitalis may do both).
- Interfering with oral function (some antidepressants may cause dry mouth).
- Causing sores or inflammation in the mouth (methotrexate may cause painful mouth ulcers).

Drugs may alter nutrient absorption by:

- Changing the acidity of the digestive tract (antacids may interfere with iron and folate absorption).
- Damaging mucosal cells (cancer chemotherapy may damage mucosal cells).
- Binding to nutrients (bile acid binders bind to fat-soluble vitamins).

Foods and nutrients may alter drug absorption by:

- Stimulating the secretion of gastric acid (the antifungal agent ketoconazole is absorbed better when taken with meals, during which gastric acid is secreted).
- Altering the rate of gastric emptying (drug absorption may be delayed when the drug is taken with food).
- Binding to drugs (calcium binds to tetracycline, reducing the absorption of both substances).
- Competing for absorption sites in the small intestine (dietary amino acids interfere with levodopa absorption).

Drugs and nutrients may interact and alter metabolism by:

- Acting as structural analogs (as do warfarin and vitamin K).
- Using similar enzyme systems (phenobarbital induces liver enzymes that increase the metabolism of folate, vitamin D, and vitamin K).
- Competing for transport on plasma proteins (fatty acids and drugs may compete for the same sites on the plasma protein albumin).

Drugs may alter nutrient excretion by:

- Altering nutrient reabsorption in the kidneys[a] (some diuretics increase the excretion of sodium and potassium).
- Causing diarrhea or vomiting (diarrhea and vomiting may cause electrolyte losses).

Food substances may alter drug excretion by:

- Inducing the activities of liver enzymes that metabolize drugs, increasing drug excretion (components of charcoal-broiled meats increase the metabolism of warfarin, theophylline, and acetaminophen).

Food substances and drugs may interact and cause drug toxicity by:

- Increasing side effects of the drug (the caffeine in beverages can increase the adverse effects of stimulants).
- Increasing drug action to excessive levels (grapefruit components inhibit the enzymes that degrade certain drugs, increasing drug concentrations in the body).

[a]When the kidneys reabsorb a substance, they retain it in the blood. Substances that are not reabsorbed are excreted in the urine.

Dietary Effects on Drug Absorption

Major influences on drug absorption include the stomach-emptying rate, the level of acidity in the stomach, and direct interactions with dietary components. The drug's formulation may also influence its absorption. The instructions included with medications typically advise whether the drug should be taken with food or on an empty stomach.

Stomach-Emptying Rate Drugs reach the small intestine more quickly when the stomach is empty. Therefore, taking a medication with meals may delay its absorption, although the total amount absorbed may not be lower. As an example, aspirin works faster when taken on an empty stomach, although taking it with food is often encouraged to reduce stomach irritation.

Slow stomach emptying can sometimes enhance drug absorption because the drug's absorption sites in the small intestine are less likely to become saturated. However, a slow drug absorption rate (due to slow stomach emptying) can be a problem if high drug concentrations are needed for effectiveness, as when a hypnotic is taken to induce sleep.

Stomach Acidity Some drugs are absorbed better in an acidic environment, whereas others are absorbed better under alkaline conditions. For example, reduced stomach acidity (due to secretory disorders or antacid medications) may reduce the absorption of ketoconazole (Nizoral, an antifungal medication) and atazanavir (an antiretroviral medication), but increase the absorption of digoxin (Lanoxin, which treats heart failure) and alendronate (Fosamax, which treats osteoporosis).[9] Some drugs can be damaged by acid and are available in coated forms that resist the stomach's acidity.

Interactions between Drugs and Dietary Components Various dietary substances can bind to drugs and inhibit their absorption. As mentioned earlier, minerals can bind to some antibiotics, reducing absorption of both the minerals and the drugs. High-fiber meals can decrease the absorption of some tricyclic antidepressants due to binding between the fiber and the drugs. Conversely, the absorption of many lipophilic drugs (those with fat-soluble structures) is improved when the drugs are taken with a fat-containing meal.[10]

Drug Effects on Nutrient Metabolism

Drugs and nutrients share similar enzyme systems in the small intestine and liver. Consequently, some drugs may enhance or inhibit the activities of enzymes needed for nutrient metabolism. For example, the **anticonvulsants** phenobarbital and phenytoin increase levels of the liver enzymes that metabolize folate, vitamin D, and vitamin K; therefore, persons using these drugs may require supplements of these vitamins.

The drug methotrexate, which treats cancer (and some inflammatory conditions), acts by interfering with folate metabolism and thus depriving rapidly dividing cancer cells of the folate they need to multiply. Methotrexate resembles folate in structure (see Figure 14-3) and competes with folate for the enzyme that converts folate to its active form. The adverse effects of using methotrexate therefore include symptoms of folate deficiency. These adverse effects can be reduced by using a preactivated form of folate (called *leucovorin*), which is often prescribed along with methotrexate to ensure that the body's rapidly dividing cells (skin cells, cells of the digestive tract, and red blood cells) receive adequate folate.

FIGURE 14-3 Folate and Methotrexate

By competing for the enzyme that activates folate, methotrexate prevents cancer cells from obtaining the folate they need to multiply. In the process, normal cells are also deprived of the folate they require.

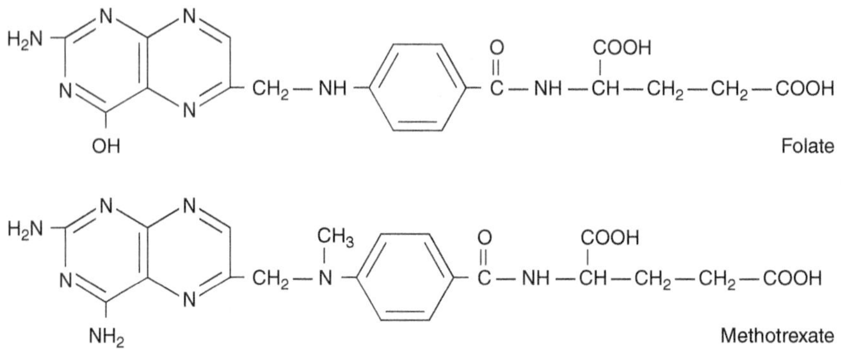

Isoniazid is an antibacterial agent that is used to treat and prevent tuberculosis. The drug inhibits the conversion of vitamin B_6 to its coenzyme form (pyridoxal phosphate), which is involved with neurotransmitter synthesis. Some patients using isoniazid therapy may develop peripheral neuropathy unless they take supplemental vitamin B_6 during the course of treatment.[11]

Dietary Effects on Drug Metabolism

Some food components alter the activities of enzymes that metabolize drugs or may counteract drug effects in other ways. Compounds in grapefruit juice (or whole grapefruit) have been found to inhibit or inactivate enzymes that metabolize a number of different drugs. As a result of the reduced enzyme action, blood concentrations of the drugs increase, leading to stronger physiological effects. The effect of grapefruit juice can last for a substantial period, possibly as long as several days after the juice is consumed[12]; thus, the interaction cannot be avoided by separating grapefruit juice consumption from drug administration. Table 14-8 provides examples of drugs that interact with grapefruit juice, as well as some drugs that are unaffected.

A number of dietary substances can alter the activity of the anticoagulant drug warfarin (Coumadin). One important interaction is with vitamin K, which is structurally similar to warfarin. Warfarin acts by blocking the enzyme that activates vitamin K, thereby preventing the synthesis of several blood-clotting factors (vitamin K is required for the synthesis of prothrombin and various other blood-clotting proteins). The amount of warfarin prescribed is dependent, in part, on how much vitamin K is in the diet. If vitamin K consumption from foods or supplements changes substantially, it can alter the effect of the drug. Individuals using warfarin are advised to consume similar amounts of vitamin K daily to keep warfarin activity stable. The dietary sources highest in vitamin K are green leafy vegetables.

TABLE 14-8   Examples of Grapefruit Juice-Drug Interactions

DRUG CATEGORY	DRUGS AFFECTED BY GRAPEFRUIT JUICE	DRUGS UNAFFECTED BY GRAPEFRUIT JUICE
Anticoagulants	—	Acenocoumarol
		Warfarin
Antidiabetic drugs	Repaglinide	Glyburide
	Saxagliptin	Metformin
Anti-infective drugs	Erythromycin	Clarithromycin
	Saquinavir	Indinivir
Cardiovascular drugs	Amiodarone	Amlodipine
	Felodipine	Digoxin
	Nicardipine	Diltiazem
Central nervous system drugs	Buspirone	Haloperidol
	Carbamazepine	Lorazepam
	Diazepam	Risperidone
Cholesterol-lowering drugs	Atorvastatin	Fluvastatin
	Lovastatin	Pravastatin
	Simvastatin	Rosuvastatin
Immunosuppressants	Cyclosporine	Prednisone
	Tacrolimus	

diuretics: drugs that promote urine production.

Several popular herbs contain natural compounds that affect blood coagulation or warfarin metabolism and therefore should be avoided during warfarin treatment. These herbs include St. John's wort, garlic, ginseng, ginkgo, dong quai, and others.[13]

Drug Effects on Nutrient Excretion

Drugs that increase urine production may reduce nutrient reabsorption in the kidneys, resulting in greater urinary losses of the nutrients. For example, some **diuretics** can increase losses of calcium, potassium, magnesium, and thiamin; thus, dietary supplements may be necessary to avoid deficiency. The risk of nutrient depletion is higher if multiple drugs with the same effect are used, if kidney function is impaired, or if the medications are used for long periods. Note that some diuretics can cause certain minerals to be retained, rather than excreted.

Corticosteroids, which are used as anti-inflammatory agents and immunosuppressants, promote sodium and water retention and increase urinary potassium excretion.[14] Long-term use of corticosteroids can have multiple adverse effects, which include muscle wasting, bone loss, weight gain, and hyperglycemia, with eventual development of osteoporosis and diabetes.

Dietary Effects on Drug Excretion

Inadequate excretion of medications can cause toxicity, whereas excessive losses may reduce the amount available for therapeutic effect. Some food components influence drug excretion by altering the amount reabsorbed in the kidneys. For example, the amount of lithium (a mood stabilizer) reabsorbed in the kidneys is similar to the amount of sodium that is reabsorbed. Consequently, both dehydration and sodium depletion, which promote sodium reabsorption, can result in lithium retention. Similarly, a person with a high sodium intake will excrete more sodium in the urine and, therefore, more lithium. Individuals using lithium are advised to maintain a consistent sodium intake from day to day to maintain stable blood concentrations of lithium.

Urine acidity can affect drug excretion due to the effects of pH on a compound's ionic (chemical) form. The medication quinidine, used to treat arrhythmias, is excreted more readily in acidic urine. Foods or drugs that cause urine to become more alkaline may reduce quinidine excretion and raise blood levels of the medication.

Drug-Nutrient Interactions and Toxicity

Interactions between food components and drugs can cause toxicity or exacerbate a drug's side effects. The combination of tyramine, a food component, and monoamine oxidase inhibitors (MAOIs), which treat depression and Parkinson's disease, can be fatal. MAOIs block an enzyme that normally inactivates tyramine, as well as the hormones epinephrine and norepinephrine. When people who take MAOIs consume excessive tyramine, the increased tyramine in the blood can induce a sudden release of stored norepinephrine. This surge in norepinephrine results in severe headaches, rapid heartbeat, and a dangerous rise in blood pressure. For this reason, people taking MAOIs are advised to restrict their intakes of foods rich in tyramine.

Tyramine occurs naturally in foods and is also formed when bacteria degrade food proteins. Thus, the tyramine content of a food usually increases when a food ages or spoils. Individuals at risk of tyramine toxicity are advised to buy mainly fresh foods and consume them promptly. Foods that often contain substantial amounts of tyramine are listed in Table 14-9.

Considering the many ways in which drugs and dietary substances can interact, health professionals should attempt to understand the mechanisms underlying diet-drug interactions, identify them when they occur, and prevent them whenever possible. Box 14-4 offers some practical advice about preventing diet-drug interactions.

| TABLE 14-9 | Examples of Foods with a High Tyramine Content[a] |

- Aged cheeses (cheddar, Gruyère)
- Aged or cured meats (sausage, salami)
- Beer
- Fermented vegetables (sauerkraut, kim chee)
- Fish or shrimp sauce
- Prepared soy foods (miso, tempeh, tofu)
- Soy sauce
- Yeast extracts (Marmite, Vegemite)

[a]The tyramine content of foods depends on storage conditions and processing; thus, the amounts in similar products can vary substantially.

Box 14-4 HOW TO Prevent Diet-Drug Interactions

The Joint Commission, an accreditation agency for health care organizations, has recommended that all patients be educated about potential diet-drug interactions. Nurses can help by informing patients of precautions related to medications and watching for signs of problems that may arise.

To prevent diet-drug interactions, first list the types and amounts of over-the-counter drugs, prescription drugs, and dietary supplements that the patient uses on a regular basis. Look up each of these substances in a drug reference and make a note of:

- The appropriate method of administration (twice daily or at bedtime, for example).
- How the drug should be administered with respect to foods, beverages, and specific nutrients (for example, take on an empty stomach, take with food, do not take with milk, or do not drink alcoholic beverages while using the medication).
- How the drug should be used with respect to other medications.
- The side effects that may influence food intake (nausea and vomiting, diarrhea, constipation, or sedation, for example) or nutrient needs (interference with nutrient absorption or metabolism, for example).

A similar process can be used to review the dietary supplements that a person is taking. A reliable reference may list their appropriate uses, possible side effects, and potential interactions with food and medications.

Patients who take multiple medications may need to time their intakes carefully to avoid drug-drug or diet-drug interactions. The nurse can use information from a patient's food and nutrition history (see Chapter 13) to help the patient coordinate meals and drugs so as to avoid interactions.

Some medications have well-known effects on nutrition status. The nurse should remain alert for signs of problems, especially when:

- Nutrition problems are a frequent result of using the medication.
- A patient requires multiple medications.
- The patient is in a high-risk group; for example, a child, a pregnant or lactating woman, an older adult, or a person who is malnourished, abuses alcohol, or has impaired liver or kidney function.
- The patient needs to use the medication for an extended period.

Check with the pharmacist for additional information about drugs and their potential adverse effects.

Review Notes

- Medications can alter food intake and affect the absorption, metabolism, or excretion of nutrients. Components of foods can similarly affect drug activity.
- Drugs can alter food intake by increasing or decreasing the appetite, altering the sense of taste, causing GI discomfort, or damaging the lining of the GI tract.
- Drugs can affect nutrient absorption by binding to nutrients, altering stomach acidity, or interfering with nutrient transport into intestinal cells. Dietary substances can influence drug absorption by altering the stomach-emptying rate, altering stomach acidity, or directly binding to the drug.
- Drugs and nutrients may interfere with each other's metabolism because they use similar enzymes in the small intestine and liver.
- Diet-drug interactions may lead to nutrient losses in urine and alter the urinary excretion of drugs. Some interactions between food components and drugs may result in toxicity.

1. A successful nutrition intervention would include a long list of:
   a. dietary changes that the patient should consider making.
   b. foods that the patient should avoid.
   c. appetizing meals and foods that the patient can include in the diet.
   d. reasons why the patient should make dietary changes.

2. Indirect calorimetry is performed by:
   a. estimating the patient's metabolic rate using a predictive equation.
   b. measuring the patient's oxygen consumption and carbon dioxide production.
   c. recording and analyzing the patient's food intake over a 24-hour period.
   d. measuring the patient's body heat losses over a 24-hour period.

3. Mechanically altered diets are often prescribed for individuals with:
   a. disorders of the liver, gallbladder, and pancreas.
   b. unusually high kcalorie and protein requirements.
   c. chewing and swallowing difficulties.
   d. malabsorptive disorders.

4. Foods permitted on the clear liquid diet include all of the following *except*:
   a. milk.
   b. fruit ices.
   c. flavored gelatin.
   d. consommé.

5. A low-fiber diet may be recommended:
   a. for patients with dysphagia.
   b. during the acute phases of some intestinal disorders.
   c. for patients who are unable to absorb fat normally.
   d. for patients with heartburn.

6. A health practitioner assisting with a tube feeding is unsure about the length of time an open can of formula can be safely stored. What resource would most likely provide this information?
   a. The manual describing the hospital's HACCP procedures.
   b. A diet manual.
   c. The diet order.
   d. The food label on the formula can.

7. Medications that reduce stomach acidity can impair the absorption of:
   a. fat-soluble vitamins.
   b. thiamin and riboflavin.
   c. sodium and potassium.
   d. vitamin B_{12}, folate, and iron.

8. Compounds in grapefruit juice can:
   a. bind to antibiotics, reducing their absorption.
   b. cause excessive drug excretion.
   c. strengthen the effects of certain drugs.
   d. alter acidity in the stomach, impairing drug absorption.

9. Individuals using the medication warfarin must maintain a consistent daily intake of:
   a. vitamin A.
   b. calcium.
   c. sodium.
   d. vitamin K.

10. People who use MAOIs must limit consumption of:
    a. aged cheeses.
    b. whole milk and yogurt.
    c. dark green leafy vegetables.
    d. grapefruit juice.

Answers: 1. c, 2. b, 3. c, 4. a, 5. b, 6. a, 7. d, 8. c, 9. d, 10. a

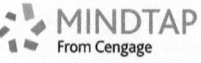 **MINDTAP** From Cengage   For more chapter resources visit **www.cengage.com** to access MindTap, a complete digital course.

Clinical Applications

1. David is a 29-year-old male who is 6 feet 2 inches tall and has a usual body weight of 180 pounds. He was admitted to the hospital following an automobile accident and was treated for minor injuries. Using the method described in Box 14-2 on p. 408, estimate an appropriate energy intake for David using both the Harris–Benedict and Mifflin–St. Jeor equations. Use the stress factor 1.25, with no additional activity factor.

2. A hospital patient with a dysphagia problem has been receiving a soft food diet. You notice that she coughs repeatedly while eating meals and eats only small portions of the foods on her plate. You suspect that the diet is inappropriate and that she may need a more restrictive dysphagia diet, but her medical chart doesn't specify the severity of the dysphagia.
   • To address these problems in your care plan, which health professionals would you need to consult, and what information would you require from each of them?

- The next meal is due within the hour, and you suspect the woman will be intolerant to the foods she is scheduled to receive. You haven't yet heard from the health practitioners you consulted while developing your care plan. What options might you consider in handling this immediate problem?

3. An elderly woman in a residential home has been losing weight since her arrival there. She has been taking several medications to treat both a heart problem and a mild case of bronchitis. You notice that she eats only a few bites at mealtimes and seems uninterested in food. Describe several steps you can take to learn whether the medications are interfering with her food intake in some way.

Notes

1. L. E. Burke and coauthors, Current theoretical bases for nutrition intervention and their uses, in A. M. Coulston, C. J. Boushey, and M. G. Ferruzzi, eds., *Nutrition in the Prevention and Treatment of Disease* (London: Academic Press/Elsevier, 2013), pp. 141–155.
2. L. M. Delahanty and J. M. Heins, Tools and techniques to facilitate nutrition intervention, in A. M. Coulston, C. J. Boushey, and M. G. Ferruzzi, eds., *Nutrition in the Prevention and Treatment of Disease* (London: Academic Press/Elsevier, 2013), pp. 169–189.
3. D. Frankenfield, Energy expenditure in the critically ill patient, in G. A. Cresci, ed., *Nutrition Support for the Critically Ill Patient* (Boca Raton, FL: CRC Press, 2015), pp. 93–110; K. M. Schlein and S. P. Coulter, Best practices for determining resting energy expenditure in critically ill adults, *Nutrition in Clinical Practice* 29 (2014): 44–55; E. Leistra and coauthors, Predictors for achieving protein and energy requirements in undernourished hospital patients, *Clinical Nutrition* 30 (2011): 484–489.
4. Schlein and Coulter, 2014.
5. J. K. Stechmiller, Understanding the role of nutrition and wound healing, *Nutrition in Clinical Practice* 25 (2010): 61–68.
6. Academy of Nutrition and Dietetics, *Nutrition Care Manual* (Chicago: Academy of Nutrition and Dietetics, 2018).
7. L.-N. Chan, Drug-nutrient interactions, in A. C. Ross and coeditors, eds., *Modern Nutrition in Health and Disease* (Baltimore: Lippincott Williams & Wilkins, 2014), pp. 1440–1452; J. I. Boullata and L. M. Hudson, Drug-nutrient interactions: A broad view with implications for practice, *Journal of the Academy of Nutrition and Dietetics* 112 (2012): 506–517.
8. J. M. Gervasio, Drug-induced changes to nutritional status, in J. I. Boullata and V. T. Armenti, eds., *Handbook of Drug-Nutrient Interactions* (New York: Humana Press, 2010), pp. 427–445.
9. E. Lahner and coauthors, Systematic review: Impaired drug absorption related to the co-administration of antisecretory therapy, *Alimentary Pharmacology and Therapeutics* 29 (2009): 1219–1229.
10. D. Fleisher and coauthors, Drug absorption with food, in J. I. Boullata and V. T. Armenti, eds., *Handbook of Drug-Nutrient Interactions* (New York: Humana Press, 2010), pp. 209–241.
11. D. H. Deck and L. G. Winston, Antimycobacterial drugs, in B. G. Katzung, ed., *Basic and Clinical Pharmacology* (New York: McGraw-Hill, 2015), pp. 815–824.
12. Chan, 2014; D. G. Bailey, Grapefruit and other fruit juices interactions with medications, in J. I. Boullata and V. T. Armenti, eds., *Handbook of Drug-Nutrient Interactions* (New York: Humana Press, 2010), pp. 267–302.
13. C. E. Dennehy and C. Tsourounis, Dietary supplements and herbal medications, in B. G. Katzung, ed., *Basic and Clinical Pharmacology* (New York: McGraw-Hill, 2015), pp. 1094–1107; L.-N. Chan, Interaction of natural products with medication and nutrients, in J. I. Boullata and V. T. Armenti, eds., *Handbook of Drug-Nutrient Interactions* (New York: Humana Press, 2010), pp. 341–366.
14. G. W. Cannon, Immunosuppressing drugs including corticosteroids, in L. Goldman and A. I. Schafer, eds., *Goldman-Cecil Medicine* (Philadelphia: Saunders, 2016), pp. 162–169.

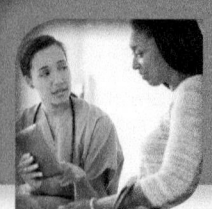

14.5 Nutrition in Practice
Complementary and Alternative Therapies

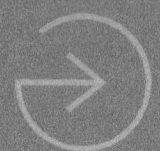

The medical treatments described in the clinical chapters are based on current scientific understanding of human physiology and biochemistry and are generally supported by well-conducted clinical research. This Nutrition in Practice examines therapies that have *not* been scientifically validated and are therefore not currently promoted by conventional health professionals; these therapies fall into a category called *complementary and alternative medicine (CAM)*. When the therapies are used together with conventional medicine, they are called *complementary*; when used in place of conventional medicine, they are called *alternative*.[1] Note that the term "alternative" may be misleading in that it inappropriately implies that unproven methods of treatment are valid alternatives to conventional treatments.

Why should mainstream health professionals learn more about CAM?

Because of significant consumer interest in trying novel treatments, health professionals need to be familiar with CAM therapies so that they can better communicate with patients regarding their medical care and advise them when an alternative approach conflicts with standard therapy or presents a danger to health. To provide medical students with objective information about CAM, many medical schools in the United States now offer elective courses about alternative forms of treatment. Physicians who practice *integrative medicine* may refer patients for complementary therapies while continuing to provide standard treatments.

How popular is CAM in the United States?

About 38 percent of adults in the United States use some form of CAM (excluding the use of prayer).[2] CAM is especially prevalent among persons with chronic pain or debilitating illness; for example, 75 percent of cancer patients reportedly use CAM.[3] Many patients use CAM as an adjunct to conventional medicine—often for symptoms or illnesses that are not sufficiently helped by conventional treatments. CAM therapies remain popular despite the dearth of evidence demonstrating their effectiveness. Reasons for their popularity include consumers' desire to maintain control over their treatments, the perception that CAM treatments are safer and easier to understand than conventional approaches, and the positive interactions consumers have with CAM practitioners.[4]

In response to the enormous popularity of CAM in the United States, in 1998 Congress established the National Center for Complementary and Integrative Health (NCCIH), which is now one of the 27 institutes that make up the National Institutes of Health (NIH). NCCIH's missions are to investigate complementary and alternative therapies by funding well-designed scientific studies and to provide authoritative information for consumers and health professionals. If enough evidence is found to support the use of a complementary or alternative therapy, it will likely become incorporated into mainstream medical practice.[5]

What kinds of practices are considered CAM therapies?

CAM encompasses any and all therapies that are not normally part of conventional medicine. Consequently, the list of CAM approaches includes hundreds of advertised therapies purchased and used by consumers. Unfortunately, terms related to alternative treatments have become marketing buzzwords and are used by unscrupulous sellers of worthless treatments. Table NP14-1 lists examples

TABLE NP14-1 Examples of Complementary and Alternative Medicine

ALTERNATIVE MEDICAL SYSTEMS
- Ayurveda
- Homeopathy
- Naturopathy
- Traditional Chinese medicine

BIOLOGICALLY BASED THERAPIES
- Aromatherapy
- Dietary supplements
- Foods and special diets
- Herbal products
- Hormones

ENERGY THERAPIES
- Bioelectrical therapies (including electric and magnetic fields)
- Biofield therapies (including acupuncture, qi gong, and therapeutic touch)

MANIPULATIVE AND BODY-BASED METHODS
- Chiropractic
- Massage therapy
- Osteopathic manipulation
- Reflexology

MIND-BODY PRACTICES
- Biofeedback
- Faith healing (prayer)
- Meditation
- Mental healing (including hypnotherapy)
- Music, art, and dance therapy

of popular CAM therapies, most of which are defined in Box NP14-1. Many other examples are discussed on the NCCIH website (nccih.nih.gov).

In what ways do alternative medical systems differ from conventional medicine?

Alternative medical systems are based on beliefs that lack the scientific basis of the theories underlying conventional medicine. Virtually all of these alternative systems were developed well over 100 years ago, before our bodies' biochemical and physiological processes were well understood. The alternative treatments may appeal to consumers because the interventions are nontechnical and seem nonthreatening. In general, however, the alternative theories and practices remain rooted in the past and have not been updated to include current knowledge. Examples of alternative medical systems include the following:

- **Naturopathy** proposes that a person's natural "life force" can foster self-healing. This life force is allegedly stimulated by certain health-promoting factors and suppressed by excesses and deficiencies. Naturopaths believe that ill health results from an internal disruption rather than from external disease-causing agents. Naturopathic therapies aim to enhance the natural healing powers of the body and may include special diets or fasting, herbal remedies and other dietary supplements, **acupuncture**, homeopathy, massage, and various other interventions.
- **Homeopathy** is based on the dubious theory that "like cures like." Homeopaths believe that a substance that causes a particular set of symptoms can be used to cure a disease that has similar symptoms. Homeopathic medicines are usually natural substances that are substantially diluted in the belief that dilution

---

Box NP14-1 Glossary

acupuncture (AK-you-PUNK-chur): a therapy that involves inserting thin needles into the skin at specific anatomical points, allegedly to correct disruptions in the flow of energy within the body.

aromatherapy: inhalation of oil extracts from plants to cure illness or enhance health.

ayurveda: a traditional medical system from India that promotes the use of diet, herbs, meditation, massage, and yoga for preventing and treating illness.

bioelectrical or **bioelectromagnetic therapies:** therapies that involve the unconventional use of electric or magnetic fields to cure illness.

biofeedback training: instruction in techniques that allow individuals to gain voluntary control of certain physiological processes, such as skin temperature or brain wave activity, to help reduce stress and anxiety.

biofield therapies: healing methods based on the belief that illnesses can be cured by manipulating energy fields that purportedly surround and penetrate the body. Examples include *acupuncture, qi gong,* and *therapeutic touch.*

chiropractic (KYE-roh-PRAK-tic): a method of treatment based on the unproven theory that spinal manipulation can restore health.

- According to chiropractic theory, a *subluxation* is a misaligned vertebra or other spinal alteration that may cause illness.
- *Adjustment* is the manipulative therapy practiced by chiropractors.

faith healing: the use of prayer or belief in divine intervention to promote healing.

homeopathy (HO-mee-AH-path-ee): a practice based on the theory that "like cures like"; that is, substances believed to cause certain symptoms are prescribed at extremely low concentrations for curing diseases with similar symptoms.

- **homeo** = like
- **pathos** = suffering

hypnotherapy: a technique that uses hypnosis and the power of suggestion to improve health behaviors, relieve pain, and promote healing.

imagery: the use of mental images of things or events to aid relaxation or promote self-healing.

massage therapy: manual manipulation of muscles to reduce tension, increase blood circulation, improve joint mobility, and promote healing of injuries.

meditation: a self-directed technique of calming the mind and relaxing the body.

naturopathy (NAY-chur-AH-path-ee): an approach to health care using practices alleged to enhance the body's natural healing abilities. Treatments may include a variety of alternative therapies including dietary supplements, herbal remedies, exercise, and homeopathy.

osteopathic (OS-tee-oh-PATH-ic) **manipulation:** a CAM technique performed by a doctor of osteopathy (D.O., or osteopath) that includes deep tissue massage and manipulation of the joints, spine, and soft tissues. A D.O. is a fully trained and licensed medical physician, although osteopathic manipulation has not been proved to be an effective treatment.

qi gong (chee-GUNG): a traditional Chinese system that combines movement, meditation, and breathing techniques and allegedly cures illness by enhancing the flow of qi (energy) within the body.

reflexology: a technique that applies pressure or massage on areas of the hands or feet to allegedly cure disease or relieve pain in other areas of the body; sometimes called *zone therapy.*

therapeutic touch: a technique of passing hands over a patient to purportedly identify energy imbalances and transfer healing power from therapist to patient; also called *laying on of hands.*

traditional Chinese medicine (TCM): an approach to health care based on the concept that illness can be cured by enhancing the flow of qi (energy) within a person's body. Treatments may include herbal therapies, physical exercises, meditation, acupuncture, and remedial massage.

---

increases potency, and most remedies are so extremely diluted that the original substance is no longer present. Homeopaths theorize that even though their remedies no longer contain a diluted substance, they still have powerful healing effects because the water structure is somehow altered during the dilution process used to prepare homeopathic medicines. This theory, however, conflicts with scientific understanding of water structure and properties.

- **Traditional Chinese medicine (TCM)** includes a large number of folk practices that originated in China. TCM is based on the theory that the body has pathways (called *meridians*) that conduct energy (called *qi*; pronounced "chee"). The interrupted flow of qi is believed to cause illness. TCM practices allegedly improve the flow of qi and include acupuncture, **qi gong**, herbal remedies, dietary practices, and massage. Ironically, the Western approach to managing illness is now the primary system of health care used in China.[6]

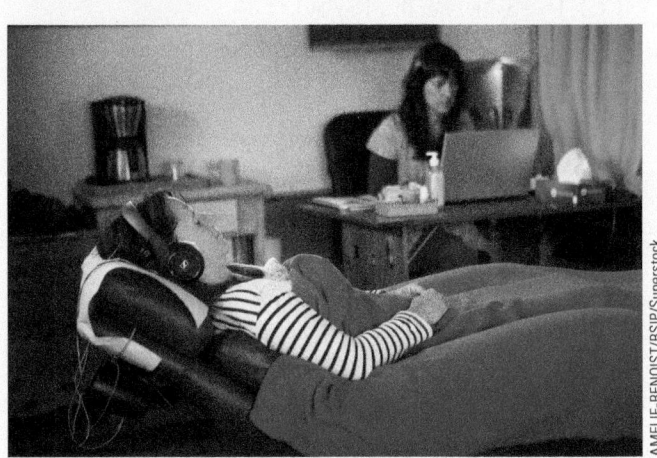

Photo NP14-1 Biofeedback Training: A Stress Reduction and Relaxation Technique

AMELIE-BENOIST/BSIP/Superstock

What is the theory underlying mind-body practices?

Mind-body practices attempt to improve a person's sense of psychological or spiritual well-being despite the presence of illness. The treatments are also used in the hope of reducing stress, dealing with pain, or lowering blood pressure. Some of these therapies have been incorporated into mainstream medicine for stress reduction or relaxation. For example, **biofeedback training**, in which individuals learn to monitor skin temperature, muscle tension, or brain wave activity while practicing relaxation techniques, is frequently taught by behavioral medicine specialists to help patients reduce stress or anxiety (see Photo NP14-1). Other techniques to reduce stress and promote relaxation include **meditation**, art and music therapy, and prayer.

The clinical applications of other mind-body practices are far more questionable. One example is guided **imagery**, in which a person tries to reverse the disease process (for example, shrink a tumor) by using mental pictures. Another example is the use of **faith healing** in place of proven conventional treatments to cure disease.

What are some examples of biologically based therapies?

Biological therapies involve the use of natural products, such as dietary supplements, herbal and plant extracts, and special foods. The most common of these treatments is the use of vitamin and mineral supplements (discussed in Nutrition in Practice 9) and herbal products. Table NP14-2 lists examples of popular herbal products

along with their common uses and potential risks associated with their use.

How effective are herbal remedies in the treatment of disease?

Despite the popularity of herbal products in the United States, the benefits of their use are uncertain. Although many medicinal herbs contain naturally occurring compounds that exert physiological effects, few herbal products have been rigorously tested, many make unfounded claims, and some may contain contaminants or produce toxic effects.[7] Only a limited number of clinical studies support the traditional uses,* and the results of studies that suggest little or no benefit are rarely publicized by the supplement industry. The NCCIH is currently funding large, controlled trials of several popular herbal treatments in an effort to obtain reliable efficacy and safety data.

Determining the effectiveness of herbal remedies can be complicated. Herbs contain numerous compounds, and it is often unclear which of these ingredients, if any, might produce the implied beneficial effects. Because the compounds in herbs vary among species and are affected by a plant's growing conditions, different samples of an herb can have different chemical compositions. Even when certain substances in an herb have been shown to be effective, the product purchased by the consumer might not provide the ingredients required for benefit. For example, a consumer group (ConsumerLab.com) that regularly analyzes dietary supplements and herbal products often reports finding lower amounts of herbal ingredients than are listed on product labels.[8] In a university study that evaluated the authenticity of 44 single-herb products, 32 percent of the

---

*For example, some studies suggest that St. John's wort may be effective for treating mild depression, ginger may help to prevent motion sickness, and garlic supplements may improve blood pressure in people with hypertension.

Popular Herbal Products, Their Common Uses, and Adverse Effects

HERB	SCIENTIFIC NAME	COMMON USES	POTENTIAL ADVERSE EFFECTS
Black cohosh	*Cimicifuga racemosa*	Relief of menopausal symptoms	Rare; stomach upset, headache, dizziness, rash, weight gain, liver damage
Chaparral	*Larrea tridentata*	General tonic, treatment of infection, cancer, and arthritis	Liver or kidney damage
Comfrey	*Symphytum officinale*	Wound healing (topical use), anti-inflammatory agent, treatment of sprains, broken bones, and arthritis	Liver damage
Echinacea	*Echinacea augustifolia, E. pallida, E. purpurea*	Prevention and treatment of upper respiratory infections	Rare; allergic reactions, gastrointestinal upset
Feverfew	*Tanacetum parthenium*	Prevention of migraine headache	Mouth and tongue sores, inflammation of oral tissues, stomach upset
Garlic	*Allium sativum*	Reduction of blood clotting, atherosclerosis, blood pressure, and blood cholesterol levels	Breath and body odor, nausea, gastrointestinal upset, hypotension, dizziness, excessive bleeding
Ginger	*Zingiber officinale*	Prevention and treatment of nausea and motion sickness	Rare; stomach upset, heartburn
Ginkgo	*Ginkgo biloba*	Treatment of dementia, memory defects, and circulatory impairment	Rare; gastrointestinal upset, allergic reactions, anxiety, excessive bleeding
Ginseng	*Panax ginseng, P. quinquefolius*	Improved energy, reduction of blood glucose levels	Rare; nervousness, insomnia, hypertension (with high doses)
Kava	*Piper methysticum*	Treatment of anxiety, stress, and insomnia	Rare; liver damage, headache, dizziness, drowsiness, allergic skin reactions
St. John's wort	*Hypericum perforatum*	Treatment of mild to moderate depression	Skin photosensitivity, stomach upset
Saw palmetto	*Serenoa repens*	Reduction of symptoms associated with enlarged prostate	Rare; gastrointestinal upset, nausea, diarrhea, fatigue, headache, decreased libido
Valerian	*Valeriana officinalis*	Sedation, treatment of insomnia	Rare; liver damage
Yohimbe	*Pausinystalia yohimbe*	Treatment of erectile dysfunction	Anxiety, dizziness, headache, nausea, rapid heartbeat, hypertension, increased urinary frequency

products were found to contain a completely different plant species than was listed on the label.[9]

How safe are the herbal products that are available in the marketplace?

Consumers often assume that because plants are "natural," herbal products must be harmless. Many herbal remedies have toxic effects, however.[10] The most common adverse effects of herbs include diarrhea, nausea, and vomiting. The popular herbs chaparral, germander, green tea, kava, and pennyroyal have caused liver damage.[11] The use of yohimbe (promoted for bodybuilding and erectile dysfunction) has been linked to heart arrhythmias, high blood pressure, anxiety, and seizures. Note that such adverse effects are rarely listed on product labels.

Contamination of herbal products is another safety concern. Many products have been found to contain lead and other toxic metals in excessive amounts.[12] Other contaminants frequently found in herbal products include molds, bacteria, and pesticides that have been banned for use on food crops.[13] Adulteration of imported products is a serious concern: chemical analyses have frequently identified synthetic drugs that were not declared on the label.[14] Illnesses or fatalities sometimes result from the intentional or accidental substitution of one plant species for another.[15] Some herbal products have been found to contain unlisted fillers made from rice, soybean, or wheat that may pose a health risk for persons with allergies to these substances.[16]

Unlike drugs, herbal products do not need FDA approval before they are marketed. According to the Dietary Supplement Health and Education Act (DSHEA) of 1994, the companies that produce or distribute dietary (including herbal) supplements are responsible for determining their safety, yet these companies are not required to provide any evidence or conduct safety studies. If a company receives reports of illness or injury related to the use of its products, it is not required to submit this information to the FDA. In addition, the FDA must show that a dietary supplement is unsafe before it can take action to remove the product from the marketplace.

Is there any risk that herbs may interact with medications like other dietary substances do?

Yes. Like drugs, herbs may either intensify or interfere with the effects of other herbs and drugs, or they may raise the risk of toxicity.[17] For example, garlic, ginger, and goldenseal contain compounds that lower blood pressure and they may therefore strengthen the effects of antihypertensive drugs. Garlic, ginkgo, and ginseng may increase the risk of bleeding when used with anticoagulant drugs. St. John's wort has been found to diminish the actions of oral contraceptives, anticoagulants, and other drugs. Information about herb-drug interactions is limited, however, and much of what is known has been obtained from case studies rather than controlled clinical trials. Table NP14-3 provides examples of herb-drug interactions.

Aside from herbal products, have other types of natural substances been found to be effective therapies?

As with herbal products, the efficacy and safety of other types of natural products are uncertain. Note that manufacturers are free to market the products even if studies fail to show measurable health benefits, and the products are not regulated or tested for safety. Natural products that are currently popular include the following:

- *Hormones.* Some hormones or hormone-like products derived from foods are considered "dietary supplements" and can be sold over the counter. One example is melatonin, a hormone made by the pineal gland and alleged to correct sleep disorders and prevent jet lag. Another example is the adrenal hormone dehydroepiandrosterone (DHEA), which is promoted to enhance immunity, increase muscle mass, improve memory, and defend against aging.
- *Glucosamine-chondroitin supplements.* Produced in the body, glucosamine and chondroitin help to

TABLE NP14-3	Examples of Herb-Drug Interactions	
HERB	**DRUGS**	**INTERACTION**
Echinacea	Immunosuppressant drugs	May reduce drug effectiveness
Feverfew	Anticoagulants, antiplatelet drugs, aspirin	May increase risk of bleeding
Garlic, ginger, ginkgo, ginseng	Anticoagulants, antiplatelet drugs	May increase risk of bleeding
Goldenseal	Anticoagulants, antihypertensives	May oppose anticoagulant effects, increasing risk of clot formation (anticoagulants); may strengthen effect of antihypertensives
Licorice	Antiarrhythmics, antihypertensives, diuretics	May cause toxicity (antiarrhythmics), oppose drug effects (antihypertensives), cause excessive potassium losses (diuretics)
St. John's wort	Various	May reduce drug effectiveness
Valerian	Sedatives	May intensify or prolong sedative effects

Sources: C. E. Dennehy and C. Tsourounis, Dietary supplements and herbal medications, in B. G. Katzung, ed., *Basic and Clinical Pharmacology* (New York: McGraw-Hill, 2015), pp. 1094–1107; P. A. Cohen and E. Ernst, Safety of herbal supplements: A guide for cardiologists, *Cardiovascular Therapeutics* 28 (2010): 246–253.

maintain joint cartilage. Early studies suggested that supplements containing glucosamine and chondroitin reduced moderate to severe symptoms of osteoarthritis better than a placebo, prompting some physicians to suggest using these supplements for pain relief.[18] More recent studies have cast doubt on the earlier findings, however, and several trials are still in progress.[19]

Is there any evidence supporting the use of various foods or supplements to cleanse or detoxify the body?

No; these practices are useless for the intended purpose. "Cleansing" practices are promoted based on the incorrect idea that the body's organs and tissues are "clogged" with toxins and undigested foods and that some types of dietary substances can rid the body of these accumulated toxins and wastes.[20] Consumers who have little or no knowledge about physiology perceive this idea as plausible and are vulnerable to deceptive claims. A common scam is the sale of supplements or recipes for liver and gallbladder "flushes," which are said to cleanse the liver, remove gallstones, or improve a wide variety of medical conditions. In many instances, the ingested substances are partially or wholly indigestible and the individual using them passes semisolid materials that resemble gallstones to the untrained eye.[21] Similarly, "colon cleanse" products are combinations of substances such as clay and gelling fibers that cause the users to pass large fecal casts claimed to represent years of accumulated wastes; such wastes are alleged to cause an array of health problems.[22] Note that there is no scientific support for the alleged benefits of products said to "flush" the liver, gallbladder, or colon.

Which alternative practices involve physical manipulation, and how do they work?

Manipulative interventions include physical touch, forceful movement of different parts of the body, and the application of pressure. Some practitioners maintain that special energy fields are manipulated during the physical treatments and that proper energy flow induces healing. Popular practices include the following:

- **Chiropractic** theory proposes that keeping the nervous system free from obstruction allows the body to heal itself, allegedly because the healing process stems from the brain and is conducted via the spinal cord and nerves to all parts of the body. Chiropractors claim to diagnose illnesses by detecting subluxations in the spine, which are variously described as misaligned vertebrae or pinched nerves that allegedly cause subtle interferences within the nervous system. The main treatment is an *adjustment*, a manual manipulation that is said to correct a subluxation and restore the body's natural healing ability. Although spinal manipulation has mainly been found to be helpful for improving back pain, many chiropractors still assert that chiropractic can cure disease rather than simply relieve symptoms. For example, many chiropractors promote spinal manipulation to treat infectious diseases and prevent cancer, even though the nervous system and spinal alignment do not play roles in the pathology of these conditions.
- **Massage therapy** is the manipulation of muscle and connective tissue to improve muscle function, reduce pain, or promote relaxation. Massage therapists may also apply heat or cold and give advice about exercises that may improve muscle tone and range of motion. Massage is often integrated into conventional physical therapy, although some massage therapists may incorrectly suggest that massage is a valid treatment for a wide range of medical conditions.

What are the alleged effects of "energy" therapies?

Two categories of therapies involve the alleged curative power of "energy":

- **Biofield therapies** are said to influence the energy that surrounds or pervades the human body, and their proponents claim that an energy therapy can strengthen or restore a person's "energy flow" and induce healing. Acupuncture, qi gong, and **therapeutic touch** are among the therapies that subscribe to these theories. Note that CAM adherents often use the term "energy" unscientifically and that there is no objective evidence of this sort of energy flow.
- **Bioelectrical** or **bioelectromagnetic therapies** use electric or magnetic fields to allegedly promote healing; for example, magnets have been marketed with claims that they can improve circulation, reduce inflammation, and speed recovery from injuries.

Acupuncture, a component of traditional Chinese medicine, is the most well known of the therapies involving "energy flow." Acupuncture is based on the theory that disease is caused by the disrupted flow of qi through the body, and the treatment allegedly corrects such disruptions and restores health. The practice involves the shallow insertion of stainless steel needles into the skin at designated points on the body, sometimes accompanied by a low-frequency current to produce greater stimulation (see Photo NP14-2).

Photo NP14-2 Acupuncture

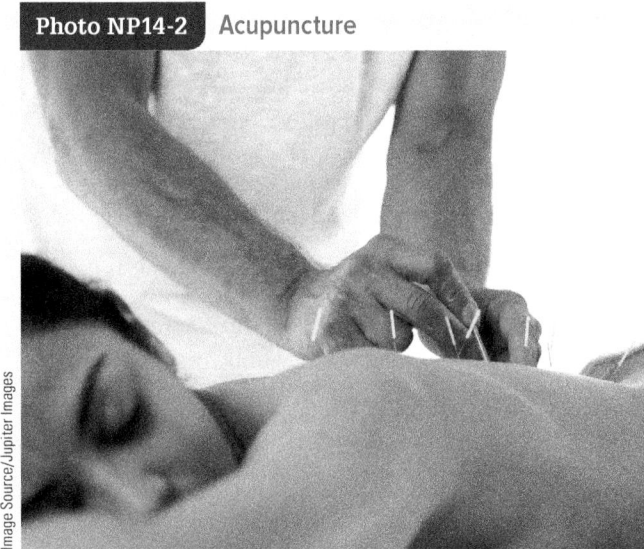

Image Source/Jupiter Images

Acupuncture involves the shallow insertion of stainless steel needles into the skin, sometimes accompanied by a low-frequency current.

Qi gong is another therapy originating in China that is said to improve the flow of qi within the body. Qi gong masters allegedly cure disease by releasing energy from their body and passing it to the person being treated. Self-help practices include deep breathing, certain types of physical exercise, and concentration and relaxation techniques.

Therapeutic touch is based on the premise that the "healing force" of a practitioner can be used to cure disease. Practitioners claim to identify and correct energy imbalances by passing their hands above a patient's body and transferring "excess energy" to the patient.

Do conventional health practitioners consider CAM treatments to be safe and effective?

As mentioned earlier, CAM treatments are generally excluded from mainstream medical practice because there is no evidence proving that they are effective for treating the diseases and medical conditions for which they are used. Many consumers think otherwise and seem satisfied that these treatments "work." How is this dichotomy to be explained?

Surveys suggest that consumers perceive their visits to CAM therapists as being far more pleasant than their visits to conventional health practitioners. CAM therapists often spend more time with patients, are more attentive, and use less invasive interventions. Self-help measures are encouraged, so the consumer has more control over the treatment. The therapies appear to be more "natural" and to have fewer side effects. Possible explanations for "cures" include the following:

- A person may seem cured because of misdiagnosis; that is, the condition diagnosed by the CAM practitioner may not have actually existed.
- The condition may have been self-limiting, or it may have gone into temporary remission after the treatment.
- Undue credit may be inappropriately assigned to the CAM therapy when the improvement was actually due to a previous or concurrent conventional treatment.
- The placebo effect may have had an influence on the course of disease.

The central question remains: Do the CAM therapies merely make people *feel* better, or do they really *get* better? This question can be answered only by well-controlled research studies.

Are any potential dangers associated with the use of CAM?

One of the attractions of alternative therapies is the assumption that they are safe. Recall, however, the concerns associated with the use of herbal products, which include the potential toxicity of herbal ingredients, product contamination or adulteration, and interactions with conventional medications. Another concern is that use of CAM therapies may delay the use of reliable treatments that have demonstrable benefits.[23] Various reports have described people with treatable medical conditions who suffered permanent disability or death when they were misdiagnosed or improperly treated by CAM practitioners. For example, a rare but well-known risk of stroke is associated with a type of cervical (neck) manipulation performed by chiropractors.[24] Unfortunately, because most CAM therapies are not regulated or monitored, there are no accurate estimates of their adverse effects.

What should health care professionals do if they think their patients are using CAM?

Health practitioners should be aware when their patients are using CAM therapies that may influence the course of a disease and its treatment. Accordingly, it is important to inquire about the use of CAM therapies in a respectful, nonjudgmental manner and to educate patients about the hazards of postponing or stopping conventional treatment. Patients should also be told about potential interactions between conventional treatments and CAM therapies. Some patients may want to learn about differences between evidence-based medical practices and untested CAM theories and may be interested in the integrative medicine options available.

All alternative therapies have one characteristic in common: their effectiveness is, for the most part, unproven. Because patients often choose CAM therapies because of positive interactions with alternative practitioners, health care professionals should realize that empathizing with patients may go a long way toward winning their trust and improving their compliance with therapy. Furthermore, health practitioners should stay informed about unconventional practices by obtaining reliable, objective resources so that they can knowledgeably discuss these options with patients.

Notes

1. S. Rosenzweig, Complementary and alternative medicine, in R. S. Porter and J. L. Kaplan, eds., *Merck Manual of Diagnosis and Therapy* (Whitehouse Station, NJ: Merck Sharp and Dohme Corp., 2011), pp. 3411–3420.

2. A. Perlman, Complementary and alternative medicine, in L. Goldman and A. I. Schafer, eds., *Goldman-Cecil Medicine* (Philadelphia: Saunders, 2016), pp. 181–184.

3. Perlman, 2016.

4. C. L. Ventola, Current issues regarding complementary and alternative medicine (CAM) in the United States, *Pharmacy and Therapeutics* 35 (2010): 461–468; A. M. McCaffrey, G. F. Pugh, and B. B. O'Connor, Understanding patient preference for integrative medical care: Results from patient focus groups, *Journal of General Internal Medicine* 22 (2007): 1500–1505.

5. S. E. Straus, Complementary and alternative medicine, in L. Goldman and D. Ausiello, eds., *Cecil Medicine* (Philadelphia: Saunders, 2008), pp. 206–209.

6. T. Liu and coauthors, Prevalence and determinants of using traditional Chinese medicine among middle-aged and older Chinese adults: Results from the China Health and Retirement Longitudinal Study, *Journal of the American Directors Association* 16 (2015): 1002.e1–1002.e5., doi: 10.1016/j.jamda.2015.07.011; D. R. Haley and coauthors, Five myths of the Chinese health care system, *Health Care Manager* 27 (2008): 147–158.

7. C. E. Dennehy and C. Tsourounis, Dietary supplements and herbal medications, in B. G. Katzung, ed., *Basic and Clinical Pharmacology* (New York: McGraw-Hill, 2015), pp. 1094–1107; M. E. Gershwin and coauthors, Public safety and dietary supplementation, *Annals of the New York Academy of Sciences* 1190 (2010): 104–117; U.S. Government Accountability Office (GAO), 2010.

8. ConsumerLab.com, Product Reviews (various reports), www.consumerlab.com, accessed 5 September 2017.

9. S. G. Newmaster and coauthors, DNA barcoding detects contamination and substitution in North American herbal products, *BMC Medicine* 11 (2013): 222–233.

10. V. J. Navarro and coauthors, Liver injury from herbal and dietary supplements, *Hepatology* 65 (2017): 363–373; Dennehy and Tsourounis, 2015; A. I. Geller and coauthors, Emergency department visits for adverse events related to dietary supplements, *New England Journal of Medicine* 373 (2015): 1531–1540.

11. Navarro and coauthors, 2017; G. Mazzanti, A. Di Sotto, and A. Vitalone, Hepatotoxicity of green tea: An update, *Archives of Toxicology* 89 (2015): 1175–1191; C. Bunchorntavakul and K. R. Reddy, Review article: Herbal and dietary supplement hepatotoxicity, *Alimentary Pharmacology and Therapeutics* 37 (2013): 3–17.

12. ConsumerLab.com, 2017; Gershwin and coauthors, 2010; U.S. Government Accountability Office (GAO), 2010.

13. U.S. Government Accountability Office (GAO), 2010; V. H. Tournas, E. Katsoudas, and E. J. Miracco, Moulds, yeasts, and aerobic plate counts in ginseng supplements, *International Journal of Food Microbiology* 108 (2006): 178–181.

14. P. A. Cohen and coauthors, Presence of banned drugs in dietary supplements following FDA recalls, *Journal of the American Medical Association* 312 (2014): 1691–1693; Z. Harel and coauthors, Frequency and characteristics of dietary supplement recalls in the United States, *JAMA Internal Medicine* 173 (2013): 929–930.

15. M. L. Coghlan and coauthors, Deep sequencing of plant and animal DNA contained within traditional Chinese medicines reveals legality issues and health safety concerns, *PLoS Genetics* 8 (2012): e1002657, doi: 10.1371/journal.pgen.1002657.

16. Bunchorntavakul and Reddy, 2013.

17. Dennehy and Tsourounis, 2015; H.-H. Tsai and coauthors, Evaluation of documented drug interactions and contraindications associated with herbs and dietary supplements: A systematic literature review, *International Journal of Clinical Practice* 66 (2012): 1056–1078.

18. O. Bruyere and J. Y. Reginster, Glucosamine and chondroitin sulfate as therapeutic agents for knee and hip osteoarthritis, *Drugs and Aging* 24 (2007): 573–580.

19. J. A. Roman-Blas and coauthors, Combined treatment with chondroitin sulfate and glucosamine sulfate shows no superiority over placebo for reduction of joint pain and functional impairment in patients with knee osteoarthritis, *Arthritis and Rheumatology* 69 (2017): 77–85; S. Yang and coauthors, Effects of glucosamine and chondroitin supplementation on knee osteoarthritis: An analysis with marginal structural models, *Arthritis and Rheumatology* 67 (2015): 714–723; D. S. Jevsevar, Treatment of osteoarthritis of the knee: Evidence-based guideline, *Journal of the American Academy of Orthopaedic Surgeons* 21 (2013): 571–576; S. Wandel and coauthors, Effects of glucosamine, chondroitin, or placebo in patients with osteoarthritis of hip or knee: Network meta-analysis, *British Medical Journal* 341 (2010): c4675, doi: 10.1136/bmj.c4675.

20. S. Gavura, The detox delusion, available at sciencebasedpharmacy.wordpress.com/2013/01/04/the-detox-delusion/, posted 4 January 2013, accessed 20 May 2017.

21. C. W. Sies and J. Brooker, Could these be gallstones? *Lancet* 365 (2005): 1388–1389.

22. S. Barrett, "Detoxification" schemes and scams, available at www.quackwatch.com/01QuackeryRelatedTopics/detox_overview.html, posted June 8, 2011.

23. Rosenzweig, 2011.

24. J. Biller and coauthors, Cervical arterial dissections and association with cervical manipulative therapy: A statement for healthcare professionals from the American Heart Association/American Stroke Association, *Stroke* 45 (2014): 3155–3174.

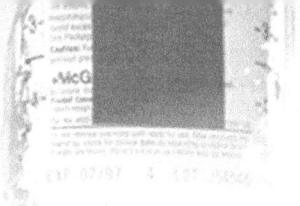

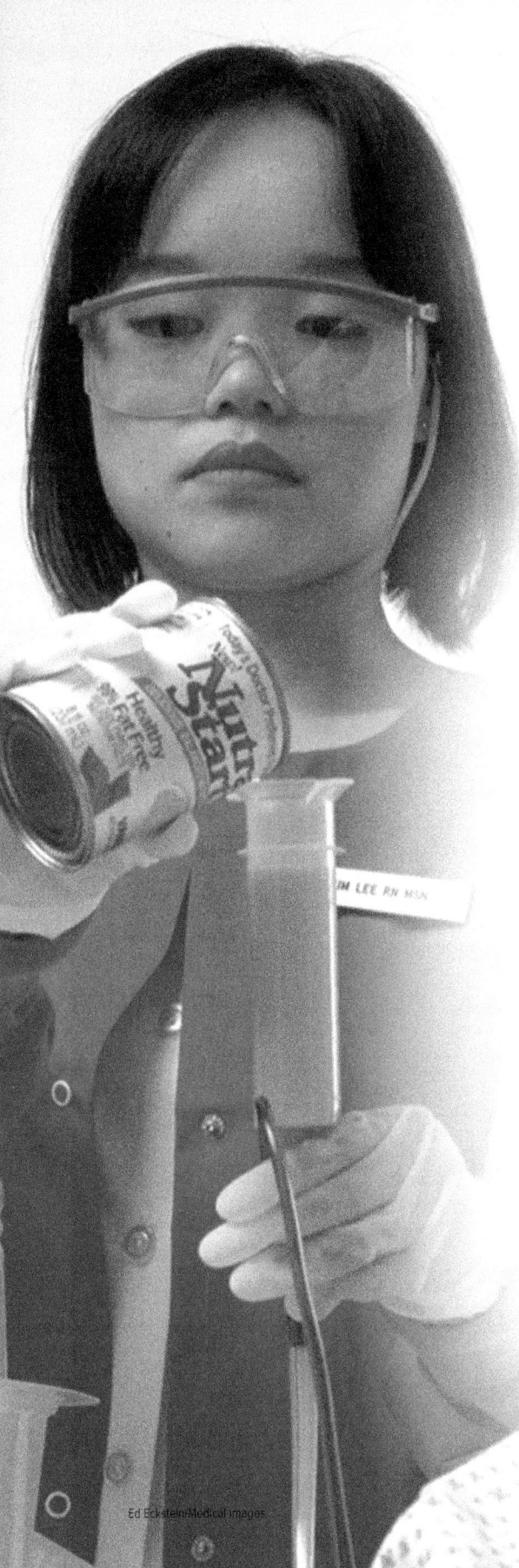

Ed Eckstein/Medical Images

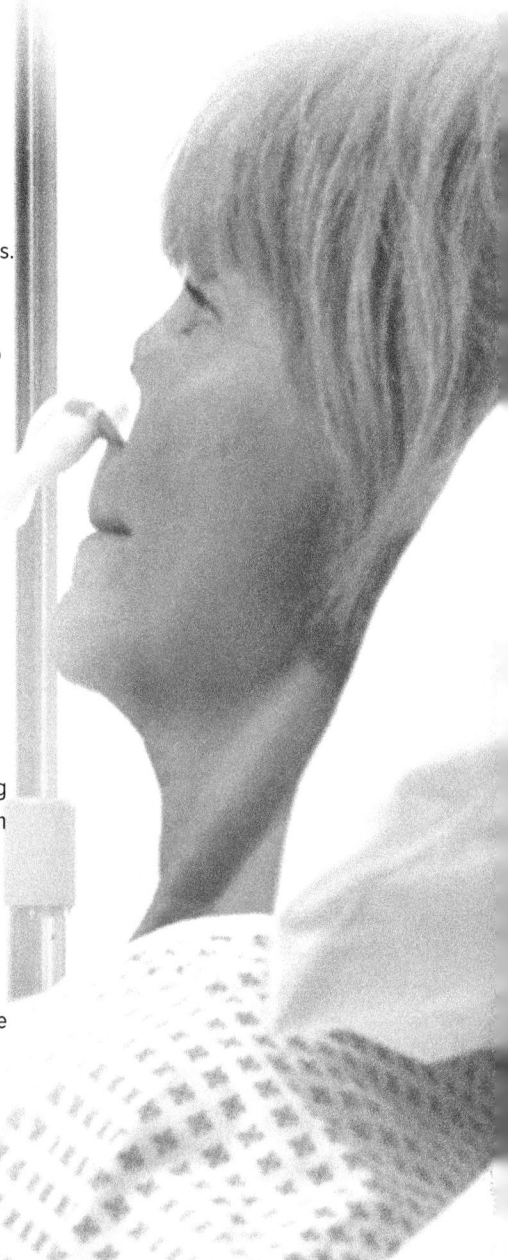

Enteral and Parenteral Nutrition Support

Chapter Sections and Learning Objectives (LOs)

15.1 Enteral Nutrition

LO 15.1 Identify patients who may benefit from enteral nutrition and describe the feeding routes, enteral formulas, and administration considerations for tube feedings.

15.2 Parenteral Nutrition

LO 15.2 Identify patients who may benefit from parenteral nutrition and describe the components of parenteral solutions and administration techniques.

15.3 Nutrition in Practice: Nutritional Genomics

LO 15.3 Give examples of individuals who may be candidates for home nutrition support and discuss the considerations involved in using enteral or parenteral nutrition in the home.

15.4 Nutrition in Practice: Inborn Errors of Metabolism

LO 15.4 Describe the possible metabolic effects of inborn errors of metabolism and discuss the complications and treatments of phenylketonuria and galactosemia.

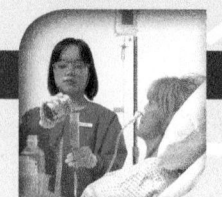

some illnesses may interfere with food consumption, digestion, or absorption to such a degree that oral intakes alone cannot supply the necessary nutrients. In such cases, **specialized nutrition support**—the delivery of nutrients using a feeding tube or intravenous infusions—can meet a patient's nutritional needs. **Enteral nutrition**, the provision of nutrients using the gastrointestinal (GI) tract, most often refers to the use of tube feedings, which deliver nutrient-dense formulas directly to the stomach or small intestine via a thin, flexible tube. **Parenteral nutrition** provides nutrients intravenously to patients who do not have adequate GI function to handle enteral feedings. If the GI tract remains functional, enteral nutrition is preferred over parenteral nutrition because it is associated with fewer infectious complications and is significantly less expensive.[1] Figure 15-1 summarizes the decision-making process for selecting the most appropriate feeding method.

15.1 Enteral Nutrition

If GI function is normal and a poor appetite is the primary nutrition problem, patients may be able to improve their diets by using oral supplements, sometimes known as **oral nutrition support**. If patients are unable to meet their nutrient needs by consuming foods and supplements, tube feedings can be used to deliver the required nutrients.

Oral Supplements

Patients who are weak or debilitated may find it easier to consume oral supplements than to consume meals (see Box 15-1 and Photo 15-1). Furthermore, a patient who

specialized nutrition support: the delivery of nutrients using a feeding tube or intravenous infusions, often referred to simply as *nutrition support*.

enteral (EN-ter-al) **nutrition:** the provision of nutrients using the GI tract; usually refers to the use of tube feedings.

parenteral (par-EN-ter-al) **nutrition:** the intravenous provision of nutrients that bypasses the GI tract.

par = beside
entero = intestine

oral nutrition support: nutrition care that allows a malnourished patient to meet nutritional requirements by mouth; may include oral nutritional supplements, nutrient-dense foods and snacks, or fortified foods.

FIGURE 15-1 Selecting a Feeding Route

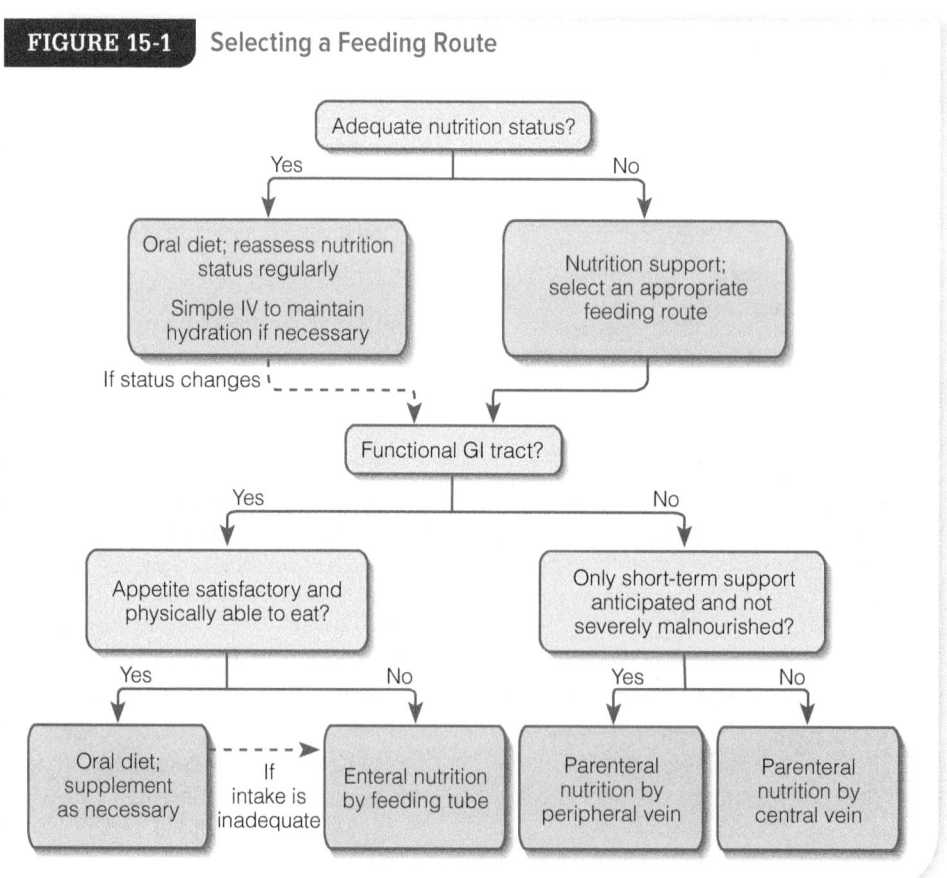

can improve nutrition status with supplements may be able to avoid the stress, complications, and expense associated with tube feedings. Hospitals usually stock a variety of nutrient-dense formulas, milkshakes, fruit drinks, and snack bars to provide to patients at risk of becoming malnourished. Note that similar products are sold in pharmacies and grocery stores for home use; examples of popular liquid supplements include Ensure, Boost, and Carnation Breakfast Essentials. These types of products can add energy and protein to the diets of patients and be a reliable source of nutrients.

When a patient uses an oral supplement, taste becomes an important consideration. Allowing patients to sample different products and select the ones they prefer helps to promote acceptance. Box 15-2 offers additional suggestions for helping patients improve their intakes using oral supplements.

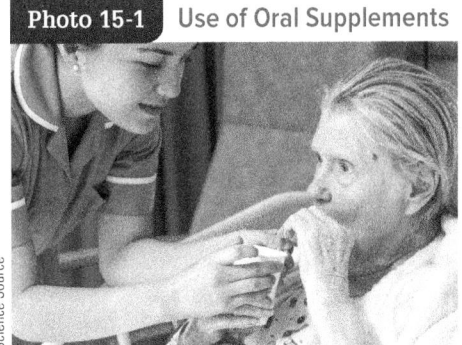

Photo 15-1 Use of Oral Supplements

Patients can drink nutrient-dense formulas when they are unable to consume enough food from a regular diet.

Candidates for Tube Feedings

Tube feedings are typically recommended for patients at risk of developing protein-energy malnutrition who are unable to consume adequate food and/or oral supplements to maintain their health. The following medical conditions or treatments may indicate the need for tube feedings:

- Severe swallowing disorders
- Impaired motility in the upper GI tract
- GI obstructions and **fistulas** that can be bypassed with a feeding tube
- Certain types of intestinal surgeries
- Little or no appetite for extended periods, especially if the patient is malnourished
- Extremely high nutrient requirements
- Mechanical ventilation
- Mental incapacitation due to confusion, neurological disorders, or coma

Contraindications for tube feedings include severe GI bleeding, high-output fistulas, **intractable** vomiting or diarrhea, and severe malabsorption. The procedure may also be contraindicated if the expected need for nutrition support is less than five to seven days in a malnourished patient or less than seven to nine days in an adequately nourished patient.[2]

fistulas (FIST-you-luz): abnormal passages between organs or tissues (or between an internal organ and the body's surface) that permit the passage of fluids or secretions.

intractable: not easily managed or controlled.

| **Box 15-2** | **HOW TO** Help Patients Improve Intakes with Oral Supplements |

Patients in hospitals are often quite ill and have poor appetites. Even when a person enjoys an oral supplement, the taste may become monotonous over time. Health practitioners may be able to motivate patients to improve intakes by trying these suggestions:

- Let the patient sample different products that are appropriate for his or her needs and provide only those that the patient enjoys.
- Serve supplements attractively. For example, a liquid formula offered in a glass on an attractive plate may be more appealing than a formula served from a can with an unfamiliar name.
- Try keeping a liquid supplement in an ice bath so that it is cool and refreshing when the patient drinks it. Check with the patient to make sure the colder temperature is suitable.

- If a patient finds the smell of a formula unappealing, it may help to cover the top of the glass with plastic wrap or a lid, leaving just enough room for a straw.
- For patients with little appetite, offer the drink or snack food in small amounts that are easy to tolerate, and serve it more frequently during the day.
- Provide easy access. Keep the supplement close to the patient's bed where it can be reached with little effort and within sight so that the patient is reminded to consume it.
- If the patient stops enjoying a particular product, suggest an alternative. Maintain an updated list of oral supplements that are available at your institution so that you can advise patients about the options.

Tube Feeding Routes

The feeding route chosen depends on the patient's medical condition, the expected duration of tube feeding, and the potential complications of a particular route. Figure 15-2 and Photo 15-2 illustrate the main feeding routes, and Box 15-3 describes each route.

FIGURE 15-2 Tube Feeding Routes

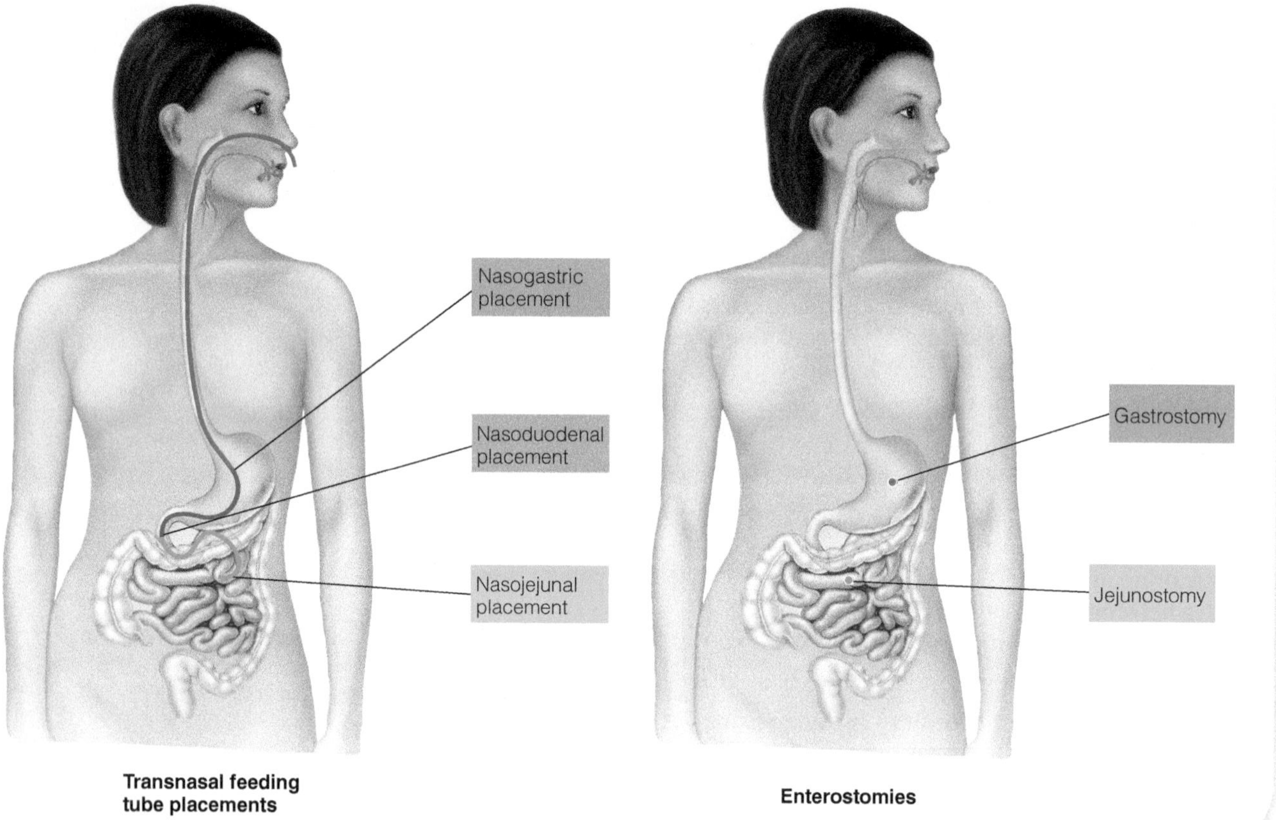

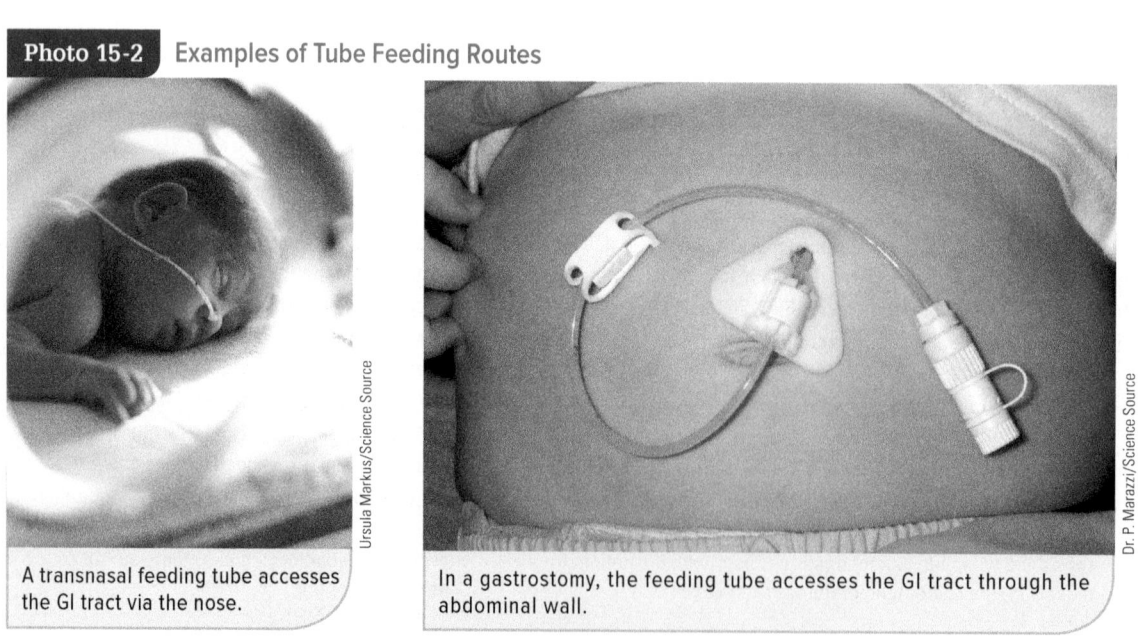

Nasogastric placement

Nasoduodenal placement

Nasojejunal placement

Gastrostomy

Jejunostomy

Transnasal feeding tube placements

Enterostomies

Photo 15-2 Examples of Tube Feeding Routes

A transnasal feeding tube accesses the GI tract via the nose.

Ursula Markus/Science Source

In a gastrostomy, the feeding tube accesses the GI tract through the abdominal wall.

Dr. P. Marazzi/Science Source

For each type of tube placement, the terms are listed in order from the upper to lower organs of the digestive system.

transnasal: a *transnasal feeding tube* is one that is inserted through the nose.

- **nasogastric (NG):** the tube is placed into the stomach via the nose.
- **nasointestinal:** the tube is placed into the GI tract via the nose; refers to *nasoduodenal* and *nasojejunal* feeding routes (also known as *nasoenteric* feeding routes).
- **nasoduodenal (ND):** the tube is placed into the duodenum via the nose.
- **nasojejunal (NJ):** the tube is placed into the jejunum via the nose.

orogastric: the tube is inserted into the stomach through the mouth. This method is often used to feed infants because a nasogastric tube may hinder the infant's breathing.

enterostomy (EN-ter-AH-stoe-mee): an opening into the GI tract through the abdominal wall.

- **gastrostomy** (gah-STRAH-stoe-mee): an opening into the stomach through which a feeding tube can be passed. A nonsurgical technique for creating a gastrostomy under local anesthesia is called *percutaneous endoscopic gastrostomy (PEG)*.
- **jejunostomy** (JEH-ju-NAH-stoe-mee): an opening into the jejunum through which a feeding tube can be passed. A nonsurgical technique for creating a jejunostomy is called *percutaneous endoscopic jejunostomy (PEJ)*. The tube can either be guided into the jejunum via a gastrostomy or passed directly into the jejunum *(direct PEJ)*.

Gastrointestinal Access When a patient is expected to be tube fed for less than four weeks, the feeding tube is generally routed into the GI tract via the nose (**nasogastric** or **nasointestinal** routes). The patient is frequently awake during **transnasal** (through-the-nose) placement of a feeding tube. While the patient is in a slightly upright position with head tilted, the tube is inserted into a nostril and passed into the stomach (nasogastric route), duodenum (**nasoduodenal** route), or jejunum (**nasojejunal** route). If the patient is awake and alert, he or she can swallow water to ease the tube's passage. The final position of the feeding tube tip is verified by X-ray or other means. In infants, **orogastric** placement, in which the feeding tube is passed into the stomach via the mouth, is sometimes preferred over transnasal routes; this placement allows the infant to breathe more normally during feedings.

When a patient will be tube fed for longer than four weeks or if the nasointestinal route is inaccessible due to an obstruction or other medical reason, a direct route to the stomach or intestine may be created by passing the tube through an **enterostomy**, an opening in the abdominal wall that leads to the stomach (**gastrostomy**) or jejunum (**jejunostomy**). An enterostomy can be made by either surgical incision or needle puncture.

Selecting a Feeding Route As mentioned, transnasal access is preferred when the tube feeding duration is expected to be less than four weeks, and enterostomies are more appropriate when tube feedings are planned for longer periods. Gastric feedings (nasogastric and gastrostomy routes) are preferred whenever possible. These feedings are more easily tolerated and less complicated to deliver than intestinal feedings because the stomach controls the rate at which nutrients enter the intestine. Gastric feedings are not possible, however, if patients have gastric obstructions, motility disorders that interfere with stomach emptying, or inadequate stomach volume due to prior gastric surgery. Gastric feedings are also avoided in patients at high risk of **aspiration** (see Box 15-4), a common complication in which substances from the GI tract (GI secretions, food, or refluxed stomach contents) are drawn into the lungs, potentially leading to **aspiration pneumonia** (note that studies have not consistently shown that gastric feedings are associated with a higher pneumonia risk[3]). Table 15-1 summarizes the advantages and disadvantages of the various tube feeding routes.

Feeding Tubes Feeding tubes are made from soft, flexible materials (usually silicone, polyurethane, or polyvinyl chloride) and come in a variety of lengths and diameters

TABLE 15-1 Comparison of Tube-Feeding Routes[a]

INSERTION METHOD OR FEEDING SITE	ADVANTAGES	DISADVANTAGES
TRANSNASAL (for short-term access, or <4 weeks duration)	Tube placement does not require surgery or incisions; tubes can be placed by a nurse or skilled dietitian.	Tubes may cause nasal, throat, or esophageal irritation; tubes are easy to remove by disoriented patients.
• **Nasogastric**	Most common route for patients with normal GI function; tubes are easy to insert and maintain; feedings can be given intermittently and without an infusion pump; least expensive method.	Risk of tube migration to the small intestine; highest risk of aspiration in compromised patients.[b]
• **Nasoduodenal and nasojejunal**	Allow enteral feedings in patients who cannot undergo gastric feedings because of obstructions, fistulas, gastric motility problems, or minimal stomach volume due to prior gastric surgery; allow for earlier tube feedings than gastric placement during critical illness; lower risk of aspiration in compromised patients.[b]	Tubes are more difficult to insert and maintain than nasogastric tubes; risk of tube migration to the stomach; infusion pump required for formula administration.
TUBE ENTEROSTOMIES (for long-term access, or >4 weeks duration)	More comfortable for patients than transnasal insertion; sites are not visible under clothing; allow the lower esophageal sphincter to remain closed, possibly lowering risk of aspiration.[b]	Tube must be placed by a physician or surgeon; tube placement may require general anesthesia; risk of complications or infection from the insertion procedure.
• **Gastrostomy**	Most common method for long-term use in patients with normal stomach emptying; easier insertion procedure than a jejunostomy; feedings can often be given intermittently and without an infusion pump.	For surgically placed tubes, feedings are often withheld for 12 to 24 hours before and 48 to 72 hours after the procedure; moderate risk of aspiration in high-risk patients.[b]
• **Jejunostomy**	Allows enteral feedings in patients who cannot undergo gastric feedings because of obstructions, fistulas, gastric motility problems, or minimal stomach volume due to prior gastric surgery; allows for earlier tube feedings than gastrostomy after tube placement or during critical illness; lowest risk of aspiration.[b]	Most difficult insertion procedure; infusion pump required for formula administration; most costly method.

[a]Relative to other tube-feeding routes. The actual advantages and disadvantages of different insertion procedures depend on the person's medical condition.
[b]The risk of aspiration associated with the different feeding routes is controversial and still under investigation.

(see Photo 15-3). The tube selected largely depends on the patient's age and size, the feeding route, and the formula viscosity. In many cases, the tube selected is the smallest-diameter tube through which the formula will flow without clogging.

The outer diameter of a feeding tube is measured in **French units**, in which each unit equals ⅓ millimeter; thus, a "12 French" feeding tube has a 4-millimeter diameter (12 × ⅓ mm = 4 mm). The inner diameter depends on the thickness of the tubing material. Double-lumen tubes are also available; these allow a single tube to be used for both intestinal feedings and **gastric decompression**, a procedure in which the stomach contents of patients with motility disorders or obstructions are removed by suction.

Enteral Formulas

Most enteral formulas can supply all of an individual's nutrient requirements when consumed in sufficient volume, a necessity for the patient who is using tube feedings for more than a few days. The formulas can be used alone or provided along with other foods.

French units: units of measure for a feeding tube's outer diameter; 1 French equals ⅓ millimeter.

gastric decompression: the removal of stomach contents (such as GI secretions, air, or blood) in patients with motility problems or obstructions that prevent stomach emptying; the procedure may be used to reduce discomfort, vomiting, or various complications during critical illness or after certain surgeries.

Types of Enteral Formulas More than 100 enteral formulas are currently marketed.[4] Appendix F lists examples of enteral formulas as well as the amounts of protein, carbohydrate, fat, and energy they provide. The main types of formulas include the following:

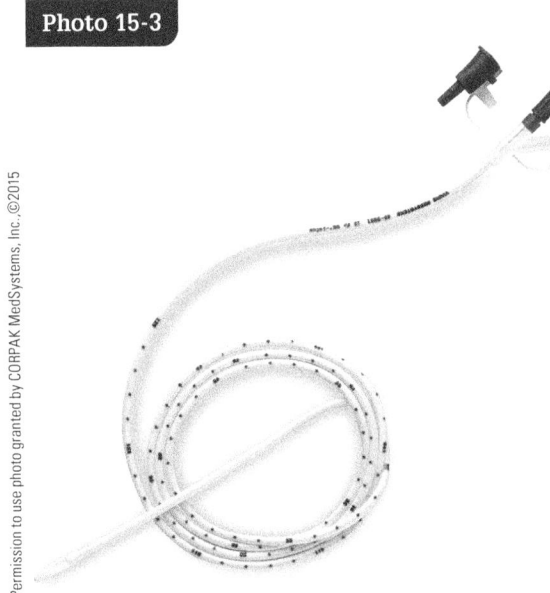

- **Standard formulas**, also called *polymeric formulas*, are provided to individuals who can digest and absorb nutrients without difficulty. They contain intact proteins extracted from milk or soybeans (called **protein isolates**) or a combination of such proteins. The carbohydrate sources include hydrolyzed cornstarch, glucose polymers (such as maltodextrin and corn syrup solids), and sugars. A few formulas, called **blenderized formulas**, are produced from whole foods such as chicken, vegetables, fruit, and oil, along with some added vitamins and minerals.
- **Elemental formulas**, also called *hydrolyzed*, *chemically defined*, or *monomeric formulas*, are prescribed for patients who have compromised digestive or absorptive functions. Elemental formulas contain proteins and carbohydrates that have been partially or fully broken down to fragments that require little (if any) digestion. The formulas are often low in fat and may provide fat from **medium-chain triglycerides (MCT)** to ease digestion and absorption.

The feeding tube shown here has centimeter marks to help with insertion and to check migration. The Y-port at the upper end of the tube allows the administration of water or medications during feedings.

- **Specialized formulas**, also called *disease-specific* or *specialty formulas*, are intended to meet the nutrient needs of patients with particular illnesses. Products have been developed for individuals with liver, kidney, and lung diseases; glucose intolerance; severe wounds; and metabolic stress (later chapters provide details). Specialized formulas are generally expensive and their effectiveness is controversial.[5]
- **Modular formulas**, created from individual macronutrient preparations called *modules*, are sometimes prepared for patients who require specific nutrient combinations. Vitamin and mineral preparations are also included in the formulas so that they can meet all of a person's nutrient needs. In some cases, one or more modules are added to other enteral formulas to adjust their nutrient composition.

Macronutrient Composition The amounts of protein, carbohydrate, and fat in enteral formulas vary substantially. The protein content of most standard formulas ranges from 12 to 20 percent of total kcalories; note that protein needs are high in patients with severe metabolic stress, whereas protein restrictions are necessary for patients with chronic kidney disease. Carbohydrate and fat provide most of the energy in enteral formulas; standard formulas generally provide 30 to 60 percent of kcalories from carbohydrate and 15 to 30 percent of kcalories from fat.

Energy Density The energy density of most enteral formulas ranges from 1.0 to 2.0 kcalories per milliliter of fluid (see Appendix F). The formulas that have lower energy densities are appropriate for patients with average fluid requirements. Formulas with higher energy densities can meet energy and nutrient needs in a smaller volume of fluid and therefore benefit patients who have high nutrient needs or fluid restrictions. Individuals with high fluid needs can be given a formula with low energy density or be supplied with additional water via the feeding tube or intravenously.

Fiber Content Fiber-containing formulas may be helpful for improving fecal bulk and colonic function, treating diarrhea or constipation, and maintaining blood glucose control. Conversely, formulas that contain fiber are avoided in patients with acute intestinal conditions or pancreatitis and before or after some intestinal examinations and surgeries.

standard formulas: enteral formulas that contain mostly intact proteins and polysaccharides; also called *polymeric formulas*.

protein isolates: proteins that have been isolated from foods.

blenderized formulas: enteral formulas that are prepared by using a food blender to mix and puree whole foods.

elemental formulas: enteral formulas that contain proteins and carbohydrates that are partially or fully hydrolyzed; also called *hydrolyzed*, *chemically defined*, or *monomeric formulas*.

medium-chain triglycerides (MCT): triglycerides that contain fatty acids that are 6 to 12 carbons in length. MCT do not require digestion and can be absorbed in the absence of lipase or bile.

specialized formulas: enteral formulas for patients with specific illnesses; also called *disease-specific formulas* or *specialty formulas*.

modular formulas: enteral formulas prepared in the hospital from *modules* that contain single macronutrients; used for people with unique nutrient needs.

osmolality (OZ-moe-LAL-ih-tee): the concentration of osmotically active solutes in a solution, expressed as milliosmoles (mOsm) per kilogram of solvent. Osmotically active solutes affect *osmosis*, the movement of water across semipermeable membranes.

isotonic formula: a formula with an osmolality similar to that of blood serum (about 300 milliosmoles per kilogram).

iso = equal
tono = pressure

hypertonic formula: a formula with an osmolality greater than that of blood serum.

Osmolality The term **osmolality** refers to the concentration of osmotically active solutes in a solution (solutes that affect water's tendency to move across cell membranes). An enteral formula with an osmolality similar to that of blood serum (about 300 milliosmoles per kilogram) is an **isotonic formula**, whereas a **hypertonic formula** has an osmolality greater than that of blood serum.

Most enteral formulas have osmolalities between 300 and 700 milliosmoles per kilogram; generally, elemental formulas and nutrient-dense formulas have higher osmolalities than standard formulas. Most people are able to tolerate both isotonic and hypertonic feedings without difficulty.[6] When medications are infused along with enteral feedings, however, the osmotic load increases substantially and may contribute to the diarrhea experienced by many tube-fed patients.

Formula Selection The formula is selected after careful assessment of the patient's medical problems, fluid and nutrition status, and ability to digest and absorb nutrients; some of the factors considered are shown in Figure 15-3. The formula chosen should

FIGURE 15-3   Selecting a Formula

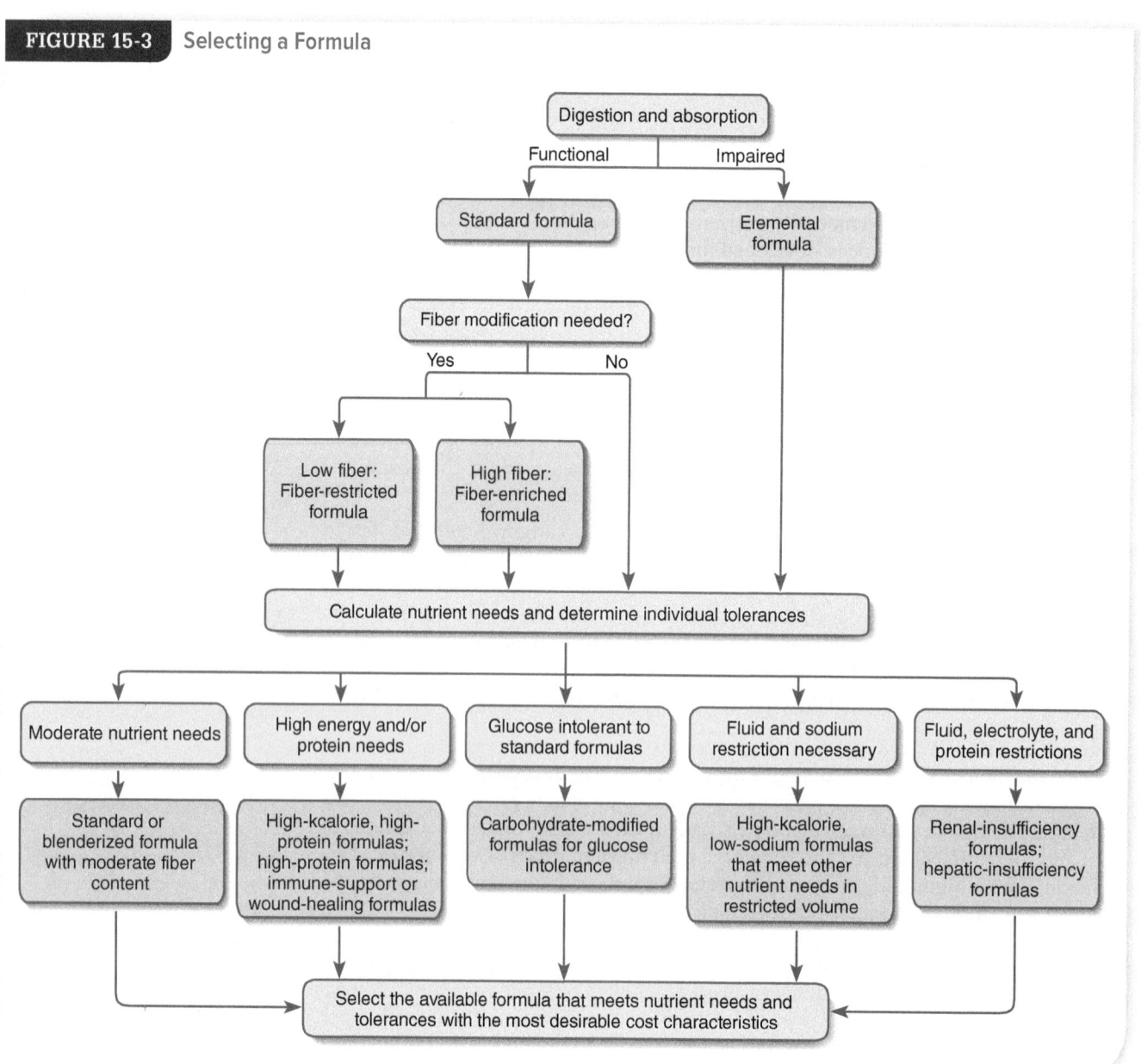

CHAPTER 15   Enteral and Parenteral Nutrition Support

meet the patient's medical and nutrient needs with the lowest risk of complications and the lowest cost. Factors that influence formula selection include:

- *GI function.* Although the vast majority of patients can use standard formulas, a person with a functional but impaired GI tract may require an elemental formula.
- *Nutrient and energy needs.* As with patients consuming regular diets, the tube-fed patient may require adjustments in nutrient and energy intakes. For example, patients with diabetes may need to control carbohydrate intake, critical-care patients may have high protein and energy requirements, and patients with chronic kidney disease may need to limit their intakes of protein and several minerals.
- *Fluid requirements.* High nutrient needs must be met using the volume of formula a patient can tolerate. If fluids need to be restricted, the formula should have adequate nutrient and energy densities to provide the required nutrients in the volume prescribed.
- *The need for fiber modifications.* Formulas that provide fiber may be helpful for managing problems such as diarrhea, constipation, and hyperglycemia. Some patients may need to avoid fiber because they have an increased risk of bowel obstruction or other complications.
- *Individual tolerances (food allergies and sensitivities).* Nearly all formulas are lactose-free and gluten-free and can accommodate the needs of patients with lactose intolerance or gluten sensitivity. For patients with food allergies, ingredient lists should be checked before providing a formula.

Health care facilities stock a limited number of formulas, so formula selection is influenced by availability. The medical staff may initially choose a formula based on the criteria previously mentioned and then reevaluate the decision according to the patient's response to the formula. Note that few research studies have confirmed the benefits of the various specialized formulas, so their additional expense may be difficult to justify.[7]

Administration of Tube Feedings

The methods of tube feeding administration vary somewhat from one health care facility to the next. The procedures presented in the following sections are suggested guidelines.

Preparing for Tube Feedings Before starting a tube feeding, health practitioners can ease fears by fully discussing the procedure with the patient and family members, who may feel anxious about the use of a feeding tube. The discussion should address the reasons why tube feeding is appropriate as well as the benefits and risks of the procedure. Box 15-5 offers suggestions that may help to ease the concerns of patients who may benefit from tube feeding.

Serious complications can develop if a transnasal tube is accidentally inserted into the respiratory tract or if formula or GI secretions are aspirated into the lungs. To minimize the risk of incorrect tube placement, clinicians verify the position of the feeding tube, usually with an X-ray, before a feeding is initiated. After the tube's placement has been confirmed, the nurse often secures the tube to the patient's nose and cheek with tape and monitors the position of the tubing throughout the day. Tube placement can also be monitored by testing the pH of a sample of bodily fluid drawn into the feeding tube, as the pH in the stomach (5 or lower) is lower than the pH in the small intestine or respiratory tract (6 or higher).

To reduce the risk of aspiration, the patient's upper body is elevated to a 30- to 45-degree angle during the feeding and for 30 to 60 minutes after the feeding whenever possible.[8] The addition of blue food coloring to formula was formerly suggested as a means of identifying aspirated formula in lung secretions; however, the practice was discontinued after it was found to be associated with various complications and even deaths.[9]

Box 15-5   **HOW TO** Help Patients Cope with Tube Feedings

Although many patients are initially apprehensive about receiving tube feedings, they may be less resistant once they understand the insertion method, the expected duration of the tube feeding, and the strategic role that nutrition plays in recovery from illness. The pointers that follow can help health practitioners prepare patients for transnasal tube feedings:

• Allow the patient to see and touch the feeding tube. Understanding that the tube is soft and narrow (often less than half the diameter of a pencil) may alleviate anxiety.

• Show the patient how the feeding equipment is attached to the feeding tube, and explain how the feeding will work. For young children, use dolls or stuffed toys to demonstrate tube insertion and feeding procedures.

• Explain that the patient remains fully alert during the procedure and helps to pass the tube by swallowing. A numbing solution sprayed on the back of the throat minimizes discomfort and prevents gagging during the procedure.

• Inform the patient that after the tube has been inserted, most people become accustomed to its presence within a few hours.

In most cases, the patient can continue to swallow foods and beverages with the tube in place.

Tube feedings may cause some patients to feel that they have lost control over an important aspect of their lives. They may also feel self-conscious about how the feeding tube looks or feel awkward when moving around with the equipment. A few measures can help:

• Assure the patient that the tube feeding is temporary, if such assurance is appropriate.

• Involve patients in the decision-making and care process whenever possible. Patients can help to arrange their daily feeding schedules and can perform some of the feeding procedures themselves.

• Show patients how to manipulate the feeding equipment so that they can get out of bed and move around.

Many patients may be relieved to know that they can receive sound nutrition without any effort. After they begin to feel better and start eating again, the enteral formula can be reduced in volume and then discontinued when food intake is adequate.

Safe Handling of Formula   Individuals who are ill or malnourished often have suppressed immune systems, making them vulnerable to infection from foodborne illness. Thus, the personnel involved with preparing or delivering formula must follow the specific protocols at their facility that prevent formula contamination, referred to as **Hazard Analysis and Critical Control Points (HACCP) systems**.

Formulas may be delivered using either an **open feeding system** or a **closed feeding system** (see Photo 15-4). With an open system, the formula needs to be transferred from its original packaging to a feeding container. Examples include formulas that are packaged in cans or bottles, concentrates that need to be diluted, and powders that require reconstitution. In a closed system, the sterile formula is prepackaged in a container that can be connected directly to a feeding tube. Closed systems are less likely to become contaminated, require less nursing time, and can hang for longer periods than open systems. Although closed systems cost more initially, they may be less expensive in the long run because they prevent bacterial contamination and thus avoid the costs of treating infections.

Formula Safety Guidelines   After the formula reaches the nursing station, the nursing staff assumes responsibility for its safe handling. Clinicians should carefully wash hands and put on disposable gloves before handling formulas and feeding containers. The following steps can reduce the risk of formula contamination when using open feeding systems[10]:

• Before opening a can of formula, clean the lid with a disposable alcohol wipe and wash the can opener (if needed) with detergent and hot water. (Check HACCP protocols for details.)

• Hang no more than an 8-hour supply of formula (or a 4-hour supply for newborn infants) when using liquid formula from a can. Formulas prepared from powders or modules should hang for no longer than 4 hours.

• If you do not use an entire can of formula at one feeding, label the can with the date and time it was opened and refrigerate the unused portion promptly. Store mixed formulas in clean, closed containers.

Hazard Analysis and Critical Control Points (HACCP) systems: management systems that address food safety by analyzing biological, chemical, and physical hazards that may arise during the preparation, storage, handling, and administration of food products; commonly referred to as *HASS-ip*.

open feeding system: a formula delivery system that requires the transfer of the formula from its original packaging to a feeding container.

closed feeding system: a formula delivery system in which the sterile formula comes prepackaged in a container that can be attached directly to the feeding tube for administration.

Photo 15-4 Comparison of Open and Closed Feeding Systems

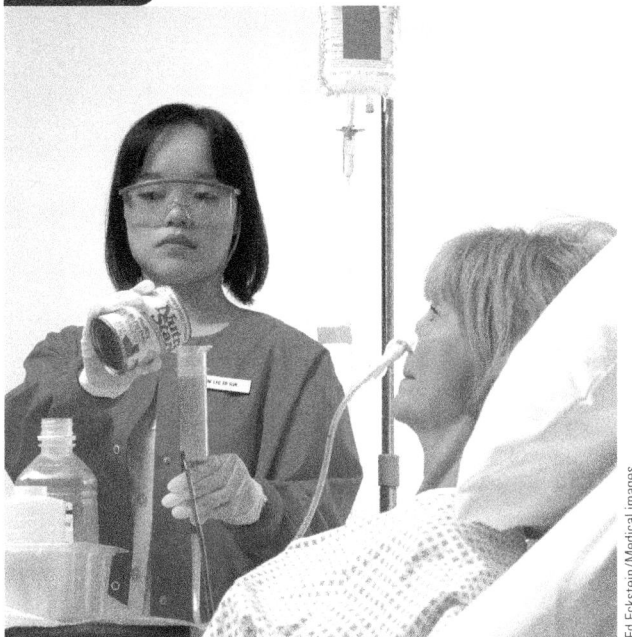

In an open feeding system, the formula is transferred from its original packaging to a feeding container.

Ed Eckstein/Medical Images

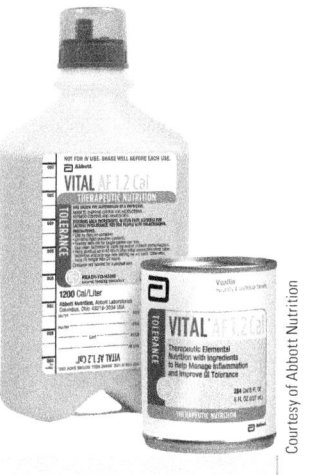

Courtesy of Abbott Nutrition

In a closed feeding system, the sterile formula is prepackaged in a container that can be attached directly to a feeding tube, such as the bottle shown on the left. The formula in the can at right can be used in an open feeding system.

- Discard all opened containers of formula that are not used within 24 to 48 hours. Discard any unlabeled or improperly labeled containers.
- When using more than one can of formula, rinse the feeding bag and tubing, and add the fresh formula to the feeding bag. A new feeding container and tubing (except for the feeding tube itself) is necessary every 24 hours.

For closed systems, the hang time should be no longer than 24 to 48 hours. Contamination is more likely with the longer time periods.

Formula Delivery Methods Nutrient needs may be met by delivering relatively large amounts of formula several times per day (**intermittent feedings** or **bolus feedings**) or smaller amounts continuously (**continuous feedings**). A patient may also start with continuous feedings and eventually transition to intermittent or bolus feedings. Each method has specific uses, advantages, and disadvantages.

Intermittent feedings are similar to the usual pattern of eating and allow the patient freedom of movement between meals. These feedings are best tolerated when they are delivered into the stomach (not the intestine). Generally, a total of about 250 to 400 milliliters of formula is delivered over 30 to 45 minutes using a gravity drip method or an infusion pump (see Photo 15-5). The exact amount is determined by dividing the required volume of formula into several daily feedings, as shown in Box 15-6. Due to the relatively high volume of formula delivered at one time, intermittent feedings may be difficult for some patients to tolerate, and the risk of aspiration may be higher than with continuous feedings.

Rapid delivery of a large volume of formula into the stomach (250 to 500 milliliters over 5 to 15 minutes) is called a *bolus feeding*; this type of feeding may be given every 3 to 4 hours using a syringe. Bolus feedings are convenient for patients and staff because they are rapidly administered, do not require an infusion pump, and allow greater independence for patients. However, bolus feedings can cause abdominal discomfort,

Courtesy of Novartis Medical Nutrition

Photo 15-5 Infusion Pump

The delivery of intermittent and continuous feedings can be controlled with an infusion pump.

intermittent feedings: feedings with delivery rates of about 250 to 400 milliliters of formula over 30 to 45 minutes.

bolus (BOH-lus) **feedings:** feedings with delivery rates of about 250 to 500 milliliters of formula over a 5- to 15-minute period.

continuous feedings: feedings that are delivered slowly and at a constant rate over an 8- to 24-hour period.

HOW TO Plan a Tube Feeding Schedule

After selecting a suitable formula, the clinician must determine the volume of formula that meets the patient's nutritional needs. Consider a patient who needs 2000 kcalories daily and is receiving a standard formula that provides 1.0 kcalorie per milliliter. The total volume of formula required would be 2000 milliliters per day:

$$x \text{ mL} \times 1.0 \text{ kcal/mL} = 2000 \text{ kcal}$$
$$x \text{ mL} = \frac{2000 \text{ kcal}}{1.0 \text{ kcal/mL}} = 2000 \text{ mL}$$

If the patient is to receive intermittent feedings six times a day, he will need about 333 milliliters of formula at each feeding:

$$2000 \text{ mL} \div 6 \text{ feedings} = 333 \text{ mL/feeding}$$

Alternatively, if he is to receive intermittent feedings eight times a day, he will need 250 milliliters (or about one can of ready-to-feed formula) at each feeding:

$$2000 \text{ mL} \div 8 \text{ feedings} = 250 \text{ mL/feeding}$$

If the patient is to receive the formula continuously over 24 hours, he will need about 83 milliliters of formula each hour:

$$2000 \text{ mL} \div 24 \text{ hours} = 83 \text{ mL/hr}$$

Appendix F lists examples of enteral formulas as well as the amounts of energy, protein, carbohydrate, and fat they provide.

---

nausea, and cramping in some patients, and the risk of aspiration is greater than with other methods of feeding. For these reasons, bolus feedings are used only in patients who are not critically ill.

Continuous feedings are delivered slowly and at a constant rate over a period of 8 to 24 hours. The slower delivery rate is easier to tolerate, so continuous feedings are generally recommended for critically ill patients or patients who cannot tolerate intermittent feedings. Continuous feedings are also the preferred delivery method for intestinal feedings. An infusion pump is usually used to ensure accurate and steady flow rates; consequently, the feedings can limit the patient's freedom of movement and are also more costly. Continuous feedings conducted for shorter periods (8 to 16 hours; called **cyclic feedings**) allow greater patient mobility and GI rest, and may be used to help patients transition to intermittent feedings or an oral diet.

Initiating and Advancing Tube Feedings Formula administration techniques vary widely among institutions, so protocols should be reviewed carefully before working with patients. In addition, patient tolerance must be considered when adjusting formula delivery rates. Some general guidelines include the following:

- Formulas are typically provided full-strength. Diluting formulas is not recommended because diluted formulas provide fewer nutrients and are more likely to become contaminated.
- Intermittent feedings may start with 60 to 120 milliliters at the initial feeding and be increased by 60 to 120 milliliters every 8 to 12 hours until the goal volume is reached. Continuous feedings may start at rates of about 10 to 40 milliliters per hour and be increased by 10 to 20 milliliters per hour every 8 to 12 hours until the goal rate is reached.[11]
- Because many patients can tolerate larger amounts than those proposed above, some institutions suggest using faster initiation and advancement rates so that patients can reach feeding goals more quickly.[12]*
- If the patient cannot tolerate an increased rate of delivery, the feeding rate is slowed until the person adapts. Goal rates can usually be achieved over

cyclic feedings: continuous feedings conducted for 8 to 16 hours daily, allowing patient mobility and bowel rest during the remaining hours of the day.

---

*For example, the University of Virginia Health System has suggested the following protocol: Intermittent feedings can begin at 125 milliliters and be advanced by 125 milliliters every 4 hours until the goal rate is reached. Continuous feedings can begin at 50 milliliters per hour and be advanced by 20 milliliters every 4 hours until the goal rate is reached.

24 to 48 hours. In some patients, formula delivery can be started at the goal rate immediately.[13]

- Slower rates of delivery may be better tolerated by critically ill patients, when concentrated formulas are used, or in patients who have undergone an extended period of bowel rest due to surgery, intestinal disease, or the use of parenteral nutrition.

Checking the Gastric Residual Volume When a patient receives a gastric feeding, the nurse may measure the **gastric residual volume**—the volume of formula and GI secretions remaining in the stomach—to ensure that the stomach is emptying properly. In this procedure, the gastric contents are gently withdrawn through the feeding tube using a syringe, usually before bolus or intermittent feedings and every 4 to 8 hours during continuous feedings in critically ill patients. Although the practice is controversial,[14]* some experts recommend that feedings be withheld and an evaluation be conducted if the gastric residual volume exceeds 500 milliliters.[15] If the tendency to accumulate fluids persists, the physician may recommend intestinal feedings or begin drug therapy to stimulate gastric emptying.

Meeting Water Needs Although water needs vary, many patients require about 30 to 40 milliliters of water per kilogram body weight daily.[16] Additional water is required in patients with severe vomiting, diarrhea, fever, excessive sweating, high urine output, high-output ostomies, blood loss, or open wounds. Fluids may be restricted in persons with kidney, liver, or heart disease (see Box 15-7).

The water in formulas meets a substantial portion of water needs: most enteral formulas contain about 70 to 85 percent water, or about 700 to 850 milliliters of water per liter of formula. In addition to the water in formulas, water can be provided by flushing water separately through the feeding tube. Water flushes are also conducted to prevent feeding tubes from clogging; the water used for flushes (20 to 30 milliliters before and after intermittent feedings and about every 4 hours during continuous feedings) should be included when estimating fluid intakes.

Medication Delivery during Tube Feedings

Patients receiving tube feedings sometimes require one or more medications that need to be delivered through feeding tubes. Because medications can interact with the components of enteral formulas in the same ways that they interact with substances in foods, potential diet-drug interactions must be considered. In addition, some medications may need to be exposed to the acidic stomach environment and thus cannot be administered via an intestinal feeding tube. Medications can also cause feeding tubes to clog. Box 15-8 provides some guidelines that may help to prevent complications.

Medications and Continuous Feedings Continuous feedings are ordinarily stopped before and after medication administration to prevent interactions that may clog the feeding tube or interfere with the medication's absorption. Some medications may require a prolonged formula-free interval; for example, feedings need to be stopped for at least one hour before and after administering phenytoin, a medication that controls seizures.[17] In such cases, the formula's delivery rate needs to be increased so that the correct amount of formula can be delivered.

gastric residual volume: the volume of formula and GI secretions remaining in the stomach after a previous feeding.

---

*High GRVs do not correlate well with incidences of aspiration or pneumonia, and withholding tube feedings on the basis of high GRVs can inappropriately reduce the volume of formula delivered.

The pharmacist is your best resource for learning how and when medications can be administered via feeding tubes, especially when you are dealing with an unfamiliar drug. Check with the pharmacist to learn the following:

- Whether a particular medication is known to be incompatible with formulas.
- The proper timing of medication administration to avoid diet-drug interactions.
- Whether a medication can be absorbed without exposure to stomach acid in patients using intestinal feedings.
- Whether a liquid form of a medication is available and, if so, the appropriate dosage of the liquid form.
- If only tablets are available, whether the tablets can be crushed and mixed with water. Enteric-coated and sustained-release medications should not be crushed due to the potential for adverse effects.

In general, it is best to give medications by mouth instead of by tube whenever possible. In some cases, the injectable form of a medication may be the best option. For medications that must be given by feeding tube:

- Do not mix medications with enteral formulas. Do not mix medications together.
- Before administering medications, ensure that the feeding tube is placed correctly, that it is not clogged, and that the gastric residual volume is not excessive.
- Position the patient in a semi-upright position (30 degrees or higher) to prevent aspiration.
- Flush the feeding tube with 15 to 30 milliliters of warm water before and after administering a medication. When more than one medication is administered, flush the feeding tube with water between medications.
- Use liquid forms of medications whenever possible. Dilute viscous or hypertonic liquid medications with at least 30 milliliters of water before administering them through the feeding tube.
- If tablets are used, crush tablets to a fine powder and mix with 30 to 60 milliliters of warm water before administering.

Diarrhea Medications are a major cause of the diarrhea that frequently accompanies tube feedings (see Box 15-9). Diarrhea is especially associated with the administration of sorbitol-containing medications, laxatives, and some types of antibiotics.[18] The high osmolality of many liquid medications can also cause diarrhea, so dilution of hypertonic medications may be helpful.

Tube Feeding Complications

Complications of tube feedings include gastrointestinal problems, such as constipation and diarrhea; mechanical problems related to the tube feeding process; and metabolic problems, such as nutrient deficiencies and changes in the body's biochemistry. Examples of the most common complications, along with some preventive and corrective measures, are summarized in Table 15-2.

Many complications of tube feeding can be prevented by choosing the most appropriate feeding route, formula, and delivery method. Attention to a patient's primary medical condition and medication use is important as well. Health practitioners responsible for the patient's day-to-day care monitor body weight, hydration status, and results of laboratory tests to detect problems before complications develop.

Transition to Table Foods

After the patient's condition improves, the volume of formula can be tapered off as the patient gradually shifts to an oral diet. The steps in the transition depend on the patient's medical condition and the type of feeding the patient is receiving. Some patients may need an evaluation of swallowing function before oral feedings begin. Individuals using continuous feedings are often switched to intermittent feedings initially. Patients receiving elemental formulas may begin the transition by using a standard formula, either orally or via tube feeding. If the patient has not consumed lactose for several weeks, a diet with minimal lactose may be better tolerated. Oral intake should supply about two-thirds of estimated nutrient needs before the tube feeding is discontinued completely.[19] The Case Study in Box 15-10 allows you to consider the many factors involved in tube feedings.

TABLE 15-2 Causes and Management of Tube Feeding Complications

COMPLICATIONS	POSSIBLE CAUSES	PREVENTIVE/CORRECTIVE MEASURES
Aspiration of formula	Inappropriate tube placement	Ensure correct placement of feeding tube.
	Delayed gastric emptying	Elevate head of bed during and after feeding; decrease formula delivery rate if gastric residual volume is excessive; consider using intestinal feedings in high-risk patients.
	Excessive sedation	Minimize use of medications that cause sedation.
Clogged feeding tube	Excessive formula viscosity	Ensure that tube size is appropriate; flush tubing with water before and after giving formula. Remedies to unclog feeding tubes include flushes with warm water or solutions that contain pancreatic enzymes and sodium bicarbonate; consult pharmacist for more options.
	Improper administration of medications	Use oral, liquid, or injectable medications whenever possible; flush tubing with water before and after a medication is given; avoid mixing medications with formula; dilute thick or sticky liquid medications before administering; crush tablets to a fine powder and mix with water (except enteric-coated or sustained-release medications).
Constipation	Inadequate dietary fiber	Use a formula with appropriate fiber content.
	Dehydration	Provide additional fluids.
	Lack of exercise	Encourage walking and other activities, if appropriate.
	Medication side effect	Consult physician about minimizing or replacing medications that cause constipation.
Diarrhea	Medication intolerance	Dilute hypertonic medications before administering; avoid using poorly tolerated medications.
	Infection in GI tract	Consult physician about specific diagnosis and appropriate treatment.
	Formula contamination	Review safety guidelines for formula preparation and delivery.
	Excessively rapid formula administration	Decrease formula delivery rate or use continuous feedings.
	Lactose or gluten intolerance	Use lactose-free or gluten-free formulas and supplements in patients with intolerances.
Fluid and electrolyte imbalances	Diarrhea	See items under *Diarrhea*.
	Inappropriate fluid intake or excessive losses	Monitor daily weights, intake and output, serum electrolyte levels, and clinical signs that indicate dehydration or overhydration; ensure that water intake and formula delivery rates are appropriate.
	Inappropriate insulin, diuretic, or other therapy	Ensure that medication doses are appropriate.
	Inappropriate nutrient intake	Use a formula with appropriate nutrient content; ensure that malnourished patients do not receive excessive nutrients.[a]
Nausea and vomiting, cramps	Delayed stomach emptying	Decrease formula delivery rate or use continuous feedings; halt feeding if gastric residual volume is excessive; evaluate for obstruction; consider use of medications to improve emptying rate.
	Formula intolerance	Ensure that formula is at room temperature, delivery rate is appropriate, and formula odor is not objectionable; consider using a formula that is low in fat, low in fiber, or elemental.
	Medication intolerance	Consult physician about replacing medications that are poorly tolerated.
	Response to disease or disease treatment	Consider use of medications that control nausea and vomiting.

[a]An excessive nutrient intake in malnourished patients may cause *refeeding syndrome*, a disorder that can lead to fluid and electrolyte imbalances; see p. 455 for details.

Sharyn Bartell is a 24-year-old student who suffered multiple fractures when she fell from a cliff while hiking. She also developed gastroparesis (delayed stomach emptying), a possible result of damage to the nerve that controls stomach muscles. As a result of her injuries, she is in traction and is immobile, although the head of her bed can be elevated 45 degrees. Sharyn weighed 140 pounds upon her arrival in the hospital two weeks ago, but she has lost 8 pounds over the course of her hospitalization. The health care team agrees that nasoduodenal tube feeding should be instituted before her nutrition status deteriorates further. A standard formula is selected for the feeding, and Sharyn's nutrient requirements can be met with 2200 milliliters of the formula per day.

1. What steps can be taken to prepare Sharyn for tube feeding? What are some reasons why nasoduodenal placement of the feeding tube might be preferred over nasogastric placement?

2. The physician's orders specify that the feeding should be given continuously over 18 hours. Using the method shown in Box 15-6, develop an appropriate tube feeding schedule.

3. Estimate Sharyn's fluid needs using the recommended intake range of 30 to 40 milliliters of water per kilogram body weight. If Sharyn's formula is 80 percent water, will she receive enough water from the formula? If not, estimate the additional fluid she would need and explain how it could be provided.

4. What steps can the health care team take to prevent aspiration? Describe precautions that should be taken if Sharyn is to receive medications through the feeding tube.

5. After three days of tube feedings, Sharyn develops diarrhea. Check Table 15-2 to determine the possible causes. What measures can be taken to correct the diarrhea?

Review Notes

- Hospitals can provide oral supplements to patients at risk of becoming malnourished; these may include nutrient-dense formulas, milkshakes, fruit drinks, and various snack food items.

- Transnasal feeding routes are preferred for short-term tube feedings, whereas enterostomies are used for longer-term feedings. Gastric feedings are preferred over intestinal feedings but may be avoided in patients at risk of aspiration.

- Patients may receive standard, elemental, specialized, or modular formulas; the formulas can be delivered intermittently, in bolus feedings, or continuously.

- Formulas can meet a substantial portion of the patient's water requirements, and additional water can be provided by flushing water through the feeding tube.

- Medications should be given separately and accompanied by water flushes to prevent tube clogging.

- Complications of tube feedings can be gastrointestinal, mechanical, or metabolic in nature.

15.2 Parenteral Nutrition

The first half of this chapter described how oral supplements and enteral formulas can improve or replace a regular diet. Because these products cannot be used when intestinal function is inadequate, the ability to meet nutrient needs intravenously is a lifesaving option for critically ill persons. The procedure is costly, however, and is associated with a number of potentially dangerous complications. As previous sections suggested, enteral nutrition support is preferred over parenteral nutrition if the GI tract is functional.

Candidates for Parenteral Nutrition

Parenteral nutrition is generally recommended for patients who are unable to digest or absorb nutrients and are either malnourished or likely to become so (review Figure 15-1 on p. 434). In addition, some medical situations require bowel rest for

peripheral veins: the small-diameter veins that carry blood from the limbs.

central veins: the large-diameter veins located close to the heart.

peripheral parenteral nutrition (PPN): the infusion of nutrient solutions into peripheral veins, usually a vein in the arm or back of the hand.

an extended period due to intestinal inflammation or tissue damage. Thus, patients with the following conditions are often considered candidates for parenteral nutrition:

- Intractable vomiting or diarrhea
- Severe GI bleeding
- Intestinal obstructions or fistulas
- Paralytic ileus (intestinal paralysis)
- Short bowel syndrome (a substantial portion of the small intestine has been removed)
- Bone marrow transplants
- Severe malnutrition and intolerance to enteral nutrition

Venous Access

Once the decision to use parenteral nutrition has been made, the access site must be selected. The access sites for intravenous nutrition fall into two main categories: the **peripheral veins** located in the forearm or hand, and the large-diameter **central veins** located near the heart. The peripheral veins may be used to deliver limited amounts of nutrients for short periods, whereas central veins can supply all of a patient's nutrient needs for longer periods.

Peripheral Parenteral Nutrition In **peripheral parenteral nutrition (PPN)**, nutrients are delivered using only the peripheral veins (see Photo 15-6). Peripheral veins can be damaged by overly concentrated solutions, however—**phlebitis** may develop, characterized by redness, swelling, and tenderness at the infusion site. To prevent phlebitis, the **osmolarity** of parenteral solutions used for PPN is generally kept below 900 milliosmoles per liter,[20] a concentration that limits the amounts of energy and protein the solution can provide. Box 15-11 compares the terms *osmolarity* and *osmolality*, both of which can be used to describe the osmolar concentration of a solution.

PPN is used most often in patients who require short-term nutrition support (less than two weeks) and who do not have high nutrient needs or fluid restrictions. The use of PPN is not possible if the peripheral veins are too weak to tolerate the procedure. In many cases, clinicians must rotate venous access sites to avoid damaging veins.

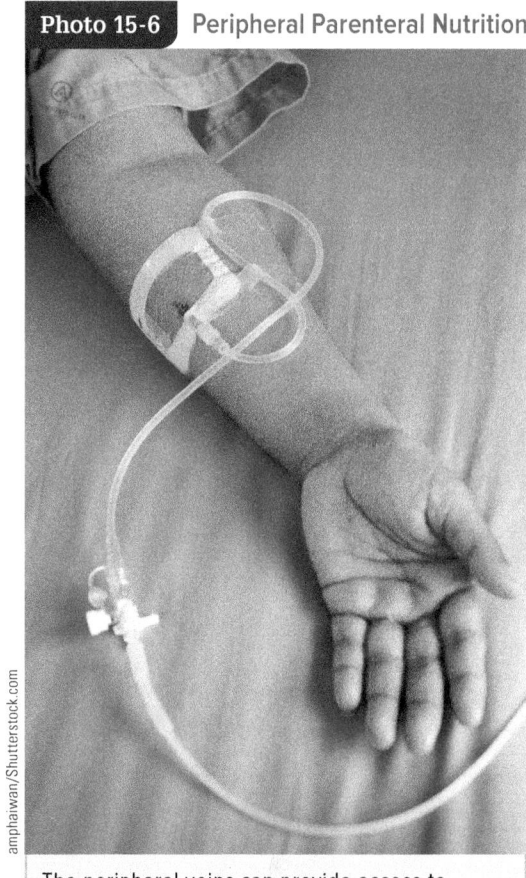

Photo 15-6 Peripheral Parenteral Nutrition

The peripheral veins can provide access to the blood for delivery of parenteral solutions.

phlebitis (fleh-BYE-tiss): inflammation of a vein.

osmolarity: the concentration of osmotically active solutes in a solution, expressed as milliosmoles per liter of solution (mOsm/L). *Osmolality* (mOsm/kg) is an alternative measure used to describe a solution's osmotic properties.

Box 15-11   ***HOW TO* Express the Osmolar Concentration of a Solution**

The movement of water across biological membranes (called osmosis) is influenced by a solution's concentration of milliosmoles, the ions and molecules that contribute to water's osmotic pressure. The terms osmolarity and osmolality are both used to express the concentration of these types of solutes:

- *Osmolarity* refers to the milliosmoles per liter of solution (mOsm/L).
- *Osmolality* refers to the milliosmoles per kilogram of solvent (mOsm/kg).

The main difference between the terms is that osmolarity refers to a volume of solution that includes the solutes of interest (milliosmoles contained in a liter of the solution), whereas osmolality refers to

the solutes separately from the solvent in which they are dissolved (milliosmoles per kilogram of solvent). A second difference is that osmolarity is expressed in terms of the solution's volume, whereas osmolality is expressed in terms of the solvent's weight. Osmolarity and osmolality are roughly equivalent when describing dilute aqueous solutions at room or body temperature; this is because 1 liter of water weighs 1 kilogram, and the solutes contribute little to the volume of the solution.

Osmolarity and osmolality are both used in clinical practice, but they are derived in different ways. Osmolarity is typically calculated using equations that account for the nutrients and electrolytes in biological solutions. Osmolality is usually a measured value obtained using an *osmometer*, a common instrument in hospital laboratories.

FIGURE 15-4 Accessing Central Veins for Total Parenteral Nutrition

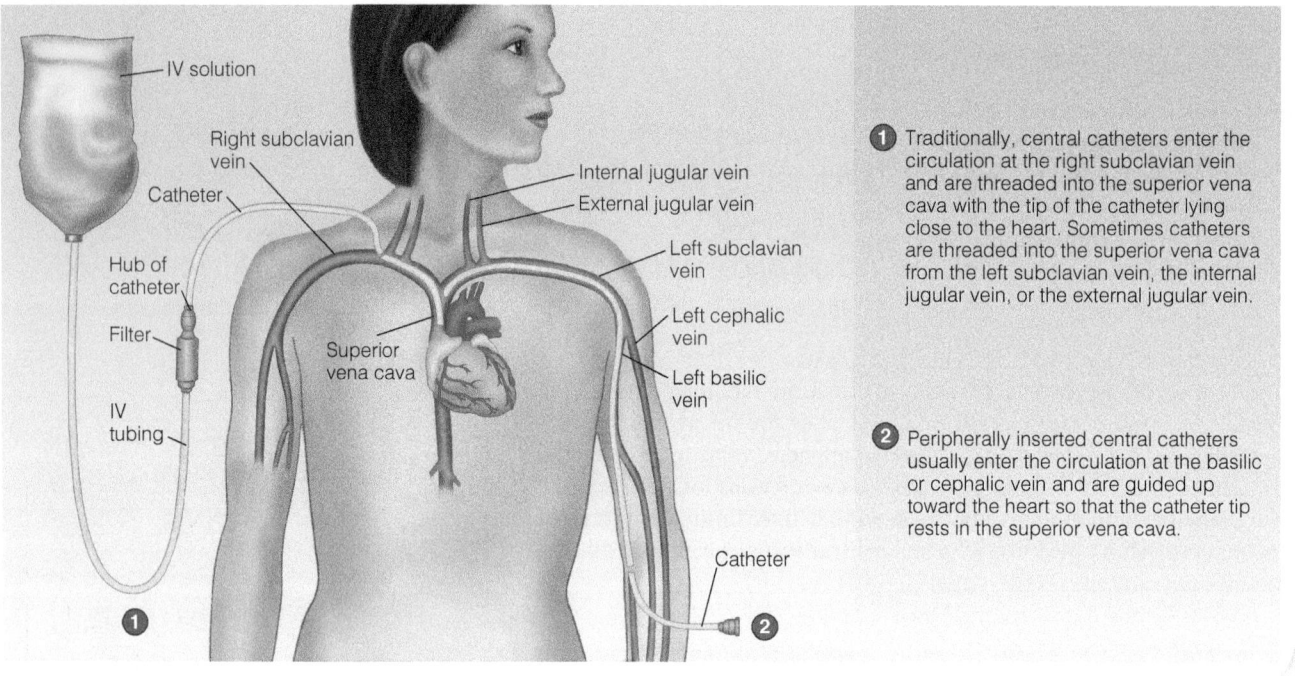

① Traditionally, central catheters enter the circulation at the right subclavian vein and are threaded into the superior vena cava with the tip of the catheter lying close to the heart. Sometimes catheters are threaded into the superior vena cava from the left subclavian vein, the internal jugular vein, or the external jugular vein.

② Peripherally inserted central catheters usually enter the circulation at the basilic or cephalic vein and are guided up toward the heart so that the catheter tip rests in the superior vena cava.

Total Parenteral Nutrition Most patients meet their nutrient needs using the larger, central veins, where blood volume is greater and nutrient concentrations do not need to be limited. This method can reliably provide all of a person's nutrient requirements and is therefore called **total parenteral nutrition (TPN)**. Because the central veins carry a large volume of blood, the parenteral solutions are rapidly diluted; thus, patients with high nutrient needs or fluid restrictions can receive the nutrient-dense solutions they require. TPN is also preferred for patients who require long-term parenteral nutrition.

To access central veins, the tip of a central venous **catheter** can either be placed directly into a large-diameter central vein or threaded into a central vein through a peripheral vein (see Figure 15-4). Peripheral insertion of central catheters is less invasive and lower in cost than direct insertion into central veins.

Parenteral Solutions

The pharmacies located within health care institutions are often responsible for preparing parenteral solutions; this arrangement is convenient because the pharmacist can customize the solutions to meet patients' nutrient needs and because the solutions have a limited shelf life. The physician typically submits an order form such as the one shown in Figure 15-5 to the pharmacy. Prescriptions for parenteral solutions are highly individualized and may need to be recalculated daily until the patient's condition is stable. Because the nutrients are provided intravenously, they must be given in forms that are safe to inject directly into the bloodstream.

Amino Acids Commercial amino acid solutions contain a mix of essential and nonessential amino acids and are available in concentrations between 3 and 20 percent (see Box 15-12); the more concentrated solutions (8.5 percent and higher) are most often

BOX 15-12

To convert nutrient concentrations to grams per milliliter:

- 10% amino acid solution = 10 g amino acids/100 mL

- 10% dextrose solution = 10 g dextrose monohydrate/100 mL

total parenteral nutrition (TPN): the infusion of nutrient solutions into a central vein, also called *central parenteral nutrition (CPN)*.

catheter: a thin tube placed within a narrow lumen (such as a blood vessel) or body cavity; can be used to infuse or withdraw fluids or to keep a passage open.

FIGURE 15-5 Sample Parenteral Nutrition Order Form

Physician Orders
PARENTERAL NUTRITION (PN) – ADULT

Primary Diagnosis: _____ Ht: _____ cm **Dosing Wt:** _____ kg

PN Indication: _____ **Allergies** _____

Instructions: This form must be completed for a new order or continuation of PN and faxed to the Pharmacy by [Insert Time] to receive same day preparation. PN administration begins at [Insert Time]. Contact the Nutrition Support Service at (XXX) XXX-XXXX for additional information.

Administration Route: CVC or PICC *Note: Proper tip placement of the CVC or PICC must be confirmed prior to PN infusion*

Peripheral IV (PIV) (*Final PN Osmolarity ≤ _____ mOsm/L*)

Monitoring: Daily weights, Strict input & output, Bedside glucose monitoring every _____ hours

Na, K, Cl, CO_2, Glucose, BUN, Scr, Mg, PO_4 every _____

T, Bili, Alk Phos, AST, ALT, Albumin, Triglycerides, Calcium every _____

Base Solution: *Parenteral nutrition MUST be administered through a dedicated infusion port and filtered with a 1.2-micron in-line*
Select one *filter at all times. Discard any unused volume after 24 hours.*

PERIPHERAL 2-in-1	**CENTRAL 2-in-1**	**CENTRAL 3-in-1**
Dextrose _____ g	Dextrose _____ g	Dextrose _____ g
Amino Acids (*Brand _____*) _____ g	Amino Acids (*Brand _____*) _____ g	Amino Acids (*Brand _____*) _____ g
For patients with PIV and established glucose tolerance; Provides _____ kcal; Maximum Rate not to exceed _____ mL/hour	*For patients with CVC or PICC and established glucose tolerance; Provides _____ kcal; Maximum Rate not to exceed _____ mL/hour*	Fat Emulsion (*Brand _____*) _____ g *For patients with CVC or PICC and established glucose/fat emulsion tolerance; Provides _____ kcal; Maximum Rate not to exceed _____ mL/hour*

RATE & VOLUME: _____ mL/hour for _____ hours = _____ mL/day
Must specify

Use of additional fat emulsion not required with 3-in-1 base solution

or **CYCLIC INFUSION:** _____ mL/hour for _____ hours, then _____ mL/hour for _____ hours = _____ mL/day

---

Fat Emulsion (*Brand _____*) – via PIV or CVC with 2-in-1 base solutions (*Select caloric density & volume*)

10%	250 mL	Infuse at _____ mL/hour over _____ hours	Frequency _____
20%	500 mL	(*Note: infusions < 4 or > 12 hours not recommended*)	*Discard any unused volume after 12 hours.*

Additives: *(per day)*		**Normal Dosages**	**Additives:** *(per day)*
Sodium Chloride	_____ mEq	*1-2 mEq Sodium/kg/day*	**Regular Insulin** _____ units
as Acetate	_____ mEq	*pH or CO_2 dependent*	*Recommend if hyperglycemic, start*
as Phosphate	_____ mmol of PO_4	*Consider if hyperkalemic*	*with 1 unit for every 10 g of dextrose*
Potassium Chloride	_____ mEq	*1-2 mEq Potassium/kg/day*	
as Acetate	_____ mEq	*pH or CO_2 dependent*	***Pharmacy Use Only:*** Ca/PO_4
as Phosphate	_____ mmol of PO_4	*20-40 mmol/day (1 mmol Phos = 1.5 mEq K)*	**Limit Checked** _____
Calcium **Gluconate**	_____ mEq	*5-15 mEq/day*	*(Note: Some brands of amino acids contain phosphate)*
Magnesium **Sulfate**	_____ mEq	*8-24 mEq/day*	
Adult **Multivitamins**	_____ mL/day	*Contains Vitamin K 150 mcg*	
Adult **Trace Elements**	_____ mL/day	*Zn ___ mg, Cu ___ mg, Mn ___ mg, Cr ___ mcg, Se ___ mcg (with normal hepatic function)*	
H_2 **Antagonist**_____	_____ mg	____ mg/day with normal renal function	
Other:			

Physician's Signature: _____ Pager Number: _____ Date/time: _____

Orders transcribed by: _____ Date/time: _____ Orders verified by: _____ Date/time: _____

SEND COMPLETED ORDERS TO PHARMACY

used for preparing parenteral solutions. Just as in regular foods, the amino acids provide 4 kcalories per gram. Disease-specific products are available for patients with liver disease, kidney disease, and metabolic stress, but they are not often used in practice because of little evidence confirming their benefit.[21]

Photo 15-7

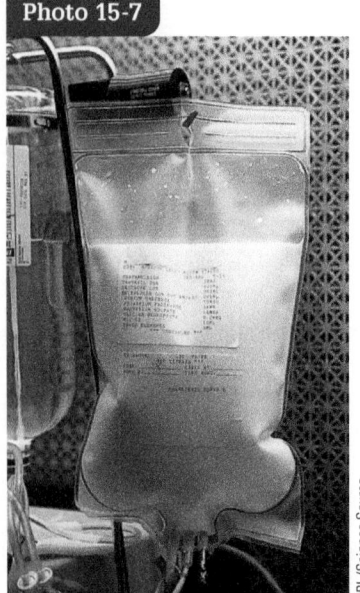

A lipid emulsion gives the parenteral solution a milky white color.

Carbohydrate Glucose is the main source of energy in parenteral solutions. It is provided in the form dextrose monohydrate, in which each glucose molecule is associated with a single water molecule. Dextrose monohydrate provides 3.4 kcalories per gram, slightly less than pure glucose, which provides 4 kcalories per gram. Commercial dextrose solutions are available in concentrations between 2.5 and 70 percent; concentrations higher than 10 percent are usually used only in TPN solutions.[22]

In parenteral solutions, the dextrose concentration is indicated by the letter D followed by its concentration in water (W) or normal saline (NS). For example, D5 or D5W indicates that a solution contains 5 percent dextrose in water. Similarly, D5NS means that a solution contains 5 percent dextrose in normal saline.

Lipids Lipid emulsions supply essential fatty acids and are a significant source of energy (see Photo 15-7). The emulsions available in the United States contain triglycerides from either soybean oil or a mixture of olive oil and soybean oil,* egg phospholipids to serve as emulsifying agents, and glycerol to make the solutions isotonic. Lipid emulsions are available in 10, 20, and 30 percent solutions, providing 1.1, 2.0, and 2.9 or 3.0† kcalories per milliliter, respectively. Therefore, a 500-milliliter container of 10 percent lipid emulsion would provide 550 kcalories; the same volume of a 20 percent lipid emulsion would provide 1000 kcalories (see Box 15-13). In the United States, the 30 percent lipid emulsion can be used for preparing mixed parenteral solutions but is not approved for direct infusion into patients.[23]

Lipid emulsions are often provided daily and may supply about 20 to 30 percent of total kcalories. Including lipids as an energy source reduces the need for energy from dextrose and thereby lowers the risk of hyperglycemia in glucose-intolerant patients. Lipid infusions must be restricted in patients with hypertriglyceridemia, however. There is also some concern that lipid emulsions that supply excessive amounts of linoleic acid (possibly including the amount contained in soybean oil) may suppress some aspects of the immune response.[24]

Fluids and Electrolytes Daily fluid needs range from 30 to 40 milliliters per kilogram body weight in stable adult patients, averaging between about 1500 and 2500 milliliters for most people.[25] The amount of fluid provided is adjusted according to daily fluid losses and the results of hydration assessment.

The electrolytes added to parenteral solutions include sodium, potassium, chloride, calcium, magnesium, and phosphate. The amounts infused differ from Dietary Reference Intake (DRI) values because they are not influenced by absorption, as they are when consumed orally. In the parenteral nutrition order, most electrolyte concentrations are expressed in *milliequivalents (mEq)*, which are units that indicate the number of ionic charges provided by the electrolyte (see Box 15-14). The body's fluids and parenteral solutions are neutral solutions that contain equal numbers of positive and negative charges.

Because electrolyte imbalances can be lethal, electrolyte management by experienced professionals is necessary whenever intravenous therapies are used. Blood tests are administered daily to monitor electrolyte levels until patients have stabilized.

Vitamins and Trace Minerals Commercial multivitamin and trace mineral preparations are added to parenteral solutions to meet micronutrient needs. All of the vitamins are usually included, although a preparation without vitamin K is available for patients using **warfarin** (Coumadin) who may need to restrict this nutrient (see

BOX 15-13

To determine the kcalories in lipid emulsions:

- 500 mL of a 10% lipid emulsion:
  500 mL × 1.1 kcal/mL = 550 kcal

- 500 mL of a 20% lipid emulsion:
  500 mL × 2 kcal/mL = 1000 kcal

BOX 15-14

Milliequivalents are determined by dividing an ion's molecular weight (MW) by its number of charges. For example:

- For calcium, MW = 40, and the ion has 2 positive charges: 40 ÷ 2 = 20. Thus, 1 mEq of Ca^{++} is equivalent to 20 mg of calcium.

- For sodium, MW = 23, and the ion has 1 positive charge: 23 ÷ 1 = 23. Thus, 1 mEq of Na^+ is equivalent to 23 mg of sodium.

- *1 mEq of Ca^{++} has the same number of charges as 1 mEq of Na^+.*

---

*Outside the United States, commercially available lipid emulsions may contain soybean oil, coconut oil (a source of medium-chain triglycerides), fish oil, and/or olive oil.

†Formulations for the 30 percent emulsions vary; check manufacturer's insert for the exact amount of energy.

Chapter 14, p. 419). The trace minerals usually added to parenteral solutions include chromium, copper, manganese, selenium, and zinc. Iron is often excluded because it can destabilize parenteral solutions that contain lipid emulsions and because some patients have allergic reactions to infused iron; therefore, special forms of iron may need to be injected separately.

Medications To avoid the need for a separate infusion site, medications are occasionally added directly to parenteral solutions or infused through a separate port in the catheter (attached via a Y-connector). The administration of a second solution using a separate port is called a **piggyback**. Insulin, for example, is sometimes added by piggyback to improve glucose tolerance. Heparin (an anticoagulant) may be added to prevent clotting at the catheter tip. In practice, few medications are added to parenteral solutions so that potential drug-nutrient interactions can be avoided.

Parenteral Formulations When a parenteral solution contains dextrose, amino acids, and lipids, it is called a **total nutrient admixture (TNA)**, a **3-in-1 solution**, or an **all-in-one solution**. A **2-in-1 solution** excludes lipids, and the lipid emulsion is administered separately, often by piggyback administration. Although the administration of TNA solutions is simpler because only one infusion pump is required, the addition of lipid emulsion to solutions may reduce their stability, potentially resulting in the formation of enlarged lipid droplets and particulates that can obstruct capillaries or have other damaging effects.[26] Thus, lipids are often administered separately when they are not a major energy source and are used only to provide essential fatty acids. Box 15-15 describes a method for calculating the macronutrient and energy content of a parenteral solution.

Osmolarity Recall that the osmolarity of PPN solutions is limited to 900 milliosmoles per liter because peripheral veins are sensitive to high nutrient concentrations, whereas TPN solutions may be as nutrient dense as necessary. The components of a parenteral solution that contribute most to its osmolarity are amino acids, dextrose, and electrolytes: as concentrations of these nutrients increase, the osmolarity of a solution increases. Because lipids contribute little to osmolarity, lipid emulsions can be used to increase the energy provided in PPN solutions.

warfarin: an anticoagulant that works by interfering with vitamin K's blood-clotting function; patients using warfarin need to maintain a consistent vitamin K intake from day to day.

piggyback: the administration of a second solution using a separate port in an intravenous catheter.

total nutrient admixture (TNA): a parenteral solution that contains dextrose, amino acids, and lipids; also called a **3-in-1 solution** or an **all-in-one solution**.

2-in-1 solution: a parenteral solution that contains dextrose and amino acids, but excludes lipids.

Box 15-15 | *HOW TO* Calculate the Macronutrient and Energy Content of a Parenteral Solution

Suppose a patient is receiving 1.25 liters (1250 milliliters) of a parenteral solution that contains 5 percent amino acids and 25 percent dextrose, supplemented with 250 milliliters of a 20 percent lipid emulsion daily. How many grams of protein and carbohydrate is the person receiving, and what is the total energy intake for the day?

Amino acids:

$$5\% \text{ amino acids} = \frac{5 \text{ g amino acids}}{100 \text{ mL}}$$

$$\frac{5 \text{ g amino acids}}{100 \text{ mL}} \times 1250 \text{ mL} = 62.5 \text{ g of amino acids}$$

$$62.5 \text{ g amino acids} \times 4.0 \text{ kcal/g} = 250 \text{ kcal}$$

Carbohydrate:

$$25\% \text{ dextrose} = \frac{25 \text{ g dextrose}}{100 \text{ mL}}$$

$$\frac{25 \text{ g dextrose}}{100 \text{ mL}} \times 1250 \text{ mL} = 312.5 \text{ g of dextrose}$$

$$312.5 \text{ g dextrose} \times 3.4 \text{ kcal/g} = 1063 \text{ kcal (rounded)}$$

Lipids:
Recall that a 20 percent lipid emulsion provides 2.0 kcalories per milliliter. If the patient is given 250 milliliters of the emulsion:

$$250 \text{ mL} \times 2.0 \text{ kcal/mL} = 500 \text{ kcal}$$

Total energy intake:

$$250 \text{ kcal} + 1063 \text{ kcal} + 500 \text{ kcal} = 1813 \text{ kcal}$$

TABLE 15-3 Potential Complications of Parenteral Nutrition

CATHETER-RELATED

- Air embolism
- Blood clotting at catheter tip
- Clogging of catheter
- Dislodgment of catheter
- Improper placement
- Infection, sepsis
- Phlebitis
- Tissue injury

METABOLIC

- Electrolyte imbalances
- Gallbladder disease
- Hyperglycemia, hypoglycemia
- Hypertriglyceridemia
- Liver disease
- Metabolic bone disease
- Nutrient deficiencies
- Refeeding syndrome

BOX 15-16 *Nursing Diagnosis*

The nursing diagnosis *risk for vascular trauma* may apply to patients undergoing intravenous therapy.

---

continuous parenteral nutrition: continuous administration of parenteral solutions over a 24-hour period.

cyclic parenteral nutrition: administration of parenteral solutions over an 8- to 14-hour period each day.

Administering Parenteral Nutrition

Parenteral nutrition is a complex treatment that requires skills from a variety of disciplines. Many hospitals organize nutrition support teams, consisting of physicians, nurses, dietitians, and pharmacists, that specialize in the provision of both enteral and parenteral nutrition. The nurse, who performs direct patient care, plays a central role in administering and monitoring parenteral infusions.

Insertion and Care of Intravenous Catheters Although skilled nurses can place catheters into peripheral veins, only qualified physicians can insert catheters directly into central veins. Patients may be awake for the procedure and given local anesthesia. Unnecessary apprehension can be avoided by explaining the procedure to the patient beforehand.

Catheter-related problems frequently cause complications (see Table 15-3 and Box 15-16). Catheters may be improperly positioned or may dislodge after placement. Air can leak into catheters and escape into the bloodstream, obstructing blood flow. Catheters in peripheral veins may cause phlebitis, necessitating reinsertion at an alternate site. A catheter may become clogged from blood clotting or from a buildup of scar tissue around the catheter tip. Catheters are also a leading cause of infection: contamination may be introduced during insertion or may develop at the placement site.

To reduce the risk of complications, nurses use aseptic techniques when inserting catheters, changing tubing, or changing the dressing that covers the catheter site. An infection may be indicated by redness and swelling around the catheter site or an unexplained fever. A sluggish infusion rate may indicate a clogged catheter or blood clotting problem. Routine inspections of equipment and frequent monitoring of patients' symptoms help to minimize the problems associated with catheter use.

Administration of Parenteral Solutions The method used to initiate and advance parenteral nutrition depends on the patient's condition and the potential for complications. One approach is to start the infusion at a slow rate (with a solution that is either full strength or nutrient dilute) and increase the rate gradually over a two- to three-day period. For example, 40 milliliters per hour can be infused during the first 24 hours of administration (supplying 960 milliliters), and the volume increased to the goal rate on the second day. Another method is to give the full volume of a nutrient-dilute solution on the first day and advance nutrient concentrations as tolerated. Solutions can often be started at full volume and full strength unless there is a risk of fluid overload, hyperglycemia, or other complications.[27]

Parenteral solutions are usually infused continuously over 24 hours (**continuous parenteral nutrition**) in acutely ill patients.[28] Patients who require long-term parenteral nutrition often receive infusions for 8- to 14-hour periods only (**cyclic parenteral nutrition**), allowing more freedom of movement during the day. For this method, patients must be able to start and stop daily infusions without complication and tolerate the nutrient-dense solutions that allow them to meet their nutritional needs in shorter time periods. Some patients may begin with continuous infusions and transition to cyclic infusions as their condition improves.

Regular monitoring can help to prevent complications. The parenteral solution and tubing are checked frequently for signs of contamination. Routine testing of glucose, lipids, and electrolyte levels helps to determine tolerance to solutions. Frequent reassessment of nutrition status may be necessary until a patient has stabilized. Rapid changes in infusion rate are discouraged in patients at risk of developing hyperglycemia or hypoglycemia.

Discontinuing Parenteral Nutrition The patient should have adequate GI function and minimal risk for aspiration before parenteral nutrition can be tapered off and enteral feedings begun. During the transition to an oral diet, a combination of methods is often necessary. Parenteral infusions are usually reduced at the same time that tube feedings or oral feedings are begun, such that the two methods can together supply the needed nutrients. A swallowing evaluation can help determine the types and textures of foods that the patient can tolerate. Once about 60 to 75 percent of nutrient needs can be provided by other means, the parenteral infusions may be discontinued.

Transitioning to oral feedings is sometimes difficult because a person's appetite remains suppressed for several weeks after parenteral nutrition is terminated. Patients receiving continuous parenteral nutrition may have better appetites during the day if they are switched to nocturnal cyclic infusions before beginning oral intakes.

Managing Metabolic Complications

As discussed previously, the catheters used for intravenous infusions may cause a number of serious complications. This section describes some metabolic complications that may result from parenteral nutrition (review Table 15-3) and some suggestions for managing them.[29]

Hyperglycemia Hyperglycemia (blood glucose levels that exceed about 180 mg/dL during parenteral infusions) most often occurs in patients who are glucose intolerant, receiving excessive energy or dextrose, undergoing severe metabolic stress, or receiving corticosteroid medications (see Box 15-17). It can be prevented by providing insulin along with parenteral solutions, avoiding overfeeding or overly rapid infusion rates, and restricting the amount of dextrose in the solution. Dextrose infusions are generally limited to less than 5 milligrams per kilogram of body weight per minute in critically ill adult patients so that the carbohydrate intake does not exceed the maximum glucose oxidation rate.

Hypoglycemia Although uncommon, hypoglycemia sometimes occurs when parenteral nutrition is interrupted or discontinued or if excessive insulin is given. In patients at risk, such as young infants, infusions may be tapered off over several hours before discontinuation. Another option is to infuse a dextrose solution at the same time that parenteral nutrition is interrupted or stopped.

Hypertriglyceridemia Hypertriglyceridemia may result from dextrose overfeeding or overly rapid infusions of lipid emulsion. Patients at risk include those with severe infection, liver disease, kidney failure, or hyperglycemia and those using immunosuppressant or corticosteroid medications. If blood triglyceride levels exceed 400 milligrams per deciliter, lipid infusions should be reduced or stopped.

Refeeding Syndrome Severely malnourished patients who are aggressively fed (parenterally or otherwise) may develop **refeeding syndrome**, characterized by fluid and electrolyte imbalances and hyperglycemia. These effects occur because dextrose infusions raise levels of circulating insulin, which promotes anabolic processes that quickly remove phosphate, potassium, and magnesium from the blood. The altered electrolyte levels can lead to fluid retention and life-threatening changes in various organ systems. Heart failure and respiratory failure are possible consequences.

The patients at highest risk of refeeding syndrome are those who have experienced chronic malnutrition or substantial weight loss. Symptoms include edema, cardiac arrhythmias, muscle weakness, and fatigue. To prevent refeeding syndrome, health practitioners may provide only half of the patient's energy requirement when they initiate nutrition support and gradually advance the dose over several days while monitoring (and possibly correcting) electrolyte levels.

Liver Disease Fatty liver often results from parenteral nutrition, but it is usually corrected after the parenteral infusions are discontinued. Long-term parenteral nutrition, however, can result in progressive liver disease and eventual liver failure (see Box 15-18).

BOX 15-17 *Nursing Diagnosis*

The nursing diagnoses *risk for unstable blood glucose level* and *risk for electrolyte imbalance* often apply to critically ill patients who begin parenteral nutrition.

BOX 15-18 *Nursing Diagnosis*

The nursing diagnosis *risk for impaired liver function* may apply to patients who undergo parenteral nutrition.

refeeding syndrome: a condition that sometimes develops when a severely malnourished person is aggressively fed; characterized by electrolyte and fluid imbalances and hyperglycemia.

Michael Reyes, a 27-year-old man with an inflammatory intestinal disease, underwent a surgical procedure in which a substantial portion of his small intestine was removed. He had received TPN prior to surgery and continued to receive it afterward. After 10 days, tube feedings were begun and initially delivered very small feedings.

1. List some reasons that the nutrition support team initially chose TPN as a means of nutrition support for this patient. How would you explain the need for parenteral nutrition to Michael?

2. Describe the components of a typical TPN solution. Calculate the energy content of 1 liter of a solution that provides 140 grams of dextrose monohydrate, 45 grams of amino acids, and 90 milliliters of 20 percent lipid emulsion. If Michael's energy requirement is 2100 kcalories per day, how many liters of solution will he need each day?

3. Why is it important that Michael begin enteral feedings as soon as possible? Assuming that Michael eventually tolerates tube feedings, in what ways can the health care team help him make the transition from parenteral nutrition to tube feedings? Consider some of the physiological problems that Michael might face when he begins a regular diet.

4. If Michael is unable to meet his nutrient needs orally, he may need to continue tube feedings or TPN at home. As you read through the section on nutrition support at home, consider the factors that would make Michael a good candidate for a home nutrition support program. Consider both the benefits of a proposed program and the problems he could encounter.

To minimize the risk, clinicians avoid giving the patient excess energy, dextrose, or lipids (which promote fat deposition in the liver) and monitor liver enzyme levels weekly. Cyclic infusions may be less problematic than continuous infusions. If appropriate, some oral feedings may be encouraged to reduce the amount of parenteral support necessary.

Gallbladder Disease When parenteral nutrition continues for more than a few weeks, sludge (thickened bile) may build up in the gallbladder and eventually lead to gallstone formation. Prevention is sometimes possible by initiating oral intakes or tube feedings before problems develop. Patients requiring long-term parenteral nutrition may be given medications to stimulate gallbladder contractions or improve bile flow or may have their gallbladders removed surgically.

Metabolic Bone Disease Long-term parenteral nutrition is associated with lower bone mineralization and bone density, which may be related to altered intakes or metabolism of calcium, phosphorus, magnesium, and vitamin D. Interventions may include adjustments in parenteral nutrients, medications, and weight-bearing physical activity.

The Case Study in Box 15-19 checks your understanding of the concepts introduced in this section.

Review Notes

- Peripheral parenteral nutrition is provided to patients who need short-term parenteral support and do not have high nutrient needs or fluid restrictions. Total parenteral nutrition supplies nutrient-dense solutions for long-term parenteral support.

- Parenteral solutions include amino acids, dextrose, electrolytes, vitamins, and minerals. Lipid emulsions may be included in the mixture or may be administered separately.

- Parenteral solutions may be initiated gradually or provided at full volume and full strength in selected patients. Critically ill patients may require continuous infusions, whereas healthier patients and long-term users may prefer cyclic infusions.

- Catheters are frequently the cause of complications, which include improper placement or dislodgment, infection, clotting, embolism, and phlebitis.

- Metabolic complications include hyperglycemia, hypoglycemia, hypertriglyceridemia, refeeding syndrome, and diseases of the liver, gallbladder, and bone.

15.3 Nutrition Support at Home

Some individuals may require nutrition support—either tube feedings or parenteral nutrition—after a medical condition has stabilized and they no longer require hospital services. For such a person, home nutrition support may be a suitable option. Current medical technology allows for the safe administration of nutrition support in the home, and insurance coverage often pays a substantial portion of the costs. Medical equipment companies and home infusion providers can provide the supplies, enteral formulas or parenteral solutions, and services necessary for home nutrition care. Most important, patients using these services can continue to receive specialized nutrition care while leading normal lives.

Candidates for Home Nutrition Support

Individuals referred for home nutrition support usually need long-term nutrition care for chronic medical conditions. Users of home nutrition services (or their families and other caregivers) must be capable of learning the required procedures and managing any complications that arise. The home should be clean and have adequate storage for formulas or solutions and equipment. The costs should be clearly explained to families who cannot get insurance reimbursement. Candidates for home nutrition support include the following:

- For home enteral nutrition, individuals who have disorders that prevent food from reaching the intestines or interfere with nutrient absorption. Examples include people with severe dysphagia, gastroparesis (delayed stomach emptying), gastric outlet or duodenal obstructions, and pancreatic or intestinal conditions that cause malabsorption.[30]
- For home parenteral nutrition, individuals who have disorders that severely impede nutrient absorption or interfere with intestinal motility. Examples include people with short bowel syndrome, radiation enteritis, certain types of motility disorders, and chronic bowel obstruction.[31]

> **BOX 15-20 Nursing Diagnosis**
>
> The nursing diagnosis *readiness for enhanced health management* may be appropriate for individuals who prepare for home nutrition support services.

Planning Home Nutrition Care

As with the nutrition support provided in health care facilities, planning for home nutrition care involves decisions about access sites, formulas, and nutrient delivery methods. Users of home services should be involved in the decision making to ensure long-term compliance and satisfaction (see Box 15-20).

Home Enteral Nutrition Access to the GI tract is possible using either transnasal feeding tubes or enterostomies. Although people can learn to place nasogastric tubes themselves, active individuals often prefer low-profile gastrostomy or jejunostomy tubes, which allow a more normal lifestyle. Jejunostomy tubes are generally less convenient because the frequent feedings required can interfere with daytime activities.

The advantages and disadvantages associated with the different administration methods should be fully discussed with patients. For gastric feedings, bolus infusions are most easily delivered. If intermittent feedings require slow or reliable delivery rates, infusion pumps may be necessary. Portable pumps can free individuals from the need to infuse formula at home and can also be used when traveling (see Photo 15-8).

The formula chosen for home use is influenced by its cost and availability. Insurance reimbursements do not always include the cost of enteral formulas, which are considered food products.

Photo 15-8 Home Nutrition Support

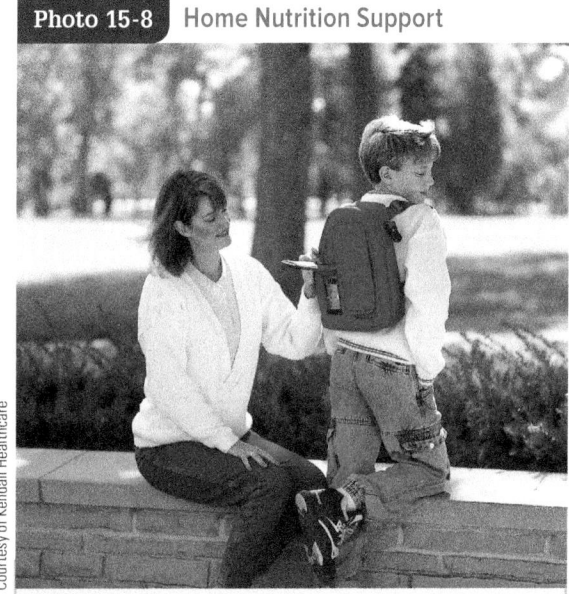

Courtesy of Kendall Healthcare

Portable pumps and convenient carrying cases allow freedom of movement for individuals using home nutrition support.

For this reason, some people choose to prepare simple formulas at home. Blenderizing home-cooked foods is possible, but the resulting mixture needs to be strained to remove particles or clumps that may obstruct the tube. Closed (ready-to-hang) feeding systems are useful for avoiding contamination risk but are not appropriate for intermittent feedings that require smaller amounts of formula.

Home Parenteral Nutrition Although both peripheral parenteral nutrition and total parenteral nutrition (TPN) can be provided at home, long-term therapy requires access to the larger, central veins that are appropriate for TPN. The catheter's exit site is typically placed on the chest wall, where it is accessible to the patient. Most people prefer cyclic infusions over continuous infusions and transition to cyclic infusions before discharge from the hospital. Because infusion pumps are required for home TPN, sufficient battery backup is necessary in case electrical service is interrupted. Portable pumps are useful for individuals who prefer to infuse during the day or have active lifestyles.

Parenteral solutions need to be sterile and aseptically prepared, and individuals who mix their own solutions must be carefully trained. Ready-made parenteral solutions require refrigeration and are stable for limited periods; for example, 3-in-1 solutions may be stable for only one week when refrigerated.

Quality-of-Life Issues

Although home nutrition support can help to improve health and extend life, consumers of these services and their families may struggle with the lifestyle adjustments required. In addition to the high costs of nutrition support, home infusions are often time-consuming and inconvenient. Activities and work schedules must be planned around feedings. Extra planning is necessary and precautions must be taken when a person wants to travel or participate in sports activities. Explaining one's medical needs to friends and acquaintances may be embarrassing.

Among physical difficulties, people receiving nocturnal feedings often cite disturbed sleep as a major problem. Disruptions may be due to multiple nighttime bathroom visits, noisy infusion pumps, or difficulty finding a comfortable sleeping position when "hooked up." People using parenteral support sometimes prefer infusing solutions during the day to improve their sleeping patterns.

Among social issues, the inability to consume meals with family and friends is often a great concern.[32] Many individuals miss the enjoyment, comfort, and socialization they previously experienced from food and mealtimes. Joining friends at restaurants and attending certain types of social events may become a source of stress for individuals who cannot consume food.

People who depend on nutrition support face many challenges that can affect quality of life. Support groups or counseling resources can help patients cope with the demands of treatment. The Oley Foundation (oley.org) is a good source of current information and emotional support for individuals who require home nutrition support.

Review Notes

- Candidates for home enteral nutrition services have disorders that interfere with swallowing ability, nutrient movement through the GI tract, or nutrient absorption. Candidates for home parenteral nutrition have disorders that severely impair nutrient absorption or intestinal motility.
- Patients and caregivers should participate in decisions about access sites, formulas, and nutrient delivery methods. Enteral formulas and parenteral solutions can be purchased or prepared in the home.
- The use of portable pumps may help individuals lead a normal lifestyle. Nevertheless, lifestyle adjustments to nutrition support may be difficult and stressful.

Nutrition Assessment Checklist for People Receiving Enteral Nutrition Support

MEDICAL HISTORY

Check the medical record for medical conditions or treatment plans that may:

- ○ Alter nutrient needs and influence formula selection
- ○ Influence the selection of the feeding route
- ○ Affect the length of time that the tube feeding will be needed

Monitor the medical record for complications or risks that may influence the formula selection or delivery technique, including:

- ○ Aspiration
- ○ Constipation
- ○ Fluid and electrolyte imbalances
- ○ Diarrhea
- ○ Hyperglycemia
- ○ Nausea and vomiting
- ○ Skin irritation

MEDICATIONS

Check medications for those that can cause side effects similar to the complications of tube feeding, such as:

- ○ Nausea and vomiting
- ○ Diarrhea
- ○ Constipation
- ○ GI discomfort

For medications delivered through the feeding tube, check:

- ○ Form of medication and possible alternatives
- ○ Viscosity of liquid medications
- ○ Potential for diet-drug interactions

DIETARY INTAKE

To assess nutritional adequacy, check to see whether:

- ○ The formula is appropriate for the patient's needs
- ○ The formula is administered as prescribed
- ○ Supplemental water is provided to meet needs
- ○ The patient is consuming food in addition to receiving tube feedings

ANTHROPOMETRIC DATA

Measure baseline height and weight, and monitor body weight regularly. If weight is not appropriate:

- ○ Determine whether energy needs have been correctly assessed
- ○ Check to see if the formula is being delivered as prescribed
- ○ Check for signs of dehydration or overhydration

LABORATORY TESTS

Check serum and urine tests for signs of:

- ○ Fluid and electrolyte imbalances
- ○ Hyperglycemia
- ○ Improvement or deterioration of the medical condition

PHYSICAL SIGNS

Look for physical signs of:

- ○ Dehydration or overhydration
- ○ Delayed gastric emptying
- ○ Malnutrition

Nutrition Assessment Checklist for People Receiving Parenteral Nutrition Support

MEDICAL HISTORY

Check the medical record for medical conditions that:

- ○ Prevent the use of enteral nutrition
- ○ Indicate the appropriate infusion route (peripheral versus central)
- ○ Suggest the length of time that parenteral nutrition will be required

Monitor the medical record for complications or risks that may influence the parenteral solution formulation or delivery technique, including:

- ○ Acid–base imbalances
- ○ Fluid and electrolyte imbalances
- ○ Hyperglycemia or hypoglycemia
- ○ Hypertriglyceridemia
- ○ Preexisting liver disease
- ○ Refeeding syndrome

MEDICATIONS

For medications added to the parenteral solution, determine the:

- ○ Medication's compatibility with the parenteral solution
- ○ Length of time that the medication can remain stable in solution

For medications infused separately, determine:

- ○ Length of time that the infusion may need to be stopped
- ○ Necessary adjustments in parenteral infusions to compensate for medication delivery

DIETARY INTAKE

To assess nutritional adequacy, check to see whether:

- ○ Patient's nutrient needs were correctly determined
- ○ Solution is administered as prescribed
- ○ Infusion pump is operating correctly

ANTHROPOMETRIC DATA

Measure baseline height and weight, and monitor daily weights. If weight is not appropriate:

- ❍ Determine whether energy needs have been correctly assessed
- ❍ Check to see if the parenteral solution is being delivered as prescribed
- ❍ Check for signs of dehydration or overhydration

LABORATORY TESTS

Check serum and urine tests for signs of:

- ❍ Fluid, electrolyte, and acid–base imbalances
- ❍ Hyperglycemia or hypoglycemia
- ❍ Hypertriglyceridemia
- ❍ Abnormal liver function
- ❍ Improvement or deterioration of the medical condition

PHYSICAL SIGNS

Routinely monitor the following:

- ❍ Catheter insertion site for signs of infection or inflammation
- ❍ Blood pressure, temperature, pulse, and respiration for signs of fluid, electrolyte, and acid–base imbalances

Look for physical signs of:

- ❍ Dehydration or overhydration
- ❍ Malnutrition

Self Check

1. For a patient who is at high risk of aspiration and is not expected to be able to eat table foods for several months, an appropriate placement of a feeding tube might be:
   a. nasogastric.
   b. nasoenteric.
   c. gastrostomy.
   d. jejunostomy.

2. In selecting an appropriate enteral formula for a patient, the primary consideration is:
   a. formula osmolality.
   b. the patient's nutrient needs.
   c. availability of infusion pumps.
   d. formula cost.

3. An important measure that may prevent bacterial contamination in tube feeding formulas is:
   a. nonstop feeding of formula.
   b. using the same feeding bag and tubing each day.
   c. discarding opened containers of formula not used within 24 hours.
   d. adding formula to the feeding container before it empties completely.

4. A difference between continuous and intermittent feedings is that continuous feedings:
   a. require an infusion pump.
   b. allow greater freedom of movement.
   c. are more similar to normal patterns of eating.
   d. are associated with more GI side effects.

5. A patient needs 1800 milliliters of formula a day. If the patient is to receive formula intermittently every four hours, how many milliliters of formula will she need at each feeding?
   a. 225
   b. 300
   c. 400
   d. 425

6. The nurse using a feeding tube to deliver medications recognizes that:
   a. medications given by feeding tube generally do not cause GI complaints.
   b. medications can usually be added directly to the feeding container.
   c. enteral formulas do not interact with medications in the same way that foods do.
   d. thick or sticky liquid medications and crushed tablets can clog feeding tubes.

7. For a patient receiving central TPN who also receives intravenous lipid emulsions two or three times a week, the lipid emulsions serve primarily as a source of:
   a. essential fatty acids.
   b. cholesterol.
   c. fat-soluble vitamins.
   d. concentrated energy.

8. Iron is typically excluded from parenteral solutions, in part, because:
   a. requirements for iron vary substantially from person to person.
   b. iron can destabilize solutions that include lipid emulsions.
   c. iron restriction is necessary in persons using warfarin therapy.
   d. iron promotes fat deposition in the liver.

9. Refeeding syndrome is associated with dangerous fluctuations in:
   a. serum electrolytes.
   b. serum liver enzyme levels.
   c. blood triglyceride levels.
   d. ketone bodies.

10. Patients using home parenteral nutrition:
    a. usually prefer continuous rather than cyclic infusions.
    b. are unable to travel or work away from home.
    c. require infusion pumps for use in the home.
    d. can only obtain 2-in-1 solutions and therefore must infuse lipids separately.

Answers: 1. d, 2. b, 3. c, 4. a, 5. b, 6. d, 7. a, 8. b, 9. a, 10. c

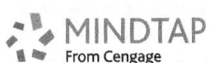
From Cengage   For more chapter resources visit **www.cengage.com** to access MindTap, a complete digital course.

Clinical Applications

1. Appendix F provides examples of enteral formulas on the market and lists their energy and macronutrient contents. Select one standard formula and one elemental formula from Tables F-1 and F-2, respectively. For the two formulas you selected, calculate the volume of formula that would meet the energy needs of a patient who requires about 1750 kcalories daily. Use these results in answering the following questions:
   a. How much protein, carbohydrate, and fat would the patient obtain from this volume of formula? Determine the percentages of kcalories that come from carbohydrate and fat. Do these percentages fall within the Acceptable Macronutrient Distribution Ranges described in Chapter 1 (p. 10)?
   b. Tables F-1 and F-2 show the formula volumes that would meet the Reference Daily Intakes (RDI). Would the volumes you obtained meet typical vitamin and mineral needs?

2. A liter of a TPN solution contains 500 milliliters of 50 percent dextrose solution and 500 milliliters of 5 percent amino acid solution. Determine the daily energy and protein intakes of a person who receives 2 liters per day of such a solution. Calculate the average daily energy intake if the person also receives 500 milliliters of a 20 percent fat emulsion three times a week.

3. Consider the clinical, financial, psychological, and social ramifications of using home parenteral nutrition, with no foods allowed by mouth, in answering the following questions:
   a. What would be the advantages of living at home instead of in a hospital or other residential facility? Can you think of some disadvantages?
   b. Think about how you, as a patient, might manage daily infusions: consider the time, cost, and commitment required to maintain the therapy.
   c. If not allowed to consume food, what possible difficulties might you encounter? How would you handle holidays and special occasions that center around food?

Notes

1. G. A. Cresci, Parenteral versus enteral nutrition, in G. A. Cresci, ed., *Nutrition Support for the Critically Ill Patient* (Boca Raton, FL: CRC Press, 2015), pp. 187–202.
2. B. Brown, Patient selection and indications for enteral feedings, in P. Charney and A. Malone, eds., *Pocket Guide to Enteral Nutrition* (Chicago: Academy of Nutrition and Dietetics, 2013), pp. 14–51.
3. S. A. McClave and coauthors, Guidelines for the provision and assessment of nutrition support therapy in the adult critically ill patient: Society of Critical Care Medicine and American Society for Parenteral and Enteral Nutrition, *Journal of Parenteral and Enteral Nutrition* 40 (2016): 159–211.
4. A. M. Malone, Enteral formulations, in G. A. Cresci, ed., *Nutrition for the Critically Ill Patient* (Boca Raton, FL: CRC Press, 2015), pp. 259–277.

5. Malone, 2015.

6. C. R. Parrish, J. Krenitsky, and K. G. Perkey, Enteral feeding challenges, in G. A. Cresci, ed., *Nutrition for the Critically Ill Patient* (Boca Raton, FL: CRC Press, 2015), pp. 291–311.

7. Malone, 2015.

8. A. Skipper, Enteral nutrition, in A. Skipper, ed., *Dietitian's Handbook of Enteral and Parenteral Nutrition* (Sudbury, MA: Jones and Bartlett Learning, 2012), pp. 259–280.

9. M. K. Russell, Complications of enteral feedings, in P. Charney and A. Malone, eds., *Pocket Guide to Enteral Nutrition* (Chicago: Academy of Nutrition and Dietetics, 2013), pp. 170–197.

10. J. I. Boullata and coauthors, ASPEN safe practices for enteral nutrition therapy, *Journal of Parenteral and Enteral Nutrition* 41 (2017): 15–103; M. Shelton, Monitoring and evaluation of enteral feedings, in P. Charney and A. Malone, eds., *Pocket Guide to Enteral Nutrition* (Chicago: Academy of Nutrition and Dietetics, 2013), pp. 153–169.

11. C. Thompson and M. Romano, Initiation, advancement, and transition of enteral feedings, in P. Charney and A. Malone, eds., *Pocket Guide to Enteral Nutrition* (Chicago: Academy of Nutrition and Dietetics, 2013), pp. 88–119; R. Bankhead and coauthors, A.S.P.E.N. enteral nutrition practice recommendations, *Journal of Parenteral and Enteral Nutrition* 33 (2009): 122–167.

12. Parrish, Krenitsky, and Perkey, 2015.

13. V. M. Zhao and T. R. Ziegler, Specialized nutrition support, in J. W. Erdman, I. A. Macdonald, and S. H. Zeisel, eds., *Present Knowledge in Nutrition* (Ames, IA: Wiley-Blackwell, 2012), pp. 982–999.

14. Boullata and coauthors, 2017; McClave and coauthors, 2016; Parrish, Krenitsky, and Perkey, 2015; T. W. Rice, Gastric residual volume: End of an era, *Journal of the American Medical Association* 309 (2013): 283–284.

15. Russell, 2013.

16. M. R. Lucarelli and coauthors, Fluid, electrolyte, and acid–base requirements in the critically ill patient, in G. A. Cresci, ed., *Nutrition for the Critically Ill Patient* (Boca Raton, FL: CRC Press, 2015), pp. 140–168.

17. R. O. Brown and R. N. Dickerson, Drug-nutrient interactions, in G. A. Cresci, ed., *Nutrition for the Critically Ill Patient* (Boca Raton, FL: CRC Press, 2015), pp. 313–327; P. D. Wohlt and coauthors, Recommendations for the use of medications with continuous enteral nutrition, *American Journal of Health-Systems Pharmacy* 66 (2009): 1458–1467.

18. Russell, 2013.

19. Thompson and Romano, 2013.

20. P. Worthington and coauthors, When is parenteral nutrition appropriate? *Journal of Parenteral and Enteral Nutrition* 41 (2017): 324–377.

21. M. Christensen, Parenteral formulations, in G. A. Cresci, ed., *Nutrition for the Critically Ill Patient* (Boca Raton, FL: CRC Press, 2015), pp. 237–258.

22. P. Ayers and coeditors, *A.S.P.E.N. Parenteral Nutrition Handbook* (Silver Spring, MD: American Society for Parenteral and Enteral Nutrition, 2014).

23. Ayers and coeditors, 2014.

24. Christensen, 2015; V. W. Vanek and coauthors, A.S.P.E.N. position paper: Clinical role for alternative intravenous fat emulsions, *Nutrition in Clinical Practice* 27 (2012): 150–192.

25. Ayers and coeditors, 2014.

26. G. Hardy and M. Puzovic, Formulation, stability, and administration of parenteral nutrition with new lipid emulsions, *Nutrition in Clinical Practice* 24 (2009): 616–625.

27. S. Roberts, Initiation, advancement, and acute complications, in P. Charney and A. Malone, eds., *ADA Pocket Guide to Parenteral Nutrition* (Chicago: American Dietetic Association, 2007), pp. 76–102.

28. P. Ayers and coauthors, A.S.P.E.N. parenteral nutrition safety consensus recommendations, *Journal of Parenteral and Enteral Nutrition* 38 (2014): 296–333.

29. M. L. Corrigan, Complications of parenteral nutrition, in G. A. Cresci, ed., *Nutrition for the Critically Ill Patient* (Boca Raton, FL: CRC Press, 2015), pp. 279–289; Ayers and coeditors, 2014; R. O. Brown, G. Minard, and T. R. Ziegler, Parenteral nutrition, in A. C. Ross and coeditors, eds., *Modern Nutrition in Health and Disease* (Baltimore: Lippincott Williams & Wilkins, 2014), pp. 1136–1161.

30. A. Pattinson and L. Epp, Home enteral nutrition, in P. Charney and A. Malone, eds., *Pocket Guide to Enteral Nutrition* (Chicago: Academy of Nutrition and Dietetics, 2013), pp. 198–229.

31. Worthington and coauthors, 2017; V. J. Kumpf and E. M. Tillman, Home parenteral nutrition: Safe transition from hospital to home, *Nutrition in Clinical Practice* 27 (2012): 749–757.

32. M. F. Winkler, Living with enteral and parenteral nutrition: How food and eating contribute to quality of life, *Journal of the American Dietetic Association* 110 (2010): 169–177.

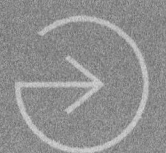

An **inborn error of metabolism** is an inherited trait, caused by a genetic **mutation**, that results in the absence, deficiency, or dysfunction of a protein that has a critical metabolic role.[1] The severity of the inborn error's effects is ultimately related to the degree of impairment caused by the missing or altered protein. This Nutrition in Practice describes some inborn errors of metabolism and discusses the role of diet in two of these disorders: phenylketonuria and galactosemia. Box NP15-1 defines some relevant terms.

What problems can result from inborn errors of metabolism?

The protein affected by an inborn error may function as an enzyme, receptor, transport protein, or structural protein. When the body fails to make a protein, the functions that depend on that protein are impaired. For example, when an enzyme is missing or malfunctioning in a metabolic pathway that typically converts compound A to compound B, compound A will accumulate and compound B will not be made. The excess of compound A and the lack of compound B may have harmful effects. Furthermore, the imbalances in one pathway may affect other pathways and ultimately cause a number of metabolic and physiologic disturbances. Table NP15-1 lists

examples of inborn errors related to defects in nutrient metabolism.

What role can diet play in treating inborn errors of metabolism?

Nutrition therapy is the primary treatment for many inborn errors that involve nutrient metabolism. Once the biochemical pathway affected by an inborn error is identified, the individual may be able to alter the diet to compensate for deficiencies and excesses. The typical dietary intervention involves restricting substances that cannot be properly metabolized and including substances that cannot be produced. Thus, dietary changes may be able to improve outcomes of some inborn errors by:

- Preventing the accumulation of toxic **metabolites** (metabolic products)
- Replacing nutrients that are deficient as a result of the defective metabolic pathway
- Providing a diet that supports normal growth and development and maintains health

Successful treatment of an inborn error of metabolism depends on the ability to screen newborns and diagnose metabolic diseases before irreversible damage occurs. After a genetic defect is identified, family members may

---

Box NP15-1 Glossary

cystic fibrosis: an inherited disorder that affects the transport of chloride across epithelial cell membranes; primarily affects the gastrointestinal and respiratory systems.

galactosemia (ga-LAK-toe-SEE-me-ah): an inherited disorder that impairs galactose metabolism; may cause damage to the brain, liver, kidneys, and lens in untreated patients.

gene therapy: treatment for inherited disorders in which DNA sequences are introduced into the chromosomes of affected cells, prompting the cells to express the protein needed to correct the disease.

genetic counseling: support for families at risk of genetic disorders; involves diagnosis of disease, identification of inheritance patterns within the family, and review of reproductive options.

hemophilia (HE-moh-FEEL-ee-ah): an inherited bleeding disorder characterized by deficiency or malfunction of a plasma protein needed for clotting blood.

inborn error of metabolism: an inherited trait (one that is present at birth) that causes the absence, deficiency, or malfunction of a protein that has a critical metabolic role.

metabolites: products of metabolism; compounds produced by a biochemical pathway.

mutation: a heritable change in the DNA sequence of a gene.

phenylketonuria (FEN-il-KEY-toe-NU-ree-ah) **or PKU:** an inherited disorder characterized by a defect in the enzyme phenylalanine hydroxylase, which normally converts the essential amino acid phenylalanine to the amino acid tyrosine. The condition is named after the phenylalanine metabolites—called *phenylketones*—that are excreted in the urine of individuals who have the disorder.

Nutrition-Related Inborn Errors of Metabolism

DISORDER	AFFECTED NUTRIENT(S) OR SUBSTANCE	METABOLIC DEFECT	NUTRITIONAL TREATMENT
AMINO ACID METABOLISM			
Maple syrup urine disease	Branched-chain amino acids (isoleucine, leucine, and valine)	Impaired metabolism of branched-chain amino acids	Restriction of branched-chain amino acids; thiamin supplementation
Phenylketonuria	Phenylalanine	Impaired conversion of phenylalanine to tyrosine	Phenylalanine-restricted diet; tyrosine supplementation
CARBOHYDRATE METABOLISM			
Galactosemia	Galactose	Impaired conversion of galactose to glucose	Galactose-restricted diet
Glycogen storage disease	Glycogen	Impaired metabolism or transport of glycogen, resulting in glycogen accumulation in tissues	Varies; may require frequent feedings, cornstarch supplementation, high-protein diet
LIPID METABOLISM			
Carnitine transporter deficiency	Fatty acids	Impaired transport of fatty acids into the mitochondria for oxidation	Carnitine supplementation; avoidance of fasting and strenuous exercise
X-linked adrenoleukodystrophy[a]	Very-long-chain fatty acids	Impaired breakdown of very-long-chain fatty acids in peroxisomes	Under investigation; limited benefit from moderate fat restriction and supplementation with a mixture of the fatty acids oleic acid and erucic acid
MINERAL METABOLISM			
Hemochromatosis	Iron	Excessive iron absorption (causes iron accumulation)	Avoidance of iron and vitamin C supplements and alcoholic beverages (routine blood draws remove excess iron from the body)
Wilson's disease	Copper	Impaired copper excretion (causes copper accumulation)	Avoidance of copper-rich foods; zinc therapy (reduces copper absorption)

[a]The disease X-linked-adrenoleukodystrophy was featured in the 1992 film *Lorenzo's Oil.*

undergo **genetic counseling** to evaluate the likelihood that they may pass on the disorder to future offspring. During counseling, couples may learn about reproductive options such as artificial insemination, *in vitro* fertilization, or prenatal monitoring after conception.

Are there treatments for inborn errors that don't involve dietary changes?

Nondietary therapies can treat some inborn errors of metabolism, although the options are somewhat limited. In some cases, the missing protein is infused; this is the primary means of treating **hemophilia**, caused by deficiency of one of the plasma proteins needed for clotting blood. Drug therapy is the main treatment for some

inborn errors, including **cystic fibrosis** (see Chapter 18), which is characterized by a defect that prevents normal chloride transport across cell membranes. Future approaches may include **gene therapy**, a treatment that introduces DNA sequences into the chromosomes of affected cells, prompting the cells to express the protein needed to correct the abnormality.

What is an example of an inborn error that benefits from dietary treatment?

A classic example is **phenylketonuria (PKU)**, a metabolic disorder that affects amino acid metabolism. PKU occurs in approximately 1 out of every 12,700 births in the United States each year.[2] In PKU, the missing or defective protein is the liver enzyme *phenylalanine hydroxylase*, which converts the essential amino acid phenylalanine to the amino acid tyrosine. This chemical reaction is also the first step in the breakdown of excess phenylalanine. Without the enzyme, phenylalanine and its by-products accumulate in the blood and tissues, resulting in severe damage to the developing brain. The impairment in the metabolic pathway also prevents the liver synthesis of tyrosine and tyrosine-derived compounds (such as the neurotransmitter epinephrine, the skin pigment melanin, and the hormone thyroxine). Under these conditions, tyrosine becomes essential: the body cannot produce tyrosine, and therefore the diet must supply it.

Although PKU's most debilitating effect is on brain development, other signs may manifest if the condition is untreated. Infants with PKU may have poor appetites and grow slowly. They may be irritable or have tremors or seizures. Their bodies and urine may have a musty odor. Their skin may be unusually pale, and they may develop skin rashes. In older children and adults who discontinue treatment, neurological and psychological problems are common. Individuals with elevated phenylalanine levels may exhibit impaired reasoning, a reduced attention span, and poor memory, among other deficits.[3]

How is PKU diagnosed?

PKU must be diagnosed soon after birth so that early treatment can prevent its devastating effects. For this reason, newborns are screened for PKU in all 50 states. A standard blood test for phenylalanine is typically conducted by heel puncture after the infant has consumed several meals containing protein (see Photo NP15-1). Abnormal results require further testing.

The screening of newborns for PKU is one of the most common genetic tests in the United States and many other countries. Before widespread newborn screening, infants with PKU demonstrated developmental delays (for example, inability to crawl) by six to nine months of age. By the time parents recognized the problem, the damage was irreversible. Most of the damaging consequences of this disorder have been eliminated due to the early detection and treatment of PKU.

What is the treatment for PKU?

The treatment for PKU is a diet that restricts phenylalanine and supplies tyrosine so that the blood levels of these amino acids are maintained within safe ranges.[4] Because phenylalanine is an essential amino acid, the diet cannot exclude it completely. Children with PKU need phenylalanine to grow, but they cannot handle excesses without detrimental effects. Therefore, their diets must provide enough phenylalanine to support growth and health, but not so much as to cause harm. The diets must also provide tyrosine, which is an essential nutrient for individuals

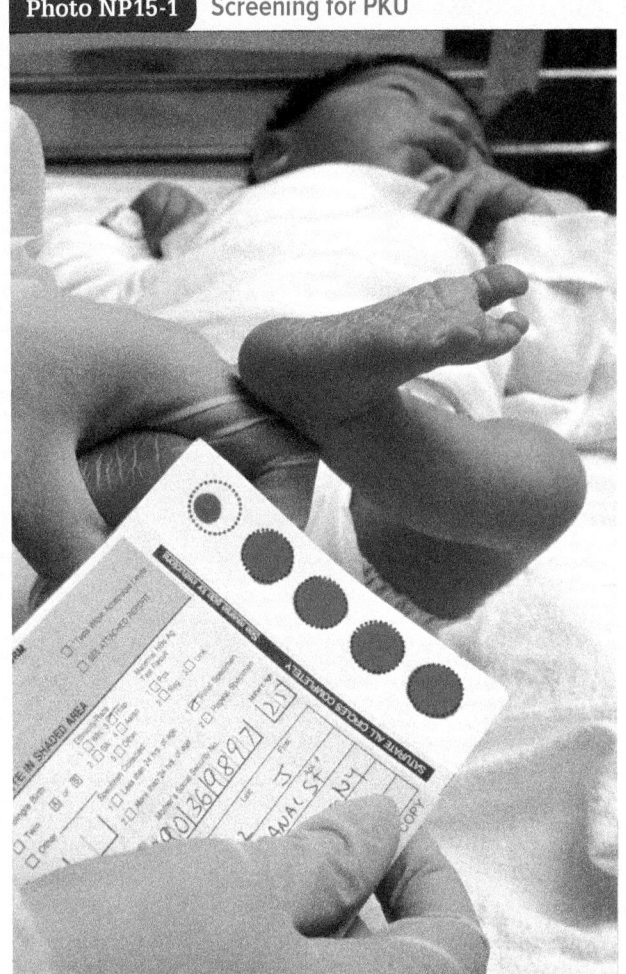

Photo NP15-1 Screening for PKU

Ted Horowitz/Flirt/Corbis

A simple blood test screens newborns for PKU—a common inborn error of metabolism.

with PKU. To ensure that blood concentrations of phenylalanine and tyrosine are close to normal, blood tests are performed periodically, and diets are adjusted when necessary. If the dietary treatment is conscientiously followed, it can prevent the effects described earlier. Older children and adults with PKU must continue to follow the PKU diet to prevent deterioration in brain function.

What are the main features of the PKU diet?

Central to the PKU diet is the use of an enteral formula that is phenylalanine-free yet supplies energy, amino acids, vitamins, and minerals (see Photo NP15-2).[5] For infants, the phenylalanine-free formula can be supplemented with measured amounts of breast milk or regular infant formula to provide the phenylalanine needed for growth. Low-phenylalanine formulas are available for infants who must meet all of their nutrient needs with formula. Formula requirements need to be

PKU Formulas

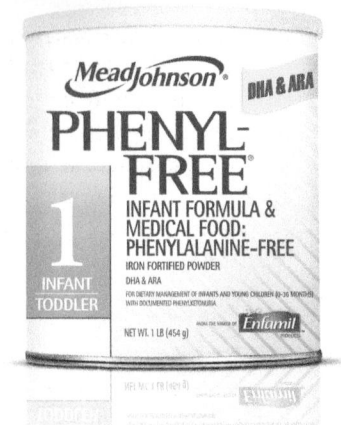
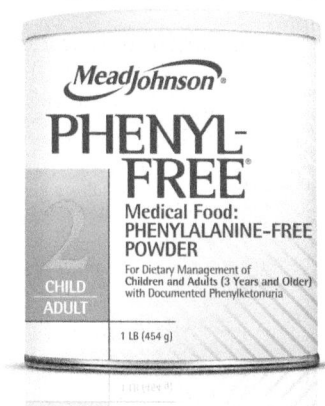

Mead Johnson Nutrition

Phenylalanine-free formulas help patients with PKU maintain safe blood levels of the amino acid phenylalanine.

recalculated periodically to accommodate the growing infant's shifting needs for protein, phenylalanine, tyrosine, and energy.

Once food consumption begins, a phenylalanine-free formula supplies the needed amino acids, and foods that contain phenylalanine are carefully monitored. All protein-containing foods provide some phenylalanine; therefore, high-protein foods such as meat, fish, poultry, milk, cheese, legumes, and nuts (including peanut butter) are omitted. Foods that contain moderate amounts of protein (potatoes, grains, some vegetables) must be restricted. Low-protein foods such as fruits and certain vegetables can be eaten more freely, although intakes may need to be limited so as not to exceed the recommended phenylalanine allowance. Low-protein flours and mixes are available for making low-phenylalanine breads, pasta, cakes, and cookies. Foods that contain little or no phenylalanine, such as jams, jellies, and most sweeteners, can help to increase energy intake. Growth rates and nutrition status are monitored to ensure that the diet is adequate. Older children, teens, and adults with PKU should continue to use the phenylalanine-free formulas to help meet their protein and energy needs.

Individuals with PKU should be encouraged to develop creative ways to make their diets enjoyable. The formula can be flavored or combined with fruit or juice to make smoothies or frozen juice bars. Sandwiches can be made with low-phenylalanine bread and fillings such as mashed bananas or avocados, shredded carrots and olives, or tomato slices with mayonnaise. Food variety can be expanded by using products made from the protein *glycomacropeptide*, which is a phenylalanine-free protein derived from whey; available products include milk substitutes, shakes, and protein bars.

How long should a person with PKU continue the dietary treatment?

Lifelong adherence to a phenylalanine-restricted diet is currently recommended for all individuals with PKU, as elevated phenylalanine levels can adversely affect cognitive function at any age.[6] In addition, women with PKU must maintain safe phenylalanine concentrations during pregnancy. Elevated phenylalanine levels, especially during the first trimester, have been associated with mental disability, birth defects, and growth retardation in the offspring of mothers with PKU who have discontinued dietary treatment.[7]

Although consuming a low-phenylalanine diet is the main treatment for patients with PKU, a number of other therapies have been investigated. The medication sapropterin dihydrochloride (Kuvan) improves phenylalanine hydroxylase function in some PKU patients, thereby allowing an increased intake of protein-containing foods.[8] Supplementation with large neutral amino acids (such as tyrosine and threonine), which compete with phenylalanine for transport across cell membranes, may improve both blood phenylalanine levels and neurologic function; different amino acid mixtures are being studied as potential therapies for patients who are unable to remain on the PKU diet long term.[9]

What is another example of an inborn error that requires dietary changes?

Galactosemia is an example of an inborn error of carbohydrate metabolism. Individuals with galactosemia are deficient in one of the enzymes needed to metabolize galactose, a sugar that is found primarily in milk products (recall that lactose molecules contain galactose). An accumulation of galactose metabolites can cause damage in multiple tissues. Infants with galactosemia who are given milk react with severe vomiting and liver jaundice within days of the initial feeding. Serious liver damage can develop and progress to symptomatic cirrhosis. Other complications may include kidney failure, cataracts, and brain damage. Treatment in the first weeks of life can prevent the most detrimental effects of galactosemia, but if treatment is delayed, the damage to the brain is irreversible.[10]

What is the dietary treatment for galactosemia?

Patients with galactosemia must consume a galactose-restricted diet. The diet is much simpler than the diet for PKU because galactose is not an essential nutrient and is not in a metabolic pathway that produces a required substance. In addition, dietary galactose is primarily obtained from lactose (the milk sugar), so the main focus of dietary treatment is the exclusion of milk and milk products. Other foods that contain galactose in substantial amounts, such as organ meats and some legumes, fruits, and vegetables, must also be avoided or restricted. Prepared foods and medications that include lactose as an additive must be avoided as well. Galactosemia patients or their caregivers are generally given food lists that identify common sources of galactose.

Infants diagnosed with galactosemia are given lactose-free formulas to meet their nutrient needs. Once a child can consume adequate amounts of regular foods, special formulas are unnecessary; however, care must be taken to ensure that the diet supplies adequate calcium. Individuals with galactosemia must remain on the galactose-restricted diet throughout their lives to avoid potential damage to the brain, liver, kidney, and lens.[11]

How effective is the dietary treatment for galactosemia?

Although the early introduction of a galactose-restricted diet can eliminate the acute toxic effects of galactosemia, complications of the disease may develop despite an individual's compliance with diet therapy. For example, many patients experience difficulties with language, abstract thinking, and visual perception. Ovarian failure and cataracts are common. The reasons for these long-term complications are not fully understood.

For many inborn errors of metabolism, effective management requires early diagnosis and treatment, as well as control of the environmental factors that may cause toxicity. In some cases, dietary changes are central to treatment and can prevent serious complications. Other inborn errors, however, may not be as easily treated. Future developments in biotechnology may allow gene therapy to assist in the medical treatment of some of these disorders.

Notes

1. O. A. Bodamer, Approach to inborn errors of metabolism, in L. Goldman and A. I. Schafer, eds., *Goldman-Cecil Medicine* (Philadelphia: Saunders, 2016), pp. 1384–1389.
2. S. A. Berry and coauthors, Newborn screening 50 years later: Access issues faced by adults with PKU, *Genetics in Medicine* 15 (2013): 591–599.
3. N. Blau, F. J. van Spronsen, and H. L. Levy, Phenylketonuria, *Lancet* 376 (2010): 1417–1427.
4. R. H. Singh and coauthors, Recommendations for the nutrition management of phenylalanine hydroxylase deficiency, *Genetics in Medicine* 16 (2014): 121–131.
5. Singh and coauthors, 2014.
6. J. Vockley and coauthors, Phenylalanine hydroxylase deficiency: Diagnosis and management guideline, *Genetics in Medicine* 16 (2014): 188–200.
7. Vockley and coauthors, 2014; Blau, van Spronsen, and Levy, 2010.
8. P. Strisciuglio and D. Concolino, New strategies for the treatment of phenylketonuria (PKU), *Metabolites* 4 (2014): 1007–1017; M. Giovannini and coauthors, Phenylketonuria: Nutritional advances and challenges, *Nutrition and Metabolism* 9 (2012): 7, doi: 10.1186/1743-7075-9-7.
9. D. Concolino and coauthors, Long-term treatment of phenylketonuria with a new medical food containing large neutral amino acids, *European Journal of Clinical Nutrition* 71 (2017): 51–55; Strisciuglio and Concolino, 2014; Giovannini and coauthors, 2012.
10. L. J. Elsas II and P. B. Acosta, Inherited metabolic disease: Amino acids, organic acids, and galactose, in A. C. Ross and coeditors, *Modern Nutrition in Health and Disease* (Baltimore: Lippincott Williams & Wilkins, 2014), pp. 906–969.
11. Elsas and Acosta, 2014.

Nutrition in Metabolic and Respiratory Stress

Chapter Sections and Learning Objectives (LOs)

John Fedele/Getty Images

chapter

16

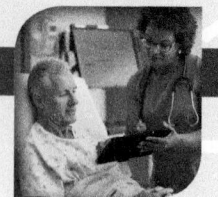
enough to threaten survival. Many patients with severe stress require life support measures and intensive monitoring. Stress also raises nutritional needs considerably—increasing the risk of malnutrition even in previously healthy individuals. **Metabolic stress**, a disruption in the body's internal chemical environment, can result from uncontrolled infections or extensive tissue damage, such as deep, penetrating wounds or multiple broken bones. As the first part of this chapter explains, the body's stress response is an attempt to restore balance, but it can have both helpful and harmful effects. Later sections of this chapter describe **respiratory stress**, characterized by insufficient oxygen and excessive carbon dioxide in the blood and tissues. Both metabolic and respiratory stress can lead to **hypermetabolism** (above-normal metabolic rate), **wasting** (loss of muscle tissue), and, in severe circumstances, life-threatening complications. Box 16-1 defines some terms related to metabolic stress.

16.1 The Body's Responses to Stress and Injury

The **stress response** is the body's *nonspecific* response to a variety of stressors, such as burns, fractures, infection, surgery, and wounds. During stress, the metabolic processes that support immediate survival are given priority, while those of lesser consequence are delayed. Energy is of primary importance, and therefore the energy nutrients are mobilized from storage and made available in the blood. Heart rate and respiration (breathing rate) increase to deliver oxygen and nutrients to cells more quickly, and

---

Box 16-1   Glossary of Terms Related to Metabolic Stress

acute-phase response: changes in body chemistry resulting from infection, inflammation, or injury; characterized by alterations in plasma proteins.

complement: a group of plasma proteins that assist the activities of antibodies and phagocytes.

C-reactive protein: an acute-phase protein produced in substantial amounts during acute inflammation; it binds dead or dying cells to activate certain immune responses. C-reactive protein is considered the best clinical indicator of the acute-phase response although it is elevated during many chronic illnesses.

cytokines (SIGH-toe-kines): signaling proteins produced by the body's cells; those produced by immune cells regulate various aspects of immune function.

eicosanoids (eye-KO-sa-noids): 20-carbon molecules derived from dietary fatty acids that help to regulate blood pressure, blood clotting, and other body functions.

- *eicosa* = twenty

hepcidin: an acute-phase protein involved in the regulation of iron metabolism.

hypermetabolism: a higher-than-normal metabolic rate.

inflammatory response: a group of nonspecific immune responses to infection or injury.

mast cells: cells within connective tissue that produce and release histamine.

metabolic stress: a disruption in the body's chemical environment due to the effects of disease or injury. Metabolic stress is characterized by changes in metabolic rate, heart rate, blood pressure, hormonal status, and nutrient metabolism.

phagocytes (FAG-oh-sites): immune cells (neutrophils and macrophages) that have the ability to engulf and destroy antigens.

- *phagein* = to eat

respiratory stress: a condition characterized by abnormal oxygen and carbon dioxide levels in body tissues due to abnormal gas exchange between the air and blood.

sepsis: a whole-body inflammatory response caused by infection; characterized by signs and symptoms similar to those of the *systemic inflammatory response syndrome* (see definition below).

shock: a severe reduction in blood flow that deprives the body's tissues of oxygen and nutrients; characterized by reduced blood pressure, raised heart and respiratory rates, and muscle weakness.

stress response: the chemical and physical changes that occur within the body during stress.

systemic (sih-STEM-ic): affecting the entire body.

systemic inflammatory response syndrome (SIRS): a whole-body inflammatory response caused by severe illness or trauma; characterized by raised heart and respiratory rates, abnormal white blood cell counts, and fever.

wasting: the breakdown of muscle tissue that results from disease or malnutrition.

---

blood pressure rises. Meanwhile, energy is diverted from processes that are not life sustaining, such as growth, reproduction, and long-term immunity. If stress continues for a long period, interference with these processes may begin to cause damage, potentially resulting in growth retardation and illness.

Hormonal Responses to Stress

The stress response is mediated by several hormones, which are released into the blood soon after the onset of injury (see Table 16-1).[1] The catecholamines (epinephrine and norepinephrine)—often called the *fight-or-flight hormones*—stimulate heart muscle, raise blood pressure, and increase metabolic rate. Epinephrine also promotes glucagon secretion from the pancreas, prompting the release of nutrients from storage. The steroid hormone cortisol enhances muscle protein degradation, raising amino acid levels in the blood and making amino acids available for conversion to glucose. All of these hormones have similar effects on glucose and fat metabolism, causing the breakdown of glycogen, the production of glucose from amino acids, and the breakdown of triglycerides in adipose tissue. Thus, the combined effects of these hormones contribute to hyperglycemia, which often accompanies critical illness. Two other hormones induced by stress, aldosterone and antidiuretic hormone, help to maintain blood volume by stimulating the kidneys to reabsorb more sodium and water, respectively.

Cortisol's effects can be detrimental when stress is prolonged (see Box 16-2). In excess, cortisol causes the depletion of protein in muscle, bone, connective tissue, and the skin. It impairs wound healing, so high cortisol levels may be especially dangerous for a patient with severe injuries. Because cortisol inhibits protein synthesis, consuming more protein cannot easily reverse tissue losses. Excess cortisol also leads to insulin resistance, contributing to hyperglycemia, and suppresses immune responses, increasing susceptibility to infection. Note that pharmaceutical forms of cortisol (such as *cortisone* and *prednisone*) are common anti-inflammatory medications; their long-term use can cause undesirable side effects such as muscle wasting, thinning of the skin, diabetes, and early osteoporosis.

> **BOX 16-2** *Nursing Diagnosis*
>
> The nursing diagnoses *impaired tissue integrity* and *risk for infection* may apply to a person who undergoes prolonged stress.

| **TABLE 16-1** | Metabolic Effects of Hormones Released during the Stress Response |

HORMONE	METABOLIC EFFECTS
Catecholamines	• Increase in metabolic rate • Glycogen breakdown in the liver and muscle • Glucose production from amino acids • Release of fatty acids from adipose tissue • Glucagon secretion from the pancreas
Glucagon	• Glycogen breakdown in the liver • Glucose production from amino acids • Release of fatty acids from adipose tissue
Cortisol	• Protein degradation • Enhancement of glucagon's action on liver glycogen • Glucose production from amino acids • Release of fatty acids from adipose tissue
Aldosterone	• Sodium reabsorption in the kidneys
Antidiuretic hormone	• Water reabsorption in the kidneys

Note: The catecholamines, glucagon, and cortisol have actions that oppose those of insulin and are therefore referred to as *counterregulatory hormones*.

The Inflammatory Response

Cells of the immune system mount a quick, nonspecific response to infection or tissue injury. This so-called **inflammatory response** serves to contain and destroy infectious agents (and their products) and prevent further tissue damage; it also triggers various events that promote healing. As in the stress response, however, there is a delicate balance between a response that protects tissues from further injury and an excessive response that can cause additional damage to tissue.

The Inflammatory Process The inflammatory response begins with the dilation of arterioles and capillaries at the site of injury, which increases blood flow to the affected area. The capillaries within the damaged tissue become more permeable, allowing some blood plasma to escape into the tissue and cause local edema (see Figure 16-1 and Box 16-3). The various changes in blood vessels attract immune cells that can destroy foreign agents and clear cellular debris. Among the first cells to arrive are the **phagocytes**, which slip through gaps between the endothelial cells that form the blood vessel walls. The phagocytes engulf microorganisms and destroy them with reactive forms of oxygen and hydrolytic enzymes. When inflammation becomes chronic, these normally useful products of phagocytes can damage healthy tissue.

Mediators of Inflammation Numerous chemical substances control the inflammatory process. These *mediators* are released from damaged tissue, blood vessel cells, and activated immune cells. Many of them help to regulate more than one step in the process. Histamine, a small molecule similar to an amino acid in structure, is released from granules within **mast cells**, causing vasodilation and capillary permeability.* Other compounds that participate in the inflammatory process include **cytokines**, produced by white blood cells (and various other cells), and **eicosanoids**, which are derived from dietary fatty acids. Note that most anti-inflammatory medications, including steroidal drugs (such as cortisone and prednisone) and nonsteroidal anti-inflammatory drugs (such as aspirin and ibuprofen), act by blocking eicosanoid synthesis.

Changing dietary fat sources may have subtle effects on the inflammatory process.[2] The major precursor for the eicosanoids is arachidonic acid, which derives from the

FIGURE 16-1 The Inflammatory Process

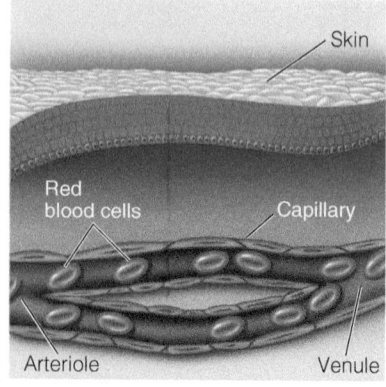

Cells lining the blood vessels lie close together, and normally do not allow the contents to cross into tissue.

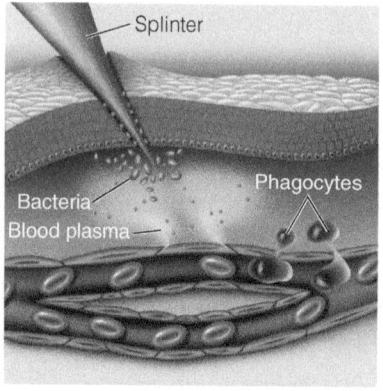

When tissues are damaged, immune cells release histamine, which dilates some blood vessels, increasing blood flow to the damaged area. Fluid leaks out of capillaries (causing swelling), and phagocytes escape between the small gaps in the blood vessel walls.

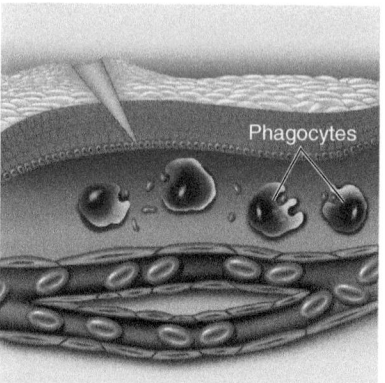

Phagocytes engulf bacteria and disable them with hydrolytic enzymes and reactive forms of oxygen.

Antihistamines are medications taken to reduce the effects of histamine.

omega-6 fatty acids in vegetable oils. Some omega-3 fatty acids compete with arachidonic acid and may inhibit the production of the most potent inflammatory mediators. Although health professionals sometimes recommend replacing some of the omega-6 fatty acids in the diet with omega-3 fatty acids to reduce inflammation, most clinical studies conducted thus far have not confirmed this benefit.[3]

Systemic Effects of Inflammation In addition to the localized effects described earlier, the cytokines released during acute inflammation produce a number of **systemic** effects, which are collectively known as the **acute-phase response**.[4] Within hours after inflammation, infection, or severe injury, the liver steps up its production of certain plasma proteins (called *acute-phase proteins*) including **C-reactive protein**, **complement**, **hepcidin**, blood-clotting proteins such as fibrinogen and prothrombin, and others. At the same time, plasma concentrations of albumin, iron, and zinc fall (recall from Chapter 13 that albumin levels are often measured to assess health status). The acute-phase response is accompanied by muscle catabolism to make amino acids available for glucose production, tissue repair, and immune protein synthesis; consequently, negative nitrogen balance (and wasting) frequently results. Other clinical features of the acute-phase response may include fever, an elevated metabolic rate, increased pulse rate and blood pressure, increased blood neutrophil levels, lethargy, and anorexia.

If inflammation does not resolve, the continued production of pro-inflammatory cytokines may lead to the **systemic inflammatory response syndrome (SIRS)**, which is diagnosed when the patient's signs and symptoms include substantial increases in heart rate and respiratory rate, abnormal white blood cell counts, and/or fever. If these problems result from a severe infection, the condition is called **sepsis**. Complications associated with severe cases of SIRS or sepsis include fluid retention and tissue edema, low blood pressure, and impaired blood flow. If the reduction in blood flow is severe enough to deprive the body's tissues of oxygen and nutrients (a condition known as **shock**; see Box 16-4), multiple organs may fail simultaneously, as discussed in Nutrition in Practice 16.

BOX 16-4 *Nursing Diagnosis*

The nursing diagnosis *risk for shock* applies to a person with SIRS or sepsis.

Review Notes

- The stress and inflammatory responses are nonspecific responses to stressors that cause infection and injury.
- The stress response is mediated by the catecholamine hormones, cortisol, and glucagon, which together raise nutrient levels in the blood, stimulate heart rate, raise blood pressure, and increase metabolic rate.
- The inflammatory process—mediated by compounds released from damaged tissues, immune cells, and blood vessels—may result in both local and systemic effects.
- Local inflammatory effects include swelling, redness, warmth, and pain in damaged tissue; systemic effects are characterized by changes in acute-phase proteins and increases in body temperature, pulse, blood pressure, metabolic rate, and blood neutrophil levels.
- Persistent, severe inflammation may lead to shock and increases the risk of multiple organ dysfunction.

16.2 Nutrition Treatment of Acute Stress

As described earlier, an excessive response to metabolic stress can worsen illness and even threaten survival. Therefore, medical personnel must manage both the acute medical condition that initiated stress and the complications that arise as a result of the stress and inflammatory responses (see Photo 16-1 and Box 16-5). Immediate concerns during severe stress are to restore lost fluids and electrolytes and remove underlying stressors.

BOX 16-5 *Nursing Diagnosis*

Nursing diagnoses that may apply to individuals undergoing metabolic stress include *risk for deficient fluid volume, risk for electrolyte imbalance,* and *risk for unstable blood glucose level.*

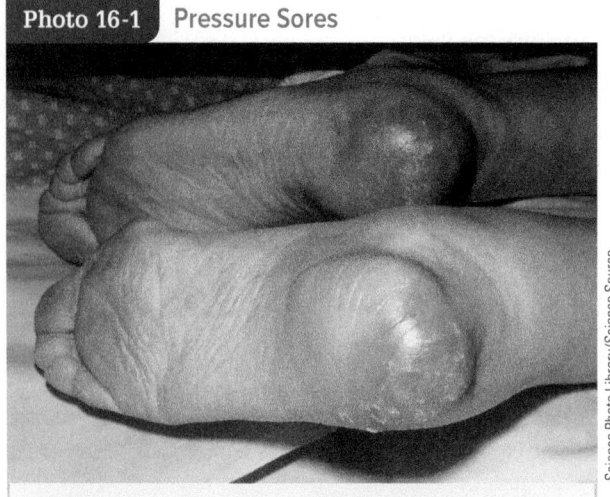

Photo 16-1 Pressure Sores

Pressure sores, wounds that develop when prolonged pressure cuts off blood circulation to the skin and underlying tissues, are a frequent source of metabolic stress in bedridden and wheelchair-bound patients. Some patients with pressure sores may be prescribed a high-protein, high-kcalorie diet to prevent malnutrition.

abscesses (AB-sess-es): accumulations of pus.

debridement: the surgical removal of dead, damaged, or contaminated tissue resulting from burns or wounds; helps to prevent infection and hasten healing.

refeeding syndrome: a group of metabolic abnormalities that may result from aggressive refeeding in severely malnourished persons; characterized by shifts in fluid and electrolyte levels that can lead to organ failure and other complications.

indirect calorimetry: a method of estimating resting energy expenditure by measuring a person's oxygen consumption and carbon dioxide production.

minute ventilation: the volume of air a person inhales or exhales each minute.

hypocaloric feeding: a reduced-kcalorie regimen that includes sufficient protein and micronutrients to maintain nitrogen balance and prevent malnutrition; also called *permissive underfeeding.*

Thus, initial treatments include administering intravenous solutions to correct fluid and electrolyte imbalances, treating infections, repairing wounds, draining **abscesses** (pus), and removing dead tissue (**debridement**). After stabilization, nutrient needs can be estimated and nutrition therapy provided.

Determining Nutritional Requirements

Notable metabolic changes in patients undergoing metabolic stress include hypermetabolism, negative nitrogen balance, insulin resistance, and hyperglycemia. Hypermetabolism and negative nitrogen balance can lead to wasting, which may impair organ function and delay recovery. Hyperglycemia increases the risk of infection, which can lead to complications and higher mortality risk. Therefore, the principal goals of nutrition therapy are to preserve lean (muscle) tissue, maintain immune defenses, and promote healing.

Feeding an acutely stressed patient is often challenging. Underfeeding can worsen negative nitrogen balance and increase lean tissue losses. Overfeeding increases the risks of **refeeding syndrome** and its associated hyperglycemia. Assessing nutritional needs can be complicated, however, because fluid imbalances prevent accurate weight measurements, and laboratory data may reflect the metabolic alterations of illness rather than the person's nutrition status.

The amounts of protein and energy to provide during acute illness are controversial and still under investigation. Research results have been mixed, in part because various conditions are associated with metabolic stress and each patient's situation is somewhat different. Moreover, protein and energy needs can vary substantially over the course of illness. Clinicians need to closely observe patients' responses to feedings and readjust nutrient intakes as necessary.

Estimating Energy Needs in Acute Stress In critically ill patients, **indirect calorimetry**— which is typically used to measure the resting metabolic rate (RMR)—can be used to determine energy requirements. This is because the RMR closely reflects total energy expenditure in bedridden, nonfasting patients.[5] If indirect calorimetry cannot be conducted, the RMR may be estimated using a predictive equation, such as those introduced in Chapter 14 (see *Energy Intakes in Hospital Patients*, pp. 408–409). In some cases, the RMR value may be multiplied by a "stress factor" to account for the increased energy requirements of stress and healing.[6] Box 16-6 reviews the use of stress factors and provides examples (note that stress factors vary among institutions, as few have been adequately validated in research studies).

Some predictive equations used for estimating energy needs include built-in factors to account for stress, injury, or intensive treatment. Table 16-2 lists examples of equations used for ventilator-dependent critical care patients and describes the use of the Penn State equation, which includes multipliers for **minute ventilation** and body temperature. Other equations in current use include factors for other pertinent variables, such as the type of injury, heart rate, and respiratory rate.[7]

Another common method for estimating energy needs during acute illness is to multiply a person's body weight by a factor considered appropriate for the medical problem. As an example, many critical care patients require between 25 and 30 kcalories per kilogram of body weight per day[8]; a patient weighing 160 pounds (72.7 kilograms) may therefore require between 1818 and 2182 kcalories per day. For critically ill obese patients (BMI >30), **hypocaloric feeding** may improve patient outcomes; the suggested energy intake is 11 to 14 kcalories per kilogram of actual body weight (or 22 to 25 kcalories per kilogram of ideal body weight) daily.[9]

Box 16-6

HOW TO Estimate Energy Needs Using Disease-Specific Stress Factors

To estimate the appropriate energy intake for a patient with an acute illness, the health practitioner may measure or calculate the patient's resting metabolic rate (RMR), and, in some cases, apply a "stress factor" to accommodate the additional energy needs imposed by the illness.

Method

Step 1. Estimate the RMR using indirect calorimetry or a predictive equation (see examples in Table 14-3, p. 408).

Step 2. Multiply the estimated RMR by an appropriate stress factor for acute illness (see Box 14-2 on p. 408; note that patients with acute illnesses are usually bedridden and do not require additional energy for activity).

Examples of Stress Factors[a]

- Intensive care: 1.0 to 1.1
- Minor surgery: 1.2
- Acute kidney injury: 1.3
- Burns (more than 20 percent of body surface): 1.3 to 1.5
- Repletion after acute inflammation: 1.3 to 1.5
- Acute pancreatitis: 1.4 to 1.8

Source: A. Skipper, ed., *Dietitian's Handbook of Enteral and Parenteral Nutrition* (Sudbury, MA: Jones & Bartlett Learning, 2012).

[a]Published values vary; energy intakes should be adjusted if the patient fails to maintain body weight at the energy level provided.

TABLE 16-2 Selected Equations for Estimating Energy Needs in Ventilator-Dependent Critical Care Patients

IRETON–JONES[a]

Energy needs (kcal/day) = $1784 + [5 \times \text{Wt (kg)}] - [11 \times \text{Age (yr)}] + [244 \times \text{Sex}] + [239 \times \text{Trauma}] + [804 \times \text{Burn}]$

where Sex is male ($\times$ 1) or female ($\times$ 0), Trauma is the presence of physical injury ($\times$ 1) or not ($\times$ 0), and Burn is the presence of a burn injury ($\times$ 1) or not ($\times$ 0).

PENN STATE[b]

Energy needs (kcal/day) = $[\text{RMR} \times 0.96] + [V_E \times 31] + [T_{max} \times 167] - 6212$

where RMR is calculated using the Mifflin–St. Jeor equation (see Table 14-3, p. 408), V_E is minute ventilation in liters per minute, and T_{max} is the patient's maximum body temperature (in degrees Celsius) in the preceding 24 hours.

Example (Penn State equation): Erin is a 27-year-old patient who is 65.0 inches (165 centimeters) tall and weighs 140 pounds (63.6 kilograms). Two days ago, she was injured in an automobile accident and is currently being cared for in a critical care unit where she is receiving mechanical ventilation. Her minute ventilation is about 8.0 liters per minute and her maximum temperature over the past day was 99.0 degrees Fahrenheit (37.2 degrees Celsius). Using the Penn State equation, her daily energy needs can be estimated as follows:

RMR (Mifflin–St. Jeor equation)

$= [9.99 \times \text{weight (kg)}] + [6.25 \times \text{height (cm)}] - [4.92 \times \text{age (years)}] - 161$

$= [9.99 \times 63.6 \text{ kg}] + [6.25 \times 165 \text{ cm}] - [4.92 \times 27 \text{ years}] - 161 = 1373 \text{ kcal}$

Energy needs (kcal/day)

$= [\text{RMR} \times 0.96] + [V_E \times 31] + [T_{max} \times 167] - 6212$

$= [1373 \times 0.96] + [8.0 \times 31] + [37.2 \times 167] - 6212 = 1566 \text{ kcal}$

[a]The Ireton-Jones equation shown here is the updated 1997 version.

[b]In overweight and obese individuals, the Penn State equation estimates energy needs more accurately than other currently used equations.

Protein Requirements in Acute Stress To maintain lean tissue, the protein intakes recommended during acute stress are higher than RDA levels (the adult RDA is 0.8 grams per kilogram of body weight per day). For example, the protein needs of nonobese critically ill patients typically range between 1.2 and 2.0 grams per kilogram of body weight per day.[10] Obese patients on a hypocaloric regimen may require 2.0 to 2.5 grams per kilogram of ideal body weight per day to maintain nitrogen balance.[11] Despite high intakes, however, nitrogen balance is difficult to achieve during acute stress because hormonal changes encourage the degradation of body protein. The bed rest required during critical illness also contributes substantially to muscle breakdown.

The amino acids glutamine and arginine are sometimes added to the diets of acutely stressed and immunocompromised patients. Although some studies have shown that glutamine supplementation may improve infection, muscle mass, and mortality rates in some critically ill patients,[12] other studies suggest that the treatment may increase mortality risk in patients with multiple organ failure and renal dysfunction.[13] Arginine supplementation has been shown to improve infection rates and wound healing in surgical patients but may have adverse effects in patients with sepsis.[14] Thus, supplementation with glutamine and arginine may be beneficial for some patient populations but harmful in others.

Carbohydrate and Fat Intakes in Acute Stress Most of the energy required is supplied by carbohydrate and fat. Carbohydrate is usually the main source of energy, providing about 50 to 60 percent of total energy requirements. When parenteral nutrition is necessary for critically ill patients, dextrose is limited to 5 milligrams per kilogram of body weight per minute to prevent hyperglycemia (see Chapter 15). In patients with severe hyperglycemia, fat may supply up to 50 percent of kcalories, although high fat intakes may suppress immune function and increase the risks of developing infections and hypertriglyceridemia. Patients with blood triglyceride levels above 500 milligrams per deciliter may require fat restriction.[15]

Micronutrient Needs in Acute Stress Acutely stressed patients are believed to have increased micronutrient needs, but specific requirements remain unknown.[16] Supplementation with antioxidants such as vitamin C, vitamin E, and selenium is sometimes recommended to counter oxidative stress. Vitamin C supplementation in patients with burn injuries has been associated with decreased infections. Zinc has critical roles in immunity and wound healing and its supplementation may speed recovery under certain circumstances.

As mentioned earlier, the acute-phase response causes a redistribution in the tissue content of some micronutrients that either raises or lowers their blood levels (for example, plasma levels of iron and zinc fall, whereas copper levels rise). Therefore, micronutrient status is often difficult to evaluate. Blood concentrations of trace minerals are monitored in patients receiving parenteral nutrition support to ensure that excessive amounts are not given intravenously.

Approaches to Nutrition Care in Acute Stress

The initial care following acute stress focuses on maintaining fluid and electrolyte balances. Simple intravenous solutions often contain dextrose, providing minimal kcalories. Once patients are stable, nutrition support may be necessary if poor appetite, the medical condition, or a medical procedure (such as mechanical ventilation) interferes with food intake. For acutely ill patients with a functional GI tract, early enteral feedings—started in the first 24 to 48 hours after hospitalization—are associated with fewer complications and shorter hospital stays as compared with delayed feedings.[17] If enteral nutrition is not possible, malnourished patients may receive parenteral nutrition support soon after admission to the hospital. In previously healthy patients, however, parenteral nutrition support may be withheld during the first seven days of hospitalization to avoid the risk of infectious complications.

Once patients can tolerate oral feedings, a high-kcalorie, high-protein diet is often prescribed, although care must be taken not to overfeed patients who are at risk of developing refeeding syndrome or hyperglycemia. Because meeting protein and energy needs may be difficult, nutrient-dense formulas or other supplements may be added to the diet (see Box 16-7). Some supplements may contain extra amounts of nutrients believed to promote healing or benefit immune function, such as the amino acids arginine and glutamine, omega-3 fatty acids, and the antioxidant nutrients. Nutrient needs should be reassessed frequently as the patient's condition improves. The Case Study in Box 16-8 reviews the nutrition care of a patient undergoing acute metabolic stress.

BOX 16-7 *Nursing Diagnosis*

The nursing diagnosis *imbalanced nutrition: less than body requirements* may apply to a patient recovering from acute stress.

Box 16-8   **Case Study: Patient with a Severe Burn**

David Bray, a 42-year-old man, has been admitted to intensive care. He suffered a severe burn covering 35 percent of his body when he was trapped inside a burning building. His wife told the nurse that Mr. Bray's height is 6 feet and that he usually weighs about 175 pounds. The physician ordered lab work, including serum protein concentrations, but the results are not yet available.

1. Identify Mr. Bray's immediate needs after the injury. Describe the initial concerns of the health care team and the measures they might take soon after Mr. Bray's arrival at the hospital.

2. Considering Mr. Bray's condition, what problems might the health care team encounter when they attempt to obtain information that can help them assess his nutrition status? What additional concerns might they have if Mr. Bray was malnourished before he experienced the burn?

3. Estimate Mr. Bray's energy and protein needs (use a protein factor of 2.0 grams per kilogram of body weight). What problems may interfere with Mr. Bray's ability to meet his nutrient needs?

4. After Mr. Bray transitions to oral feedings, he is able to obtain only 65 percent of his energy requirements. What other feeding options may be considered?

Review Notes

- Severe metabolic stress can cause hypermetabolism, negative nitrogen balance, hyperglycemia, and wasting. The objectives of nutrition care are to preserve muscle tissue, maintain immune defenses, and promote healing.

- To determine the energy needs of patients with acute illness, indirect calorimetry is recommended; otherwise, predictive equations may be used to estimate RMR or energy requirements.

- Protein recommendations during acute stress are higher than RDA levels to help prevent tissue losses and allow the healing of damaged tissue. Carbohydrates and lipids provide most of the patient's energy needs.

- Enteral or parenteral nutrition support or oral supplements may be used to meet the high nutrient needs of acutely stressed patients.

16.3 Nutrition and Respiratory Stress

Some medical problems upset the process of gas exchange between the air and blood and result in respiratory stress, which is characterized by a reduction in the blood's oxygen supply and an increase in carbon dioxide levels. Excessive carbon dioxide in the blood may disturb the breathing pattern enough to interfere with food intake. Moreover, the labored breathing caused by many respiratory disorders entails a higher energy cost than normal breathing does, raising energy needs and increasing carbon dioxide production further. Lung diseases make physical activity difficult and can lead to muscle wasting. Weight loss and malnutrition therefore become dangerous outcomes of some types of respiratory illnesses.

Chronic Obstructive Pulmonary Disease

Chronic obstructive pulmonary disease (COPD) refers to a group of conditions characterized by the persistent obstruction of airflow through the lungs. Figure 16-2 illustrates the main airways (**bronchi** and **bronchioles**) and air sacs (**alveoli**) of the normal respiratory system, and Figure 16-3 shows how they are altered in **chronic bronchitis** and **emphysema**,

chronic obstructive pulmonary disease (COPD): a group of lung diseases characterized by persistent obstructed airflow through the lungs and airways; includes chronic bronchitis and emphysema.

bronchi (BRON-key), **bronchioles** (BRON-key-oles): the main airways of the lungs. The singular form of bronchi is *bronchus*.

alveoli (al-VEE-oh-lee): air sacs in the lungs. One air sac is an *alveolus*.

chronic bronchitis (bron-KYE-tis): a lung disorder characterized by persistent inflammation and excessive secretions of mucus in the main airways of the lungs.

emphysema (EM-fih-ZEE-mah): a progressive lung disease characterized by the breakdown of the lungs' elastic structure and destruction of the walls of the respiratory bronchioles and alveoli, reducing the surface area involved in respiration.

FIGURE 16-2 The Respiratory System

Inhaled air travels via the trachea to the bronchi and bronchioles, the major airways of the lungs. Oxygen and carbon dioxide are exchanged across the thin-walled alveoli, which are surrounded by capillaries.

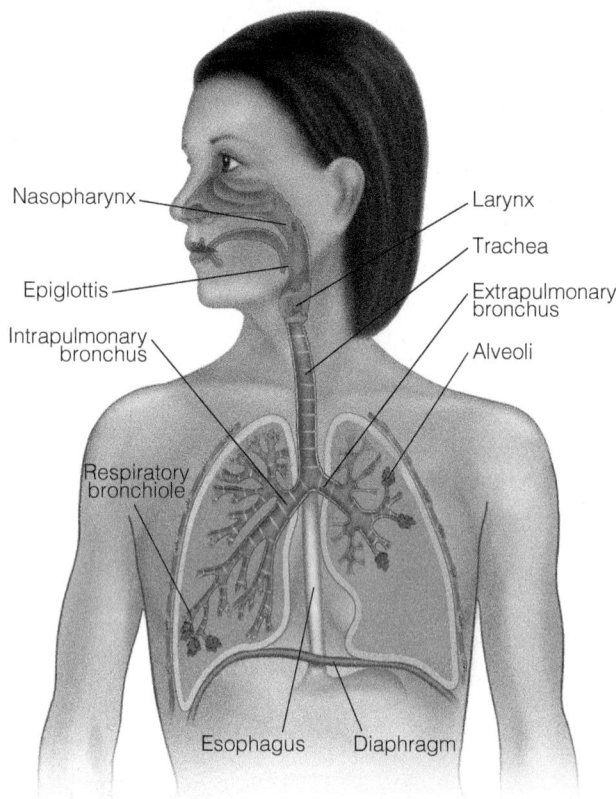

- Nasopharynx
- Epiglottis
- Intrapulmonary bronchus
- Respiratory bronchiole
- Larynx
- Trachea
- Extrapulmonary bronchus
- Alveoli
- Esophagus
- Diaphragm

Source: Based on a drawing in Carol Mattson Port, *Pathophysiology,* 5th ed. (Lippincott Williams & Wilkins, 1998). From Rolfes/Pinna/Whitney, *Understanding Normal and Clinical Nutrition,* 9E. © 2012 Cengage Learning.

the two main types of COPD. Note that most COPD patients display features of both of these conditions:[18]

- *Chronic bronchitis* is characterized by persistent inflammation and excessive secretions of mucus in the airways of the lungs, which may ultimately thicken and become too narrow for adequate mucus clearance. Chronic bronchitis may be diagnosed when a chronic, productive cough persists for at least three consecutive months in at least two consecutive years.
- *Emphysema* is characterized by the breakdown of the lungs' elastic structure and destruction of the walls of the smallest bronchioles and alveoli, changes that significantly reduce the surface area available for respiration. Emphysema is diagnosed on the basis of clinical signs and the results of lung function tests.

Both chronic bronchitis and emphysema are associated with abnormal levels of oxygen and carbon dioxide in the blood and shortness of breath (**dyspnea**). COPD may eventually lead to respiratory or heart failure and, together with other chronic respiratory illnesses, ranks as the third leading cause of death in the United States.[19]

COPD is a debilitating condition. Generally, dyspnea worsens as the disease progresses, resulting in dramatic reductions in physical activity and quality of life (see Box 16-9). Activities of daily living such as bathing or dressing may cause exhaustion or breathlessness. Weight loss and wasting are common in the advanced stages of disease and may result from hypermetabolism, poor food intake, and the actions of various inflammatory proteins.

FIGURE 16-3 Chronic Obstructive Pulmonary Disease

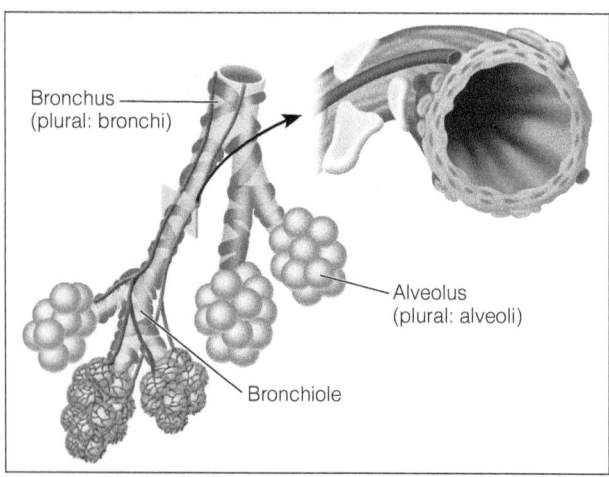

- Bronchus (plural: bronchi)
- Alveolus (plural: alveoli)
- Bronchiole

Healthy bronchi provide an open passageway for air. Healthy alveoli permit gas exchange between the air and blood.

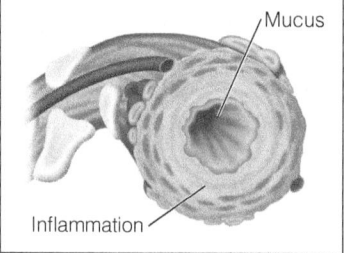

- Mucus
- Inflammation

Chronic bronchitis is characterized by inflammation, excessive secretion of mucus, and narrowing of the airways—factors that reduce normal airflow.

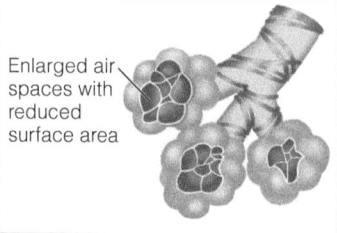

- Enlarged air spaces with reduced surface area

Emphysema is characterized by gradual destruction of the walls separating the alveoli and reduced lung elasticity.

© Wadsworth, Cengage Learning

Causes of COPD Cigarette smoking is the primary risk factor for COPD; about 35 to 50 percent of heavy smokers develop the condition.[20] Other risk factors include the repeated exposure to environmental or occupational pollutants and various genetic factors. Alpha-1-antitrypsin deficiency, an inherited disorder, accounts for 1 to 2 percent of COPD cases; individuals with this defect have inadequate blood levels of a plasma protein (alpha-1-antitrypsin) that normally inhibits the enzymatic break-down of lung tissue.[21]

Treatment of COPD The primary objectives of COPD treatment are to prevent the disease from progressing and to relieve major symptoms (dyspnea and coughing). Individuals with COPD are encouraged to quit smoking to prevent disease progression and to get vaccinated against influenza and pneumonia to avoid complications. The most frequently prescribed medications are bronchodilators, which improve airflow, and corticosteroids (anti-inflammatory medications), which help to relieve symptoms and prevent exacerbations; note that corticosteroids promote catabolic processes and can exacerbate the muscle loss that often accompanies COPD. For people with severe COPD, supplemental oxygen therapy (18 hours daily) can maintain normal oxygen levels in the blood and reduce mortality risk (see Photo 16-2). Box 16-10 lists nutrition-related effects of the medications used to treat COPD.

Nutrition Therapy for COPD The main goals of nutrition therapy for COPD are to correct malnutrition (which affects up to 60 percent of COPD patients[22]), promote the maintenance of a healthy body weight, and prevent muscle wasting. Energy needs of COPD patients are usually increased because of hypermetabolism (about 20 percent above normal), which results from chronic inflammation and the increased work-load of respiratory muscles.[23] Because underweight COPD patients have higher mortality rates, encouraging adequate food intake is generally the main focus of the nutrition care plan. Conversely, excess body weight places an additional strain on the respiratory system, and so COPD patients who are overweight or obese may benefit from energy restriction and gradual weight reduction.

Food intake often declines as COPD progresses, although the causes of poor intake vary among patients. Dyspnea may interfere with chewing or swallowing. Physical changes in the lungs and diaphragm may reduce abdominal volume, leading to early satiety. Appetite may be reduced by medications, depression, or altered taste perception (which may be due to the use of bronchodilators or the mouth dryness caused by chronic mouth breathing). Some patients may become too

dyspnea (DISP-nee-ah): shortness of breath.

Photo 16-2 Oxygen Therapy

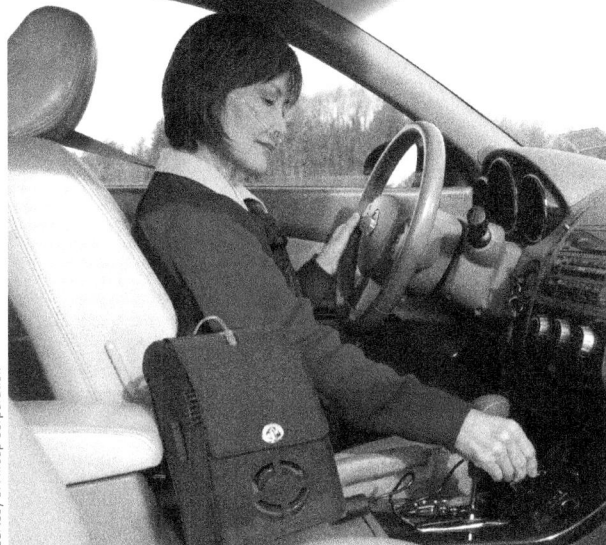

Courtesy of Airsep Corporation

Patients who need supplemental oxygen can use lightweight, portable equipment that allows them to move around freely. Although many patients use pre-filled oxygen tanks when traveling, portable oxygen concentrators—which produce oxygen from the surrounding air—are also available.

Box 16-10 Diet-Drug Interactions

Check this table for notable nutrition-related effects of the medications discussed in this chapter.

Bronchodilators (albuterol, salmeterol, ipratropium, tiotropium)	**Gastrointestinal effects:** dry mouth (ipratropium, tiotropium), altered taste sensation
	Metabolic effect: mild hypokalemia (albuterol, salmeterol)
Corticosteroids (inhaled) (fluticasone, beclomethasone)	**Gastrointestinal effect:** altered taste sensation
	Metabolic effect: low bone density

disabled to shop or prepare food or may lack adequate support at home. The clinician must assess the unique needs of a COPD patient before proposing a nutrition care plan.

Some patients may benefit from eating small, frequent meals spaced throughout the day rather than two or three large ones. The lower energy content of small meals reduces the carbon dioxide load, and the smaller meals may produce less abdominal discomfort and dyspnea. Some individuals may eat better if they receive supplemental oxygen at mealtimes. Consuming adequate fluids should be encouraged to help prevent the secretion of overly thick mucus; however, some patients should consume liquids between meals so as not to interfere with food intake. For undernourished persons, a high-kcalorie, high-protein diet may be helpful, but excessive energy intakes increase the amount of carbon dioxide produced and can increase respiratory stress. Oral supplements may be recommended as between-meal snacks to improve weight gain or endurance, but patients should be cautioned not to consume amounts that reduce energy intake at mealtime.

Pulmonary Formulas Enteral formulas designed for use in COPD provide more kcalories from fat and fewer from carbohydrate than standard formulas. The ratio of carbon dioxide production to oxygen consumption is lower when fat is consumed, so theoretically these formulas should lower respiratory requirements. However, research studies have not confirmed that the reduced-carbohydrate formulas improve clinical outcomes more than moderate energy intakes.[24]

Incorporating an Exercise Program Loss of muscle can be more readily prevented or reversed if the treatment plan includes an effective exercise program. With exercise, patients are likely to see improvements in their strength, endurance, and ability to perform activities of daily living. Both aerobic training and resistance exercise can be beneficial.[25] Some patients may need to increase activity gradually over a period of four to six weeks before reaching exercise goals.[26] The Case Study in Box 16-11 allows you to review the nutrition care for a patient with COPD.

Respiratory Failure

In **respiratory failure**, the gas exchange between the air and circulating blood is severely impaired, resulting in abnormal levels of tissue gases that can be life-threatening. Any of a large number of conditions that cause lung injury or impair lung function can be the underlying cause of failure; examples include infection (such as pneumonia or sepsis), physical trauma, neuromuscular disorders, aspiration of stomach contents, smoke inhalation, and airway obstruction.[27]

If an acute lung injury causes enough damage that emergency care is required to restore normal oxygen and carbon dioxide levels, the condition is known as **acute respiratory distress syndrome (ARDS)**. In ARDS, the lungs exhibit extensive

---

Box 16-11 | Case Study: Elderly Man with Emphysema

John Todaro is an 84-year-old man who has severe emphysema that affects both lungs. He is 5 feet 9 inches tall and currently weighs 150 pounds, about 20 pounds less than his weight in earlier years. He lives with a daughter and son-in-law and eats meals with their family. He becomes breathless when eating and when walking around the house, and he feels tired much of the time. A medical clinic recently ordered oxygen therapy for home use, but supplies have not yet arrived. Mr. Todaro's daughter is concerned about her father's recent weight loss and breathlessness.

1. Assess Mr. Todaro's risk of malnutrition, using information from Table 13-8 in Chapter 13 (p. 392). What factors may have contributed to his weight loss?

2. What are possible reasons for Mr. Todaro's difficulty with eating? List some dietary suggestions that may help to improve his appetite and food intake. How might the use of oxygen therapy help?

3. Based on the history given, what factors may account for Mr. Todaro's tiredness? What suggestions would you give Mr. Todaro and his daughter regarding physical activity?

inflammation and fluid buildup (called *pulmonary edema*) that interfere with lung ventilation and damage the alveoli. Later stages of ARDS are associated with a proliferation of lung cells, resulting in fibrosis and disrupted lung structure. A dangerous complication of ARDS is the progression to multiple organ dysfunction syndrome, described in the Nutrition in Practice following this chapter.

Consequences of Respiratory Failure Respiratory failure is characterized by severe **hypoxemia** (insufficient oxygen in the blood) and **hypercapnia** (excessive carbon dioxide in the blood). Inadequate oxygen in body tissues (**hypoxia**) can impede cellular function and lead to cell death. Severe hypercapnia can cause **acidosis**, which interferes with normal functioning of the central nervous system. To compensate for respiratory failure, a person breathes more rapidly, and the heart rate increases. The skin may become sweaty and develop a bluish cast (**cyanosis**). Headache, confusion, and drowsiness may occur. Severe cases of respiratory failure can cause heart arrhythmias and, ultimately, coma.

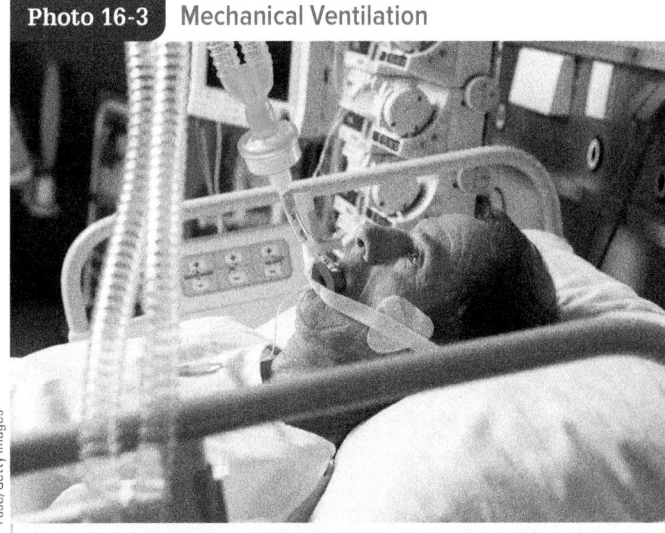

Photo 16-3 Mechanical Ventilation

Mechanical ventilation assists or replaces spontaneous breathing, thereby substituting for a patient's failing lungs. In this photo, a tube has been inserted into the patient's trachea via the mouth, and the ventilator controls the rate of breathing and volume of oxygen supplied to the patient's lungs.

Treatment of Respiratory Failure The treatment of respiratory failure focuses on supporting lung function and correcting the underlying disorder. Because respiratory failure can be caused by a number of different conditions, treatment plans vary considerably. Individuals with chronic lung disorders may be provided with oxygen therapy via a face mask or nasal tubing to relieve symptoms, whereas patients with ARDS receive mechanical ventilation until they are able to breathe independently (see Photo 16-3). Diuretics may be prescribed to help remove the fluid that has accumulated in lung tissue; other medications are provided to treat infections, keep airways open, or relieve inflammation. Complications are common in ARDS and must be forestalled to prevent multiple organ dysfunction.

Nutrition Therapy for Respiratory Failure Patients with lung injuries or ARDS are frequently hypermetabolic and/or catabolic and at high risk of muscle wasting.[28] The primary concerns are therefore to provide enough energy and protein to sustain muscle tissue and lung function without overtaxing the respiratory system. Fluid restrictions may be necessary to help correct pulmonary edema. As usual, when nutrition support is necessary, enteral nutrition is preferred over parenteral nutrition. Specific recommendations for respiratory failure include the following:

- *Energy*. Energy needs can be estimated using either indirect calorimetry or predictive equations such as those described earlier in this chapter; the body weight used in predictive equations may need to be corrected for pulmonary edema. Overfeeding should be avoided because it can cause excessive carbon dioxide production and worsen respiratory function.
- *Protein*. Protein requirements are increased in patients with lung inflammation or ARDS. For mild or moderate lung injury, protein recommendations range from 1.0 to 1.5 grams of protein per kilogram of body weight per day. Patients with ARDS may require 1.5 to 2 grams of protein per kilogram of body weight daily.[29]
- *Fluids*. Although most patients have normal fluid requirements, fluid status should be monitored daily to prevent fluid imbalances. Some patients may require fluid restriction to prevent or correct edema in lung tissue, whereas others may become

hypoxemia (high-pock-SEE-me-ah): insufficient oxygen in the blood.

hypercapnia (high-per-CAP-nee-ah): excessive carbon dioxide in the blood.

hypoxia (high-POCK-see-ah): insufficient oxygen in body tissues.

acidosis: acid accumulation in body tissues; depresses the central nervous system and may lead to disorientation and, eventually, coma.

cyanosis (sigh-ah-NOH-sis): a bluish cast in the skin due to the color of deoxygenated hemoglobin. Cyanosis is most evident in individuals with lighter, thinner skin; it is mostly seen on lips, cheeks, and ears and under the nails.

dehydrated because of diuretic therapy, an increase in bronchial secretions, or a low fluid intake. The presence of edema can make it difficult to assess whether a critically ill patient is maintaining weight.

Nutrition Support in Respiratory Failure Patients with severe cases of respiratory failure may be unable to eat meals and may require nutrition support. Enteral nutrition is used if the intestine is functional, and intestinal feedings may be preferred over gastric feedings because they reduce the risk of aspiration. Nutrient-dense formulas (1.5 to 2.0 kcalories per milliliter) are prescribed for patients with fluid restrictions.[30] Patients with acute lung injuries or ARDS are sometimes given enteral formulas fortified with omega-3 fatty acids and antioxidant nutrients in an effort to reduce inflammation and promote healing; however, some research suggests that the formulas are unlikely to improve clinical endpoints and may possibly increase mortality.[31] If the risk of aspiration is too high to continue enteral feedings, parenteral nutrition support may be considered.

Review Notes

- Chronic obstructive pulmonary disease (COPD) is a debilitating, progressive type of illness that can lead to malnutrition, muscle wasting, and activity intolerance. The main categories of COPD are chronic bronchitis and emphysema.
- The goals of nutrition therapy for COPD are to improve food intake, maintain proper weight, preserve muscle tissue, and improve exercise endurance.
- Respiratory failure, characterized by severe hypoxemia and hypercapnia, can result from conditions that cause lung injury or impair lung function. Acute respiratory distress syndrome is a severe form of respiratory failure that requires emergency care.
- Goals of nutrition therapy for respiratory failure are to provide enough energy and protein to support lung function without burdening the respiratory system. Fluid restrictions may be necessary to prevent or reverse pulmonary edema.

Nutrition Assessment Checklist for People Undergoing Metabolic or Respiratory Stress

MEDICAL HISTORY

Check the medical record to determine:

- ○ Cause of stress
- ○ Severity of stress
- ○ Whether any organ system is compromised
- ○ Whether nutrition support is required

For patients with COPD, check to determine:

- ○ Degree of breathing difficulty
- ○ Use of oxygen therapy
- ○ Activity tolerance

Review the medical record for complications related to underfeeding or overfeeding, such as:

- ○ Dehydration or fluid overload
- ○ Electrolyte imbalances
- ○ Fatty liver
- ○ Hyperglycemia
- ○ Hypertriglyceridemia

MEDICATIONS

Record all medications and note:

- ○ Side effects that may alter food intake or nutrition status

DIETARY INTAKE

If the patient is not meeting nutrition goals:

- ○ Monitor intakes to ensure that the patient is receiving the diet prescribed.
- ○ Investigate appetite problems or difficulties with eating.
- ○ Consider interventions to improve food intake.
- ○ Consider the need for oral supplements.

○ In patients with COPD, consider problems that may hamper the patient's ability to prepare or consume foods.

ANTHROPOMETRIC DATA

Measure baseline height and weight, and monitor daily weights. Remember that body weight can fluctuate in acutely ill patients who undergo fluid resuscitation. After the patient's weight has stabilized:

○ Reevaluate protein and energy needs.
○ Consider the need to alter the energy prescription to meet weight goals.

LABORATORY TESTS

Laboratory tests that may be affected by stress and therefore require careful interpretation include:

○ Albumin
○ C-reactive protein
○ Serum iron and zinc
○ Transferrin
○ Transthyretin
○ White blood cell count

Monitor laboratory tests for signs of:

○ Dehydration or fluid overload
○ Electrolyte and acid–base imbalances
○ Hyperglycemia
○ Hypertriglyceridemia
○ Nutrient deficiencies
○ Negative nitrogen balance
○ Organ dysfunction or organ function that has normalized

PHYSICAL SIGNS

Regularly assess vital signs, including:

○ Blood pressure
○ Body temperature
○ Pulse
○ Respiratory rate

Look for physical signs of:

○ Protein-energy malnutrition
○ Dehydration or fluid overload
○ Nutrient deficiencies and excesses

Self Check

1. Which of the following metabolic changes accompanies acute stress?
   a. Hypoglycemia
   b. Reduced heart and respiratory rates
   c. Elevated immune responses
   d. Muscle protein catabolism

2. After an injury occurs, typical changes in the damaged tissue include all of the following *except*:
   a. reduced capillary permeability.
   b. increased blood flow.
   c. warmth.
   d. fluid accumulation.

3. How do nonsteroidal anti-inflammatory drugs suppress inflammatory processes?
   a. They interfere with histamine secretion.
   b. They inhibit eicosanoid synthesis.
   c. They impair the actions of certain cytokines.
   d. They inhibit the absorption of omega-6 fatty acids.

4. Examples of acute-phase proteins include all of the following *except*:
   a. C-reactive protein.
   b. hepcidin.
   c. albumin.
   d. fibrinogen.

5. Which of the following statements concerning protein and energy recommendations during acute metabolic stress is true?
   a. Protein and energy recommendations are similar to those for healthy people.
   b. Protein and energy requirements are reduced because a stressed individual cannot metabolize nutrients normally.
   c. Acutely stressed individuals can benefit from as much protein and energy as can be provided.
   d. Protein and energy requirements are often increased to minimize muscle tissue losses.

6. Hypocaloric feedings may benefit critical care patients who are:
   a. elderly.
   b. obese.
   c. receiving mechanical ventilation.
   d. accumulating fluid.

7. The primary risk factor for COPD is:
   a. alpha-1-antitrypsin deficiency.
   b. occupational exposure to dusts or chemicals.
   c. cigarette smoking.
   d. frequent respiratory infections.

8. A primary feature of emphysema is:
   a. obstruction within the bronchi.
   b. a chronic, productive cough.
   c. destruction of the walls separating the alveoli.
   d. excessive lung elasticity.

9. The weight loss and wasting that often occur in COPD can be caused by:
   a. reduced food intake.
   b. increased metabolic rate.
   c. reduced exercise tolerance.
   d. all of the above.

10. Nutrition therapy for a person with respiratory failure includes:
    a. careful attention to providing enough, but not too much, energy.
    b. a generous fluid intake to facilitate mucus clearance.
    c. a high fat intake to help prevent weight loss and wasting.
    d. a high carbohydrate intake to increase carbon dioxide production.

Answers: 1.d, 2.a, 3.b, 4.c, 5.d, 6.b, 7.c, 8.c, 9.d, 10.a

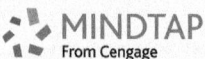

For more chapter resources visit **www.cengage.com** to access MindTap, a complete digital course.

Clinical Applications

1. Adam is a 29-year-old male who is 6 feet 2 inches tall and has a usual body weight of 180 pounds. He underwent emergency surgery following a serious injury and is now being cared for in the intensive care unit, where he is receiving mechanical ventilation. His minute ventilation is about 9.0 liters per minute and his maximum temperature over the past day was 98.6 degrees Fahrenheit. Using the Penn State equation shown in Table 16-2, estimate Adam's energy requirement. Estimate his protein requirement, using the factor 1.5 grams per kilogram of body weight.

2. Ayesha is a 23-year-old law student who was admitted to the hospital following an automobile accident in which she broke several bones and ruptured part of her small intestine. She has been in the hospital for several weeks and has just begun eating table foods. Her brother, who was driving the vehicle, was also seriously injured and nearly lost his life. Aside from the increased nutritional needs imposed by the stress of the accident, discuss how the following factors might interfere with Ayesha's ability to improve her nutrition status:
   • Ayesha's injuries are painful.
   • Ayesha's medications cause drowsiness.
   • Ayesha is depressed.
   • Ayesha is often out of her room for X-rays and other diagnostic tests when the menus and food trays arrive.
   • Ayesha's food intake is sometimes restricted due to the procedures she is undergoing.

   How might these problems be resolved to improve Ayesha's food intake?

Notes

1. S. F. Lowry and S. M. Coyle, Hypercatabolic states, in A. C. Ross and coeditors, *Modern Nutrition in Health and Disease* (Baltimore: Lippincott Williams & Wilkins, 2014), pp. 1261–1272; P. A. Fitzgerald, Adrenal medulla and paraganglia, in D. G. Gardner and D. Shoback, eds., *Greenspan's Basic & Clinical Endocrinology* (New York: McGraw-Hill, 2011), pp. 345–393; T. B. Carroll and coauthors, Glucocorticoids and adrenal androgens, in D. G. Gardner and D. Shoback, eds., *Greenspan's Basic & Clinical Endocrinology* (New York: McGraw-Hill, 2011), pp. 285–327.

2. P. C. Calder, Mechanisms of action of (n-3) fatty acids, *Journal of Nutrition* 142 (2012): 592S–599S.

3. G. H. Johnson and K. Fritsche, Effect of dietary linoleic acid on markers of inflammation in healthy persons: A systematic review of randomized controlled trials, *Journal of the Academy of Nutrition and Dietetics* 112 (2012): 1029–1041.

4. V. Kumar, A. K. Abbas, and J. C. Aster, Inflammation and repair, in V. Kumar and coeditors, *Robbins and Cotran Pathologic Basis of Disease* (Philadelphia: Saunders, 2015), pp. 69–111; D. S. Pisetsky,

Laboratory testing in the rheumatic diseases, in L. Goldman and A. I. Schafer, eds., *Goldman's Cecil Medicine* (Philadelphia: Saunders, 2012), pp. 1651–1656.

5. K. M. Schlein and S. P. Coulter, Best practices for determining resting energy expenditure in critically ill adults, *Nutrition in Clinical Practice* 29 (2014): 44–55.

6. D. Frankenfield, Energy expenditure in the critically ill patient, in G. A. Cresci, ed., *Nutrition for the Critically Ill Patient* (Boca Raton, FL: CRC Press, 2015), pp. 93–110.

7. K. R. Maday, Energy estimation in the critically ill: A literature review, *Universal Journal of Clinical Medicine* 1 (2013): 39–43.

8. S. A. McClave and coauthors, Guidelines for the provision and assessment of nutrition support therapy in the adult critically ill patient: Society of Critical Care Medicine (SCCM) and American Society for Parenteral and Enteral Nutrition (A.S.P.E.N.), *Journal of Parenteral and Enteral Nutrition* 40 (2016): 159–211.

9. McClave and coauthors, 2016; P. Choban and coauthors and the American Society for Parenteral and Enteral Nutrition, A.S.P.E.N. clinical guidelines:

Nutrition support of hospitalized adult patients with obesity, *Journal of Parenteral and Enteral Nutrition* (2013): 714–744.

10. McClave and coauthors, 2016.

11. McClave and coauthors, 2016; P. Choban and coauthors and the American Society for Parenteral and Enteral Nutrition, 2013.

12. L. Bollhalder and coauthors, A systematic literature review and meta-analysis of randomized clinical trials of parenteral glutamine supplements, *Clinical Nutrition* 32 (2013): 213–223.

13. D. K. Heyland and coauthors, Glutamine and antioxidants in the critically ill patient: A post hoc analysis of a large-scale randomized trial, *Journal of Parenteral and Enteral Nutrition* 39 (2015): 401–409.

14. P. E. Wischmeyer, Evolution of nutrition in critical care: How much, how soon? *Critical Care* 17 (2013): S7, doi: 10.1186/cc11505.

15. K. A. Kudsk, Nutrition support for the patient with surgery, trauma, or sepsis, in A. C. Ross and coeditors, *Modern Nutrition in Health and Disease* (Baltimore: Lippincott Williams & Wilkins, 2014), pp. 1273–1288.

16. K. Sriram, Micronutrient and antioxidant therapy in adult critically ill patients, in G. A. Cresci, ed., *Nutrition for the Critically Ill Patient* (Boca Raton, FL: CRC Press, 2015), pp. 124–137; Kudsk, 2014.

17. McClave and coauthors, 2016.

18. A. N. Husain, The lung, in V. Kumar and coeditors, *Robbins and Cotran Pathologic Basis of Disease* (Philadelphia: Saunders, 2015), pp. 669–726.

19. National Center for Health Statistics, *Health, United States, 2016: With Chartbook on Long-Term Trends in Health* (Hyattsville, MD: National Center for Health Statistics, 2017).

20. Husain, 2015.

21. D. E. Niewoehner, Chronic obstructive pulmonary disease, in L. Goldman and A. I. Schafer, eds., *Goldman-Cecil Medicine* (Philadelphia: Saunders, 2016), pp. 555–562.

22. N. M. Patel and M. M. Johnson, Nutrition in respiratory diseases, in A. C. Ross and coeditors, *Modern Nutrition in Health and Disease* (Baltimore: Lippincott Williams & Wilkins, 2014), pp. 1385–1395.

23. C. C. Kao, Resting energy expenditure and protein turnover are increased in patients with severe chronic obstructive pulmonary disease, *Metabolism* 60 (2011): 1449–1455; R. A. Wise, Chronic obstructive pulmonary disease, in R. S. Porter and J. L. Kaplan, eds., *Merck Manual of Diagnosis and Therapy* (Whitehouse Station, NJ: Merck Sharp and Dohme Corp., 2011), pp. 1889–1902.

24. A. A. Matos, W. Manzanares, and V. S. Nava, Nutrition support for pulmonary failure, in G. A. Cresci, ed., *Nutrition for the Critically Ill Patient* (Boca Raton, FL: CRC Press, 2015), pp. 467–482; A. Malone, Enteral formula selection, in P. Charney and A. Malone, eds., *Pocket Guide to Enteral Nutrition* (Chicago: Academy of Nutrition and Dietetics, 2013), pp. 120–152.

25. F. Maltais and coauthors, An official American Thoracic Society/European Respiratory Society statement: Update on limb muscle dysfunction in chronic obstructive pulmonary disease, *American Journal of Respiratory and Critical Care Medicine* 189 (2014): e15–e62; W. D. Reid and coauthors, Exercise prescription for hospitalized people with chronic obstructive pulmonary disease and comorbidities: A synthesis of systematic reviews, *International Journal of COPD* 7 (2012): 297–320.

26. Wise, 2011.

27. M. A. Matthay and A. S. Slutsky, Acute respiratory failure, in L. Goldman and A. I. Schafer, eds., *Goldman-Cecil Medicine* (Philadelphia: Saunders, 2016), pp. 655–664.

28. Patel and Johnson, 2014.

29. Academy of Nutrition and Dietetics, *Nutrition Care Manual* (Chicago: Academy of Nutrition and Dietetics, 2018); Matos, Manzanares, and Nava, 2015.

30. McClave and coauthors, 2016.

31. A. R. H. van Zanten and coauthors, High-protein enteral nutrition enriched with immune-modulating nutrients vs. standard high-protein enteral nutrition and nosocomial infections in the ICU, *Journal of the American Medical Association* 312 (2014): 514–524.

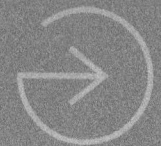

16.4 Nutrition in Practice

Multiple Organ Dysfunction Syndrome

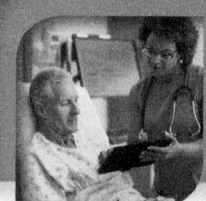

Multiple organ dysfunction syndrome (MODS), also called *multiple organ failure*, is a frequent cause of death in critically ill patients. Described as the progressive dysfunction of two or more of the body's organ systems, MODS most often involves the lungs, kidneys, and liver. MODS is not a disease *per se*, but rather a late stage of severe illness or injury that results from a severe inflammatory response (discussed in Chapter 16). MODS can be initiated by a number of very different critical illnesses and conditions, including respiratory failure, sepsis, burn injuries, trauma, and pancreatitis. This Nutrition in Practice discusses how MODS develops, the manner in which it is treated, and the importance of its prevention.

How long has MODS been a major clinical problem?

MODS was recognized as a clinical entity only after World War II. Prior to the mid-20th century, patients with severe illnesses or multiple injuries frequently died of shock or circulatory failure. After fluid replacement and blood transfusions became standard treatments, the kidneys became the organs at highest risk, and kidney failure became the most common cause of death. Eventually, physicians learned to better support kidney function by providing appropriate electrolyte solutions and improving urine output. With improved kidney care, the lungs became the most vulnerable organ after severe injury. Improved treatment of respiratory failure eventually led to the current situation: advances in critical care allow patients to survive severe illnesses and injuries, but the body's defenses often overburden organs that were not originally injured.

Why does critical illness sometimes lead to MODS?

As discussed earlier in Chapter 16, injury and infection cause the release of chemical mediators that have systemic (whole body) effects. A severe, persistent inflammatory response can lead to the systemic inflammatory response syndrome (SIRS), which is associated with a constellation of signs and symptoms including fever, raised heart and respiratory rates, and abnormal white blood cell counts. SIRS is a normal adaptive response to a severe insult, but if not reversed quickly enough it can progress to shock, which is characterized by extremely low blood pressure

and an inadequate blood supply for the tissues and organs of the body.[1]

As might be expected from a systemic reduction in blood availability, shock can impair numerous organ systems. The abnormal delivery of oxygen and nutrients to tissues and insufficient removal of wastes result in irreversible injury to cells and tissues. Although each organ system is affected differently, ultimately one or more organs may begin to fail. The failure of one organ may place excessive demands on another, causing the second to fail as well. The progression of SIRS to MODS reflects the inability of the body's defenses and medical treatments to counter the detrimental effects of a sustained and potent inflammatory response.

The specific pathophysiology of MODS is poorly understood. Although early reports attempted to link the development of MODS directly to sepsis, sepsis is not present in all cases. Infection often results from impaired immune function and therefore is a frequent consequence of MODS, but it is not necessarily the underlying trigger of organ dysfunction. Recall from this chapter that sepsis gives rise to signs and symptoms identical to those seen in SIRS. Figure NP16-1 illustrates the relationships among SIRS, infection, sepsis, and MODS.

Do organs fail in a specific pattern?

Although the clinical course of MODS differs substantially among patients, the sequence of organ dysfunction often follows a similar pattern: first the lungs fail, then the heart, and finally the liver, kidneys, and gastrointestinal tract.[2] Other organs or systems may also become involved, and each additional failure reduces the likelihood of survival. Table NP16-1 lists the organs and systems most often involved in MODS and the potential consequences of their failure.

Are there any risk factors for MODS?

Epidemiological studies have identified a number of factors that increase risk. For example, people who develop MODS are often older, have multiple or severe injuries, or are obese.[3] Table NP16-2 lists the major risk factors associated with MODS, some of which are discussed below:

- *Age.* Patients over 55 years old are several times more likely to develop MODS than are younger patients. In elderly patients, the increased risk may be due to the

FIGURE NP16-1 Relationships among SIRS, Sepsis, and Multiple Organ Dysfunction Syndrome

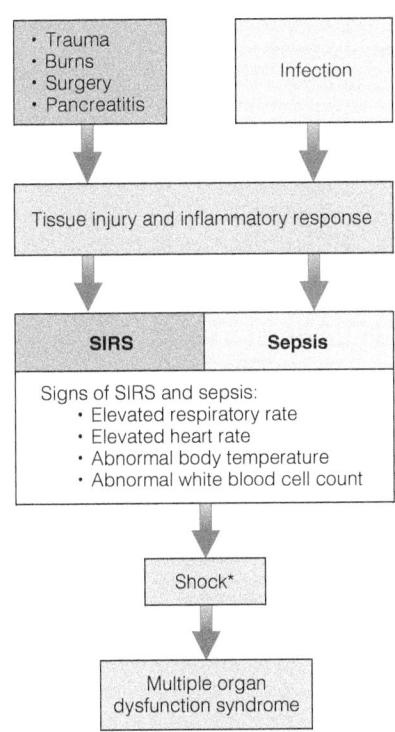

*After critical injury, shock may sometimes precede and be the cause of SIRS.

TABLE NP16-1 Physiological Effects of Organ or System Failure

ORGAN OR SYSTEM	EFFECTS OF FAILURE
Lungs	Inability to maintain gas exchange
Heart	Low cardiac output, low blood pressure, inadequate circulation, shock
Liver	Altered metabolic processes
Kidneys	Inability to regulate blood volume, maintain electrolytes, remove wastes
GI tract	Impaired digestion and absorption, abnormal bleeding, bacterial translocation
Immune system	Infection, sepsis
Coagulation system	Excessive bleeding or blood clotting
Central nervous system	Decreased perceptions, brain injury, coma

TABLE NP16-2 Factors That Influence Risk of Multiple Organ Dysfunction Syndrome

- Age over 55 years
- Obesity
- Prior chronic illness
- Persistent SIRS
- Major infection
- Blood transfusions
- Severity of tissue injury
- Length of time between injury and arrival at hospital
- Malnutrition

presence of chronic illnesses that directly affect organ function, such as heart disease, lung disease, diabetes, or liver damage. Aging also decreases the functional reserve of organs, thereby reducing an older patient's ability to deal with the additional stress that arises during critical illness.

- *Severity of SIRS.* The length of time that SIRS persists is related to the development of MODS. Patients who have SIRS that persists for more than three days are more likely to develop MODS than patients who have SIRS for less than two days.
- *Infection.* Prolonged SIRS can suppress immune function and increase the risk of developing an infection. During hospital stays, critically ill patients often contract pneumonia—the principal infection associated with MODS. The risks of infection and sepsis greatly increase with the use of invasive catheters, which are frequently needed during intensive care to provide oxygen support, intravenous fluid resuscitation, nutrition support, and urine clearance.
- *Blood transfusions.* Blood transfusions are immunosuppressive and may increase a patient's risks of developing infection or sepsis. Blood transfusions frequently have adverse effects that can add further stress; they may cause acute lung injury, allergic reactions, red blood cell hemolysis (breakdown), and other complications.

What is the treatment for MODS?

Once MODS has developed, extensive medical support is needed until the inflammatory response has abated. Unfortunately, aggressive treatments can have damaging effects of their own and may cause further injury to organs that are already weakened by illness. Health practitioners should therefore be aware of the adverse effects of aggressive therapies and remain alert to a patient's responses to treatments. Therapies that are often used to manage MODS include the following:[4]

- *Lung support.* Mechanical ventilation is used to assist injured lungs and sustain gas exchange.
- *Fluid resuscitation.* Fluids and electrolytes are supplied to restore blood volume and maintain electrolyte balance.
- *Support of heart and blood vessel function.* Medications help to sustain or increase cardiac output and maintain adequate blood pressure.
- *Kidney support.* Hemofiltration or dialysis helps to prevent the buildup of toxic metabolites in the blood.
- *Protection against infection.* Antibiotic therapy may reverse or prevent infections.
- *Nutrition support.* Enteral and parenteral nutrition support provide nutrients, help to prevent excessive wasting, and promote recovery.

What can be done to reduce the incidence of MODS?

Because mortality rates for MODS are so high, prevention must be considered at the earliest stages of injury and treatment, before an excessive inflammatory response can cause further damage. Health practitioners have learned to identify the conditions that can increase organ stress whether they are due to a disease process, an inflammatory response, or an aggressive treatment that is intended to provide organ support. Although improvements in care over the past few decades have reduced some of the complications that arise during intensive care, rates of mortality from MODS have not changed. Thus, a focus on prevention is critical until a better understanding of the pathophysiology of MODS is achieved, which may lead to additional therapeutic options.

Notes

1. J. A. Russell, Shock syndromes related to sepsis, in L. Goldman and A. I. Schafer, eds., *Goldman-Cecil Medicine* (Philadelphia: Saunders, 2016), pp. 685–691.
2. D. C. Dewar and coauthors, Post-injury multiple organ failure, *Trauma* 13 (2011): 81–91.
3. Dewar and coauthors, 2011.
4. Russell, 2016; D. J. Cook, Approach to the patient in a critical care setting, in L. Goldman and A. I. Schafer, eds., *Goldman-Cecil Medicine* (Philadelphia: Saunders, 2016), pp. 650–652.

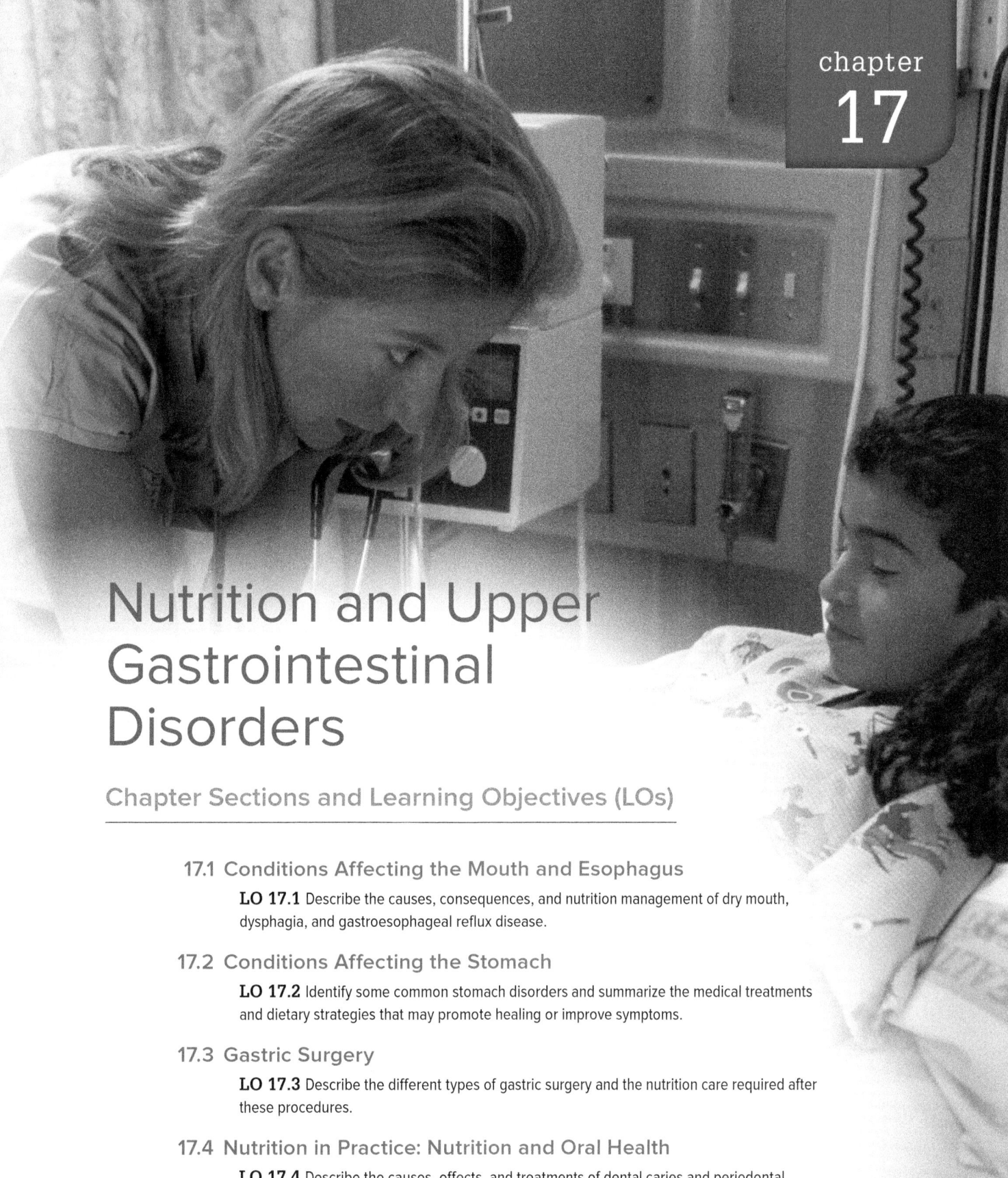

Chapter 17

Nutrition and Upper Gastrointestinal Disorders

Chapter Sections and Learning Objectives (LOs)

17.1 Conditions Affecting the Mouth and Esophagus

LO 17.1 Describe the causes, consequences, and nutrition management of dry mouth, dysphagia, and gastroesophageal reflux disease.

17.2 Conditions Affecting the Stomach

LO 17.2 Identify some common stomach disorders and summarize the medical treatments and dietary strategies that may promote healing or improve symptoms.

17.3 Gastric Surgery

LO 17.3 Describe the different types of gastric surgery and the nutrition care required after these procedures.

17.4 Nutrition in Practice: Nutrition and Oral Health

LO 17.4 Describe the causes, effects, and treatments of dental caries and periodontal disease and discuss the relationships between these conditions and chronic diseases.

Ryan McVay/Digital Vision/Getty Images

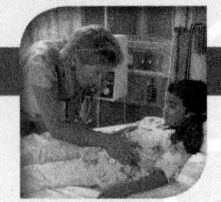

fraction of hospital admissions and visits to health practitioners each year. Diagnosis is not always straightforward, however, because many patients with GI complaints exhibit no physical abnormalities. Evaluation therefore requires a detailed review of a patient's symptoms and responses to dietary adjustments. Because GI complications frequently accompany other illnesses, the medical history can sometimes uncover the underlying source of distress.

17.1 Conditions Affecting the Mouth and Esophagus

Chapter 14 described several types of mechanically altered diets that can be used by individuals who have difficulty chewing and swallowing (see pp. 409–410). This section describes how to relieve the discomfort of dry mouth and examines the causes and treatments of the two most common disorders involving the esophagus: dysphagia (difficulty swallowing) and gastroesophageal reflux disease.

Dry Mouth

Dry mouth (**xerostomia**), caused by reduced salivary flow, is a side effect of many medications and is associated with a number of diseases and disease treatments.[1] Anticholinergics, antidepressants, antihistamines, antihypertensives, and other medications can cause dry mouth. Poorly controlled diabetes mellitus is often associated with dry mouth, as are conditions that directly affect salivary gland function, such as **Sjögren's syndrome**. Radiation therapy that treats head and neck cancers often damages salivary glands, sometimes permanently. Excessive mouth breathing is also a common cause of dry mouth.

Dry mouth can impair health in a variety of ways (see Box 17-1).[2] It can interfere with speaking and swallowing. Mouth infections, bad breath, and dental diseases are more common. Dentures may be uncomfortable to wear, and ulcerations may develop where they contact the mouth. Taste sensation is often diminished, and salty or spicy foods may cause pain. Dry mouth may cause a person to reduce food intake and may thereby increase malnutrition risk. Table 17-1 offers suggestions that can help to manage dry mouth.

Dysphagia

The act of swallowing involves multiple processes. In the initial, or **oropharyngeal**, phase of swallowing, muscles in the mouth and tongue propel the bolus of food through the pharynx and into the esophagus. At the same time, tissues of the soft palate prevent food from entering the nasal cavity, and the epiglottis blocks the opening to the trachea to prevent aspiration of food substances or saliva into the lungs. In the second, or **esophageal**, phase of swallowing, peristalsis forces the bolus through the esophagus, and the lower esophageal sphincter relaxes to allow passage of the bolus into the stomach. Because of the many tasks involved in swallowing, **dysphagia** can result from a number of different physical or neurological problems (see Box 17-2). Table 17-2 lists some potential causes of dysphagia, which are categorized according to the phase of swallowing that is impaired.[3]

A person with **oropharyngeal dysphagia** has difficulty transferring food from the mouth and pharynx to the esophagus. The condition is typically due to a neuromuscular or structural disorder that inhibits the swallowing reflex or impairs the strength or coordination of the muscles involved with swallowing. Symptoms include an inability to initiate swallowing, coughing during or after swallowing (due to aspiration), and

xerostomia (ZEE-roh-STOE-me-ah): dry mouth caused by reduced salivary flow.

xero = dry
stomia = mouth

Sjögren's (SHOW-grenz) **syndrome:** an autoimmune disease characterized by the destruction of secretory glands, resulting in dry mouth and dry eyes.

oropharyngeal (OR-row-fah-ren-JEE-al): involving the mouth and pharynx.

esophageal (eh-SOF-ah-JEE-al): involving the esophagus.

dysphagia (dis-FAY-jah): difficulty swallowing.

oropharyngeal dysphagia: difficulty transferring food from the mouth and pharynx to the esophagus to initiate the swallowing process; usually due to a neurological, muscular, or structural disorder.

TABLE 17-1 Suggestions for Managing Dry Mouth

FOOD AND BEVERAGE TIPS
- Take frequent sips of water or another sugarless beverage.
- Suck on ice cubes or frozen fruit juice bars (unless their coldness causes discomfort).
- Consume foods that have a high fluid content, such as soups, stews, sauces and gravies, yogurt, and pureed fruit.
- Avoid dry foods such as toast, chips, and crackers.
- Avoid citrus juices and spicy or salty foods if they cause mouth irritation.

LIFESTYLE PRACTICES
- Chew sugarless gum to help stimulate salivary flow.
- Avoid caffeine, alcohol, and smoking, which may dry the mouth.
- Use a humidifier during the night.

SALIVA SUBSTITUTES
- Use over-the-counter saliva substitutes (available as gels, sprays, and tablets), especially just before meals and at bedtime.
- Try rinsing the mouth with a teaspoonful of vegetable oil or softened margarine.

DENTAL CARE
- Pay strict attention to oral hygiene, brushing teeth and flossing at least twice daily. Try to brush immediately after each meal.
- Avoid alcohol- and detergent-containing mouthwashes that may dry and irritate the mouth.
- Ask your dentist about fluoride treatments that help to prevent tooth decay.

MEDICATIONS
- If dry mouth is caused by a medication, ask your physician about possible alternatives.
- Ask your physician whether using a medication to stimulate saliva secretion may be of benefit; examples include cevimeline (Evoxac) and pilocarpine (Salagen).

TABLE 17-2 Selected Causes of Dysphagia

OROPHARYNGEAL DYSPHAGIA
- Alzheimer's disease (advanced stages)
- Amyotrophic lateral sclerosis (Lou Gehrig's disease)
- Brain injury
- Cerebral palsy
- Multiple sclerosis
- Muscular dystrophy
- Myasthenia gravis
- Parkinson's disease
- Poliomyelitis
- Stroke

ESOPHAGEAL DYSPHAGIA
- Achalasia
- Esophageal cancer
- Esophageal spasm
- External compression (from a tumor, enlarged thyroid gland, or enlarged left atrium)
- Scleroderma
- Strictures (from inflammation, scarring, or a congenital abnormality)

nasal regurgitation. Other signs include a gurgling noise after swallowing, a hoarse or "wet" voice, or a speech disorder. Oropharyngeal dysphagia is common in older adults and frequently follows a stroke.

A person with **esophageal dysphagia** has difficulty passing materials through the esophageal lumen and into the stomach, usually due to an obstruction in the esophagus or a motility disorder. The main symptom is the sensation of food "sticking" in the esophagus after it is swallowed. An obstruction can be caused by a **stricture** (abnormal narrowing), tumor, or compression of the esophagus by surrounding tissues. Whereas an obstruction can prevent the passage of solid foods but may not affect liquids, a motility disorder hinders the passage of both solids and liquids. **Achalasia**, the most common motility disorder, is a degenerative nerve condition affecting the esophagus; it is characterized by the absence of peristalsis and impaired relaxation of the lower esophageal sphincter when swallowing.

Complications of Dysphagia Health practitioners should be alert to the various complications that may accompany dysphagia (see Box 17-3). If the condition restricts food consumption, malnutrition and weight loss may develop. Individuals who cannot swallow liquids are at increased risk of dehydration. If aspiration occurs, it may cause choking, airway obstruction, or respiratory infections, including pneumonia. If a person lacks a normal cough reflex, aspiration is more difficult to diagnose and may go unnoticed.

Nutrition Intervention for Dysphagia To compensate for swallowing difficulties, a person with dysphagia may need to consume foods and beverages that have been physically modified so that they are easier to swallow. Because a wide variety of defects can cause dysphagia, finding the best diet is often a challenge. Furthermore, a person's swallowing ability can fluctuate over time, so the dietary plan needs frequent reassessment.

BOX 17-3 Nursing Diagnosis

The nursing diagnoses *imbalanced nutrition: less than body requirements* and *risk for aspiration* often apply to a patient with dysphagia.

esophageal dysphagia: difficulty passing food through the esophagus; usually caused by an obstruction or a motility disorder.

stricture: abnormal narrowing of a passageway; often due to inflammation, scarring, or a congenital abnormality.

achalasia (ack-ah-LAY-zhah)**:** an esophageal disorder characterized by the absence of peristalsis and impaired relaxation of the lower esophageal sphincter.

a = without
chalasia = relaxation

The National Dysphagia Diet, developed in 2002 by a panel of dietitians, speech and language therapists, and a food scientist, has helped to standardize the nutrition care of dysphagia patients.[4] Table 17-3 presents brief descriptions of the different levels of the diet and some sample meals. After the appropriate dietary level is selected,

---

TABLE 17-3 National Dysphagia Diet

LEVEL 1: DYSPHAGIA PUREED

Foods should be pureed or well mashed, smooth (lump-free), and cohesive. This diet is for patients with moderate to severe dysphagia and poor oral or chewing ability.

Sample menus:

- *Breakfast:* Cream of Wheat, slurried muffins or pancakes,[a] pureed scrambled eggs, plain or vanilla yogurt, well-mashed bananas, fruit juice without pulp (thickened as needed), coffee or tea (if thin liquids are acceptable).

- *Lunch or dinner:* Pureed tomato soup, slurried crackers, pureed meat or poultry, zucchini soufflé, mashed potatoes with gravy, pureed carrots or green beans, smooth applesauce, pureed peaches, chocolate pudding.

Foods to avoid: Dry breads and cereals, oatmeal, rice, fruit yogurt, cheese (including cottage cheese), peanut butter, nuts and seeds, raw fruits and vegetables that have not been pureed, chunky applesauce, fruit preserves with chunks or seeds, tomato sauce with seeds, beverages with pulp, coarsely ground pepper, herbs.

LEVEL 2: DYSPHAGIA MECHANICALLY ALTERED

Foods should be moist, cohesive, and ground or soft-textured and should easily form a bolus. This diet is for patients with mild to moderate dysphagia; some chewing ability is required.

Sample menus:

- *Breakfast:* Moist oatmeal, cornflakes or puffed rice cereal with milk (thickened as needed), moist pancakes or muffins (with butter, margarine, or jam; without nuts or seeds), soft scrambled eggs, cottage cheese, ripe bananas or cooked fruit without skin or seeds, fruit juice (thickened as needed), coffee or tea (if thin liquids are allowed).

- *Lunch or dinner:* Soup with easy-to-chew meat and vegetables; slurried bread or crackers; minced, tender-cooked meat; well-cooked pasta with moist meatballs and tomato sauce; baked potato with gravy; soft, tender-cooked vegetables (not fibrous or rubbery); canned peach slices; soft fruit pie (with bottom crust only); soft, smooth chocolate bar.

Foods to avoid: Dry or coarse foods; breads and cereals with nuts, seeds, or dried fruit; frankfurters and sausages; hard-cooked eggs; corn and clam chowders; sandwiches; pizza; sliced cheese; rice; French fries; potato skins; undercooked vegetables; fibrous, rubbery, or non-tender cooked vegetables such as asparagus, broccoli, brussels sprouts, cabbage, celery, corn, and peas; peanut butter; coconut; nuts and seeds; fresh or frozen fruit (except banana); cooked fruit with skin or seeds; pineapple; mango; uncooked dried fruit; popcorn; chewy candies (such as caramel or licorice).

LEVEL 3: DYSPHAGIA ADVANCED

Foods should be moist and in bite-sized pieces when swallowed; foods with mixed textures are included. This diet is for patients with mild dysphagia and adequate chewing ability.

Sample menus:

- *Breakfast:* Cereal with milk, moist pancakes or muffins (with butter, margarine, or jam; without nuts or seeds), poached or scrambled eggs, fruit yogurt, soft fresh fruit (peeled) or berries, coffee or tea (if thin liquids are tolerated).

- *Lunch or dinner:* Chicken noodle soup; moistened crackers or moist bread; thin-sliced tender meat; cheese; moist, soft-cooked potatoes or rice; tender-cooked vegetables; shredded lettuce with dressing; fresh, peeled peach or melon; canned fruit salad; moist chocolate chip cookie (without nuts).

Foods to avoid: Dry or coarse foods; tough, crusty breads such as French bread or baguettes; breads and cereals with nuts, seeds, or dried fruit; corn and clam chowders; potato skins; raw vegetables (except shredded lettuce); corn; chunky peanut butter; coconut; nuts and seeds; hard fruit (such as apples or pears); fruit with skin, seeds, or a stringy texture (such as mango or pineapple); uncooked dried fruit; fruit leather; popcorn; potato chips; chewy candies (such as caramel or licorice).

LIQUID CONSISTENCIES (ONLY THOSE TOLERATED ARE ALLOWED IN THE DIET)

- *Thin:* Watery fluids; may include milk, coffee, tea, juice, carbonated beverages, gelatin desserts, ice cream or sherbet.

- *Nectar-like:* Fluids thicker than water that can be sipped through a straw; may include buttermilk, eggnog, tomato juice, cream soup.

- *Honey-like:* Fluids that can be eaten with a spoon but do not hold their shape; may include honey, some yogurt products, tomato sauce.

- *Spoon-thick:* Thick fluids that must be eaten with a spoon and can hold their shape; may include milk pudding, thickened applesauce.

[a] Slurried foods are foods that have been mixed with liquid to achieve an appropriate consistency; they may be gelled and shaped to improve their appearance.

the diet must be adjusted to suit the person's swallowing abilities and tolerances. In many cases, the most appropriate foods may be determined only by trial and error. A consultation with a swallowing expert, such as a speech and language therapist, is often necessary.

Food Properties and Preparation Foods included in dysphagia diets should have easy-to-manage textures and consistencies. Soft, cohesive foods are easier to swallow than hard or crumbly foods. Moist foods are better tolerated than dry foods. Some foods within a category may be acceptable and others may not; for example, some cookies are soft and tender, whereas others are hard and brittle. Sticky or gummy foods, such as peanut butter and cream cheese, may be difficult to clear from the mouth and throat.

The textures of foods are usually altered to make them easier to swallow. Solid foods are often pureed, mashed, ground, or minced (review Table 14-5 on p. 410). Foods that have more than one texture, such as vegetable soup or cereal with milk, are difficult to manage, so ingredients may be blended to a single consistency with items such as nuts and seeds omitted. Semi-liquid foods such as sauces and gravies may be thickened with food starches (such as cornstarch or potato flakes) during cooking or mixed with commercial food thickeners after cooking until the desired consistency is reached. A variety of pre-thickened food products, including pureed meats, eggs, vegetables, and pasta, are commercially available.

Consuming foods that have a similar consistency can quickly become monotonous. Including a variety of flavors and colors can make a meal more appealing. Box 17-4 and Photo 17-1 present suggestions for improving the acceptance of pureed and other mechanically altered foods.

Properties of Liquids Thickened liquids are easier to swallow than thin liquids such as water or juice. Table 17-3 describes the four levels of liquid consistencies prescribed for dysphagia patients, referred to as thin, nectar-like, honey-like, and spoon-thick. To increase viscosity, commercial thickeners can be stirred into beverages and other liquid foods, such as soup broths. Some beverages may lose their appeal when thickened; for example, individuals may find thickened coffee and tea unacceptable. Moreover, hydration is more difficult to maintain when a patient has access to only thickened beverages, which are often less acceptable for quenching thirst.[5]

Alternative Feeding Strategies for Dysphagia Some patients may be able to learn alternative feeding techniques to help them compensate for their swallowing problem. For example, changing the position of the head and neck while eating and drink-

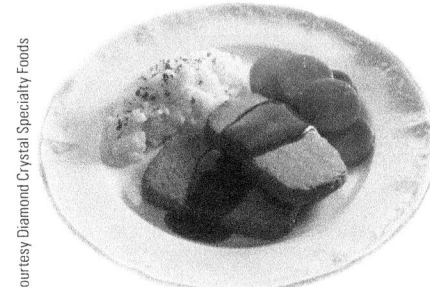

Photo 17-1 Meal of Pureed Foods

Courtesy Diamond Crystal Specialty Foods

Pureed foods can be formed into attractive shapes using commercial thickeners and food molds. Most commercial thickening agents are gels or powders made from modified food starches or food gums.

Box 17-4   *HOW TO* Improve Acceptance of Mechanically Altered Foods

Take a moment to think about a meal of pureed or ground foods. A typical dinner of baked chicken, potatoes, carrots, and green beans can look like mounds of differently colored mush. The foods may taste great, but a person may have little appetite before trying a first bite. To improve appetite, be creative when preparing and serving meals:

- Help to stimulate the appetite by preparing favorite foods and foods with pleasant smells. Enliven food flavors with aromatic spices and seasonings.

- Substitute brightly colored vegetables for white vegetables; for example, replace mashed potatoes with mashed sweet potatoes. If serving more than one vegetable, place contrasting colors (such as spinach and carrots) side by side or swirl the two together.

- Shape pureed and ground foods so they resemble traditional dishes; for example, meat can be flattened to form a patty or rounded to resemble meatballs. Use food molds to restore slurried breads and pureed meats to their traditional shapes.

- Try layering ingredients so that the food looks like a fancy casserole or popular hors d'oeuvre. For example, food items can resemble lasagna, moussaka, tamales, or sushi.

- Use attractive plates and silverware to improve the visual appeal of a meal. Colorful garnishes can add interest and eye appeal.

Efforts to improve the appearance of foods can go a long way toward helping people eat nourishing meals and maintain a healthy weight.

Conditions Affecting the Mouth and Esophagus   **493**

ing can minimize some swallowing difficulties. (As an example, cups designed for dysphagia patients allow drinking without tilting the head back.) Individuals with oropharyngeal dysphagia can be taught exercises that strengthen the jaws, tongue, or larynx, or they can learn new methods of swallowing that allow them to consume a normal diet. Speech and language therapists are often responsible for teaching patients these techniques.

Gastroesophageal Reflux Disease

Gastroesophageal reflux disease (GERD) is characterized by frequent reflux (backward flow) of the stomach's acidic contents into the esophagus, leading to pain, inflammation, and, possibly, tissue damage. People who suffer from GERD often refer to these symptoms as *heartburn* or *acid indigestion*. The reflux itself does not necessarily cause symptoms or injury—it occurs occasionally in healthy people and is a problem only if it creates complications and requires lifestyle changes or medical treatment.

Causes of GERD The lower esophageal sphincter is the main barrier to gastric reflux, so GERD can result if the sphincter muscle is weak or relaxes inappropriately. Other factors that predispose a person to GERD include high stomach pressures and inadequate acid clearance from the esophagus.[6] Conditions associated with high rates of GERD include obesity, pregnancy, and **hiatal hernia**, in which a portion of the stomach protrudes above the diaphragm (see Figure 17-1). During pregnancy, nearly two-thirds of women report heartburn, which typically worsens during the third trimester.[7] Many medications can increase the risk of reflux, as does the use of nasogastric tubes in tube feedings. Various other conditions or substances can exacerbate GERD by increasing stomach pressures or weakening the lower esophageal sphincter; Table 17-4 lists examples.[8]

FIGURE 17-1 The Upper GI Tract, Acid Reflux, and Hiatal Hernia

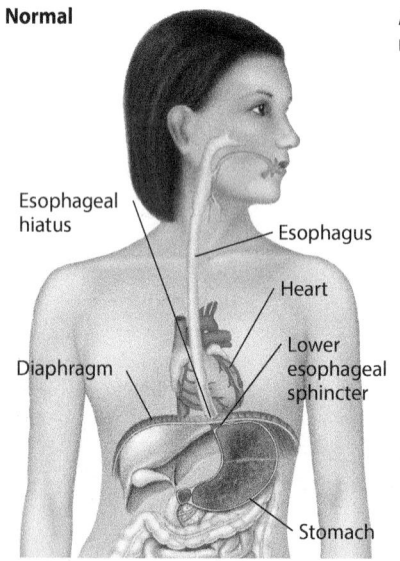

Normal

Esophageal hiatus
Esophagus
Heart
Lower esophageal sphincter
Diaphragm
Stomach

The stomach normally lies below the diaphragm, and the esophagus passes through the esophageal hiatus. The lower esophageal sphincter prevents reflux of stomach contents.

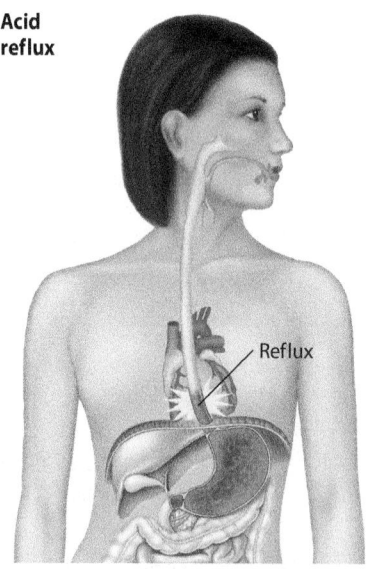

Acid reflux

Reflux

Whenever the pressure in the stomach exceeds the pressure in the esophagus, as can occur with overeating and overdrinking, the chance of reflux increases. The resulting "heartburn" is so-named because it is felt in the area of the heart.

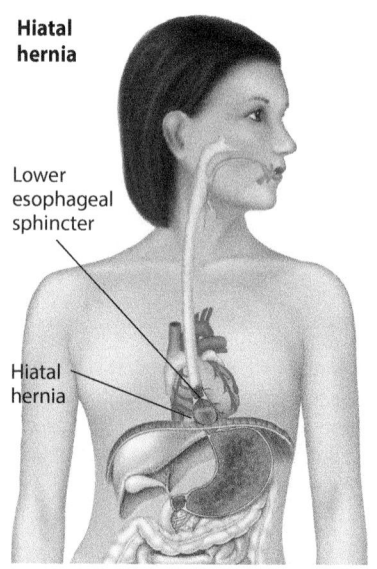

Hiatal hernia

Lower esophageal sphincter
Hiatal hernia

Risk of acid reflux may increase as a consequence of a hiatal hernia. A "sliding" hiatal hernia occurs when part of the stomach, along with the lower esophageal sphincter, rises into the area above the diaphragm.

Consequences of GERD The primary symptoms associated with GERD are **acid regurgitation** and **heartburn**, which generally occur after meals. If gastric acid remains in the esophagus long enough to damage the esophageal lining, the resulting inflammation is called **reflux esophagitis**. Severe and chronic inflammation may lead to esophageal ulcers, with consequent bleeding. After healing begins, the scar tissue may narrow the inner diameter of the esophagus, causing esophageal stricture. A slowly progressive dysphagia for solid foods sometimes results, and swallowing occasionally becomes painful. Pulmonary disease may develop if gastric contents are aspirated into the lungs (see Box 17-5). Chronic reflux is also associated with **Barrett's esophagus**, a condition in which damaged esophageal cells are gradually replaced by cells that resemble those in gastric or intestinal tissue; such cellular changes increase the risk of developing esophageal cancer. GERD can also damage tissues in the mouth, pharynx, and larynx, resulting in eroded tooth enamel, sore throat, and laryngitis.[9]

Treatment of GERD Treatment objectives are to alleviate symptoms and facilitate the healing of damaged tissue. Severe ulcerative disease may require immediate acid-suppressing medication, whereas a mild case may be managed with dietary and lifestyle changes. Box 17-6 lists lifestyle modifications that may help to prevent the recurrence of gastroesophageal reflux.

Medications that suppress gastric acid secretion help the healing process by reducing the damaging effects of acid on esophageal tissue. **Proton-pump inhibitors** are the most effective of the antisecretory agents and are used both for rapid healing of esophagitis and as a maintenance treatment. Other antisecretory drugs include the **histamine-2 receptor blockers** (often referred to as *H2 blockers*). Antacids, which neutralize stomach acid, are frequently used to relieve occasional heartburn, but they are not necessarily appropriate for GERD because they have only short-term effects and are ineffective for healing esophagitis.

Surgery may be required in severe cases of GERD that are unresponsive to medications and lifestyle changes. In one popular procedure (called *fundoplication*), the upper section of the stomach (the fundus) is gathered up around the lower esophagus and sewn in such a way that the lower esophagus and sphincter are surrounded by stomach muscle; this technique increases pressure within the esophagus and fortifies the sphincter muscle. Esophageal strictures are often treated by dilating the esophagus with an inflatable balloon-like device or a fixed-size dilator. The Case Study in Box 17-7 will help you to review the treatments available for a patient with GERD.

TABLE 17-4	Conditions and Substances Associated with Esophageal Reflux

Conditions/Substances That Increase Pressure Within the Stomach

- Ascites (abdominal fluid accumulation)
- Bending over
- Carbonated beverages
- Delayed stomach emptying
- Eating large meals
- Lifting heavy objects
- Lying down after eating
- Obesity
- Pregnancy
- Wearing tight-fitting clothing around the waist or abdomen

Conditions/Substances That Weaken the Lower Esophageal Sphincter

- Alcohol
- Anticholinergic drugs
- Caffeinated beverages
- Calcium channel blockers
- Chocolate
- Cigarette smoking
- Diazepam
- Estrogen, progesterone
- Fatty foods
- Peppermint
- Theophylline
- Tricyclic antidepressants

BOX 17-5 *Nursing Diagnosis*

The nursing diagnoses *acute pain* and *risk for aspiration* may apply to a person with GERD.

Review Notes

- Dry mouth can diminish taste sensation, lead to reduced food intake, and increase the risk of developing oral infections. It can be managed with oral hygiene, dietary changes, and saliva substitutes.
- Dysphagia may interfere with food intake and increase the risk of aspiration. Treatment may include dietary adjustments, strengthening exercises, and using different swallowing techniques.
- Gastroesophageal reflux disease (GERD) may lead to inflammation, esophageal ulcers, bleeding, and stricture. Treatment includes lifestyle changes and use of acid-suppressing drugs.

proton-pump inhibitors: a class of drugs that inhibit the enzyme that pumps hydrogen ions (protons) into the stomach. Examples include omeprazole (Prilosec) and lansoprazole (Prevacid).

histamine-2 receptor blockers: a class of drugs that suppress acid secretion by inhibiting receptors on acid-producing cells; commonly called *H2 blockers*. Examples include cimetidine (Tagamet), ranitidine (Zantac), and famotidine (Pepcid).

Box 17-6

HOW TO Manage Gastroesophageal Reflux Disease

Management of GERD may require modifications in diet and lifestyle to reduce the recurrence of acid reflux or minimize discomfort. Recommendations typically include the following:

- Consume only small meals and drink liquids between meals so that the stomach does not become overly distended, which can exert pressure on the lower esophageal sphincter.

- Limit foods or substances that increase gastric acid secretion (such as coffee, beer, and wine) or weaken the pressure of the lower esophageal sphincter (such as alcoholic beverages, chocolate, fried or fatty foods, and peppermint).

- During periods of esophagitis, avoid foods and beverages that may irritate the esophagus, such as citrus fruits and juices, tomato products, garlic, onions, pepper, spicy foods, carbonated beverages, and very hot or very cold foods (depending on individual tolerances).

- Avoid eating bedtime snacks or lying down after meals. Meals should be consumed at least three hours before bedtime.

- Reduce nighttime reflux by elevating the head of the bed on 6-inch blocks, inserting a foam wedge under the mattress, or propping pillows under the head and upper torso.

- Avoid bending over and wearing tight-fitting garments; both can cause pressure in the stomach to increase, heightening the risk of reflux.

- Avoid cigarette smoking, which relaxes the lower esophageal sphincter.

- Avoid using nonsteroidal anti-inflammatory drugs (NSAIDs) such as aspirin, naproxen, and ibuprofen, which can damage the esophageal mucosa.

Food tolerances among people with GERD can vary markedly. Health practitioners can help patients pinpoint food intolerances by advising them to keep a record of the foods and beverages they consume, as well as any resulting symptoms.

Box 17-7

Case Study: Woman with GERD

Joanne Rinaldi is a 39-year-old accountant who is 5 feet 4 inches tall and weighs 165 pounds. During a recent physical examination, she mentioned to her physician that she had been feeling fairly well until she began experiencing heartburn, which has progressively become more frequent and painful. The heartburn often occurs after she eats a large meal and is particularly bad after she goes to bed at night. By directly examining the esophageal lumen using an endoscope (a thin, flexible tube equipped with an optical device), the physician found evidence of reflux esophagitis and a slight narrowing throughout the length of the esophagus.

Ms. Rinaldi's medical history does not indicate any significant health problems. During her last physical exam, her physician advised her to stop smoking cigarettes and to try to lose some weight, but she has not attempted

to do either. The nutrition assessment reveals that Ms. Rinaldi is feeling stressed because it is the middle of the tax season. She usually has little time for breakfast, eats a lunch of fast foods while continuing to work at her desk, and eats a large dinner at around 8 P.M. She generally has wine with dinner and another alcoholic beverage later in the evening.

1. Explain to Ms. Rinaldi the meaning of the medical diagnoses *reflux esophagitis* and *esophageal stricture*.

2. Based on the brief history provided, list the factors and behaviors that increase Ms. Rinaldi's risks of experiencing reflux. What recommendations can you make to help her change these behaviors?

3. What medications might the physician prescribe, and why?

BOX 17-8 *Nursing Diagnosis*

The nursing diagnoses *acute pain* and *nausea* may be appropriate for a person with dyspepsia.

dyspepsia: symptoms of pain or discomfort in the upper abdominal area, often called "indigestion"; a symptom of illness rather than a disease itself.

dys = bad; impaired
pepsis = digestion

bloating: the sensation of swelling in the abdominal area; often due to the accumulation of stomach or intestinal gas, or fluid.

17.2 Conditions Affecting the Stomach

Stomach disorders range from occasional bouts of discomfort to severe conditions that require surgery. This section begins with a discussion of *dyspepsia* (often called "indigestion"), the sensation of pain or discomfort in the upper abdomen that occurs after food consumption. More serious stomach conditions that may benefit from dietary adjustments include *gastritis* and *peptic ulcers*, which most often result from bacterial infection or the use of medications that damage the stomach lining.

Dyspepsia

Dyspepsia refers to general symptoms of pain or discomfort in the upper abdominal region, which may include stomach pain, gnawing sensations, early satiety, nausea, vomiting, and **bloating** (see Box 17-8). These symptoms sometimes indicate the presence of more serious diseases, such as GERD or peptic ulcer disease. Although about 25 percent of the population experiences dyspepsia, only half of those affected seek medical attention.[10]

Causes of Dyspepsia Abdominal symptoms don't always lead to a clear diagnosis. Various medical problems can cause abdominal discomfort, including foodborne illness,

GERD, peptic ulcers, gastric motility disorders, gallbladder and pancreatic diseases, and tumors in the upper GI tract. Chronic diseases such as diabetes mellitus, heart disease, and hypothyroidism are sometimes accompanied by gastric symptoms. Various medications and dietary supplements can cause gastrointestinal problems. Intestinal conditions such as irritable bowel syndrome or lactose intolerance may mimic dyspepsia. Although pinpointing the cause of gastric symptoms can be difficult, a complete examination is in order if the individual experiences unintentional weight loss, dysphagia, persistent vomiting, GI bleeding, or anemia, which suggest the presence of serious illness.[11]

Potential Food Intolerances Although many people believe that their symptoms are caused by consuming certain types of foods, meals, or spices, controlled studies have been unable to associate specific food intolerances with dyspepsia.[12] Foods often reported to cause problems include chocolate, citrus fruits, coffee, fish, onions, peppers, and spicy foods.[13] Fatty foods and high-fat meals, which slow gastric emptying, may exacerbate symptoms in some individuals. To minimize discomfort, people with dyspepsia are typically advised to avoid large or fatty meals, highly spiced foods, and the specific foods or substances believed to trigger symptoms.[14]

Bloating and Stomach Gas The feeling of bloating may be caused by excessive gas in the stomach, which accumulates when air is swallowed. Air swallowing often accompanies gum chewing, smoking, rapid eating, drinking carbonated beverages, and using a straw. Omitting these practices generally helps to correct the problem.

Nausea and Vomiting

Nausea and vomiting accompany many illnesses and are common side effects of medications. Although occasional vomiting is not dangerous, prolonged vomiting can cause esophagitis and fluid and electrolyte imbalances and may require medical care. Chronic vomiting can reduce food intake and lead to malnutrition and nutrient deficiencies.

The symptoms that accompany vomiting may give clues about its cause.[15] If abdominal pain is present, a GI disorder or obstruction is usually the cause. If abdominal pain is not present, possible causes of vomiting include medications, foodborne illness, pregnancy, motion sickness, neurological disease, inner ear disorders, hepatitis, and various chronic illnesses.

Treatment of Nausea and Vomiting Most cases are short-lived and require no treatment. When treatment is necessary, the main goal is to find and correct the underlying disorder. Restoring hydration may also be necessary in some individuals. If a medication is the cause, taking it with food may help. If the cause is unknown or the underlying disorder cannot be corrected, medications that suppress nausea and vomiting can be prescribed. People with **intractable vomiting**—severe vomiting that is not easily controlled—may require intravenous nutrition support.

Dietary Interventions Sometimes nausea can be prevented or improved with dietary measures.[16] To minimize stomach distention, patients should consume small meals and drink beverages between meals rather than during a meal. Dry, starchy foods such as toast, crackers, and pretzels may help to reduce nausea, whereas fatty foods and foods with strong odors may worsen symptoms. Foods that are cold or at room temperature may be better tolerated than hot foods. Individuals often have strong food aversions when nauseated, and tolerances vary greatly.

Gastroparesis

Gastroparesis is a motility disorder characterized by delayed stomach emptying. It is often a consequence of diabetes or gastric surgery, but may also be caused by various stomach disorders, neuromuscular diseases, spinal cord injuries, and thyroid diseases; in 40 percent of cases, the cause is unknown.[17] Symptoms of gastroparesis include nausea, vomiting, early satiety, stomach pain or discomfort, and acid reflux; in addition, many patients lose weight or exhibit signs of nutrient deficiency.

intractable vomiting: vomiting that is not easily managed or controlled.

gastroparesis: delayed stomach emptying; most often a consequence of diabetes, gastric surgery, or neurological disorders.

CHEMICAL SUBSTANCES
- Alcoholic beverages
- Cancer chemotherapy
- Drugs (especially aspirin and other NSAIDs)
- Ingestion of toxins or corrosive materials

INFECTION
- Bacterial: *Helicobacter pylori*
- Fungal: *Candida albicans*
- Parasitic: *Anisakis* (nematode infection)
- Viral: *Cytomegalovirus*

INTERNAL (BODILY) CAUSES
- Autoimmune disease
- Bile reflux
- Severe stress or sepsis

MISCELLANEOUS
- Foreign bodies
- High salt intake
- Radiation therapy

gastritis: inflammation of stomach tissue. (The suffix -*itis* refers to the presence of inflammation in an organ or tissue.)

atrophic gastritis: chronic gastritis characterized by destruction of gastric mucosal tissue due to chronic inflammation; eventually the gastric epithelium may be replaced with another type of tissue.

Helicobacter pylori (*H. pylori*): a species of bacterium that colonizes the GI mucosa; a primary cause of gastritis and peptic ulcer disease.

hypochlorhydria (HIGH-poe-clor-HIGH-dree-ah): abnormally low gastric acid secretions.

achlorhydria (AY-clor-HIGH-dree-ah): absence of gastric acid secretions.

pernicious anemia: vitamin B_{12} deficiency that results from lack of intrinsic factor; may be evidenced by macrocytic anemia, muscle weakness, and neurological damage.

peptic ulcer: an open sore in the GI mucosa; may develop in the esophagus, stomach, or duodenum.

peptic = related to digestion

Medical treatments for gastroparesis include drug therapies, which improve stomach motility or reduce nausea and vomiting, and electrical stimulation of stomach tissue, which promotes muscle contractions. Dietary practices that may improve stomach emptying include drinking fluids with meals, chewing foods well, and remaining upright or walking after meals are consumed. Patients are encouraged to eat small, frequent meals, as small meals empty from the stomach more quickly. Meals that are high in fat or soluble fibers are discouraged because they may delay stomach emptying. Patients who cannot tolerate solid foods may be able to consume blenderized or liquid meals. In severe cases of gastroparesis, tube feedings may be necessary.[18]

Gastritis

Gastritis is a general term that refers to inflammation of the gastric mucosa. Acute cases of gastritis usually result from irritating substances or treatments that damage stomach tissue, resulting in tissue erosion, ulcers, or hemorrhaging (severe bleeding). Chronic gastritis is frequently caused by long-term infection or autoimmune disease and may progress to **atrophic gastritis**, which is characterized by widespread gastric inflammation and tissue atrophy. In most cases, gastritis results from ***Helicobacter pylori* (*H. pylori*)** infection or the use of non-steroidal anti-inflammatory drugs (NSAIDs), which are both primary causes of peptic ulcer disease as well. Table 17-5 lists some potential causes of gastritis.[19]

Complications of Gastritis The extensive tissue damage that develops in long-term gastritis may disrupt gastric secretory functions and increase the risk of cancer. If hydrochloric acid secretions become abnormally low (**hypochlorhydria**) or absent (**achlorhydria**), absorption of nonheme iron and vitamin B_{12} can be impaired, increasing the risk of deficiency. Lack of intrinsic factor (a protein secreted by stomach cells) can result in vitamin B_{12} malabsorption and the vitamin B_{12}–deficiency condition known as **pernicious anemia** (see p. 221); possible consequences include macrocytic anemia and neurological damage.[20]

Dietary Interventions for Gastritis Dietary recommendations depend on an individual's symptoms. In asymptomatic cases, no dietary adjustments are needed. If pain or discomfort is present, the patient should avoid irritating foods and beverages; these often include alcoholic beverages, coffee (including decaffeinated), acidic beverages, and fried or fatty foods. If hypochlorhydria or achlorhydria is present, supplementation of iron and vitamin B_{12} may be warranted.

Peptic Ulcer Disease

A **peptic ulcer** is an open sore that develops in the GI mucosa when gastric acid and pepsin overwhelm mucosal defenses and destroy mucosal tissue (see Photo 17-2). A primary factor in peptic ulcer development is *H. pylori* infection, which is present in up to 30 to 60 percent of patients with gastric ulcers and 70 to 90 percent of those with duodenal ulcers.[21] Another major factor is the use of NSAIDs, which have both topical and systemic effects that can damage the GI lining. In rare cases, ulcers may develop from disorders that cause excessive acid secretion. Ulcer risk can also be increased by cigarette smoking and psychological stress. Note that the specific reasons why ulcers develop are unknown; only 5 to 15 percent of people with chronic *H. pylori* infection actually develop a peptic ulcer.[22]

Effects of Psychological Stress Although most ulcers are associated with *H. pylori* infection or NSAID use, about 20 to 30 percent of ulcers develop for other reasons.[23] Psychological stress by itself is not believed to cause ulcers, but it has effects on physiological processes and behaviors that may increase a person's vulnerability. The physiological effects of stress vary among individuals but may include hormonal changes that impair immune responses and wound healing, increased secretions of hydrochloric acid and pepsin, and rapid stomach emptying (which increases the acid load in the duodenum). Stress may also lead to behavioral changes, including the increased use of cigarettes, alcohol, and NSAIDs—all potential risk factors for ulcers. Thus, stress may play a contributory role in ulcer development, although its precise effects are not fully understood.

Symptoms of Peptic Ulcers Peptic ulcer symptoms vary. Some people are asymptomatic or experience only mild discomfort. In others, ulcer "pain" may be experienced as a hunger pain, a sensation of gnawing, or a burning pain in the stomach region (see Box 17-9). The pain or discomfort of ulcers may be relieved by food and recur several hours after a meal, especially if the ulcer is duodenal. Gastric ulcers may be aggravated by food and can cause loss of appetite and eventual weight loss. Ulcer symptoms tend to go into remission regularly and recur every few weeks or months.[24]

Complications of Peptic Ulcers Peptic ulcers are a major cause of GI bleeding, which occurs in up to 15 percent of ulcer cases.[25] Bleeding is a potential cause of death and, if severe, may indicate the need for surgical intervention. Severe bleeding is evidenced by black, tarry stools or, occasionally, vomit that resembles coffee grounds. Other serious complications of ulcers include perforations of the stomach or duodenum (sometimes leading directly into the peritoneal cavity), penetration of the ulcer into an adjacent organ, and **gastric outlet obstruction** due to scarring or inflammation.

Drug Therapy for Peptic Ulcers The goals of ulcer treatment are to relieve pain, promote healing, and prevent recurrence. In most cases, treatment requires using a combination of antibiotics to eradicate *H. pylori* infection and/or discontinuing the use of aspirin and other NSAIDs, which can irritate the gastric mucosa and delay healing. The antibiotics used to treat *H. pylori* infection most often include amoxicillin, clarithromycin, levofloxacin, metronidazole, and tetracycline. Antisecretory drugs (either proton-pump inhibitors or H2 blockers) are prescribed to relieve pain and allow healing (as used in GERD; see the section *Treatment of GERD* on p. 495). The most frequently prescribed drug regimen is a "triple therapy" that includes two antibiotics and an antisecretory drug. Bismuth preparations (such as Pepto-Bismol) and the medication sucralfate may also help to heal ulcers by coating ulcerated tissue and preventing further tissue erosion. Box 17-10 provides examples of the nutrition-related effects of some of these medications.

Nutrition Care for Peptic Ulcers The goals of nutrition care are to correct nutrient deficiencies, if necessary, and encourage dietary and lifestyle practices that minimize symptoms.[26] Patients should avoid dietary items that increase acid secretion or irritate the GI lining; examples include alcoholic beverages, chocolate, caffeine-containing beverages, noncaffeinated coffee and tea, and pepper, although individual tolerances vary. Small meals may be better tolerated than large ones. Patients should avoid food consumption for at least two hours before bedtime. There is no evidence that dietary adjustments alter the rate of healing or prevent recurrence.[27]

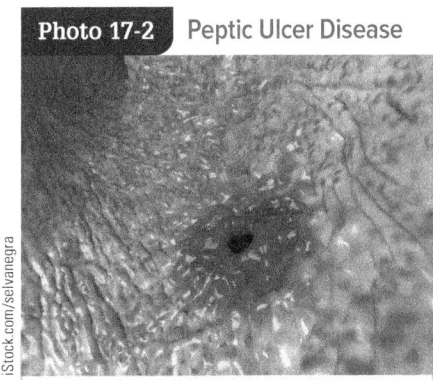

Photo 17-2 — Peptic Ulcer Disease

iStock.com/selvanegra

A peptic ulcer, such as the gastric ulcer shown here, damages mucosal tissue and may cause pain and bleeding. Duodenal ulcers are more common than gastric ulcers in the United States and other Western countries.

BOX 17-9 *Nursing Diagnosis*

Nursing diagnoses for people with peptic ulcers may include *acute pain* and *nausea*. For patients with bleeding ulcers, appropriate diagnoses may include *risk for deficient fluid volume, imbalanced nutrition: less than body requirements*, and *fatigue*.

Review Notes

- *Dyspepsia* refers to general symptoms of pain or discomfort in the upper abdominal region; dietary measures may include avoiding large meals, fatty or spicy foods, and foods that trigger symptoms.

- Gastritis and peptic ulcer disease are most often associated with *H. pylori* infection, which can be eradicated by antibiotic therapy. NSAID use may promote gastritis and peptic ulcer disease by damaging the mucosal lining.

- Nutrition care for gastritis and peptic ulcer disease includes correcting any nutritional deficiencies that develop and eliminating dietary substances that cause pain or discomfort.

gastric outlet obstruction: an obstruction that prevents the normal emptying of stomach contents into the duodenum.

Conditions Affecting the Stomach   **499**

Box 17-10 Diet-Drug Interactions

Check this table for notable nutrition-related effects of the medications discussed in this chapter.

Antacids (aluminum hydroxide, magnesium hydroxide, calcium carbonate)	**Gastrointestinal effects:** Constipation (aluminum- or calcium-containing antacids), diarrhea (magnesium-containing antacids)
	Dietary interactions: May decrease iron, calcium, folate, and vitamin B_{12} absorption
	Metabolic effects: Electrolyte imbalances
Antibiotics (for *H. pylori* infection; include amoxicillin, metronidazole, tetracycline)	**Gastrointestinal effects:** Diarrhea, nausea and vomiting (tetracycline, metronidazole), altered taste sensation (metronidazole)
	Dietary interactions: Avoid alcohol with metronidazole; tetracycline can bind to calcium, iron, magnesium, and zinc, reducing absorption of both the tetracycline and the minerals
Antisecretory drugs (proton-pump inhibitors, H2 blockers)	**Gastrointestinal effects:** Diarrhea, constipation, nausea and vomiting, abdominal pain (proton-pump inhibitors)
	Dietary interactions: May decrease iron, calcium, folate, and vitamin B_{12} absorption
Octreotide	**Gastrointestinal effects:** Abdominal cramps, diarrhea, nausea and vomiting, flatulence
	Dietary interactions: May decrease absorption of fat, fat-soluble vitamins, and vitamin B_{12}
	Metabolic effects: Hyperglycemia, hypothyroidism

17.3 Gastric Surgery

Gastric surgery is sometimes necessary for treating stomach cancer, some ulcer complications, and ulcers that are resistant to drug therapy. In recent years, gastric surgeries have also become popular treatments for severe obesity. This section describes **gastrectomy**, the surgery that removes diseased regions of the stomach, and **bariatric surgery**, the type of surgery that treats severe obesity. Because gastric surgeries can interfere with stomach function either temporarily or permanently, patients generally need to make significant dietary adjustments afterward.

Gastrectomy

Figure 17-2 illustrates some typical gastrectomy procedures. In a partial gastrectomy, only part of the stomach is removed, and the remaining portion is connected to the duodenum or jejunum. In a total gastrectomy, the surgeon removes the entire stomach and connects the esophagus directly to the small intestine. After the surgery, many patients must alter their diet because of reduced (or absent) stomach capacity and more rapid stomach emptying.

Nutrition Care after a Gastrectomy The primary goals of nutrition care after a gastrectomy are to meet the nutritional needs of the postsurgical patient and promote the healing of stomach tissue. Another goal is to prevent discomfort or nutrient deficiencies that may arise due to reduced stomach capacity or altered stomach function. As the next section describes, some gastric surgeries increase the risk of **dumping syndrome**, a group of symptoms that result when a large amount of food passes rapidly into the small intestine.

Following a gastrectomy, the oral ingestion of fluids and foods is suspended until some healing has occurred, and fluids are supplied intravenously. Oral intakes may begin with small sips of water, ice chips (melted in the mouth), and broth. Once fluids are tolerated, patients may be offered liquid meals (with no sugars) at first; after solid foods are started, meals may contain only one or two food items at a time so that

gastrectomy (gah-STREK-ta-mie): the surgical removal of part of the stomach (partial gastrectomy) or the entire stomach (total gastrectomy).

bariatric (BAH-ree-AH-trik) **surgery:** surgery that treats severe obesity.

baros = weight

dumping syndrome: a cluster of symptoms that result from the rapid emptying of an osmotic load from the stomach into the small intestine.

FIGURE 17-2   Gastrectomy Procedures

Gastrectomies are performed to treat stomach cancers, some ulcer complications, and ulcers that do not respond to drug therapy. Part or all of the stomach may be surgically removed. The dashed lines show the removed sections.

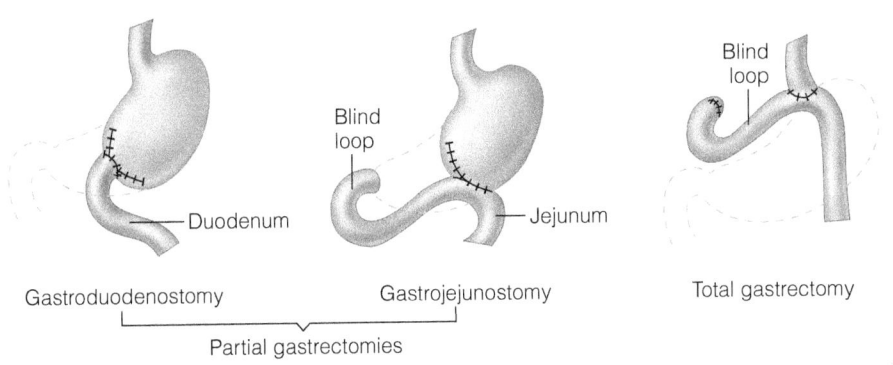

tolerance can be evaluated. Tube feedings may be necessary if complications prevent a normal progression to solid foods.[28]

Dietary measures after a gastrectomy are determined by the size of the remaining stomach, which influences meal size, and the stomach emptying rate, which affects food tolerances. Depending on the amount of food tolerated, the patient may require as many as five to eight small meals and snacks per day; a protein food (fish, lean meat, eggs, or cheese) should be included in each meal so that adequate protein is obtained. Patients should avoid sweets and sugars because they increase osmolarity in the small intestine and thereby increase the risk of dumping syndrome (discussed on p. 502). Patients with lactose intolerance may need to limit their intake of milk products. Soluble fibers may be added to meals to slow stomach emptying and reduce the risk of diarrhea. Liquids are restricted during meals (and for up to 30 to 60 minutes after meals) due to limited stomach capacity and because liquids can increase the stomach emptying rate. Table 17-6 lists foods that are often permitted or limited in postgastrectomy diets.

TABLE 17-6   Postgastrectomy Diet

FOOD CATEGORY	FOODS RECOMMENDED (AS TOLERATED)	FOODS TO LIMIT (UNLESS TOLERATED)
Meat and meat alternatives	Lean tender meat, fish, poultry, and shellfish; eggs; smooth nut butters	Fried, tough, or chewy meat, fish, poultry, and shellfish; frankfurters and sausages; bacon; luncheon meat; dried peas and beans; nuts; chunky nut butters
Milk and milk products	Milk, plain yogurt, cheese	Milkshakes, chocolate milk, sweetened yogurt
Breads and cereals	Bread, crackers, bagels, pasta, and breakfast cereals made from enriched white flour (cereals should contain no added sugars)	Breads and cereals with more than 2 grams of fiber per serving; baked goods with dried fruit, nuts, or seeds; granola; frosted cereals; pastry; doughnuts
Vegetables	Tender-cooked vegetables without peels, skin, or seeds; raw lettuce	Raw vegetables (except lettuce), beets, broccoli, brussels sprouts, cabbage, cauliflower, collard and mustard greens, corn, potato skin
Fruit	Canned fruit without added sugar, bananas, melon	Canned fruit in syrup, raw fruit (except bananas and melons), dried fruit, fruit juice
Beverages	Decaffeinated coffee and tea, beverages sweetened with artificial sweeteners	Caffeinated beverages; alcoholic beverages; beverages sweetened with sugar, corn syrup, or honey; fruit juices and fruit drinks

TABLE 17-7	Symptoms of Dumping Syndrome

EARLY DUMPING SYNDROME

Symptoms may begin within 30 minutes after eating[a]

- Abdominal cramps, bloating
- Diarrhea
- Flushing, sweating
- Light-headedness
- Nausea and vomiting
- Rapid heartbeat
- Weakness, feeling faint

LATE DUMPING SYNDROME

Symptoms may begin 1 to 3 hours after eating[b]

- Anxiety
- Confusion
- Headache, dizziness
- Hunger
- Palpitations
- Sweating
- Weakness, feeling faint

[a]Symptoms are due to rapid gastric emptying, which leads to a fluid shift from the bloodstream to the intestinal lumen, intestinal distention, and decreased blood volume.

[b]Symptoms are due to rapid glucose absorption and the excessive release of insulin, resulting in hypoglycemia.

Dumping Syndrome Dumping syndrome, a common complication of a gastrectomy, is characterized by a group of symptoms resulting from rapid gastric emptying.[29] Ordinarily, the pyloric sphincter controls the rate of flow from the stomach into the duodenum. After some types of stomach surgery, stomach emptying is no longer regulated, and the stomach's hyperosmolar contents rush into the small intestine more quickly after meals, causing a number of unpleasant effects. Early symptoms can occur within 30 minutes after eating and may include nausea, vomiting, abdominal cramping, diarrhea, light-headedness, rapid heartbeat, and others (see Table 17-7). These symptoms are due to a shift of fluid from the bloodstream to the intestinal lumen that increases intestinal distention and lowers blood volume; in addition, the accelerated release of GI hormones may alter both intestinal motility and blood flow. Several hours later, symptoms of hypoglycemia may occur because the unusually large spike in blood glucose following the meal (due to rapid nutrient influx and absorption) can result in an excessive insulin response.

Dietary adjustments can greatly minimize or prevent the symptoms of dumping syndrome. The goals are to slow the rate of gastric emptying, limit the amount of food material that reaches the intestine, and reduce foods that increase osmolarity. Therefore, fluids are restricted during meals, meal size is limited, and sugars (including milk sugar) are restricted. In some cases, octreotide—a medication that inhibits GI motility and insulin release—may be prescribed to lessen symptoms. Box 17-11 lists practical suggestions for reducing the occurrence of dumping syndrome. The Case Study in Box 17-12 provides the opportunity to design a menu for a postgastrectomy patient who is at risk of dumping syndrome.

Nutrition Problems following a Gastrectomy After a gastrectomy, it may take time for the patient to learn the amount of food that can be consumed without discomfort. The symptoms associated with meals may lead to food avoidance, substantial weight loss, and eventually, malnutrition. Other nutrition problems that may occur after a gastrectomy include the following:

- *Fat malabsorption.* Fat digestion and absorption may become impaired for a number of reasons after a gastrectomy. The accelerated transit of food material may prevent the normal mixing of fat with lipase and bile. If the duodenum has been removed or is bypassed, less lipase is available for

Box 17-11	*HOW TO* Alter the Diet to Reduce Symptoms of Dumping Syndrome

Dietary adjustments can greatly minimize or prevent the symptoms of dumping syndrome. The following suggestions may help:

- Eat smaller meals that suit the reduced capacity of the stomach. Increase the number of meals consumed daily so that energy intake is adequate.
- Eat in a relaxed setting. Eat slowly, and chew food thoroughly.
- Include fiber-rich foods in each meal. Adding soluble fibers like pectin or guar gum to meals may help to control symptoms.
- If symptoms of hypoglycemia continue, try including a protein-rich food in each meal.
- Limit the amount of fluid included in meals. Avoid drinking beverages within 30 to 60 minutes before and after meals, but be sure to consume adequate fluid to avoid dehydration.

- Avoid juices, sweetened beverages, and foods that contain high amounts of sugar. Use artificial sweeteners to sweeten beverages and desserts.
- Avoid milk and most milk products, which are high in lactose. Avoid enzyme-treated milk as well, because the breakdown products of lactose (glucose and galactose) can also cause dumping symptoms. Cheese may be better tolerated than milk because its lactose content is low. Make an effort to consume nonmilk calcium sources such as green leafy vegetables, fish with bones, and tofu.
- Avoid carbonated beverages if they cause bloating.
- Avoid foods and beverages that are very hot or very cold, unless tolerated.
- Lie down for 20 to 30 minutes (or longer) after eating to help slow the transit of food to the small intestine. While eating a meal, sit upright.

Ed Hanson, a 58-year-old biology teacher, was admitted to the hospital for gastric surgery after numerous medical treatments failed to manage severe complications related to his peptic ulcer disease. A gastrojejunostomy was performed, and after about 24 hours, Mr. Hanson was able to take small sips of warm water. The health care team anticipates multiple nutrition-related problems and is taking measures to prevent them.

1. Review Figure 17-2 to better understand Mr. Hanson's surgical procedure. Consider the possibility that he might experience the following problems:

early satiety, nausea and vomiting, weight loss, dumping syndrome, fat malabsorption, anemia, and bone disease. Explain why each of these conditions may occur.

2. What type of diet will the physician prescribe for Mr. Hanson after he begins eating solid foods? Create a day's worth of menus, using foods from Table 17-6.

3. What advice can you give Mr. Hanson that will help to prevent dumping syndrome? List several foods from each major food group that may cause symptoms of dumping syndrome.

---

fat digestion. **Bacterial overgrowth**, a common consequence of gastric surgeries, can lead to changes in bile acids that upset bile function. The fat malabsorption that results from these changes can eventually cause deficiencies of fat-soluble vitamins and some minerals. Supplemental pancreatic enzymes are sometimes provided to improve fat digestion. Medium-chain triglycerides, which are more easily digested and absorbed, can be used to supply additional fat kcalories.

- *Bone disease.* Osteoporosis and osteomalacia are common outcomes following a gastrectomy.[30] The fat malabsorption described above can cause malabsorption of both vitamin D and calcium*; furthermore, patients at risk of dumping syndrome may need to avoid most milk products, which are among the best sources of these nutrients. Bone density should be monitored during the years following surgery, and supplementation of calcium and vitamin D is often recommended.
- *Anemia.* After a gastrectomy, the reduced secretion of gastric acid and intrinsic factor impairs the absorption of both iron and vitamin B_{12}, often leading to anemia. If the duodenum has been removed or is bypassed, the risk of iron deficiency increases because the duodenum is a major site of iron absorption. Supplementation of both iron and vitamin B_{12} is usually warranted after surgery.

Bariatric Surgery

Bariatric surgery is currently considered the most effective and durable treatment for morbid obesity.[31] Candidates for bariatric surgery are obese individuals who have a body mass index (BMI) greater than 40, or a BMI between 35 and 40 accompanied by severe weight-related problems such as diabetes, hypertension, or debilitating osteoarthritis (a healthy BMI usually falls between 18.5 and 25). In addition, the patient should have attempted a variety of nonsurgical weight-loss measures—such as dietary adjustments, exercise, medications, and behavior modification—prior to seeking surgery. Patients preparing for bariatric surgery should have realistic expectations about the amount of weight they are likely to lose, the diet they will need to follow, and the complications that may ensue (see Box 17-13). Some types of bariatric surgery can dramatically affect health and nutrition status, and many patients require lifelong management.

Bariatric Surgical Procedures Figure 17-3 illustrates the most popular surgical options for weight reduction. The *gastric bypass* operation, which accounts for about 45 to 50 percent of bariatric surgeries,[32] constructs a small gastric pouch that reduces stomach capacity and thereby restricts meal size. In addition, the gastric pouch is connected directly to the jejunum, resulting in significant nutrient malabsorption because the flow of food bypasses a large portion of the small intestine. In the *gastric banding*

BOX 17-13 *Nursing Diagnosis*

Nursing diagnoses appropriate for the ideal bariatric surgery candidate may include *readiness for enhanced health management* and *readiness for enhanced knowledge.*

---

bacterial overgrowth: excessive bacterial colonization of the stomach and small intestine; may be due to reduced gastric acid secretions, altered motility of intestinal contents, or changes in intestinal anatomy due to surgical reconstruction. (Chapter 18 describes bacterial overgrowth in detail.)

---

*Fat malabsorption reduces calcium absorption because the negatively charged fatty acids combine with calcium (which is positively charged) and prevent its absorption.

FIGURE 17-3   Surgical Procedures for Severe Obesity

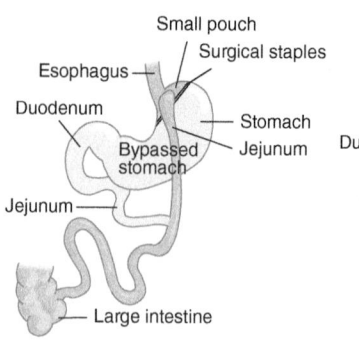

In the gastric bypass operation, the surgeon constructs a small gastric pouch and connects it directly to the jejunum so that the flow of food bypasses a substantial portion of the small intestine. The dark pink area highlights the altered flow of food through the GI tract. The pale pink area indicates the bypassed sections.

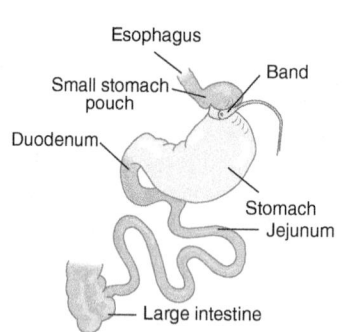

In the gastric banding procedure, the surgeon creates a small gastric pouch using an inflatable band placed near the top of the stomach. The band is tightened or loosened by adding or removing fluid via an access port placed under the skin.

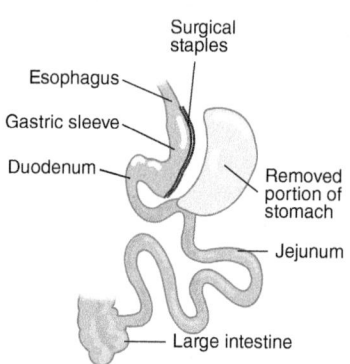

In the sleeve gastrectomy procedure, the surgeon removes 70 to 85 percent of stomach tissue and staples the remaining portions together to create a vertical, tube-shaped stomach with limited capacity. The sleeve gastrectomy is often a stand-alone procedure but may also be performed as the first stage of a more complex surgery if greater weight loss is desired.

procedure, a fluid-filled inflatable band is placed around the uppermost portion of the stomach; adjusting the band's fluid level can tighten or loosen the band and alter the size of the opening to the rest of the stomach. A smaller opening slows the rate at which the upper region is emptied and prolongs the sense of fullness after a meal. The *sleeve gastrectomy* procedure removes a large portion of the stomach, leaving a narrow gastric tube (or "sleeve") that holds only about 3 to 5 ounces (about ½ cup) of food. This operation may be converted to a gastric bypass or other type of malabsorptive surgery if weight loss is inadequate. Whereas the gastric bypass and sleeve gastrectomy operations are permanent, the gastric banding procedure is fully reversible. Clinical studies indicate that the gastric bypass and sleeve gastrectomy surgeries usually result in greater weight loss than the gastric banding procedure.[33]

Nutrition Care after Bariatric Surgery   The objectives of nutrition care after bariatric surgery are to maximize and maintain weight loss, ensure appropriate nutrient intakes, maintain hydration, and avoid complications such as nausea and vomiting or dumping syndrome.[34] Note that patients who have had gastric bypass surgery are at risk of multiple nutrient deficiencies due to malabsorption, whereas the gastric banding and sleeve gastrectomy procedures have little impact on nutrient absorption because none of the small intestine is bypassed. In addition, individuals who have had gastric bypass surgery are at risk of dumping syndrome. Thus, the precise dietary guidelines vary depending on the type of procedure performed.

After bariatric surgery, patients initially consume only sugar-free, noncarbonated clear liquids and low-fat broths; they then progress to a liquid diet (high in protein, low in sugars and fat), followed by pureed and/or soft foods and then solid foods (see Box 17-14).[35] The diet is advanced as tolerated. Once the diet progresses to solid foods, patients consume between three and six small meals and snacks per day. Only small portions of food can be consumed at each meal because overeating can stretch the gastric region or result in vomiting or regurgitation. Similarly, fluids must be consumed separately from meals to avoid excessive distention. Other dietary recommendations include the following:[36]

- *Protein intake.* Recommendations range from about 1.0 to 1.5 grams of protein per kilogram of ideal body weight per day; however, intakes are often lower than recommended. Patients are generally instructed to consume liquid protein supplements regularly and to eat high-protein foods before consuming other foods in a meal.

- *Vitamin and mineral supplementation*. Daily multivitamin/mineral supplements help to prevent nutrient deficiencies. To compensate for nutrient malabsorption, patients who have had gastric bypass surgery usually require additional supplementation of vitamin B_{12}, vitamin D, calcium, and iron.
- *Foods to avoid*. Some foods may obstruct the gastric outlet; these include doughy or sticky breads and pasta products; rice; melted cheese; raw vegetables; fibrous or stringy vegetables such as asparagus and celery; foods with seeds, hulls, peels, or skins; nuts; popcorn; and tough, chewy meats.
- *Dumping syndrome*. To avoid symptoms of dumping syndrome, patients who have had the gastric bypass procedure must carefully control food portions, avoid foods high in sugars, and consume liquids between meals (review Box 17-11).

After bariatric surgery, patient education and counseling are critical for weight loss and weight management, and patients also need to learn the elements of a healthy diet. Box 17-15 includes additional dietary suggestions for patients who have undergone bariatric surgery.

Postsurgical Concerns Common complaints after bariatric surgery include nausea, vomiting, and constipation.[37] Although the cause of these problems varies among patients, dietary noncompliance and inadequate fluid intake are often contributing factors, and improved dietary intakes can help in resolving these conditions. The long-term complications that may develop after gastric bypass surgery are similar to those that arise after a gastrectomy and may include fat malabsorption, bone disease, and anemia. Rapid weight loss increases a person's risk of developing gallbladder disease; patients at especially high risk sometimes have their gallbladders removed while undergoing bariatric surgery. After weight loss, plastic surgery may be necessary to remove extra skin, especially on the abdomen, buttocks, hips, and thighs.

Box 17-15 | *HOW TO* Alter Dietary Habits to Achieve and Maintain Weight Loss after Bariatric Surgery

Patients need to learn new dietary habits after bariatric surgery. The following recommendations may help:

- Consume only small portions of food and chew food thoroughly. Use a small spoon, and take small bites. Relax and enjoy the meal, taking at least 15 to 20 minutes to eat.

- Understand that, at first, the appropriate amount of each food served at mealtime may be only a few spoonfuls. Learn to recognize the sensations that occur when the gastric region is full. Signs of fullness may include pressure in the stomach region, a slight feeling of nausea, or pain in the upper chest or shoulder.

- To control vomiting, try eating smaller volumes of food, eating more slowly, and avoiding foods known to cause difficulty. Continued vomiting may be a sign that some food choices or amounts are inappropriate.

- Consume food only during designated mealtimes (usually three to six small meals and snacks per day), and avoid consuming foods at other times of the day. Snacking throughout the day can become a bad habit that causes weight to be regained.

- Learn to recognize foods that cause problems. Foods that are dry, sticky, or fibrous may be difficult to tolerate during the weeks after surgery.

- Wait at least 30 minutes after meals before consuming liquids. Avoid high-kcalorie drinks such as sweetened soda, milkshakes, and alcoholic beverages. Avoid drinking carbonated beverages or using a straw, as these practices can increase stomach gas and cause bloating.

- Sip water and other beverages throughout the day to obtain sufficient fluids. Aim to consume between 6 and 8 cups of water and other noncaloric beverages daily. Remember that most people meet a significant fraction of their fluid needs by eating food, but a person who has undergone bariatric surgery must limit food intake.

- Engage in regular physical activity. Activity is a valuable aid to weight maintenance and can help to maintain muscle tissue while weight is being lost.

Nutrition Assessment Checklist for People with Disorders of the Upper GI Tract

MEDICAL HISTORY

Check the medical history to uncover conditions or treatments that may:

- ○ Interfere with chewing or swallowing
- ○ Lead to dry mouth
- ○ Lead to dyspepsia, nausea, or vomiting

Check for a medical diagnosis of:

- ○ Gastritis or peptic ulcer
- ○ GERD
- ○ Hiatal hernia
- ○ Pernicious anemia

For a patient who has undergone gastric surgery, check for the following complications:

- ○ Anemia
- ○ Bone disease
- ○ Dumping syndrome
- ○ Fat malabsorption

MEDICATIONS

Record all medications and note:

- ○ Aspirin or NSAID use in patients with gastritis or peptic ulcer disease
- ○ Medications that may cause dry mouth
- ○ Medications that may cause nausea and vomiting

To help alleviate nausea, suggest that medications be taken with food, when possible.

DIETARY INTAKE

To devise an acceptable meal plan, obtain:

- ○ An accurate and thorough record of food intake
- ○ A thorough record of dietary supplement intake, including both vitamin/mineral supplements and herbal products

- ○ A record of food allergies and intolerances, as well as food preferences
- ○ A record of foods that provoke symptoms of GERD, dyspepsia, gastritis, peptic ulcers, or dumping syndrome

For patients on long-term dysphagia diets, monitor appetite, food tolerances, and the variety of foods consumed.

ANTHROPOMETRIC DATA

Measure baseline height and weight. Address weight loss early to prevent malnutrition in patients with:

- ○ Difficulty chewing or swallowing
- ○ Dumping syndrome
- ○ Dyspepsia
- ○ Frequent nausea and vomiting
- ○ Malabsorption

LABORATORY TESTS

Check laboratory test results for signs of dehydration for patients with:

- ○ Constipation
- ○ Dumping syndrome
- ○ Persistent vomiting

Check laboratory test results for nutrition-related anemia in patients with:

- ○ Gastritis
- ○ Long-term use of antisecretory drugs
- ○ Previous gastric surgeries

PHYSICAL SIGNS

Look for physical signs of:

- ○ Dehydration—in patients with constipation, dumping syndrome, or persistent vomiting
- ○ Iron and vitamin B_{12} deficiencies—in patients with hypochlorhydria or achlorhydria

Self Check

1. If a patient with dysphagia has difficulty swallowing solids but can easily swallow liquids:
   a. the problem is most likely a motility disorder.
   b. the patient may have achalasia.
   c. the problem is probably an esophageal obstruction.
   d. the patient most likely has oropharyngeal dysphagia.

2. The clinician working with a patient with dysphagia should recognize that:
   a. the patient should eat only pureed foods to minimize the risk of aspiration.
   b. the foods allowed are those that can be comfortably and safely chewed and swallowed.
   c. highly seasoned foods are often restricted.
   d. regular diets do not meet nutrient needs, so supplements are required.

3. Possible consequences of GERD include all of the following *except*:
   a. reflux esophagitis.
   b. dysphagia.
   c. Barrett's esophagus.
   d. gastric ulcer.

4. Treating GERD with proton-pump inhibitors is effective because they:
   a. reduce gastric acid secretion.
   b. reduce pressure within the stomach.
   c. strengthen the lower esophageal sphincter.
   d. provide a protective barrier between gastric acid and the esophageal mucosa.

5. For the patient with persistent vomiting, the major nutrition-related concern(s) is/are:
   a. dehydration and malnutrition.
   b. reflux esophagitis.
   c. dyspepsia.
   d. peptic ulcers.

6. Chronic gastritis may increase risk of:
   a. dumping syndrome.
   b. bone disease.
   c. iron and vitamin B_{12} deficiencies.
   d. gallbladder disease.

7. The primary cause of most peptic ulcers is:
   a. consumption of spicy foods.
   b. psychological stress.
   c. smoking cigarettes.
   d. *Helicobacter pylori* infection.

8. The main dietary recommendation for patients with gastritis or peptic ulcers is to consume foods that:
   a. neutralize stomach acidity.
   b. are well tolerated and do not cause discomfort.
   c. coat the stomach lining.
   d. promote healing of mucosal tissue.

9. Following a gastrectomy, patients can greatly minimize the risk of dumping syndrome by:
   a. increasing intake of carbohydrates and avoiding fatty foods.
   b. consuming liquids between meals and avoiding foods that supply sugars.
   c. consuming a high-fiber diet and minimizing meat and cheese intake.
   d. including milk products with each meal to provide protein.

10. After a gastric bypass operation, the patient should be monitored for all of the following conditions *except*:
    a. anemia.
    b. bone disease.
    c. hiatal hernia.
    d. fat-soluble vitamin deficiencies.

Answers: 1. c, 2. b, 3. d, 4. a, 5. a, 6. c, 7. d, 8. b, 9. b, 10. c

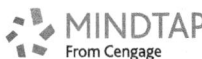 **From Cengage** For more chapter resources visit **www.cengage.com** to access MindTap, a complete digital course.

Clinical Applications

1. Although some individuals require a mechanically altered diet for just a few weeks, others have medical problems that require long-term use of such diets. Consider the difference between working with a person who has had a swallowing problem for years and a person who recently had mouth surgery and is just beginning to eat again.
   - Explain how the needs of these individuals may differ. What nutrition-related problems may develop if a person has been following a restrictive dysphagia diet for several years?
   - Using Table 17-3 (p. 492) and Box 17-4 (p. 493), create a day's worth of menus for a person who requires long-term use of a pureed dysphagia diet and tolerates only liquids that have a honey-like or spoon-thick consistency.

2. Jillian, a 38-year-old woman who is 5 feet 4 inches tall and weighs 227 pounds, has had severe hip and knee osteoarthritis for several years and was recently diagnosed with type 2 diabetes. After trying numerous weight-loss programs without success, she finally visits a bariatric surgeon to learn about the surgical options for treating her obesity.

- Calculate Jillian's BMI, and explain why Jillian would or would not be a good candidate for bariatric surgery.
- Should Jillian decide to undergo gastric bypass surgery, she will need to permanently change her dietary habits. Describe the dietary recommendations and nutrition concerns following bariatric surgery. Summarize the measures necessary for preventing vomiting, distention of the gastric pouch, gastric outlet obstruction, and dumping syndrome.
- Explain why dehydration is a frequent complication following bariatric surgery. What tips can you give Jillian to help her avoid this problem?

Notes

1. G. W. Mirowski, J. Leblanc, and L. A. Mark, Oral disease and oral-cutaneous manifestations of gastrointestinal and liver disease, in M. Feldman and coeditors, *Sleisenger and Fordtran's Gastrointestinal and Liver Disease* (Philadelphia: Saunders, 2016), pp. 377–396; T. E. Daniels and R. C. Jordan, Diseases of the mouth and salivary glands, in L. Goldman and A. I. Schafer, eds., *Goldman-Cecil Medicine* (Philadelphia: Saunders, 2016), pp. 2579–2585.

2. Academy of Nutrition and Dietetics, *Nutrition Care Manual* (Chicago: Academy of Nutrition and Dietetics, 2018.

3. H. Mashimo, Oropharyngeal and esophageal motility disorders, in N. J. Greenberger, ed., *Current Diagnosis and Treatment: Gastroenterology, Hepatology, and Endoscopy* (New York: McGraw-Hill, 2016), pp. 174–192.

4. Academy of Nutrition and Dietetics, 2018.

5. J. A. Y. Cichero, Thickening agents used for dysphagia management: effect on bioavailability of water, medication and feelings of satiety, *Nutrition Journal* 12 (2013): 54.

6. J. E. Richter and F. K. Friedenberg, Gastroesophageal reflux disease, in M. Feldman and coeditors, *Sleisenger and Fordtran's Gastrointestinal and Liver Disease* (Philadelphia: Saunders, 2016), pp. 733–754.

7. S. Friedman and J. R. Agrawal, Gastrointestinal and biliary complications of pregnancy, in N. J. Greenberger, ed., *Current Diagnosis and Treatment: Gastroenterology, Hepatology, and Endoscopy* (New York: McGraw-Hill, 2016), pp. 84–111.

8. W. W. Chan and J. R. Saltzman, Gastroesophageal reflux disease, in in N. J. Greenberger, ed., *Current Diagnosis and Treatment: Gastroenterology, Hepatology, and Endoscopy* (New York: McGraw-Hill, 2016), pp. 157–166.

9. Chan and Saltzman, 2016; G. W. Falk and D. A. Katzka, Diseases of the esophagus, in L. Goldman and A. I. Schafer, eds., *Goldman-Cecil Medicine* (Philadelphia: Saunders, 2016), pp. 896–908.

10. W. W. Chan and R. Burakoff, Functional (nonulcer) dyspepsia, in N. J. Greenberger, ed., *Current Diagnosis and Treatment: Gastroenterology, Hepatology, and Endoscopy* (New York: McGraw-Hill, 2016), pp. 215–226.

11. Chan and Burakoff, Functional (nonulcer) dyspepsia, 2016.

12. J. Tack, Dyspepsia, in M. Feldman and coeditors, *Sleisenger and Fordtran's Gastrointestinal and Liver Disease* (Philadelphia: Saunders, 2016), pp. 194–206; B. E. Lacy and coauthors, Review article: Current treatment options and management of functional dyspepsia, *Alimentary Pharmacology and Therapeutics* 36 (2012): 3–15.

13. Chan and Burakoff, Functional (nonulcer) dyspepsia, 2016.

14. Chan and Burakoff, Functional (nonulcer) dyspepsia, 2016; Tack, 2016.

15. K. McQuaid, Approach to the patient with gastrointestinal disease, in L. Goldman and A. I. Schafer, eds., *Goldman-Cecil Medicine* (Philadelphia: Saunders, 2016), pp. 850–866.

16. Academy of Nutrition and Dietetics, 2018.

17. K. L. Koch, Gastric neuromuscular function and neuromuscular disorders, in M. Feldman and coeditors, *Sleisenger and Fordtran's Gastrointestinal and Liver Disease* (Philadelphia: Saunders, 2016), pp. 811–838.

18. Academy of Nutrition and Dietetics, 2018; M. Camilleri and coauthors, Clinical guideline: Management of gastroparesis, *American Journal of Gastroenterology* 108 (2013): 18–37.

19. M. Feldman and E. L. Lee, Gastritis, in M. Feldman and coeditors, *Sleisenger and Fordtran's Gastrointestinal and Liver Disease* (Philadelphia: Saunders, 2016), pp. 868–883.

20. A. C. Antony, Megaloblastic anemias, in L. Goldman and A. I. Schafer, eds., *Goldman-Cecil Medicine* (Philadelphia: Saunders, 2016), pp. 1104–1114; J. R. Turner, Gastrointestinal Tract, in V. Kumar and coeditors, *Robbins and Cotran Pathologic Basis of Disease* (Philadelphia: Saunders, 2015), pp. 749–819.

21. E. Lew, Peptic ulcer disease, in N. J. Greenberger, ed., *Current Diagnosis and Treatment: Gastroenterology, Hepatology, and Endoscopy* (New York: McGraw-Hill, 2016), pp. 197–208.

22. E. J. Kuipers and M. J. Blaser, Acid peptic disease, in L. Goldman and A. I. Schafer, eds., *Goldman-Cecil Medicine* (Philadelphia: Saunders, 2016), pp. 908–918.

23. F. K. L. Chan and J. Y. W. Lau, Peptic ulcer disease, in M. Feldman and coeditors, *Sleisenger and Fordtran's Gastrointestinal and Liver Disease* (Philadelphia: Saunders, 2016), pp. 884–900.

24. Lew, 2016.

25. Lew, 2016.

26. Academy of Nutrition and Dietetics, 2018.

27. S. Cohen, Gastritis and peptic ulcer disease, in R. S. Porter and J. L. Kaplan, eds., *Merck Manual of Diagnosis and Therapy* (Whitehouse Station, NJ: Merck Sharp and Dohme, 2011), pp. 128–138.

28. Academy of Nutrition and Dietetics, 2018.

29. W. W. Chan and R. Burakoff, Disorders of gastric and small bowel motility, in N. J. Greenberger, ed., *Current Diagnosis and Treatment: Gastroenterology, Hepatology, and Endoscopy* (New York: McGraw-Hill, 2016), pp. 227–237; M. A. Schattner and E. B. Grossman, Nutritional management, in M. Feldman and coeditors, *Sleisenger and Fordtran's Gastrointestinal and Liver Disease* (Philadelphia: Saunders, 2016), pp. 83–101.

30. S. Carey, Bone health after major upper gastrointestinal surgery, *Practical Gastroenterology* (March 2013): 46–55.

31. M. K. Robinson and N. J. Greenberger, Treatment of obesity: The impact of bariatric surgery, in N. J. Greenberger, ed., *Current Diagnosis and Treatment: Gastroenterology, Hepatology, and Endoscopy* (New York: McGraw-Hill, 2016), pp. 238–250; S.-H. Chang and coauthors, Effectiveness and risks of bariatric surgery: An updated systematic review and meta-analysis, 2003–2012, *JAMA Surgery* 149 (2014): 275–287.

32. S. S. Dagan and coauthors, Nutritional recommendations for adult bariatric surgery patients: Clinical practice, *Advances in Nutrition* 8 (2017): 382–394; Robinson and Greenberger, 2016.

33. Robinson and Greenberger, 2016; Chang and coauthors, 2014.

34. Academy of Nutrition and Dietetics, 2018.

35. Dagan and coauthors, 2017; Weight Management Dietetic Practice Group, *Pocket Guide to Bariatric Surgery* (Chicago: Academy of Nutrition and Dietetics, 2015), pp. 41–85.

36. K. Tymitz, T. Magnuson, and M. Schweitzer, Bariatric surgery, in A. C. Ross and coeditors, *Modern Nutrition in Health and Disease* (Baltimore: Lippincott Williams & Wilkins, 2014), pp. 800–807; J. I. Mechanick and coauthors, Clinical practice guidelines for the perioperative nutritional, metabolic, and nonsurgical support of the bariatric surgery patient—2013 update, *Endocrine Practice* 19 (2013): 337–372.

37. Robinson and Greenberger, 2016.

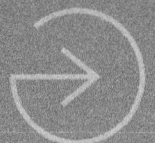

17.4 Nutrition in Practice

Nutrition and Oral Health

Various aspects of nutrition and oral health have been discussed in this book. Chapters 3 and 9 describe the effects of carbohydrates and fluoride, respectively, on the development of dental caries. Chapter 11 discusses the development of tooth decay in babies who are given bottles for prolonged periods. This Nutrition in Practice provides additional information about dental caries and introduces other problems related to oral health. The glossary in Box NP17-1 defines related terms.

What is dental caries, and what factors influence its development?

Dental caries is an oral infectious disease that affects the structures and integrity of the teeth. Caries develops when the bacteria that reside in **dental plaque** metabolize dietary carbohydrates and produce acids that attack tooth enamel. If allowed to progress, the decay can penetrate the dentin and destroy other structures that support and maintain the tooth (see Figure NP17-1). The development of dental caries is influenced by the type of carbohydrate consumed, the frequency of carbohydrate intake, the stickiness of the foods that contain carbohydrate, and the availability of saliva to rinse the teeth and neutralize acid. Other factors include oral hygiene, fluoride intake, and the composition of tooth enamel, which together influence a person's susceptibility to caries. Poor nutrition during pregnancy, infancy, or early childhood can impair the development of healthy teeth and increase vulnerability to dental caries. Table NP17-1 lists examples of nutrient deficiencies that influence the development of dental caries.[1]

FIGURE NP17-1 Development of Dental Caries

Dental caries begins when acid dissolves the enamel that covers the tooth. If not repaired, the decay may penetrate the dentin and spread into the pulp of the tooth, causing inflammation, abscess, and possible loss of the tooth.

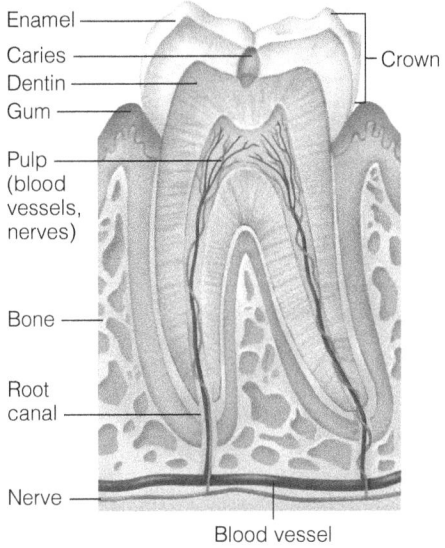

Which foods promote caries development?

The most **cariogenic** foods are carbohydrate-containing foods that remain in contact with the teeth for prolonged periods, are difficult to clear from the mouth, or are consumed frequently or over an extended time period.[2]

Box NP17-1 Glossary

cariogenic (KAH-ree-oh-JEN-ic): conducive to the development of dental caries.

dental calculus: mineralized dental plaque, often associated with inflammation and progressive gum disease.

dental caries (KAH-reez): tooth decay caused by the acidic by-products of carbohydrate fermentation by bacteria residing in dental plaque.

dental plaque (PLACK): a film of bacteria and bacterial by-products that accumulates on the tooth surface.

gingiva (jin-JYE-va, JIN-jeh-va): the gums.

gingivitis (jin-jeh-VYE-tus): inflammation of the gums, characterized by redness, swelling, and bleeding.

periodontal disease: disease that involves the connective tissues that support the teeth.

periodontitis: inflammation or degeneration of the tissues that support the teeth.

periodontium: the tissues that support the teeth, including the gums, cementum (bonelike material covering the dentin layer of the tooth), periodontal ligament, and underlying bone.

- *peri* = around, surrounding
- *odont* = tooth

TABLE NP17-1	Nutrient Deficiencies Affecting Development of Dental Caries
NUTRIENT DEFICIENCY	**EFFECT ON DENTAL TISSUES**
Protein	Delayed tooth development, decreased tooth size, increased solubility of tooth enamel, degradation of salivary glands
Vitamin A	Impaired formation of tooth enamel, degradation of salivary glands
Vitamin D, calcium, and phosphorus	Impaired formation of tooth enamel, reduced enamel mineralization, decreased resistance to dental caries
Fluoride	Increased susceptibility to enamel demineralization, reduced protection against decay-causing bacteria

Examples include hard candies or lozenges that dissolve slowly in the mouth; sticky or chewy foods such as dried fruit or chewy bread; starchy snack foods such as pretzels or chips; and sweetened beverages that are repeatedly sipped. These foods can be eaten without provoking tooth decay if they are consumed quickly and removed from tooth surfaces promptly.

Acidic foods and beverages—such as cola drinks, citrus fruits and juices, pickles, and some herbal teas—also contribute to the erosion of tooth enamel. Acidic food items are more cariogenic when consumed after or between meals because they are less likely to be rinsed away by saliva or neutralized by alkaline foods that may be consumed during the meal.[3]

Do any foods help to prevent caries?

Yes, foods that stimulate saliva flow, neutralize mouth acidity, or induce the clearance of food particles from the teeth can help to prevent caries formation. Examples include cheese, which increases salivary secretions and contains nutrients that neutralize acid; milk, which reduces mouth acidity due to its nearly neutral pH; and raw vegetables, which require vigorous chewing and therefore stimulate saliva flow. Some foods contain substances that reduce enamel solubility, such as the fluoride in tea and an unidentified compound in cocoa. The sequence in which foods are eaten influences caries development; for example, eating cheese after consuming an acidic fruit dessert can raise plaque pH and reduce caries risk, whereas drinking sugared coffee at the end of the meal can prolong plaque acidity. Chewing sugarless gum after or between meals can help to prevent caries by stimulating salivary flow, pushing saliva into hard-to-reach crevices in and around teeth, and removing food particles from the teeth.[4]

How does saliva protect against caries formation?

In addition to rinsing away the sugars and food particles that remain on the teeth, saliva contains substances (such as proteins, bicarbonate, and phosphates) that dilute and neutralize mouth acidity. Furthermore, saliva contains antimicrobial proteins (immunoglobulins and lysozyme) that defend against bacteria and fungi. Finally, the calcium, phosphate, and fluoride ions in saliva help to prevent dissolution of enamel and promote remineralization. If salivary secretions are low or absent, the risk of developing dental caries and other dental diseases greatly increases.[5]

Does dental plaque contribute to other dental diseases?

Yes, the deposits of plaque can thicken and lead to other dental problems. As plaque accumulates on the tooth surface, it fills with calcium and phosphate, eventually forming **dental calculus**.[6] Calculus develops either at the gum surface or in the crevice between the gum and a tooth; its presence may lead to additional plaque retention. The buildup of plaque and calculus increases the likelihood of infection and subsequent inflammation.

Periodontal disease is the name given to inflammatory conditions that involve the **periodontium**, the structures that support the tooth in its bony socket (see Photo NP17-1). The periodontium includes the gums (called **gingiva**), other connective tissues surrounding the tooth, and the bone underneath. Inflammation of the gums, called **gingivitis**, is characterized by redness, bleeding, and

Photo NP17-1	Periodontal Disease

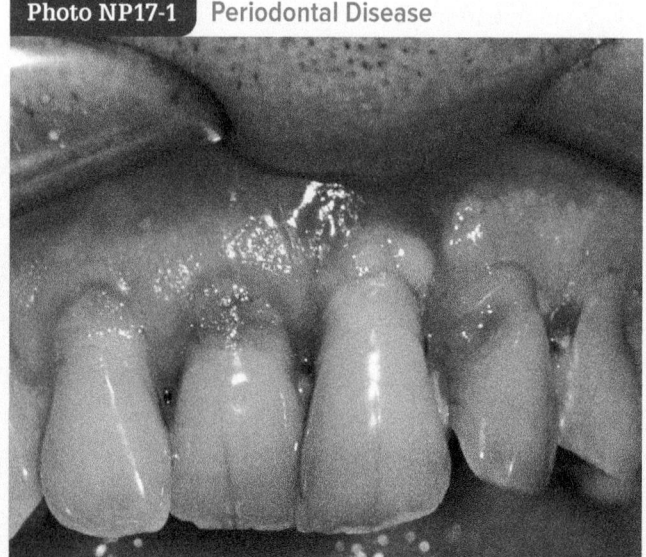

CNRI/Science Source

Periodontal disease destroys the tissues and bones that hold teeth in place.

swelling of gum tissue. **Periodontitis** is an inflammation of the other tissues surrounding the tooth. As plaque invades the space below the gum line, the combination of toxic bacterial by-products and the body's immune responses can damage the tissues holding a tooth in place. Left untreated, the tissues and bone of the periodontium may ultimately be destroyed, leading to permanent tooth loss.

What are the risk factors for periodontal disease, and how is it treated?

Dental plaque is the primary risk factor associated with periodontal disease, and the severity of disease is related to the amount of plaque present. Tobacco smoking is another factor, possibly due to its destructive effects on cellular immune responses.[7] The likelihood of developing periodontal disease is increased if a person has a chronic illness that impairs immune status, such as diabetes mellitus or HIV infection. Other risk factors include stress, pregnancy, use of certain medications (including oral contraceptives, antiepileptic drugs, and anticancer drugs), and dental conditions that increase plaque accumulation, such as poorly aligned teeth or ill-fitting bridges. Strategies for reducing risk focus on improving oral hygiene (proper brushing and flossing) and encouraging smoking cessation. Table NP17-2 provides suggestions that may help to decrease the risk of developing oral diseases.

Treatment of periodontal disease depends on the extent of damage. In mild cases, deep cleaning (removal of plaque and calculus deposits) and proper oral hygiene may reverse the condition. Antimicrobial mouth rinses and topical antibiotics may be prescribed to control infection. Surgical approaches may be used to eliminate gum pockets (by reshaping tooth and bone surfaces) or to replace tissues that have been destroyed.

How do chronic diseases influence a person's risk for dental and oral diseases?

Some chronic diseases can alter the structure and function of dental tissues, impair immune responses, or cause reduced salivary flow. Furthermore, certain medications can reduce salivary secretions, along with the immune protection that saliva provides. Examples of conditions that may upset oral health and increase the risks of developing dental problems include the following:

- *Diabetes mellitus.* Periodontal disease is more prevalent among people with diabetes mellitus, especially those whose diabetes is poorly controlled.[8] People with diabetes often have impaired immune responses and a greater susceptibility to infection. Diabetes also favors the growth of bacteria that infect periodontal tissues. Compared with healthy individuals, people with diabetes tend to have increased plaque accumulations

TABLE NP17-2 Suggestions for Preventing Oral Diseases

PERSONAL HYGIENE

- Brush your teeth twice daily for at least 2 minutes with a fluoride toothpaste. Replace your toothbrush every 3 or 4 months or whenever the bristles become frayed.
- Floss between your teeth at least once a day.
- Avoid smoking. If you smoke, look into tobacco cessation programs in your area.
- Avoid consuming excessive amounts of alcohol.

DIETARY PRACTICES

- Reduce your consumption of sugary foods. Avoid consuming sugary and starchy snacks between meals.
- After consuming carbohydrate-containing foods, sugary beverages, or acidic soft drinks or teas, rinse your mouth or clean your teeth.
- If you chew gum, use a sugarless gum.
- Avoid putting an infant or child to bed with a nursing bottle containing anything except plain water.
- In communities that do not provide fluoridated water, provide children at high risk of dental caries with a fluoride supplement.

PROFESSIONAL DENTAL CARE

- Visit a dentist at least once a year to have your teeth and mouth examined and teeth cleaned. Visit the dentist more often if necessary.
- Ask the dentist if you are a candidate for topical fluoride treatments or tooth sealants, which protect susceptible tooth surfaces.

and reduced salivary flow. In addition, the damaging effects of hyperglycemia weaken the collagen structure of dental tissues, making them more vulnerable to destruction.

- *Human immunodeficiency virus (HIV)/AIDS.* HIV infection is characterized by compromised immunity, and the risk of developing periodontal disease is closely linked to the degree of immunosuppression present. Those at greatest risk include smokers and individuals with poor oral hygiene.[9] In untreated persons, fungal and viral infections are common and may cause burning in the mouth and painful ulcerations. Many HIV-infected individuals develop dry mouth as a result of medications or salivary gland dysfunction.
- *Radiation treatment for oral cancers.* The radiation treatment required for oral cancers often causes serious oral and dental complications.[10] Inflammation and tissue damage can be so severe that the radiation treatment may need to be halted or the intensity significantly reduced. Other complications include dry

mouth, changes in taste sensation, fungal and viral infections, and tissue and muscle scarring (which often reduces chewing ability). To minimize complications, dental care is often initiated before radiation therapy begins.

Can dental diseases have adverse effects on health beyond their effects on the teeth?

Yes, the bacteria that reside on dental tissues can enter the bloodstream and travel to other tissues; therefore, they may be able to trigger immune responses or cause infections elsewhere in the body.[11] Some evidence supports a link between dental bacteria and other medical conditions, including the following:

- *Atherosclerosis and heart disease.* The inflammatory process induced by periodontal pathogens may increase levels of cytokines and other mediators that accelerate the progression of atherosclerosis. In addition, periodontal bacteria may enter the bloodstream and contribute to the processes of arterial plaque formation or blood clotting.[12]

- *Diabetes mellitus.* The chronic inflammation caused by periodontal disease can exacerbate insulin resistance and provoke events leading to type 2 diabetes. Severe periodontal disease has also been linked to poor glycemic control in persons with diabetes.[13]
- *Respiratory illnesses.* Clinical studies suggest a link between pneumonia and poor oral health. In addition, dental treatment and improvements in oral health have been associated with significant reductions in respiratory diseases in institutionalized older adults.[14]

Research studies are in progress to confirm cause-and-effect relationships between oral bacteria and the medical conditions described above, as well as the specific mechanisms involved.

Nutrition status and health status have strong influences on oral health. Developing sound eating habits and maintaining good dental hygiene are practices that can promote dental health and possibly reduce the risk of developing other medical problems. Additional studies will help to clarify the complex interactions between dental disease and chronic illnesses.

Notes

1. R. Touger-Decker, D. R. Radler, and D. P. DePaola, Nutrition and dental medicine, in A. C. Ross and coeditors, eds., *Modern Nutrition in Health and Disease* (Baltimore: Lippincott Williams & Wilkins, 2014), pp. 1016–1040.
2. P. Gupta and coauthors, Role of sugar and sugar substitutes in dental caries: A review, ISRN Dentistry 2013 (2013): doi.org/10.1155/2013/519421.
3. Touger-Decker, Radler, and DePaola, 2014.
4. Touger-Decker, Radler, and DePaola, 2014; S. K. Stookey, The effect of saliva on dental caries, *Journal of the American Dental Association* 139 (2008): 11S–17S.
5. S. Ruhl, The scientific exploration of saliva in the past-proteomic era: From database back to basic function, *Expert Review of Proteomics* 9 (2012): 85–96.
6. M. W. Lingen, Head and neck, in V. Kumar and coeditors, *Robbins and Cotran Pathologic Basis of Disease* (Philadelphia: Saunders, 2015), pp. 727–748.
7. J. B. C. Neto and coauthors, Smoking and periodontal tissues: A review, *Brazilian Oral Research* 26 (2012): 25–31.
8. Touger-Decker, Radler, and DePaola, 2014.

9. C. N. John, L. X. Stephen, and C. W. J. Africa, Is human immunodeficiency virus (HIV) stage an independent risk factor for altering the periodontal status of HIV-positive patients? A South African study, *BMC Oral Health* 13 (2013): 69, doi: 10.1186/1472-6831-13-69.
10. Touger-Decker, Radler, and DePaola, 2014; Academy of Nutrition and Dietetics, Position of the Academy of Nutrition and Dietetics: Oral health and nutrition, *Journal of the Academy of Nutrition and Dietetics* (2013): 693–701.
11. R. V. Oppermann, P. Weidlich, and M. L. Musskopf, Periodontal disease and systemic complications, *Brazilian Oral Research* 26 (2012): 39–47.
12. P. B. Lockhart and coauthors, Periodontal disease and atherosclerotic vascular disease: Does the evidence support an independent association? *Circulation* 125 (2012): 2520–2544.
13. P. M. Preshaw and coauthors, Periodontitis and diabetes: A two-way relationship, *Diabetologia* 55 (2012): 21–31.
14. A. Azarpazhooh and H. C. Tenenbaum, Separating fact from fiction: Use of high-level evidence from research syntheses to identify diseases and disorders associated with periodontal disease, *Journal of the Canadian Dental Association* 78 (2012): c25.

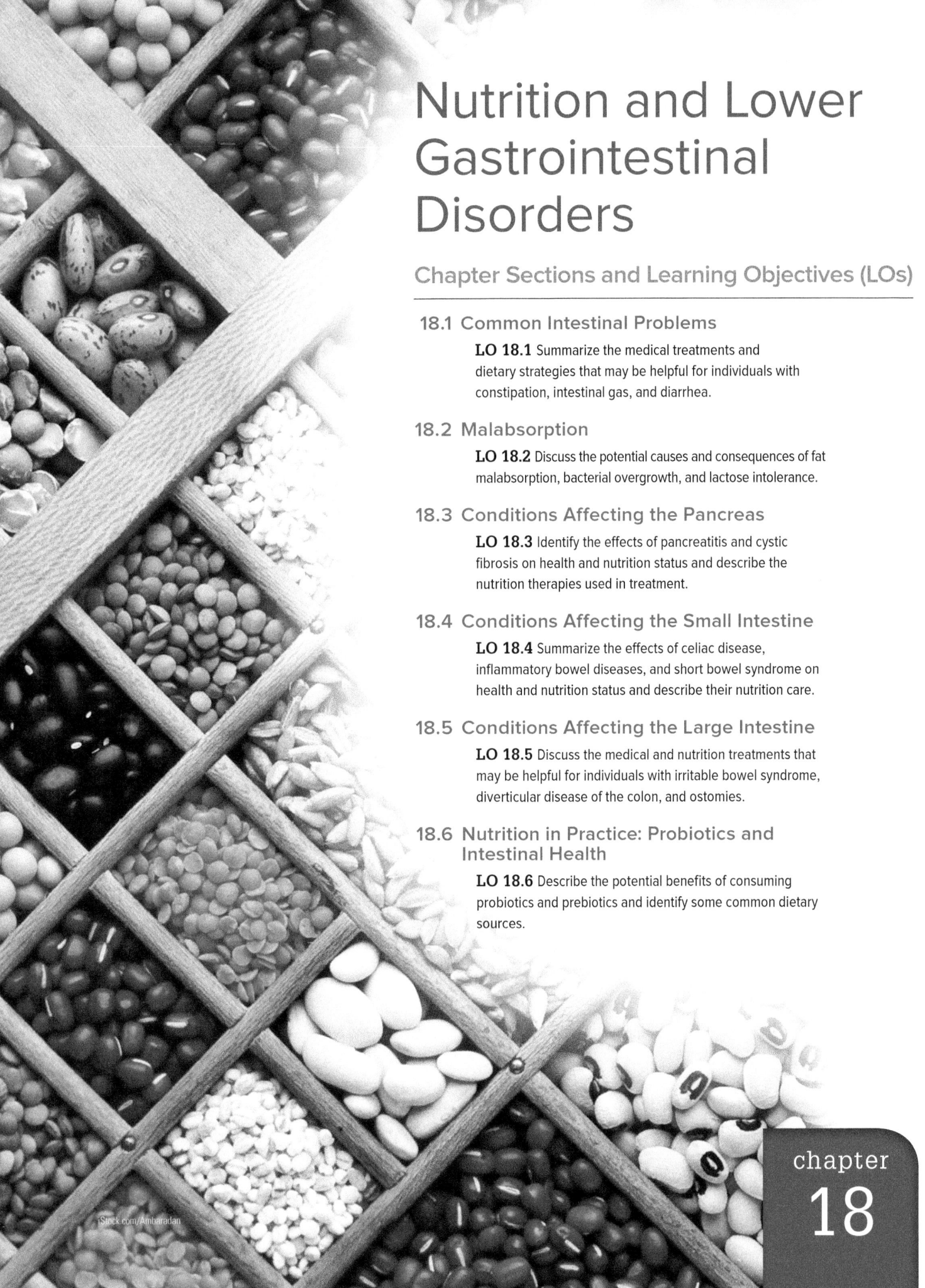

Chapter 18

Nutrition and Lower Gastrointestinal Disorders

Chapter Sections and Learning Objectives (LOs)

18.1 Common Intestinal Problems

LO 18.1 Summarize the medical treatments and dietary strategies that may be helpful for individuals with constipation, intestinal gas, and diarrhea.

18.2 Malabsorption

LO 18.2 Discuss the potential causes and consequences of fat malabsorption, bacterial overgrowth, and lactose intolerance.

18.3 Conditions Affecting the Pancreas

LO 18.3 Identify the effects of pancreatitis and cystic fibrosis on health and nutrition status and describe the nutrition therapies used in treatment.

18.4 Conditions Affecting the Small Intestine

LO 18.4 Summarize the effects of celiac disease, inflammatory bowel diseases, and short bowel syndrome on health and nutrition status and describe their nutrition care.

18.5 Conditions Affecting the Large Intestine

LO 18.5 Discuss the medical and nutrition treatments that may be helpful for individuals with irritable bowel syndrome, diverticular disease of the colon, and ostomies.

18.6 Nutrition in Practice: Probiotics and Intestinal Health

LO 18.6 Describe the potential benefits of consuming probiotics and prebiotics and identify some common dietary sources.

iStock.com/Ambaradan

chapter
18

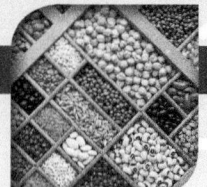

small intestine, disorders of the lower gastrointestinal (GI) tract can interfere substantially with a person's diet and lifestyle. Some of the diets required for these conditions are complicated and difficult to follow, and the foods that are tolerated can vary considerably. In visits with patients, health professionals should ensure that patients understand the nutrition prescription and help to pinpoint difficult foods. They can also suggest ways to make restrictive diets more acceptable.

18.1 Common Intestinal Problems

Nearly all people experience occasional intestinal problems, which usually clear up without medical treatment. Intestinal discomfort can sometimes drive a person to seek medical attention, however, and the symptoms may be evidence of a serious intestinal disorder or other illness. Common intestinal problems and their causes and treatments are discussed below.

Constipation

A diagnosis of constipation is based, in part, on a defecation frequency of fewer than three bowel movements per week.[1] Other symptoms may include excessive straining during defecation, the passage of hard stools, and incomplete evacuation. In some cases, a person's perception of constipation may be due to a mistaken notion of what constitutes "normal" bowel habits, so the person's expectations about bowel function may need to be addressed (see Box 18-1).

The prevalence of constipation is higher in women than in men and is especially high in older adults (65 years and older). Older adults tend to report problems with excessive straining and hard stools rather than infrequent defecation.[2]

Causes of Constipation The risk of constipation is increased in individuals with a low-fiber diet, low food intake, inadequate fluid intake, or low level of physical activity. All of these factors can extend transit time, leading to increased water reabsorption within the colon and dry, hard stools that are difficult to pass. Medical conditions often associated with constipation include diabetes mellitus and hypothyroidism (see Box 18-2). Neurological conditions such as Parkinson's disease, spinal cord injury, and multiple sclerosis may cause motor problems that lead to constipation. During pregnancy, women often experience constipation because of hormonal changes and the pressure of the enlarged uterus on the intestines. Constipation is also a common side effect of several classes of medications and some dietary supplements, including opiate-containing analgesics, anticholinergics, diuretics, calcium channel blockers, and calcium and iron supplements.

Treatment of Constipation In individuals with a low fiber intake, the primary treatment for constipation is a gradual increase in fiber intake to at least 20 to 25 grams per day.[3] High-fiber diets increase stool weight and fecal water content and promote a more rapid transit of materials through the colon. Foods that increase stool weight the most include wheat bran, fruits, and vegetables (see Photo 18-1). Bran intake can be increased by adding bran cereals and whole-wheat bread to the diet or by mixing bran powder with beverages or foods. The transition to a high-fiber diet may be

BOX 18-1 *Nursing Diagnosis*

The nursing diagnosis *perceived constipation* may apply to people with adequate bowel movements who self-diagnose constipation.

BOX 18-2 *Nursing Diagnosis*

The nursing diagnoses *constipation and risk for constipation* may apply to persons with medical problems that predispose them to constipation.

Photo 18-1

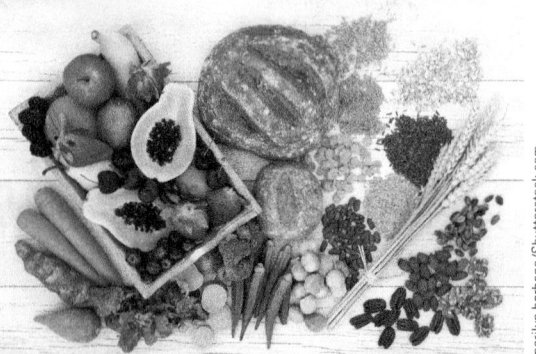

marilyn barbone/Shutterstock.com

High-fiber foods promote regular bowel movements. The fiber DRI for women and men aged 19 to 50 years are 25 and 38 grams, respectively.

difficult for some people because it can increase intestinal gas, so high-fiber foods should be added gradually, as tolerated. Fiber supplements such as methylcellulose (Citrucel), psyllium (Metamucil, Fiberall), and polycarbophil (Fiber-Lax) are also effective (see Table 18-1); these supplements can be mixed with beverages and taken several times daily. Unlike other fibers, methylcellulose and polycarbophil do not increase intestinal gas.

Several other dietary or lifestyle measures may help to relieve constipation. Consuming adequate fluid (1.5 to 2 liters daily) enhances the effect of an increased fiber intake on stool frequency, and an appropriate fluid intake prevents excessive reabsorption of water from the colon, resulting in wetter stools. Consuming prunes or prune juice is often recommended because prunes contain compounds that have a mild laxative effect. Skipping breakfast is discouraged, as colonic motility is highest after a morning meal. Inactive individuals are generally encouraged to increase physical activity, although clinical studies have not confirmed that increasing exercise improves constipation symptoms.[4]

Laxatives Laxatives may improve a constipation problem by increasing stool weight, increasing the water content of stool, or stimulating peristaltic contractions. Table 18-1 includes examples of common laxatives and describes their modes of

TABLE 18-1	Laxatives and Bulk-Forming Agents			
LAXATIVE TYPE	**ACTIVE INGREDIENTS**	**PRODUCT EXAMPLES**	**METHOD OF ACTION**	**CAUTIONS**
Chloride channel activators	Lubiprostone, linaclotide	Amitiza, Linzess	Activate chloride channels in the intestines to increase fluid secretions, which help in passing stools.	May cause diarrhea, nausea, and abdominal discomfort; available by prescription only.
Fiber (bulk-forming agents)	Malt soup extract, methylcellulose, polycarbophil, psyllium	Citrucel, Fiberall, Fiber-Lax, Metamucil	Increase stool weight and aid in the formation of soft, bulky stools. Similar effects may be achieved by consuming a high-fiber diet. For mild to moderate constipation. Safe for long-term use.	Some fiber supplements may increase flatulence. Psyllium may cause an allergic reaction.
Osmotic laxatives: poorly absorbed salts	Magnesium citrate, magnesium hydroxide	Epsom salts, milk of magnesia, Citromag	Attract water and increase the liquidity of stools, which stimulates contractions.	May cause bloating and watery stools or diarrhea. Should be used with caution. Avoid using in patients with kidney disease and in children.
Osmotic laxatives: poorly absorbed sugars	Lactulose, polyethylene glycol, sorbitol	Cephulac, Chronulac, CoLyte	Attract water and increase the liquidity of stools, which stimulates contractions. Must be used for several days to take effect. Safe for long-term use.	May cause flatulence and cramps. Can lose effectiveness over time.
Stimulant or irritant laxatives	Bisacodyl, cascara, castor oil, senna	Correctol, Dulcolax, Ex-Lax	Act as local irritants to colonic tissue; stimulate peristalsis and mucosal secretions. For moderate to severe constipation. Long-term use is discouraged.	Usually given only after milder treatments fail. May alter fluid and electrolyte balances. May lead to laxative dependency.
Stool surfactant agents (stool softeners)	Docusate sodium, docusate calcium	Colace, Surfak	Promote the mixing of water with stools; prevent formation of dry, hard stools.	Do not increase stool weight. Limited effectiveness.

TABLE 18-2 Foods That May Increase Intestinal Gas[a]

- Apples
- Artichokes
- Asparagus
- Beans and peas
- Brussels sprouts
- Carbonated beverages
- Cabbage
- Cauliflower
- Fructose-sweetened products
- Fruit juices
- Garlic
- Milk products (if lactose intolerant)
- Mushrooms
- Onions
- Pears
- Wheat

[a]Responses to individual foods vary; tolerances are best determined by trial and error.

Note: The quantity of food consumed influences the amount of gas produced and the corresponding symptoms.

action. Enemas and suppositories (chemicals introduced into the rectum) are also used to promote defecation; they work by distending and stimulating the rectum or by lubricating the stool.

Medical Interventions For patients with severe constipation who do not respond to dietary or laxative treatments, physicians may prescribe medications (called *prokinetic agents*) that stimulate colonic contractions. Physical therapy and biofeedback techniques are sometimes successful in training patients to relax their pelvic muscles more effectively. Surgical interventions are a last resort and include colonic resections and colostomy operations, which are discussed later in the chapter.

Intestinal Gas

As mentioned previously, increased intestinal gas (**flatulence**) may be an unpleasant side effect of consuming a high-fiber diet. Because dietary fibers are not digested, they pass into the colon and are fermented by bacteria, which produce gas as a by-product (soluble fibers are more readily fermented than insoluble fibers). Other incompletely digested or poorly absorbed carbohydrates have similar effects; these include the indigestible carbohydrates in beans (raffinose and stachyose), lactose (in lactose-intolerant individuals), fructose, some sugar alcohols (such as sorbitol, xylitol, and mannitol), and some forms of resistant starch, found in grain products and potatoes. For purposes of nutrition therapy, fermentable dietary carbohydrates are often referred to as **FODMAPs**, which is an acronym for *fermentable oligosaccharides, disaccharides, monosaccharides, and polyols*. Restricting food sources of FODMAPs has been found to improve intestinal discomfort in individuals with certain GI diseases, such as irritable bowel syndrome (see p. 534).[5]

Table 18-2 lists examples of foods commonly associated with excessive gas production, although individual responses vary. With the exception of carbonated beverages, the foods in Table 18-2 are sources of FODMAPs; wheat is also a source of resistant starch. Carbonated beverages contain dissolved carbon dioxide gas, which contributes to intestinal gas. Similarly, swallowed air that is not expelled by belching may travel to the intestines and be a source of intestinal gas. Malabsorption disorders (discussed later in this chapter) can also cause considerable flatulence because the undigested macronutrients can be metabolized by colonic bacteria.

Although many people attribute their symptoms of bloating and abdominal pain to excessive gas, these symptoms do not correlate well with an increase in intestinal gas.[6] Most people who self-diagnose a flatulence problem have no more intestinal gas than others. Some individuals who experience recurrent bloating and abdominal pain are later diagnosed with irritable bowel syndrome (discussed later in this chapter) or dyspepsia (discussed in Chapter 17).

flatulence: the condition of having excessive intestinal gas, which causes abdominal discomfort.

FODMAPs: an acronym for *fermentable oligosaccharides, disaccharides, monosaccharides, and polyols*, which are incompletely digested or poorly absorbed carbohydrates that are fermented in the large intestine; a low-FODMAP diet may help to reduce flatulence, abdominal distention, and diarrhea.

Diarrhea

Diarrhea is characterized by the passage of frequent, watery stools. In most cases, it lasts for only a day or two and subsides without complication. Severe or persistent diarrhea, however, can cause dehydration and electrolyte imbalances. If chronic, it may lead to weight loss and malnutrition. Diarrhea may be accompanied by other symptoms, such as fever, abdominal cramps, dyspepsia, or bleeding, which help in diagnosing the cause.

Causes of Diarrhea Diarrhea is a complication of multiple GI disorders and may also be caused by infections, medications, and dietary substances.[7] It results from inadequate fluid reabsorption in the intestines, sometimes in conjunction with an increase in intestinal secretions. In *osmotic diarrhea*, unabsorbed nutrients or other substances attract water to the colon and increase fecal water content; common causes include high intakes of poorly absorbed sugars (such as sorbitol, mannitol, or fructose), lactase deficiency (which causes lactose malabsorption), and ingestion of laxatives that contain magnesium or phosphates. In *secretory diarrhea*, the fluid secreted by the intestines exceeds the amount that can be reabsorbed by intestinal cells. Secretory diarrhea is often due to foodborne illness but can also be caused by intestinal inflammation and various chemical substances, such as medications or unabsorbed bile acids. *Motility disorders* that cause rapid intestinal transit may also result in diarrhea because they reduce the contact time available for fluid reabsorption.

Acute cases of diarrhea start abruptly and may persist for several weeks; they are most often caused by viral, bacterial, parasitic, or protozoal infections but may also occur as a side effect of medications. Chronic diarrhea, which persists for about four weeks or longer, can result from malabsorptive disorders, inflammatory diseases, motility disorders, chronic infections, radiation treatment, and many other conditions. As mentioned in earlier chapters, diarrhea is a frequent complication of tube feedings and may also occur when oral or enteral feedings are resumed after a period of bowel rest (see Chapter 15).

Medical Treatment of Diarrhea Correcting the underlying medical problem is the first step in treating diarrhea. For example, antibiotics are prescribed to treat intestinal infections. If a medication is the cause of diarrhea, a different drug may be prescribed. If certain foods are responsible, they can be omitted from the diet. Bulk-forming agents such as psyllium (Metamucil) or methylcellulose (Citrucel) can help to reduce the liquidity of the stool. If chronic diarrhea does not respond to treatment, antidiarrheal drugs may be prescribed to slow GI motility or reduce intestinal secretions. **Probiotics** may be beneficial for treating certain types of diarrhea (especially infectious diarrhea) but standard treatment protocols have not been developed.[8] People with severe, **intractable** diarrhea sometimes require total parenteral nutrition.

Oral Rehydration Therapy Severe diarrhea requires the replacement of lost fluid and electrolytes. Oral rehydration solutions can be purchased or easily mixed using water, salts, and a source of glucose (see Box 18-3); the presence of glucose in the solution enhances sodium and water absorption.[9] Commercial sports drinks are not ideal fluids for rehydration because their sodium content is too low, but they can be used if accompanied by salty snack foods.[10] When diarrhea results in extreme dehydration, intravenous solutions are used to quickly replenish fluid and electrolytes.

Nutrition Therapy for Diarrhea Nutrition care depends on the cause of diarrhea and its severity and duration. The dietary treatment initially recommended is often a low-fiber, low-fat, lactose-free diet,[11] which limits foods that contribute to stool volume, such as those with significant amounts of fiber, resistant starch, fructose, sugar alcohols, and lactose (in lactose-intolerant individuals). Fructose and sugar alcohols, which are poorly absorbed, retain fluids in the colon and contribute to osmotic diarrhea. Similarly, milk products may worsen osmotic diarrhea in persons who are lactose intolerant. Avoidance of fatty foods may be advised if they aggravate diarrhea. Gas-producing foods (those with poorly digested or absorbed carbohydrates) can increase intestinal distention and cause additional discomfort. Although fluid intakes must usually be increased to replace fluid losses, patients should avoid caffeinated coffee and tea because caffeine stimulates GI motility and can thereby reduce water reabsorption. Apple pectin or banana flakes are sometimes added to foods or baby formulas to help thicken stool consistency. Table 18-3 lists examples of foods that may worsen diarrhea, although individual tolerances vary.

BOX 18-3

An oral rehydration solution can be mixed from the following ingredients:

- ½ tsp table salt (sodium chloride)
- ⅓ tsp salt substitute (potassium chloride)
- ½ tsp baking soda (sodium bicarbonate)
- 1½ tbs sugar
- 1 liter drinking water

probiotics: live microorganisms from foods or supplements that confer a health benefit when taken in sufficient amounts. Nutrition in Practice 18 provides additional information about probiotics.

intractable: not easily managed or controlled.

TABLE 18-3 Foods That May Worsen Diarrhea

FOODS TO AVOID	RATIONALE	SELECTED EXAMPLES[a]
High-fiber foods	They increase colonic residue.	Breads and cereals with more than 2 g fiber per serving, fruits and vegetables with peels or skin
Foods with indigestible carbohydrates	They contribute to osmotic diarrhea.	Artichokes, asparagus, broccoli, brussels sprouts, cabbage, dried beans and peas, garlic, leeks, okra, onions, wheat
Foods that contain fructose or sugar alcohols	They contribute to osmotic diarrhea.	Dried fruit, fresh fruit (except bananas), fruit juices, fructose-sweetened soft drinks, sugar-free gums and candies
Milk products, if person is lactose intolerant	They contribute to osmotic diarrhea.	Milk and milk products
Gas-producing foods	They increase abdominal discomfort.	Foods with poorly digested or absorbed carbohydrates (including foods listed in the three rows directly above)
Caffeine-containing beverages	They increase intestinal motility.	Coffee, tea, cola beverages, energy drinks

[a]Individual tolerances vary; the foods to avoid are best determined by trial and error.

Review Notes

- Constipation accompanies many health problems but generally correlates with low-fiber diets, low food or fluid intakes, and physical inactivity; a high-fiber diet or fiber supplements may improve symptoms.
- Most intestinal gas is associated with nutrient malabsorption; individuals with excessive gas can avoid foods that cause symptoms.
- Diarrhea may result from malabsorption, intestinal infections, motility disorders, or medications; a low-fiber, low-fat, lactose-free diet can help to reduce symptoms. Some patients with diarrhea require oral rehydration therapy to replace fluid and electrolyte losses.

18.2 Malabsorption

To digest and absorb nutrients, we depend on normal digestive secretions and healthy intestinal mucosa. Malabsorption can therefore be caused by pancreatic disorders that cause enzyme or bicarbonate deficiencies, disorders that result in bile deficiency, and inflammatory diseases or medical treatments that damage intestinal tissue. In some cases, the treatment of an intestinal disease requires surgical removal of a section (**resection**) of the small intestine, leaving minimal absorptive capacity in the portion that remains. Table 18-4 lists examples of diseases and treatments that are frequently associated with malabsorption.

Malabsorption rarely involves a single nutrient. When malabsorption is caused by pancreatic enzyme deficiencies, all macronutrients—protein, carbohydrate, and fat—may be affected. When fat is malabsorbed, fat-soluble nutrients and some minerals are usually malabsorbed as well. Malabsorption disorders and their treatments can tax

resection: the surgical removal of part of an organ or body structure.

steatorrhea (stee-AT-or-REE-ah): excessive fat in the stool due to fat malabsorption; characterized by stools that are loose, frothy, and foul smelling because of a high fat content.

- *steat* = fat
- *rheo* = flow

soaps: chemical compounds formed from fatty acids and positively charged minerals.

nutrition status further by causing complications that alter food intake, raise nutrient needs, or promote additional nutrient losses.

Fat Malabsorption

Fat is the nutrient most frequently malabsorbed because both digestive enzymes and bile must be present for its digestion. Thus, fat malabsorption often develops when an illness reduces either pancreatic or bile secretions. For example, both chronic pancreatitis and cystic fibrosis can decrease the secretion of pancreatic lipase, whereas severe liver disease can cause bile insufficiency. Motility disorders that accelerate gastric emptying or intestinal transit can cause fat malabsorption because they prevent the normal mixing of dietary fat with lipase and bile. Fat malabsorption can also be caused by conditions or treatments that damage the intestinal mucosa, such as inflammatory bowel diseases, AIDS, and radiation treatments for cancer.

Fat malabsorption is often evidenced by **steatorrhea**, the presence of excessive fat in the stools. Steatorrhea can be evaluated by placing the patient on a high-fat diet (80 to 100 grams per day), performing a 48- to 72-hour stool collection, and measuring the stool's fat content. Elimination of more than 7 to 8 percent of the fat intake generally indicates fat malabsorption.[12]

Consequences of Fat Malabsorption Fat malabsorption is associated with losses of food energy, essential fatty acids, fat-soluble vitamins, and some minerals (see Figure 18-1). Weight loss may result if the individual fails to consume alternative sources of energy (see Box 18-4). Deficiencies of fat-soluble vitamins and essential fatty acids are common in chronic conditions. Malabsorption of some minerals, including calcium, magnesium, and zinc, often occurs because the minerals form **soaps** with the unabsorbed fatty acids

| TABLE 18-4 | Potential Causes of Malabsorption |

GENETIC DISORDERS
- Enzyme deficiencies

INTESTINAL DISORDERS
- AIDS-related enteropathy
- Bacterial overgrowth
- Celiac disease
- Crohn's disease
- Radiation enteritis

INTESTINAL INFECTIONS
- Giardiasis
- Nematode (roundworm) infections

LIVER DISEASE (BILE INSUFFICIENCY)

PANCREATIC DISORDERS
- Chronic pancreatitis
- Cystic fibrosis

SURGERIES
- Gastric or intestinal bypass surgery
- Intestinal resection (short bowel syndrome)

| FIGURE 18-1 | The Consequences of Fat Malabsorption

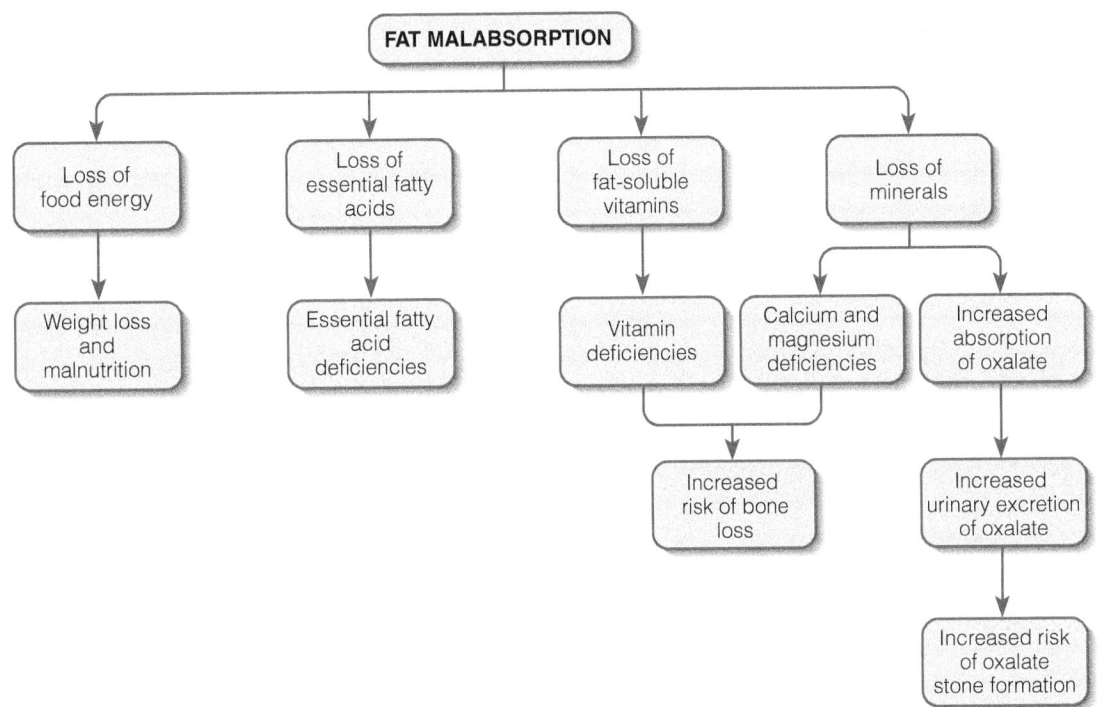

oxalates: plant compounds found in green leafy vegetables and some other foods; these compounds can bind to minerals in the GI tract and form complexes that cannot be absorbed.

and bile acids. Calcium deficiency may lead to bone loss, which is further aggravated by the vitamin D deficiency that may develop as a result of fat malabsorption.

Another consequence of fat malabsorption is an increased risk of kidney stones, which are most often composed of calcium oxalate. The **oxalates** in foods ordinarily bind to calcium in the small intestine and are eliminated in the stool. If calcium instead binds to fatty acids or bile acids, the oxalates are free to be absorbed into the blood and are ultimately excreted in the urine. The risk of developing kidney stones composed of oxalates increases when urinary oxalate levels are high. Kidney stones are discussed further in Chapter 22.

Nutrition Therapy for Fat Malabsorption If steatorrhea does not improve, a fat-restricted diet may be recommended (see Table 18-5). The diet may help to relieve intestinal symptoms that are aggravated by fat intake (such as diarrhea and flatulence) and reduce vitamin and mineral losses. Because fat is a primary energy

TABLE 18-5 Fat-Restricted Diet

A fat-restricted diet includes mostly low-fat and fat-free foods. For a fat intake of 50 grams per day, limit meats and meat substitutes to 6 ounces per day, and limit fats and oils to 8 teaspoons per day.[a] Foods from other food groups should provide less than 1 gram of fat per serving.

FOOD CATEGORY	FOODS RECOMMENDED	FOODS TO AVOID
Meat and meat alternatives	Lean meat, fish, and skinless poultry prepared by broiling, roasting, grilling, or boiling; low-fat luncheon meat such as sliced turkey breast; meat alternatives such as dried beans or peas; low-fat egg substitutes; egg whites	Meat with visible fat, ground beef (unless extra lean), sausage, bacon, frankfurters, spareribs, duck, tuna packed in oil, whole eggs and egg yolks
Milk and milk products	Fat-free milk, fat-free yogurt, fat-free sour cream substitutes, fat-free half-and-half and cream substitutes, fat-free cheese; low-fat milk products can be used in moderation	Milk products that are not fat-free or low-fat
Breads, cereals, rice, and pasta	Whole-grain and enriched breads, cooked cereals and most cold breakfast cereals, plain tortillas, bagels, English muffins, fat-free muffins, saltine crackers, graham crackers, pretzels, plain rice, plain noodles and pasta	Biscuits, pancakes, waffles, granola, snack crackers made with fat, cornbread, doughnuts, corn chips, fried rice, buttered or butter-flavored popcorn
Vegetables	All vegetables prepared without added fat	Buttered, creamed, breaded, or fried vegetables; vegetables prepared au gratin style; french-fried potatoes; potato chips, olives
Fruit	All types of fruit except avocados	Avocados; fruit dishes prepared with fat, nuts, or coconut
Desserts	Sherbet; fruit ices; flavored gelatin; fat-free pudding; angel food cake; meringue; fat-free bakery products; fat-free ice cream or frozen yogurt; fat-free candy such as marshmallows, jelly beans, and hard candy	Cake, cookies, pie, and pastries made with fat; pudding made with whole milk or eggs; ice cream; candy made with fat, such as caramel or chocolate
Fats and oils	Vegetable oils, soft or liquid margarines and spreads, limited amounts of butter or stick margarine (1 tsp provides about 3½–4½ g fat) Each of these foods can replace 1 tsp fat in the amounts specified: 1 tbs salad dressing, 2 tbs low-fat salad dressing, ½ tbs peanut butter, 1 tbs chopped nuts, 2 tbs mashed avocado	Dietary fat that exceeds the amount specified in the nutrition prescription
Beverages	Fruit juice, soft drinks, fat-free milk, coffee, tea, coffee substitutes	Beverages made with milk (unless fat-free) or added cream, chocolate milk, eggnog, milkshakes

[a]To achieve a fat intake that is less than 50 grams, additional reductions may be necessary. For example, for a fat intake of 25 grams per day, limit meats and meat substitutes to 4 ounces per day, and limit fats and oils to 2 teaspoons per day.

source, it should not be restricted more than necessary. **Medium-chain triglycerides (MCT)**, which do not require lipase or bile for digestion and absorption, can be used as an alternative source of dietary fat, although MCT oil does not provide essential fatty acids. Figure 18-2 presents an example of a menu for a fat-restricted diet, and Box 18-5 offers suggestions for following a fat-restricted diet and for using MCT oil.

Bacterial Overgrowth

Ordinarily, the GI tract is protected from **bacterial overgrowth** by gastric acid, which destroys bacteria; peristalsis, which flushes bacteria through the small intestine before they multiply; and immunoglobulins that are secreted into the GI lumen.[13] When bacterial overgrowth does occur, it can lead to fat malabsorption because the bacteria dismantle the bile acids needed for fat emulsification. Deficiencies of the fat-soluble vitamins A, D, and E may eventually develop. The bacteria also produce enzymes and toxins that injure the intestinal mucosa, destroying some mucosal enzymes (especially lactase) and increasing the risk of **bacterial translocation**.[14] Some types of bacteria metabolize vitamin B_{12}, reducing its absorption and increasing the risk of deficiency. Although symptoms of bacterial overgrowth are often minor and nonspecific, severe cases may lead to chronic diarrhea, steatorrhea, flatulence, bloating, and weight loss.

Causes of Bacterial Overgrowth Conditions that impair intestinal motility and allow material to stagnate can greatly increase susceptibility to bacterial overgrowth. For example, intestinal motility can be reduced by strictures, obstructions, or diverticula (protrusions) in the small intestine, as well as by **blind loops** created in certain types of gastrectomy procedures (see the blind loop in Figure 17-2 on p. 501). Some chronic diseases may lead to impaired intestinal motility, including diabetes mellitus (due to the development of neuropathy), scleroderma, and muscular dystrophy.[15]

Reduced secretions of gastric acid can also lead to bacterial overgrowth. Possible causes include atrophic gastritis, use of acid-suppressing medications, and some gastrectomy procedures.

Treatment for Bacterial Overgrowth Treatment may include antibiotics to suppress bacterial growth and surgical correction of the anatomical defects that contribute to a motility disorder. Use of acid-suppressing medications should be discontinued. A lactose-restricted diet may reduce flatulence and diarrhea in some individuals. Dietary supplements can correct nutrient deficiencies, especially deficiencies of the fat-soluble vitamins, calcium and magnesium (which combine with malabsorbed fatty acids), and vitamin B_{12}.[16]

Lactose Intolerance

Approximately 75 percent of people worldwide have some degree of **lactose intolerance**, which is caused by the loss or reduction of lactase, the intestinal enzyme that digests the lactose in milk products.[17] Lactose intolerance is especially prevalent among individuals of certain ethnic groups, including Asians, African Americans, Native Americans, Ashkenazi Jews, and Hispanic/Latino populations. It may also result from GI disorders, medications, or medical treatments that damage the small intestinal mucosa. The primary symptoms of lactose intolerance are diarrhea, bloating, and increased intestinal gas.

FIGURE 18-2 Sample Menu for a Fat-Restricted Diet

The menu shown here contains approximately 50 grams of fat.

❦〜 *Breakfast* 〜❦

6 oz orange juice
1 c oatmeal with raisins and nonfat milk
1 slice whole-wheat toast with 1 tsp margarine
Coffee with fat-free half and half

❦〜 *Lunch* 〜❦

Turkey breast sandwich (includes 2 slices whole-wheat bread, 2 oz lean turkey breast, 2 tomato slices, lettuce leaf, and 2 tsp mayonnaise)
2 c salad greens with 1 tbs salad dressing
Fruit cup (includes 1 c peaches and ½ c berries) with ½ c orange sherbet

❦〜 *Snack* 〜❦

6 oz nonfat fruit yogurt
6 saltine crackers with 1 tbs peanut butter and ½ tbs honey

❦〜 *Dinner* 〜❦

4 oz cod with sliced lemon and dill
1 slice French bread with 1 tsp butter
1 c steamed rice with herbs and walnut oil (includes ½ tsp oil)
1 c steamed broccoli and carrots with ½ tsp margarine
1 piece angel food cake with fat-free whipped cream

medium-chain triglycerides (MCT): triglycerides with fatty acids that are 6 to 12 carbons in length. MCT do not require digestion and can be absorbed in the absence of lipase or bile.

bacterial overgrowth: excessive bacterial colonization of the stomach and small intestine; may be due to low gastric acidity, altered GI motility, mucosal damage, or contamination.

bacterial translocation: the migration of viable bacteria and/or bacterial products from the GI tract to normally sterile tissues such as the bloodstream, lymph nodes, or internal organs, potentially causing infection or tissue injury.

blind loops: bypassed sections of small intestine that are cut off from the normal flow of food material, allowing bacteria to flourish; created in certain types of gastrectomy procedures.

Box 18-5

HOW TO Follow a Fat-Restricted Diet

For some individuals, fat-restricted diets can be difficult to follow. Fats add flavors, aromas, and textures to foods—characteristics that make foods more enjoyable. Unlike dietary changes that can be introduced gradually, fat restriction is often implemented immediately, allowing little time for adaptation. These suggestions may help:

- Fat is better tolerated if provided in small portions. Divide the day's allotment into several servings that can be consumed throughout the day.
- Use variety to enhance enjoyment of meals: vary flavors, textures, colors, and seasonings.
- Look for fat-free items when grocery shopping. Incorporate fat-free ingredients when preparing favorite recipes.
- Try fat-free and low-fat condiments to improve the diet's palatability. Experiment with herbs and spices. Instead of butter, use fruit butter on toast. Use butter-flavored granules on vegetables.

Replace the mayonnaise in sandwiches with a spicy mustard. Replace salad dressing with a flavored vinegar.

If patients are interested in using medium-chain triglyceride (MCT) oil:

- Explain that MCT products are expensive but that the cost is sometimes covered by medical insurance.
- Advise patients to add MCT oil to the diet gradually. Diarrhea and abdominal cramps may result if too much is used at once. Tolerance to MCT oil may improve in time.
- Advise patients that MCT oil may have an unpleasant taste when used alone. Suggest using MCT oil in recipes as a substitute for regular oil. MCT oil can replace the oil in salad dressings, be incorporated into sauces, and be used in cooking or baking. It can also be added to fat-free milk products to make milkshakes.
- Explain that MCT oil should not be used to fry foods because it decomposes at lower temperatures than most cooking oils.

Photo 18-2 Milk and Lactose Intolerance

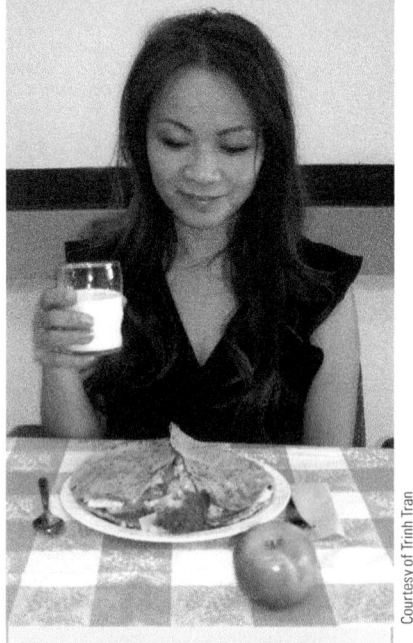

Courtesy of Trinh Tran

Most people with lactose intolerance can drink milk, especially if they drink it along with other foods and limit the amount they consume at any one time.

lactose intolerance: intolerance to lactose-containing foods due to the loss or reduction of intestinal lactase; symptoms may include flatulence, bloating, and diarrhea.

Lactose intolerance is rarely serious and is easily managed by simple dietary adjustments. Although people with the condition are sometimes reluctant to consume milk products, clinical studies have found that individuals with lactose intolerance can tolerate up to 2 cups of milk daily without significant symptoms.[18] In addition, the regular consumption of milk products increases the amount of lactose metabolized by intestinal bacteria, which improves lactose tolerance.[19] People who avoid milk for fear of intestinal discomfort can be urged to gradually increase their consumption of lactose-containing foods. They may more readily tolerate milk when intake is divided throughout the day and the milk is taken with food (see Photo 18-2). Some people tolerate chocolate milk better than plain milk. Most aged cheeses are well tolerated because they contain little lactose. Yogurts that contain live bacterial cultures are often acceptable because the bacteria contain lactase, which may aid in lactose digestion. Other options are to add a lactase preparation to milk or to take enzyme tablets before consuming milk products. Lactose-free milk is also commercially available.

People who develop lactose intolerance as a result of intestinal illness are generally advised to temporarily restrict milk and milk products. Foods that contain lactose can be reintroduced in small amounts once the condition improves. Individuals who restrict milk products should be encouraged to consume alternative food sources of calcium and vitamin D (see Chapters 8 and 9).

Review Notes

- Nutrient malabsorption can result from an undersupply of digestive secretions, motility disorders, or damaged intestinal mucosa.
- Fat malabsorption, which is usually indicated by steatorrhea, can cause losses of food energy and deficiencies of essential fatty acids, fat-soluble vitamins, and some minerals. In severe cases, nutrition therapy may include a fat-restricted diet and use of MCT oil.
- Bacterial overgrowth may result from conditions that reduce gastric acidity or intestinal motility; it typically causes malabsorption of fat and some essential nutrients.
- Lactose intolerance, caused by lactase deficiency, can be managed by adjusting the amount and timing of lactose consumption.

18.3 Disorders of the Pancreas

As mentioned previously, pancreatic disorders can lead to maldigestion and malabsorption because the secretion of digestive enzymes is impaired. This section describes several diseases that disrupt pancreatic function and cause widespread malabsorption.

Pancreatitis

Pancreatitis is an inflammatory disease of the pancreas. Although mild cases may subside in a few days, other cases can persist for weeks or months. Chronic pancreatitis can result in irreversible damage to pancreatic tissue and permanent loss of function.

Acute Pancreatitis In acute pancreatitis, the digestive enzymes within pancreatic cells become prematurely activated, causing destruction of pancreatic tissue and subsequent inflammation. About 70 to 80 percent of acute cases are caused by gallstones or alcohol abuse; less frequent causes include elevated blood triglyceride levels (greater than 1000 milligrams per deciliter) or exposure to various drugs and toxins.[20] Common symptoms include severe abdominal pain, nausea and vomiting, and abdominal distention (see Box 18-6). In most patients, the condition resolves within a week with no complications. More severe cases may lead to chronic pancreatitis, infection, the systemic inflammatory response syndrome (see Chapter 16, p. 473), or multiple organ failure.

Nutrition Therapy for Acute Pancreatitis The initial treatment for acute pancreatitis is supportive and includes pain control and intravenous hydration. In cases of mild-to-moderate pancreatitis, oral fluids and food are withheld until the patient is pain-free and experiences no nausea or vomiting.[21] Afterward, patients are usually prescribed a regular, low-fat diet; the fat restriction may be gradually lifted if the diet is well tolerated and symptoms of fat malabsorption (such as steatorrhea and abdominal pain) remain absent. In severe pancreatitis, continuous tube feedings, started within the initial 48 hours of treatment, may lead to improved outcomes compared with withholding intakes; the use of elemental formulas (formulas that contain hydrolyzed nutrients) may improve patient tolerance.[22] Protein needs are generally high in pancreatitis patients (between 1.2 and 1.5 grams per kilogram of body weight per day[23]) due to the catabolic effects of inflammation. Patients should be given multivitamin/mineral supplements until food intakes can meet their nutritional needs.

Chronic Pancreatitis Chronic pancreatitis is characterized by progressive, permanent damage to pancreatic tissue, resulting in the impaired secretion of digestive enzymes and bicarbonate. Up to 60 to 70 percent of chronic pancreatitis cases are associated with excessive alcohol consumption; other risk factors include cigarette smoking and repeated episodes of acute pancreatitis.[24] Most patients with chronic pancreatitis experience persistent abdominal pain, which may worsen with eating and be accompanied by nausea and vomiting. Although all macronutrients are maldigested, the symptoms of fat malabsorption are typically the most severe. Food avoidance (due to pain associated with eating) and malabsorption may lead to weight loss and malnutrition (see Box 18-7). Long-term illness is associated with reduced secretion of insulin and glucagon, and diabetes frequently develops in the later stages of disease.

Nutrition Therapy for Chronic Pancreatitis The main objectives of nutrition therapy are to reduce malabsorption and correct malnutrition. Pancreatic enzyme replacement may be prescribed to treat steatorrhea and other symptoms of malabsorption. Some enzyme preparations are **enteric-coated** to resist the acidity of the stomach and do not dissolve until they reach the small intestine. If nonenteric-coated preparations are used, acid-suppressing drugs are also required (Box 18-8 lists nutrition-related side effects of these medications). Fecal fat concentrations may be monitored

BOX 18-6 *Nursing Diagnosis*

Nursing diagnoses for people with acute pancreatitis may include *acute pain, nausea,* and *risk for deficient fluid volume.*

BOX 18-7 *Nursing Diagnosis*

The nursing diagnosis *imbalanced nutrition: less than body requirements* may be appropriate for some individuals with chronic pancreatitis.

enteric-coated: refers to medications or enzyme preparations that are coated to withstand stomach acidity and dissolve only at the higher pH of the small intestine.

Box 18-8 Diet-Drug Interactions

Check this table for notable nutrition-related effects of the medications discussed in this chapter.

Antidiarrheal drugs	**Gastrointestinal effect:** Constipation
Anti-inflammatory drugs (sulfasalazine, corticosteroids)	**Gastrointestinal effects:** Nausea, vomiting (sulfasalazine)
	Dietary interactions: Sulfasalazine may decrease folate absorption; supplementation is recommended
	Metabolic effects: Anemia (sulfasalazine); fluid retention, hyperglycemia, hypocalcemia, hypokalemia, hypophosphatemia, increased appetite, protein catabolism (corticosteroids)
Antisecretory drugs (proton-pump inhibitors, H2 blockers)	**Gastrointestinal effects:** Diarrhea, constipation, nausea and vomiting, abdominal pain (proton-pump inhibitors)
	Dietary interactions: May decrease iron, calcium, folate, and vitamin B_{12} absorption
Laxatives	**Gastrointestinal effects:** Diarrhea, flatulence, abdominal discomfort
	Metabolic effects: Dehydration, electrolyte imbalances, laxative dependency
Pancreatic enzyme replacements	**Gastrointestinal effects:** Constipation, nausea and vomiting, diarrhea, abdominal cramps, irritation of GI mucosa
	Dietary interactions: May decrease folate and iron absorption
	Metabolic effects: Elevated serum or urinary uric acid levels (with high doses), allergic reactions (rare)

to determine whether the enzyme treatment has been effective. Patients who cannot be successfully treated with enzyme replacement may be prescribed a low-fat diet to reduce their symptoms.

Patients with chronic pancreatitis who are hypermetabolic and underweight have high protein and energy requirements; a protein intake of 1.0 to 1.5 grams per kilogram of body weight per day is usually sufficient, while energy needs may be about 35 kcalories per kilogram of body weight daily.[25] Dietary supplements are used to correct nutrient deficiencies, which may be due to malabsorption or to the alcohol abuse that caused the disease. Patients should avoid consuming alcohol and quit smoking cigarettes, as these practices can exacerbate illness and interfere with healing.[26]

Cystic Fibrosis

Cystic fibrosis is the most common life-threatening genetic disorder among Caucasians, with an incidence of approximately 1 in 2500 to 3200 white births.[27] The condition is characterized by a mutation in the protein that regulates chloride transport across epithelial cell membranes. The abnormality alters the ion concentration and/or viscosity of **exocrine** secretions, causing a broad range of serious complications (see Box 18-9). Until a few decades ago, few infants born with cystic fibrosis survived to adulthood. Now, with early detection and advances in medical treatment, the median life span has reached nearly 40 years of age, with many patients surviving into their 50s.[28]

Consequences of Cystic Fibrosis Cystic fibrosis is characterized by abnormal chloride and sodium levels in exocrine secretions. These altered secretions ultimately disrupt the functioning of multiple tissues and organs. Common complications

BOX 18-9 *Nursing Diagnosis*

Nursing diagnoses that may apply to people with cystic fibrosis include *ineffective airway clearance, risk for infection, risk for deficient fluid volume, risk for delayed development,* and *imbalanced nutrition: less than body requirements.*

cystic fibrosis: a genetic disorder characterized by abnormal chloride and sodium levels in exocrine secretions; often leads to respiratory illness and pancreatic insufficiency.

exocrine: pertains to external secretions, such as those of the mucous membranes or the skin. Opposite of *endocrine*, which pertains to hormonal secretions into the blood.

exo = outside
krinein = to secrete

of cystic fibrosis involve the lungs, pancreas, and sweat glands.

- *Lung disease.* Changes in bronchial secretions lead to an impaired ability to clear airway mucus, resulting in chronic respiratory infections, progressive inflammation, and airway obstruction (see Photo 18-3). The eventual lung damage causes breathing difficulties, chronic coughing, and lower exercise tolerance. As with other obstructive airway diseases (see Chapter 16), nutrition status may become impaired because of hypermetabolism, the greater energy cost of labored breathing, and anorexia (loss of appetite). The chronic respiratory infections raise metabolic rate (and therefore, energy needs) further.
- *Pancreatic disease.* About 85 to 90 percent of cystic fibrosis patients show evidence of exocrine pancreatic dysfunction.[29] Most patients produce thickened pancreatic secretions that obstruct the pancreatic ducts; the trapped pancreatic enzymes eventually damage pancreatic tissue, leading to progressive atrophy and scarring. Inadequate amounts of digestive enzymes and bicarbonate are delivered to the small intestine, resulting in severe malabsorption of protein, fat, and fat-soluble vitamins. Other problems that may develop over time include pancreatitis and glucose intolerance or diabetes (due to destruction of the insulin-producing cells).
- *Sweat glands.* Salt losses in sweat are usually excessive, increasing the risk of dehydration.
- *Other complications.* Because cystic fibrosis affects all exocrine secretions, complications may develop in many other tissues or organs. Intestinal obstruction is a common problem in newborn infants and may also occur in older patients. Gallbladder and liver diseases may result from bile duct obstructions. Abnormalities in genital tissues cause sterility in men and reduced fertility in women.

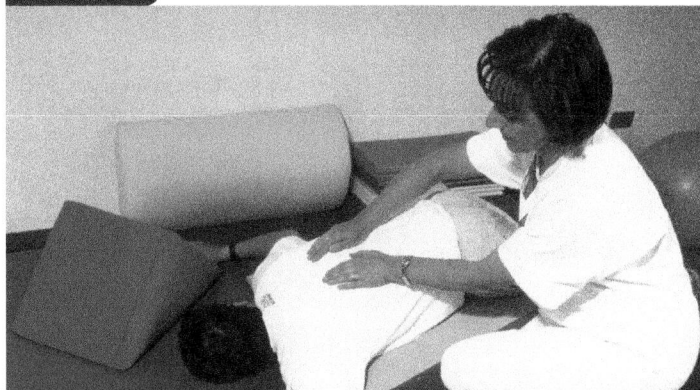

Photo 18-3 Postural Drainage Therapy

Postural drainage, a type of physical therapy used in cystic fibrosis, helps to clear the thick, sticky secretions that block airways and increase infection risk. The therapy involves maintaining a position that helps fluid drain out of the lungs, sometimes helped by soft claps or vibration over the areas that require drainage.

Nutrition Therapy for Cystic Fibrosis Children with cystic fibrosis are chronically undernourished, grow poorly, and have difficulty maintaining normal body weight. Their energy and protein needs are high because of increased metabolism and nutrient malabsorption, yet their appetites are usually poor. Energy requirements may range from 120 to 150 percent of DRI values; however, intakes are often much lower than these levels.[30] To achieve normal growth and appropriate weight, patients are encouraged to eat a high-kcalorie, high-protein, high-fat diet (with about 20 percent of kcalories from protein and 35 to 40 percent of kcalories from fat), eat frequent meals and snacks, and supplement meals with milkshakes or oral supplements. Supplemental tube feedings can help to improve nutrition status if energy intakes are inadequate.

Pancreatic enzyme replacement therapy is a central feature of cystic fibrosis treatment. Supplemental enzymes must be included with every meal or snack. For young children, the contents of capsules are mixed in small amounts of liquid or a soft food (such as applesauce) and administered with a spoon. Enzyme dosages may need to be adjusted if malabsorption continues, as evidenced by poor growth or GI symptoms such as steatorrhea, intestinal gas, or abdominal pain.

The risk of nutrient deficiency depends on the degree of malabsorption; nutrients of greatest concern include the fat-soluble vitamins, essential fatty acids, calcium, iron, and zinc. Multivitamin/mineral and fat-soluble vitamin supplements are routinely recommended. The liberal use of table salt and salty foods is encouraged to make up for sodium losses in sweat.

18.4 Disorders of the Small Intestine

When the intestinal mucosa is damaged by inflammation, infection, or other causes, malabsorption is the likely outcome. This section discusses *celiac disease* and the *inflammatory bowel diseases*, which are intestinal diseases that can damage the intestinal mucosa, and *short bowel syndrome*, the malabsorption disorder that results when a substantial portion of the small intestine is surgically removed.

Celiac Disease

Celiac disease is an immune disorder characterized by an abnormal immune response to a protein fraction in **wheat gluten** and to related proteins in barley and rye. The reaction to gluten causes severe damage to the intestinal mucosa and subsequent malabsorption. Celiac disease affects approximately 1 percent of Caucasian persons in the United States and elsewhere, although it is less common in other ethnic groups.[31]

Consequences of Celiac Disease The immune reaction to gluten can cause striking changes in intestinal tissue (see Photo 18-4). In affected areas, the villi may be

Photo 18-4 Effect of Celiac Disease on Intestinal Tissue

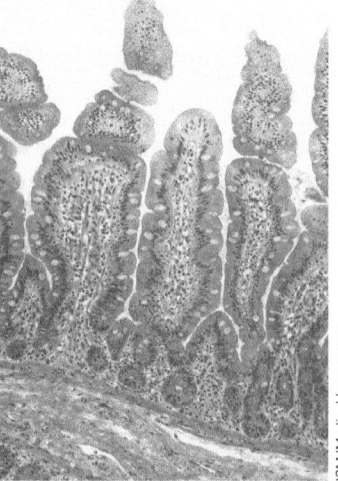

ISM/Medical Images.com

In the healthy intestine, the villi greatly increase the absorptive surface area.

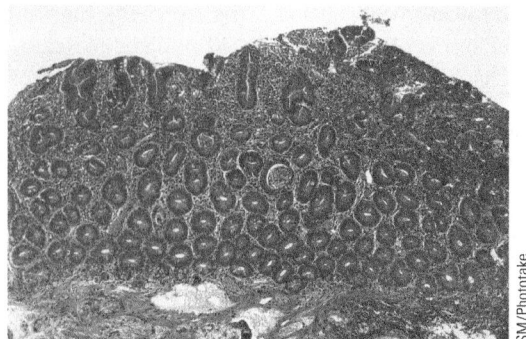

ISM/Phototake

In celiac disease, the villi may be shortened or absent, resulting in substantial reductions in nutrient absorption.

celiac (SEE-lee-ack) **disease:** an immune disorder characterized by an abnormal immune response to wheat gluten and related proteins; also called *gluten-sensitive enteropathy* or *celiac sprue.*

wheat gluten (GLU-ten): a family of water-insoluble proteins in wheat; includes the gliadin (GLY-ah-din) fractions that are toxic to persons with celiac disease.

shortened or absent, resulting in a significant reduction in mucosal surface area (and, therefore, in the number of cells that digest and absorb nutrients). The damage may be restricted to the duodenum or may involve the full length of the small intestine. Individuals with severe disease may malabsorb all nutrients to some degree; in mild cases, the nutrients malabsorbed vary according to the extent of damage and portion of intestine affected.

Symptoms of celiac disease may include GI disturbances such as diarrhea, steatorrhea, and flatulence (see Box 18-10). Because lactase deficiency can result from the mucosal damage, milk products may exacerbate GI symptoms. As a result of nutrient malabsorption, children with celiac disease often exhibit poor growth, low body weight, muscle wasting, and anemia. Adults may develop anemia, bone disorders, neurological symptoms, and fertility problems. Individuals with celiac disease are at risk of developing a wide variety of other diseases, including type 1 diabetes, autoimmune thyroid diseases, inflammatory bowel diseases, and intestinal cancers.[32]

Some gluten-sensitive individuals may have few GI symptoms but react to gluten by developing a severe, itchy rash. This condition is called **dermatitis herpetiformis** and requires dietary adjustments similar to those for celiac disease.

Nutrition Therapy for Celiac Disease The treatment for celiac disease is lifelong adherence to a gluten-free diet. Improvement in symptoms often occurs within a few weeks, although mucosal healing can sometimes take years. If lactase deficiency is suspected, patients should avoid lactose-containing foods until the intestine has recovered. Dietary supplements can be used to meet micronutrient needs and reverse deficiencies.

The gluten-free diet eliminates foods that contain wheat, barley, and rye (see Table 18-6, p. 528). Because many foods contain ingredients derived from these grains, foods that are problematic are not always obvious. Even small amounts of gluten may cause symptoms in some people, so patients need to check ingredient lists on food labels carefully. Gluten sources that may be overlooked include beer, brewer's yeast, caramel coloring, coffee substitutes, communion wafers, imitation meats, malt syrup, medications, salad dressings, and soy sauce. Gluten-free products can be purchased to replace common food items such as bread, pasta, and cereals. Patients should also be instructed in food preparation methods that prevent cross-contamination from utensils, cutting boards, and toasters. Figure 18-3 shows an example of a menu for a gluten-free diet.

Although most people with celiac disease can safely consume moderate amounts of oats, most oats grown in the United States are contaminated with wheat, barley, or rye. Oats are usually grown in rotation with other grains and may become contaminated during harvesting or processing. Some oat manufacturers now produce oats in dedicated facilities and test the products to ensure that they are gluten-free. Individuals who wish to include oats in their diet should purchase only uncontaminated oats and limit intakes to the amounts found to be safe (about ½ cup of dry rolled oats or ¼ cup of dry steel-cut oats per day).

A gluten-free diet may become monotonous unless care is taken to diversify food choices. The diet can also be a social liability by restricting food choices when individuals eat in restaurants, visit friends, or travel. Nonadherence is common when individuals eat away from home. Nutrition education can help patients with celiac disease learn how to meet their nutrient needs and expand meal options despite dietary constraints.

BOX 18-10 *Nursing Diagnosis*

Nursing diagnoses for people with celiac disease may include *diarrhea* and *imbalanced nutrition: less than body requirements.*

dermatitis herpetiformis (HER-peh-tih-FOR-mis): a gluten-sensitive disorder characterized by a severe skin rash.

FIGURE 18-3 Sample Menu for a Gluten-Free Die

❀❧ *Breakfast* ❧❀

Orange juice
Gluten-free pancake with maple syrup
Plain yogurt with banana and strawberries
Coffee with half-and-half

❀❧ *Lunch* ❧❀

Grilled chicken breast with cranberry chutney
Baked potato topped with grated cheddar cheese
Sliced tomato with chopped basil
Raspberry sherbet

❀❧ *Snack* ❧❀

Tortilla chips and guacamole
Hot cocoa (made with cocoa powder)

❀❧ *Dinner* ❧❀

Sauteed catfish with sliced lemon and dill
Wild rice pilaf
Collard greens and garlic sauteed in olive oil
Green salad with oil and vinegar dressing
Vanilla egg custard

TABLE 18-6 Gluten-Free Diet

FOOD CATEGORY	GLUTEN-FREE CHOICES	POTENTIAL GLUTEN SOURCES
Meat and meat alternatives	Fresh meat, fish, and poultry; shellfish; dried peas and beans; tofu; nuts and seeds; eggs	Luncheon meats, frankfurters, sausages, meatloaf, meatballs, poultry injected with broth, imitation meat products, imitation seafood, meat extenders, veggie burgers, miso, egg substitutes, dried egg products, dry roasted nuts, peanut butter *Avoid*: products made with hydrolyzed vegetable protein (HVP), marinades, and soy sauce; breaded foods; foods prepared with cream sauces or gravies
Milk and milk products	Milk, buttermilk, half-and-half, cream, plain yogurt, cheese, cottage cheese, cream cheese	Chocolate milk, milkshakes, frozen yogurt, flavored yogurt, cheese spreads, cheese sauces *Avoid*: malted milk, malted milk powder
Breads, cereals, rice, and pasta	Breads, bakery products, and cereals made with amaranth, arrowroot, buckwheat, corn, flax, hominy grits, millet, potato flour or potato starch, quinoa, rice, sorghum, soybean flour, tapioca, and teff; pasta and noodles made with the grains or starches listed above; corn tacos and corn tortillas	Oatmeal and oat bran (due to possible contamination), rice crackers, rice cakes, corn cakes *Avoid:* breads, bakery products, cereals, tortillas, matzo, pasta, and pancake or baking mixes made with wheat, rye, barley, and triticale. *Wheat products* include bulghur, couscous, durum flour, einkorn, emmer, farina, farro, graham flour, kamut, orzo, semolina, spelt, wheat bran, and wheat germ. *Barley products* include malt, malt flavoring, and malt extract.
Fruits and vegetables	Any fresh, frozen, or canned fruits and vegetables	French fries from fast-food restaurants, commercial salad dressings, fruit pie fillings, dried fruit (may be dusted with flour) *Avoid:* scalloped potatoes (usually made with wheat flour), creamed vegetables, vegetables dipped in batters
Desserts	Bakery products made with gluten-free flours, most ice creams, sherbet, sorbet, Italian ices, popsicles, gelatin desserts, egg custard, some chocolate bars, chocolate chips, hard candies, marshmallows, whipped toppings	Some ice creams (especially if made with cookie dough, brownies, nuts, and other added ingredients), candies, and candy bars *Avoid:* bakery products or doughnuts made with wheat, rye, or barley; pudding made with wheat flour; ice cream or sherbets that contain gluten stabilizers; ice cream cones; licorice; chocolate bars that contain barley malt, wheat flour, or food starch
Beverages	Coffee; tea; cocoa made with pure cocoa powder; soft drinks; wine; distilled alcoholic beverages such as rum, gin, whiskey, and vodka	Instant tea or coffee, coffee substitutes, chocolate drinks, hot cocoa mixes *Avoid:* beer, ale, lager, malt beverages, cereal beverages, beverages that contain nondairy cream substitutes, herbal teas that contain roasted barley

Inflammatory Bowel Diseases

Inflammatory bowel diseases are chronic inflammatory disorders characterized by abnormal immune responses to microbes that inhabit the GI tract.[33] Although both genetic and environmental factors contribute to the development of these diseases, the exact triggers are unknown. Table 18-7 compares the two major forms of inflammatory bowel disease, **Crohn's disease** and **ulcerative colitis**.* Crohn's disease usually involves the small intestine and may lead to nutrient malabsorption, whereas ulcerative colitis affects the large intestine, where little nutrient absorption occurs. Both diseases are characterized by periods of active disease interspersed with periods of remission. Nutrient losses can result from tissue damage, bleeding, and diarrhea.

Crohn's disease: an inflammatory bowel disease that usually occurs in the lower portion of the small intestine and the colon; the inflammation may pervade the entire intestinal wall.

ulcerative colitis (ko-LY-tis): an inflammatory bowel disease that involves the rectum and colon; the inflammation affects the mucosa and submucosa of the intestinal wall.

---

*Although ulcerative colitis affects the large intestine, the condition is included in this section because it is one of the major subtypes of inflammatory bowel disease.

TABLE 18-7	Comparison of Crohn's Disease and Ulcerative Colitis	
	CROHN'S DISEASE	**ULCERATIVE COLITIS**
Location of inflammation	Approximately 40% of cases involve the ileum and colon, 30% are in the ileum only, and 30% are confined to the colon	Confined to the rectum and colon; always involves the rectum but often extends into the colon
Pattern of inflammation	Discrete areas separated by normal tissue ("skip" lesions)	Continuous inflammation throughout the affected region
Depth of damage	Damage throughout all layers of tissue; causes deep fissures that give intestinal tissue a "cobblestone" appearance	Damage primarily in the mucosa and submucosa (the layers of intestinal tissue closest to the lumen)
Fistulas	Common	Usually do not occur
Cancer risk	Increased	Greatly increased

fistulas (FIST-you-luz): abnormal passages between organs or tissues that allow the passage of fluids or secretions.

Complications of Crohn's Disease Crohn's disease may occur in any region of the GI tract, but most cases involve the ileum and/or large intestine (see Photo 18-5). Lesions may develop in different areas in the intestine, with normal tissue separating affected regions (called "skip" lesions). During exacerbations, the inflammation may extend deeply into intestinal tissue and be accompanied by ulcerations, fissures, and **fistulas** (abnormal passages between tissues). Loops of intestine may become matted together. The resultant scar tissue can eventually thicken, narrowing the lumen and possibly causing strictures or obstructions. Nearly half of patients require surgery within 10 years of diagnosis.[34] Patients with Crohn's disease are also at increased risk of developing intestinal cancers.

Malnutrition may result from poor food intake, malabsorption, diarrhea, bleeding, nutrient losses (especially of protein) from inflamed tissues, increased needs due to inflammation, and surgical resections that shorten the small intestine. If the ileum is affected, bile acids may become depleted,* causing malabsorption of fat, fat-soluble vitamins, calcium, magnesium, and zinc (the minerals bind to the unabsorbed fatty acids). Because the ileum is the site of vitamin B_{12} absorption, deficiency can develop unless the patient is given vitamin B_{12} injections. Anemia may result from bleeding, inadequate absorption of the nutrients involved in blood cell formation (iron, folate,

Photo 18-5 Comparison of Crohn's Disease and Ulcerative Colitis

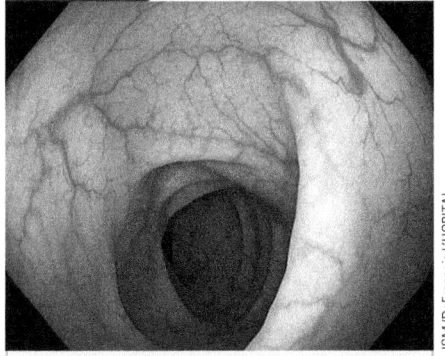

The healthy colon has a smooth surface with a visible pattern of fine blood vessels.

ISM/Dr François L'HOPITAL

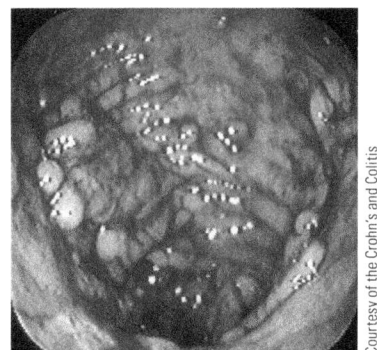

In Crohn's disease, the mucosa has a "cobblestone" appearance due to deep fissuring in the inflamed mucosal tissue.

Courtesy of the Crohn's and Colitis Foundation of America Inc.

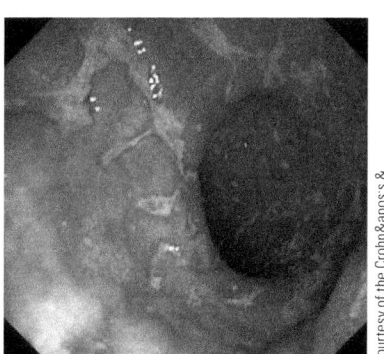

In ulcerative colitis, the colon appears inflamed and reddened, and ulcers are visible.

Courtesy of the Crohn's & Colitis Foundation of America, Inc.

*Most of the bile used during digestion is eventually reabsorbed in the ileum and returned to the liver.

and vitamin B_{12}), or the metabolic effects of chronic illness. Anorexia often develops because of abdominal pain and the effects of cytokines produced during the inflammatory process.

Complications of Ulcerative Colitis Ulcerative colitis always involves the rectum and usually extends into the colon. Tissue inflammation is continuous along the length of intestine affected, ending abruptly at the area where healthy tissue begins. The erosion or ulceration affects the mucosa and submucosa only (the tissue layers closest to the lumen). In early stages, the mucosa appears reddened and swollen; advanced stages may feature mucosal atrophy, thin colon walls, and, in some cases, colon dilation (known as *toxic megacolon*). During active episodes, patients may have frequent, urgent bowel movements that are small in volume and contain blood and mucus. Symptoms vary among patients but may include diarrhea, constipation, rectal bleeding, and abdominal pain (see Box 18-11).

Although mild disease may cause few complications, weight loss, fever, and weakness are common when much of the colon is involved. Severe disease is often associated with anemia (due to blood loss), dehydration, and electrolyte imbalances. Protein losses from the inflamed tissue can be substantial. A **colectomy** (removal of the colon) is performed in 25 to 45 percent of patients and prevents future recurrence.[35] Colon cancer risk is substantially increased in patients with ulcerative colitis.

Drug Treatment of Inflammatory Bowel Diseases Medications help to reduce inflammation, control symptoms, and minimize complications. The drugs prescribed may include immunosuppressants, anti-inflammatory drugs (usually corticosteroids and salicylates), biological therapies, and antibiotics. Although these medications may allow the patient to achieve and maintain remission, some may cause side effects that are detrimental to nutrition status. Box 18-8 (p. 524) lists some nutrition-related effects of the medications used in inflammatory bowel diseases.

Nutrition Therapy for Crohn's Disease Crohn's disease often requires aggressive dietary management because it can lead to protein-energy malnutrition, nutrient deficiencies, and growth failure in children. Food avoidance is common because of abdominal pain, anorexia, and diarrhea. Specific dietary measures depend on the functional status of the GI tract and the symptoms and complications that develop; thus, nutrition care varies among patients and throughout the course of illness.

High-kcalorie, high-protein diets may be prescribed to prevent or treat malnutrition or promote healing. Oral supplements can help to increase energy intake and improve weight gain. Vitamin and mineral supplements are usually necessary, especially if nutrient malabsorption is present; nutrients at risk include iron, zinc, magnesium, calcium, vitamin D, folate, and vitamin B_{12}.[36] In some instances, tube feedings are used to supplement the diet or may be the sole means of providing nutrients.

During disease exacerbations, a low-fiber, low-fat diet provided in small, frequent feedings can minimize stool output and reduce symptoms of malabsorption. If diarrhea or flatulence is present, a restricted intake of lactose, fructose, and sorbitol may improve symptoms. Patients with diarrhea should make sure they obtain adequate fluids to prevent dehydration. Individuals with partial obstructions may need to restrict high-fiber foods. Table 18-8 includes examples of the various dietary adjustments that may be beneficial for patients with Crohn's disease.

Nutrition Therapy for Ulcerative Colitis In most cases, the diet for ulcerative colitis requires few adjustments. As in Crohn's disease, the symptoms and complications that arise are managed with the appropriate dietary measures (review Table 18-8). During disease exacerbations, emphasis is given to restoring fluid and electrolyte balances and correcting deficiencies that result from protein and blood losses; dietary adjustments are based on the extent of bleeding and diarrhea output. Thus, adequate protein, energy, fluid, and electrolytes need to be provided. A low-fiber diet may reduce irritation by minimizing fecal volume. If colon function becomes severely impaired, food

colectomy: removal of a portion or all of the colon.

TABLE 18-8 Management of Symptoms and Complications in Crohn's Disease

SYMPTOM OR COMPLICATION	POSSIBLE DIETARY MEASURES
Growth failure, weight loss, or muscle wasting	• High-kcalorie, high-protein diet • Oral supplements • Tube feedings
Anorexia or pain with eating	• Small, frequent meals • Oral supplements, as tolerated • Tube feedings if long term (>5 to 7 days)
Malabsorption	• High-kcalorie diet • Nutrient supplementation
Steatorrhea (fat malabsorption)	• Low-fat diet • Medium-chain triglycerides • Nutrient supplementation
Diarrhea	• Fluid and electrolyte replacement • Nutrient supplementation • Restricted intake of fructose and sugar alcohols
Lactose intolerance	• Avoidance of lactose-containing foods
Nutrient deficiencies	• Nutrient-dense diet • Nutrient supplementation
Strictures, partial obstruction, or fistulas	• Low-fiber diet • Liquid supplements
Severe bowel obstruction, high-output fistulas, or severe exacerbations of disease	• Total parenteral nutrition

and fluids may be withheld and fluids and electrolytes supplied intravenously until colon function is restored.

Short Bowel Syndrome

The treatment of Crohn's disease, intestinal cancers, and other intestinal conditions may include the surgical resection (removal) of a major portion of the small intestine. **Short bowel syndrome** is the malabsorption syndrome that results when the absorptive capacity of the remaining intestine is insufficient for meeting nutritional needs. Without appropriate dietary adjustments, short bowel syndrome can result in fluid and electrolyte imbalances and multiple nutrient deficiencies. Symptoms of short bowel syndrome include diarrhea, steatorrhea, dehydration, weight loss, and growth impairment in children.

Figure 18-4 reviews nutrient absorption in the GI tract and describes how absorption is affected by surgical resections. Generally, up to 50 percent of the small intestine can be resected without serious nutritional consequences.[37] More extensive resections lead to generalized malabsorption, and patients may need lifelong parenteral nutrition to supplement oral intakes.

Intestinal Adaptation After an intestinal resection, the remaining intestine undergoes **intestinal adaptation**, which dramatically improves the intestine's absorptive capacity. Adaptation—which depends on the presence of nutrients and GI secretions in the

short bowel syndrome: the malabsorption syndrome that follows resection of the small intestine; characterized by inadequate absorptive capacity in the remaining intestine.

intestinal adaptation: physiological changes in the small intestine that increase its absorptive capacity after resection.

About 90 to 95% of nutrient absorption takes place in the first half of the small intestine. After a resection, nutrient absorption may be reduced.

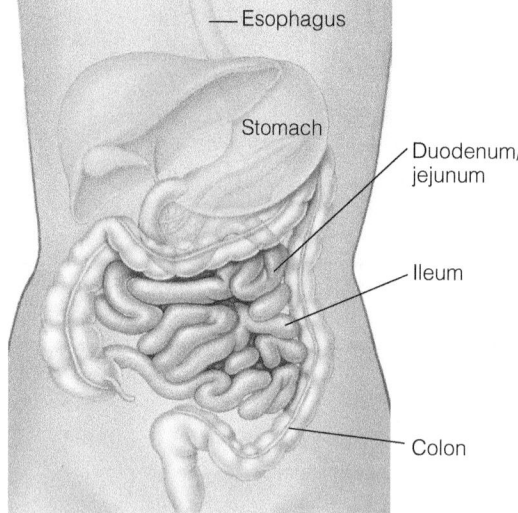

WHAT IS ABSORBED

Duodenum/jejunum
- Simple carbohydrates
- Fats
- Amino acids
- Vitamins[a]
- Minerals[a]
- Water

Ileum
- Bile salts
- Vitamin B_{12}
- Water
(Can adapt to assume absorptive functions of the duodenum and jejunum)

Colon
- Water
- Electrolytes
- Short-chain fatty acids

POSSIBLE CONSEQUENCES OF RESECTION

Duodenum/jejunum
- Minimal consequences if the ileum remains intact
- Calcium and iron malabsorption if the duodenum is resected

Ileum
- Fat malabsorption
- Protein malabsorption
- Malabsorption of fat-soluble vitamins and vitamin B_{12}
- Reduced calcium, magnesium, and zinc absorption
- Fluid losses
- Diarrhea/steatorrhea

Colon
- Fluid and electrolyte losses
- Diarrhea
(Losses are compounded if the ileum is also resected)

Labels on figure: Esophagus, Stomach, Duodenum/jejunum, Ileum, Colon

[a]The absorption of vitamins and minerals begins in the duodenum and continues throughout the length of the small intestine.

lumen—begins soon after surgery and continues for several years. During this period, the remaining section of intestine develops taller villi and deeper crypts and also grows in length and diameter; these changes dramatically increase the absorptive surface area of the remaining intestine. The ileum has a greater capacity for adaptation than the jejunum; thus, removal of the ileum has more severe consequences than removal of the jejunum. Loss of the ileum permanently disrupts both vitamin B_{12} and bile acid absorption, and depletion of bile acids exacerbates fat malabsorption. Adaptation is achieved more easily if the colon is present because the colon's resident bacteria can metabolize unabsorbed carbohydrates and produce some usable nutrients. An intact colon also helps to reduce losses of fluids and electrolytes.

Nutrition Therapy for Short Bowel Syndrome Immediately after a resection, fluids and electrolytes must be supplied intravenously. In the first few weeks after surgery, the fluid losses from diarrhea can be substantial, so appropriate rehydration therapy is critical to recovery. The diarrhea gradually lessens as intestinal adaptation progresses.

Total parenteral nutrition meets nutritional needs after surgery and is gradually replaced by tube feedings and/or oral feedings. To promote intestinal adaptation, the feedings may be started within a week after surgery, after diarrhea subsides somewhat and some bowel function is restored. Initial oral intake may consist of sips of clear, sugar-free liquids, progressing to larger amounts of liquid formulas and then to solid foods, as tolerated. Very small, frequent feedings can utilize the remaining intestine most effectively. To compensate for malabsorption and reduce the need for nutrition support, a high-kcalorie diet is typically encouraged.[38]

The exact diet prescribed for short bowel syndrome depends on the portion of intestine removed, the length of remaining intestine, and whether the colon is still intact; moreover, dietary readjustments may be required as intestinal adaptation progresses. If fat is well tolerated, a high-fat, low-carbohydrate diet may help to increase

Box 18-12 Case Study: Patient with Short Bowel Syndrome

Judi Morel is a 30-year-old economist with an eight-year history of Crohn's disease. Judi is 5 feet 7 inches tall. Three years ago, she underwent a small bowel resection and remained free of active disease for two years. During that time, her symptoms subsided; she was able to tolerate most foods without any problem and gained weight. Ten months ago, Judi experienced a severe flare-up of her Crohn's disease. Since that time, she has lost 15 pounds and currently weighs 118 pounds. She has experienced severe abdominal pain and fatigue that have persisted despite aggressive medical management that included intravenous nutrition. Five days ago, Judi underwent another resection, which left her with 40 percent of healthy small intestine. Her colon is intact. She is experiencing extensive diarrhea.

1. Describe the manifestations of Crohn's disease, and explain why surgery is sometimes performed as part of the treatment. Describe the complications of the disease that may affect nutrient needs.

2. Using the BMI table in the back of the book, check the ideal weight range for a person of Judi's height. What nutrition-related concerns are suggested by Judi's recent weight loss? What other nutrition problems did Judi probably experience as a consequence of Crohn's disease?

3. Discuss the complications that may follow an extensive intestinal resection. What factors may affect a person's ability to meet nutrient needs with an oral diet?

4. Describe the dietary progression recommended after an extensive intestinal resection. After Judi is able to eat solid foods, what factors may affect the type of diet that is recommended for her?

energy intakes. Conversely, a high-complex-carbohydrate, low-fat diet may be suggested for patients who have an intact colon, because the colon bacteria can metabolize the unabsorbed carbohydrate and produce short-chain fatty acids (which are absorbed and used in the colon), and the fat restriction may improve steatorrhea. In most cases, the extremely high energy requirement permits a high intake of all three macronutrients, so if tolerated, high intakes of protein, complex carbohydrates, and fat may all be encouraged.[39]

Dietary choices are tailored according to individual symptoms and tolerances. Some patients may need to drink oral rehydration solutions to stay sufficiently hydrated and obtain adequate electrolytes. Concentrated sweets (which attract fluids) should be avoided if they worsen diarrhea. Patients who have developed lactose intolerance may need to limit milk consumption. Because calcium malabsorption increases the risk of developing kidney stones, a low-oxalate diet may be recommended (see Chapter 22). Vitamin and mineral supplementation can prevent deficiencies from developing due to malabsorption. The Case Study in Box 18-12 can help you review the material on Crohn's disease and short bowel syndrome.

Review Notes

- Disorders of the small intestine that cause damage to mucosal tissue, such as celiac disease and Crohn's disease, often result in malabsorption.

- Celiac disease is characterized by an abnormal immune response to wheat gluten and to related proteins in barley and rye; a gluten-free diet is the primary treatment.

- Crohn's disease is an inflammatory disorder associated with extensive damage to intestinal tissue. Treatment includes medications that suppress inflammation and relieve symptoms, dietary adjustments that reduce symptoms and correct deficiencies, and intestinal resection to remove damaged tissue.

- Ulcerative colitis is an inflammatory disease that affects the rectum and colon only; severe cases may require colectomy.

- Short bowel syndrome may result from major intestinal resections. Although intestinal adaptation can improve absorptive capacity over time, individuals with extensive resections may require lifelong parenteral nutrition support.

18.5 Disorders of the Large Intestine

In the large intestine, the colon moves undigested materials to the rectum and has a central role in maintaining fluid and electrolyte balances. Its bacterial population ferments undigested nutrients and produces short-chain fatty acids and some vitamins that our bodies can absorb and use. This section describes several conditions that may impair the function or structure of the large intestine.

Irritable Bowel Syndrome

People with **irritable bowel syndrome** experience chronic and recurring intestinal symptoms that cannot be explained by specific physical abnormalities. The symptoms usually include disturbed defecation (diarrhea and/or constipation), bloating, and abdominal discomfort or pain; the pain is often aggravated by eating and relieved by defecation (see Box 18-13). In some patients, symptoms are mild; in others, the disturbances in colonic function can interfere with work and social activities enough to dramatically alter the person's lifestyle and sense of well-being. Irritable bowel syndrome affects 10 to 20 percent of the adult population in the United States; it occurs most often in individuals between 20 and 40 years of age.[40]

Although the causes of irritable bowel syndrome remain elusive, people with the disorder tend to have excessive colonic responses to meals, gastrointestinal hormones, and psychological stress.[41] Intestinal transit after meals may be accelerated, leading to diarrhea, or be delayed, causing constipation. Many individuals exhibit hypersensitivity to a normal degree of intestinal distention and feel discomfort when experiencing normal meal transit or typical amounts of intestinal gas. Some patients show signs of low-grade intestinal inflammation; others may have had a bacterial infection that initiated their GI problems. Coexisting psychiatric disorders, such as anxiety and depression, can exacerbate symptoms. Diagnosing irritable bowel syndrome is difficult because its symptoms are typical of other GI disorders and laboratory tests for the condition are nonexistent.

Treatment of Irritable Bowel Syndrome Medical treatment of irritable bowel syndrome often includes dietary adjustments, stress management, and behavioral therapies. Medications may be prescribed to manage symptoms but they are not always helpful. The drugs prescribed may include antidiarrheal agents, laxatives, antidepressants, antispasmotics (which reduce pain by relaxing GI muscles), and antibiotics (which alter bacterial populations in the colon).

Nutrition Therapy for Irritable Bowel Syndrome Although dietary adjustments may reduce symptoms, responses among patients vary considerably. Foods that aggravate symptoms may include gas-producing foods, wheat and other grains, milk products, caffeine-containing beverages, and carbonated beverages; however, individual tolerances are best determined by trial and error.[42] Consuming a low-FODMAP diet (see *Intestinal Gas*, p. 516) has been found to be helpful for reducing flatulence, abdominal pain, bloating, and diarrhea.[43] Some individuals have less discomfort when they consume small, frequent meals instead of larger ones. Supplementation with psyllium (Metamucil or Fiberall) may help to improve constipation and, possibly, other symptoms. Note that high-fiber diets are often recommended for individuals with irritable bowel syndrome, but clinical studies suggest that these diets are ineffective for improving symptoms and may worsen flatulence.[44] Because psychological associations have a strong influence on food tolerance, patients should carefully identify the foods and habits that cause intestinal symptoms so that they avoid restricting their diet unnecessarily.

Treatments under investigation for irritable bowel syndrome include peppermint oil, which relaxes smooth muscle, and various types of probiotics.[45] The Case Study in Box 18-14 can help you apply your knowledge about irritable bowel syndrome to a clinical situation.

irritable bowel syndrome: an intestinal disorder of unknown cause that disturbs the functioning of the large intestine; symptoms include abdominal pain, flatulence, diarrhea, and constipation.

Case Study: Young Adult with Irritable Bowel Syndrome

Hannah Tran is a 22-year-old recent college graduate who began her first professional job in a bank six months ago. As a college student, she occasionally experienced abdominal pain and cramping after eating. She also had frequent bouts of diarrhea and felt somewhat better after bowel movements. Once Hannah began her new job, her symptoms occurred more frequently. At first, she attributed her symptoms to job stress, but when the symptoms continued for several months, she decided to see her physician. After taking a careful history and conducting tests to rule out other bowel disorders, the physician diagnosed irritable bowel syndrome. The physician suggested a trial of psyllium and advised Hannah to keep a record of her food intake and symptoms for one week. Hannah was then referred to a dietitian for a review of her dietary record. The dietitian noticed that Hannah routinely drank several cups of coffee in the morning and had large meals for lunch and dinner. Hannah often ate out in Mexican restaurants and favored spicy foods, refried beans, and fatty desserts. Between meals, she drank fruit juice or soda and snacked on candies sweetened with sugar alcohols.

1. Describe the characteristics of irritable bowel syndrome to Hannah, and indicate the role that stress might play in her illness.

2. Explain how the record of food intake and symptoms might be helpful in devising an appropriate dietary plan for Hannah.

3. Could any of the foods that are currently in Hannah's diet be aggravating her symptoms? Give examples of dietary measures that are typically suggested for individuals with irritable bowel syndrome.

Diverticular Disease of the Colon

Diverticulosis refers to the presence of pebble-sized herniations (outpockets) in the intestinal mucosa, known as diverticula (see Figure 18-5). Most people with diverticulosis are symptom-free and remain unaware of the condition until a complication develops. The prevalence of diverticulosis increases with age, occurring in 50 to 65 percent of 80-year-old individuals.[46]

Although the cause of diverticulosis is unclear, changes in connective tissue proteins that occur with aging may contribute to its development.[47] Epidemiological studies have suggested that low-fiber diets may increase risk due to fiber's influence on transit time, stool volume, and intraluminal pressures[48]; however, some recent clinical studies were unable to find an association between low-fiber intakes and the incidence of diverticulosis.[49] Other potential risk factors for diverticulosis include genetic factors, high red meat or alcohol intakes, obesity, smoking, and physical inactivity.

FIGURE 18-5 Diverticula in the Colon

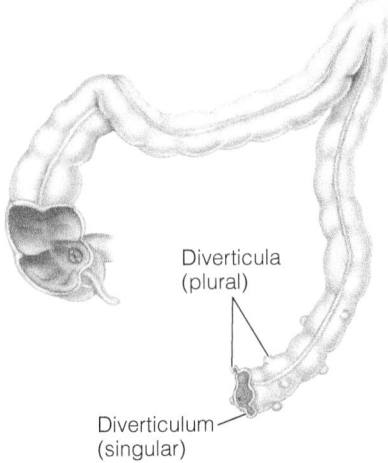

Diverticula (plural)

Diverticulum (singular)

Diverticula are small pouches that develop in weakened areas of the intestinal wall. The condition of having diverticula is known as *diverticulosis*.

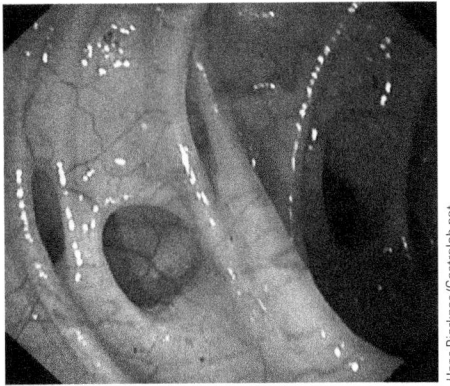

Hans Bjorknas/Gastrolab.net

Diverticula are frequently seen during a colonoscopy, a procedure that uses a flexible, lighted tube to examine the inside of the colon.

diverticulosis (DYE-ver-tic-you-LOH-sis): an intestinal condition characterized by the presence of small herniations (called diverticula) in the intestinal wall.

Diverticulitis Inflammation or infection sometimes develops in the area around a diverticulum. This condition, called **diverticulitis**, is the most common complication of diverticulosis, affecting 10 to 25 percent of individuals with the condition.[50] It is thought to result from erosion of the diverticular wall by thickened fecal matter, leading to inflammation and eventually a microperforation that causes subsequent infection. Later developments may include a larger perforation, abscess, extension of disease to adjacent organs, and fistula formation. In some cases, the infection spreads to the peritoneal cavity, causing life-threatening illness. Symptoms of diverticulitis may include persistent abdominal pain, tenderness in the affected area, fever, nausea, and vomiting. Constipation or diarrhea may also occur (see Box 18-15).

Treatment for Diverticular Disease Medical treatment for diverticulosis is necessary only if symptoms develop. Patients are often advised to increase fiber intake to relieve constipation and other symptoms, although high-fiber diets have not been shown to reverse diverticulosis or prevent disease progression.[51] Fiber should be increased gradually to ensure tolerance; the emphasis should be on insoluble fiber sources such as wheat bran, whole grains, fruits, and vegetables. Bulk-forming agents, such as psyllium, can help to increase fiber intake if food sources are insufficient. In the past, clinicians often recommended that patients avoid nuts, seeds, and popcorn to prevent complications, but these restrictions have not been supported by current research.[52]

Patients with diverticulitis may need antibiotics to treat infections and, possibly, pain-control medications. In mild cases, patients may need to reduce oral intakes until symptoms subside, and then increase food intake as tolerated.[53] In severe cases, oral fluids and food are withheld and fluids are provided intravenously. After pain and diarrhea have resolved, an oral diet is reintroduced, beginning with clear liquids and progressing to a low-fiber diet (about 10 grams of fiber per day). Once inflammation has subsided, fiber intakes should be increased by about 5 grams each week until recommended intakes (about 25 to 35 grams per day) are achieved.[54] Surgical interventions are sometimes necessary to treat complications of diverticulitis and may include removal of the affected portion of the colon.

Colostomies and Ileostomies

An *ostomy* is a surgically created opening (called a **stoma**) in the abdominal wall through which dietary wastes can be eliminated. Whereas a permanent ostomy is necessary after a partial or total colectomy, a temporary ostomy is sometimes constructed to bypass the colon after injury or extensive surgery. To create the stoma, the cut end of the remaining segment of functional intestine is routed through an opening in the abdominal wall and stitched in place so that it empties to the exterior. The stoma can be formed from a section of the colon (**colostomy**) or ileum (**ileostomy**), as shown in Figure 18-6. Conditions that may require these procedures include inflammatory bowel diseases, diverticulitis, and colorectal cancers.

To collect wastes, a disposable bag is affixed to the skin around the stoma and emptied during the day as needed. In some cases, an internal pouch is constructed from ileal tissue and attached to the anus so that the anal sphincter can control output. Stool consistency varies according to the length of colon that is functional. If a small portion of the colon is absent or bypassed, the stools may continue to be semisolid. If the entire colon has been removed or is bypassed, the ability to reabsorb fluid and electrolytes is substantially reduced, and the output is liquid (see Box 18-16).

Nutrition Care for Patients with Ostomies Dietary adjustments are individualized according to the surgical procedure and symptoms that develop afterward. Following surgery, the diet may progress from clear liquids (low in sugars) to regular foods, as tolerated. To reduce stool output, a low-fiber diet may be recommended. Small, frequent meals may be more acceptable than larger ones. To determine food tolerances, patients should try small amounts of questionable foods and assess their effects; a food

diverticulitis (DYE-ver-tic-you-LYE-tis): inflammation or infection involving diverticula.

stoma (STOE-ma): a surgically created opening in a body tissue or organ.

colostomy (co-LAH-stoe-me): a surgical passage through the abdominal wall into the colon.

ileostomy (ill-ee-AH-stoe-me): a surgical passage through the abdominal wall into the ileum.

FIGURE 18-6 Colostomy and Ileostomy

Colostomy

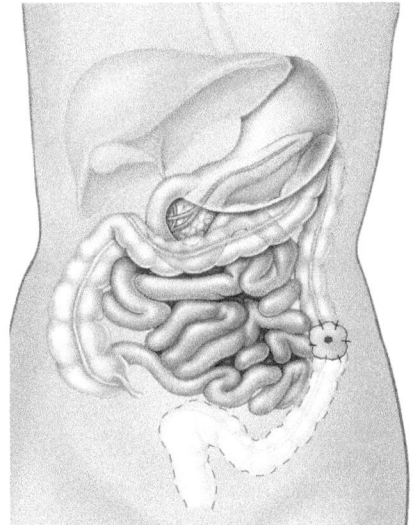

Ileostomy

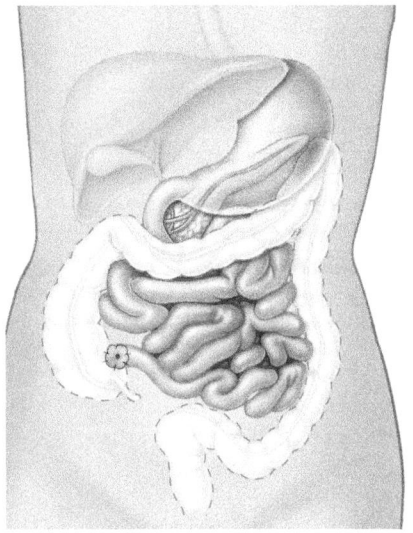

In a colostomy, a portion of the colon is removed or bypassed, and the stoma is formed from the remaining section of functional colon.

In an ileostomy, the entire colon is removed or bypassed, and the stoma is formed from the ileum.

that causes problems can be tried again later. Appropriate fluid and electrolyte intakes should be encouraged when a large portion of the colon has been removed.[55]

People with ileostomies need to chew thoroughly to ensure that foods are adequately digested and to prevent obstructions, a common complication due to the small diameter of the ileal lumen. Foods high in insoluble fibers are sometimes discouraged because they reduce transit time, may cause obstructions, and increase stool output. To replace electrolyte losses, patients are encouraged to use salt liberally and to ingest beverages with added electrolytes (such as sports drinks and oral rehydration beverages), if necessary. If a large portion of the ileum has been removed—reducing both bile acid reabsorption and vitamin B_{12} absorption—fat malabsorption may develop and vitamin B_{12} injections may be required.

Dietary concerns after colostomies depend on the length of colon remaining. Most patients have no dietary restrictions and can return to a regular diet. Patient concerns may include stool odors, excessive gas, and diarrhea. If a large portion of colon was removed, recommendations may be similar to those given to ileostomy patients.

Obstructions As mentioned, foods that are incompletely digested can cause obstructions, a primary concern of ileostomy patients. Although these patients can consume almost any food that is cut into small pieces and carefully chewed, the following foods may cause difficulty: celery, coconut, coleslaw, corn, cucumbers, dried fruit, fruits or vegetables with peels or skins, mushrooms, nuts, peas, pineapple, popcorn, salad greens, sausages, seeds, and tough, chewy meats.[56]

Reducing Gas and Odors Persons with ostomies are often concerned about foods that may increase gas production or cause strong odors. Foods and practices that may cause excessive gas were discussed earlier (see *Intestinal Gas*, p. 516). Foods that sometimes produce unpleasant odors include asparagus, beer, broccoli, brussels sprouts, cabbage, cauliflower, dried beans and peas, eggs, fish, onions, and turnips. Foods that may help to reduce odors include buttermilk, cranberry juice, parsley, and yogurt.[57]

Diarrhea Examples of foods that aggravate diarrhea are listed in Table 18-3 (p. 518). Foods that may thicken stool include applesauce, banana, cheese, oatmeal, pasta, potatoes, smooth peanut butter, tapioca, and white rice.[58] What works may differ for each individual, however, and is best determined by trial and error.

Review Notes

- Irritable bowel syndrome is characterized by chronic, recurring intestinal symptoms such as diarrhea and/or constipation, bloating, and abdominal pain. Although the causes are unknown, the disorder is influenced by food intake, stress, and psychological factors.
- Diverticulosis is often asymptomatic until complications develop; its prevalence increases with advancing age. Diverticulitis, which involves inflammation or infection of the diverticula, may require medical treatment and temporary bowel rest.
- Colostomies and ileostomies are surgically created openings in the abdominal wall using the cut end of the colon or ileum. Fluid and electrolyte requirements are greater after an ostomy if colon function is reduced or absent.

Nutrition Assessment Checklist | for People with Lower GI Tract Disorders

MEDICAL HISTORY
Check the medical record for diseases that:

○ Cause chronic GI symptoms, such as irritable bowel syndrome or an inflammatory bowel disease
○ Interfere with pancreatic enzyme secretion, such as chronic pancreatitis or cystic fibrosis
○ Interfere with nutrient absorption, such as Crohn's disease or celiac disease

Check for surgical procedures involving the lower GI tract, such as:

○ Intestinal resections or bypass surgeries
○ Ileostomy or colostomy

Check for the following symptoms or complications:

○ Anemia
○ Bacterial overgrowth
○ Bone disease
○ Constipation
○ Diarrhea, dehydration
○ Fistulas
○ Lactose intolerance
○ Nutrient deficiencies
○ Obstructions
○ Oxalate kidney stones
○ Poor growth, in children
○ Steatorrhea

MEDICATIONS
Check for medications or dietary supplements that may:

○ Cause constipation or diarrhea
○ Interfere with food intake by causing nausea, vomiting, abdominal discomfort, dry mouth, or drowsiness
○ Alter appetite or nutrient needs

DIETARY INTAKE
Note the following problems, and contact the dietitian if you suspect difficulties such as:

○ Poor appetite or food intake
○ Food intolerances
○ Inadequate fiber intake, in patients with constipation
○ Inadequate fluid intake
○ Malabsorbed carbohydrates, in patients with diarrhea

ANTHROPOMETRIC DATA
Measure baseline height and weight. Address weight loss early to prevent malnutrition in patients with:

○ Severe or persistent diarrhea
○ Nutrient malabsorption

LABORATORY TESTS

Check laboratory test results for signs of dehydration, electrolyte imbalances, nutrient deficiencies, and anemia in patients with:

○ Severe or persistent diarrhea or steatorrhea
○ Nutrient malabsorption
○ Intestinal resections

PHYSICAL SIGNS

Look for physical signs of:

○ Dehydration
○ Essential fatty acid and fat-soluble vitamin deficiencies
○ Folate and vitamin B_{12} deficiencies
○ Mineral deficiencies
○ Protein-energy malnutrition

Self Check

1. The health practitioner advising an elderly patient with constipation encourages the patient to:
   a. consume a low-fat diet low in sodium.
   b. consume a high-protein diet rich in calcium.
   c. eliminate gas-forming foods from the diet.
   d. gradually add high-fiber foods to the diet.

2. Osmotic diarrhea often results from:
   a. excessive colonic contractions.
   b. excessive fluid secretion by the intestines.
   c. nutrient malabsorption.
   d. viral, bacterial, or protozoal infections.

3. Nutrition problems that may result from fat malabsorption include all of the following *except*:
   a. weight loss.
   b. essential amino acid deficiencies.
   c. bone loss.
   d. oxalate kidney stones.

4. Common nutrition problems associated with bacterial overgrowth in the stomach and small intestine include:
   a. sensitivity to gluten.
   b. fat malabsorption and vitamin B_{12} deficiency.
   c. constipation.
   d. permanent loss of digestive enzymes.

5. Chronic pancreatitis and cystic fibrosis are both treated with:
   a. intestinal resection.
   b. postural drainage.
   c. enzyme replacement therapy.
   d. stool softeners.

6. A person with celiac disease must avoid products containing:
   a. wheat, barley, and rye.
   b. lactose.
   c. excessive fat.
   d. corn, rice, and millet.

7. Despite the intestine's capacity for adaptation, removal of which section of the intestine will likely result in fat malabsorption and multiple nutrient deficiencies?
   a. Duodenum
   b. Jejunum
   c. Ileum
   d. Colon

8. Symptoms of irritable bowel syndrome most often include:
   a. nausea and vomiting.
   b. weight loss and malnutrition.
   c. strong odors and obstructions.
   d. constipation and/or diarrhea and abdominal discomfort.

9. Diverticulosis is most often associated with:
   a. aging.
   b. inadequate exercise.
   c. intestinal surgery.
   d. a high-fiber diet.

10. After an ileostomy, the most serious concern is that:
    a. the diet is too restrictive to meet nutrient needs.
    b. waste disposal causes frequent daily interruptions.
    c. fluid restrictions prevent patients from drinking beverages freely.
    d. incompletely digested foods may cause obstructions.

Answers: 1. d, 2. c, 3. b, 4. b, 5. c, 6. a, 7. c, 8. d, 9. a, 10. d

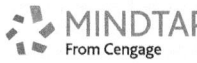 MINDTAP From Cengage For more chapter resources visit **www.cengage.com** to access MindTap, a complete digital course.

Clinical Applications

1. A health practitioner working with a patient with a constipation problem provides him with detailed information about a high-fiber diet. At a follow-up appointment, the patient reports no change in symptoms. His food diary for that day shows that he consumed an omelet and toast for breakfast and a sandwich with juice for lunch.

   • Considering these two meals only, what additional information would help the health practitioner evaluate the man's compliance with the diet he was given?

- Review the discussion about fiber in Chapter 3, and create a one-day menu that provides the DRI for fiber for an adult male, using the fiber values listed in a food composition table.

2. Using Table 18-5 on p. 520 as a guide, plan a day's menus for a diet containing approximately 50 grams of fat. Take care to make the meals both palatable and nutritious. How can these menus be improved using the suggestions in Box 18-5 (p. 522)?

3. As stated in this chapter, the treatment of celiac disease is deceptively simple—eliminate wheat, barley, and rye, and possibly oats. Remaining on a gluten-free diet is more challenging than it appears, however.
- Randomly select 10 of your favorite snack and convenience foods. Take a trip to the grocery store, and check the labels of the products you selected to see if they would be allowed on a gluten-free diet. Keep in mind that the labels may not list all offending ingredients.
- Find acceptable substitutes for the products that are not allowed, either by substituting other foods or by checking for gluten-free products in the grocery store. You can also investigate websites that advertise gluten-free products to get an idea of what is available.

Notes

1. A. J. Lembo, Constipation, in M. Feldman and coeditors, *Sleisenger and Fordtran's Gastrointestinal and Liver Disease* (Philadelphia: Saunders, 2016), pp. 270–296.
2. Lembo, 2016; B. G. Schuster, L. K. Kosar, and R. Kamrul, Constipation in older adults, *Canadian Family Physician* 61 (2015): 152–158.
3. Lembo, 2016; Schuster, Kosar, and Kamrul, 2015.
4. Lembo, 2016.
5. P. R. Gibson and S. J. Shepherd, Evidence-based dietary management of functional gastrointestinal symptoms: The FODMAP approach, *Journal of Gastroenterology and Hepatology* 25 (2010): 252–258.
6. F. Azpiroz, Intestinal gas, in M. Feldman and coeditors, *Sleisenger and Fordtran's Gastrointestinal and Liver Disease* (Philadelphia: Saunders, 2016), pp. 242–250.
7. L. R. Schiller and J. H. Sellin, Diarrhea, in M. Feldman and coeditors, *Sleisenger and Fordtran's Gastrointestinal and Liver Disease* (Philadelphia: Saunders, 2016), pp. 221–241; J. S. Trier, Acute diarrheal disorders, in N. J. Greenberger, ed., *Current Diagnosis and Treatment: Gastroenterology, Hepatology, and Endoscopy* (New York: McGraw-Hill, 2016), pp. 51–72.
8. M. E. Sanders and coauthors, An update on the use and investigation of probiotics in health and disease, *Gut* 62 (2013): 787–796; D. Wolvers and coauthors, Guidance for substantiating the evidence for beneficial effects of probiotics: Prevention and management of infections by probiotics, *Journal of Nutrition* 140 (2010): 698S–712S.
9. H. J. Binder and coauthors, Oral rehydration therapy in the second decade of the twenty-first century, *Current Gastroenterology Reports* 16 (2014): 376; doi: 10.1007/s11894-014-0376-2.
10. Schiller and Sellin, 2016.
11. Academy of Nutrition and Dietetics, *Nutrition Care Manual* (Chicago: Academy of Nutrition and Dietetics, 2018.
12. J. S. Trier, Intestinal malabsorption, in N. J. Greenberger, ed., *Current Diagnosis and Treatment: Gastroenterology, Hepatology, and Endoscopy* (New York: McGraw-Hill, 2016), pp. 251–273.
13. Trier, Intestinal malabsorption, 2016.
14. E. M. M. Quigley, Small intestinal bacterial overgrowth, in M. Feldman and coeditors, *Sleisenger and Fordtran's Gastrointestinal and Liver Disease* (Philadelphia: Saunders, 2016), pp. 1824–1831.
15. Quigley, 2016.
16. Quigley, 2016; C. E. Semrad, Approach to the patient with diarrhea and malabsorption, in L. Goldman and A. I. Schafer, eds., *Goldman-Cecil Medicine* (Philadelphia: Saunders, 2016), pp. 918–935.
17. S. Hertzler and coauthors, Nutrient considerations in lactose intolerance, in A. M. Coulston and coeditors, *Nutrition in the Prevention and Treatment of Disease* (London: Academic Press/Elsevier, 2017), pp. 875–892.
18. Hertzler and coauthors, 2017.
19. Hertzler and coauthors, 2017; A. Szilagyi and coauthors, Differential impact of lactose/lactase phenotype on colonic microflora, *Canadian Journal of Gastroenterology* 24 (2010): 373–379.
20. C. E. Forsmark, Pancreatitis, in L. Goldman and A. I. Schafer, eds., *Goldman-Cecil Medicine* (Philadelphia: Saunders, 2016), pp. 959–967.
21. Forsmark, Pancreatitis, 2016; D. L. Conwell and P. A. Banks, Acute pancreatitis, in N. J. Greenberger, ed., *Current Diagnosis and Treatment: Gastroenterology, Hepatology, and Endoscopy* (New York: McGraw-Hill, 2016), pp. 335–351.
22. Forsmark, Pancreatitis, 2016; J. M. Mirtallo, International consensus guidelines for nutrition therapy in pancreatitis, *Journal of Parenteral and Enteral Nutrition* 36 (2012): 284–291.
23. R. F. Meier, Nutritional support in acute pancreatitis, in G. A. Cresci, ed., *Nutrition Support for the Critically Ill Patient* (Boca Raton, FL: CRC Press, 2015), pp. 535–548; Mirtallo, 2012.
24. D. L. Conwell and P. A Banks, Chronic pancreatitis, in N. J. Greenberger, ed., *Current Diagnosis and Treatment: Gastroenterology, Hepatology, and Endoscopy* (New York: McGraw-Hill, 2016), pp. 343–351.
25. S. N. Duggan and K. C. Conlon, A practical guide to the nutritional management of chronic pancreatitis, *Practical Gastroenterology* (June 2013): 24–32.
26. C. E. Forsmark, Chronic pancreatitis, in M. Feldman and coeditors, *Sleisenger and Fordtran's Gastrointestinal and Liver Disease* (Philadelphia: Saunders, 2016), pp. 994–1026.
27. D. C. Whitcomb and M. E. Lowe, Hereditary, familial, and genetic disorders of the pancreas and pancreatic disorders in childhood, in M. Feldman and coeditors, *Sleisenger and Fordtran's Gastrointestinal and Liver Disease* (Philadelphia: Saunders, 2016), pp. 944–968.
28. M. Wilschanski, Novel therapeutic approaches for cystic fibrosis, *Discovery Medicine* 15 (2013): 127–133; C. L. Rogers, Nutritional management of the adult with cystic fibrosis—part I, *Practical Gastroenterology* (January 2013): 10–24.
29. Whitcomb and Lowe, 2016.
30. Rogers, 2013; J. L. Matel, Nutritional management of cystic fibrosis, *Journal of Parenteral and Enteral Nutrition* 36 (2012): 60S–67S.
31. Trier, Intestinal malabsorption, 2016; A. Rubio-Tapia and coauthors, Prevalence of celiac disease in the United States, *American Journal of Gastroenterology* 107 (2012): 1538–1544.
32. C. P. Kelly, Celiac disease, in M. Feldman and coeditors, *Sleisenger and Fordtran's Gastrointestinal and Liver Disease* (Philadelphia: Saunders, 2016), pp. 1849–1872.
33. R. S. Blumberg and S. B. Snapper, Inflammatory bowel disease: Immunologic considerations and therapeutic implications, in N. J. Greenberger, ed., *Current Diagnosis and Treatment: Gastroenterology, Hepatology, and Endoscopy* (New York: McGraw-Hill, 2016), pp. 14–25.

34. G. R. Lichtenstein, Inflammatory bowel disease, in L. Goldman and A. I. Schafer, eds., *Goldman-Cecil Medicine* (Philadelphia: Saunders, 2016), pp. 935–943.

35. J. L. Irani and R. Bleday, Inflammatory bowel disease: Surgical considerations, in N. J. Greenberger, ed., *Current Diagnosis and Treatment: Gastroenterology, Hepatology, and Endoscopy* (New York: McGraw-Hill, 2016), pp. 40–50.

36. Academy of Nutrition and Dietetics, 2018; A. S. Naik and N. Venu, Nutritional care in adult inflammatory bowel disease, *Practical Gastroenterology* (June 2012): 18–27.

37. A. L. Buchman, Short bowel syndrome, in M. Feldman and coeditors, *Sleisenger and Fordtran's Gastrointestinal and Liver Disease* (Philadelphia: Saunders, 2016), pp. 1832–1848.

38. Buchman, 2016; K. N. Jeejeebhoy, Short bowel syndrome, in A. C. Ross and coeditors, *Modern Nutrition in Health and Disease* (Baltimore: Lippincott Williams & Wilkins, 2014), pp. 1069–1079.

39. Jeejeebhoy, 2014.

40. S. Friedman, Irritable bowel syndrome, in N. J. Greenberger, ed., *Current Diagnosis and Treatment: Gastroenterology, Hepatology, and Endoscopy* (New York: McGraw-Hill, 2016), pp. 316–327.

41. Friedman, 2016; A. C. Ford and N. J. Talley, Irritable bowel syndrome, in M. Feldman and coeditors, *Sleisenger and Fordtran's Gastrointestinal and Liver Disease* (Philadelphia: Saunders, 2016), pp. 2139–2153.

42. P. A. Hayes, M. H. Fraher, and E. M. M. Quigley, Irritable bowel syndrome: The role of food in pathogenesis and management, *Gastroenterology and Hepatology* 10 (2014): 164–174.

43. A. Lenhart and W. D. Chey, A systematic review of the effects of polyols on gastrointestinal health and irritable bowel syndrome, *Advances in Nutrition* 8 (2017): 587–596; Ford and Talley, 2016; Friedman, 2016.

44. Hayes, Fraher, and Quigley, 2014; L. Ruepert and coauthors, Bulking agents, antispasmodics and antidepressants for the treatment of irritable bowel syndrome, *Cochrane Database of Systematic Reviews* 8 (2011), doi: 10.1002/14651858.CD003460.

45. Ford and Talley, 2016; Hayes, Fraher, and Quigley, 2014.

46. A. C. Travis, Diverticular disease of the colon, in N. J. Greenberger, ed., *Current Diagnosis and Treatment: Gastroenterology, Hepatology, and Endoscopy* (New York: McGraw-Hill, 2016), pp. 274–287.

47. Travis, 2016; T. P. Bhuket and N. H. Stollman, Diverticular disease of the colon, in M. Feldman and coeditors, *Sleisenger and Fordtran's Gastrointestinal and Liver Disease* (Philadelphia: Saunders, 2016), pp. 2123–2138.

48. Travis, 2016; Bhuket and Stollman, 2016.

49. A. F. Peery and coauthors, Constipation and a low-fiber diet are not associated with diverticulosis, *Clinical Gastroenterology and Hepatology* 11 (2013): 1622–1627; A. F. Peery and coauthors, A high-fiber diet does not protect against asymptomatic diverticulosis, *Gastroenterology* 142 (2012): 266–272; L. L. Strate, Lifestyle factors and the course of diverticular disease, Digestive Diseases 30 (2012): 35–45.

50. Travis, 2016; Bhuket and Stollman, 2016.

51. C. Ünlü and coauthors, A systematic review of high-fibre dietary therapy in diverticular disease, *International Journal of Colorectal Disease* 27 (2012): 419–427.

52. Bhuket and Stollman, 2016; L. L. Strate, A. F. Peery, and I. Neumann, American Gastroenterological Association Institute technical review on the management of acute diverticulitis, *Gastroenterology* 149 (2015): 1950–1976.

53. S. Tarleton and J. K. DiBaise, Low-residue diet in diverticular disease: Putting an end to a myth, *Nutrition in Clinical Practice* 26 (2011): 137–142.

54. L. Schwartz and C. E. Semrad, Irritable bowel syndrome and diverticular disease, in A. C. Ross and coeditors, *Modern Nutrition in Health and Disease* (Baltimore: Lippincott Williams & Wilkins, 2014), pp. 1096–1102.

55. Academy of Nutrition and Dietetics, 2018.

56. Academy of Nutrition and Dietetics, 2018.

57. Academy of Nutrition and Dietetics, 2018.

58. Academy of Nutrition and Dietetics, 2018.

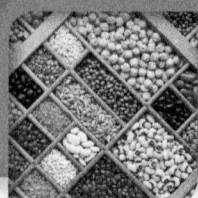

18.6 Nutrition in Practice

Probiotics and Intestinal Health

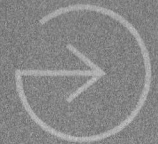

Soon after birth, the warm, nutrient-rich environment within the gastrointestinal tract is colonized by a wide variety of bacterial species. In fact, the approximately 10 trillion bacterial cells inhabiting our bodies represent more than 90 percent of the cells in the body. Most bacterial cells reside in our colon, which harbors over 500 different species.[1] Although the exact composition of intestinal bacteria varies among individuals, the pattern within an individual tends to remain constant over time, fluctuating somewhat due to age, illness, antibiotic treatment, and, to some extent, dietary factors. Table NP18-1 lists examples of the dominant types of bacteria that colonize the human intestines, and Table NP18-2 shows how the bacterial populations vary within different regions of the GI tract.

Over the past several decades, nutritional scientists and microbiologists have tried to determine whether **probiotics**—live, **nonpathogenic** microorganisms supplied in sufficient numbers to possibly benefit our health—can be useful for

TABLE NP18-2	Bacterial Populations in the Gastrointestinal Tract
ORGAN	**TOTAL BACTERIA (PER mL OF CONTENTS)**
Stomach, duodenum	10–1000
Jejunum, ileum	10^4–10^8
Colon	10^{10}–10^{12}

preventing or treating various medical conditions. Although the diseases of interest include gastrointestinal disorders, researchers have also been studying the effects of bacterial probiotics on cancer, immune system disorders, and other diseases. This Nutrition in Practice discusses some of the research and explains some of the issues involved in selecting and consuming probiotics. The glossary in Box NP18-1 defines some relevant terms.

How do our intestinal bacteria influence health?

Intestinal bacteria can benefit our health in a number of different ways. First, the bacteria degrade much of our undigested or unabsorbed dietary carbohydrate, including certain dietary fibers, starch that is resistant to digestion, and poorly absorbed sugars and sugar alcohols. In turn, the bacteria produce some vitamins, as well as short-chain fatty acids that our colonic epithelial cells and other body cells can use as an energy source. Intestinal bacteria also assist in the development and maintenance of mucosal tissue, protect intestinal tissue from **pathogenic** bacteria, and stimulate immune defenses in mucosal cells and other body tissues.[2]

TABLE NP18-1	Intestinal Bacteria
PREDOMINANT TYPES ($>10^9$ CFU/mL)	**SUBDOMINANT TYPES ($<10^9$ CFU/mL)**
• Bacteroides	• Enterobacteria
• Bifidobacteria	• Enterococci
• Clostridia	• Escherichia
• Eubacteria	• Fusobacteria
• Peptostreptococci	• Lactobacilli
• Ruminococci	• Streptococci

Note: CFU = colony-forming units (number of viable bacteria)

Box NP18-1 Glossary

bacterial translocation: movement of bacteria across the intestinal mucosa, allowing access to body tissues.
nonpathogenic: not capable of causing disease.
pathogenic: capable of causing disease.

prebiotics: indigestible substances in foods that stimulate the growth of nonpathogenic bacteria within the large intestine.
probiotics: live microorganisms provided in foods and dietary supplements that confer a health benefit when taken in sufficient amounts.

Certain nondigestible substances in food, called **prebiotics**, can stimulate the growth or activity of the resident bacteria within the large intestine. Prebiotics include some of the carbohydrates found in artichokes, asparagus, beetroot, chicory root, garlic, Jerusalem artichokes, leeks, onions, and other foods.[3] Because the intestinal bacteria that degrade these substances produce gas as a by-product, people who consume high amounts of these foods may experience more flatulence than usual.

Why are certain types of bacteria considered "probiotic"?

For microbes to be "probiotic"—that is, beneficial to health—they must be nonpathogenic when consumed. They must survive their transit through the digestive tract; therefore, they must be resistant to destruction by stomach acid, bile, and digestive enzymes. They should be able to alter the intestinal environment in some way that is beneficial to the human host, either by producing antimicrobial substances, altering immune responses, metabolizing undigested foodstuffs, or protecting the intestinal walls.[4]

Probiotic bacteria must be consumed in large amounts—at least 1 billion live bacteria per day—to survive in sufficient numbers to influence the bacterial populations in the large intestine; a serving of yogurt usually provides these amounts. Carefully controlled studies have not found that probiotic bacteria actually *colonize* the intestine, however, as they are no longer detected in fecal or intestinal samples once ingestion of the probiotic product stops. Note that only a few different types of bacteria are used in foods, and the relatively small amounts consumed cannot compete with the huge populations that normally reside in our digestive tract.

What types of medical problems are helped by probiotics?

Although the results of research studies vary, probiotics may help to prevent and treat some gastric and intestinal disorders (such as inflammatory bowel diseases and irritable bowel syndrome), alter susceptibility to food allergens and alleviate some allergy symptoms, and improve the availability and digestibility of various nutrients. Other potential benefits include improved immune responses, reduced symptoms of lactose intolerance, and reduced cancer risk.[5]

Much of the research investigating probiotics and intestinal illness has focused on the prevention and treatment of infectious diarrhea. For example, controlled trials have suggested that certain strains of probiotic bacteria may shorten the duration of diarrhea caused by rotavirus infection in infants and children, decrease the incidence of traveler's diarrhea in tourists visiting high-risk areas,

and prevent the recurrence of infectious diarrhea in hospitalized patients.[6] In studies of children and adults using antibiotics, some strains of probiotic bacteria have been shown to reduce the incidence and duration of antibiotic-associated diarrhea.[7] As another example, some studies have suggested that probiotic treatment may help to reduce the recurrence of *pouchitis*, an inflammation of the surgical pouch created in some patients who have had an ileostomy or colostomy.[8]

Despite promising research results thus far, there are no clear conclusions about the appropriate probiotic doses or durations of treatment for many of these conditions. Moreover, the beneficial effects of one bacterial strain cannot be extrapolated to other strains of the same species, as different strains can have contrasting effects.[9] Thus, individuals who decide to consume probiotic-containing foods and supplements to benefit their health cannot be certain that the substances they use will help their condition. At best, probiotics should be considered an adjunct therapy rather than a primary treatment for a disease.

What are the main dietary sources of probiotics?

Probiotics are available from fermented milk products such as yogurt and kefir, which are produced using various species of lactobacilli and bifidobacteria; note that the bacterial strains are chosen for their ability to produce desirable food products rather than for their potential health benefits (see Photo NP18-1). Probiotics are added to many other types of foods as well, including cereals, cookies, snack bars, candies, protein powders, drink mixes, and lozenges. Although fermented food products

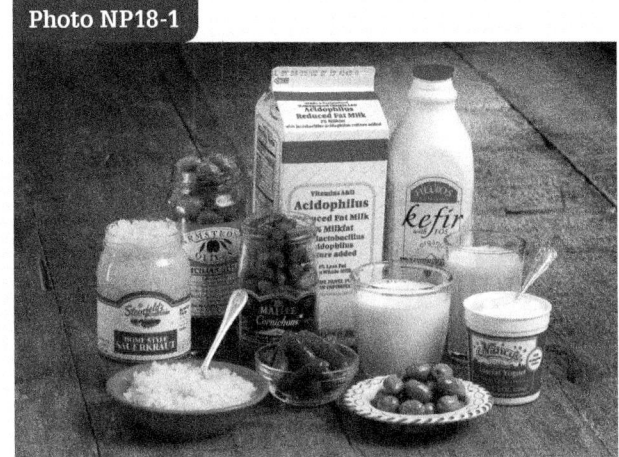

Photo NP18-1

Various species of *Lactobacillus* are used in the production of fermented food products, such as the foods shown in this photo.

© Polara Studios, Inc.

such as sauerkraut, pickles, and olives are produced using lactobacilli, these foods retain few, if any, live bacteria after they undergo typical food processing methods.

A number of companies market probiotic supplements, which are available in capsules, tablets, and powders. Because probiotic products contain living organisms, storage conditions may affect viability—heat, moisture, and oxygen can reduce survival times—and therefore consumers should check the expiration date before purchasing a product. When a consumer group (ConsumerLab.com) tested 18 probiotic supplements, they found that 2 of the products contained only 47 and 49 percent of the organisms claimed on the label.[10] Thus, there is no guarantee that a dietary supplement will contain the numbers of microbes expected.

Are there any potential problems associated with the use of probiotics?

Although adverse effects are rare, one concern is the possibility that probiotic bacteria may cause infection in immune-compromised individuals.[11] Various species of probiotic bacteria, including *Lactobacillus* species, have been isolated from the infection sites of severely ill individuals who were consuming the probiotic. Risk may be increased by the use of antibiotic therapy (which reduces bacterial populations), diseases or medications that suppress immunity, and diseases that increase risk of **bacterial translocation** (including inflammatory bowel diseases and intestinal infections).[12] Care should be taken to inquire about probiotic use in these patients.

Other safety concerns include the potential for allergic reactions to ingredients in probiotic supplements and possible exposure to undesirable yeasts and molds in contaminated products. In addition, the amounts and types of probiotic bacteria in a product may vary considerably from those declared on the label; therefore, the consumer cannot be certain that the product they purchase will help them achieve the desired effect.

The microbes that inhabit the GI tract have critical roles in maintaining the integrity of intestinal tissues and influence health in various other ways. Preliminary research suggests that altering our bacterial populations by consuming probiotics or prebiotics may help to improve our defenses against certain illnesses. Additional studies are needed to verify the beneficial effects of probiotics and prebiotics and to develop standard protocols that can be used for treating illness.

Notes

1. C. M. C. Maranduba and coauthors, Intestinal microbiota as modulators of the immune system and neuroimmune system: Impact on the host health and homeostasis, *Journal of Immunology Research* 2015 (2015): dx.doi.org/10.1155/2015/931574.
2. C. Hill and F. Shanahan, Enteric microbiota, in M. Feldman and coeditors, *Sleisenger and Fordtran's Gastrointestinal and Liver Disease* (Philadelphia: Saunders, 2016), pp. 28–35; T. Peregrin, Inside tract: What RDs need to know about the gut microbiome, *Journal of the Academy of Nutrition and Dietetics* 113 (2013): 1019–1023.
3. E. M. M. Quigley, Prebiotics and probiotics: Their role in the management of gastrointestinal disorders in adults, *Nutrition in Clinical Practice* 27 (2012): 195–200.
4. S. Tejero and coauthors, Probiotics and prebiotics as modulators of the gut microbiota, in A. C. Ross and coeditors, *Modern Nutrition in Health and Disease* (Baltimore: Lippincott Williams & Wilkins, 2014), pp. 506–512.
5. M. W. Ariefdjohan, O. N. Brown-Esters, and D. A. Savaiano, Intestinal microflora and diet in health, in A. M. Coulston, C. J. Boushey, and M. G. Ferruzzi, eds., *Nutrition in the Prevention and Treatment of Disease* (London: Academic Press/Elsevier, 2013), pp. 719–738; M. E. Sanders and

coauthors, An update on the use and investigation of probiotics in health and disease, *Gut* 62 (2013): 787–796.
6. Ariefdjohan, Brown-Esters, and Savaiano, 2013.
7. C. M. Surawicz and L. J. Brandt, Probiotics and fecal microbiota transplantation, in M. Feldman and coeditors, *Sleisenger and Fordtran's Gastrointestinal and Liver Disease* (Philadelphia: Saunders, 2016), pp. 2339–2343; Tejero and coauthors, 2014.
8. Surawicz and Brandt, 2016; Tejero and coauthors, 2014.
9. C. Hill and coauthors, International Scientific Association for Probiotics and Prebiotics consensus statement on the scope and appropriate use of the term probiotic, *Nature Reviews Gastroenterology and Hepatology* 11 (2014): 506–514; Quigley, 2012.
10. ConsumerLab.com, Product review: Probiotics (for Adults, Children and Pets) and Kefirs (30 August 2017), available at www.consumerlab.com.
11. Surawicz and Brandt, 2016.
12. K. Whelan and C. E. Myers, Safety of probiotics in patients receiving nutritional support: A systematic review of case reports, randomized controlled trials, and nonrandomized trials, *American Journal of Clinical Nutrition* 91 (2010): 687–703.

Nutrition and Liver Diseases

Chapter Sections and Learning Objectives (LOs)

chapter

19

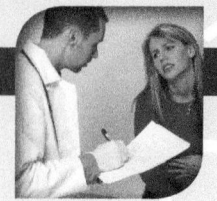

THE LIVER IS THE MOST METABOLICALLY ACTIVE ORGAN IN THE BODY.

It plays a central role in processing, storing, and redistributing the nutrients provided by the foods we eat. The liver produces most of the proteins that circulate in plasma, including albumin, blood clotting proteins, and transport proteins; it also produces the bile that emulsifies fat during digestion. In addition, the liver detoxifies drugs and alcohol and processes excess nitrogen so that it can be safely excreted as urea. If damage or disease hinders the liver's ability to perform its various functions, the effects on health and nutrition status can be profound.

Liver disease progresses slowly. Its primary symptom, fatigue, often goes unnoticed. Other symptoms may be so mild that complications develop before liver disease is diagnosed. Once liver disease is recognized, health practitioners emphasize the need to preserve remaining liver function, as the liver can regenerate some healthy tissue, improving the prognosis. Preventing additional damage is the principal means of avoiding liver failure or a liver transplant.

19.1 Fatty Liver and Hepatitis

Fatty liver and hepatitis are the two most common disorders affecting the liver. Although both conditions may be mild and are usually reversible, each may progress to more serious illness and eventually cause liver damage.

Fatty Liver

Fatty liver is an accumulation of fat in liver tissue. It represents an imbalance between the amount of fat produced in the liver or picked up from the blood and the amount the liver uses or exports to the blood via very-low-density lipoproteins (VLDL).[1] Fatty liver may be caused by defects in metabolism, excessive alcohol ingestion, or exposure to various drugs and toxins. In cases unrelated to alcohol (a condition known as *nonalcoholic fatty liver disease*), **insulin resistance** is the primary risk factor; thus, fatty liver frequently accompanies type 2 diabetes mellitus, metabolic syndrome, and obesity. Other causes of fatty liver include protein-energy malnutrition and long-term total parenteral nutrition. Fatty liver is estimated to affect about 24 percent of the adult population in the United States, and nearly 90 percent of heavy drinkers.[2]

Consequences of Fatty Liver In many individuals, fatty liver is asymptomatic and causes no harm. In other cases, it may be associated with inflammation (**steatohepatitis**), liver enlargement (**hepatomegaly**), and fatigue. If inflammation and scarring develop, fatty liver may progress to cirrhosis (discussed in a later section), liver failure, and liver cancer.[3]

Fatty liver is the most common cause of abnormal liver enzyme levels in the blood. Laboratory findings typically include elevated concentrations of the liver enzymes alanine aminotransferase (ALT) and aspartate aminotransferase (AST), as well as increased blood levels of triglycerides, cholesterol, and glucose. Table 19-2 (p. 550) provides normal ranges for these liver enzymes.

Treatment of Fatty Liver The usual treatment for fatty liver is to eliminate the factors that cause it.[4] For example, if fatty liver is due to alcohol abuse or drug treatment, it may improve after the patient discontinues use of the substance. In patients with elevated blood lipids, fatty liver may improve after blood lipid levels are lowered. An appropriate treatment for obese or diabetic patients might be weight reduction, increased physical activity, or medications that improve insulin sensitivity. Rapid weight loss should be discouraged, however, because it may accelerate the progression

fatty liver: an accumulation of fat in liver tissue; also called *hepatic steatosis*.

insulin resistance: the reduced sensitivity to insulin in liver, muscle, and adipose cells.

steatohepatitis (STEE-ah-to-HEP-ah-TYE-tis): liver inflammation that is associated with fatty liver.

hepatomegaly (HEP-ah-toe-MEG-ah-lee): enlargement of the liver.

TABLE 19-1 Features of Hepatitis Viruses

HEPATITIS VIRUS	MAJOR MODE OF TRANSMISSION	NEW CASES (UNITED STATES, 2015)	CHRONIC DISEASE RATE (% OF CASES)	CHRONIC CASES[a] (UNITED STATES, 2015)	VACCINE
A	Fecal-oral	2,800	None	0	Available
B	Bloodborne, sexual transmission	21,900	Newborn infants: 90% Children (1 to 5 years): 30–50% Adults: 5%	0.85–2.2 million	Available
C	Bloodborne	33,900	75–85%	3.5 million	None

[a]Chronic cases of hepatitis are those that last 6 months or longer.

Note: A much larger percentage of HCV cases become chronic than HBV cases, so there are significantly more HCV carriers than HBV carriers.

Source: Centers for Disease Control and Prevention, *Viral Hepatitis Surveillance: United States, 2015* (Atlanta: U.S. Department of Health and Human Services, 2017).

of liver disease.[5] Note that lifestyle modifications are not always successful in reversing fatty liver, especially in patients who lack the usual risk factors.

Hepatitis

Hepatitis, a condition of liver inflammation, results from damage to liver tissue. Most often, the damage is caused by infection with specific viruses, designated by the letters *A, B, C, D,* and *E*. Other causes include excessive alcohol intake, exposure to some drugs and toxic chemicals, fatty liver disease, and autoimmune disease. A number of herbal remedies are reported to cause hepatitis; these include chaparral, germander, jin bu huan, kava, ma huang, pennyroyal, senna, and skullcap.[6] Long-term hepatitis can lead to cirrhosis (discussed in a later section) and liver cancer.

Viral Hepatitis In the United States, acute hepatitis is most often caused by infection with hepatitis viruses A, B, or C (see Table 19-1). Specific features of these viruses include the following:

- *Hepatitis A virus* (HAV) is primarily spread via fecal-oral transmission, which usually involves the ingestion of foods or beverages that have been contaminated with fecal material. Outbreaks of HAV infection are often associated with floods and other natural disasters, when inadequately treated sewage contaminates water supplies. Vaccinations against HAV are recommended for high-risk individuals, such as international travelers, children living in communities with high disease rates, people who inject illicit drugs, and persons with unsafe sexual behaviors.[7] In addition, routine vaccination is recommended for all children at 1 year of age. HAV infection usually resolves within a few months and does not cause chronic infection or permanent liver damage.
- *Hepatitis B virus* (HBV) is transmitted by infected blood or needles, by sexual contact with an infected person, and from mother to infant during childbirth. A major global health concern, HBV has infected as much as one-half of the world population (as evidenced by HBV antibodies), although chronic illness develops in less than 10 percent of cases.[8] Vaccinations are currently recommended for newborn infants, unvaccinated children and adolescents, health care workers, recipients of certain blood products, dialysis patients, sexually active adults, and people who inject illicit drugs.[9]
- *Hepatitis C virus* (HCV) is spread via infected blood or needles but is not readily spread by sexual contact or childbirth. HCV infection is currently the most common bloodborne infection in the United States and is a leading cause of

hepatitis (hep-ah-TYE-tis): inflammation of the liver.

jaundice (JAWN-dis): yellow discoloration of the skin and eyes due to an accumulation of bilirubin, a breakdown product of hemoglobin that normally exits the body via bile secretions.

Photo 19-1 Jaundice

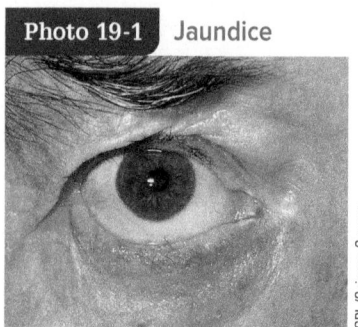

Jaundice is a yellow discoloration of the tissues that is most easily seen in the sclera. Jaundice results when liver dysfunction impairs the metabolism of bilirubin, a breakdown product of hemoglobin that is normally excreted in bile and urine. Accumulation of bilirubin in the bloodstream leads to yellow discoloration of tissues.

SPL/Science Source

BOX 19-1 *Nursing Diagnosis*

Nursing diagnoses appropriate for people with hepatitis may include *fatigue, risk for deficient fluid volume (due to vomiting and diarrhea), imbalanced nutrition: less than body requirements, acute pain,* and *risk for impaired liver function.*

BOX 19-2 *Nursing Diagnosis*

Nursing diagnoses appropriate for people with cirrhosis may include *fatigue, nausea, ineffective protection, risk for impaired skin integrity, chronic pain,* and *imbalanced nutrition: less than body requirements.*

cirrhosis (sih-ROE-sis): an advanced stage of liver disease in which extensive scarring replaces healthy liver tissue, causing impaired liver function and liver failure.

chronic liver disease.[10] No vaccine is available to protect against HCV infection. Preventive measures include blood donor screening, HCV inactivation in blood products, infection control practices in health care settings, and risk reduction counseling to high-risk individuals.

Symptoms and Signs of Hepatitis The effects of hepatitis depend on the cause and severity of the condition. Individuals with mild or chronic cases are often asymptomatic. The onset of acute hepatitis may be accompanied by fatigue, malaise, nausea, occasional vomiting, anorexia, and pain in the liver area (see Box 19-1). The liver is often slightly enlarged and tender. **Jaundice** (yellow discoloration of tissues) may develop, causing yellowing of the skin, urine, and sclera (see Photo 19-1). Other symptoms of hepatitis may include fever, muscle weakness, joint pain, and skin rashes. Serum levels of the liver enzymes ALT and AST are typically elevated. Chronic hepatitis can cause complications that are typical of liver cirrhosis and may lead to liver cancer.

Treatment of Hepatitis Hepatitis is treated with supportive care, such as bed rest (if necessary) and an appropriate diet. Hepatitis patients should avoid substances that irritate the liver, such as alcohol, drugs, and dietary supplements that cause liver damage. Hepatitis A infection usually resolves without the use of medications. Antiviral agents may be used to treat HBV and HCV infections; examples include lamivudine and ribavirin, which block viral replication, and interferon alfa, which both inhibits viral replication and enhances immune responses.[11] Nonviral forms of hepatitis may be treated with anti-inflammatory and immunosuppressant drugs. Hospitalization is not required for hepatitis unless other medical conditions or complications hamper recovery.

Nutrition Therapy for Hepatitis Nutrition care varies according to a patient's symptoms and nutrition status.[12] Most individuals require no dietary changes. Those who have difficulty eating due to anorexia or abdominal discomfort may find four to six small meals per day easier to tolerate than three larger ones. Patients with persistent vomiting may require fluid and electrolyte replacement. Alcohol should be avoided because it can increase liver damage. Oral supplements may be helpful for improving nutrient intakes.

Review Notes

- Fatty liver can result from metabolic defects, exposure to some drugs and toxins, or excessive alcohol intake. Insulin resistance is a primary risk factor for fatty liver; thus, the condition often accompanies type 2 diabetes mellitus, metabolic syndrome, and obesity.
- Hepatitis is frequently caused by viral infection but can also result from alcohol abuse, drug toxicity, fatty liver disease, and other causes. Hepatitis B and C viruses may lead to chronic hepatitis.
- Fatty liver can be treated by eliminating the factors that cause it. Hepatitis treatment involves supportive care, such as bed rest, elimination of liver toxins, and dietary measures that maintain or improve nutrition status.

19.2 Cirrhosis

Cirrhosis is a late stage of chronic liver disease. Long-term liver disease gradually destroys liver tissue, leading to scarring (fibrosis) in some regions and small areas of regenerated, healthy tissue in others (see Photo 19-2). As the disease progresses, the scarring becomes more extensive, leaving fewer areas of healthy tissue. A cirrhotic liver is often shrunken and has an irregular, nodular appearance. Cirrhosis is characterized

Photo 19-2 Cirrhosis of the Liver

Normal liver tissue is smooth and has a regular texture.

Martin Rotker/Phototake

A cirrhotic liver has an irregular, nodular appearance. The nodules represent clusters of regenerating cells within the damaged liver tissue.

Dr. Joseph William/Phototake

by impaired liver function and may eventually result in liver failure. Together, chronic liver disease and cirrhosis rank as the 12th leading cause of death in the United States.[13]

The chief causes of cirrhosis in the United States are chronic hepatitis C infection and alcoholic liver disease, followed by nonalcoholic fatty liver disease and chronic hepatitis B infection.[14] Additional causes include other types of chronic hepatitis, drug-induced liver injury, some inherited metabolic disorders, and bile duct blockages, which cause bile acids to accumulate to toxic levels in the liver.

Consequences of Cirrhosis

Many patients with liver disease remain asymptomatic for years. Because liver damage progresses slowly, the effects of chronic liver disease may be subtle at first (see Box 19-2). Initial symptoms are usually nonspecific and may include fatigue, malaise, anorexia, and weight loss. Later, the decline in liver function can lead to metabolic disturbances: patients may develop anemia, bruise easily, and be more susceptible to infection. If bile obstruction occurs, jaundice, fat malabsorption, and **pruritis** (itchy skin) are likely. The physical changes in liver tissue may interfere with blood flow, causing fluid to accumulate in blood vessels and body tissues. Advanced cirrhosis can disrupt kidney, lung, and brain function, and is usually associated with malnutrition. Figure 19-1 illustrates some common clinical effects of liver cirrhosis.

Table 19-2 lists laboratory tests that are used to monitor the extent of liver damage. Serum liver enzyme levels are elevated in liver disease because the injured liver tissue releases the enzymes into the bloodstream. Serum levels of bilirubin may be elevated if the liver is too damaged to process the bilirubin or if bile ducts are blocked and prevent its excretion. The impaired synthesis of plasma proteins in the liver reduces albumin levels and extends blood-clotting time. Liver damage also impairs the conversion of ammonia to urea, causing ammonia levels in the blood to rise.

Portal Hypertension A large volume of blood normally flows through the liver. The **hepatic portal vein** and hepatic artery together supply approximately 1500 milliliters (about 1.5 quarts) of blood each minute to the extensive network of vessels in the liver. The scarred tissue of a cirrhotic liver impedes the flow of blood, three-fourths of which is supplied by the portal vein. The restricted blood flow within the liver

FIGURE 19-1 Clinical Effects of Liver Cirrhosis

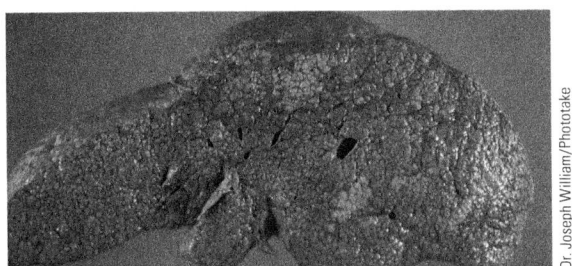

- Neurological disturbances
- Jaundice
- Altered breath
- Esophageal varices
- Feminization (altered sex hormones)
- Extensively scarred liver
- Portal hypertension
- Enlarged collateral vessels
- Ascites
- Hand tremor
- Hypogonadism
- Easy bruisability
- Muscle wasting
- Edema

pruritis: itchy skin.

hepatic portal vein: the blood vessel that conducts nutrient-rich blood from the digestive tract to the liver; also known simply as the *portal vein*.

TABLE 19-2	Laboratory Tests for Evaluation of Liver Disease	
LABORATORY TEST	**NORMAL LEVELS (SERUM)**	**VALUES IN LIVER DISEASE**
Alanine aminotransferase (ALT)	Male: <45 U/L Female: <34 U/L	Elevated
Albumin	3.4–4.8 g/dL	Low
Alkaline phosphatase	Male (>20 yr): 53–128 U/L Female (>20 yr): 42–98 U/L	Normal or elevated
Ammonia	15–45 μg N/dL	Elevated
Aspartate aminotransferase (AST)	Male: <35 U/L Female: <31 U/L	Elevated
Bilirubin (total)	0–2.0 mg/dL	Elevated
Blood urea nitrogen (BUN)	6–20 mg/dL	Normal or low
Gamma-glutamyl transferase (GGT)	Male: <55 U/L Female: <38 U/L	Elevated
Prothrombin time[a] (plasma)	11–16 seconds	Prolonged

[a] The test for prothrombin time evaluates the clotting ability of blood.

Note: U/L = units per liter; dL = deciliter; μg = micrograms; N = nitrogen

Source: L. Goldman and A. I. Schafer, eds., *Goldman-Cecil Medicine* (Philadelphia: Saunders, 2016).

Photo 19-3 Esophageal Varices

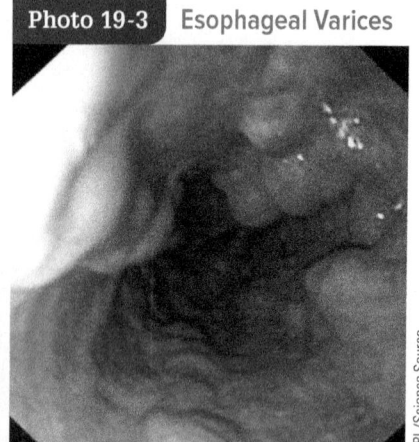

SPL/Science Source

Esophageal varices, such as those shown here, may protrude into the lumen and be vulnerable to rupture and bleeding.

stimulates the release of vasodilators (and therefore, increased blood flow) in nearby arterioles, leading to a greater volume of portal blood. The increased portal blood coupled with resistance to blood flow within the liver causes a rise in blood pressure within the portal vein, called **portal hypertension**.[15]

Collateral Vessels and Gastroesophageal Varices When blood flow through the portal vein is impeded, the blood is forced backward into the veins that normally supply the portal vein with blood. This blood is then diverted to the systemic circulation via **collateral vessels**, which develop and expand throughout the gastrointestinal (GI) tract and in regions near the abdominal wall. As portal pressure builds, some of these collaterals can become enlarged and engorged with blood, forming abnormally dilated vessels called **varices** (see Photo 19-3). The varices that develop in the esophagus (*esophageal varices*) and stomach (*gastric varices*) are vulnerable to rupture because they have thin walls and often bulge into the lumen. If ruptured, they can cause massive bleeding that is sometimes fatal (see Box 19-3). The blood loss is exacerbated by the liver's reduced production of blood-clotting factors.

Ascites Within 10 years of disease onset, about 50 percent of cirrhosis patients develop **ascites**, a large accumulation of fluid in the abdominal cavity (see Photo 19-4 and Box 19-4). The development of ascites indicates that liver damage has reached a critical stage, as up to half of patients with ascites die within five years.[16] Ascites is primarily a consequence of portal hypertension, sodium and water retention in the kidneys, and reduced albumin synthesis in the diseased liver.[17] As a result of portal hypertension, the distorted blood flow elsewhere in the body alters kidney function, leading to sodium and water retention and an accumulation of body fluid. The elevated pressure within the liver's small blood vessels (**sinusoids**) causes fluid to leak into lymphatic vessels and, ultimately, the abdominal cavity.

The movement of water into the abdomen is exacerbated by low levels of serum albumin, a protein that helps to retain fluid in blood vessels. Ascites can cause abdominal discomfort and early satiety, which contribute to malnutrition. Because ascites can raise the body's water weight considerably, weight changes may be difficult to interpret.

Hepatic Encephalopathy Advanced liver disease often leads to **hepatic encephalopathy**, a disorder characterized by abnormal neurological functioning. Signs of hepatic encephalopathy include adverse changes in mental abilities, mood, personality, behavior, and motor functions (see Table 19-3 and Box 19-5). At worst, amnesia, unresponsiveness, and **hepatic coma** may develop. Although hepatic encephalopathy is reversible with medical treatment, its presence suggests a poor prognosis for liver disease, especially when the neurological changes are more pronounced.

The exact causes of hepatic encephalopathy remain elusive, although elevated blood ammonia levels (also known as *hyperammonemia*) are thought to play a key role in its development due to ammonia's neurotoxicity. Other substances that may accumulate in brain tissue and disturb brain function include sulfur compounds, naturally occurring benzodiazepines, short-chain fatty acids, and manganese.[18] Some research shows that severe liver damage may lead to reduced serum levels of the **branched-chain amino acids** and increased levels of the **aromatic amino acids**, which may alter the types of neurotransmitters produced in the brain.[19] Most likely, a combination of abnormalities contributes to the disruption in neurological functioning.

Elevated Ammonia Levels Much of the body's free ammonia is produced by bacterial action on unabsorbed dietary protein in the colon. Normally, the liver extracts this ammonia from portal blood and converts it to urea, which is then excreted by the kidneys. In advanced liver disease, the liver is unable to process the ammonia sufficiently. In addition, much of the ammonia-laden portal blood bypasses the liver by way of collateral vessels and reaches the general blood circulation, causing a substantial increase in the ammonia that reaches brain tissue. Although blood ammonia levels do not correlate well with the degree of neurological impairment in hepatic encephalopathy, ammonia-reducing medications can successfully reverse the neurological symptoms.[20]

Malnutrition and Wasting Most patients with advanced cirrhosis develop protein-energy malnutrition and experience some degree of wasting.[21] Malnutrition is usually

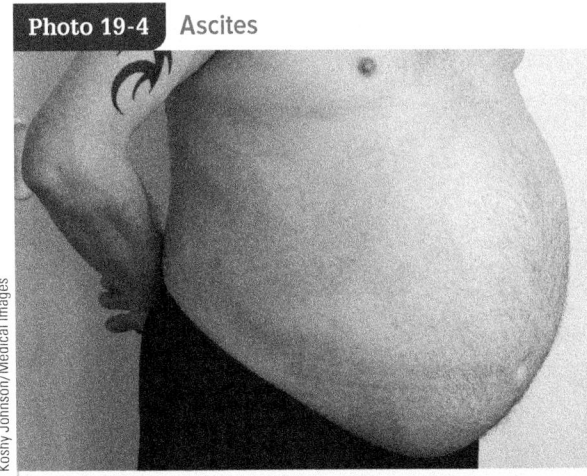

Photo 19-4 | Ascites

Koshy Johnson/Medical Images

Ascites can be caused by various illnesses, but cirrhosis is the underlying cause in most patients with the condition. In addition to ascites, this patient displays an extensive network of collateral vessels in the abdominal region.

BOX 19-4 *Nursing Diagnosis*

Nursing diagnoses appropriate for people with ascites may include *excess fluid volume, impaired comfort*, and *imbalanced nutrition: less than body requirements*.

BOX 19-5 *Nursing Diagnosis*

Nursing diagnoses appropriate for people with hepatic encephalopathy may include *chronic confusion, impaired memory*, and *disturbed sleep pattern*.

hepatic encephalopathy (en-sef-ah-LOP-ah-thie): a neurological complication of advanced liver disease that is characterized by changes in personality, mood, behavior, mental ability, and motor functions.

encephalo = brain
pathy = disease

hepatic coma: loss of consciousness resulting from severe liver disease.

branched-chain amino acids: the essential amino acids leucine, isoleucine, and valine, which have side groups with a branched structure.

aromatic amino acids: the amino acids phenylalanine, tyrosine, and tryptophan, which have carbon rings in their side groups.

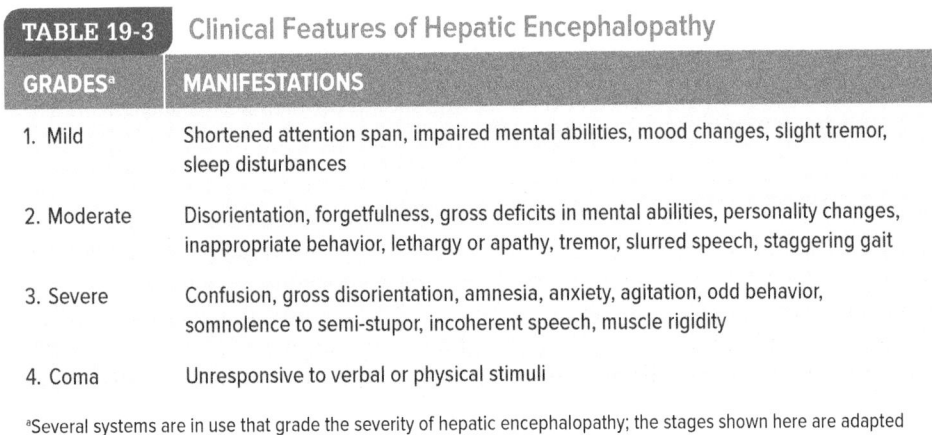

TABLE 19-3	Clinical Features of Hepatic Encephalopathy
GRADES[a]	**MANIFESTATIONS**
1. Mild	Shortened attention span, impaired mental abilities, mood changes, slight tremor, sleep disturbances
2. Moderate	Disorientation, forgetfulness, gross deficits in mental abilities, personality changes, inappropriate behavior, lethargy or apathy, tremor, slurred speech, staggering gait
3. Severe	Confusion, gross disorientation, amnesia, anxiety, agitation, odd behavior, somnolence to semi-stupor, incoherent speech, muscle rigidity
4. Coma	Unresponsive to verbal or physical stimuli

[a]Several systems are in use that grade the severity of hepatic encephalopathy; the stages shown here are adapted from the West Haven Grading System.

TABLE 19-4	Possible Causes of Malnutrition in Liver Disease
MECHANISM	**EXAMPLES**
Reduced nutrient intake	Abdominal discomfort, altered mental status, altered taste sensation, anorexia, dietary restrictions, early satiety (due to ascites), effects of medications (including GI disturbances and taste changes), fasting for medical procedures, fatigue, nausea, and vomiting
Malabsorption or nutrient losses	Diarrhea, effects of medications (including malabsorption and nutrient losses from diuretic use), fat malabsorption (due to reduced bile flow), GI bleeding, vomiting
Altered metabolism or increased nutrient needs	Hypermetabolism, impaired protein synthesis, infections or inflammation, muscle catabolism, reduced nutrient storage and metabolism in the liver, reduced synthesis of nutrient transport proteins

caused by a combination of factors (see Table 19-4). Patients may consume less food due to reduced appetite, GI symptoms, early satiety associated with ascites, or fatigue. If the diet is restricted in sodium (to treat ascites), foods may seem unpalatable. Reduced bile availability can result in fat malabsorption, which may lead to steatorrhea and deficiencies of the fat-soluble vitamins and some minerals. Additional nutrient losses may result from diarrhea, vomiting, and GI bleeding. If cirrhosis is a consequence of alcohol abuse, multiple nutrient deficiencies may be present.

Treatment of Cirrhosis

Medical treatment for cirrhosis aims to correct the underlying cause of disease and prevent or treat complications. Supportive care, including an appropriate diet and avoidance of liver toxins, promotes recovery and helps to prevent further damage. Abstinence from alcohol is critical for preserving remaining liver function and extending survival. Antiviral medications may be prescribed to treat viral infections. Patients should be screened and treated for life-threatening complications, such as gastroesophageal varices and liver cancer. A liver transplant may be necessary for patients with advanced cirrhosis.

Medications can effectively treat many of the complications that accompany cirrhosis. Individuals with portal hypertension and varices may be given beta-blockers such as propranolol (Inderal) and nadolol (Corgard), which reduce portal blood pressure and bleeding risk. Diuretics help to control portal hypertension and ascites; common examples include spironolactone (Aldactone) and furosemide (Lasix). Lactulose, a nonabsorbable disaccharide, treats hepatic encephalopathy by reducing ammonia production and absorption in the colon. The antibiotic rifaximin is an alternative treatment for elevated ammonia that works by altering bacterial populations. To stimulate the appetite and promote weight gain, megestrol acetate (Megace) or dronabinol (Marinol) may be prescribed. Box 19-6 lists potential nutritional problems associated with some of these medications.

Nutrition Therapy for Cirrhosis

Nutrition care for cirrhosis depends on the patient's general health, extent of liver damage, and accompanying complications. As common problems include protein-energy malnutrition and muscle wasting, a high-kcalorie, high-protein diet may be advised for maintaining nitrogen balance and body weight. Dietary substances that may cause additional liver injury should be avoided; examples include alcohol, some herbal supplements, and vitamin or mineral megadoses. If esophageal varices are present, a soft diet (which contains only moist, soft-textured foods; see Chapter 14) may be prescribed to reduce the risk of bleeding. Table 19-5 lists the general dietary guidelines for cirrhosis.

Box 19-6 Diet-Drug Interactions

Check this table for notable nutrition-related effects of the medications discussed in this chapter.

Appetite stimulants (megestrol acetate, dronabinol)	**Gastrointestinal effects:** Nausea, vomiting, diarrhea
	Dietary interaction: Dronabinol potentiates the effects of alcohol
	Metabolic effect: Hyperglycemia (megestrol acetate)
Diuretics (furosemide, spironolactone[a])	**Gastrointestinal effects:** Dry mouth, anorexia, decreased taste perception
	Dietary interactions: Furosemide's bioavailability is reduced when taken with food; licorice root may interfere with the effects of diuretics
	Metabolic effects: Fluid and electrolyte imbalances,[a] hyperglycemia, hyperlipidemias, thiamin deficiency (furosemide), elevated uric acid levels (furosemide)
Immunosuppressants (cyclosporine, tacrolimus)	**Gastrointestinal effects:** Nausea, vomiting, abdominal discomfort, diarrhea, constipation, anorexia
	Dietary interactions: Alcohol intake should be limited due to the potential for toxic effects; grapefruit juice can raise serum concentrations of these drugs to toxic levels; the bioavailability of tacrolimus is reduced when the drug is taken with food
	Metabolic effects: Electrolyte imbalances, hyperglycemia, hyperlipidemias, anemia, hypertension
Lactulose	**Gastrointestinal effects:** Nausea, vomiting, diarrhea, flatulence
	Dietary interactions: Calcium and magnesium supplements may reduce the effectiveness of lactulose
	Metabolic effects: Fluid and electrolyte imbalances

[a] *Furosemide* is a "potassium-wasting" diuretic; patients should increase intakes of potassium-rich foods. *Spironolactone* is a "potassium-sparing" diuretic; patients should avoid supplemental potassium and potassium-containing salt substitutes.

TABLE 19-5 Nutrition Therapy for Liver Cirrhosis

Energy	• Estimates of energy needs range from 25 to 40 kcal/kg body weight per day; patients with stable cirrhosis usually require 25 to 35 kcal/kg per day, whereas those with multiple complications or malnutrition may require 30 to 40 kcal/kg per day. • In patients with ascites, a value for "dry body weight" should be used for calculating nutrition needs. • Energy requirements may be higher in patients with hypermetabolism, catabolism, infection, malabsorption, or recent unintentional weight loss. Energy requirements may be lower in patients who would benefit from weight loss.
Meal frequency	• To improve food intake, patients should consume small meals and snacks four to six times daily. A bedtime snack may help to reduce muscle catabolism during the night.
Protein	• Estimates of protein needs range from 1.0 to 1.5 g of protein/kg dry body weight per day to maintain or improve nitrogen balance. • In patients with hepatic encephalopathy, the protein intake should be spread throughout the day; protein restriction is rarely recommended as it may worsen malnutrition.
Carbohydrate and fat	• Carbohydrate and fat recommendations are similar to those for the general population. • Persons with insulin resistance or diabetes should monitor carbohydrate intakes and consume a diet that maintains blood glucose control. • If fat is malabsorbed, patients should restrict fat to 30% of total kcalories or as necessary to control steatorrhea and use medium-chain triglycerides (MCT) to increase kcalories.
Sodium	• Patients should restrict sodium as necessary to control ascites; 2000 mg sodium per day is adequate restriction in most cases.
Vitamins and minerals	• Patients may require dietary supplements to obtain adequate amounts of vitamins and minerals.

Energy Estimates of energy needs range from 25 to 40 kcalories per kilogram of body weight per day; recommendations for patients with stable cirrhosis usually fall in the lower part of this range, whereas patients with malnutrition or multiple complications usually require higher intakes.[22] Requirements may be increased by hypermetabolism, catabolism, infection, nutrient malabsorption, or recent unintentional weight loss. In patients with ascites, a value for "dry body weight" should be used for calculating nutritional needs; this value can be obtained after diuretic therapy or after a medical procedure that directly removes excess abdominal fluid.

Many patients with cirrhosis have difficulty consuming enough food to achieve good nutrition status.[23] Some individuals may find four to six small meals and snacks easier to tolerate than three large meals each day. Oral supplements, including liquid formulas and energy bars, can help to improve energy intakes. Box 19-7 offers additional suggestions that can help a patient meet energy needs.

Protein Estimates of protein needs range from 1.0 to 1.5 grams of protein per kilogram of body weight per day based on dry weight or an appropriate weight for height (the protein RDA for healthy adults is 0.8 g/kg).[24] Protein requirements are higher in patients who are malnourished or have complications that promote muscle wasting, such as infection, GI bleeding, or severe ascites. In patients with hepatic encephalopathy, the protein intake should be spread throughout the day so that only modest amounts are consumed at each meal. Protein restriction is rarely recommended because an inadequate protein intake can worsen malnutrition and wasting.

Clinical studies have suggested that oral supplementation with branched-chain amino acids (BCAA) may improve neurological functioning in patients with hepatic

---

Box 19-7   *HOW TO* Help the Cirrhosis Patient Eat Enough Food

Individuals with cirrhosis often have difficulty consuming enough food to prevent malnutrition and its consequences. Ascites and GI symptoms such as nausea and vomiting may interfere with food intake. Fatigue may cause a lack of interest in food preparation. Sodium restrictions may make foods unpalatable. Measures that may improve food intake include the following:

- If nutrient restrictions are necessary, make sure the patient fully understands how to modify the diet so that food intake is not restricted unnecessarily. Provide lists of acceptable foods and menus. Explain how recipes can be altered so that favorite foods can still be incorporated into the diet.

- Suggest between-meal snacks during the day and a snack at bedtime. A liquid supplement like Boost or Ensure can substitute for a snack and requires no preparation. Snacks should not be consumed within two hours of meals because they may reduce appetite at mealtime.

- If the patient has little appetite or is quickly satiated, suggest foods that are higher in food energy, such as whole milk instead of reduced-fat milk or canned fruit that is packed in heavy syrup instead of fruit juice. Suggest that beverages be consumed separately from meals.

- Recommend energy boosters. Cream sauces and gravies can add kcalories to entrées. Fruit juices and fruit nectars can substitute for drinking water. The following additions can boost the energy content of meals:

  - Sour cream and butter—on vegetables and potatoes

  - Mayonnaise—in sandwiches and salads

- Half-and-half and light cream—in soups and on cereal

- Hard-cooked eggs—in casseroles and meat loaf

- Cheese—in salads and casseroles and melted on steamed vegetables

- Avocados—in sandwiches, tacos, and salads

- Peanut butter, nut butters, and cream cheese—on crackers or celery and in milkshakes

- Chopped nuts—in salads, cooked cereals, and bakery products

Sodium-restricted diets are recommended for treating ascites and other medical conditions, including kidney and heart disorders. Box 21-11 (p. 613) and Table 22-1 (p. 629) provide information about restricting dietary sodium. To improve the palatability of low-sodium meals:

- Suggest that patients replace salt with strong-flavored herbs and spices such as chili powder, coriander, cumin, curry powder, garlic, ginger, lemon, mint, and parsley.

- Advise patients to check food labels to learn the sodium content of packaged foods. Similar products may be available that are lower in sodium. (Persons using potassium-sparing diuretics should be cautioned to avoid salt substitutes that replace sodium with potassium.)

Offer support and encouragement to the patient with cirrhosis. Significant malnutrition is less likely to occur if dietary advice is provided before problems progress.

---

encephalopathy.[25] BCAA supplementation has also been associated with fewer disease complications and improved nutrition status in patients with cirrhosis.[26] Whether BCAA supplementation improves survival rates of cirrhosis patients, however, is still in question.

Carbohydrate and Fat Carbohydrate and fat recommendations for cirrhosis patients are similar to those for the general population. Many patients with cirrhosis are insulin resistant, however, and require medications or insulin to manage their hyperglycemia.[27] These individuals should follow the dietary guidelines for diabetes: monitor carbohydrate intakes and consume a diet that maintains blood glucose levels within a normal range (see Chapter 20). In addition, carbohydrate intakes should be fairly consistent from day to day for improved blood glucose control. In patients with fat malabsorption, fat intake may be restricted to less than 30 percent of total kcalories or as necessary to control steatorrhea; medium-chain triglycerides (MCT) can be used to provide additional energy. Severe steatorrhea warrants supplementation of the fat-soluble vitamins, calcium, magnesium, and zinc (see Chapter 18).

Sodium Restriction for Ascites Patients with ascites are generally advised to restrict sodium. Because ascites is partly caused by sodium and water retention in the kidneys, treatment usually includes both sodium restriction (to no more than 2000 milligrams of sodium per day) and diuretic therapy to promote fluid loss.[28] Potassium intake should be monitored if a potassium-wasting diuretic (such as furosemide) is used. Note that fluid restrictions are occasionally implemented when ascites is accompanied by severe **hyponatremia** (serum sodium less than about 125 milliequivalents per liter) but other methods of reducing the body's water volume are preferable.[29]

Many patients find low-sodium diets unpalatable, so some health practitioners may allow a more liberal sodium intake and depend on diuretics to remove excess fluid. If patients do not respond to sodium restriction and diuretic therapy, excess fluid may be removed from the abdomen by surgical puncture (**paracentesis**). To prevent recurrent ascites, a **transjugular intrahepatic portosystemic shunt** may be performed; this procedure relieves portal pressure (which contributes to the development of ascites) by creating a passage between the portal vein and the hepatic vein using a stent.

Vitamins and Minerals Vitamin and mineral deficiencies are common in patients with cirrhosis because of poor oral intakes, malabsorption, metabolic changes, or the alcohol abuse that may have induced liver disease. Therefore, vitamin/mineral supplementation is often necessary. If steatorrhea is present, fat-soluble nutrients can be provided in water-soluble forms. Patients with esophageal varices may find it easier to ingest supplements in liquid form.

Enteral and Parenteral Nutrition Support In hospitalized patients who are unable to consume enough food, tube feedings may be infused overnight as a supplement to oral intakes or may replace oral feedings entirely. Although standard formulas are often appropriate, an energy-dense formula (supplying at least 1.5 kcalories per milliliter) should be provided for patients with ascites.[30] In patients with esophageal varices, the feeding tube should be as narrow and flexible as possible to prevent rupture and bleeding. Parenteral nutrition support should be considered for patients who are unable to tolerate enteral feedings due to intestinal obstruction, GI bleeding, or uncontrollable vomiting. To avoid excessive fluid delivery, patients with ascites typically require concentrated parenteral solutions, which are infused into central veins.

The Case Study in Box 19-8 can help you apply your knowledge of cirrhosis to a clinical situation.

hyponatremia: abnormally low sodium levels in the blood; a possible result of fluid overload.

paracentesis (pah-rah-sen-TEE-sis): the surgical puncture of a body cavity with an aspirator to draw out excess fluid.

transjugular intrahepatic portosystemic shunt: a passage within the liver that connects a portion of the portal vein to the hepatic vein using a stent; access to the liver is gained via the jugular vein in the neck.

Box 19-8   **Case Study: Man with Cirrhosis**

Lenny Levitt, a 49-year-old carpenter, has just been diagnosed with cirrhosis, which is a consequence of his alcohol abuse over the past 25 years. Although he understands that he has an alcohol problem and recently entered an alcohol rehabilitation program, he is still drinking. At 5 feet 8 inches tall, Mr. Levitt, who formerly weighed 160 pounds, now weighs 130 pounds. According to family members, he is showing signs of mental deterioration, such as forgetfulness and an inability to concentrate. He is jaundiced and appears thin, although his abdomen is distended with ascites. Laboratory findings indicate elevated serum concentrations of AST, ALT, and ammonia; low albumin levels; and hyperglycemia.

1. Do Mr. Levitt's laboratory values suggest liver disease? Compare the results of his laboratory tests with the values shown in Table 19-2 (p. 550).

2. From the limited information available, evaluate Mr. Levitt's nutrition status. What medical problem makes it difficult to interpret his present weight? Describe the development of that type of problem in liver disease, and explain how the diet is usually adjusted for such a patient.

3. Estimate Mr. Levitt's energy and protein needs. Describe the general diet you might recommend for him. What suggestions do you have for increasing his energy intake?

4. Explain the significance of Mr. Levitt's elevated blood ammonia levels. What signs may indicate that he is undergoing mental decline?

5. Describe each of the following complications of liver disease: portal hypertension, jaundice, and gastroesophageal varices. What complication may result if the esophageal varices are not treated?

Review Notes

- Liver cirrhosis is characterized by extensive fibrosis and progressive liver dysfunction. The primary causes of cirrhosis in the United States are chronic hepatitis C infection and alcoholic liver disease.

- Symptoms of cirrhosis include fatigue, GI disturbances, anorexia, and weight loss; eventually, patients may bruise easily and be more susceptible to infections.

- Complications of cirrhosis include portal hypertension, gastroesophageal varices, ascites, hepatic encephalopathy, and malnutrition.

- Treatment of cirrhosis is highly individualized and depends on the accompanying symptoms and complications; both drug therapies and dietary adjustments are usually necessary. Many patients with cirrhosis need to consume a high-kcalorie, high-protein diet to prevent weight loss and wasting. Patients with ascites may be advised to restrict sodium.

19.3 Liver Transplantation

Acute or chronic liver disease can lead to liver failure, in which case liver transplantation is the only remaining treatment option. The most common illnesses that precede liver transplants are chronic hepatitis C infection and alcoholic liver disease, which account for about 50 percent of liver transplant cases.[31] Five-year survival rates among transplant recipients may be as high as 85 to 90 percent, depending on the cause of illness.[32] Complications such as ascites and hepatic encephalopathy worsen the prognosis.

Nutrition Status of Transplant Patients As mentioned earlier, advanced liver disease is usually associated with malnutrition, which can increase the risk of complications following a liver transplant. Evaluating nutrition status in transplant candidates can be difficult, however, because liver dysfunction and malnutrition often have similar metabolic effects. In addition, the presence of edema or ascites can alter anthropometric values and mask weight loss. Correcting malnutrition prior to transplant surgery can help to speed recovery after the surgery.[33]

Posttransplant Concerns The concerns immediately following a transplant are organ rejection and infection. Immunosuppressive drugs, including prednisone, cyclosporine, and tacrolimus, help to reduce the immune responses that cause rejection, but they also raise the risk of infection. Infections are a potential cause of death following a liver transplant; therefore, antibiotics and antiviral medications are prescribed to reduce infection risk.

Immunosuppressive drugs can affect nutrition status in numerous ways (see Box 19-9 and review Box 19-6). Gastrointestinal side effects include nausea, vomiting, diarrhea, abdominal pain, and mouth sores. Some medications may alter appetite and taste perception. Some of the drugs may cause hyperglycemia or outright diabetes, which may need to be controlled with insulin. Electrolyte and fluid imbalances are common. Other possible effects include hypertension, hyperlipidemias, kidney toxicity, protein catabolism, and increased osteoporosis risk.[34]

The stress associated with transplant surgery increases protein and energy requirements. High-kcalorie, high-protein snacks and oral supplements can help the transplant patient meet postsurgical needs. Vitamin and mineral supplementation is also an integral part of nutrition care. To help transplant patients avoid developing foodborne illnesses, health practitioners should provide information about food safety measures, such as cooking foods adequately, washing fresh produce, and avoiding foods that may be contaminated. Nutrition in Practice 2 provides additional information about food safety.

BOX 19-9 *Nursing Diagnosis*

Nursing diagnoses for people with liver transplants may include *ineffective protection*, *risk for infection*, and *imbalanced nutrition: less than body requirements*.

Review Notes

- Liver transplantation has improved the long-term outlook for patients with advanced liver disease. Transplant patients are typically malnourished, however, and may have medical problems that affect transplant success.
- Immunosuppressive drugs are prescribed after an organ transplant to avoid the potential for organ rejection. Use of these drugs increases the risk of infection, and the drugs have side effects that can impair nutrition status and general health.

Nutrition Assessment Checklist for People with Liver Disorders

MEDICAL HISTORY

Check the medical record to determine:

- ○ Type of liver disorder
- ○ Cause of the liver disorder
- ○ Whether the patient has received a liver transplant

Review the medical record for complications that may alter nutritional needs, including:

- ○ Abdominal pain
- ○ Anemia
- ○ Ascites
- ○ Esophageal varices
- ○ Hepatic encephalopathy
- ○ Impaired kidney or lung function
- ○ Infections
- ○ Insulin resistance or diabetes mellitus
- ○ Malabsorption
- ○ Malnutrition
- ○ Pancreatitis

MEDICATIONS

In patients with liver dysfunction, the risk of diet-drug interactions is high because most drugs are metabolized in the liver. The risk of interactions is intensified for patients with:

- ○ Ascites (medications may take a long time to reach the liver)
- ○ Renal failure (medications often undergo further metabolism in the kidneys and are excreted in the urine)
- ○ Malnutrition
- ○ Multiple prescriptions
- ○ Long-term medication use

DIETARY INTAKE

In patients with fatty liver, pay special attention to:

- ○ Energy intake, if the patient is overweight or malnourished, has diabetes, or is receiving total parenteral nutrition
- ○ Carbohydrate intake, if the patient has diabetes or is receiving total parenteral nutrition
- ○ Alcohol abuse

In patients with hepatitis, cirrhosis, or ascites:
- ○ Check appetite.
- ○ Ensure that energy and nutrient intakes are appropriate.
- ○ Determine whether alcohol is being consumed.
- ○ Determine whether sodium restriction is warranted.
- ○ Base energy intakes on desirable weight or an estimated dry weight to avoid overfeeding.

ANTHROPOMETRIC DATA

Take baseline height and weight measurements, and monitor weight regularly. In patients with ascites and edema:

- ○ Monitor weight changes to evaluate the degree of fluid retention.
- ○ Remember that the patient may be malnourished, and weight may be deceptively high.

LABORATORY TESTS

Note that albumin and serum proteins are often reduced in people with liver disease and are not appropriate indicators of nutrition status. Review the following laboratory test results to assess liver function:

- ○ Albumin
- ○ Alkaline phosphatase
- ○ ALT and AST
- ○ Ammonia
- ○ Bilirubin
- ○ Gamma-glutamyl transpeptidase
- ○ Prothrombin time

Check laboratory test results for complications associated with liver failure, including:

- ○ Anemia
- ○ Decreased renal function
- ○ Fluid retention
- ○ Hyperglycemia

PHYSICAL SIGNS

Look for physical signs of:

- ○ Fluid retention (ascites and edema)
- ○ Protein-energy malnutrition (muscle wasting and unintentional weight loss)
- ○ Nutrient deficiencies

Self Check

1. In cases of fatty liver that are unrelated to excessive alcohol intakes, the primary risk factor is:
   a. following a high-protein diet.
   b. use of illicit drugs.
   c. following a high-fat diet.
   d. insulin resistance.

2. Which of the following statements about hepatitis is true?
   a. Chronic hepatitis can progress to cirrhosis.
   b. Whatever the cause of hepatitis, symptoms are typically severe.
   c. Vaccines are available to protect against hepatitis A, B, and C viruses.
   d. HCV infection can be spread through contaminated foods and water.

3. Which blood test values often indicate the presence of liver disease?
   a. Increased albumin levels
   b. Increased liver enzyme levels
   c. Decreased bilirubin levels
   d. Decreased alkaline phosphatase levels

4. Esophageal varices are a dangerous complication of liver disease primarily because they:
   a. interfere with food intake.
   b. divert blood flow from the GI tract.
   c. can lead to massive bleeding.
   d. contribute to hepatic encephalopathy.

5. A complication of cirrhosis that contributes to the development of ascites is:
   a. portal hypertension.
   b. insulin resistance.
   c. elevated serum albumin levels.
   d. bile obstruction.

6. Lactulose, a nonabsorbable disaccharide, is generally prescribed to patients who develop which complication of cirrhosis?
   a. Portal hypertension
   b. Hepatic encephalopathy
   c. Bile insufficiency
   d. Ascites

7. With respect to protein intake, patients with hepatic encephalopathy should:
   a. consume a high-protein diet.
   b. restrict protein intake to avoid elevations in serum ammonia.
   c. spread protein intake evenly throughout the day.
   d. use formulas enriched with aromatic amino acids to meet their protein needs.

8. People with ascites must often restrict dietary intake of:
   a. fat.
   b. protein.
   c. sugars.
   d. sodium.

9. After a liver transplant, the major health concern is:
   a. jaundice.
   b. bile insufficiency.
   c. infection.
   d. hepatic coma.

10. Dietary concerns after a liver transplant include all of the following *except*:
    a. severe protein restrictions that are difficult to adhere to.
    b. increased risk of foodborne illness.
    c. gastrointestinal side effects of medications.
    d. altered appetite and taste perception from medications.

Answers: 1. d, 2. a, 3. b, 4. c, 5. a, 6. b, 7. c, 8. d, 9. c, 10. a

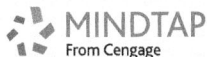

For more chapter resources visit **www.cengage.com** to access MindTap, a complete digital course.

Clinical Applications

1. Vijaya Reddy is a college student who visited relatives near her parents' birthplace in Anantapur, India, during summer vacation. Although her relatives provided boiled or purified water at their home, they occasionally took Vijaya to local restaurants, where she drank tap water. Several weeks after Vijaya returned home, she developed flu-like symptoms and started feeling extremely tired. She also experienced upper abdominal pain and felt nauseated after meals. After her roommate told her that her eyes and skin appeared yellow, she knew something was definitely wrong. A physician at the student health center diagnosed hepatitis.

   • Which type of hepatitis did Vijaya most likely have?
   • What additional symptoms may develop? Is Vijaya's condition likely to become chronic?
   • What medical treatment is suggested for Vijaya's condition? Describe the dietary modifications that may be necessary in some cases.

2. As discussed in the section on cirrhosis, many patients develop protein-energy malnutrition and wasting during the course of illness. Review Table 19-4 on p. 552 to find examples of problems that may lead to malnutrition. Select three nutrition or medical problems (from the "Examples" column), and discuss the complications of liver disease that may cause the problems you selected. What dietary or medical treatments can help in managing these problems?

Notes

1. D. M. Torres and S. A. Harrison, Nonalcoholic fatty liver disease, in M. Feldman and coeditors, *Sleisenger and Fordtran's Gastrointestinal and Liver Disease* (Philadelphia: Saunders, 2016), pp. 1428–1441.

2. Z. M. Younossi and coauthors, Global epidemiology of nonalcoholic fatty liver disease—Meta-analytic assessment of prevalence, incidence, and outcomes, *Hepatology* 64 (2016): 73–84; R. L. Carithers, Jr., and C. J. McClain, Alcoholic liver disease, in M. Feldman and coeditors, *Sleisenger and Fordtran's Gastrointestinal and Liver Disease* (Philadelphia: Saunders, 2016), pp. 1409–1427.

3. N. Chalasani and coauthors, Diagnosis and management of nonalcoholic fatty liver disease: Practice guideline from the American Association for the Study of Liver Diseases, *Hepatology* 142 (2017), doi: 10.1002/hep.29367.

4. Chalasani and coauthors, 2017; D. E. Cohen and F. A. Anania, Nonalcoholic fatty liver disease, in N. J. Greenberger, ed., *Current Diagnosis and Treatment: Gastroenterology, Hepatology, and Endoscopy* (New York: McGraw-Hill, 2016), pp. 536–542.

5. J. M. Kneeman, J. Misdraji, and K. E. Corey, Secondary causes of nonalcoholic fatty liver disease, *Therapeutic Advances in Gastroenterology* 5 (2012): 199–207.

6. C. Bunchorntavakul and K. R. Reddy, Review article: Herbal and dietary supplement hepatotoxicity, *Alimentary Pharmacology and Therapeutics* 37 (2013): 3–17.

7. Centers for Disease Control and Prevention, *Viral Hepatitis Surveillance: United States, 2015* (Atlanta: U.S. Department of Health and Human Services, 2017).

8. A. Rutherford and J. L. Dienstag, Viral hepatitis, in N. J. Greenberger, ed., *Current Diagnosis and Treatment: Gastroenterology, Hepatology, and Endoscopy* (New York: McGraw-Hill, 2016), pp. 480–507.

9. Centers for Disease Control and Prevention, 2017.

10. Rutherford and Dienstag, 2016.

11. S. Safrin, Antiviral agents, in B. G. Katzung, ed., *Basic and Clinical Pharmacology* (New York: McGraw-Hill, 2015), pp. 835–864.

12. Academy of Nutrition and Dietetics, *Nutrition Care Manual* (Chicago: Academy of Nutrition and Dietetics, 2018).

13. N. D. Grace and M. A. Minor, Portal hypertension and esophageal variceal hemorrhage, in N. J. Greenberger, ed., *Current Diagnosis and Treatment: Gastroenterology, Hepatology, and Endoscopy* (New York: McGraw-Hill, 2016), pp. 562–573.

14. G. Garcia-Tsao, Cirrhosis and its sequelae, in L. Goldman and A. I. Schafer, eds., *Goldman-Cecil Medicine* (Philadelphia: Saunders, 2016), pp. 1023–1031.

15. V. H. Shah and P. S. Kamath, Portal hypertension and variceal bleeding, in M. Feldman and coeditors, *Sleisenger and Fordtran's Gastrointestinal and Liver Disease* (Philadelphia: Saunders, 2016), pp. 1524–1552.

16. N. J. Greenberger, Ascites and spontaneous bacterial peritonitis, in N. J. Greenberger, ed., *Current Diagnosis and Treatment: Gastroenterology, Hepatology, and Endoscopy* (New York: McGraw-Hill, 2016), pp. 549–556.

17. N. D. Theise, Liver and gallbladder, in V. Kumar and coeditors, *Robbins and Cotran Pathologic Basis of Disease* (Philadelphia: Saunders, 2015), pp. 821–881.

18. N. J. Greenberger, Portal systemic encephalopathy and hepatic encephalopathy, in N. J. Greenberger, ed., *Current Diagnosis and Treatment: Gastroenterology, Hepatology, and Endoscopy* (New York: McGraw-Hill, 2016), pp. 543–548.

19. K. Tajiri and Y. Shimizu, Branched-chain amino acids in liver diseases, *World Journal of Gastroenterology* 19 (2013): 7620–7629.

20. Greenberger, Portal systemic encephalopathy and hepatic encephalopathy, 2016.

21. J. Krenitsky, Nutrition update in hepatic failure, *Practical Gastroenterology* (April 2014): 47–55.

22. M. Albeldawi, P. Hipskind, and D. J. Chiang, Nutrition for the critically ill patient with hepatic failure, in G. A. Cresci, ed., *Nutrition for the Critically Ill Patient* (Boca Raton, FL: CRC Press, 2015), pp. 497–509; T. M. Johnson and coauthors, Nutrition assessment and management in advanced liver disease, *Nutrition in Clinical Practice* 28 (2013): 15–29.

23. Krenitsky, 2014.

24. Albeldawi, Hipskind, and Chiang, 2015; Johnson and coauthors, 2013.

25. L. R. Anastácio and M. I. T. D. Correia, Nutrition therapy: Integral part of liver transplant care, *World Journal of Gastroenterology* 22 (2016): 1513–1522.

26. Anastácio and Correia, 2016; P. Amodio and coauthors, Nutritional management of hepatic encephalopathy in patients with cirrhosis: International Society for Hepatic Encephalopathy and Nitrogen Metabolism consensus, *Hepatology* 58 (2013): 325–336.

27. L. Elkrief and coauthors, Diabetes mellitus in patients with cirrhosis: Clinical implications and management, *Liver International* 36 (2016): 936–948.

28. B. A. Runyon, Ascites and spontaneous bacterial peritonitis, in M. Feldman and coeditors, *Sleisenger and Fordtran's Gastrointestinal and Liver Disease* (Philadelphia: Saunders, 2016), pp. 1553–1576.

29. Johnson and coauthors, 2013; B. A. Runyon, Management of adult patients with ascites due to cirrhosis: Update 2012, *Hepatology* 57 (2013): 1651–1653.

30. Johnson and coauthors, 2013.

31. G. T. Everson, Hepatic failure and liver transplantation, in L. Goldman and A. I. Schafer, eds., *Goldman-Cecil Medicine* (Philadelphia: Saunders, 2016), pp. 1031–1038.

32. A. A. Qamar, Liver transplantation, in N. J. Greenberger, ed., *Current Diagnosis and Treatment: Gastroenterology, Hepatology, and Endoscopy* (New York: McGraw-Hill, 2016), pp. 593–604.

33. A. F. Carrion and P. Martin, Liver transplantation, M. Feldman and coeditors, *Sleisenger and Fordtran's Gastrointestinal and Liver Disease* (Philadelphia: Saunders, 2016), pp. 1628–1646.

34. Qamar, 2016.

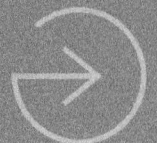

19.4 Nutrition in Practice

Alcohol in Health and Disease

As Chapter 19 described, excessive alcohol consumption is a primary cause of liver disease. Alcohol can be toxic to other organs as well, including the brain, gastrointestinal (GI) tract, and pancreas. In addition, **alcohol abuse** can lead to a number of nutrient deficiencies. Moderate use of alcohol, however, has been associated with some health benefits, such as lower heart disease risk in middle-aged and older adults. This Nutrition in Practice discusses current recommendations concerning alcohol and the health problems and benefits associated with its use. The Glossary in Box NP19-1 defines the relevant terms.

What are the current guidelines for alcohol consumption?

For those who choose to drink alcoholic beverages, the *Dietary Guidelines for Americans* recommend that women and men limit their daily intakes of alcohol to one drink and two drinks per day, respectively. In addition, women should avoid consuming more than three drinks in a single day, whereas men should consume no more than four drinks in one day.[1] One **drink** is defined as 12 ounces of beer, 5 ounces of wine, 10 ounces of wine cooler, or 1½ ounces of 80-proof distilled spirits such as gin, rum, vodka, and whiskey (see Photo NP19-1). Some people should not consume alcohol at all, such as pregnant women, individuals younger than the legal drinking age, individuals who are unable to control their alcohol intake, people using medications that can interact with alcohol, and individuals with certain medical conditions. Alcohol should also be avoided by anyone who is involved in an activity that requires attention or coordination, such as driving or operating machinery.

Photo NP19-1

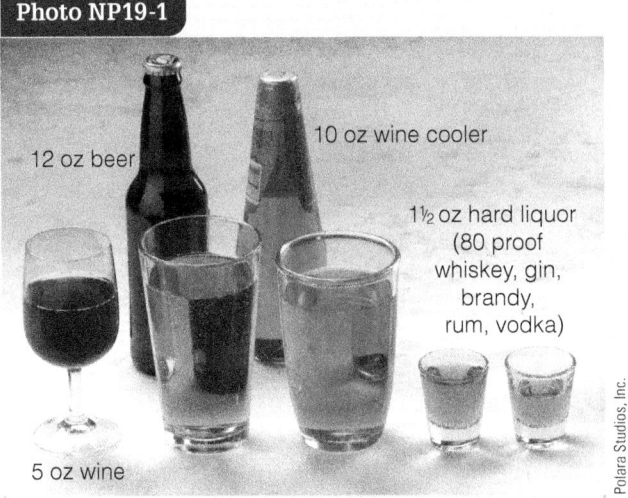

12 oz beer

10 oz wine cooler

1½ oz hard liquor (80 proof whiskey, gin, brandy, rum, vodka)

5 oz wine

Polara Studios, Inc.

Each of the amounts shown is equivalent to one drink.

About 73 percent of adults in the United States drink alcoholic beverages regularly.[2] The prevalence of alcohol abuse is estimated to be between 7.4 and 9.7 percent in the general population.[3]

What happens to alcohol in the body?

Recall that alcohol is a source of food energy, providing 7 kcalories per gram. Although a small amount of alcohol is metabolized in the stomach, most of the alcohol consumed is quickly absorbed in the stomach or small intestine and passes readily into the body's cells, where alcohol concentrations reach levels similar to those in the blood. The liver is the site of most alcohol metabolism,

---

Box NP19-1 Glossary

acetaldehyde (ah-set-AL-deh-hide): an intermediate in alcohol metabolism that, in excess, can damage the body's tissues and interfere with cellular functions.
acetate (AH-seh-tate): the product of alcohol metabolism that is used as a source of energy by many tissues in the body.
alcohol abuse: the continued use of alcohol despite the development of health, psychological, social, or legal problems; also known as *alcohol misuse or alcohol use disorder.*

alcoholic liver disease: liver disease that is related to excessive alcohol consumption. Disorders that may develop include fatty liver, hepatitis, and cirrhosis, which may lead to liver failure.
drink: an alcoholic beverage that contains about half an ounce of pure alcohol. One drink is equivalent to 12 ounces of beer, 5 ounces of wine, 10 ounces of wine cooler, or 1½ ounces of 80-proof distilled spirits.

although its ability to metabolize alcohol is somewhat limited: the average adult metabolizes only 7 to 10 grams of alcohol per hour, about the amount in one drink.[4] The main product of alcohol metabolism is **acetate**, which can be used as a source of energy by most tissues.

Because there is no storage pool for alcohol and it can be toxic to cells, the metabolism of alcohol in the liver takes priority over that of other substances. Thus, alcohol suppresses the breakdown of fat for energy, leading to fat accumulation in the liver and the increased release of triglyceride-carrying lipoproteins (very-low-density lipoproteins, or VLDL). An excessive alcohol intake inhibits both the storage of glycogen and the liver's production of glucose between meals. Heavy drinkers are at risk of developing hypoglycemia, an effect that is accentuated in people with diabetes who use insulin or medications to reduce glucose levels. Alcohol ingestion can also impair the synthesis and secretion of a number of liver proteins, including albumin and fibrinogen (a blood-clotting protein).

How is alcohol toxic to cells?

Alcohol can damage cells either directly, or indirectly via the metabolite **acetaldehyde** that is created during alcohol metabolism. High alcohol concentrations change the structure of cell membranes, increasing membrane permeability. Cell membrane proteins may become damaged, interfering with the transport of substances across the membrane. The presence of alcohol also activates inflammatory responses in cells, which can eventually lead to cell death and tissue damage. Acetaldehyde can cause numerous adverse effects: it binds to other molecules and interferes with their functions, alters immune responses, causes oxidative damage, inhibits DNA repair, and prevents the formation of microtubules within cells.

How does alcohol affect brain function?

Alcohol acts as a central nervous system depressant. It can cause sedation, slow reaction times, and relieve anxiety. In excess, it impairs judgment, reduces inhibitions, and impairs speech and motor functions. Extremely high blood alcohol levels can lead to coma, respiratory depression, and death.

Chronic heavy drinking can cause certain types of neurological damage. The most common abnormality is injury to the peripheral nerves, which is evidenced by tingling in the hands and feet, lack of muscular coordination, and changes in a person's manner of walking. Visual impairments, such as blurred vision and optic nerve degeneration, can also occur.

Chronic drinkers who are forced to discontinue their use of alcohol may experience withdrawal symptoms, which include anxiety, irritability, and palpitations. In severe cases, symptoms may include nausea and vomiting, delirium, and seizures.

What are some other long-term consequences of drinking too much alcohol?

Alcoholic liver disease is the most common complication of alcohol abuse, occurring in about 15 to 30 percent of chronic heavy drinkers.[5] The disease develops in a manner similar to the disease progression described in Chapter 19: fatty liver, hepatitis, and, eventually, cirrhosis and liver failure. In addition to liver damage, alcohol can cause damage to the GI tract, pancreas, and heart (see Figure NP19-1). In the GI tract, alcohol's eventual effects may include gastritis, ulcers, nutrient malabsorption, diarrhea, and GI cancers. Chronic alcohol ingestion frequently injures pancreatic tissue and may lead to chronic pancreatitis. Heavy drinking is also associated with heart arrhythmias, impaired heart muscle contractility, and hypertension.

What are the effects of excessive alcohol consumption on nutrition status?

An excessive alcohol intake can cause multiple nutrient deficiencies. Because alcohol supplies 7 kcalories per gram, it displaces other energy sources along with the essential nutrients such foods would provide. As mentioned earlier, alcohol consumption can cause nutrient malabsorption as a result of direct damage to the GI mucosa. Alcohol also interferes with the way the body processes nutrients. Examples of common deficiencies in persons who abuse alcohol include:[6]

- *Vitamin A.* Alcohol and vitamin A are metabolized by similar enzymes, so heavy drinking—which induces the enzymes that break down alcohol—increases the degradation of vitamin A.
- *Thiamin.* Alcohol abuse is the most common cause of thiamin deficiency in the United States. Heavy drinking is associated with low thiamin intakes, and alcohol ingestion dramatically reduces thiamin absorption.
- *Folate.* Alcohol reduces the absorption of folate in the small intestine and increases folate degradation. Because folate has a central role in cell division (and cells of the GI tract are rapidly dividing cells), folate deficiency contributes to the malabsorption of other nutrients as well.

Can alcohol have disruptive effects on the metabolism of medications?

Yes. Alcohol consumption activates enzymes that metabolize certain drugs, so alcohol ingestion can alter drug metabolism. For example, the consumption of several drinks daily activates enzymes that convert acetaminophen (Tylenol) to chemicals that are toxic to the liver; thus, alcohol drinkers should avoid combining alcohol and acetaminophen. In contrast, impaired drug metabolism is likely

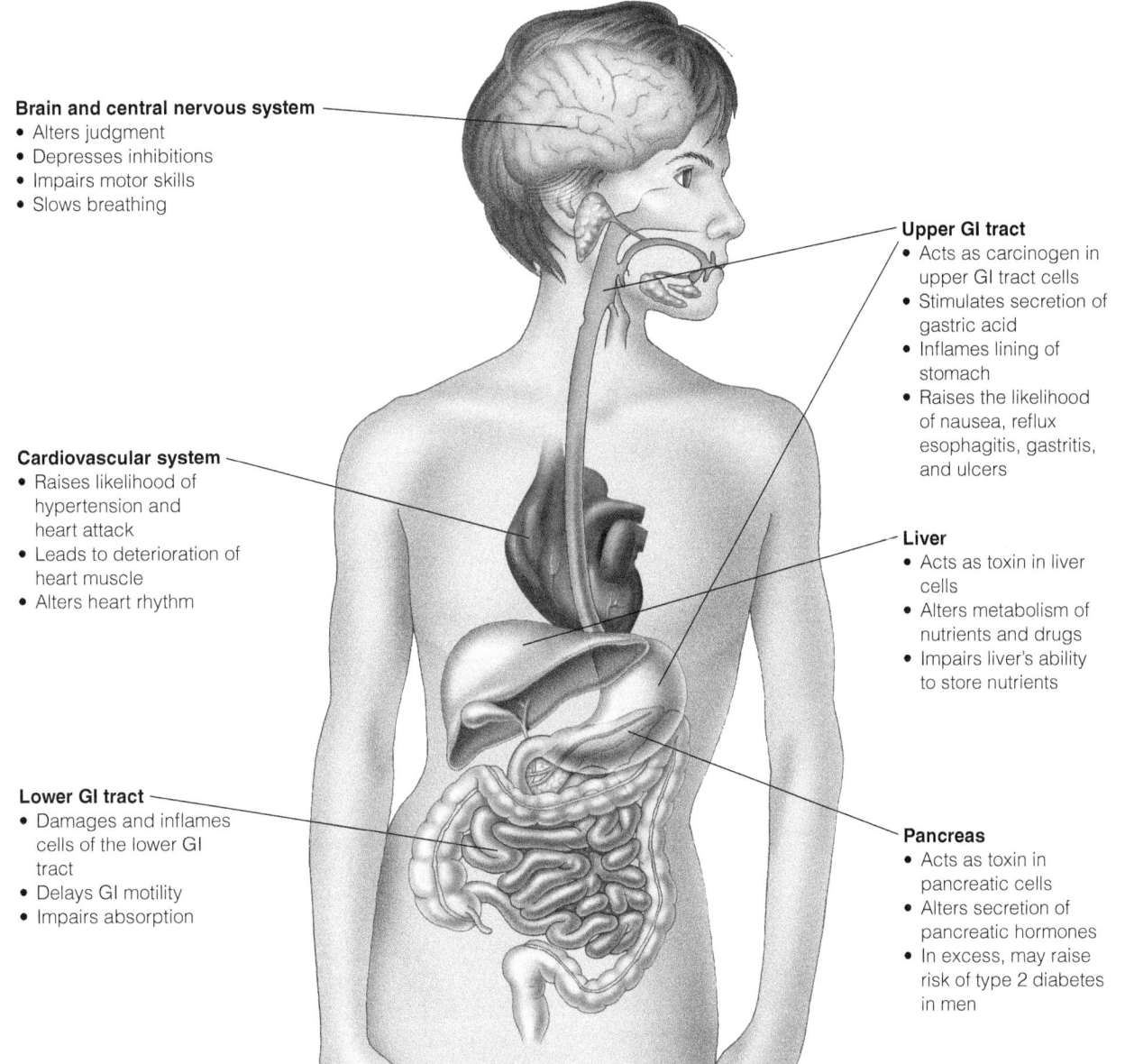

Brain and central nervous system
- Alters judgment
- Depresses inhibitions
- Impairs motor skills
- Slows breathing

Upper GI tract
- Acts as carcinogen in upper GI tract cells
- Stimulates secretion of gastric acid
- Inflames lining of stomach
- Raises the likelihood of nausea, reflux esophagitis, gastritis, and ulcers

Cardiovascular system
- Raises likelihood of hypertension and heart attack
- Leads to deterioration of heart muscle
- Alters heart rhythm

Liver
- Acts as toxin in liver cells
- Alters metabolism of nutrients and drugs
- Impairs liver's ability to store nutrients

Lower GI tract
- Damages and inflames cells of the lower GI tract
- Delays GI motility
- Impairs absorption

Pancreas
- Acts as toxin in pancreatic cells
- Alters secretion of pancreatic hormones
- In excess, may raise risk of type 2 diabetes in men

when the drugs and alcohol require similar enzymes for their metabolism. As an example, when alcohol is ingested at the same time that some sedative drugs are taken, drug metabolism is delayed until the alcohol is degraded, prolonging the drugs' effects.[7]

Does alcohol consumption have any beneficial effects on health?

Yes. Epidemiological studies in Western countries have consistently shown that a moderate alcohol intake reduces total mortality among middle-aged and older men and women. In addition, researchers have learned that moderate alcohol drinking can help reduce risks of developing the following chronic diseases:[8]

- *Heart disease.* Individuals with a light to moderate intake of alcohol—from beer, wine, or liquor—have a lower risk of heart disease than nondrinkers. Alcohol helps to protect against the development of atherosclerosis, increases levels of high-density lipoproteins (HDLs), and reduces the tendency for blood clotting. Its protective effects are seen mainly in older persons who have one or more classic risk factors for heart disease.

- *Stroke.* Moderate alcohol consumption may reduce the risk of stroke, especially ischemic stroke (caused by blood clotting in arteries that supply blood to the brain). Conversely, heavy drinking increases the risk of all forms of stroke.
- *Diabetes.* The risk of type 2 diabetes may be lower in moderate drinkers than in individuals who abstain from alcohol. In addition, some studies have found that a moderate alcohol intake may improve insulin sensitivity and reduce fasting glucose concentrations.

Note that unlike other recommendations for disease prevention, medical personnel rarely recommend that a nondrinker begin drinking to reduce disease risk, due to the potential for addiction and the adverse effects caused by excessive intakes.

Notes

1. P. D. Friedmann, Alcohol use in adults, *New England Journal of Medicine* 368 (2013): 365–373; P. M. Guenther, E. L. Ding, and E. B. Rimm, Alcoholic beverage consumption by adults compared to dietary guidelines: Results of the National Health and Nutrition Examination Survey, 2009–2010; *Journal of the Academy of Nutrition and Dietetics* 113 (2013): 546–550.
2. B. F. Grant and coauthors, Prevalence of 12-month alcohol use, high-risk drinking, and DSM-IV alcohol use disorder in the United States, 2001–2002 to 2012–2013, *JAMA Psychiatry* 74 (2017): 911–923.
3. P. G. O'Connor, Alcohol use disorders, in L. Goldman and A. I. Schafer, eds., *Goldman-Cecil Medicine* (Philadelphia: Saunders, 2016), pp. 149–156.
4. S. B. Masters and A. J. Trevor, The alcohols, in B. G. Katzung, ed., *Basic and Clinical Pharmacology* (New York: McGraw-Hill, 2015), pp. 384–395.
5. Masters and Trevor, 2015.
6. P. M. Suter, Alcohol: Its role in nutrition and health, in J. W. Erdman, I. A. Macdonald, and S. H. Zeisel, eds., *Present Knowledge in Nutrition* (Ames, IA: Wiley-Blackwell, 2012): pp. 912–938.
7. Masters and Trevor, 2015.
8. K. D. Shield, C. Parry, and J. Rehm, Chronic diseases and conditions related to alcohol use, *Alcohol Research: Current Reviews* 35, No. 2 (2013): 155–171.

Nutrition and Diabetes Mellitus

Chapter Sections and Learning Objectives (LOs)

20.1 Overview of Diabetes Mellitus

LO 20.1 Characterize type 1 and type 2 diabetes and discuss the complications associated with these conditions.

20.2 Treatment of Diabetes Mellitus

LO 20.2 Explain how diabetes can be managed using dietary adjustments, medications, and physical activity.

20.3 Diabetes Management in Pregnancy

LO 20.3 Describe the possible effects of diabetes on pregnancy outcomes and the approaches used to maintain glycemic control in pregnant women with diabetes.

20.4 Nutrition in Practice: Metabolic Syndrome

LO 20.4 Identify the features and possible consequences of the metabolic syndrome and describe the current treatment approaches for this condition.

chapter
20

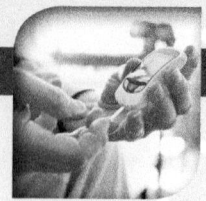

United States and many other countries. It now affects an estimated 12.2 percent of adults aged 18 and older in the United States, or about 30 million people.[1] About 24 percent of persons with diabetes are unaware that they have it,[2] a danger because its damaging effects often occur before symptoms develop. Diabetes ranks seventh among the leading causes of death in the United States. It also contributes to the development of other life-threatening diseases, including heart disease and kidney failure, which are discussed in the two chapters that follow.

diabetes (DYE-ah-BEE-teez) **mellitus:** a group of metabolic disorders characterized by hyperglycemia and disordered insulin metabolism.

diabetes = siphon (in Greek), referring to the excessive passage of urine that is characteristic of untreated diabetes

mellitus = sweet, honeylike

insulin: a pancreatic hormone that regulates glucose metabolism; its actions are countered mainly by the hormone *glucagon*.

renal threshold: the blood concentration of a substance that exceeds the kidneys' capacity for reabsorption, causing the substance to be passed into the urine.

20.1 Overview of Diabetes Mellitus

The term **diabetes mellitus** refers to metabolic disorders characterized by elevated blood glucose concentrations and disordered **insulin** metabolism. People with diabetes may be unable to produce sufficient insulin or use insulin effectively, or they may have both types of abnormalities. These impairments result in defective glucose uptake and utilization in muscle and adipose cells and unrestrained glucose production in the liver. The result is **hyperglycemia**, a marked elevation in blood glucose levels that can ultimately cause damage to blood vessels, nerves, and tissues. Box 20-1 defines diabetes-related symptoms and complications.

Symptoms of Diabetes Mellitus

Symptoms of diabetes are usually related to the degree of hyperglycemia present (see Table 20-1 and Box 20-2). When the plasma glucose concentration rises above about 200 milligrams per deciliter (mg/dL), it exceeds the **renal threshold**, the concentration

---

Box 20-1   Glossary of Diabetes-Related Symptoms and Complications

acetone breath: a distinctive fruity odor on the breath of a person with ketosis.

albuminuria: the presence of albumin (a blood protein) in the urine, a sign of diabetic nephropathy.

claudication (CLAW-dih-KAY-shun): pain in the legs while walking; usually due to an inadequate supply of blood to muscles.

diabetic coma: a coma that occurs in uncontrolled diabetes; may be due to diabetic ketoacidosis, the hyperosmolar hyperglycemic syndrome, or severe hypoglycemia. Diabetic coma was a frequent cause of death before insulin was routinely used to manage diabetes.

diabetic nephropathy (neh-FRAH-pah-thee): kidney damage that results from long-term diabetes.

diabetic neuropathy (nur-RAH-pah-thee): nerve damage that results from long-term diabetes.

diabetic retinopathy (REH-tih-NAH-pah-thee): retinal damage that results from long-term diabetes.

gangrene: death of tissue due to a deficient blood supply and/or infection.

gastroparesis (GAS-troe-pah-REE-sis): delayed stomach emptying, often caused by nerve damage in a person with diabetes.

glycosuria (GLY-co-SOOR-ee-ah): the presence of glucose in the urine.

hyperglycemia: elevated blood glucose concentrations. Normal fasting plasma glucose levels are less than 100 mg/dL. Fasting

plasma glucose levels between 100 and 125 mg/dL suggest prediabetes; values of 126 mg/dL and above suggest diabetes.

hyperosmolar hyperglycemic syndrome: a condition of extreme hyperglycemia associated with dehydration, hyperosmolar blood, and altered mental status; sometimes called the *hyperosmolar hyperglycemic nonketotic state*.

hypoglycemia: abnormally low blood glucose concentrations. In diabetes, hypoglycemia is treated when plasma glucose falls below 70 mg/dL.

ketoacidosis (KEY-toe-ass-ih-DOE-sis): an acidosis (lowering of blood pH) that results from the excessive production of ketone bodies.

ketonuria (KEY-toe-NOOR-ee-ah): the presence of ketone bodies in the urine.

ketosis (key-TOE-sis): elevated levels of ketone bodies in body tissues.

macrovascular complications: disorders that affect large blood vessels, including the coronary arteries and arteries of the limbs.

microvascular complications: disorders that affect small blood vessels, including those in the retina and kidneys.

peripheral vascular disease: a condition characterized by impaired blood circulation in the limbs.

polydipsia (POL-ee-DIP-see-ah): excessive thirst.

polyphagia (POL-ee-FAY-jee-ah): excessive hunger or food intake.

polyuria (POL-ee-YOOR-ree-ah): excessive urine production.

---

at which the kidneys begin to pass glucose into the urine (**glycosuria**). The presence of glucose in the urine draws additional water from the blood, increasing the amount of urine produced. Thus, the symptoms that arise in diabetes may include excessive urine production (**polyuria**), dehydration, and excessive thirst (**polydipsia**). Some people lose weight and have excessive hunger (**polyphagia**) as a result of the nutrient depletion that occurs when insulin is deficient. Another potential consequence of hyperglycemia is blurred vision, caused by the exposure of eye tissues to **hyperosmolar** fluids. Increased infections are common in individuals with diabetes and may be due to weakened immune responses and impaired circulation. In some cases, constant fatigue is the only symptom and may be related to altered energy metabolism, dehydration, or other effects of the disease.

Diagnosis of Diabetes Mellitus

The diagnosis of diabetes is based primarily on plasma glucose levels, which can be measured under fasting conditions or at random times during the day. In some cases, an **oral glucose tolerance test** is given: the individual ingests a 75-gram glucose load, and plasma glucose is measured at one or more time intervals following glucose ingestion. **Glycated hemoglobin (HbA$_{1c}$)** levels, which reflect hemoglobin's exposure to glucose over the preceding two to three months, are an indirect assessment of blood glucose levels. The following criteria are currently used to diagnose diabetes:[3]

- The plasma glucose concentration is 126 mg/dL or higher after at least 8 hours of fasting (normal fasting plasma glucose levels are 75 to 100 mg/dL).
- In a person with classic symptoms of hyperglycemia, the plasma glucose concentration of a random, or casual, blood sample (that is, obtained from a nonfasting individual) is 200 mg/dL or higher.
- The plasma glucose concentration measured two hours after a 75-gram glucose load is 200 mg/dL or higher.
- The HbA$_{1c}$ level is 6.5 percent or higher.

Following a preliminary diagnosis of diabetes by clinical testing, confirmation is required either by the presence of overt symptoms or a follow-up blood test that yields similar results.

The term **prediabetes** is used when an individual's blood glucose levels are above normal but not high enough to be classified as diabetes; that is, between 100 and 125 mg/dL when fasting or between 140 and 199 mg/dL when measured two hours after ingesting a 75-gram glucose load.[4] HbA$_{1c}$ levels between 5.7 and 6.4 percent also suggest prediabetes. Although people with prediabetes are usually asymptomatic, they are at high risk of eventually developing type 2 diabetes (described in a later section) and cardiovascular diseases. Prediabetes affects approximately 34 percent of adults in the United States[5] and 23 percent of adolescents aged 12 to 19 years,[6] and it is especially prevalent among those who are overweight or obese.

Types of Diabetes Mellitus

Table 20-2 lists features of the two main types of diabetes, type 1 and type 2 diabetes. Pregnancy can lead to abnormal glucose tolerance and the condition known as *gestational diabetes* (discussed later in this chapter), which often resolves after pregnancy but is a risk factor for type 2 diabetes. Diabetes can also be caused by medications that cause glucose intolerance (such as steroids) and medical conditions that damage the pancreas or interfere with insulin function.

Type 1 Diabetes **Type 1 diabetes** accounts for about 5 to 10 percent of diabetes cases.[7] It is usually caused by **autoimmune** destruction of the pancreatic beta cells,

TABLE 20-1	Symptoms of Diabetes Mellitus

- Excessive urine production (polyuria)
- Dehydration, dry mouth
- Excessive thirst (polydipsia)
- Weight loss
- Excessive hunger (polyphagia)
- Blurred vision
- Increased infections
- Fatigue

BOX 20-2 *Nursing Diagnosis*

Nursing diagnoses for people with diabetes may include *risk for unstable blood glucose level*, *risk for deficient fluid volume*, and *risk for infection*.

hyperosmolar: having an abnormally high osmolarity; osmolarity refers to the concentration of osmotically active particles in solution. Hyperglycemia may cause some body fluids to become hyperosmolar.

oral glucose tolerance test: a test that evaluates a person's ability to tolerate an oral glucose load.

glycated hemoglobin (HbA$_{1c}$): hemoglobin that has nonenzymatically attached to glucose; the level of HbA$_{1c}$ in the blood helps to diagnose diabetes and evaluate long-term glycemic control. Also called *glycosylated hemoglobin*.

prediabetes: the state of having plasma glucose levels that are higher than normal but not high enough to be diagnosed as diabetes; occurs in individuals who have metabolic defects that often lead to type 2 diabetes.

type 1 diabetes: diabetes that is characterized by absolute insulin deficiency, usually resulting from the autoimmune destruction of pancreatic beta cells.

autoimmune: refers to an immune response directed against the body's own tissues.

auto = self

TABLE 20-2 Features of Type 1 and Type 2 Diabetes Mellitus

FEATURE	TYPE 1 DIABETES	TYPE 2 DIABETES
Prevalence in diabetic population	5–10% of cases	90–95% of cases
Age of onset	<30 years	>40 years[a]
Associated conditions	Autoimmune diseases, viral infection, inherited factors	Obesity, aging, inactivity, inherited factors
Major defect	Destruction of pancreatic beta cells; insulin deficiency	Insulin resistance; insulin deficiency relative to needs
Insulin secretion	Little or none	Varies; may be normal, increased, or decreased
Requirement for insulin therapy	All cases	Some cases
Former names	Juvenile-onset diabetes Insulin-dependent diabetes	Adult-onset diabetes Noninsulin-dependent diabetes

[a]Incidence of type 2 diabetes is increasing in children and adolescents; in more than 90% of these cases, it is associated with overweight or obesity and a family history of type 2 diabetes.

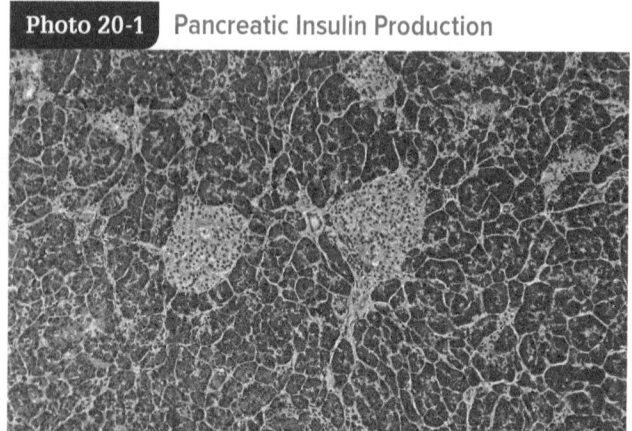

Photo 20-1 Pancreatic Insulin Production

Cross-sections of the pancreas reveal small clusters of cells known as the islets of Langerhans; these regions contain the beta cells that produce insulin.

Ed Reschke/Peter Arnold/Getty Images

which produce and secrete insulin (see Photo 20-1). By the time symptoms develop, the damage to the beta cells has progressed so far that insulin must be provided exogenously, most often by injection. Although the reason for the autoimmune attack is usually unknown, environmental toxins or infections are likely triggers. People with type 1 diabetes often have a genetic susceptibility for the disorder and are at increased risk of developing other autoimmune diseases.

Type 1 diabetes typically develops during childhood or adolescence, although it may occur at any age. Diagnosis often follows an unrelated illness, which increases insulin requirements and stresses the limited reserve of the defective pancreatic beta cells.[8] Hence, classic symptoms of hyperglycemia (polyuria, polydipsia, weight loss, and weakness or fatigue) may appear abruptly in a previously healthy child or young adult. Disease onset tends to be more gradual in individuals who develop type 1 diabetes in later years. Blood tests that detect antibodies to insulin, pancreatic islet cells, and pancreatic enzymes can confirm the diagnosis and help to predict risk of the disease in close relatives.

Type 2 Diabetes **Type 2 diabetes** is the most prevalent form of diabetes, accounting for 90 to 95 percent of cases.[9] It is often asymptomatic for many years before diagnosis. The defect in type 2 diabetes is **insulin resistance**, the reduced sensitivity to insulin in muscle, adipose, and liver cells, coupled with relative insulin deficiency, the lack of sufficient insulin to manage glucose effectively. Normally, the pancreatic beta cells secrete more insulin to compensate for insulin resistance. In type 2 diabetes, insulin levels are often abnormally high (**hyperinsulinemia**) but the additional insulin is insufficient to compensate for its diminished effect in cells. Thus, the hyperglycemia that develops represents a mismatch between the amount of insulin required and the amount produced by beta cells. Beta cell function tends to worsen over time in people with type 2 diabetes, and insulin production gradually declines as the condition progresses.

type 2 diabetes: diabetes that is characterized by insulin resistance coupled with insufficient insulin secretion.

insulin resistance: reduced sensitivity to insulin in muscle, adipose, and liver cells.

hyperinsulinemia: abnormally high levels of insulin in the blood.

Although the precise causes of type 2 diabetes are unknown, risk is substantially increased by obesity (especially abdominal obesity), aging, and physical inactivity. More than 80 percent of individuals with type 2 diabetes are obese, and obesity itself can directly cause some degree of insulin resistance (see Nutrition in Practice 20).[10] Prevalence increases with age and exceeds 25 percent in persons aged 65 years or older; however, many cases remain undiagnosed.[11] Genetic factors strongly influence risk, as type 2 diabetes is more prevalent in certain ethnic groups, including African Americans, Hispanic/Latino populations, Native Americans, Asian Indians, and Pacific Islanders.

Type 2 Diabetes in Children and Adolescents Although most cases of type 2 diabetes are diagnosed in individuals who are over 40 years old, children and teenagers who are overweight or obese or have a family history of diabetes are at increased risk. Because type 2 diabetes is frequently asymptomatic, it is generally identified in youths only when high-risk groups are screened for the disease.

Increased rates of both type 1 and type 2 diabetes have been documented in children in past decades and correlate with the rise in childhood obesity. Type 1 and type 2 diabetes are sometimes difficult to distinguish in children, however, and a few studies have found that some children diagnosed with one of these types of diabetes actually had the other type.[12] Note that type 2 diabetes is still extremely rare in children; for example, its estimated incidence in 10- to 19-year-old African-American and Hispanic-American youths—two groups at high risk—is about 33 and 18 cases per 100,000 individuals per year, respectively.[13] Its increasing prevalence, however, indicates that routine screening and diabetes prevention programs may be important safeguards for children at risk.

Prevention of Type 2 Diabetes Mellitus

Clinical trials have shown that intensive lifestyle changes can prevent or delay the development of type 2 diabetes in individuals at risk for as long as 10 to 20 years.[14] Based on the results of these studies, guidelines for diabetes prevention include the following strategies:

- *Weight management.* A sustained weight loss of at least 7 percent of body weight is recommended for overweight and obese individuals with prediabetes. Individuals who cannot achieve weight loss should avoid gaining additional weight.
- *Dietary modifications.* Diets rich in whole grains, fruits, vegetables, legumes, and nuts and low in refined grains, red meat, and sugar-sweetened beverages may reduce diabetes risk.[15] In addition, individuals who attempt weight loss may need to reduce dietary fat to avoid consuming excessive energy.
- *Physical activity.* At least 150 minutes of moderate physical activity (such as brisk walking) is recommended weekly; the activity should be conducted in at least three separate sessions during the week.
- *Regular monitoring.* Individuals with prediabetes should be monitored yearly to check for the development of diabetes.*

Acute Complications of Diabetes Mellitus

Untreated or poorly controlled diabetes may result in life-threatening complications. Insulin deficiency can cause significant disturbances in energy metabolism, and severe hyperglycemia can lead to dehydration and electrolyte imbalances. In treated diabetes, **hypoglycemia** (low blood glucose) is a possible complication of inappropriate disease management. Figure 20-1 presents an overview of some of the effects of insulin insufficiency on energy metabolism.

---

*The antidiabetic medication metformin may be beneficial for preventing diabetes in high-risk individuals, such as those who are very obese, have severe or worsening hyperglycemia, or have a history of gestational diabetes.

FIGURE 20-1 Effects of Insulin Insufficiency

The effects of insulin insufficiency can be grouped according to the changes in carbohydrate, protein, and fat metabolism.

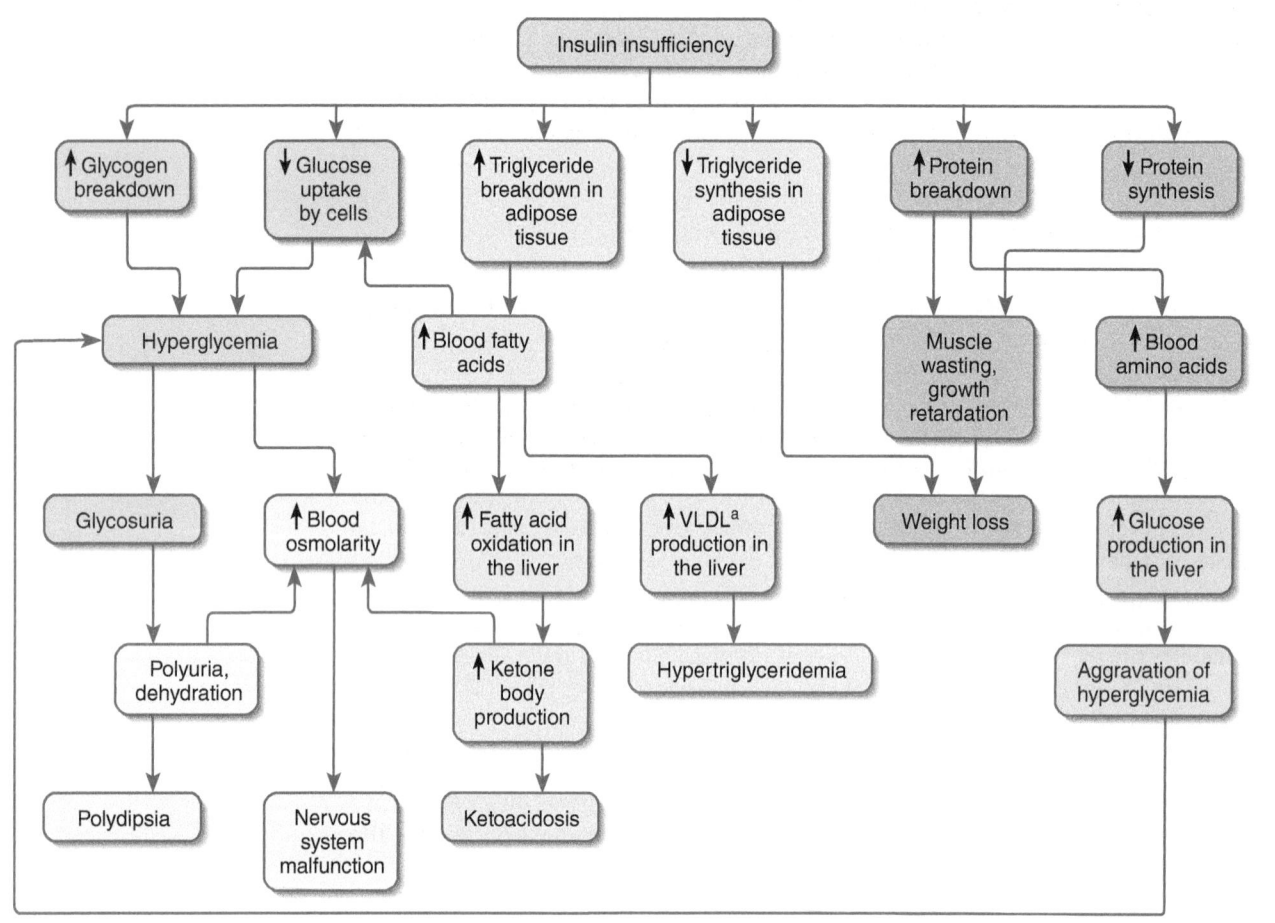

aVery-low-density lipoproteins; these lipoproteins transport triglycerides from the liver to other tissues.

Diabetic Ketoacidosis in Type 1 Diabetes A severe lack of insulin causes diabetic keto-acidosis. Without insulin, glucagon's effects become more pronounced, leading to the unrestrained breakdown of the triglycerides in adipose tissue and the protein in muscle. As a result, an increased supply of fatty acids and amino acids arrives in the liver, fueling the production of ketone bodies and glucose. Ketone bodies, which are acidic, can reach dangerously high levels in the bloodstream (ketoacidosis) and spill into the urine (**ketonuria**). Blood pH typically falls below 7.30 (blood pH normally ranges between 7.35 and 7.45). Blood glucose levels usually exceed 250 mg/dL and rise above 1000 mg/dL in severe cases. The main features of diabetic ketoacidosis therefore include severe **ketosis** (abnormally high levels of ketone bodies), acidosis, and hyperglycemia.[16]

Patients with ketoacidosis may exhibit symptoms of both acidosis and dehydration (see Box 20-3). Acidosis is partially corrected by exhalation of carbon dioxide, so rapid or deep breathing is characteristic.* Ketone accumulation is sometimes evident by a fruity odor on a person's breath (**acetone breath**). Significant urine loss (polyuria) accompanies the hyperglycemia, lowering blood volume and blood pressure and depleting electrolytes. In response, patients may demonstrate marked fatigue,

BOX 20-3 *Nursing Diagnosis*

Nursing diagnoses for people with diabetic ketoacidosis or hyperosmolar hyperglycemic syndrome may include *ineffective health management, deficient fluid volume, risk for electrolyte imbalance,* and *acute confusion.*

---

*Bicarbonate is a buffer in the blood that corrects acidosis. The acid (H^+) combines with bicarbonate (HCO_3^-) to form carbonic acid (H_2CO_3), which breaks down to water (H_2O) and carbon dioxide (CO_2). The carbon dioxide is then exhaled.

lethargy, nausea, and vomiting. The mental state may vary from alert to comatose (**diabetic coma**). Treatment of diabetic ketoacidosis includes insulin therapy to correct the hyperglycemia, intravenous fluid and electrolyte replacement, and, in some cases, bicarbonate therapy to treat acidosis.

Diabetic ketoacidosis is sometimes the earliest sign that leads to a diagnosis of type 1 diabetes, but more often it results from inadequate insulin treatment, illness or infection, alcohol abuse, or other physiological stressors. The condition usually develops quickly, within one to two days. Mortality rates are generally less than 5 percent but may exceed 20 percent among very old individuals or patients with profound coma.[17] Although diabetic ketoacidosis can occur in type 2 diabetes—usually due to severe stressors such as infection, trauma, or surgery—it develops less often because even relatively low insulin concentrations are able to suppress ketone body production.

Hyperosmolar Hyperglycemic Syndrome in Type 2 Diabetes The **hyperosmolar hyperglycemic syndrome** is a condition of severe hyperglycemia and dehydration that develops in the absence of significant ketosis. As mentioned earlier, the hyperglycemia that develops in poorly controlled diabetes leads to polyuria, which results in substantial fluid and electrolyte losses. In the hyperosmolar hyperglycemic syndrome, patients are unable to recognize thirst or adequately replace fluids due to age, illness, sedation, or incapacity. The profound dehydration that eventually develops exacerbates the rise in blood glucose levels, which often exceed 600 mg/dL and may climb above 1000 mg/dL. Blood plasma may become so hyperosmolar as to cause neurological abnormalities, such as confusion, speech or vision impairments, muscle weakness, abnormal reflexes, and seizures; about 10 percent of patients lapse into coma.[18] Treatment includes intravenous fluid and electrolyte replacement and insulin therapy.

The hyperosmolar hyperglycemic syndrome is sometimes the first sign of type 2 diabetes in persons with undiagnosed diabetes. It is usually precipitated by an infection, serious illness, or drug treatment that impairs insulin action or secretion. Unlike diabetic ketoacidosis, the condition often evolves slowly, over one week or longer; the absence of clinical symptoms can delay its diagnosis. The mortality rate may be as high as 20 percent, in part because the condition occurs more often in older patients with cardiovascular disease or other major illnesses.[19]

Hypoglycemia Hypoglycemia, or low blood glucose, is the most frequent complication of type 1 diabetes and may occur in type 2 diabetes as well. It is due to the inappropriate management of diabetes rather than to the disease itself, and is usually caused by excessive dosages of insulin or antidiabetic drugs, prolonged exercise, skipped or delayed meals, inadequate food intake, or the consumption of alcohol without food. Hypoglycemia is the most frequent cause of coma in insulin-treated patients and is believed to account for 4 to 10 percent of deaths in this population.[20]

Symptoms of hypoglycemia include sweating, heart palpitations, shakiness, hunger, weakness, dizziness, and irritability. Mental confusion may prevent a person from recognizing the problem and taking corrective action such as ingesting glucose tablets, juice, or candy (see Box 20-9 on p. 582). If hypoglycemia occurs during the night, patients may be completely unaware of its presence.

Chronic Complications of Diabetes Mellitus

Prolonged exposure to high glucose concentrations can damage cells and tissues. Glucose nonenzymatically combines with proteins, producing molecules that eventually break down to form reactive compounds known as **advanced glycation end products (AGEs)**; in diabetes, these AGEs accumulate to such high levels that they alter the structures of proteins and stimulate metabolic pathways that are damaging to tissues. In addition, excessive glucose promotes the production and accumulation of sorbitol, which increases oxidative stress within cells and causes cellular injury.

Chronic complications of diabetes typically involve the large blood vessels (**macrovascular complications**), smaller vessels such as arterioles and capillaries

advanced glycation end products (AGEs): reactive compounds formed after glucose combines with protein; AGEs can damage tissues and lead to diabetic complications.

(**microvascular complications**), and the nerves (**diabetic neuropathy**). Other tissues adversely affected include the lens of the eye and the skin; cataracts, glaucoma, and various types of skin lesions sometimes develop. Infections are common in diabetes, a possible consequence of hyperglycemia, impaired circulation, and/or depressed immune responses (see Box 20-4). Many of these complications appear 15 to 20 years after the onset of diabetes.[21] In individuals with type 2 diabetes, complications often develop before diabetes is diagnosed.

Macrovascular Complications The damage caused by diabetes accelerates the development of atherosclerosis in the arteries of the heart, brain, and limbs. Moreover, type 2 diabetes is frequently accompanied by multiple risk factors for cardiovascular disease, including hypertension and blood lipid abnormalities. People with diabetes also have increased tendencies for thrombosis (blood clot formation) and abnormal ventricle function, both of which can worsen the clinical course of heart disease. As a result of cardiovascular complications, the most common causes of death in individuals with long-term diabetes are heart attack and stroke.[22]

About 20 to 30 percent of individuals with diabetes develop **peripheral vascular disease** (impaired blood circulation in the limbs),[23] which increases the risk of **claudication** (pain while walking) and contributes to the development of foot ulcers (see Photo 20-2). Left untreated, foot ulcers can lead to **gangrene** (tissue death), and some patients require foot amputation, a major cause of disability in individuals with diabetes.

Photo 20-2 | Diabetic Foot Ulcer

SPL/Science Source

Foot ulcers are a common complication of diabetes because blood circulation is impaired, which slows healing, and nerve damage dampens foot pain, delaying recognition and treatment of cuts and bruises.

Microvascular Complications Long-term diabetes is associated with detrimental changes in capillary structure and function, including the thickening of basement membranes, growth of fibrous tissue (scarring), increased capillary permeability, and proliferation of vessels that function abnormally. The primary microvascular complications involve the retina of the eye and the kidneys.

In **diabetic retinopathy**, the weakened capillaries of the retina leak fluid, lipids, or blood, causing local edema or hemorrhaging. The defective blood flow also leads to damage and scarring within retinal tissue. New blood vessels eventually form, but they are fragile and bleed easily, releasing blood and proteins that obscure vision. About 60 to 80 percent of diabetes patients develop retinopathy 15 to 20 years after diagnosis.[24] Retinopathy progresses most rapidly when diabetes is poorly controlled, and intensive diabetes management substantially reduces the risk.

In **diabetic nephropathy**, damage to the kidneys' specialized capillaries prevents adequate blood filtration, resulting in abnormal urinary protein losses (**albuminuria**). As the kidney damage worsens, urine production decreases and nitrogenous wastes accumulate in the blood; eventually, the individual requires dialysis (artificial filtration of blood) to survive. Because the kidneys normally regulate blood volume and blood pressure, inadequate kidney function may also result in hypertension. At least 20 to 40 percent of persons with diabetes develop some degree of nephropathy, although a greater fraction of type 1 patients progress to kidney failure.[25] As with diabetic retinopathy, intensive diabetes management can help slow the progression of kidney damage.

Diabetic Neuropathy Diabetic neuropathy often involves the peripheral nerves (*peripheral neuropathy*) and nerves that control body organs and glands (*autonomic neuropathy*). Peripheral neuropathy—the most common form of neuropathy in diabetes—may be experienced as pain, numbness, or tingling in the hands, feet, and legs or weakness of the limbs. Peripheral neuropathy also contributes to the development of foot ulcers because cuts and bruises may go unnoticed until wounds are severe. Autonomic neuropathy may be indicated by sweating abnormalities, disturbed bladder function, erectile dysfunction, delayed stomach emptying (**gastroparesis**), constipation, and cardiac arrhythmias. Neuropathy occurs in about 50 percent of patients with diabetes;[26] the extent of nerve damage depends on the severity and duration of hyperglycemia.

20.2 Treatment of Diabetes Mellitus

Diabetes is a chronic and progressive illness that requires lifelong treatment. Managing blood glucose levels is a delicate balancing act that involves meal planning, proper timing of medications, and physical exercise. Frequent adjustments in treatment are often necessary to establish good **glycemic** control. Individuals with type 1 diabetes require insulin therapy for survival. Type 2 diabetes may initially be treated with nutrition therapy and exercise, but most patients eventually need to add antidiabetic medications or insulin. Diabetes management becomes even more difficult once complications develop. Although the health care team must determine the appropriate therapy, the individual with diabetes ultimately assumes much of the responsibility for treatment and therefore requires education in self-management of the disease.

Treatment Goals

The main goal of diabetes treatment is to maintain blood glucose levels within a desirable range to prevent or reduce the risk of complications. Several multicenter clinical trials have shown that *intensive* diabetes treatment, which keeps blood glucose levels tightly controlled, can greatly reduce the incidence and severity of some chronic complications.*[27] Therefore, maintenance of near-normal glucose levels has become the fundamental objective of diabetes care plans. Other goals of treatment include maintaining healthy blood lipid concentrations, controlling blood pressure, and managing weight—measures that can help to prevent or delay diabetes complications as well. Table 20-3 provides examples of some major differences between conventional and intensive therapies for type 1 diabetes. For type 2 diabetes, intensive therapy involves the addition of certain medications or insulin to standard dietary and lifestyle modifications. Note that intensive therapy is recommended only if the benefits of therapy outweigh the potential risks, and it may be inappropriate for some individuals (including those with limited life expectancies, history of hypoglycemia, or previous heart disease).

Diabetes education provides an individual with the knowledge and skills necessary to implement treatment. The primary instructor is often a **Certified Diabetes Educator**, a

*Studies that evaluated the benefits of intensive treatment include the Diabetes Control and Complications Trial and the United Kingdom Prospective Diabetes Study.

glycemic (gly-SEE-mic): pertaining to blood glucose.

Certified Diabetes Educator: a health care professional who specializes in diabetes management education; certification is obtained from the National Certification Board for Diabetes Educators.

	CONVENTIONAL THERAPY	**INTENSIVE THERAPY**
TABLE 20-3	Comparison of Conventional and Intensive Therapies for Type 1 Diabetes[a]	
Blood glucose monitoring	Monitored daily	Monitored at least three times daily
Insulin therapy[b]	One or two daily injections; no daily adjustments	Three or more daily injections or use of an external insulin pump; dosage adjusted according to the results of blood glucose monitoring and expected carbohydrate intake
Advantages	Fewer incidences of severe hypoglycemia; less weight gain	Delayed progression of retinopathy, nephropathy, and neuropathy
Disadvantages	More rapid progression of retinopathy, nephropathy, and neuropathy	Twofold to threefold increase in severe hypoglycemia; weight gain; increased risk of becoming overweight

[a]The therapies shown here were compared in the *Diabetes Control and Complications Trial*, which was conducted in patients with type 1 diabetes. For type 2 diabetes, intensive therapy involves the addition of certain medications or insulin to standard dietary and lifestyle modifications.
[b]In the Diabetes Control and Complications Trial, insulin therapy was conducted using various mixtures of short-acting, intermediate-acting, and long-acting insulins. Since the study, a variety of other insulin therapies have been developed (including rapid-acting insulin and long-acting insulin analogs), allowing for treatments associated with less risk of hypoglycemia.

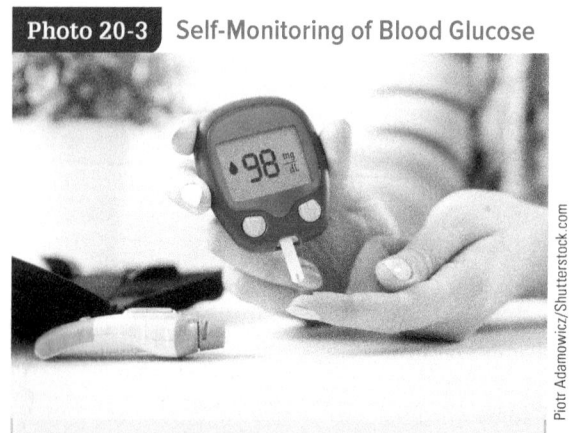

Photo 20-3 Self-Monitoring of Blood Glucose

Self-monitoring of blood glucose involves applying a drop of blood from a finger prick to a chemically treated paper strip, which is then analyzed for glucose.

Piotr Adamowicz/Shutterstock.com

health care professional (often a nurse or dietitian) who has specialized knowledge about diabetes treatment and the health education process. To manage diabetes, patients need to learn about appropriate meal planning, medication administration, blood glucose monitoring, weight management, appropriate physical activity, and prevention and treatment of diabetic complications.

Evaluating Diabetes Treatment

Diabetes treatment is largely evaluated by monitoring glycemic status. Good glycemic control requires frequent testing of blood glucose levels using a glucose meter, referred to as **self-monitoring of blood glucose** (see Box 20-5 and Photo 20-3). Glucose testing provides valuable feedback when the patient adjusts food intake, medications, and physical activity and is helpful for preventing hypoglycemia. Ideally, patients with type 1 diabetes should measure blood glucose levels prior to meals and snacks, at bedtime, prior to exercise or critical tasks such as driving, whenever they suspect hypoglycemia, and after treating hypoglycemia.[28] Some patients may achieve better glycemic control by also using a **continuous glucose monitoring** system, which measures tissue glucose levels every few minutes using a tiny sensor placed under the skin. Although self-monitoring of blood glucose is also useful in type 2 diabetes, the recommended frequency varies according to the specific needs of individual patients.

Long-Term Glycemic Control Health care providers periodically evaluate long-term glycemic control by measuring HbA$_{1c}$ levels. The glucose in blood freely enters red blood cells and attaches to hemoglobin in direct proportion to the amount of glucose present. The percentage of HbA$_{1c}$ in hemoglobin reflects glycemic control over the preceding two to three months, the average age of circulating red blood cells

self-monitoring of blood glucose: home monitoring of blood glucose levels using a glucose meter.

continuous glucose monitoring: continuous monitoring of tissue glucose levels using a small sensor placed under the skin.

(Box 20-6 shows how HbA_{1c} correlates with average plasma glucose levels). The goal of diabetes treatment is usually an HbA_{1c} value less than 7 percent, but the percentage is often markedly higher in people with diabetes, even those who are maintaining near-normal blood glucose levels. Less stringent HbA_{1c} goals (for example, a value less than 8 percent) may be suitable for some patients, including those with limited life expectancy, advanced diabetic complications, or a history of severe hypoglycemia. HbA_{1c} testing is typically conducted two to four times yearly.

The **fructosamine test** is sometimes conducted to determine glycemic control over the preceding two to three weeks. This test determines the nonenzymatic glycation of serum proteins (primarily albumin), which have a shorter half-life than hemoglobin. Most often, the fructosamine test is used to evaluate recent adjustments in diabetes treatment or glycemic control during pregnancy. The test cannot be used if the patient has a liver or kidney disorder that lowers serum protein levels.

Ketone Testing Ketone testing, which checks for the development of ketoacidosis, should be performed if symptoms are present or if risk has increased due to acute illness, stress, or pregnancy. Both blood and urine tests are available for home use, although the blood tests are generally more reliable. Ketone testing is most useful for patients who have type 1 diabetes or are pregnant. Individuals with type 2 diabetes may produce excessive ketone bodies when severely stressed by infection or trauma.

Monitoring for Long-Term Complications Individuals with diabetes are routinely monitored for signs of long-term complications. Blood pressure is measured at each checkup. Annual lipid screening is suggested for adult patients. Routine checks for urinary protein (albuminuria) can determine whether nephropathy has developed. Physical examinations generally screen for signs of retinopathy, neuropathy, and foot problems.

Nutrition Therapy: Dietary Recommendations

Nutrition therapy can improve glycemic control and slow the progression of diabetic complications. As always, the nutrition care plan must consider personal preferences and lifestyle habits. In addition, dietary intakes must be modified to accommodate growth, lifestyle changes, aging, and any complications that develop. Although all members of the diabetes care team should understand the principles of dietary treatment, a registered dietitian is best suited to design and implement the nutrition therapy provided to diabetes patients. This section presents the dietary recommendations for diabetes; a later section describes meal-planning strategies.

Macronutrient Intakes The recommended macronutrient distribution (percent of kcalories from carbohydrate, fat, and protein) depends on food preferences and metabolic factors (for example, insulin sensitivity, blood lipid levels, and kidney function).[29] Intakes suggested for the general population are often used as a guideline (see Box 20-7). Day-to-day consistency in carbohydrate intake is associated with better glycemic control, unless the patient is undergoing intensive insulin therapy that matches insulin doses to mealtime carbohydrate intakes.

Total Carbohydrate Intake The amount of carbohydrate consumed has the greatest influence on blood glucose levels after meals—the more grams of carbohydrate ingested, the greater the glycemic response. The carbohydrate recommendation is based in part on the person's metabolic needs (which are related to the type of diabetes, degree of glucose tolerance, and blood lipid levels), the type of insulin or other medications used to manage the diabetes, and individual preferences. For optimal health, the carbohydrate sources should be vegetables, fruits, whole grains, legumes, and milk products, whereas foods made with refined grains and added sugars should be limited.[30]

BOX 20-6

Comparison of HbA_{1c} and plasma glucose levels:

HbA_{1c} (%)	Average glucose levels (mg/dL)
6[a]	126
7	154
8	183
9	212

[a]HbA_{1c} is typically <6% in nondiabetics.

BOX 20-7

Macronutrient DRI for adults:
Macronutrient ranges (% of total kcal):

- Carbohydrate: 45–65%
- Fat: 20–35%
- Protein: 10–35%

Carbohydrate RDA: 130 g/day

Fiber AI: 21–38 g/day

Protein RDA: 0.8 g/kg body weight

fructosamine test: a measurement of glycated serum proteins that reflects glycemic control over the preceding two to three weeks; also known as the *glycated albumin test* or the *glycated serum protein test*.

Glycemic Index Different carbohydrate-containing foods have different effects on blood glucose levels after they are ingested; for example, consuming a portion of white rice causes blood glucose to increase more than would a similar portion of barley. A food's glycemic effect is influenced by the type of carbohydrate in a food, the food's fiber content, the preparation method, the other foods included in a meal, and individual tolerances (see Nutrition in Practice 3 for details). For individuals with diabetes, choosing foods with a low **glycemic index (GI)** over those with a high GI may modestly improve glycemic control.[31] A food's glycemic effect is not usually a primary consideration when treating diabetes, however, because clinical studies investigating the potential benefits of low-GI diets on glycemic control have had mixed results.[32] Nonetheless, high-fiber, minimally processed foods—which typically have lower glycemic effects than do highly processed, starchy foods—are among the foods frequently recommended for persons with diabetes.

Sugars A common misperception is that people with diabetes need to avoid sugar and sugar-containing foods. In reality, table sugar (sucrose), made up of glucose and fructose, has a lower glycemic effect than starch. Because moderate consumption of sugar has not been shown to adversely affect glycemic control,[33] sugar recommendations for people with diabetes are similar to those for the general population, which advise minimizing foods and beverages that contain added sugars. However, sugars and sugary foods must be counted as part of the daily carbohydrate allowance.

Although fructose has a minimal glycemic effect, its use as an added sweetener should be limited because excessive dietary fructose may adversely affect blood lipids and lipid metabolism (note that it is not necessary to avoid the naturally occurring fructose in fruits and vegetables).[34] Sugar alcohols (such as sorbitol and maltitol) have lower glycemic effects than glucose or sucrose and may be used as sugar substitutes. Artificial sweeteners (such as aspartame, saccharin, and sucralose) contain no digestible carbohydrate and can be safely used in place of sugar.

Whole Grains and Fiber Recommendations for whole grain and fiber intakes are similar to those for the general population. People with diabetes are encouraged to include fiber-rich foods such as whole-grain cereals, legumes, fruits, and vegetables in their diet. Although some studies have suggested that very high intakes of fiber (more than 50 grams per day) may improve glycemic control, many individuals have difficulty enjoying or tolerating such large amounts of fiber.[35]

Dietary Fat A Mediterranean-style dietary pattern that emphasizes unsaturated fats may benefit both glycemic control and cardiovascular disease (CVD) risk.[36] In addition, increased intakes of omega-3 fatty acids from fatty fish or plant sources may improve the lipoprotein profile and various other CVD risk factors (see Chapter 4). Other guidelines related to fat intake are similar to those suggested for the general population: saturated fat should be less than 10 percent of total kcalories and *trans* fats should be avoided.

Protein Protein recommendations for people with diabetes are similar to those for the general population (see Box 20-7). In the United States, the average protein intake is about 16 percent of the energy intake. Although several small, short-term studies have suggested that higher protein intakes (28 to 40 percent of total kcalories) may improve glycemic control or lipoprotein levels in diabetic individuals, other studies did not show any benefit.[37] In addition, high protein intakes are sometimes discouraged because they may be detrimental to kidney function in patients with nephropathy.

Alcohol Use in Diabetes Guidelines for alcohol intake are similar to those for the general population, which recommend that women and men limit their average daily intakes of alcohol to one **drink** and two drinks per day, respectively. In addition, individuals using insulin or medications that promote insulin secretion should consume

glycemic index (GI): a ranking of carbohydrate foods based on their effect on blood glucose levels after ingestion; foods with a low GI have a lesser glycemic effect whereas those with a high GI have a greater glycemic effect. The website *www .glycemicindex.com* provides GI values for a wide variety of foods.

drink: volume of an alcoholic beverage that contains about ½ ounce of pure ethanol; equivalent to 12 oz of beer, 5 oz of wine, or 1½ oz of 80-proof distilled spirits such as gin, rum, vodka, and whiskey.

food when they ingest alcoholic beverages to avoid hypoglycemia (alcohol can cause hypoglycemia by interfering with glucose production in the liver).[38] Conversely, an excessive alcohol intake (three or more drinks per day) can worsen hyperglycemia and raise triglyceride levels in some individuals. People who should avoid alcohol include pregnant women and individuals with advanced neuropathy, abnormally high triglyceride levels, or a history of alcohol abuse.

Micronutrients Micronutrient recommendations for people with diabetes are the same as for the general population. Vitamin and mineral supplementation is not recommended unless nutrient deficiencies develop; those at risk include elderly individuals, pregnant or lactating women, strict vegetarians, and individuals on kcalorie-restricted diets. Although various micronutrients (including chromium and antioxidant nutrients such as vitamins C and E) have been tested for their potential benefits in managing diabetes or diabetes complications, results have not been promising.[39]

Excess Body Weight and Type 2 Diabetes Because excessive body fat can worsen insulin resistance, weight loss is recommended for overweight or obese individuals who have diabetes. Even moderate weight loss (5 to 10 percent of body weight) can help to improve insulin resistance, glycemic control, blood lipid levels, and blood pressure. Weight loss is most beneficial early in the course of diabetes, before insulin secretion has diminished.[40]

Nutrition Therapy: Meal-Planning Strategies

Dietitians provide a number of meal-planning strategies to help people with diabetes maintain glycemic control. These strategies emphasize control of carbohydrate intake and portion sizes. Initial dietary instructions may include guidelines for maintaining a healthy diet, improving blood lipids, and reducing cardiovascular risk factors. Sample menus that include commonly eaten foods can help to illustrate general principles. People using intensive insulin therapy must learn to coordinate insulin injections with meals and to match insulin dosages to carbohydrate intake, as discussed later.

Carbohydrate Counting Carbohydrate-counting techniques are simpler and more flexible than other menu-planning approaches and are widely used for planning diabetes diets. Carbohydrate counting works as follows: After an interview in which the dietitian learns about the patient's usual food intake and calculates nutrient and energy needs, the patient is given a daily carbohydrate allowance, divided into a pattern of meals and snacks according to individual preferences. The carbohydrate allowance can be expressed in grams or as the number of carbohydrate portions allowed per meal (see Table 20-4). The user of the plan need only be concerned about meeting carbohydrate goals and can select from any of the carbohydrate-containing food groups when planning meals (see Table 20-5 and Figure 20-2). Although encouraged to make healthy food choices, the individual has the freedom to choose the foods desired at each meal without risking loss of glycemic control. Some people may also need guidance about consuming a diet that improves blood lipids or energy intakes. Box 20-8 shows how to implement carbohydrate counting in clinical practice.

Carbohydrate counting is taught at different levels of complexity depending on a person's needs and abilities. The basic carbohydrate-counting method just described can be helpful for most people, although it requires a consistent carbohydrate intake from day to day to match the medication or insulin regimen. Advanced carbohydrate counting allows more flexibility but is best suited for patients using intensive insulin therapy. With this method, a person can determine the specific dose of insulin needed to cover the amount of carbohydrate consumed in a meal. The person is then free to choose the types and portions of food desired without sacrificing glycemic control. Advanced carbohydrate counting requires some training and should be attempted only after an individual has mastered more basic methods.

Box 20-8

HOW TO Use Carbohydrate Counting in Clinical Practice

1. The first step in basic carbohydrate counting is to determine an appropriate carbohydrate allowance and suitable distribution pattern; an example is shown in Table 20-4. To ensure that the carbohydrate level will be acceptable to the person using the plan, the dietitian can conduct a nutrition assessment to estimate the person's usual carbohydrate intake and food habits. Frequent monitoring of blood glucose levels can help to determine whether additional carbohydrate restriction would be helpful.

   The example given in Table 20-4 illustrates a meal pattern for a person consuming 2000 kcalories daily with a carbohydrate allowance of 50 percent of kcalories. This is calculated as follows:

   $$2000 \text{ kcal} \times 50\% = 1000 \text{ kcal of carbohydrate}$$

   $$\frac{1000 \text{ kcal carbohydrate}}{4 \text{ kcal/g carbohydrate}} = 250 \text{ g carbohydrate/day}$$

   $$\frac{250 \text{ g carbohydrate}}{15 \text{ g/1 carbohydrate portion}} = 16.7 \text{ carbohydrate portions/day}$$

2. The distribution of carbohydrates among meals and snacks is based on both individual preferences and metabolic needs. In type 1 diabetes, the insulin regimen must coordinate with the individual's dietary and lifestyle choices. People using conventional insulin therapy must maintain a consistent carbohydrate intake from day to day to match their particular insulin prescription, whereas those using intensive therapy can alter insulin dosages when carbohydrate intakes change. People with type 2 diabetes are encouraged to develop dietary patterns that suit their lifestyle and medication schedules. For all types of diabetes, the carbohydrate recommendation may need to be altered periodically to improve blood glucose control.

3. Carbohydrate counting can be done in one of two ways:
   - Count the grams of carbohydrate provided by foods.
   - Count carbohydrate portions, expressed in terms of servings that contain about 15 grams of carbohydrate each.

TABLE 20-4 Sample Carbohydrate Distribution for a 2000-kCalorie Diet

MEALS	CARBOHYDRATE ALLOWANCE	
	GRAMS	PORTIONS[a]
Breakfast	60	4
Lunch	60	4
Afternoon snack	30	2
Dinner	75	5
Evening snack	30	2
Totals	**255 g**	**17**

[a]1 portion = 15 g carbohydrate = 1 portion of starchy food, milk, or fruit.

Note: The carbohydrate allowance in this example is approximately 50% of total kcalories.

Success with carbohydrate counting requires knowledge about the food sources of carbohydrates and an understanding of portion control. As shown in Table 20-5, food selections that contain about

TABLE 20-5 Carbohydrate-Containing Food Groups and Sample Portion Sizes

Bread, cereal, rice, and pasta: 1 portion = 15 g carbohydrate
- 1 slice of bread or 1 small tortilla
- ½ English muffin
- ¾ c unsweetened, ready-to-eat cereal
- ½ c cooked oatmeal
- ⅓ c cooked rice or pasta

Starchy vegetables: 1 portion = 15 g carbohydrate
- 1 small (3 oz) potato
- ½ c canned or frozen corn
- ½ c cooked beans
- 1 c winter squash, cubed

Fruit: 1 portion = 15 g carbohydrate
- 1 small (4 oz) apple
- 1 medium (6 oz) peach
- ¾ c blueberries
- ½ c apple or orange juice

Milk products: 1 portion = 12 g carbohydrate; may be rounded up to 15 g for ease in counting carbohydrate portions
- 1 c milk (whole, low-fat, or fat-free)
- 1 c buttermilk
- 6 oz plain yogurt

Sweets and desserts:[a] Carbohydrate content varies; portions listed contain approximately 15 g
- ½ c ice cream
- 2 sandwich cookies (with cream filling)
- 1 small (¾ oz) granola bar
- 5 chocolate kisses
- 1 tbs honey

Nonstarchy vegetables: 1 portion = approximately 5 g carbohydrate; 3 servings are equivalent to 1 carbohydrate portion; can be disregarded if fewer than 3 servings are consumed
- ½ c cooked cauliflower
- ½ c cooked cabbage, collards, or kale
- ½ c cooked okra
- ½ c diced or raw tomatoes

[a]Products sweetened with artificial sweeteners or sugar alcohols contain fewer grams of carbohydrate than products sweetened with sugar or honey.

Note: Unprocessed meats, fish, and poultry contain negligible amounts of carbohydrate.

(Continued)

Box 20-8 HOW TO Use Carbohydrate Counting in Clinical Practice (*continued*)

15 grams of carbohydrate are interchangeable. The portions of foods that contain 15 grams may vary substantially, however, even among foods in a single food group. Accurate carbohydrate counting often requires instruction and practice in portion control using measuring cups, spoons, and a food scale. Food lists that indicate the carbohydrate content of common foods are available from the American Diabetes Association and the Academy of Nutrition and Dietetics; these are helpful resources for learning carbohydrate-counting methods.

When using packaged foods, individuals should check the Nutrition Facts panel of food labels to find the carbohydrate content of a serving. If the fiber content is more than 5 grams per serving, it should be subtracted from the *Total Carbohydrate* value, as fiber does not contribute to blood glucose (some clinicians may suggest subtracting only half of the grams of fiber). If the sugar alcohol content is greater than 5 grams per serving, half of the grams of sugar alcohols can be subtracted from the *Total Carbohydrate* value.

4. Once they have learned the basic carbohydrate counting method, individuals can select whatever foods they wish as long as they do not exceed their carbohydrate goals. Figure 20-2 shows a day's menu that provides the carbohydrate allowance shown in Table 20-4. Although carbohydrate counting focuses on a single macronutrient, people using this technique should be encouraged to follow a healthy eating plan that meets other dietary objectives as well.

FIGURE 20-2 Translating Carbohydrate Portions into a Day's Meals

SAMPLE MENU

Breakfast	Carbohydrate Portions
Carbohydrate goal = 4 portions or 60 g	
¾ c unsweetened, ready-to-eat cereal	1
½ c low-fat milk	½
1 scrambled egg	–
1 slice whole-wheat toast (with margarine or butter)	1
6 oz orange juice	1½
Coffee (without milk or sugar)	–

Lunch	Carbohydrate Portions
Carbohydrate goal = 4 portions or 60 g	
1 tuna salad sandwich (includes 2 slices whole-grain bread, mayonnaise)	2
6 oz yogurt (plain) with ¾ c blueberries and artificial sweetener	2
Diet cola	–

Afternoon snack	Carbohydrate Portions
Carbohydrate goal = 2 portions or 30 g	
2 sandwich cookies	1
1 c low-fat milk	1

Dinner	Carbohydrate Portions
Carbohydrate goal = 5 portions or 75 g	
4 oz grilled steak	–
1 small baked potato (with margarine or butter)	1
Corn on cob, 1 large ear	2
½ c steamed collard greens[a]] 1 c sliced, raw tomatoes[a]]	1
½ c ice cream	1

Evening snack	Carbohydrate Portions
Carbohydrate goal = 2 portions or 30 g	
1 small apple	1
¾ oz granola bar	1

[a]Three servings of nonstarchy vegetables are equivalent to 1 carbohydrate portion.

Food Lists for Diabetes A meal-planning system originally developed for persons with diabetes allows individuals to create an eating plan by choosing foods with specified portions from a variety of food lists. The different food lists group foods according to their proportions of carbohydrate, fat, and protein so that all items on a particular list have similar macronutrient and energy contents (see Appendix C, pp. C-1 to C-2). Thus, each food on a food list can be substituted for any other food on the same list without affecting the macronutrient balance in a day's meals. Although the food list system may be helpful for individuals who want to maintain a diet with specific macronutrient percentages, it is less flexible than carbohydrate counting and offers no advantages for maintaining glycemic control. However, the food lists may be helpful resources for individuals using carbohydrate-counting methods because the portions are similar to the portions used in carbohydrate counting, providing about 15 grams of carbohydrate per food item (see pp. C-3 to C-6; note that the carbohydrates in foods on the *Milk and Milk Substitutes* list can be rounded up to 15 grams).

Insulin Therapy

Insulin therapy is necessary for individuals who cannot produce enough insulin to meet their metabolic needs. It is therefore required by people with type 1 diabetes and those with type 2 diabetes who cannot maintain glycemic control with medications, diet, and exercise. The pancreas normally secretes insulin in relatively low amounts between meals and during the night (called *basal insulin*) and in much higher amounts when meals are ingested. Ideally, the insulin treatment should reproduce the natural pattern of insulin secretion as closely as possible.

Insulin Preparations The forms of insulin that are commercially available differ by their onset of action, timing of peak action, and duration of effects. Table 20-6 and Figure 20-3 show how insulin preparations are classified: they may be rapid acting (lispro, aspart, glulisine, and inhaled insulin), short acting (regular), intermediate acting (NPH), or long acting (glargine, detemir, and degludec), thereby allowing substantial flexibility in establishing a suitable insulin regimen.[41] The rapid- and short-acting insulins are typically used at mealtimes, whereas the intermediate- and long-acting insulins provide basal insulin for the periods between meals and during the night. Thus, mixtures of several types of insulin can produce greater glycemic control than any one type alone. Several premixed formulations are also available; examples are listed in Table 20-6.

Insulin Delivery Insulin is most often administered by **subcutaneous** injection, either self-administered or provided by caregivers (note that insulin is a protein, and would be destroyed by digestive processes if taken orally). Disposable **syringes**, which are filled from vials that contain multiple doses of insulin, are the most common devices

TABLE 20-6 Insulin Preparations

FORM OF INSULIN	COMMON PREPARATIONS	ONSET OF ACTION	PEAK ACTION	DURATION OF ACTION
Rapid acting	Lispro (Humalog) Aspart (Novolog) Glulisine (Apidra) Inhaled insulin (Afrezza)[a]	5–15 minutes	60–90 minutes	3–5 hours
Short acting	Regular (Humulin R, Novolin R)	30–60 minutes	2–3 hours	5–8 hours
Intermediate acting	NPH (Humulin N, Novolin N)	2–4 hours	6–8 hours	10–18 hours
Long acting	Glargine (Lantus) Detemir (Levemir) Degludec (Tresiba)	1–2 hours	Steady effects	24 hours or longer
Insulin mixtures (with sample ratios)	NPH/regular (70:30) NPL (modified lispro)/lispro (75:25)	Variable; depends on formulation	Variable; depends on formulation	Variable; depends on formulation

[a]Afrezza is a powdered insulin administered by inhalation; its peak action (53 minutes) occurs earlier than that of other rapid-acting insulin products.

FIGURE 20-3 Effects of Insulin Preparations

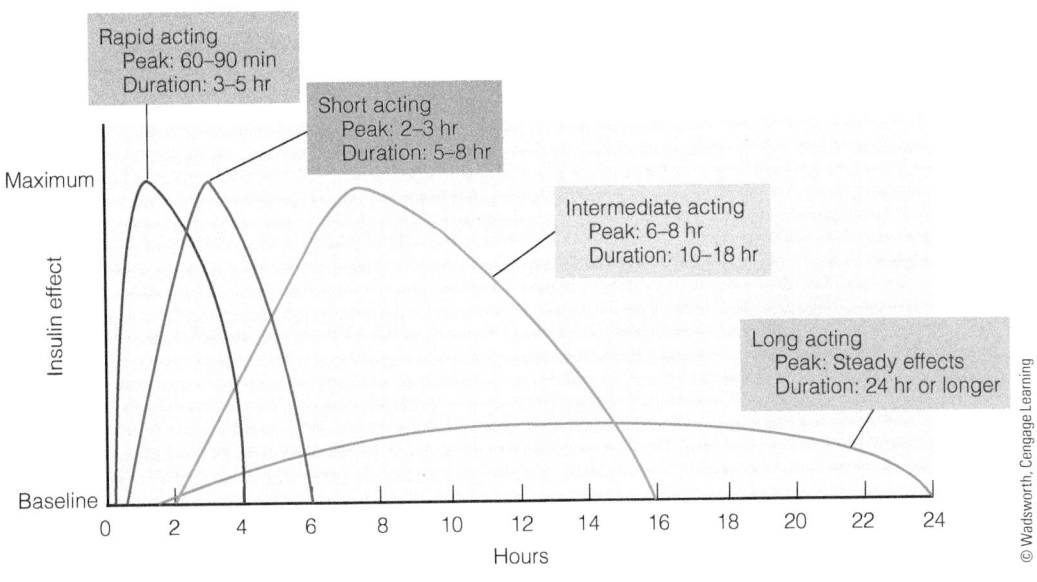

Rapid acting
Peak: 60–90 min
Duration: 3–5 hr

Short acting
Peak: 2–3 hr
Duration: 5–8 hr

Intermediate acting
Peak: 6–8 hr
Duration: 10–18 hr

Long acting
Peak: Steady effects
Duration: 24 hr or longer

Maximum

Insulin effect

Baseline

0 2 4 6 8 10 12 14 16 18 20 22 24

Hours

© Wadsworth, Cengage Learning

used for injecting insulin (see Photo 20-4). Another option is to use insulin pens, injection devices that resemble permanent marking pens. Disposable insulin pens are prefilled with insulin and are used one time only, whereas reusable pens can be fitted with prefilled insulin cartridges and replaceable needles. A rapid-acting inhalation powder is available for use before meals, although it cannot be used by patients with lung disease. Some individuals use insulin pumps, computerized devices that infuse insulin through thin, flexible tubing that remains in the skin; the pump can be attached to a belt or kept in a pocket (see Photo 20-5). Some of the newer insulin pumps include built-in continuous glucose monitoring systems.

Insulin Regimen for Type 1 Diabetes Type 1 diabetes is best managed with intensive insulin therapy, which typically involves three or four daily injections of several types of insulin or the use of an insulin pump.[42] Insulin pumps are usually programmed to deliver low amounts of rapid-acting insulin continuously (to meet basal insulin needs) and bolus doses of rapid-acting insulin at mealtimes. In persons who inject insulin, intermediate- or long-acting insulin meets basal insulin needs, and rapid- or short-acting insulin is injected (or in some cases, administered via inhalation*) before meals. Simpler regimens involve twice-daily injections of a mixture of intermediate- and short-acting insulin. Regimens that include three or more injections allow for greater flexibility in carbohydrate intake and meal timing. With fewer injections, the timing of both meals and injections must be similar from day to day to avoid periods of insulin deficiency or excess.

A person using intensive therapy must learn to accurately determine the amount of insulin to inject before each meal. The amount required depends on the pre-meal blood glucose level, the carbohydrate content of the meal, and the person's body weight and sensitivity to insulin. To determine insulin sensitivity, the individual

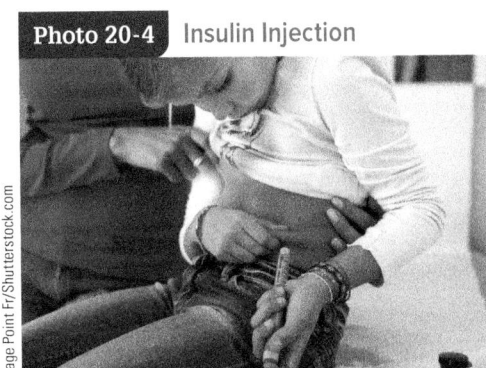

Photo 20-4 Insulin Injection

Image Point Fr/Shutterstock.com

Children with diabetes often become adept at administering the insulin they require.

---

*The inhalation powder *Afrezza* is the only form of inhaled insulin on the market; it has not become a popular alternative to injectable forms of insulin.

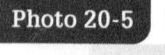
Photo 20-5 | Insulin Pump

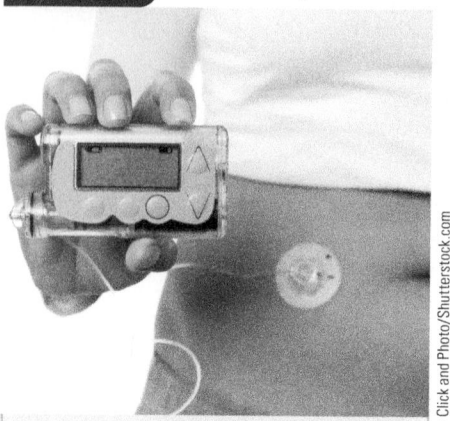

An external insulin pump delivers a low dosage of insulin continuously and bolus doses at mealtimes. Insulin therapy using an insulin pump is also known as *continuous subcutaneous insulin infusion*.

keeps careful records of food intake, insulin dosages, and blood glucose levels. Eventually, these records are analyzed by medical personnel to determine the appropriate **carbohydrate-to-insulin ratio** for that individual, which assists in calculating insulin doses at mealtime. Intensive therapy allows for substantial variation in food intake and lifestyle, but it requires frequent testing of blood glucose levels and a good understanding of carbohydrate counting.

After insulin therapy is initiated, persons with type 1 diabetes may experience a temporary remission of disease symptoms and a reduced need for insulin, known as the *honeymoon period*. The remission is due to a temporary improvement in pancreatic beta-cell function and may last for several weeks or months. It is important to anticipate this period of remission to avoid insulin excess. In all cases, the honeymoon period eventually ends, and the patient must reinstate full insulin treatment.[43]

Insulin Regimen for Type 2 Diabetes Although initial treatment of type 2 diabetes usually involves nutrition therapy, physical activity, and oral antidiabetic medications, long-term results with these treatments are often disappointing. As the disease progresses, pancreatic function worsens, and many individuals require insulin therapy to maintain glycemic control.

Many possible regimens can be used to control type 2 diabetes.[44] Most persons use insulin in combination with one or more antidiabetic drugs, although some individuals may be treated with insulin alone. Many patients need only one or two daily injections. In some cases, an injection of an intermediate- or long-acting form of insulin may be needed once or twice a day. Other regimens may involve two or more daily injections of an insulin mixture that includes both a rapid- or short-acting insulin and an intermediate- or long-acting insulin. Doses and timing are adjusted according to the results of blood glucose self-monitoring.

Insulin Therapy and Hypoglycemia Hypoglycemia (blood glucose levels below 70 mg/dL) is the most common complication of insulin treatment, although it may also result from the use of some oral antidiabetic drugs. It most often results from intensive insulin therapy because the attempt to attain near-normal blood glucose levels increases the risk of overtreatment. Other potential causes include skipped meals or snacks or prolonged exercise.

Hypoglycemia can be corrected by consuming glucose or a glucose-containing food. Usually, 15 to 20 grams of carbohydrate (see Box 20-9) can relieve hypoglycemia in about 15 minutes, although patients should monitor their blood glucose levels in case additional treatment is necessary.[45] Foods that provide pure glucose yield a better response than foods that contain other sugars, such as sucrose or fructose. Individuals who use insulin are usually advised to carry glucose tablets or a source of carbohydrate that can be easily ingested. After blood glucose normalizes, patients should consume a meal or snack to prevent recurrence. Those at risk of severe hypoglycemia (blood glucose levels below 54 mg/dL) are often given prescriptions for the hormone glucagon, which can be injected by caregivers in case of unconsciousness.

Insulin Therapy and Weight Gain Weight gain is sometimes an unintentional side effect of insulin therapy, especially in individuals undergoing intensive insulin treatment. Although the exact causes of the weight gain are unclear, it may partly be due to insulin's stimulatory effect on fat synthesis. Patients may be able to avoid weight gain by reducing the ratio of basal to mealtime insulin and improving carbohydrate-counting skills to obtain better estimates of mealtime insulin requirements.[46] Concerns about weight should not discourage the use of intensive therapy, which is associated with longer life expectancy and fewer complications than occur with conventional therapy.

BOX 20-9

Each of the following sources provides about 15 g of carbohydrate:

- Glucose tablets: 4 tablets
- Table sugar: 1 tbs
- Honey: 1 tbs
- Hard candy: 3 pieces
- Orange juice: ½ c

carbohydrate-to-insulin ratio: the amount of carbohydrate that can be handled per unit of insulin; on average, every 15 grams of carbohydrate requires about 1 unit of rapid- or short-acting insulin.

Fasting Hyperglycemia Insulin therapy must sometimes be adjusted to prevent **fasting hyperglycemia**, which typically develops in the early morning after an overnight fast of at least eight hours. The usual cause is a waning of insulin action during the night due to insufficient insulin dosing the evening before. A second possibility, known as the **dawn phenomenon**, is an increase of blood glucose in the morning due to the early-morning secretion of growth hormone, which reduces insulin sensitivity. Less frequently, fasting hyperglycemia develops as a result of nighttime hypoglycemia, which causes the secretion of hormones that stimulate glucose production; the resulting condition is known as **rebound hyperglycemia** (also called the *Somogyi effect*). Whatever the cause, fasting hyperglycemia can be treated by adjusting the dosage or formulation of insulin administered in the evening.[47]

Antidiabetic Drugs

Treatment of type 2 diabetes often requires the use of oral medications and injectable drugs other than insulin. As shown in Table 20-7, these drugs can improve hyperglycemia by various modes of action. Treatment may involve the use of a single medication (monotherapy) or a combination of several medications (combination therapy). By utilizing several mechanisms at once, combination therapy achieves more rapid and sustained glycemic control than is possible with monotherapy. Box 20-10 lists some nutrition-related effects of several antidiabetic drugs.

TABLE 20-7 Antidiabetic Drugs

DRUG CATEGORY	COMMON EXAMPLES	MODE OF ACTION
Alpha-glucosidase inhibitors	Acarbose (Precose) Miglitol (Glyset)	Delay carbohydrate digestion and absorption
Amylin analogs (injected)	Pramlintide (Smylin)	Suppress glucagon secretion, delay stomach emptying, increase satiety
Biguanides	Metformin (Glucophage)	Inhibit liver glucose production, improve glucose utilization
Bile acid sequestrants	Colesevelam (Welchol)	Unknown; may inhibit liver glucose production
Dipeptidyl peptidase 4 (DPP-4) inhibitors	Saxagliptin (Onglyza) Sitagliptin (Januvia)	Improve insulin secretion, suppress glucagon secretion, delay stomach emptying
Dopamine D2 receptor agonists	Bromocriptine (Cycloset)	Increase insulin sensitivity
GLP-1 receptor agonists (injected)	Exenatide (Byetta) Liraglutide (Victoza)	Improve insulin secretion, suppress glucagon secretion, delay stomach emptying, increase satiety
Meglitinides	Nateglinide (Starlix) Repaglinide (Prandin)	Stimulate insulin secretion from pancreatic beta cells
Sodium-glucose cotransporter 2 (SGLT2) inhibitors	Canagliflozin (Invokana) Dapagliflozin (Farxiga) Empagliflozin (Jardiance)	Inhibit glucose reabsorption in the kidneys, thereby increasing urinary glucose excretion
Sulfonylureas	Glipizide (Glucotrol) Glyburide (Diabeta)	Stimulate insulin secretion from pancreatic beta cells
Thiazolidinediones	Pioglitazone (Actos) Rosiglitazone (Avandia)	Increase insulin sensitivity

fasting hyperglycemia: hyperglycemia that typically develops in the early morning after an overnight fast of at least eight hours.

dawn phenomenon: morning hyperglycemia that is caused by the early-morning release of growth hormone, which reduces insulin sensitivity.

rebound hyperglycemia: hyperglycemia that results from the release of counterregulatory hormones following nighttime hypoglycemia; also called the *Somogyi effect*.

Box 20-10 Diet-Drug Interactions

Check this table for notable nutrition-related effects of the medications discussed in this chapter.

Alpha-glucosidase inhibitors	**Gastrointestinal effects:** Flatulence, abdominal cramps, diarrhea
	Metabolic effects: May decrease blood concentrations of calcium and vitamin B_6
Biguanides (metformin)	**Gastrointestinal effects:** Metallic taste, nausea, vomiting, anorexia, flatulence, abdominal cramps, diarrhea
	Dietary interaction: Excessive alcohol intake may cause lactic acidosis, which requires emergency treatment
	Metabolic effects: Decreased folate and vitamin B_{12} absorption, which may lead to deficiency
Meglitinides	**Metabolic effects:** Hypoglycemia, weight gain
Sulfonylureas	**Gastrointestinal effects:** Nausea, abdominal cramps, diarrhea, constipation
	Dietary interaction: Alcohol may delay drug absorption and prolong hypoglycemia (if hypoglycemia occurs)
	Metabolic effects: Hypoglycemia, weight gain, allergic skin reactions
Thiazolidinediones	**Metabolic effects:** Weight gain, fluid retention, edema, anemia, decreased bone density and increased risk of fractures (women)

Physical Activity and Diabetes Management

Regular physical activity can improve insulin sensitivity, muscle glucose uptake, and overall glycemic control and is therefore a central feature of diabetes management. Physical activity also benefits other aspects of health, including cardiovascular risk factors and body weight. Children with diabetes or prediabetes should engage in at least 60 minutes of aerobic activity each day. Adults with diabetes are advised to perform at least 150 minutes of moderate-to-vigorous aerobic activity each week, spread over at least three days of the week. Both children and adults should participate in two or three sessions of muscle-strengthening exercises weekly.[48]

Medical Evaluation before Exercise Before a person with diabetes begins a new exercise program, a medical evaluation should screen for problems that may be aggravated by certain activities. Complications involving the heart and blood vessels, eyes, kidneys, feet, and nervous system may limit the types of activity recommended. For individuals with a low level of fitness who have been relatively inactive, only mild or moderate exercise may be prescribed at first; a short walk at a comfortable pace may be the first activity suggested. People with severe retinopathy should avoid vigorous aerobic or resistance exercise, which may lead to retinal detachment and damage to eye tissue. Individuals with peripheral neuropathy should ensure that they wear proper footwear during exercise; those with a foot injury or open sore should avoid weight-bearing activity.

Maintaining Glycemic Control during Exercise Individuals who use insulin or medications that increase insulin secretion must carefully adjust food intake and medication dosages to prevent hypoglycemia during physical activity. Medication dosages that precede exercise often need to be reduced substantially. Blood glucose levels should be checked both before and after an activity. If blood glucose is below 100 mg/dL, carbohydrate should be consumed before the exercise begins.* Additional carbohydrate may

---

*As an example, about 15 grams of carbohydrate may be needed for 30 minutes of moderate-intensity exercise, such as swimming or jogging.

be needed during or after prolonged activity or even several hours after the activity is completed. Individuals with type 1 diabetes who have hyperglycemia and ketosis should delay exercise until blood glucose falls below 250 mg/dL, as even mild exercise may cause additional increases in blood glucose and ketone levels.[49]

Sick-Day Management

Illness, infection, or injury can cause hormonal changes that raise blood glucose levels and increase the risk of developing diabetic ketoacidosis or the hyperosmolar hyperglycemic syndrome (see Box 20-11). During illness, individuals with diabetes should measure blood glucose and ketone levels several times daily. They should continue to use antidiabetic drugs, including insulin, as prescribed; adjustments in dosages may be necessary if they alter their diet or have persistent hyperglycemia. If appetite is poor, patients should select easy-to-manage foods and beverages that provide the prescribed amount of carbohydrate at each meal. To prevent dehydration, especially if vomiting or diarrhea is present, patients should make sure they consume adequate amounts of liquids throughout the day.

The Case Study in Box 20-12 provides an opportunity to review the treatment for diabetes.

BOX 20-11 *Nursing Diagnosis*

The nursing diagnosis *risk for unstable blood glucose level* may apply to an individual with diabetes who has an illness or injury.

Review Notes

- Diabetes treatment includes nutrition therapy, the use of insulin and/or other antidiabetic medications, and appropriate physical activity. Glycemic control is evaluated by monitoring blood glucose levels and glycated hemoglobin.
- The quantity of carbohydrate consumed has the most significant influence on blood glucose levels after meals and is more important than the type of carbohydrate consumed.
- Carbohydrate counting is widely used in menu planning and can be taught at different levels of complexity, depending on individual needs and abilities.
- Insulin therapy is required for patients who are unable to produce sufficient insulin and may be used in both type 1 and type 2 diabetes. Antidiabetic drugs prescribed for type 2 diabetes improve hyperglycemia by various modes of action.
- Physical activity can improve glycemic control and enhance various aspects of general health. Illness can worsen glycemic status and often requires medication adjustments.

Box 20-12 Case Study: Child with Type 1 Diabetes

Nora is a 12-year-old girl who was diagnosed with type 1 diabetes two years ago. She practices intensive therapy and has had the support of her parents and an excellent diabetes management team. With their help, Nora has been able to assume the bulk of the responsibility for her diabetes care and has managed to control her blood glucose remarkably well. In the past few months, however, Nora has been complaining bitterly about the impositions diabetes has placed on her life and her interactions with friends. Sometimes she refuses to monitor her blood glucose levels, and she has skipped insulin injections a few times. Recently, Nora was admitted to the emergency room complaining of fever, nausea, vomiting, and intense thirst. The physician noted that Nora was confused and lethargic. A urine test was

positive for ketones, and her blood glucose levels were 400 mg/dL. The diagnosis was diabetic ketoacidosis.

1. Describe the metabolic events that lead to ketoacidosis. Were Nora's symptoms and laboratory tests consistent with the diagnosis?

2. Review Table 20-3 on p. 574, and consider the advantages and disadvantages that intensive therapy might have for Nora. Describe the complications associated with long-term diabetes.

3. Discuss how Nora's age might influence her ability to cope with and manage her diabetes. Why might she feel that diabetes is disrupting her life? List suggestions that may help. How might you explain the importance of glycemic control to a 12-year-old girl?

BOX 20-14

Goals for glycemic control in pregnant women:

- Before meals: <95 mg/dL
- 1 hour after the start of a meal: <140 mg/dL
- 2 hours after the start of a meal: <120 mg/dL
- HbA$_{1c}$: 6–6.5%

20.3 Diabetes Management in Pregnancy

Women with diabetes face new challenges during pregnancy. Due to hormonal changes, pregnancy increases insulin resistance and the body's need for insulin, so maintaining glycemic control may be more difficult. In addition, 4 to 14 percent of nondiabetic women in the United States develop gestational diabetes (the prevalence depends on the patient population).[50] Women with gestational diabetes are at greater risk of developing type 2 diabetes later in life, and their children are at increased risk of developing obesity and type 2 diabetes as they enter adulthood.

A pregnancy complicated by diabetes increases health risks for both mother and fetus (see Box 20-13). Uncontrolled diabetes is linked with increased incidences of miscarriage, birth defects, and fetal deaths. Newborns are more likely to suffer from respiratory distress and to develop metabolic problems such as hypoglycemia, jaundice, and hypocalcemia. Women with diabetes often deliver babies with **macrosomia** (abnormally large bodies), which makes delivery more difficult and can result in birth trauma or the need for a cesarean section. Macrosomia results because maternal hyperglycemia induces excessive insulin production by the fetal pancreas, which stimulates growth and fat deposition.[51] Box 20-14 shows the glycemic goals for pregnant women with diabetes.

Pregnancy in Type 1 or Type 2 Diabetes

Women with diabetes who achieve glycemic control at conception and during the first trimester of their pregnancy substantially reduce the risks of birth defects and spontaneous abortion (see Photo 20-6). For this reason, women contemplating pregnancy should receive preconception care to avoid complications that can result from uncontrolled diabetes. Maintaining glycemic control during the second and third trimesters minimizes the risks of macrosomia and morbidity in newborn infants.

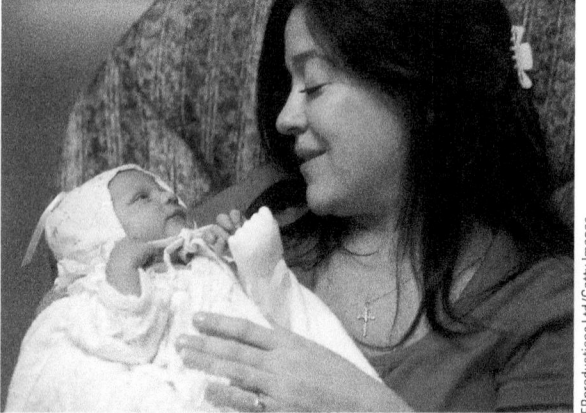

Photo 20-6   Diabetic Pregnancy

Glycemic control during pregnancy offers the best chance of a safe delivery and a healthy infant.

Women with type 1 diabetes require intensive insulin therapy during pregnancy. Insulin adjustments may be necessary every few weeks due to changes in insulin sensitivity. Patients with type 2 diabetes are usually switched from their usual medications to insulin therapy to prevent possible toxicity to the fetus.[52] Although metformin and the sulfonylurea glyburide may be safe to use at conception and during early pregnancy in pregnant women with type 2 diabetes, research data are limited in this population so physicians may be reluctant to prescribe the drugs.[53]

Nutrient requirements during pregnancy are similar for women with and without diabetes. In women with diabetes, however, carbohydrate intakes must be balanced with insulin treatment and physical activity to avoid hypoglycemia and hyperglycemia. To help with this goal, women should consume meals and snacks at similar times each day, and select carbohydrate sources that facilitate glucose control after meals, such as whole grains, fruits, and vegetables. An evening snack is usually required to prevent overnight hypoglycemia and ketosis. When insulin dosages are adjusted, the diabetic woman will need to modify her carbohydrate intake as well.

Gestational Diabetes

Risk of gestational diabetes is highest in women who have a family history of diabetes, are obese, are in a high-risk ethnic group (for example, African American, Hispanic/Latino, Native American, or Pacific Islander), or have previously given birth to an infant

macrosomia (Mak-roh-SOH-mee-ah): the condition of having an abnormally large body; in infants, refers to birth weights of 4000 grams (8 pounds, 13 ounces) and above.

Teresa Cordova is a 41-year-old Mexican-American woman recently diagnosed with type 2 diabetes. Mrs. Cordova developed gestational diabetes while she was pregnant with her second child. Her blood glucose levels returned to normal following pregnancy, and she was advised to get regular checkups, maintain a desirable weight, and engage in regular physical activity. Although she reports that she does not overeat and that she exercises regularly, she has been unable to maintain a healthy weight. At 5 feet 3 inches tall, Mrs. Cordova currently weighs 165 pounds. She has decided to lose weight and join a gym because she is concerned about the long-term effects of diabetes and the possibility that she may need insulin injections. She is also concerned about her husband and children because they are overweight and not very active. The physician refers Mrs. Cordova to a dietitian to help her with her weight-management goals.

1. What factors in Mrs. Cordova's medical history increase her risk for diabetes? Are her husband and children also at risk?

2. Describe the general characteristics of a diet and exercise program that would be appropriate for Mrs. Cordova. How might weight loss and physical activity benefit her diabetes?

3. If Mrs. Cordova is unable to control her blood glucose with diet and physical activity, what treatment might be suggested? Explain to Mrs. Cordova why she would probably not require insulin at this time.

4. What dietary and lifestyle changes may help to prevent diabetes in Mrs. Cordova's husband and children?

weighing over 9 pounds. To ensure that appropriate treatment is offered, physicians routinely test women for gestational diabetes between 24 and 28 weeks of gestation. In high-risk women, testing may begin prior to pregnancy or soon after conception; note that some women may be found to have undiagnosed type 2 diabetes at the earlier time points. Even mild hyperglycemia can have adverse effects on a developing fetus and may lead to complications during pregnancy.

Weight loss is not recommended during pregnancy. For women with gestational diabetes who are overweight or obese, a modest caloric reduction (about 30 percent less than the total energy requirement) may be recommended to slow weight gain.[54] Limiting the carbohydrate intake to less than 45 percent of total energy intake may improve blood glucose levels after meals. Carbohydrate is usually poorly tolerated in the morning; therefore, restricting carbohydrate (to about 30 grams) at breakfast may be helpful. The remaining carbohydrate intake should be spaced throughout the day in several meals and snacks, including an evening snack to prevent ketosis during the night. Regular aerobic activity is recommended because it can help to improve glycemic control. Women who fail to achieve glycemic goals through diet and exercise alone may need to use insulin or an antidiabetic drug that is safe to use during pregnancy (such as metformin or glyburide).[55] The Case Study in Box 20-15 reviews the connections between gestational diabetes and type 2 diabetes.

Review Notes

- Careful management of blood glucose levels before and during pregnancy may prevent complications in mother and infant. Women with diabetes who become pregnant may need to adjust their insulin therapy or medications, consume meals and snacks at similar times each day, and consume an evening snack to prevent overnight ketosis.

- Women with gestational diabetes may need to restrict energy and/or carbohydrate intakes to maintain appropriate blood glucose levels; insulin or an antidiabetic drug may be prescribed to help them maintain glycemic control.

Nutrition Assessment Checklist for People with Diabetes

MEDICAL HISTORY

Check the medical record to determine:

- ○ Type of diabetes
- ○ Duration of diabetes
- ○ Acute and chronic complications
- ○ Conditions, including pregnancy, that may alter treatment

MEDICATIONS

In people with preexisting diabetes who use antidiabetic drugs (including insulin), note:

- ○ Type of medication
- ○ Administration schedule

Check for use of other medications, including:

- ○ Medications that affect blood glucose levels
- ○ Cholesterol- and triglyceride-lowering medications
- ○ Antihypertensive medications

DIETARY INTAKE

To devise an acceptable meal plan and coordinate medications, obtain:

- ○ An accurate and thorough record of food intake and meal patterns
- ○ An account of usual physical activities

At medical checkups, reassess the person's ability to:

- ○ Maintain an appropriate carbohydrate intake
- ○ Maintain an appropriate energy intake

- ○ Monitor blood glucose levels at home
- ○ Adjust insulin and diet to accommodate sick days
- ○ Use appropriate foods to treat hypoglycemia

ANTHROPOMETRIC DATA

Take accurate baseline height and weight measurements as a basis for:

- ○ Appropriate energy intake
- ○ Initial insulin therapy

Periodically reassess height and weight in children and weight in adults and pregnant women to ensure that the meal plan provides an appropriate energy intake.

LABORATORY TESTS

Monitor the success of diabetes treatment using these tests:

- ○ Blood lipid concentrations
- ○ Blood or urinary ketones
- ○ Glycated hemoglobin
- ○ Urinary protein (albuminuria)

PHYSICAL SIGNS

Look for physical signs of:

- ○ Dehydration, especially in older adults
- ○ Foot ulcers
- ○ Nerve damage
- ○ Vision problems

Self Check

1. Which of the following is characteristic of type 1 diabetes?
   a. Abdominal obesity increases risk.
   b. The pancreas makes little or no insulin.
   c. It is the predominant form of diabetes.
   d. It often arises during pregnancy.

2. Which of the following is true about type 2 diabetes?
   a. It is usually an autoimmune disease.
   b. The pancreas makes little or no insulin.
   c. Diabetic ketoacidosis is a common complication.
   d. Chronic complications may develop before it is diagnosed.

3. Most chronic complications associated with diabetes result from:
   a. altered kidney function.
   b. infections that deplete nutrient reserves.
   c. weight gain and hypertension.
   d. damage to blood vessels and nerves.

4. Long-term glycemic control is usually evaluated by:
   a. self-monitoring of blood glucose.
   b. testing urinary ketone levels.
   c. measuring glycated hemoglobin.
   d. testing urinary protein levels (albuminuria).

5. Regarding dietary carbohydrate, a patient with diabetes should be most concerned about:
   a. consuming an appropriate quantity of carbohydrate at each meal or snack.
   b. consuming the correct proportion of sugars, starches, and fiber in meals.
   c. avoiding added sugars and kcaloric sweeteners.
   d. choosing meals with ideal proportions of protein, carbohydrate, and fat.

6. Which of the following is true regarding the general use of alcohol in diabetes?
   a. A serving of alcohol is considered part of the carbohydrate allowance.

b. Alcohol contributes to hyperglycemia and should be avoided completely.

c. Alcohol can cause hypoglycemia and should therefore be consumed with food if patients use insulin or medications that stimulate insulin secretion.

d. Patients can use alcohol in unlimited quantities unless they are pregnant.

7. The most effective meal-planning strategy for managing diabetes is:

a. carbohydrate counting.

b. an eating plan based on food lists created for persons with diabetes.

c. following menus and recipes provided by a registered dietitian.

d. the approach that best helps the patient control blood glucose levels.

8. A patient using intensive insulin therapy is likely to follow a regimen that involves:

a. twice-daily injections that combine short-, intermediate-, and long-acting insulin in each injection.

b. a mixture of intermediate- and long-acting insulin injected between meals.

c. multiple daily injections that supply basal insulin and precise insulin doses at each meal and snack.

d. the use of both insulin and oral antidiabetic agents.

9. In a person who has previously maintained good glycemic control, hyperglycemia can be precipitated by:

a. infections or illness.

b. chronic alcohol ingestion.

c. undertreatment of hypoglycemia.

d. prolonged exercise.

10. Which dietary adjustment may be helpful for women with gestational diabetes?

a. Consuming most of the day's carbohydrate allotment in the morning.

b. Restricting carbohydrate to about 30 grams at breakfast.

c. Avoiding food intake after dinner.

d. Reducing energy intake to about 50 percent of the calculated requirement.

Answers: 1. b, 2. d, 3. d, 4. c, 5. a, 6. c, 7. d, 8. c, 9. a, 10. b

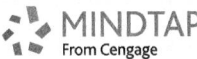 **MINDTAP** From Cengage   For more chapter resources visit **www.cengage.com** to access MindTap, a complete digital course.

Clinical Applications

1. Using the carbohydrate-counting method described in Box 20-8 on pp. 578–579, determine an appropriate carbohydrate intake (in both grams and portions) for a man with type 2 diabetes who requires approximately 2600 kcalories daily. Assume he would benefit from a carbohydrate allowance that is 50 percent of his energy intake. Using information from Tables 20-4 and 20-5 on p. 578, develop a one-day sample menu that is likely to meet his carbohydrate goals. Use the food lists in Appendix C to find additional examples of foods to include in your menu.

2. A diabetes educator typically meets with patients who have a wide variety of problems, concerns, and abilities. What suggestions can be offered to patients who have the problems listed below?

   - An 18-year-old college woman with type 1 diabetes has a date at an unfamiliar restaurant and is uncertain how she will calculate the correct dose of rapid-acting insulin before the meal.

   - A 45-year-old man with an HbA$_{1c}$ value of 8.5 percent states that he is unable to improve his diet because his job keeps him busy all day and his wife handles the food shopping and meal preparations.

   - A 75-year-old man with type 2 diabetes has developed retinopathy and can no longer read the digital display on his blood glucose monitor.

Notes

1. Centers for Disease Control and Prevention, *National Diabetes Statistics Report, 2017: Estimates of Diabetes and its Burden in the United States* (Atlanta, GA: Centers for Disease Control and Prevention, U.S. Department of Health and Human Services, 2017).

2. Centers for Disease Control and Prevention, 2017.

3. American Diabetes Association, Classification and diagnosis of diabetes: Standards of medical care in diabetes—2018, *Diabetes Care* 41 (2018): S13–S27.

4. American Diabetes Association, Classification and diagnosis of diabetes: Standards of medical care in diabetes—2018, 2018.

5. Centers for Disease Control and Prevention, 2017.

6. A. L. May, E. V. Kuklina, and P. W. Yoon, Prevalence of cardiovascular disease risk factors among U.S. adolescents, 1999–2008, *Pediatrics* 129 (2012): 1035–1041.

7. A. Maitra, Endocrine system, in V. Kumar and coeditors, *Robbins Basic Pathology* (Philadelphia: Elsevier, 2018), pp. 749–796.

8. J. Crandall and H. Shamoon, Diabetes mellitus, in L. Goldman and A. I. Schafer, eds., *Goldman-Cecil Medicine* (Philadelphia: Saunders, 2016), pp. 1527–1548.

9. Maitra, 2018.

10. A. M. Kanaya and C. Vaisse, Obesity, in D. G. Gardner and D. Shoback, eds., *Greenspan's Basic and Clinical Endocrinology* (New York: McGraw-Hill/Lange, 2018), pp. 731–741; T. Ota, Chemokine systems link obesity to insulin resistance, *Diabetes and Metabolism Journal* 37 (2013): 165–172.

11. Centers for Disease Control and Prevention, 2017.

12. J. E. von Oettingen and coauthors, Utility of diabetes-associated autoantibodies for classification of new onset diabetes in children and adolescents, *Pediatric Diabetes* 17 (2016): 417–425; R. B. Lipton and coauthors, Onset features and subsequent clinical evolution of childhood diabetes over several years, *Pediatric Diabetes* 12 (2011): 326–334.

13. E. J. Mayer-Davis and coauthors, Incidence trends of type 1 and type 2 diabetes among youths, 2002–2012, *New England Journal of Medicine* 376 (2017): 1419–1429.

14. American Diabetes Association, Prevention or delay of type 2 diabetes: Standards of medical care in diabetes—2018, *Diabetes Care* 41 (2018): S51–S54.

15. S. H. Ley and coauthors, Prevention and management of type 2 diabetes: Dietary components and nutritional strategies, *Lancet* 383 (2014): 1999–2007.

16. Crandall and Shamoon, 2016.

17. U. Masharani and M. S. German, Pancreatic hormones and diabetes mellitus, in D. G. Gardner and D. Shoback, eds., *Greenspan's Basic and Clinical Endocrinology* (New York: McGraw-Hill/Lange, 2018), pp. 595–682.

18. Crandall and Shamoon, 2016.

19. D. G. Gardner, Endocrine emergencies, in D. G. Gardner and D. Shoback, eds., *Greenspan's Basic and Clinical Endocrinology* (New York: McGraw-Hill/Lange, 2018), pp. 783–807.

20. Crandall and Shamoon, 2016.

21. Maitra, 2018.

22. Maitra, 2018.

23. C. J. White, Atherosclerotic peripheral arterial disease, in L. Goldman and A. I. Schafer, eds., *Goldman-Cecil Medicine* (Philadelphia: Saunders, 2016), pp. 497–504.

24. Maitra, 2018.

25. Maitra, 2018.

26. Masharani and German, 2018; Crandall and Shamoon, 2016.

27. American Diabetes Association, Implications of the United Kingdom Prospective Diabetes Study, *Diabetes Care* 25 (2002): S28–S32; Diabetes Control and Complications Trial Research Group, The effect of intensive treatment of diabetes on the development and progression of long-term complications in insulindependent diabetes mellitus, *New England Journal of Medicine* 329 (1993): 977–986.

28. American Diabetes Association, Glycemic targets: Standards of medical care in diabetes—2018, *Diabetes Care* 41 (2018): S55–S64.

29. American Diabetes Association, Lifestyle management: Standards of medical care in diabetes—2018, *Diabetes Care* 41 (2018): S38–S50.

30. American Diabetes Association, Lifestyle management: Standards of medical care in diabetes—2018, 2018.

31. A. B. Evert and coauthors, Nutrition therapy recommendations for the management of adults with diabetes, *Diabetes Care* 37 (2014): S120–S143.

32. J. MacLeod and coauthors, Academy of Nutrition and Dietetics nutrition practice guideline for type 1 and type 2 diabetes in adults: Nutrition intervention evidence reviews and recommendations, *Journal of the Academy of Nutrition and Dietetics* 117 (2017): 1637–1658; Evert and coauthors, 2014.

33. MacLeod and coauthors, 2017; Evert and coauthors, 2014.

34. Evert and coauthors, 2014.

35. Evert and coauthors, 2014.

36. American Diabetes Association, Lifestyle management: Standards of medical care in diabetes—2018, 2018; MacLeod and coauthors, 2017.

37. Evert and coauthors, 2014.

38. Evert and coauthors, 2014.

39. MacLeod and coauthors, 2017; Evert and coauthors, 2014.

40. Evert and coauthors, 2014.

41. M. S. N. Kennedy and U. Masharani, Pancreatic hormones and antidiabetic drugs, in B. G. Katzung, ed., *Basic and Clinical Pharmacology* (New York: McGraw-Hill/Lange, 2018), pp. 747–771.

42. American Diabetes Association, Pharmacologic approaches to glycemic treatment: Standards of medical care in diabetes—2018, Diabetes Care 41 (2018): S73–S85.

43. Kennedy and Masharani, 2018.

44. S. E. Inzucchi and coauthors, Management of hyperglycemia in type 2 diabetes, 2015: A patient-centered approach, *Diabetes Care* 38 (2015): 140–149.

45. American Diabetes Association, Glycemic targets: Standards of medical care in diabetes—2018, 2018.

46. C. Boucher-Berry, E. A. Parton, and R. Alemzadeh, Excess weight gain during insulin pump therapy is associated with higher basal insulin doses, *Journal of Diabetes and Metabolic Disorders* 15 (2016): 47; R. J. Brown and coauthors, Uncoupling intensive insulin therapy from weight gain and hypoglycemia in type 1 diabetes, *Diabetes Technology and Therapeutics* 13 (2011): 457–460.

47. Masharani and German, 2018.

48. American Diabetes Association, Lifestyle management: Standards of medical care in diabetes—2018, 2018; MacLeod and coauthors, 2017.

49. S. R. Colberg and coauthors, Physical activity/exercise and diabetes: A position statement of the American Diabetes Association, *Diabetes Care* 39 (2016): 2065–2079.

50. K. Rosene-Montella, Common medical problems in pregnancy, in L. Goldman and A. I. Schafer, eds., *Goldman-Cecil Medicine* (Philadelphia: Saunders, 2016), pp. 1610–1623.

51. Masharani and German, 2018.

52. American Diabetes Association, Management of diabetes in pregnancy: Standards of medical care in diabetes—2018, *Diabetes Care* 41 (2018): S137–S143.

53. Masharani and German, 2018; R. I. Holt and K. D. Lambert, Use of oral hypoglycaemic agents in pregnancy, *Diabetic Medicine* 31 (2014): 282–291.

54. Academy of Nutrition and Dietetics, *Nutrition Care Manual* (Chicago: Academy of Nutrition and Dietetics, 2018).

55. American Diabetes Association, Management of diabetes in pregnancy: Standards of medical care in diabetes—2018, 2018.

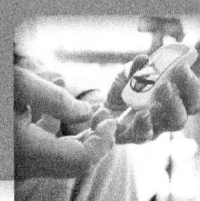

20.4 Nutrition in Practice
The Metabolic Syndrome

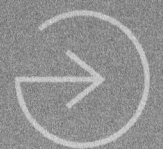

Chapter 20 described how insulin resistance—a reduced sensitivity to insulin in muscle, adipose, and liver cells—can contribute to hyperglycemia and hyperinsulinemia and, eventually, to type 2 diabetes. Insulin resistance is also a central feature of several other conditions, including the **metabolic syndrome**, a cluster of metabolic abnormalities that are associated with an increased risk of developing cardiovascular diseases (CVD) and type 2 diabetes. This Nutrition in Practice describes how the metabolic syndrome is diagnosed, how and why it might develop, its potential consequences, and current treatment approaches. Box NP20-1 defines the relevant terms.

How is the metabolic syndrome diagnosed, and how common is it in the United States?

Table NP20-1 lists the laboratory values used to identify the metabolic syndrome, which is diagnosed when at least three of the following disorders are present: hyperglycemia, abdominal obesity, **hypertriglyceridemia** (elevated blood triglyceride levels), reduced high-density lipoprotein (HDL) cholesterol levels, and hypertension (high blood pressure). Although published values vary, an estimated 23 percent of adults in the United States may meet the criteria for the metabolic syndrome.[1] Prevalence of the metabolic syndrome greatly increases with age, ranging from about 18 percent in people who are 20 to 39 years old to about 53 percent in those who are 60 years old or older. In addition, risk varies according to ethnicity and gender: Mexican-American men have the highest incidence of the metabolic syndrome in the United

States, with an overall prevalence of nearly 35 percent (see Figure NP20-1).[2]

Because the disorders that identify the metabolic syndrome are considered independent risk factors for heart disease or diabetes, some medical experts have questioned whether the diagnosis of metabolic syndrome is a useful one.[3] The main benefit of grouping the disorders may be to

TABLE NP20-1	Features of the Metabolic Syndrome

The metabolic syndrome is diagnosed when three or more of the following abnormalities are present.

MEASURE	REFERENCE VALUE
Hyperglycemia	Fasting plasma glucose ≥100 mg/dL, or undergoing drug treatment for elevated glucose
Abdominal obesity	Waist circumference >40" in men, >35" in women
Hypertriglyceridemia	VLDLs ≥150 mg/dL, or undergoing drug treatment for elevated triglycerides
Reduced HDL cholesterol	HDLs <40 mg/dL in men, <50 mg/dL in women
Hypertension	Blood pressure ≥130/85 mm Hg, or undergoing drug treatment for hypertension

Box NP20-1 Glossary

adiponectin (AH-dih-poe-NECK-tin): a hormone produced by adipose cells that promotes insulin sensitivity.
cytokines (SIGH-toe-kines): signaling proteins produced by the body's cells; many cytokines are produced by immune cells and regulate immune responses.
fibrinogen (fye-BRIN-oh-jen): a liver protein that promotes blood clot formation.
hypertriglyceridemia: elevated blood triglyceride levels. Blood triglycerides are transported in *very-low-density lipoproteins (VLDL).*

metabolic syndrome: a cluster of interrelated disorders, including abdominal obesity, insulin resistance, high blood pressure, and abnormal blood lipids, which together increase the risk of diabetes and cardiovascular disease; also known as *insulin resistance syndrome* or *syndrome X.*
plasminogen activator inhibitor-1: a protein that promotes blood clotting by inhibiting blood clot degradation within blood vessels.
resistin (re-ZIST-in): a hormone produced by adipose cells that promotes insulin resistance.

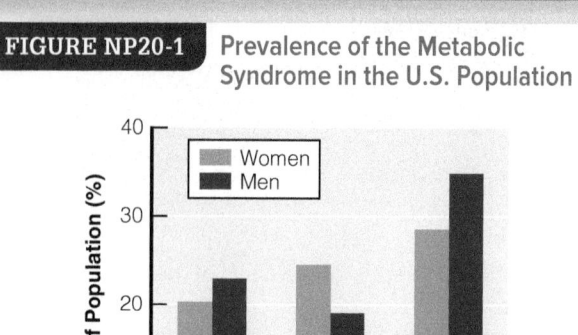

FIGURE NP20-1 Prevalence of the Metabolic Syndrome in the U.S. Population

Source: E. J. Benjamin and coauthors, Heart disease and stroke statistics—2017 update: A report from the American Heart Association, *Circulation* 135 (2017): e146–e603.

guide clinical management of these interrelated metabolic problems.[4] In addition, some studies indicate that heart disease risk actually varies substantially among individuals with the metabolic syndrome, suggesting that further screening is needed to identify those who would benefit from aggressive treatment.[5]

What causes the metabolic syndrome?

Both genetic and environmental factors probably contribute to the development of the metabolic syndrome. However, the close relationship between abdominal obesity and insulin resistance suggests that the current obesity crisis in the United States may be largely responsible for its high prevalence. Visceral fat is thought to induce a number of metabolic changes that promote insulin resistance, which then leads to hyperglycemia and other abnormalities.

How does obesity lead to insulin resistance?

Various theories have been proposed to explain the relationship between obesity and insulin resistance. The enlarged adipose cells of obese individuals have a limited capacity to store triglyceride. Instead, these cells increase their release of fatty acids into the bloodstream, resulting in the abnormal accumulation of triglycerides in the muscle, liver, and other tissues; the high fat content of these tissues may alter cellular responses to insulin that lead to insulin resistance.[6] In addition, enlarged adipose cells alter the hormones and proteins they release into the blood, promoting a state of insulin resistance.[7] For example, obesity is associated with the reduced secretion

of **adiponectin**, an adipocyte hormone that promotes insulin sensitivity and glucose tolerance. Conversely, the adipose cells release larger amounts of the hormone **resistin**, which promotes insulin resistance. Enlarged adipose cells also activate local macrophages (immune cells), which secrete a number of **cytokines** (signaling proteins) that induce inflammation; the inflammatory process leads to multiple metabolic changes that reduce insulin responsiveness.[8]

Can obesity lead to other problems related to the metabolic syndrome?

Abdominal obesity is frequently associated with blood lipid abnormalities. Because the insulin-resistant adipose cells release more fatty acids into the blood, the liver must accelerate its production of very-low-density lipoproteins (VLDL), and hypertriglyceridemia develops.[9] At the same time, insulin resistance hinders the ability of adipose cells to extract and store triglycerides from chylomicrons and VLDL. Excessive body fatness is also associated with elevated low-density lipoprotein (LDL) cholesterol levels and reduced HDL levels.

Several mechanisms may play a role in promoting the hypertension associated with obesity.[10] The hyperinsulinemia that typically accompanies obesity promotes sodium reabsorption in the kidneys, resulting in fluid retention and an expanded blood volume. Elevated fatty acid levels may lead to increased vasoconstriction and reduced vasorelaxation. Some obese individuals have increased sympathetic nervous system activity, which could contribute to hypertension. Finally, adipocytes produce angiotensinogen, a precursor of the vasoconstrictor angiotensin II, which raises blood pressure.

How does the metabolic syndrome contribute to cardiovascular disease risk?

The disorders that characterize the metabolic syndrome—obesity, lipid abnormalities, and hypertension—are all independent risk factors for CVD. In addition, the condition is often associated with blood vessel dysfunction and the tendency to form blood clots, characteristics that favor the development of atherosclerosis and raise the risk of heart attack or stroke. For example, individuals with the metabolic syndrome exhibit reduced production of the vasodilator nitric oxide and increased secretion of the vasoconstrictor endothelin-1—changes that enhance vasoconstriction and stimulate the release of pro-inflammatory cytokines. These cytokines release factors that increase endothelial permeability, recruit immune cells, and increase oxidative stress, thereby promoting atherosclerosis. Inflammation of endothelial tissue, obesity, and insulin resistance may all promote the increased production of procoagulant proteins such as **fibrinogen** and **plasminogen activator inhibitor-1**.[11] Individuals with the metabolic syndrome are also at increased risk of developing diabetes, which is another major risk factor for CVD.

What is the usual treatment for the metabolic syndrome?

The usual treatment goals for the metabolic syndrome are to correct the abnormalities that increase CVD and diabetes risk. In most individuals, a combination of weight loss and physical activity can improve insulin resistance, blood pressure, and blood lipid levels.[12] Even a moderate weight loss (7 to 10 percent of body weight) can improve the abnormalities, although many people find this difficult to achieve. Additional dietary strategies depend on a patient's specific problems. If dietary and lifestyle modifications are not successful, medications may be prescribed. Because effective treatment requires lifelong commitment, health care providers should work with patients to develop a treatment plan that they are willing to adopt.

What dietary strategies, other than weight loss, are suggested for people with the metabolic syndrome?

In individuals with hypertriglyceridemia, the general recommendations are to reduce intakes of added sugars and refined grain products (sugar-sweetened beverages, juices, white bread, sweetened cereal, and desserts) and increase servings of whole grains and foods high in fiber (whole-wheat bread, oatmeal, legumes, fruits, and vegetables).[13] In some people, carbohydrate restriction may help to reduce blood triglyceride levels and improve hyperglycemia. Including fish in the diet each week may also improve triglyceride levels. Individuals with hypertension are encouraged to reduce sodium intake and increase consumption of fruits and vegetables and low-fat milk products. A diet low in saturated and *trans* fats can help to reduce LDL cholesterol levels. Chapter 21 describes additional dietary modifications that may reduce CVD risk.

Why is physical activity recommended for people with the metabolic syndrome?

Regular physical activity helps with weight management and may also improve blood lipid concentrations, hypertension, and insulin resistance—all changes that can reduce the risk of developing CVD.[14] A regular exercise program can also prevent or delay the onset of diabetes in persons at risk (see Photo NP20-1). About 150 minutes per week (about 30 minutes of activity on five days of the week) of moderate-intensity aerobic activity is often suggested,

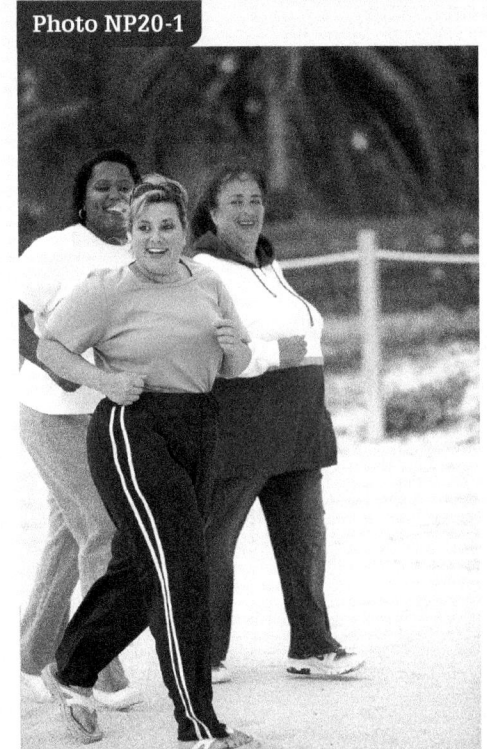

Photo NP20-1

Regular exercise can reduce the risks of developing the metabolic syndrome, cardiovascular diseases, and type 2 diabetes.

Rolf Bruderer/Flirt/Corbis

although longer periods (one hour daily) are recommended for weight control.[15] Resistance exercise, using free weights or weight machines, is beneficial for improving insulin sensitivity and should be performed at least twice weekly. A sedentary lifestyle can worsen the progression of metabolic syndrome and should be discouraged.

What types of medications are used to treat the metabolic syndrome?

If dietary and lifestyle changes are unsuccessful, medications may be prescribed to correct hypertriglyceridemia and hypertension (Chapter 21 provides details). At present, antidiabetic drugs are not routinely used to treat insulin resistance in patients with the metabolic syndrome due to insufficient evidence that the drugs can improve long-term outcomes better than lifestyle changes.

As explained in this Nutrition in Practice, the metabolic syndrome consists of a cluster of interrelated disorders that may increase the risk of developing CVD and type 2 diabetes. Whereas most of the features of the metabolic syndrome are individual risk factors for CVD, in combination they may raise risk twofold to threefold. Treatment of the metabolic syndrome emphasizes dietary and lifestyle changes.

Notes

1. E. Benjamin and coauthors, Heart disease and stroke statistics—2017 update: A report from the American Heart Association, *Circulation* 135 (2017): e146–e603.
2. Benjamin and coauthors, 2017.
3. A. M. Kanaya and C. Vaisse, Obesity, in D. G. Gardner and D. Shoback, eds., *Greenspan's Basic and Clinical Endocrinology* (New York: McGraw-Hill/Lange, 2018), pp. 731–741; S. N. Magge, E. Goodman, and S. C. Armstrong, The metabolic syndrome in children and adolescents: Shifting the focus to cardiometabolic risk factor clustering, *American Academy of Pediatrics* 140 (2017): doi: 10.1542/peds.2017-1603.
4. U. Masharani and M. S. German, Pancreatic hormones and diabetes mellitus, in D. G. Gardner and D. Shoback, eds., *Greenspan's Basic and Clinical Endocrinology* (New York: McGraw-Hill/Lange, 2018), pp. 595–682.
5. S. Malik and coauthors, Impact of subclinical atherosclerosis on cardiovascular disease events in individuals with metabolic syndrome and diabetes, *Diabetes Care* 34 (2011): 2285–2290.
6. Masharani and German, 2018.
7. Kanaya and Vaisse, 2018.
8. Masharani and German, 2018.
9. D. N. Reeds, Metabolic syndrome: Definition, relationship with insulin resistance, and clinical utility, in A. C. Ross and coeditors, *Modern Nutrition in Health and Disease* (Baltimore: Lippincott Williams & Wilkins, 2014), pp. 828–836.
10. M. D. Jensen, Obesity, in L. Goldman and A. I. Schafer, eds., *Goldman-Cecil Medicine* (Philadelphia: Saunders, 2016): 1458–1466.
11. E. Kassi and coauthors, Metabolic syndrome: Definitions and controversies, *BMC Medicine* 9 (May 5, 2011): doi: 10.1186/1741-7015-9-48.
12. Academy of Nutrition and Dietetics, *Nutrition Care Manual* (Chicago: Academy of Nutrition and Dietetics, 2018).
13. L. Berglund and coauthors, Evaluation and treatment of hypertriglyceridemia, *Journal of Clinical Endocrinology and Metabolism* 97 (2012): 2969–2989; M. Miller and coauthors, Triglycerides and cardiovascular disease: A scientific statement from the American Heart Association, *Circulation* 123 (2011): 2292–2333.
14. B. Strasser, Physical activity in obesity and metabolic syndrome, *Annals of the New York Academy of Sciences* 1281 (2013): 141–159.
15. Academy of Nutrition and Dietetics, 2018.

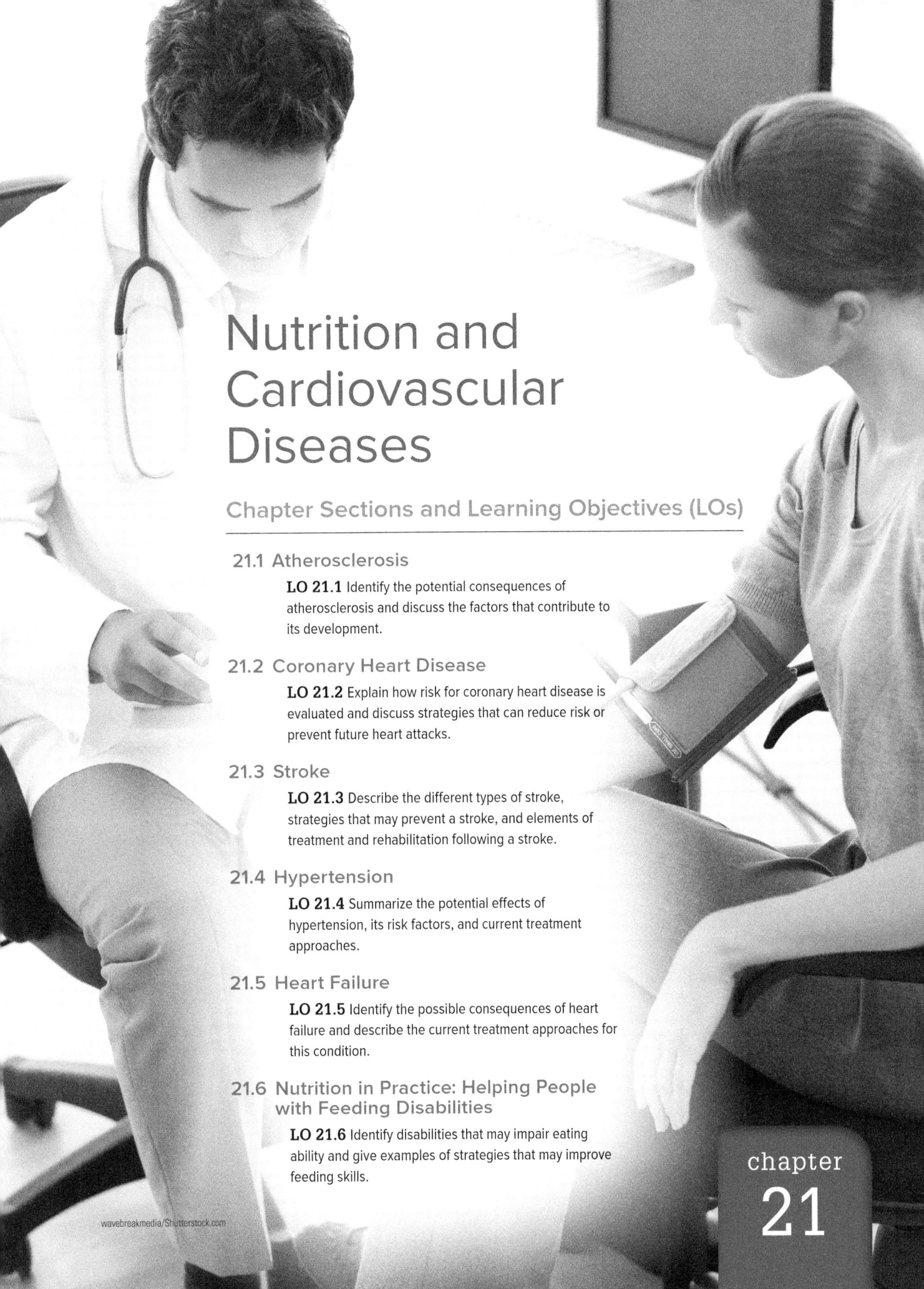

Nutrition and Cardiovascular Diseases

Chapter Sections and Learning Objectives (LOs)

21.1 Atherosclerosis

LO 21.1 Identify the potential consequences of atherosclerosis and discuss the factors that contribute to its development.

21.2 Coronary Heart Disease

LO 21.2 Explain how risk for coronary heart disease is evaluated and discuss strategies that can reduce risk or prevent future heart attacks.

21.3 Stroke

LO 21.3 Describe the different types of stroke, strategies that may prevent a stroke, and elements of treatment and rehabilitation following a stroke.

21.4 Hypertension

LO 21.4 Summarize the potential effects of hypertension, its risk factors, and current treatment approaches.

21.5 Heart Failure

LO 21.5 Identify the possible consequences of heart failure and describe the current treatment approaches for this condition.

21.6 Nutrition in Practice: Helping People with Feeding Disabilities

LO 21.6 Identify disabilities that may impair eating ability and give examples of strategies that may improve feeding skills.

chapter
21

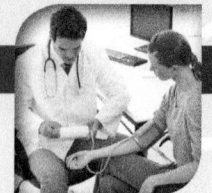

the heart and blood vessels, is responsible for nearly 31 percent of deaths in the United States.[1] Although many people assume that heart conditions are men's diseases, death rates from CVD are similar in men and women. Furthermore, CVD is a global health issue; it is the leading cause of death worldwide.[2] Figure 21-1 shows the percentages of deaths in the United States resulting from the various types of CVD.

The most common form of CVD is **coronary heart disease (CHD)**, which is usually caused by **atherosclerosis** in the coronary arteries that supply blood to heart muscle. If atherosclerosis restricts blood flow in these arteries, the resulting deprivation of oxygen and nutrients can destroy heart tissue and cause a **myocardial infarction**—a **heart attack**. When the blood supply to brain tissue is blocked, a **stroke** occurs. Both heart attack and stroke may result in disablement or death. Box 21-1 defines common terms related to CVD.

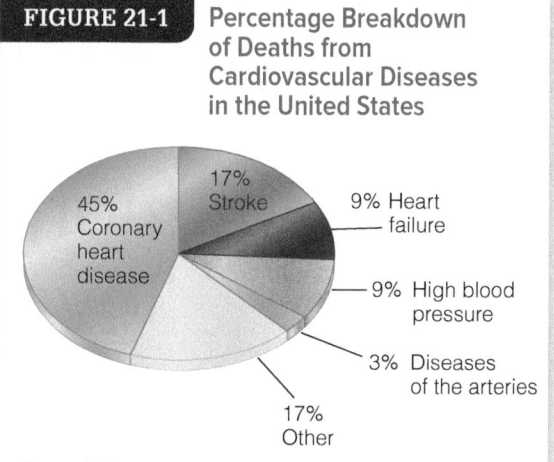

FIGURE 21-1 Percentage Breakdown of Deaths from Cardiovascular Diseases in the United States

- 45% Coronary heart disease
- 17% Stroke
- 9% Heart failure
- 9% High blood pressure
- 3% Diseases of the arteries
- 17% Other

Source: E. Benjamin and coauthors, Heart disease and stroke statistics—2017 update: A report from the American Heart Association, *Circulation* 135 (2017): e146–e603.

Box 21-1 Glossary of Terms Related to Cardiovascular Diseases

aneurysm (AN-you-rih-zum): an abnormal enlargement or bulging of a blood vessel (usually an artery) caused by weakness in the blood vessel wall.

angina (an-JYE-nah or AN-ji-nah) **pectoris:** a condition caused by ischemia in the heart muscle that results in discomfort or dull pain in the chest region. The pain often radiates to the left shoulder, arms, neck, back, or jaw.

atherosclerosis (ATH-er-oh-scler-OH-sis): an arterial disease characterized by a buildup of lipids and fibrous scar tissue on the inner walls of arteries.

cardiovascular disease (CVD): a general term describing diseases of the heart and blood vessels.

- *cardio* = heart
- *vascular* = blood vessels

coronary heart disease (CHD): a chronic, progressive disease characterized by obstructed blood flow in the coronary arteries; also called *coronary artery disease*.

embolism (EM-boh-lizm): the obstruction of a blood vessel by an embolus, causing sudden tissue death.

- *embol* = to insert, plug

embolus (EM-boh-lus): an abnormal particle, such as a blood clot or air bubble, that travels in the blood.

ischemia (iss-KEE-mee-a): inadequate blood supply within a tissue due to obstructed blood flow.

myocardial (MY-oh-CAR-dee-al) **infarction** (in-FARK-shun): death of heart muscle caused by a sudden obstruction in blood flow to the heart; also called a **heart attack**.

- *myo* = muscle
- *cardial* = heart
- *infarct* = tissue death

peripheral artery disease: impaired blood flow in the arteries of the legs; may cause pain and weakness in the legs and feet, especially during exercise. The presence of pain or discomfort while walking is known as *intermittent claudication*.

plaque (PLACK): an accumulation of fatty deposits, fibrous connective tissue, and smooth muscle cells in the walls of blood vessels.

stroke: sudden death of brain cells due to impaired blood flow to the brain or rupture of an artery in the brain; also called a *cerebrovascular accident*.

- *cerebro* = brain

thrombosis (throm-BOH-sis): the formation or presence of a blood clot in blood vessels. A *coronary thrombosis* occurs in a coronary artery, and a *cerebral thrombosis* occurs in an artery that supplies blood to the brain.

- *thrombo* = clot

thrombus: a blood clot formed within a blood vessel that remains attached to its place of origin.

21.1 Atherosclerosis

In atherosclerosis, the artery walls become progressively thickened due to an accumulation of fatty deposits, fibrous connective tissue, and smooth muscle cells, collectively known as **plaque**. Atherosclerosis initially arises in response to minimal but chronic injuries that damage the inner arterial wall.[3] The first lesions tend to occur in regions where the arteries branch or bend due to the disturbed blood flow in those areas (see Figure 21-2). The subtle damage elicits an inflammatory response, attracting immune cells and increasing the permeability of the artery wall. **Low-density lipoproteins (LDL)** slip under the artery's thin layer of **endothelial cells**, become oxidized by local enzymes, and accumulate. Eventually, the plaque thickens and hardens as additional lipids, fibrous proteins, calcium, and cellular debris accumulate. Atherosclerosis begins to develop as early as childhood or adolescence and typically progresses over several decades before symptoms develop.

Consequences of Atherosclerosis

As atherosclerosis worsens, it may eventually narrow the lumen of an artery and interfere with blood flow. Some types of plaque are highly susceptible to rupture, which promotes blood clotting within the artery (**thrombosis**). A blood clot (**thrombus**) may enlarge in time and ultimately obstruct blood flow. A portion of a clot can also break free (**embolus**) and travel through the circulatory system until it lodges in a narrowed artery and shuts off blood flow to the surrounding tissue (**embolism**). Most complications of atherosclerosis result from the deficiency of blood and oxygen within the tissue served by an obstructed artery (**ischemia**).

Atherosclerosis can affect almost any organ or tissue in the body and, accordingly, is a major cause of disability or death. Obstructed blood flow in the coronary arteries can cause pain or discomfort in the chest and surrounding regions (**angina pectoris**) or lead to a heart attack. As mentioned earlier, obstructed blood flow to the brain can injure or destroy brain tissue, causing a stroke. Impaired blood flow in the arteries of the legs (**peripheral artery disease**) can cause pain and weakness in the legs and feet, especially while walking. Blockage of the arteries that supply the kidneys can result in kidney disease or even kidney failure.

Atherosclerosis is the most common cause of an **aneurysm**—the abnormal dilation of a blood vessel. Plaque can weaken the blood vessel wall, and eventually the pressure of blood flow can cause the damaged region to stretch and balloon outward. Aneurysms can rupture and lead to massive bleeding and death, particularly when a large vessel such as the aorta is affected. In the arteries of the brain, an aneurysm may lead to bleeding within the brain, coma, or a stroke.

Causes of Atherosclerosis

The factors that initiate atherosclerosis either cause direct damage to the artery wall or allow lipid materials to penetrate its surface. Factors that generally worsen atherosclerosis or lead to complications are those that cause plaque rupture or blood coagulation. The development of advanced atherosclerosis is a long-term process that involves recurrent plaque rupture, thrombosis, and healing at sites in the artery wall.

Shear Stress/Hypertension The stress of blood flow along artery walls—called **shear stress**—can cause physical damage to arteries.[4] Hypertension (high blood pressure)

FIGURE 21-2 Plaque Formation in Atherosclerosis

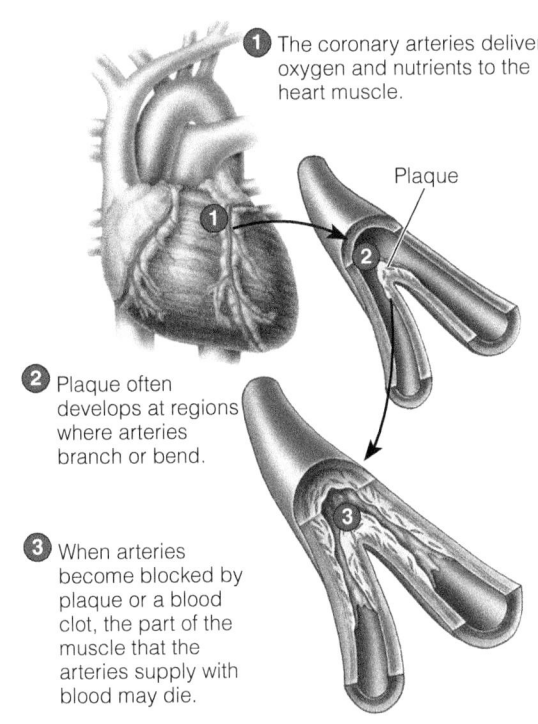

1 The coronary arteries deliver oxygen and nutrients to the heart muscle.

Plaque

2 Plaque often develops at regions where arteries branch or bend.

3 When arteries become blocked by plaque or a blood clot, the part of the muscle that the arteries supply with blood may die.

low-density lipoproteins (LDL): lipoproteins that transport cholesterol in the blood.

endothelial cells: cells that line the inner surfaces of blood vessels, lymphatic vessels, and body cavities.

shear stress: a stress that occurs sideways against a surface rather than perpendicular to a surface. In blood vessels, disturbed blood flow can be harmful to endothelial cells, whereas regular blood flow is protective against atherosclerosis.

intensifies the stress of blood flow on arterial tissue, provoking a low-grade inflammatory state that may stimulate plaque formation or progression.[5]

Abnormal Blood Lipids When LDL levels are high, they are actively taken up and retained in susceptible regions in the artery wall. Elevated levels of **very-low-density lipoproteins (VLDL)** can also promote atherosclerosis, either by influencing the production of other **atherogenic** lipoproteins or by causing molecular changes in endothelial cells and macrophages that promote inflammation or plaque development.[6] Because **high-density lipoproteins (HDL)** remove cholesterol from circulation and contain proteins that inhibit inflammation, LDL oxidation, and plaque accumulation, low HDL levels can contribute to the development of atherosclerosis as well.[7]

LDL vary in size and density, and these LDL subtypes have differing effects on heart disease risk. The smallest, most dense LDL can slip into artery walls easily and are more atherogenic than the larger, less dense LDL.[8] Furthermore, people who have small, dense LDL frequently have elevated VLDL and low HDL levels. This lipoprotein profile is especially prevalent in individuals with the metabolic syndrome and type 2 diabetes.

Elevated concentrations of a variant form of LDL called *lipoprotein(a)* have been found to speed the progression of atherosclerosis and to raise the risk of various types of CVD.[9] Lipoprotein(a) levels are primarily genetically determined and are influenced to only a minor degree by age and environmental factors.

Cigarette Smoking Compounds in cigarette smoke (including nicotine) are toxic to endothelial cells and contribute to arterial injury. Other damaging effects of smoking include chronic inflammation, vasoconstriction, enhanced blood coagulation, increased LDL cholesterol, and decreased HDL cholesterol—all effects that can promote the progression of atherosclerosis.[10]

Diabetes Mellitus Chronic hyperglycemia leads to the accumulation of **advanced glycation end products (AGEs)**, which promote inflammation and oxidative stress, induce the production of compounds that favor plaque progression, and disturb blood vessel function. By various other mechanisms, diabetes increases tendencies for vasoconstriction, endothelial permeability, plaque rupture, and blood clotting.[11]

Age and Sex As a person ages, arterial cells tend to degenerate, and risk factors for CVD accumulate. The risk of atherosclerosis increases significantly in men and women older than 45 and 55 years of age, respectively. After menopause, women's risk increases, in part, because the decline in estrogen has unfavorable effects on lipoprotein levels and arterial function.*[12] Elevated levels of the amino acid **homocysteine**, which may impair endothelial cell function, have been associated with aging and are more prevalent in men; however, it is unclear whether the increased homocysteine levels directly contribute to the disease process or are merely an indicator of abnormal metabolism.[13]

very-low-density lipoproteins (VLDL): lipoproteins that transport triglycerides from the liver to other tissues; in clinical practice, VLDL are commonly referred to as *blood triglycerides*.

atherogenic: able to initiate or promote atherosclerosis.

high-density lipoproteins (HDL): lipoproteins that help to remove cholesterol from the bloodstream by transporting it to the liver for reuse or disposal.

advanced glycation end products (AGEs): reactive compounds formed after glucose combines with protein; AGEs can damage tissues and lead to diabetic complications.

homocysteine: an amino acid produced during the conversion of methionine to cysteine; blood homocysteine levels are influenced by intakes of folate, vitamin B_{12}, and vitamin B_6.

Review Notes

- Atherosclerosis, characterized by the buildup of arterial plaque, can lead to complications such as angina pectoris, heart attack, stroke, peripheral artery disease, kidney disease, and aneurysms.
- Plaque develops in response to long-term, chronic inflammation at susceptible sites in artery walls. Leading causes of plaque development include disturbed blood flow, hypertension, elevated LDL and VLDL levels, cigarette smoking, diabetes, and aging.

*Estrogen replacement therapy after menopause has mixed effects on heart disease risk: it can improve endothelial function and reduce LDL levels, but it also promotes blood clotting.

21.2 Coronary Heart Disease

Coronary heart disease (CHD), also called *coronary artery disease*, is the most common type of cardiovascular disease. As discussed earlier, CHD is characterized by impaired blood flow through the coronary arteries, which may lead to angina pectoris, heart attack, or even sudden death. CHD is most often caused by atherosclerosis but occasionally results from a **spasm** or inflammatory condition that causes narrowing of the coronary arteries.

Symptoms of Coronary Heart Disease

Symptoms of CHD usually arise only after many years of disease progression (see Box 21-2). In angina pectoris and heart attacks, pain or discomfort most often occurs in the chest region and may be perceived as a feeling of heaviness, constriction, or squeezing; the pain may radiate to the left shoulder, arms, neck, back, or jaw.[14] In angina pectoris, the symptoms are often triggered by exertion and subside with rest; in a heart attack, the pain may be severe, last longer, and occur without exertion. Other symptoms of CHD include shortness of breath, unusual weakness or fatigue, nausea, vomiting, and abdominal discomfort. Women are more likely than men to have a heart condition (or even a heart attack) that is unaccompanied by chest pain or acute symptoms.

Evaluating Risk for Coronary Heart Disease

Because heart disease develops over many years, prevention should begin well before symptoms appear. The American Heart Association (AHA) and American College of Cardiology (ACC) recommend a review of CHD risk factors every four to six years in individuals who are 20 to 79 years of age.[15] The major risk factors for CHD are listed in Table 21-1; most of those listed can be modified by changes in diet and lifestyle. The AHA and ACC have developed an online calculator to predict 10-year and lifetime atherosclerotic CVD risk that includes some of these variables (available at tools.acc.org/ASCVD-Risk-Estimator-Plus/#!/calculate/estimate/).

Clinical Measures CHD risk assessment requires several key laboratory measures, as shown in Table 21-2. A typical lipoprotein profile (also called a *blood lipid profile*) includes measures of total cholesterol, LDL and HDL cholesterol, and blood triglycer-

TABLE 21-1 Major Risk Factors for CHD

NONMODIFIABLE RISK FACTORS

- Advancing age
- Family history of heart disease

MODIFIABLE RISK FACTORS

- High LDL cholesterol
- High blood triglyceride (VLDL) levels
- Low HDL cholesterol
- Hypertension (high blood pressure)
- Diabetes mellitus
- Obesity (especially abdominal obesity)
- Physical inactivity
- Cigarette smoking
- Alcohol overconsumption (≥3 drinks per day)
- An atherogenic diet (high in saturated fat and *trans* fats; low in fruits and vegetables)

Note: Risk factors highlighted in the darker blue shade have relationships with diet.

TABLE 21-2 Laboratory Measures for CHD Risk Assessment

CLINICAL MEASURES	ACCEPTABLE	BORDERLINE HIGH RISK	HIGH RISK
Total blood cholesterol (mg/dL)	<200	200–239	≥240
LDL cholesterol (mg/dL)	<100[a]	130–159	160–189[b]
HDL cholesterol (mg/dL)[c]	≥60	Men: 40–59 Women: 50–59	Men: <40 Women: <50
Triglycerides, fasting (mg/dL)	<150	150–199	200–499[d]
Blood pressure (systolic/diastolic)	<120/<80	130–139/80–89[e]	≥140/≥90[f]
Body mass index (BMI)[g]	18.5–24.9	25–29.9	≥30

[a]<70 mg/dL is a desirable goal for very high-risk persons.
[b]LDL levels ≥190 mg/dL indicate a very high risk.
[c]To estimate non-HDL cholesterol, subtract the HDL level from the total cholesterol level; non-HDL cholesterol risk levels are 30 mg/dL higher than the LDL risk levels
[d]Triglyceride levels ≥500 mg/dL indicate a very high risk.
[e]These values are classified as stage 1 hypertension.
[f]These values are classified as stage 2 hypertension. (Physicians use these classifications to determine medical treatment).
[g]Body mass index (BMI) was defined in Chapter 6; BMI standards are found on the inside back cover.

spasm: a sudden, forceful, and involuntary muscle contraction.

ides (VLDL). Some clinicians may use the ratio of total cholesterol to HDL cholesterol or LDL cholesterol to HDL cholesterol to help assess CHD risk. In persons with high blood triglycerides, the non-HDL cholesterol level (total cholesterol value minus the HDL value) may be more accurate than the LDL level for predicting CHD risk.[16] Blood pressure and body weight measurements are also regularly included in risk assessment.

In some individuals, a CHD risk assessment may include tests that provide additional detail about blood lipids or suggest the presence of atherosclerosis.[17] Blood lipid status is sometimes evaluated by measuring LDL and HDL subclasses, the LDL particle number, lipoprotein(a) levels, or levels of proteins or enzymes associated with lipoproteins (especially apolipoprotein B—a component of LDL, lipoprotein(a), and VLDL). Atherosclerosis may be evaluated using the coronary artery calcium score, a value obtained from a computed tomography (CT) scan that analyzes the calcium content of plaque in the coronary arteries. Levels of C-reactive protein, a marker of inflammation, may identify some patients at risk for CHD. The ankle-brachial index, a ratio of blood pressure measurements taken at the ankles and the upper arms, can help to determine the presence or severity of peripheral artery disease.

Blood Cholesterol Levels and CHD Risk Once a person's level of risk has been identified, much of the treatment focuses on lowering LDL cholesterol. Elevated LDL levels are directly related to the development of atherosclerosis, and clinical studies have confirmed that LDL-lowering treatments can successfully reduce the rates of cardiovascular events.[18] CHD is seldom seen in populations that maintain desirable LDL levels.

As mentioned earlier, HDL help to protect against atherosclerosis, and low HDL levels often coexist with other lipid abnormalities; thus, a low HDL level is highly predictive of CHD risk. In addition, low HDL levels are usually associated with other CHD risk factors, such as obesity, smoking, inactivity, and insulin resistance. Although having adequate HDL is beneficial, high HDL levels do not necessarily confer additional benefit.[19]

Lifestyle Management to Reduce CHD Risk

People at significant risk of heart attack, stroke, or other complications of atherosclerosis are typically advised to modify their health behaviors to reduce their risk (see Box 21-3). The main features of lifestyle management include a healthy dietary pattern, regular physical activity, nonsmoking status, and a healthy body weight (see Table 21-3). The following sections describe lifestyle practices that have been found to improve the lipoprotein profiles of individuals with elevated LDL levels.

Healthy Dietary Pattern People with elevated LDL levels have been found to benefit from diets that emphasize vegetables, fruit, and whole grains; include fat-free or low-fat milk products, lean meat, poultry, fish, legumes, nontropical vegetable oils, and nuts; and limit intakes of sweets, sugar-sweetened beverages, and foods high in solid fats.[20] Acceptable diets include the USDA Food Patterns (described in Chapter 1) and the DASH Eating Plan described later in this chapter (see p. 611–612).

Saturated Fat Of the dietary lipids, saturated fat has the strongest effect on blood cholesterol levels, and replacing saturated fats with polyunsaturated or monounsaturated fats can generally lower LDL levels. For individuals with elevated LDL, current guidelines suggest limiting saturated fat intake to less than 7 percent of the total kcalories consumed.[21] The response to a reduced saturated fat intake varies among individuals, however, and may depend on the dietary sources of saturated fat, other nutrients in the diet, body fatness, and genetic factors.[22] The average saturated fat intake in the United States is about 11 percent of the energy intake.[23]

For most people, cutting down on saturated fat involves more than just switching from butter to vegetable oil, as the main sources of saturated fat in the United States include cheese, hamburgers, meat and poultry dishes, and various types of desserts.

BOX 21-3 *Nursing Diagnosis*

The nursing diagnosis *readiness for enhanced health management* applies to people who wish to alter their health behaviors to reduce risk of CHD.

TABLE 21-3 Lifestyle Management to Reduce CVD Risk

Ideal cardiovascular health is defined by the absence of CVD and presence of the following attributes: a healthy dietary pattern, appropriate physical activity, nonsmoking status, a healthy body weight, total blood cholesterol <200 mg/dL, blood pressure <120/<80 mm Hg, and fasting plasma glucose <100 mg/dL.[a] The strategies in this table may allow an individual at significant risk of CVD to achieve these goals.

DIETARY STRATEGIES

- Adopt a healthy dietary pattern such as the USDA Food Patterns or the DASH Eating Plan.
- Limit saturated fat to less than 7 percent of total kcalories and cholesterol to less than 200 milligrams per day. Replace saturated fats with unsaturated fats from fish, vegetable oils, and nuts or with carbohydrates from whole grains, legumes, fruits, and vegetables.
- Avoid food products that contain *trans* fat. The *trans* fat content in packaged foods is shown on the Nutrition Facts panel.
- Choose foods high in soluble fibers, including oats, barley, legumes, and fruit. Use dietary supplements that contain psyllium seed husks to help lower LDL cholesterol levels.
- Regularly consume food products that contain added plant sterols or stanols.
- Fish can be consumed regularly as part of a CVD risk-reduction diet.
- If alcohol is consumed, it should be limited to one drink daily for women and two drinks daily for men.
- To reduce blood pressure, consume a low-sodium diet that is high in fruits and vegetables, whole grains, nuts, and low-fat milk products.

LIFESTYLE CHOICES

- Physical activity: Engage in at least 30 minutes of moderate-intensity aerobic activity on most days of the week.
- Tobacco avoidance: Exposure to any form of tobacco smoke should be minimized.

WEIGHT REDUCTION

- In overweight or obese individuals, weight reduction may improve some CVD risk factors. The general goals of a weight-management program should be to prevent weight gain, reduce body weight, and maintain a lower body weight over the long term.
- The initial goal of a weight-loss program should be to lose no more than 5 to 10 percent of the original body weight.

[a]The concept of *ideal cardiovascular health* was defined and developed by the American Heart Association.

Thus, choosing fat-free or low-fat milk products,* selecting lean meat or fish, and avoiding certain types of desserts are usually more effective ways of reducing saturated fat. Some people may find that limiting their total fat intake can indirectly help them reduce their saturated fat intake.

Replacing saturated fats with carbohydrates can also lower LDL cholesterol, but such a change may raise blood triglyceride (VLDL) levels as well.[24] The effect on blood triglycerides can be minimized by limiting added sugars and including fiber-rich foods; ideally, the diet should include generous amounts of whole grains, legumes, fruits, and vegetables.

Polyunsaturated and Monounsaturated Fat As described in the previous section, replacing saturated fat with either monounsaturated or polyunsaturated fat helps to lower LDL levels; a switch to polyunsaturated fat tends to have the greater effect. In addition, replacing saturated fat with polyunsaturated fat has been associated with reductions in morbidity and mortality from CHD.[25] Note that most polyunsaturated fat in the diet consists of omega-6 fatty acids such as linoleic acid; omega-3 fatty acids may also have beneficial effects on heart disease risk, as described in a later section.

Total Fat As mentioned previously, limiting the total fat intake may indirectly reduce saturated fat; the general recommendation is a fat intake of about 25 to 35 percent of the energy intake.[26] Individuals with elevated blood triglycerides may benefit from achieving a fat intake at the upper end of this range (30 to 35 percent) so that their carbohydrate intakes are not excessive. Fat intakes higher than 35 percent of kcalories are discouraged because they may promote weight gain in some people.

Trans **Fats** *Trans* fats can raise LDL levels, and when they replace saturated fats in the diet (as when stick margarine replaces butter), they may also reduce HDL levels.[27] Furthermore,

*Note that some research suggests that consumption of cheese (and perhaps, other dairy products) may not have adverse effects on CVD risk.

trans fats may raise CHD risk by promoting inflammation and endothelial dysfunction. Thus, the *trans* fat intake should be kept as low as possible.

Most sources of *trans* fats are products made with partially hydrogenated vegetable oils; examples include baked goods such as crackers, cookies, and doughnuts; snack foods such as potato chips and corn chips; and fried foods such as french fries and fried chicken. In recent years, food manufacturers have reformulated many food products so that they contain little or no *trans* fat. In some cases, however, the *trans* fats have been replaced with saturated fat sources, so consumers should read labels carefully to avoid both types of cholesterol-raising fats.

Dietary Cholesterol The influence of dietary cholesterol on CHD risk is somewhat unclear; although some research studies have found a relationship between dietary cholesterol and CHD risk, others have not.[28] Due to concerns about the potential adverse effects of excessive dietary cholesterol in some people, some guidelines recommend cholesterol intakes of less than 200 milligrams per day for high-risk individuals.[29] Cholesterol intakes of women and men in the United States average about 242 and 348 milligrams per day, respectively.[30] Eggs contribute about one-quarter of the cholesterol in the U.S. diet, followed by chicken, beef, and cheese.

The effect of eggs on CHD risk is controversial. While egg intakes have not been linked to CHD risk in healthy populations, a number of observational studies have found an association in persons with diabetes.[31] The optimal number of eggs to include in a heart-healthy diet is undetermined, and different guidelines may be necessary for healthy and high-risk populations.

Soluble Fibers Soluble, viscous fibers can reduce LDL cholesterol levels by inhibiting cholesterol and bile absorption in the small intestine and reducing cholesterol synthesis in the liver. Good sources of soluble fibers include oats, barley, legumes, and some fruits and vegetables. The soluble fiber in psyllium seed husks, frequently used to treat constipation, is effective for lowering cholesterol levels when used as a dietary supplement.

Plant Sterols Foods or supplements that contain significant amounts of **plant sterols** (or *plant stanols*) can help to lower LDL cholesterol levels by interfering with cholesterol and bile absorption. These plant compounds are added to various food products, such as margarine and orange juice, or supplied in dietary supplements. About 2 grams of plant sterols daily (provided by 2 to 2½ tablespoons of sterol-enriched margarines) can lower LDL cholesterol by 5 to 10 percent.[32]

Fish and Omega-3 Fatty Acids The omega-3 fatty acids in fatty fish, eicosapentaenoic acid (EPA) and docosahexaenoic acid (DHA), may benefit people at risk of CHD by suppressing inflammation, lowering blood triglyceride levels, reducing blood clotting, and stabilizing heart rhythm. In addition, including fish in the diet can reduce CHD risk because fish is low in saturated fat and often replaces meat dishes that contain saturated fat. The American Heart Association and several other health organizations recommend consuming two or more servings of fish per week, with an emphasis on fatty fish.[33]

It is not clear whether fish oil supplements have effects similar to those of fish consumption. Some of the more recent clinical trials of EPA and DHA supplementation did not result in lower numbers of heart attacks or heart disease deaths, and researchers have suggested that the benefits of supplementation may be difficult to distinguish from those of other treatments or lifestyle practices.[34]

Alcohol Light to moderate consumption of alcohol—from beer, wine, or liquor—has favorable effects on atherosclerosis, HDL levels, blood-clotting activity, insulin resistance, and overall CHD risk.[35] Consumption should be limited to one drink daily for women and two for men, however, because higher intakes may promote plaque formation and increase blood triglyceride levels and blood pressure. Because alcohol consumption increases the risk of various cancers and may have other detrimental effects on health (see Nutrition in Practice 19), nondrinkers are not encouraged to start drinking in an effort to decrease their risk for CHD.

plant sterols: steroid compounds produced in plants; those added to commercial food products are extracted from soybeans and pine tree oils. Plant sterols can be hydrogenated to produce *plant stanols*, which have LDL-lowering effects similar to those of plant sterols.

Blood Pressure Reduction Excessive dietary sodium may raise blood pressure, whereas potassium can help to lower blood pressure. A low-sodium diet that contains generous amounts of fruits and vegetables, whole grains, nuts, and low-fat milk products has been found to substantially reduce blood pressure, largely due to the diet's content of potassium and several other minerals that have blood pressure–lowering effects. This diet (the *DASH Eating Plan*) and other lifestyle modifications that may reduce blood pressure are discussed in a later section of this chapter.

Regular Physical Activity Regular aerobic activity reverses a number of risk factors for CHD: it can lower LDL levels, reduce blood pressure, improve insulin sensitivity, promote weight loss, strengthen heart muscle, and increase coronary artery size and tone (see Photo 21-1). Current guidelines recommend at least 30 minutes of moderate-intensity activity on most days of the week.[36] Activities that use large muscle groups provide the greatest benefits; such activities include brisk walking, swimming, cycling, stair stepping, and cross-country skiing. If preferred, physical activity can be divided into several sessions during the day. Note that vigorous activity increases the risk of a heart attack or sudden death in individuals with diagnosed heart disease, so sedentary adults may be advised to increase their activity levels gradually.

Smoking Cessation Cigarette smoking is a major risk factor for CHD and other types of cardiovascular disease. In addition to promoting atherosclerosis, cigarette smoking decreases the oxygen supplied to heart tissue, raises the heart rate, inhibits vasodilation, promotes blood clotting, and reduces exercise tolerance, among other effects. Smoking just one or two cigarettes daily—even low-tar, low-nicotine cigarettes—increases CHD risk. Quitting smoking improves CHD risk quickly; the incidence of CHD drops to levels near those of nonsmokers within three years.[37] Currently, about 17 percent of men and 14 percent of women in the United States are cigarette smokers.[38] Although cigar and pipe smoking can also increase the risk of CHD, the risk may not be quite as great because the smoke is less likely to be inhaled.

Weight Reduction Obesity—especially abdominal obesity—is often associated with a number of metabolic abnormalities that increase CHD risk, such as insulin resistance, hypertension, elevated blood triglycerides, low HDL levels, and reduced LDL size. In addition, the adipose tissue of obese individuals produces various types of inflammatory mediators and blood clotting factors, raising the risks of both atherosclerosis and heart attack.[39] Obesity also strains the heart and blood vessels because **cardiac output** is greater, resulting in a greater workload for the left ventricle, which pumps blood to the major arteries.

In persons who are obese, weight reduction can improve such CHD risk factors as hypertension, blood lipid abnormalities, and insulin resistance. The goal of a typical weight-reduction program is a loss of 5 to 10 percent of a person's initial body weight over the ensuing 6 months, followed by additional periods of weight loss until an acceptable weight is reached.[40] For some, maintaining smaller amounts of weight loss may be a desirable starting point.

Managing Lifestyle Changes Adopting multiple lifestyle changes at once is challenging. Health practitioners can help to motivate patients by explaining the reasons for each change, setting obtainable goals, and providing practical suggestions. In some individuals, high LDL levels may persist despite adjustments in health behaviors, and drug therapy may be the only effective treatment. Review Table 21-3 for a summary of the recommendations discussed in this section. Box 21-4 offers suggestions for implementing a heart-healthy diet.

Vitamin Supplementation and CHD Risk

Patients are often interested in the potential benefits of using certain types of dietary supplements for reducing CHD risk, particularly B vitamin and antioxidant

Photo 21-1

Regular aerobic activity can reduce CHD risk by strengthening the cardiovascular system, promoting weight loss, reducing blood pressure, and improving blood glucose and lipid levels.

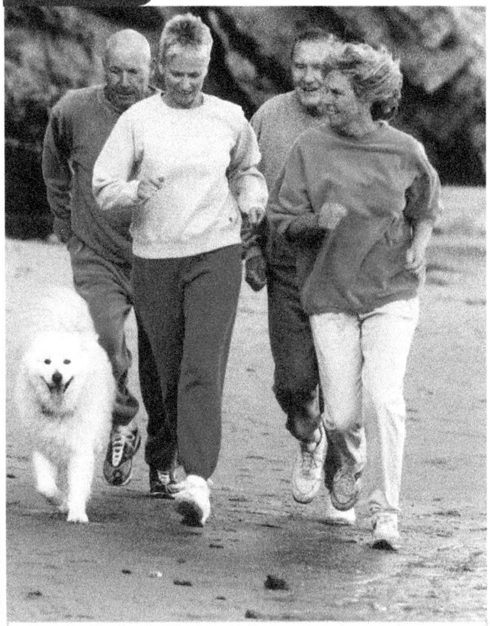

Ronnie Kaufman/Flirt/Corbis

cardiac output: the volume of blood pumped by the heart within a specified period of time.

Box 21-4
HOW TO Implement a Heart-Healthy Diet

For many people, following a heart-healthy diet may require significant changes in food choices. It is often easier to adopt a new diet if only a few changes are made at a time. Discussing positive choices (what to eat) first, rather than negative ones (what not to eat), may improve compliance. These suggestions can help patients implement their diet:

Breads, Cereals, and Pasta

- Choose whole-grain breads and cereals. Make sure the first ingredient on bread and cereal labels is "whole wheat flour" rather than "enriched wheat flour." Consume oats and barley regularly, as they are good sources of soluble fiber.

- Bakery products and snack foods often contain *trans* fat. Buy only food products that list 0 grams of *trans* fat on the Nutrition Facts panel. Ingredient lists should not include any "partially hydrogenated vegetable oil," the main source of *trans*-fatty acids.

Fruits and Vegetables

- Incorporate at least one or two servings of fruits and vegetables into each meal. Keep the refrigerator stocked with a variety of ready-to-eat fruits and vegetables (baby carrots, blueberries, grapes) for snacks.

- Check food labels on canned products carefully. Canned vegetables (especially tomato-based products) are often high in sodium. Fruit that is canned in juice is higher in nutrient density than that canned in syrup.

- Avoid french fries from fast-food restaurants, which are often prepared with *trans* fat. Restrict high-sodium foods such as pickles, olives, sauerkraut, and kimchee.

Lunch and Dinner Entrées

- Prepare plant-based entrees whenever possible. Use soybean products and other legumes as sources of protein in soups, stews, and stir-fry dishes.

- Plan to eat fish twice a week, preferably fatty fish such as salmon, tuna, and mackerel.

- When purchasing meat or poultry, select lean cuts of beef, such as sirloin tip and round steak; lean cuts of pork, such as loin chops and tenderloin; and skinless poultry pieces. Trim visible fat before cooking.

- Select extra-lean ground meat and drain well after cooking. Use lean ground turkey, without skin added, in place of ground beef.

- If you have been advised to reduce cholesterol intake, limit cholesterol-rich organ meats (liver, brain, sweetbreads) and shrimp. Replace whole eggs in recipes with egg whites or commercial egg substitutes.

- Restrict these high-sodium foods: cured or smoked meat such as beef jerky, bologna, corned beef, frankfurters, ham, luncheon meat, salt pork, and sausage; salty or smoked fish such as anchovies, caviar, salted or dried cod, herring, and smoked salmon; and canned, frozen, or packaged soups, sauces, and entrées.

Milk Products

- Select fat-free or low-fat milk products only. Use yogurt or fat-free sour cream to make dips or salad dressings. Substitute fat-free evaporated milk for heavy cream.

- Limit foods high in saturated fat or sodium, such as butter, sour cream, processed cheese, and ice cream or other milk-based desserts.

Fats and Oils

- Prepare salad dressings and other foods with vegetable oils rich in omega-3 fatty acids, such as canola, soybean, flaxseed, and walnut oil. Select other unsaturated vegetable oils—such as corn, olive, peanut, sesame, safflower, and sunflower oil—instead of saturated fat sources such as butter and lard.

- Select only margarine products that list 0 grams of *trans* fat on the Nutrition Facts panel, and avoid products that list "partially hydrogenated vegetable oil" as an ingredient. To help lower LDL cholesterol levels, use margarines with added plant sterols or stanols.

- Add unsalted nuts, seeds, or avocados to meals to make them more appetizing; these foods are good sources of unsaturated fat.

Spices and Seasonings

- Use salt only at the end of cooking, and you will need to add much less. Use salt substitutes at the table.

- Check the sodium content on food labels. Flavorings and sauces that are usually high in sodium include bouillon cubes, soy sauce, hoisin sauce, steak and barbecue sauces, relishes, mustard, and catsup.

- Spices and herbs can improve food flavor without adding sodium. Try using more garlic, ginger, basil, curry or chili powder, cumin, pepper, lemon, mint, oregano, rosemary, and thyme.

Snacks and Desserts

- Select snacks that are low in sodium and saturated fat, such as unsalted pretzels and nuts, plain popcorn, and unsalted chips and crackers. Avoid products that include *trans* fat.

- Select low-fat frozen desserts such as sherbet, sorbet, fruit bars, and some low-fat ice creams.

- Snack on canned or dried fruit and crunchy raw vegetables to boost fruit and vegetable intake.

supplements. Most clinical trials have not been able to confirm any benefits from using these supplements, as described in this section.

B Vitamin Supplements and Homocysteine As mentioned earlier, elevated blood homocysteine is a risk factor for atherosclerosis, but the exact role of homocysteine in the disease process remains unknown. Although increased intakes of folate, vitamin B_6, and vitamin B_{12} can lower homocysteine levels, clinical trials have not demonstrated that supplementation with these vitamins can reduce the incidence of heart attacks in those at risk.[41] Hence, B vitamin supplements are not currently recommended for patients at risk for CHD.

Antioxidant Supplements Because oxidative stress promotes atherosclerosis, researchers have hypothesized that antioxidant supplementation may inhibit atherosclerosis progression and reduce CHD risk. Several epidemiological studies have suggested that antioxidant-rich diets can protect against CHD, but because persons who consume such diets usually maintain a healthy lifestyle and body weight as well, it has been difficult to determine whether the antioxidants were responsible for the effect. Most studies that have tested supplementation with single antioxidants (such as vitamins C or E) or combinations of antioxidants have produced weak or inconsistent results, and several studies suggested possible harm.[42] Until more data are available, the use of antioxidant supplements is not recommended for heart disease prevention.

Lifestyle Changes for Hypertriglyceridemia

Hypertriglyceridemia (see Box 21-5) affects about 24 percent of adults in the United States.[43] It is common in people with diabetes mellitus, obesity, and the metabolic syndrome and may also result from other disorders. Elevated blood triglycerides may coexist with elevated LDL cholesterol or occur separately. Whereas mild or moderate hypertriglyceridemia is often associated with increased CHD risk, more serious cases (blood triglycerides above 500 mg/dL) can cause additional complications, including fatty deposits in the skin and soft tissues and acute pancreatitis.[44]

Nutrition Therapy for Hypertriglyceridemia Dietary and lifestyle changes can improve most cases of mild hypertriglyceridemia.[45] Excessive weight gain and an inactive lifestyle may both raise triglyceride levels. Dietary factors that increase triglyceride levels include high intakes of alcohol and refined carbohydrates; sucrose and fructose are the carbohydrates with the strongest effect. Thus, controlling body weight, being physically active, restricting alcohol, and limiting intakes of refined carbohydrates (especially sweetened beverages and food items made with white flour and added sugars) are basic treatments for hypertriglyceridemia. As mentioned earlier, high triglyceride levels are often associated with low HDL, and the lifestyle changes listed here are likely to improve HDL levels as well.

Severe Hypertriglyceridemia Extreme elevations in blood triglycerides are usually caused by genetic mutations that upset lipoprotein metabolism. In addition to dietary and lifestyle changes, medications are usually necessary for lowering blood triglyceride levels above about 500 milligrams per deciliter. If blood triglycerides exceed 1000 milligrams per deciliter, a very low-fat diet, providing 10 to 15 percent of kcalories from fat, may be required.[46] Patients must also eliminate consumption of alcoholic beverages.

Fish Oil Supplements and Hypertriglyceridemia Fish oil supplements are sometimes recommended for treating hypertriglyceridemia. Clinical trials suggest that a daily intake of 4 grams of EPA and DHA (combined) may reduce elevated triglyceride levels by 25 to 30 percent.[47] Although fish oil supplements can be effective for reducing blood triglyceride levels, the studies have not shown that their use in hypertriglyceridemia patients can improve cardiovascular disease outcomes.[48] In addition, fish oil therapy should be monitored by a physician due to the potential for adverse effects.

Drug Therapies for CHD Prevention

Individuals who cannot improve CHD risk with dietary and lifestyle changes alone may be prescribed one or more medications.[49] The drugs most often prescribed for lowering LDL levels are the *statins* (such as Lipitor and Crestor), which reduce cholesterol synthesis in the liver. Although less effective than the statins, *bile acid sequestrants* (such as Colestid or Questran) can reduce LDL levels by interfering with bile acid reabsorption in the small intestine. For lowering triglyceride levels and increasing HDL, both *fibrates* (such as Lopid and Tricor) and *nicotinic acid* (a form of niacin) are effective; nicotinic acid can also reduce LDL and lipoprotein(a) levels. Individuals using these medications should continue their dietary and lifestyle modifications so that they can use the minimum effective doses of the drugs they require.

In addition to lipid-lowering medications, some people may require drugs that suppress blood clotting (such as anticoagulants and aspirin) or reduce blood

hypertriglyceridemia: elevated blood triglyceride levels.

pressure. Nitroglycerin (a vasodilator) may be given to alleviate angina as needed. Some medications may affect nutrition status or food intake (see Box 21-6); the interactions can be even more complicated when multiple medications are used.

Box 21-6 Diet-Drug Interactions

Check this table for notable nutrition-related effects of the medications discussed in this chapter.

Anticoagulants (warfarin)	**Dietary interactions:** Warfarin requires a consistent vitamin K intake to maintain effectiveness. Drug effects may be enhanced with supplementation of vitamin E, fish oils, garlic, ginkgo, and glucosamine. Drug effects may be reduced with coenzyme Q, St. John's wort, and green tea. Avoid alcohol.
Antihypertensives Calcium channel blockers	**Gastrointestinal effects:** Nausea, GI discomfort, flatulence, constipation, diarrhea
	Dietary interactions: Avoid herbal supplements that contain natural licorice. Avoid grapefruit juice, which may enhance drug effects (depends on specific drug used). Avoid alcohol.
	Metabolic effects: Edema, flushing
ACE inhibitors[a]	**Gastrointestinal effects:** Reduced taste sensation
	Dietary interactions: Food intake and certain mineral supplements may interfere with absorption (depends on specific drug used). Avoid herbal supplements that contain natural licorice.
	Metabolic effects: Elevated serum potassium levels
Antilipimics Statins	**Gastrointestinal effects:** Constipation, flatulence, GI discomfort
	Dietary interactions: Avoid grapefruit juice and red yeast rice, which may enhance drug effects, and St. John's wort, which may reduce drug effects (interactions depend on specific drug used).
	Metabolic effects: Elevated serum liver enzymes
Bile acid sequestrants	**Gastrointestinal effects:** Constipation, flatulence, GI discomfort
	Dietary interactions: May reduce absorption of fat, fat-soluble vitamins, and some minerals.
	Metabolic effects: Electrolyte imbalances, nutrient deficiencies
Nicotinic acid	**Gastrointestinal effects:** GI discomfort (unless taken with milk or food), nausea, diarrhea, flatulence
	Dietary interactions: Alcoholic beverages may increase side effects.
	Metabolic effects: Elevated serum liver enzymes, elevated uric acid levels, hyperglycemia, flushing
Digoxin	**Gastrointestinal effects:** Anorexia, nausea, vomiting, diarrhea
	Dietary interactions: Antacids or magnesium supplements can reduce drug absorption. St. John's wort may reduce drug efficacy.
	Metabolic effects: Electrolyte imbalances
Diuretics (furosemide, spironolactone)	**Gastrointestinal effects:** Dry mouth, anorexia, decreased taste perception
	Dietary interactions: Furosemide's bioavailability is reduced when taken with food. Licorice root may interfere with the effects of diuretics.
	Metabolic effects: Fluid and electrolyte imbalances,[b] hyperglycemia, hyperlipidemias, thiamin deficiency (furosemide), elevated uric acid levels (furosemide)

[a]ACE is an abbreviation for *angiotensin-converting enzyme*. An ACE inhibitor interferes with the conversion of angiotensin I to angiotensin II, a peptide that helps to regulate blood pressure.

[b]*Furosemide* is a potassium-wasting diuretic; patients should increase intakes of potassium-rich foods. *Spironolactone* is a potassium-sparing diuretic; patients should avoid supplemental potassium and potassium-containing salt substitutes.

Treatment of Heart Attack

As explained earlier, a heart attack occurs when the blood supply to heart muscle is blocked, causing death of heart tissue (see Photo 21-2 and Box 21-7). The damage to heart muscle may result in **cardiac arrhythmias** or even heart failure. Drug therapies given immediately after a heart attack may include thrombolytic drugs (sometimes called *clot-busting drugs*), aspirin, anticoagulants, painkillers, and medications that regulate heart rhythm and reduce blood pressure. Patients are not given food or beverages, except for sips of water or clear liquids, until their condition stabilizes.[50] Once able to eat, they are offered a heart-healthy diet, limited to 2000 milligrams of sodium per day, in small portions or as tolerated. The sodium restriction helps to limit fluid retention but may be lifted after several days if the patient shows no signs of heart failure.

A heart attack patient needs to regain strength and learn strategies that can reduce the risk of a future heart attack; such strategies are similar to the lifestyle changes described earlier. Thus, the cardiac rehabilitation programs in hospitals and outpatient clinics include exercise therapy, instruction about heart-healthy food choices, help with smoking cessation, and medication counseling. These programs often last several months. Home-based rehabilitation programs are also beneficial but they are more limited in scope and lack the benefit of group interaction.

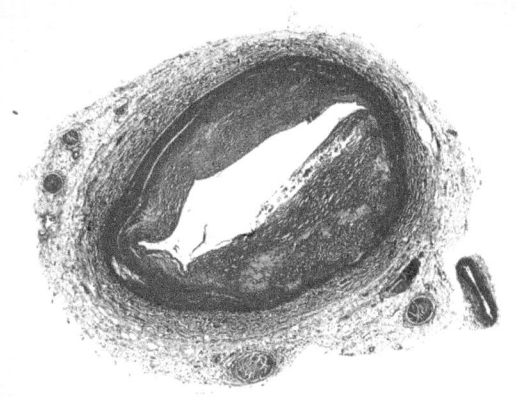

Photo 21-2 Development of a Heart Attack

In a coronary artery narrowed by atherosclerotic plaque, as shown here, a blood clot may form and stop the flow of blood, resulting in a heart attack.

Dr. Gladden Willis/Encyclopedia/Corbis

Review Notes

- Long-term CHD management emphasizes risk reduction. Modifiable risk factors include elevated LDL and triglyceride levels, low HDL levels, hypertension, diabetes, obesity, an inactive lifestyle, cigarette smoking, and various dietary factors.

- Dietary and lifestyle modifications can help to correct blood lipid abnormalities and eliminate other risk factors. Dietary recommendations are to reduce saturated fat, *trans* fats, and cholesterol; increase soluble fiber; and incorporate plant sterols (or stanols) and fish into the diet. Other recommendations include regular physical activity, smoking cessation, and weight reduction.

- Treatment for mild hypertriglyceridemia emphasizes weight control, regular physical activity, and restriction of refined carbohydrates (especially foods with added sugars) and alcohol. More severe cases of hypertriglyceridemia require drug therapies and dietary fat restriction.

- Medications given after a heart attack suppress blood clotting, regulate heart rhythm, and reduce blood pressure. To reduce the risk of a future heart attack, patients can use strategies similar to those recommended for CHD risk reduction.

cardiac arrhythmias: abnormal heart rhythms.

ischemic strokes: strokes caused by the obstruction of blood flow to brain tissue.

hemorrhagic strokes: strokes caused by bleeding within the brain, which destroys or compresses brain tissue.

21.3 Stroke

Stroke is the fifth most common cause of death in the United States and a leading cause of long-term disability in adults. About 87 percent of strokes are **ischemic strokes**, caused by the obstruction of blood flow to brain tissue.[51] **Hemorrhagic strokes** occur in

13 percent of cases and result from bleeding within the brain, which damages brain tissue. Most ischemic strokes are a result of blood clotting within an artery narrowed by atherosclerosis, but an embolism may also cause a stroke. Hemorrhagic strokes often result from the rupture of a blood vessel that has been weakened by atherosclerosis and chronic hypertension. Hemorrhagic strokes are generally more deadly: more than 33 percent of cases result in death within 30 days.[52]

Strokes that occur suddenly and are short-lived (lasting several minutes to several hours) are called **transient ischemic attacks (TIAs)**. These brief strokes are a warning sign that a more severe stroke may follow, and they need to be evaluated and treated quickly. TIAs typically cause short-term neurological symptoms, such as confusion, slurred speech, numbness, paralysis, or difficulty speaking. Treatment includes the use of aspirin and other drugs that inhibit blood clotting.

Stroke Prevention

Stroke is largely preventable by recognizing its risk factors and making lifestyle choices that reduce risk. Many of the risk factors are similar to those for heart disease and include hypertension, elevated LDL cholesterol, diabetes mellitus, cigarette smoking, physical inactivity, aging, and genetic influences.[53] Medications that suppress blood clotting reduce the risk of ischemic stroke, especially in people who have suffered a first stroke or a TIA. The drugs typically prescribed include antiplatelet drugs (including aspirin) and anticoagulants such as warfarin (Coumadin). Anticoagulant therapy requires regular follow-up and occasional adjustments in dosage to prevent excessive bleeding.

Stroke Management

The effects of a stroke vary according to the area of the brain that has been injured (see Box 21-8). Body movements, senses, and speech are often impaired, and one side of the body may be weakened or paralyzed. Early diagnosis and treatment are necessary to preserve brain tissue and minimize long-term disability. Ideally, thrombolytic (clot-busting) drugs should be used within 4½ hours following an ischemic stroke to restore blood flow and prevent further brain damage.[54] After patients have stabilized, they are usually started on medications that help to prevent stroke recurrence or complications, including anticoagulants or antiplatelet drugs, antihypertensives, and blood lipid-lowering drugs.

Rehabilitation programs typically start as soon as possible after stabilization. Patients must be evaluated for neurological deficits, sensory loss, mobility impairments, bowel and bladder function, communication ability, and psychological problems. Rehabilitation services often include physical therapy, occupational therapy, speech and language pathology, and kinesiotherapy (training to improve strength and mobility).

The focus of nutrition care is to help patients maintain nutrition status and overall health despite the disabilities caused by the stroke. The initial assessment should determine the nature of the patient's self-feeding difficulty (if any) and the adjustments required for appropriate food intake. Some patients may need to learn about dietary treatments that improve blood lipid levels and blood pressure. Dysphagia (difficulty swallowing) is a frequent complication and is associated with a poorer prognosis. Difficulty with speech may prevent patients from communicating food preferences or describing the problems they may be having with eating. Coordination problems can make it hard for patients to grasp utensils or bring food from table to mouth. In some cases, tube feedings may be necessary until the patient has regained these skills. Nutrition in Practice 21 describes additional options for people who have disabilities that impair eating ability as a result of a stroke or other condition.

transient ischemic attacks (TIAs): brief ischemic strokes that cause short-term neurological symptoms.

21.4 Hypertension

Although people cannot feel the physical effects of hypertension (high blood pressure), it is a primary risk factor for atherosclerosis and cardiovascular diseases. In addition to hypertension's damaging effect on arteries, elevated blood pressure forces the heart to work harder to eject blood into the arteries; this effort weakens heart muscle and increases the risk of developing heart arrhythmias, heart failure, and even sudden death. Hypertension is also a primary cause of stroke and kidney failure, and reducing blood pressure can dramatically reduce the incidence of these diseases. Photo 21-3 shows a common technique for measuring blood pressure, and Box 21-9 explains how to interpret blood pressure readings.

Hypertension affects about 46 percent of adults in the United States.[55] Prevalence is especially high in African Americans, who develop hypertension earlier in life and sustain higher average blood pressures throughout their lives than other ethnic groups. An estimated 16 percent of people with hypertension are unaware that they have it.[56]

Factors That Influence Blood Pressure

As shown in Figure 21-3, blood pressure depends on the volume of blood pumped by the heart (cardiac output) and the resistance the blood encounters in the arterioles (peripheral resistance). When either cardiac output or peripheral resistance increases, blood pressure rises. Cardiac output is raised when heart rate or blood volume increases; peripheral resistance is affected mainly by the diameters of the arterioles and blood viscosity. Blood pressure is therefore influenced by the nervous system, which regulates heart muscle contractions and arteriole diameters, and hormonal signals, which may cause fluid retention or blood vessel constriction. The kidneys also play a role in regulating blood pressure by controlling the secretion of the hormones involved in vasoconstriction and retention of sodium and water.

Factors That Contribute to Hypertension

In 90 to 95 percent of hypertension cases, the cause is unknown (called **primary hypertension**).[57] In other cases, hypertension is caused by a known physical or metabolic disorder (**secondary hypertension**), such as an abnormality in an organ or hormone involved in blood pressure regulation. For example, conditions characterized by the narrowing of renal arteries often result in the increased production of proteins and hormones that stimulate water retention and vasoconstriction, thereby raising blood pressure. A number of hormonal disorders and medications may also cause secondary hypertension.

BOX 21-9

Blood pressure is measured both when heart muscle contracts (*systolic* blood pressure) and when it relaxes (*diastolic* blood pressure). Measurements are expressed as millimeters of mercury (mm Hg).

	SYSTOLIC	DIASTOLIC
• Normal	<120	<80
• Elevated	120–129	<80
• Stage 1 hypertension	130–139	80–89
• Stage 2 hypertension	≥140	≥90

primary hypertension: hypertension with an unknown cause; also known as *essential hypertension*.

secondary hypertension: hypertension that results from a known physiological abnormality.

Photo 21-3 Hypertension Screening

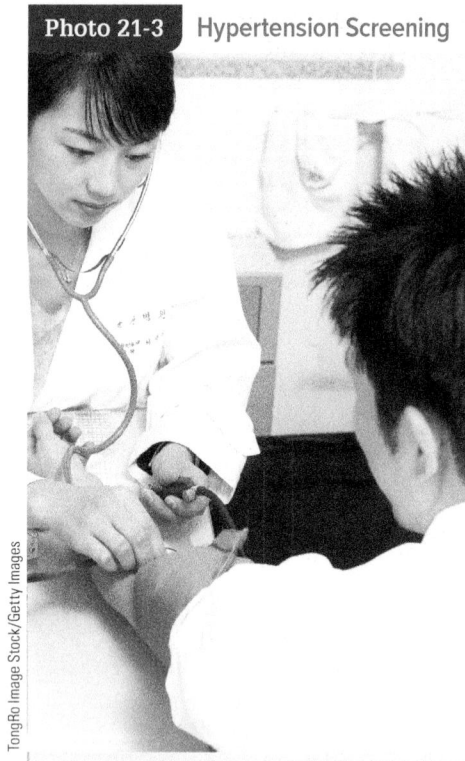

To determine blood pressure, the clinician restricts blood flow in the brachial artery using an inflatable cuff, and then slowly releases air from the cuff until blood flow resumes, indicating that blood pressure in the artery has matched or exceeded the air pressure in the cuff.

FIGURE 21-3 Determinants of Blood Pressure

Blood pressure is influenced by both cardiac output and peripheral resistance as expressed by the formula *Blood Pressure = Cardiac Output × Peripheral Resistance*.

Cardiac output is the volume of blood pumped by the heart within a specified period of time.

Peripheral resistance refers to the resistance to pumped blood by the small arterial branches (arterioles) that carry blood to tissues.

BOX 21-10 *Nursing Diagnosis*

The nursing diagnosis *ineffective health maintenance* may apply to some individuals with hypertension.

A number of risk factors for hypertension have been identified, and some can be modified by changes in diet or lifestyle (see Box 21-10). The major risk factors include the following:

- *Increased age.* Hypertension risk increases with age. In the United States, about 76 percent of persons aged 65 years or older have hypertension.[58] Moreover, at least 90 percent of individuals who live long enough are likely to develop hypertension during their lifetimes.[59]
- *Genetic factors.* Risk of hypertension is similar among family members. It is also more prevalent and severe in certain ethnic groups; for example, the prevalence in African-American adults is about 58 percent, compared with a prevalence of about 44 percent in whites, 43 percent in Hispanics, and 41 percent in non-Hispanic Asians.[60]
- *Obesity.* Numerous clinical studies have confirmed a strong relationship between excess body fat and increased blood pressure.[61] Obesity raises blood pressure, in part, by stimulating the sympathetic nervous system and activating hormonal processes that promote sodium reabsorption and blood vessel constriction.[62]
- *Salt sensitivity.* More than half of the adults in the United States have blood pressure that is sensitive to salt intake.[63] Salt sensitivity (also called *sodium sensitivity*) is influenced by age, sex, genetic factors, body fatness, and the presence of diabetes, kidney disease, or hypertension itself.[64]
- *Alcohol.* Heavy drinking (three or more drinks daily) increases the incidence and severity of hypertension. The mechanisms involved are unclear but probably include activation of the sympathetic nervous system and altered responses of endothelial tissue in the presence of alcohol.[65] Alcohol's effects are transient, as blood pressure falls quickly after consumption is stopped.

- *Dietary factors.* A person's diet may influence hypertension risk. As explained later, diets that emphasize vegetables, fruit, and whole grains and include low-fat milk products have been shown to reduce blood pressure.

Treatment of Hypertension

Controlling hypertension improves CVD risk considerably: a 10 mm Hg reduction in systolic blood pressure (or a 5 mm Hg reduction in diastolic blood pressure) may lower the risks of death from CHD and stroke by about 45 and 55 percent, respectively.[66] Both lifestyle modifications and medications are used to treat hypertension. For many people with stage 1 hypertension (review Box 21-9), changes in diet and lifestyle alone may lower blood pressure to a normal level.

Table 21-4 lists lifestyle modifications that can reduce blood pressure and the expected decrease in systolic blood pressure for each change. The recommendations include reducing weight if overweight or obese, adopting a healthy dietary pattern, engaging in regular physical activity, and limiting alcohol intake, if one chooses to drink.[67] Combining two or more of these modifications can enhance results. As Table 21-4 shows, weight reduction and dietary adjustments generally have the most significant effects on blood pressure.

Weight Reduction In obese individuals, weight reduction may lower blood pressure significantly. Clinical studies suggest that systolic blood pressure can be decreased by about 1 mm Hg for each kilogram of weight loss and that the blood pressure reduction may be sustained for several years.[68] In the long term, however (more than three years), blood pressure tends to revert to initial levels, even when weight loss is partially maintained. Weight reduction is most beneficial for blood pressure control during periods when the body weight is actually decreasing.[69] Moreover, larger amounts of weight loss seem to provide more substantial improvements in blood pressure than smaller amounts.[70]

Dietary Approaches for Blood Pressure Reduction A number of research studies have shown that a significant reduction in blood pressure can be achieved by following a diet

TABLE 21-4 Lifestyle Modifications for Blood Pressure Reduction

LIFESTYLE MODIFICATION	RECOMMENDATION	EXPECTED DECREASE IN SYSTOLIC BLOOD PRESSURE
Weight reduction if overweight or obese	Reduce weight to achieve a healthy body weight (BMI 18.5–24.9).	1 mm Hg for every 1 kg of weight loss
Healthy diet, such as the DASH Eating Plan[a]	Consume a diet rich in vegetables, fruit, and whole grains that includes low-fat milk products and limits saturated fat, sugars, and red meat.	11 mm Hg
Reduced intake of dietary sodium	Reduce sodium intake by at least 1000 mg per day; the ideal intake is <1500 mg of sodium per day.	5–6 mm Hg
Increased intake of dietary potassium	Consume 3500–5000 mg of potassium per day, preferably by consuming a potassium-rich diet.	4–5 mm Hg
Physical activity	Participate in 90–150 minutes of moderate-to-vigorous aerobic activity and three sessions of resistance exercise each week.	4–8 mm Hg
Moderate alcohol consumption	Men: Limit alcohol intake to two drinks daily. Women and lighter-weight men: Limit alcohol intake to one drink daily.	4 mm Hg

[a]The DASH Eating Plan was tested in a study called *Dietary Approaches to Stop Hypertension.*

Source: P. K. Whelton and coauthors, 2017 ACC/AHA/AAPA/ABC/ACPM/AGS/APhA/ASH/ASPC/NMA/PCNA guideline for the prevention, detection, evaluation, and management of high blood pressure in adults, *Journal of the American College of Cardiology* (2017): doi: 10.1016/j.jacc.2017.11.006.

that emphasizes fruit, vegetables, and whole grains and includes low-fat milk products, poultry, fish, and nuts.[71] This type of dietary pattern provides more fiber, potassium, magnesium, and calcium than the typical American diet. The most popular diet tested in these studies, known as the DASH Eating Plan (see Table 21-5), also limits red meat, sweets, sugar-containing beverages, saturated fat (to 7 percent of kcalories), and cholesterol (to 150 milligrams per day), so it is beneficial for reducing CHD risk as well.[72] During the eight-week study period when hypertensive subjects consumed the DASH diet, their systolic blood pressures fell by 11.4 mm Hg more than the blood pressures of subjects who remained on the standard American control diet.[73]

The DASH Eating Plan is even more effective when accompanied by a low sodium intake. In a research study that tested the blood pressure-lowering effects of the DASH dietary pattern in combination with sodium restriction, the best results were achieved when sodium was reduced to 1500 milligrams daily—a level much lower than the amounts typically consumed in the United States (average sodium intakes for men and women are about 4100 milligrams and 3000 milligrams per day, respectively[74]). Note that a sodium intake as low as 1500 mg per day may lead to health problems in some individuals;* thus, the optimal sodium intake for hypertensive patients is still in question.[75]

TABLE 21-5 The DASH Eating Plan

FOOD GROUP	RECOMMENDED SERVINGS FOR DIFFERENT ENERGY INTAKES (SERVINGS PER DAY EXCEPT AS NOTED)			
	1600 kcal	2000 kcal	2600 kcal	3100 kcal
Grains and grain products[a] (1 serving = 1 slice bread, 1 oz dry cereal,[b] or ½ c cooked rice, pasta, or cereal)	6	6–8	10–11	12–13
Vegetables (1 serving = ½ c cooked vegetables, 1 c raw leafy vegetables, or ½ c vegetable juice)	3–4	4–5	5–6	6
Fruit (1 serving = 1 medium fruit; ½ c fresh, frozen, or canned fruit; ¼ c dried fruit; or ½ c fruit juice)	4	4–5	5–6	6
Milk products (low fat or fat free) (1 serving = 1 c milk or yogurt, or 1½ oz cheese)	2–3	2–3	3	3–4
Meat, poultry, and fish (1 serving = 1 oz cooked lean meat, poultry, or fish; or 1 egg)	3–4 oz or less	6 oz or less	6 oz or less	6–9 oz or less
Nuts, seeds, and legumes (1 serving = ⅓ c nuts, 2 tbs peanut butter, 2 tbs seeds, or ½ c cooked dry beans or peas)	3–4 per week	4–5 per week	1	1
Fats and oils (1 serving = 1 tsp vegetable oil or soft margarine, ½ tbs mayonnaise, or 1 tbs salad dressing)	2	2–3	3	4
Sweets and added sugars (1 serving = 1 tbs sugar, jelly, or jam; ½ c sorbet; or 1 c lemonade)	3 or less per week	5 or less per week	≤2	≤2

[a]Whole grains are recommended for most servings consumed.

[b]One ounce of dry cereal may be equivalent to ½ to 1¼ cups, depending on the cereal. Check the food label for the portion size.

Source: U.S. Department of Agriculture and U.S. Department of Health and Human Services, *Dietary Guidelines for Americans, 2010* (Washington, D.C.: U.S. Government Printing Office, 2010).

---

*As an example, sodium intakes lower than 2 grams per day have been associated with increased hospital readmissions and mortality rates in some heart failure patients. Other examples of adverse effects are described in the references listed.

Box 21-11

HOW TO Reduce Sodium Intake

- Select fresh, unprocessed foods. Packaged foods, canned goods, and frozen meals are often high in sodium.
- Do not use salt at the table or while cooking. Salt substitutes may be useful for some people. Salt substitutes often contain potassium, however, and are not appropriate for people using diuretics that promote potassium retention in the blood.
- Avoid eating in fast-food restaurants; most menu choices are very high in sodium.
- Check food labels. The labeling term *low sodium* is a better guide than the terms *reduced sodium* (contains 25 percent less sodium than the regular product) or *light in sodium* (contains 50 percent less sodium). To be labeled *low sodium*, a food product must contain less than 140 milligrams of sodium per serving. Keep your sodium goal in mind when you read labels.
- Recognize the high-sodium foods in each food category, and purchase only unsalted or low-sodium varieties of these products if they are available. High-sodium foods include the following:
  - Snack foods made with added salt, such as tortilla chips, popcorn, and nuts.

- Processed meat, such as ham, corned beef, bologna, salami, sausage, bacon, frankfurters, and pastrami.
- Processed fish, such as salted fish and canned fish.
- Tomato-based products, such as tomato sauce, tomato juice, pizza, canned tomatoes, and catsup.
- Canned soup or broth; note that even reduced-sodium varieties may contain excessive sodium.
- Cheese, such as cottage cheese, American cheese, and Parmesan and most other hard cheeses.
- Bakery products made with baking powder or baking soda (sodium bicarbonate), such as cake, cookies, doughnuts, and muffins.
- Condiments and relishes, such as bouillon cubes, olives, and pickled vegetables.
- Flavoring sauces, such as soy sauce, hoisin sauce, barbecue sauce, and steak sauce.
- Check for the word *sodium* on medication labels. Sodium is often an ingredient in some types of antacids and laxatives.

Sodium restriction by itself can have a modest blood pressure-lowering effect (review Table 21-4), but some people are more responsive than others. Although a low-sodium diet may improve blood pressure to some extent, it should be combined with other lifestyle modifications for greater effect. Box 21-11 lists practical suggestions for restricting sodium intake; additional detail is provided in Table 22-1 on p. 629.

Drug Therapies People with hypertension usually require two or more medications to meet their blood pressure goals. Using a combination of drugs with different modes of action can reduce the doses of each drug needed and minimize side effects. Most treatments include diuretics, which lower blood pressure by reducing blood volume. Other medications commonly prescribed include calcium channel blockers, angiotensin-converting enzyme (ACE) inhibitors, and angiotensin-receptor blockers (see Box 21-12); some of these drugs are also used to treat various heart conditions. Drug dosages may need regular adjustment until the blood pressure goal is reached.

BOX 21-12

Medications that lower blood pressure:

- *ACE inhibitors* interfere with the production of angiotensin II, a vasoconstrictor.
- *Angiotensin-receptor blockers* interfere with angiotensin II activity.
- *Calcium channel blockers* inhibit calcium's entry into arterial cells, promoting vasodilation.
- *Diuretics* increase urine output, reducing blood volume.

Review Notes

- About 46 percent of adults in the United States have hypertension, which increases the risk of developing CHD, stroke, heart failure, and kidney failure.
- Blood pressure is elevated by factors that increase blood volume, heart rate, or resistance to blood flow. Although the underlying cause of most hypertension cases is unknown, risk factors include increased age, genetic factors, obesity, and various dietary practices.
- Treatment of hypertension usually includes a combination of lifestyle modifications and drug therapies.

The Case Study in Box 21-13 (p. 614) provides an opportunity to review the risk factors and treatments for CHD and hypertension.

| Box 21-13 | **Case Study: Patient with Cardiovascular Disease** |

Robert Reid, a 48-year-old African-American computer programmer, is 5 feet 9 inches tall and weighs 240 pounds. He sits for long hours at work and is too tired to exercise when he gets home at night. His meals usually include fatty meat, eggs, and cheese, and he likes dairy desserts such as pudding and ice cream. He has a family history of CHD and hypertension. His recent laboratory tests show that his blood pressure is 160/100 mm Hg, and his LDL and HDL levels are 160 mg/dL and 35 mg/dL, respectively. He smokes a pack of cigarettes each day and usually has two glasses of wine at both lunch and dinner.

1. Identify Mr. Reid's major risk factors for CHD and hypertension. Which can be modified? What complications might occur if he delays treatment for his blood lipids and blood pressure?

2. What dietary changes would you recommend that could help to improve Mr. Reid's blood pressure and LDL cholesterol level? Explain the rationale for each dietary change. Prepare a day's menu for Mr. Reid using the DASH Eating Plan as an outline for your choices.

3. What other laboratory tests or measurements would you need to better assess Mr. Reid's condition? Why?

4. Describe several benefits that Mr. Reid might obtain from a program that includes weight reduction and regular physical activity. Explain why the use of alcohol can be both a protective and a damaging lifestyle habit.

5. Assuming that Mr. Reid does not make any changes in his diet and lifestyle and suffers a heart attack, identify the elements of a cardiac rehabilitation program that would be critical for his long-term survival.

21.5 Heart Failure

Heart failure is characterized by the heart's inability to pump enough blood, resulting in inadequate blood delivery and a buildup of fluids in the veins and tissues. Heart failure has various causes, but it is often a consequence of chronic disorders that create extra work for the heart muscle, such as hypertension or CHD. To accommodate the extra workload, the heart enlarges or pumps faster or harder, but eventually it may weaken enough to fail completely (see Photo 21-4). Heart failure develops mainly in older adults and is the leading cause of hospitalization in individuals over 65 years of age.[76]

Consequences of Heart Failure

The effects of heart failure depend on the severity of illness: mild cases may be asymptomatic, but severe cases may cause considerable damage to health (see Box 21-14). Heart failure may begin on the left or the right side of the heart, or both sides may fail simultaneously.

- *Left-sided heart failure.* The left side of the heart normally receives blood from the lungs and pumps it to peripheral tissues. A weakened left heart may allow fluid to build up in the lungs (a condition called *pulmonary edema*), resulting in extreme shortness of breath, limited oxygen for activity, and, in severe cases, respiratory failure. The inadequate blood flow to tissues can result in organ dysfunction. In addition, fluid accumulation within the lungs increases fluid pressure in the right side of the heart, potentially damaging heart tissue and leading to right-sided heart failure.

- *Right-sided heart failure.* The right side of the heart normally receives blood from the peripheral tissues and pumps blood to the lungs. With impaired pumping, fluids can back up into the abdomen and peripheral tissues, potentially causing **ascites**, liver and spleen enlargement, impaired liver and gastrointestinal function, and swelling in the legs, ankles, and feet.

heart failure: a condition characterized by the heart's inability to pump adequate blood to the body's cells, resulting in fluid accumulation in the tissues; also called *congestive heart failure.*

ascites: (ah-SIGH-teez): an abnormal accumulation of fluid in the abdominal cavity.

cardiac cachexia: severe malnutrition that develops in heart failure patients; characterized by weight loss and tissue wasting.

Heart failure often affects a person's food intake and level of physical activity. In persons with abdominal bloating and liver enlargement, pain and discomfort may worsen with meals. Limb weakness and fatigue can limit physical activity. End-stage heart failure is often accompanied by **cardiac cachexia**, a condition of severe malnutrition characterized by significant weight loss and tissue wasting. Cardiac cachexia may develop due to increased levels of pro-inflammatory cytokines (which promote catabolism), elevated metabolic rate, reduced food intake, and malabsorption. The resultant weakness further lowers the person's strength, functional capacity, and activity levels.

Photo 21-4 Heart Failure

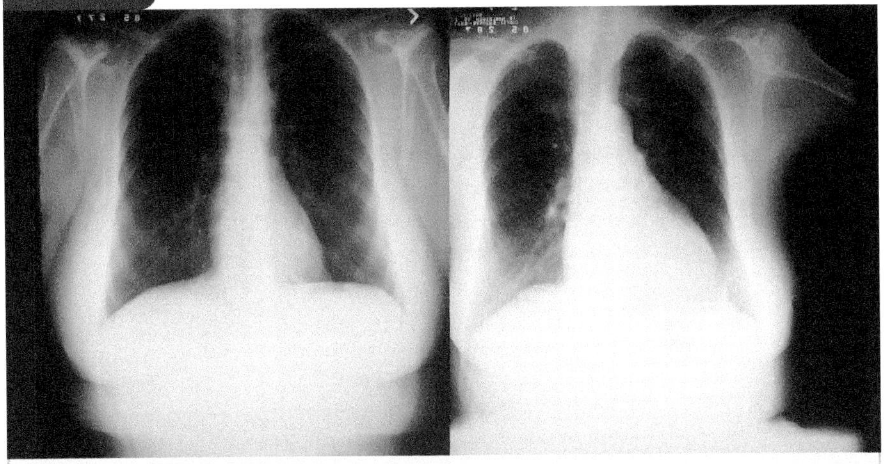

In heart failure, the overburdened heart enlarges in an effort to supply blood to the body's tissues.

Susan Leavines/Science Source

Medical Management of Heart Failure

Heart failure is a chronic, progressive illness that may require frequent hospitalizations. Many patients face a combination of debilitating symptoms, complex treatments, and an uncertain outcome. Important goals of medical therapy are to slow disease progression and enhance the patient's quality of life.

The specific treatment for heart failure depends on the nature and severity of the illness. Medications help to manage fluid retention and improve heart function. Dietary sodium and fluid restrictions can help to prevent fluid accumulation. Vaccinations for influenza and pneumonia reduce the risk of developing respiratory infections. Treatment of CHD risk factors, such as hypertension and lipid disorders, may slow disease progression. Heart failure patients are encouraged to participate in exercise programs to avoid becoming physically disabled and to improve endurance.

Drug Therapies for Heart Failure The medications prescribed for heart failure include diuretics, ACE inhibitors, angiotensin receptor blockers, beta blockers, vasodilators, and digitalis.[77] The diuretics are given to reverse or prevent fluid retention. The patient must monitor fluid fluctuations with daily weight measurements and can make small adjustments in the diuretic dose as needed. The other drugs listed help to improve heart and blood vessel function and blood flow.

Nutrition Therapy for Heart Failure For patients using diuretics, a modest sodium restriction is often advised to help reduce fluid retention. Sodium recommendations typically fall between 1500 and 3000 milligrams per day, depending on the patient's stage of illness, symptoms, and response to diuretic therapy.[78] (Note that some research studies have linked sodium intakes lower than 2000 milligrams per day to increased hospital readmissions and mortality rates in heart failure patients, and the ideal sodium intake for this population remains unknown.[79]) In patients with persistent or recurrent fluid retention, fluid intakes may be restricted to 2 liters per day or less.[80]

Patients with heart failure may be prone to constipation due to diuretic use and reduced physical activity. Maintaining an adequate fiber intake can help to minimize constipation problems. Because alcohol consumption can worsen heart function, some patients may need to restrict or avoid alcoholic beverages. Individuals who have difficulty eating due to nausea or abdominal bloating may tolerate small, frequent meals better than large meals.

No known therapies can reverse cardiac cachexia, and the prognosis is poor. For some patients, liquid supplements, tube feedings, or parenteral nutrition support can be supportive additions to treatment.

Review Notes

- Heart failure is usually a chronic, progressive condition that results from other cardiovascular illnesses.
- In heart failure, the heart is unable to pump adequate blood to tissues. Consequences may include fluid accumulation in the lungs, abdomen, and limbs and impaired organ function.
- Drug therapies can reduce fluid accumulation and improve heart function. Nutrition therapy may include sodium, fluid, and alcohol restrictions.

Nutrition Assessment Checklist for People with Cardiovascular Diseases

MEDICAL HISTORY

Check the medical record for a diagnosis of:

○ Coronary heart disease
○ Stroke
○ Hypertension
○ Heart failure

Review the medical record for complications related to cardiovascular diseases:

○ Heart attack
○ Transient ischemic attack
○ Cardiac cachexia

Note risk factors for CHD or stroke that are related to diet, including:

○ Elevated LDL or triglyceride levels
○ Obesity or overweight
○ Diabetes
○ Hypertension

MEDICATIONS

In patients using drug treatments for cardiovascular diseases, note:

○ Side effects that may alter food intake
○ Medications that may interact with grapefruit juice
○ Use of warfarin, which requires a consistent vitamin K intake
○ Use of diuretics or other drugs associated with potassium imbalances
○ Potential diet-drug or herb-drug interactions

DIETARY INTAKE

In patients with CHD, a previous stroke, or hypertension, assess the diet for:

○ Energy intake
○ Saturated fat, *trans* fat, cholesterol, and sodium content
○ Soluble fiber and plant sterol or plant stanol content
○ Intakes of fruit, vegetables, whole grains, legumes, and nuts
○ Alcohol content

In patients with complications resulting from cardiovascular diseases:

○ Check physical disabilities that may interfere with food preparation or consumption following a stroke.
○ Check adequacy of food and nutrient intake in patients with heart failure.

ANTHROPOMETRIC DATA

Measure baseline height and weight, and reassess weight at each medical checkup. Note whether patients are meeting weight goals, including:

○ Weight loss or maintenance in patients who are overweight
○ Weight maintenance in patients with advanced heart failure

Remember that weight may be deceptively high in people who are retaining fluids, especially individuals with heart failure.

LABORATORY TESTS

Monitor the following laboratory tests in people with cardiovascular diseases:

○ LDL cholesterol, blood triglycerides, and HDL cholesterol
○ Blood glucose in patients with diabetes
○ Serum potassium in patients using diuretics, antihypertensive medications, or digoxin
○ Blood-clotting time in patients using anticoagulants
○ Indicators of fluid retention in patients with heart failure

PHYSICAL SIGNS

Blood pressure measurement is routine in physical exams but is especially important for people who:

○ Have cardiovascular diseases
○ Have experienced a heart attack or stroke
○ Have risk factors for CHD or hypertension

Look for signs of:

○ Potassium imbalances (muscle weakness, numbness and tingling, irregular heartbeat) in those using diuretics, antihypertensive medications, or digoxin
○ Fluid overload in patients with heart failure

Self Check

1. Ischemia in the coronary arteries is a frequent cause of:
   a. angina pectoris.
   b. hemorrhagic stroke.
   c. aneurysm.
   d. hypertension.

2. Risk factors for atherosclerosis include all of the following *except*:
   a. smoking.
   b. hypertension.
   c. diabetes mellitus.
   d. elevated HDL cholesterol.

3. Which clinical test can help to diagnose peripheral artery disease?
   a. Lipoprotein profile
   b. Coronary artery calcium score
   c. Ankle-brachial index
   d. C-reactive protein levels

4. Dietary lipids with the strongest LDL cholesterol-raising effects are:
   a. saturated fats.
   b. polyunsaturated fats.
   c. monounsaturated fats.
   d. plant sterols.

5. Moderate alcohol consumption can improve heart disease risk, in part, because it:
   a. lowers blood pressure.
   b. increases HDL cholesterol levels.
   c. offsets the damage from smoking.
   d. improves nutrition status.

6. Patients with mild hypertriglyceridemia may improve their triglyceride levels by:
   a. reducing sodium intake.
   b. reducing cholesterol intake.
   c. consuming moderate amounts of alcohol.
   d. limiting intakes of refined carbohydrates.

7. Which medications reduce cholesterol synthesis in the liver?
   a. Bile acid sequestrants
   b. Statins
   c. ACE inhibitors
   d. Fibrates

8. Hemorrhagic stroke:
   a. is the most common type of stroke.
   b. results from obstructed blood flow within brain tissue.
   c. comes on suddenly and usually lasts for up to 30 minutes.
   d. results from bleeding within the brain, which damages brain tissue.

9. Hypertensive patients can benefit from all of the following dietary and lifestyle modifications *except*:
   a. including fat-free or low-fat milk products in the diet.
   b. reducing total fat intake.
   c. consuming generous amounts of fruit, vegetables, legumes, and nuts.
   d. reducing sodium intake.

10. Nutrition therapy for a patient with heart failure often includes:
    a. weight loss.
    b. reducing total fat intake.
    c. sodium restriction.
    d. cholesterol restriction.

Answers: 1. a, 2. d, 3. c, 4. a, 5. b, 6. d, 7. b, 8. d, 9. b, 10. c

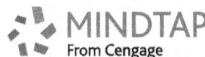 From Cengage   For more chapter resources visit **www.cengage.com** to access MindTap, a complete digital course.

Clinical Applications

1. List risk factors for coronary heart disease, and identify possible interrelationships among the factors. For example, a woman over 55 years of age is also at risk for diabetes; a person with diabetes is more likely to have hypertension.

2. Review the DASH Eating Plan shown in Table 21-5. As the chapter describes, the DASH dietary pattern is helpful for lowering blood pressure and for reducing CHD risk as well.
   - List elements of the DASH Eating Plan that are consistent with the dietary recommendations for CHD risk reduction.
   - Suggest ways in which a person following the DASH Eating Plan might accomplish the following additional dietary modifications: consume a higher percentage of fat from unsaturated sources, reduce intake of *trans* fat, and include EPA/DHA and plant sterols in the diet.

Notes

1. D. E. Benjamin and coauthors, Heart disease and stroke statistics—2017 update: A report from the American Heart Association, *Circulation* 135 (2017): e146–e603.

2. Benjamin and coauthors, 2017.

3. R. N. Mitchell, Blood vessels, in V. Kumar and coeditors, *Robbins Basic Pathology* (Philadelphia: Elsevier, 2018), pp. 361–398.

4. K.-S. Heo, K. Fujiwara, and J. Abe, Shear stress and atherosclerosis, *Molecules and Cells* 37 (2014): 435–440.

5. Mitchell, 2018.

6. M. Miller and coauthors, Triglycerides and cardiovascular disease: A scientific statement from the American Heart Association, *Circulation* 123 (2011): 2292–2333.

7. Y. He, V. Kothari, and K. E. Bornfeldt, High-density lipoprotein function in cardiovascular disease and diabetes mellitus, *Arteriosclerosis, Thrombosis, and Vascular Biology* 38 (2018): e10–e16.

8. G. K. Hansson and A. Hamsten, Atherosclerosis, thrombosis, and vascular biology, in L. Goldman and A. I. Schafer, eds., *Goldman-Cecil Medicine* (Philadelphia: Saunders, 2016), pp. 417–419.

9. T. A. Jacobson, Lipoprotein(a), cardiovascular disease, and contemporary management, *Mayo Clinic Proceedings* 88 (2013): 1294–1311; J. B. Dubé and coauthors, Lipoprotein(a): More interesting than ever after 50 years, *Current Opinion in Lipidology* 23 (2012): 133–140.

10. N. Chalouhi and coauthors, Cigarette smoke and inflammation: Role in cerebral aneurysm formation and rupture, *Mediators of Inflammation* 2012 (2012): 271582, doi: 10.1155/2012/271582.

11. J. Crandall and H. Shamoon, Diabetes mellitus, in L. Goldman and A. I. Schafer, eds., *Goldman-Cecil Medicine* (Philadelphia: Saunders, 2016), pp. 1527–1548; C. E. Tabit and coauthors, Endothelial dysfunction in diabetes mellitus: Molecular mechanisms and clinical implications, *Reviews in Endocrine and Metabolic Disorders* 11 (2010): 61–74.

12. F. Lenfant and coauthors, Timing of the vascular actions of estrogens in experimental and human studies: Why protective early, and not when delayed? *Maturitas* 68 (2011): 165–173.

13. P. Ganguly and S. F. Alam, Role of homocysteine in the development of cardiovascular disease, *Nutrition Journal* 14 (2015): 6.

14. W. E. Boden, Angina pectoris and stable ischemic heart disease, in L. Goldman and A. I. Schafer, eds., *Goldman-Cecil Medicine* (Philadelphia: Saunders, 2016), pp. 420–432.

15. D. C. Goff and coauthors, 2013 ACC/AHA guideline on the assessment of cardiovascular risk: A report of the American College of Cardiology/American Heart Association Task Force on Practice Guidelines, *Circulation* 129 (2014): S49–S73.

16. P. S. Jellinger and coauthors, American Association of Clinical Endocrinologists and American College of Endocrinology guidelines for management of dyslipidemia and prevention of cardiovascular disease, *Endocrine Practice* 23 (2017): 479–497.

17. Jellinger and coauthors, 2017; Boden, 2016.

18. C. F. Semenkovich, Disorders of lipid metabolism, in L. Goldman and A. I. Schafer, eds., *Goldman-Cecil Medicine* (Philadelphia: Saunders, 2016), pp. 1389–1397; J. A. Jarcho and J. F. Keaney, Proof that lower is better—LDL cholesterol and IMPROVE-IT, *New England Journal of Medicine* 372 (2015): 2448–2450.

19. B. F. Voight and coauthors, Plasma HDL cholesterol and risk of myocardial infarction: A mendelian randomization study, *Lancet* 380 (2012): 572–580.

20. C. Richter, A. Skulas-Ray, and P. Kris-Etherton, The role of diet in the prevention and treatment of cardiovascular disease, in A. M. Coulston amd coeditors, *Nutrition in the Prevention and Treatment of Disease* (London: Academic Press/Elsevier, 2017), pp. 595–623; R. H. Eckel and coauthors, 2013 AHA/ACC guideline on lifestyle management to reduce cardiovascular risk: A report of the American College of Cardiology/American Heart Association Task Force on Practice Guidelines, *Circulation* 129 (2014): S76–S99.

21. Jellinger and coauthors, 2017; Eckel and coauthors, 2014.

22. O. M. C. de Oliveira and coauthors, Dietary intake of saturated fat by food source and incident cardiovascular disease: The Multi-Ethnic Study of Atherosclerosis, *American Journal of Clinical Nutrition* 96 (2012): 397–404; M. R. Flock, M. H. Green, and P. M. Kris-Etherton, Effects of adiposity on plasma lipid response to reductions in dietary saturated fatty acids and cholesterol, *Advances in Nutrition* 2 (2011): 261–274;

23. P. W. Siri-Tarino and coauthors, Saturated fatty acids and risk of coronary heart disease: Modulation by replacement nutrients, *Current Atherosclerosis Reports* 12 (2010): 384–390.

23. U.S. Department of Agriculture, Agricultural Research Service, Energy intakes: Percentages of energy from protein, carbohydrate, fat, and alcohol, by gender and age, *What We Eat in America, NHANES 2013–2014* (2016), available at www.ars.usda.gov/nea/bhnrc/fsrg.

24. Richter, Skulas-Ray, and Kris-Etherton , 2017.

25. F. M. Sacks and coauthors, Dietary fats and cardiovascular disease: A presidential advisory from the American Heart Association, *Circulation* 136 (2017): e1–e23; P. M. Kris-Etherton and J. A. Fleming, Emerging nutrition science on fatty acids and cardiovascular disease: Nutritionists' perspectives, *Advances in Nutrition* 6 (2015): 326S–337S.

26. Jellinger and coauthors, 2017.

27. D. D. Wang and F. B. Hu, Dietary fat and risk of cardiovascular disease: Recent controversies and advances, *Annual Review of Nutrition* 37 (2017): 423–446.

28. Richter, Skulas-Ray, and Kris-Etherton , 2017; S. Berger and coauthors, Dietary cholesterol and cardiovascular disease: A systematic review and meta-analysis, *American Journal of Clinical Nutrition* 102 (2015): 276–294.

29. Jellinger and coauthors, 2017; T. A. Jacobson and coauthors, National Lipid Association recommendations for patient-centered management of dyslipidemia: Part 2, *Journal of Clinical Lipidology* 9 (2015): S1–S122.

30. U.S. Department of Agriculture, Agricultural Research Service, Nutrient intakes from food and beverages: Mean amounts consumed per individual, by gender and age, *What We Eat in America, NHANES 2013–2014* (2016), available at www.ars.usda.gov/nea/bhnrc/fsrg.

31. Jacobson and coauthors, 2015; N. L. Tran and coauthors, Egg consumption and cardiovascular disease among diabetic individuals: A systematic review of the literature, *Diabetes, Metabolic Syndrome and Obesity: Targets and Therapy* 7 (2014): 121–137.

32. Jacobson and coauthors, 2015.

33. Jellinger and coauthors, 2017; Jacobson and coauthors, 2015.

34. T. Aung and coauthors, Associations of omega-3 fatty acid supplement use with cardiovascular disease risks, *JAMA Cardiology* 3 (2018): doi:10.1001/jamacardio.2017.5205; Richter, Skulas-Ray, and Kris-Etherton, 2017; Jacobson and coauthors, 2015; H. K. Maehre and coauthors, ω-3 fatty acids and cardiovascular diseases: Effects, mechanisms and dietary relevance, *International Journal of Molecular Sciences* 16 (2015): 22636–22661.

35. A. J. Trevor, The alcohols, in B. G. Katzung, ed., *Basic and Clinical Pharmacology* (New York: McGraw-Hill, 2018), pp. 396–407; D. Mozaffarian, Dietary and policy priorities for cardiovascular disease, diabetes, and obesity: A comprehensive review, *Circulation* 133 (2016): 187–225.

36. Jellinger and coauthors, 2017.

37. J. J. Prochaska and N. L. Benowitz, Smoking cessation and the cardiovascular patient, *Current Opinion in Cardiology* 30 (2015): 506–511.

38. A. Jamal and coauthors, Current cigarette smoking among adults—United States, 2005–2015, *Morbidity and Mortality Weekly Report* 65 (2016): 1205–1211.

39. A. M. Kanaya and C. Vaisse, Obesity, in D. G. Gardner and D. Shoback, eds., *Greenspan's Basic and Clinical Endocrinology* (New York: McGraw-Hill/Lange, 2018), pp. 731–741; H. E. Bays and coauthors, Obesity, adiposity, and dyslipidemia: A consensus statement from the National Lipid Association, *Journal of Clinical Lipidology* 7 (2013): 304–383.

40. M. D. Jensen and coauthors, 2013 AHA/ACC/TOS guideline for the management of overweight and obesity in adults: a report of the American College of Cardiology/American Heart Association Task Force on Practice Guidelines and The Obesity Society, *Circulation* 129 (2014): S102–S138.

41. Jellinger and coauthors, 2017; Mozaffarian, 2016; M. J. Jardine and coauthors, The effect of folic acid based homocysteine lowering on cardiovascular events in people with kidney disease: Systematic review and meta-analysis, *British Medical Journal* 344 (2012): e3533.

42. Mozaffarian, 2016; V. A. Moyer on behalf of the U.S. Preventive Services Task Force, Vitamin, mineral, and multivitamin supplements for the primary prevention of cardiovascular disease and cancer, *Annals of Internal Medicine* 160 (2014): 558–564.

43. Benjamin and coauthors, 2017.

44. M. J. Malloy and J. P. Kane, Disorders of lipoprotein metabolism, in D. G. Gardner and D. Shoback, eds., *Greenspan's Basic and Clinical Endocrinology* (New York: McGraw-Hill/Lange, 2018), pp. 705–729.

45. Jellinger and coauthors, 2017; Jacobson and coauthors, 2015; L. Berglund and coauthors, Evaluation and treatment of hypertriglyceridemia, *Journal of Clinical* Endocrinology *and Metabolism* 97 (2012): 2969–2989; Miller and coauthors, 2011.

46. Jacobson and coauthors, 2015.

47. Jellinger and coauthors, 2017.

48. Berglund and coauthors, 2012; Miller and coauthors, 2011.

49. M. J. Malloy and J. P. Kane, Agents used in dyslipidemia, B. G. Katzung, ed., *Basic and Clinical Pharmacology* (New York: McGraw-Hill/Lange, 2018), pp. 626–641.

50. J. L. Anderson, ST segment elevation acute myocardial infarction and complications of myocardial infarction, in L. Goldman and A. I. Schafer, eds., *Goldman-Cecil Medicine* (Philadelphia: Saunders, 2016), pp. 441–456.

51. Benjamin and coauthors, 2017.

52. A. González-Pérez and coauthors, Mortality after hemorrhagic stroke: Data from general practice, *Neurology* 81 (2013): 559–565.

53. J. F. Meschia and coauthors, Guidelines for the primary prevention of stroke: A statement for healthcare professionals from the American Heart Association/American Stroke Association, *Stroke* 45 (2014): 3754–3832.

54. L. B. Goldstein, Ischemic cerebrovascular disease, in L. Goldman and A. I. Schafer, eds., *Goldman-Cecil Medicine* (Philadelphia: Saunders, 2016), pp. 2434–2445.

55. G. Bakris and M. Sorrentino, Redefining hypertension—assessing the new bloodpressure guidelines, *New England Journal of Medicine* 378 (2018): 497–499.

56. Benjamin and coauthors, 2017.

57. R. G. Victor, Arterial hypertension, in L. Goldman and A. I. Schafer, eds., *Goldman-Cecil Medicine* (Philadelphia: Saunders, 2016), pp. 381–397.

58. P. K. Whelton and coauthors, 2017 ACC/AHA/AAPA/ABC/ACPM/AGS/APhA/ASH/ASPC/NMA/PCNA guideline for the prevention, detection, evaluation, and management of high blood pressure in adults, *Journal of the American College of Cardiology* (2017): doi: 10.1016/j.jacc.2017.11.006.

59. Whelton and coauthors, 2017; Victor, 2016.

60. Whelton and coauthors, 2017.

61. Whelton and coauthors, 2017.

62. L. Landsberg and coauthors, Obesity-related hypertension: Pathogenesis, cardiovascular risk, and treatment, *Journal of Clinical Hypertension* 15 (2013): 14–33.

63. Whelton and coauthors, 2017.

64. F. Elijovich and coauthors, Salt sensitivity of blood pressure: A scientific statement from the American Heart Association, *Hypertension* 68 (2016): e7–e46.

65. M. R. Piano, Alcohol's effects on the cardiovascular system, *Alcohol Research: Current Reviews* 38 (2017): 219–241; K. Husain, R. A. Ansari, and L. Ferder, Alcohol-induced hypertension: Mechanism and prevention, *World Journal of Cardiology* 6 (2014) 245–252.

66. C. Rosendorff and coauthors, Treatment of hypertension in patients with coronary artery disease: A scientific statement from the American Heart Association, American College of Cardiology, and American Society of Hypertension, *Circulation* 131 (2015): e435–e470.

67. Whelton and coauthors, 2017.

68. Whelton and coauthors, 2017; C. C. Tyson and coauthors, Impact of 5-year weight change on blood pressure, *Journal of Clinical Hypertension* 15 (2013): 458–464.

69. Tyson and coauthors, 2013; V. Savica, G. Bellinghieri, and J. D. Kopple, The effect of nutrition on blood pressure, *Annual Review of Nutrition* 30 (2010): 365–401.

70. C. D. Sjöström, T. Kystig, and A. K. Lindroos, Impact of weight change, secular trends and ageing on cardiovascular risk factors: 10-year experiences from the SOS study, *International Journal of Obesity* 35 (2011): 1413–1420.

71. R. N. Ndanuko and coauthors, Dietary patterns and blood pressure in adults: A systematic review and meta-analysis of randomized controlled trials, *Advances in Nutrition* 7 (2016): 76–89.

72. F. M. Sacks and coauthors, Effects on blood pressure of reduced dietary sodium and the Dietary Approaches to Stop Hypertension (DASH) Diet, *New England Journal of Medicine* 344 (2001): 3–10; L. J. Appel and coauthors, A clinical trial on the effects of dietary patterns on blood pressure, *New England Journal of Medicine* 336 (1997): 1117–1124.

73. Appel and coauthors, 1997.

74. U.S. Department of Agriculture, Agricultural Research Service, Nutrient intakes from food and beverages: Mean amounts consumed per individual, by gender and age, 2016.

75. A. Mente and coauthors, Associations of urinary sodium excretion with cardiovascular events in individuals with and without hypertension: A pooled analysis of data from four studies, *Lancet* 388 (2016) 465–475; M. H. Alderman, The science upon which to base dietary sodium policy, *Advances in Nutrition* 5 (2014): 764–769; Institute of Medicine, *Sodium Intake in Populations: Assessment of Evidence* (Washington, D.C.: National Academies Press, 2013).

76. C. M. O'Connor and J. G. Rogers, Heart failure: Pathophysiology and diagnosis, in L. Goldman and A. I. Schafer, eds., *Goldman-Cecil Medicine* (Philadelphia: Saunders, 2016), pp. 298–305.

77. B. G. Katzung, Drugs used in heart failure, in B. G. Katzung, ed., *Basic and Clinical Pharmacology* (New York: McGraw-Hill/Lange, 2018), pp. 212–227.

78. C. W. Yancy and coauthors, 2013 ACCF/AHA guideline for the management of heart failure, *Circulation* 128 (2013): e240–e327; T. A. Lennie, M. L. Chung, and D. K. Moser, What should we tell patients with heart failure about sodium restriction and how should we counsel them? *Current Heart Failure Reports* 10 (2013): 219–226; D. Gupta and coauthors, Dietary sodium intake in heart failure, *Circulation* 126 (2012): 479–485.

79. B. D. Weiss, Sodium restriction in heart failure: How low should you go? *American Family Physician* 89 (2014): 509–510; Lennie, Chung, and Moser, 2013; Gupta and coauthors, 2012.

80. J. J. V. McMurray and M. A. Pfeffer, Heart failure: Management and prognosis, in L. Goldman and A. I. Schafer, eds., *Goldman-Cecil Medicine* (Philadelphia: Saunders, 2016), pp. 305–320.

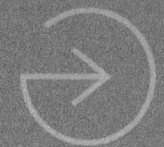

21.6 Nutrition in Practice

Helping People with Feeding Disabilities

Chapter 21 referred to difficulties following a stroke that can interfere with the ability to eat independently. This Nutrition in Practice discusses the problems faced by individuals who must cope with various disabilities that interfere with the process of eating, including those that interfere with chewing, swallowing, or bringing food to the mouth. These obstacles can arise at any time during a person's life and from any number of causes. An infant may be born with a physical impairment such as cleft palate; an adolescent may lose motor control following injuries sustained in an automobile accident; an older adult may struggle with the pain of arthritis or the mental deterioration of dementia. Table NP21-1 lists examples of conditions that may lead to feeding problems.

In what ways can disabilities impair a person's ability to eat?

Eating and drinking require a considerable number of individual coordinated motions. Consider an infant learning the skills required for feeding: each step—sitting, grasping cups and utensils, bringing food to the mouth, biting, chewing, and swallowing—requires coordinated movements. An injury or disability that interferes with any of these movements can lead to feeding problems and inadequate food intake. Total food intake is often significantly reduced when individuals with inefficient motor function take a long time to eat.[1] Difficulties that affect the procurement of food, such as the inability to drive, walk, or carry groceries, can also lower food intake and lead to malnutrition and weight loss.

Can disabilities alter a person's energy needs?

Yes, certain disabilities may either lower or raise energy requirements. Disabilities that affect muscle tension or mobility—such as cerebral palsy—are typically associated with reduced muscle mass and physical activity; consequently, energy requirements tend to be lower.[2] Loss of a limb due to amputation reduces energy needs in proportion to the weight and metabolism represented by the missing limb, but energy needs may be higher if an individual increases activity to compensate for the loss, as is necessary when using a prosthesis.[3] Because the effects of disabilities are often unpredictable, the health care practitioner may find it difficult to assess energy requirements until weight gain or loss has occurred.

Overweight and obesity often accompany conditions that limit mobility or result in short stature; examples include Down syndrome and spina bifida.[4] Obesity may also develop if the individual is unable to regulate food intake adequately or is using a medication that promotes weight gain. In these cases, the health practitioner may need to counsel the patient or caregiver about appropriate food choices and portion sizes.

Can disease symptoms cause problems with food intake and nutrition status?

Yes, physical symptoms of disease can sometimes create feeding problems; examples include difficulty with swallowing or breathing, frequent coughing or choking, and gastroesophageal reflux. Individuals with speech problems may have difficulty communicating with caregivers about thirst and hunger. Mobility problems and physical weakness can interfere with food preparation and the physical movements required for eating meals.

Which health professionals typically work with people who have feeding problems?

Evaluating and treating feeding problems may involve the joint efforts of health care professionals from a

---

TABLE NP21-1 Conditions That May Lead to Feeding Problems

The following conditions may lead to feeding problems by interfering with a person's ability to suck, bite, chew, swallow, or coordinate hand-to-mouth movements.

- Accidents
- Amputations
- Arthritis
- Birth defects
- Brain tumors
- Cerebral palsy
- Cleft palate
- Down syndrome
- Head injuries

- Huntington's chorea
- Language or visual impairments
- Multiple sclerosis
- Muscle weakness
- Muscular dystrophy
- Parkinson's disease
- Spinal cord injuries
- Stroke

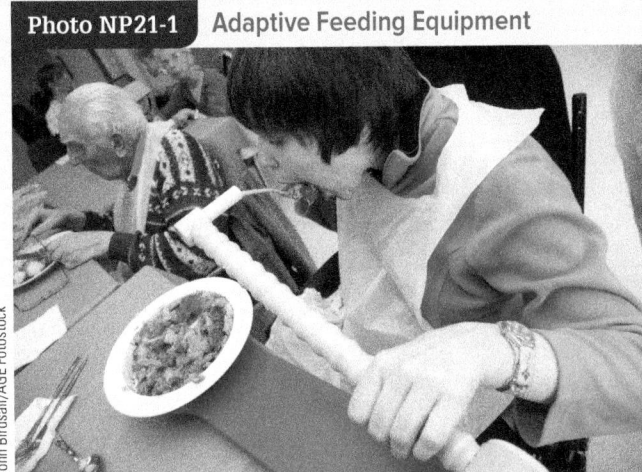

The device shown here is a Neater Eater®, a feeding aid that allows individuals with limited mobility to feed themselves. The extension arm can be moved easily by people with reduced hand and wrist strength, and can also dampen extraneous movements, such as tremors.

variety of disciplines, including nurses, dietitians, occupational therapists, speech-language pathologists, and gastroenterologists.[5] Together, these professionals can evaluate the patient's dietary needs and assess abilities to grasp and use utensils, bring foods from the plate to the mouth, chew, sip, and swallow. A speech-language pathologist or occupational therapist may evaluate chewing and swallowing abilities and self-feeding skills; these professionals can also demonstrate alternative feeding strategies, including changes in body position that improve feeding ability, techniques for handling utensils and food, and the use of special feeding devices (see Photo NP21-1). Gastroenterologists can use various noninvasive techniques to evaluate relevant gastrointestinal functions. Direct observation of the patient during mealtimes allows these health practitioners to assess current eating behaviors, demonstrate feeding techniques, monitor the patient's or caregiver's understanding of the techniques, and evaluate how well the care plan is working.

To illustrate one type of strategy used to treat feeding problems, consider a child with feeding difficulties caused by hypersensitivity to oral stimulation. The therapist may start by teaching the caregiver to gently stroke the child's face with a hand, washcloth, or soft toy. Once the child tolerates touch on less sensitive areas of the face, the therapist may encourage the caregiver to slowly begin to rub the child's lips, gums, palate, and tongue. With time, the child may be better able to tolerate the presence of food in the mouth. Examples of other strategies that can help feeding problems are listed in Table NP21-1.

TABLE NP21-2   Interventions for Feeding-Related Problems

Inability to Suck

- Use squeeze bottles, which do not require sucking, to express liquids into the mouth.
- Place a spoon on the center of the tongue and apply downward pressure to stimulate sucking.
- Apply rhythmic, slow strokes on the tongue to alter tongue position and improve the sucking response.

Inability to Chew

- Place foods between teeth to promote chewing.
- Improve chewing skills with foods of different textures; for example, fruit leathers stimulate jaw movements but dissolve quickly enough to minimize choking.
- Provide soft foods that require minimal chewing or are easily chewed.

Inability to Swallow

- Provide thickened liquids, pureed foods, and moist foods that form boluses easily.
- Provide cold formulas, frozen fruit juice bars, and ice; cold substances promote swallowing movements by the tongue and soft palate.
- Make sure the patient's jaw and lips are closed to facilitate swallowing action.
- Correct posture and head position if they interfere with swallowing ability.

Inability to Grasp or Coordinate Movements

- Provide utensils that have modified handles, or are smaller or larger as necessary.
- Encourage the use of hands for feeding if utensils are difficult to maneuver.
- Provide plates with food guards to prevent spilling.
- Supply clothing protection.

Impaired Vision

- Place foods (meats, vegetables) in similar locations on the plate at each meal.
- Provide plates with food guards to prevent spilling.

Can special equipment be used to help people with certain feeding difficulties?

Yes. Adaptive feeding devices can make a remarkable difference in a person's ability to eat independently. Figure NP21-1 shows a few of the many special feeding devices that are available and describes their uses. Other examples of adaptive equipment include specialized chairs to improve posture, bolsters inserted under arms to improve elbow stability, and raised trays or eating surfaces to simplify hand-to-mouth movements.

Utensils

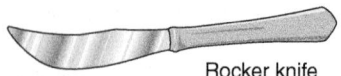

Rocker knife

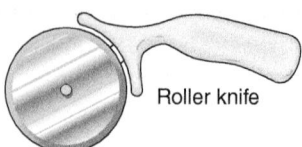

Roller knife

People with only one arm or hand may have difficulty cutting foods and may appreciate using a *rocker knife* or a *roller knife.*

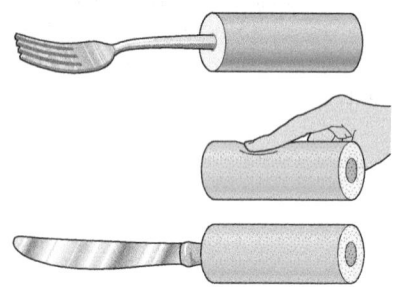

People with a limited range of motion can feed themselves better when they use *flatware with built-up handles.*

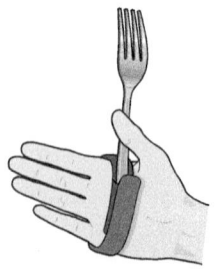

People with extreme muscle weakness may be able to eat with a *utensil holder.*

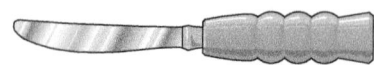

For people with tremors, spasticity, and uneven jerky movements, *weighted utensils* can aid the feeding process.

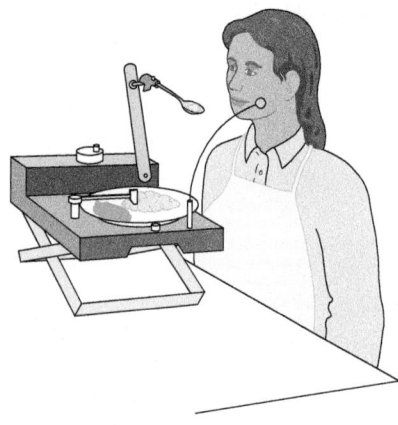

Battery-powered feeding machines enable people with severe limitations to eat with less assistance from others.

Plates

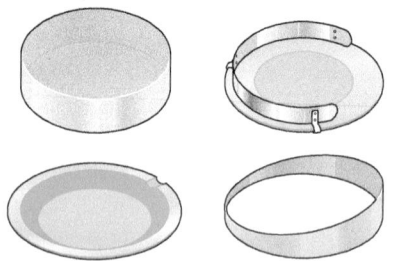

People who have limited dexterity and difficulty maneuvering food find *scoop dishes* or *food guards* useful.

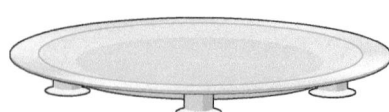

People with uncontrolled or excessive movements might move dishes around while eating and may benefit from using *unbreakable dishes with suction cups.*

Cups

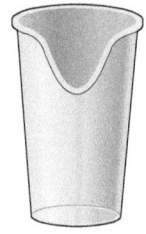

People with limited neck motion can use a *cutout plastic cup.*

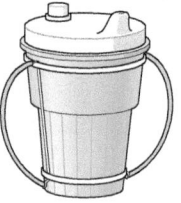

Two-handed cups enable people with moderate muscle weakness to lift a cup with two hands.

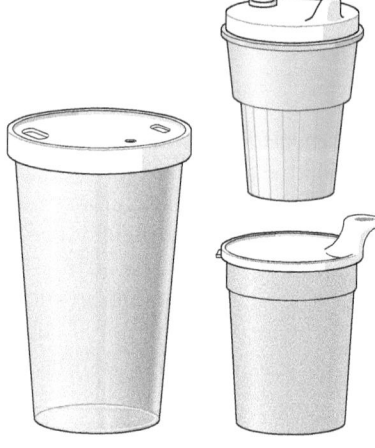

People with uncontrolled or excessive movements might prefer to drink liquids from a *covered cup* or glass with a *slotted opening* or *spout.*

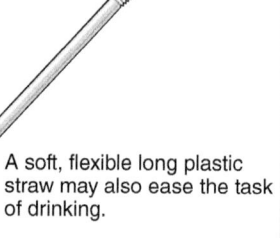

A soft, flexible long plastic straw may also ease the task of drinking.

Sometimes, despite the best efforts of all involved, a patient is unable to maintain adequate weight or hydration with oral feedings. In such a case, tube feedings can help to improve nutrition status. Tube feedings are also recommended for patients who have significant dysphagia (difficulty swallowing) with aspiration.[6]

In what ways can feeding difficulties affect family life?

Mealtimes are a critical time for social interaction, and therefore individuals with feeding problems may encounter emotional and social problems if they are unable to participate. Children may fail to develop social skills, whereas adults may miss the social stimulation that mealtimes provide. Individuals should be encouraged to sit with family and friends during meals so that they are not deprived of the social and cultural aspects of eating.

The responsibility of caring for a person with a feeding problem can frequently overwhelm a caregiver.[7] Caring for a person with disabilities requires time and patience—and many new therapies to be learned and administered. The caregiver may spend many hours preparing special foods, monitoring the use of adaptive feeding equipment, and helping with feedings. Moreover, a person with disabilities may need help with other tasks as well, and all may require a considerable amount of time. In many cases, a caregiver receives little or no assistance. These conditions may lead to strained interactions between caregiver and patient and cause stress and frustration. The members of the health care team can assist patients or caregivers by offering emotional support and practical suggestions that may relieve caregivers' difficulties and frustrations.

With the help of health professionals, people with feeding disabilities may be able to learn strategies that allow them to prepare and consume appropriate amounts of food without assistance. The ideal intervention would also educate patients about dietary choices that promote good nutrition status and reduce the risk of malnutrition and its associated complications.

Notes

1. Position of the Canadian Paediatric Society: Nutrition in neurologically impaired children, *Paediatrics and Child Health* 14 (2009): 395–401.
2. K. L. Bell and L. Samson-Fang, Nutritional management of children with cerebral palsy, *European Journal of Clinical Nutrition* 67 (2013): S13–S16.
3. T. Chin and coauthors, Energy consumption during prosthetic walking and physical fitness in older hip disarticulation amputees, *Journal of Rehabilitation Research and Development* 49 (2012): 1255–1260.
4. Position of the Academy of Nutrition and Dietetics: Nutrition services for individuals with intellectual and developmental disabilities and special health care needs, *Journal of the Academy of Nutrition and Dietetics* 115 (2015): 593–608.
5. R. M. Katz, J. K. Hyche, and E. K. Wingert, Pediatric feeding problems, in A. C. Ross and coeditors, eds., *Modern Nutrition in Health and Disease* (Baltimore: Lippincott Williams & Wilkins, 2014), pp. 887–893.
6. Position of the Academy of Nutrition and Dietetics, 2015.
7. Katz, Hyche, and Wingert, 2014; G. M. Craig, Psychosocial aspects of feeding children with neurodisability, *European Journal of Clinical Nutrition* 67 (2013): S17–S20.

Nutrition and Renal Diseases

Chapter Sections and Learning Objectives (LOs)

22.1 Nephrotic Syndrome

LO 22.1 Identify the potential causes and consequences of the nephrotic syndrome and describe the medical and nutrition therapies used in treatment.

22.2 Acute Kidney Injury

LO 22.2 Discuss the potential causes and effects of acute kidney injury and describe the approaches to treatment for this condition.

22.3 Chronic Kidney Disease

LO 22.3 Describe the potential causes and consequences of chronic kidney disease, its medical treatment, and nutrition therapy for this condition.

22.4 Kidney Stones

LO 22.4 Compare the different types of kidney stones and explain how kidney stones can be prevented or treated.

22.5 Nutrition in Practice: Dialysis

LO 22.5 Explain how dialysis removes fluids and wastes from the blood and compare the different types of dialysis procedures.

chapter
22

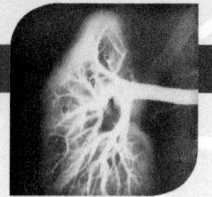

spinal column. As part of the urinary system, they are responsible for filtering the blood and removing excess fluid and wastes for elimination in urine. Because the kidneys are so proficient at this task, disturbances in body fluids that result from water intake, physical activity, and metabolism are normally corrected within hours.

Figure 22-1 shows the kidneys' placement and structure and one of their functional units, the **nephron**. Within each nephron, the **glomerulus**, a ball-shaped tuft of capillaries, serves as a gateway through which blood components must pass to form **filtrate**. The glomerulus and surrounding **Bowman's capsule** function like a sieve, retaining blood cells and most plasma proteins in the blood while allowing fluid and small solutes to enter the nephron's system of **tubules**. As the filtrate moves through the tubules, its composition continuously changes as some of its components are reabsorbed and returned to the blood via capillaries surrounding the tubules; the remaining substances contribute to the final urine product. By filtering the blood and forming urine, the kidneys regulate the extracellular fluid volume and osmolarity, electrolyte concentrations, and acid–base balance. They also excrete metabolic waste products such as urea and **creatinine**, as well as various drugs and toxicants. Other roles of the kidneys include the following:

- Secretion of the enzyme *renin*, which helps to regulate blood pressure
- Production of the hormone **erythropoietin**, which stimulates the production of red blood cells in the bone marrow
- Conversion of vitamin D to its active form, thereby helping to regulate calcium balance and bone formation

Subsequent sections of this chapter explain how **renal** diseases can interfere with the kidneys' various functions and severely disrupt health.

nephron (NEF-ron): the functional unit of the kidneys, consisting of a glomerulus and tubules.

nephros = kidney

glomerulus (gloh-MEHR-yoo-lus): a tuft of capillaries within the nephron that filters water and solutes from the blood as urine production begins (plural: *glomeruli*).

filtrate: the substances that pass through the glomerulus and travel through the nephron's tubules, eventually forming urine.

Bowman's (BOE-minz) **capsule**: a cuplike component of the nephron that surrounds the glomerulus and collects the filtrate that is passed to the tubules.

FIGURE 22-1   The Kidneys and Nephron Function

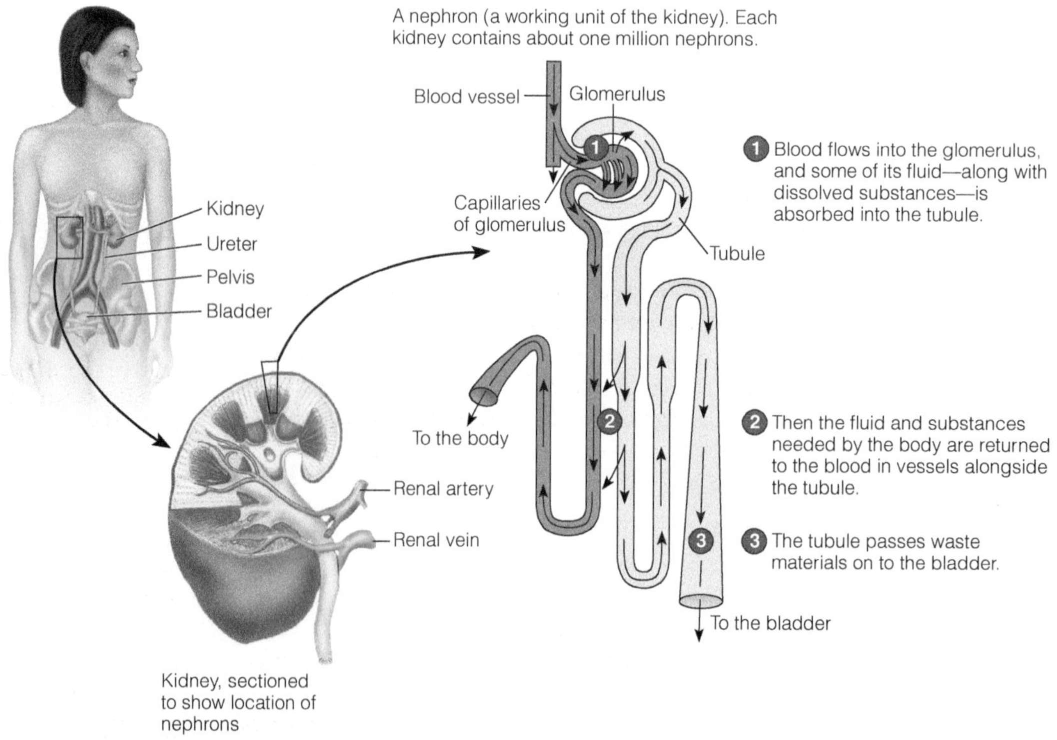

A nephron (a working unit of the kidney). Each kidney contains about one million nephrons.

Blood vessel — Glomerulus

Kidney
Ureter
Pelvis
Bladder

Capillaries of glomerulus

Tubule

1 Blood flows into the glomerulus, and some of its fluid—along with dissolved substances—is absorbed into the tubule.

To the body

Renal artery

Renal vein

2 Then the fluid and substances needed by the body are returned to the blood in vessels alongside the tubule.

3 The tubule passes waste materials on to the bladder.

To the bladder

Kidney, sectioned to show location of nephrons

22.1 Nephrotic Syndrome

The **nephrotic syndrome** is not a specific disease; rather, the term refers to a syndrome caused by significant urinary protein losses (**proteinuria**) that result from severe glomerular damage. The condition arises because damage to the glomeruli increases their permeability to plasma proteins, allowing the proteins to escape into the urine. The loss of these proteins (typically more than 3 to 3½ grams daily) may cause serious consequences, including edema, blood lipid abnormalities, blood coagulation disorders, and infections. In some cases, the nephrotic syndrome can progress to renal failure.

Causes of the nephrotic syndrome include glomerular disorders, diabetic nephropathy, immunological and hereditary diseases, infections (involving the kidneys or elsewhere in the body), chemical damage (from medications or illicit drugs), and some cancers.[1] Depending on the underlying condition, some patients may experience one or more relapses and require additional treatment to prevent proteinuria from recurring.

Consequences of the Nephrotic Syndrome

Although protein losses vary, proteinuria in adult patients may average as much as 10 grams daily.[2] The liver tries to compensate by increasing its synthesis of various plasma proteins, but some of the proteins are produced in excessive amounts. The imbalance in plasma protein concentrations contributes to a number of complications (see Box 22-1).

Edema Albumin is the most abundant plasma protein, and it is the protein with the most significant urinary losses as well. The **hypoalbuminemia** characteristic of the nephrotic syndrome contributes to a fluid shift from blood plasma to the interstitial spaces and, thus, edema. Impaired sodium excretion also contributes to edema: the nephrotic kidney tends to reabsorb sodium in greater amounts than usual, causing sodium and water retention within the body.[3]

Blood Lipid and Blood Clotting Abnormalities Individuals with the nephrotic syndrome frequently have elevated levels of low-density lipoproteins (LDL), very-low-density lipoproteins (VLDL), and the more atherogenic LDL variant known as lipoprotein(a). Furthermore, blood clotting risk is increased due to urinary losses of proteins that inhibit blood clotting and elevated levels of plasma proteins that favor clotting. The blood clotting abnormalities increase the risk of **deep vein thrombosis** and similar disorders. The nephrotic syndrome is associated with accelerated atherosclerosis and a sharply increased risk of heart disease and stroke.

Other Effects of the Nephrotic Syndrome The proteins lost in urine include immunoglobulins (antibodies) and vitamin D–binding protein. Depletion of immunoglobulins increases susceptibility to infection. Loss of vitamin D–binding protein results in lower vitamin D and calcium levels and increases the risk of rickets in children. If proteinuria continues, protein-energy malnutrition (PEM) and muscle wasting may develop. Figure 22-2 summarizes the effects of urinary protein losses in the nephrotic syndrome.

Treatment of the Nephrotic Syndrome

Medical treatment of the nephrotic syndrome requires diagnosis and management of the underlying disorder responsible for the proteinuria. Complications are managed with medications and nutrition therapy. The drugs prescribed may include diuretics, angiotensin-converting enzyme (ACE) inhibitors and angiotensin-receptor blockers (which reduce protein losses), lipid-lowering drugs, anti-inflammatory drugs (usually corticosteroids, such as prednisone), and immunosuppressants (such as

---

BOX 22-1 *Nursing Diagnosis*

The nursing diagnoses *impaired urinary elimination, excess fluid volume, risk for infection,* and *imbalanced nutrition: less than body requirements* may apply to people with nephrotic syndrome.

---

tubules: tubelike structures of the nephron that process filtrate during urine production. The tubules are surrounded by capillaries that reabsorb substances retained by tubule cells.

creatinine: the waste product of creatine, a nitrogen-containing compound in muscle cells that supplies energy for muscle contraction.

erythropoietin (eh-RITH-ro-POY-eh-tin): a hormone made by the kidneys that stimulates red blood cell production.

renal (REE-nal): pertaining to the kidneys.

nephrotic (neh-FROT-ik) **syndrome:** a syndrome caused by significant urinary protein losses (more than 3 to 3½ grams daily), as a result of severe glomerular damage.

proteinuria (PRO-teen-NOO-ree-ah): the presence of protein in the urine. When only urinary albumin is measured, the term used is *albuminuria.*

hypoalbuminemia: low plasma albumin concentrations. Plasma proteins such as albumin help to maintain fluid balance within the blood; thus, low levels contribute to edema.

deep vein thrombosis: formation of a stationary blood clot (thrombus) in a deep vein, usually in the leg, which causes inflammation, pain, and swelling, and is potentially fatal.

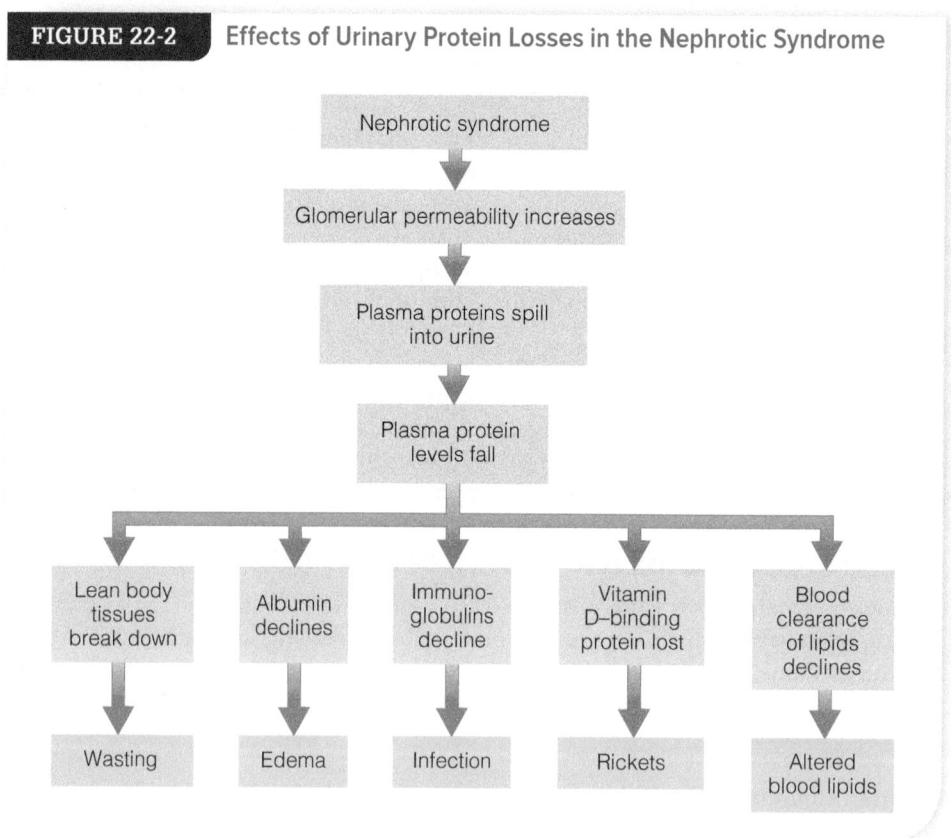

FIGURE 22-2 Effects of Urinary Protein Losses in the Nephrotic Syndrome

Nephrotic syndrome
↓
Glomerular permeability increases
↓
Plasma proteins spill into urine
↓
Plasma protein levels fall

- Lean body tissues break down → Wasting
- Albumin declines → Edema
- Immuno-globulins decline → Infection
- Vitamin D–binding protein lost → Rickets
- Blood clearance of lipids declines → Altered blood lipids

cyclosporine). Nutrition therapy can help to prevent PEM, alleviate edema, and correct lipid abnormalities.

Protein and Energy Meeting protein and energy needs helps to minimize losses of muscle tissue. High-protein diets are not advised, however, because they can exacerbate urinary protein losses and result in further damage to the kidneys. Instead, the protein intake should fall between 0.8 and 1.0 gram per kilogram of body weight per day.[4] An adequate energy intake (about 35 kcalories per kilogram of body weight daily) sustains weight and spares protein. Weight loss or infections suggest the need for additional energy.

Lipids As Chapter 21 explains, a diet low in saturated fat, *trans* fats, and refined sugars may help to control elevated LDL and VLDL levels. Dietary measures are usually inadequate for controlling blood lipids, however, so physicians may prescribe lipid-lowering medications as well. In some cases, treating the underlying cause of nephrotic syndrome is sufficient for correcting the lipid disorders.[5]

Sodium and Potassium Controlling sodium intake helps to control edema; therefore, the sodium intake may be limited to 1000 to 2000 milligrams daily.[6] Table 22-1 provides guidelines for following a diet restricted to 2000 milligrams of sodium. If diuretics prescribed for the edema cause potassium losses, patients are encouraged to select foods rich in potassium (see Chapter 9).

Vitamins and Minerals Multivitamin/mineral supplementation can help patients avoid nutrient deficiencies; nutrients at risk include iron and vitamin D. To reduce risk of bone loss, calcium supplementation (about 1000 to 1500 milligrams per day) may also be advised.[7]

TABLE 22-1 Low-Sodium Diet

An individual with the nephrotic syndrome may need to restrict sodium intakes to less than 2000 milligrams per day to help control edema. Similar sodium restrictions may be recommended for individuals with hypertension, heart failure, and ascites.

GENERAL GUIDELINES

About 75 percent of the sodium in a typical diet comes from processed foods, about 10 percent from unprocessed natural foods, and about 15 percent from table salt. With this in mind:

- Whenever possible, select fresh foods, which are usually low in sodium.
- Select frozen and canned food products that have been prepared without added salt.
- Avoid adding salt to foods while cooking or at the table. In restaurants, ask that meals be prepared without salt.

SODIUM IN FOODS

All foods contain sodium, but some contain more than others. Use the information below to plan low-sodium meals.

FOOD GROUP	SERVING	SODIUM PER SERVING (mg)
Milk products	1 cup milk or yogurt, 1 oz hard cheese (cheddar, Swiss, jack)	150–200
	Avoid: buttermilk, cottage cheese, cheese spreads, processed cheese (such as American cheese)	
Meat, fish, poultry, and eggs	3 oz fresh meat, fish, or poultry; 1 large egg	60
	Avoid: luncheon meat, corned beef, salt pork, sausage, frankfurters, bacon, canned meat or fish, fresh meat or poultry prepared with injected broth	
Fruits and vegetables	½ cup fresh vegetables, ½ cup fresh or frozen fruit, 6 oz fruit juice, 6 oz tomato or vegetable juice without added salt	10–20
	Avoid: pickled vegetables, olives, tomato or vegetable juices with added salt; dried fruit with added sodium sulfite	
Breads and cereals	½–⅔ cup dry or cooked cereal without added salt, ½ cup cooked rice or pasta	0–10
	½–⅔ cup dry or cooked cereal prepared with salt, 1 slice bread, 1 roll or tortilla	150
	Avoid: pancakes, waffles, muffins, biscuits, and quick breads made with baking powder or baking soda; instant or ready-to-eat cereals with >175 mg sodium; salted snack foods	
Condiments	½ tbs unsalted butter, 1 tsp no-salt mustard, 1 tbs no-salt ketchup, 1 tsp sodium-free bouillon, onion or garlic powders without added salt	0–10
	Avoid: commercial salad dressings; gravy and soup mixes; barbeque sauce; steak sauce; soy sauce; spice, herb, or bouillon products made with salt; meat tenderizer; monosodium glutamate	

A SAMPLE DIET RESTRICTED TO 2000 mg OF SODIUM

Using the guidelines provided here, an individual can develop a variety of menus. A possible plan for a day might look like this:

FOOD GROUP	SODIUM (mg)
Meat, 6 oz (2 servings × 60 mg)	120
Milk, 3 c (3 servings × 150 mg)	450
Fruit, 2 servings	negligible
Vegetables, 3 servings	45
Whole-grain bread, 4 slices (4 × 150 mg)	600
Salt, ¼ tsp (used lightly at meals)	600
Total	**1815**

Individuals can use the remainder of the sodium allowance for whatever foods they desire. The sodium content of most foods can be obtained by reading food labels or using food composition tables. See additional information about reducing sodium intake in Chapter 21 (Box 21-11, p. 613).

Review Notes

- The nephrotic syndrome is characterized by significant proteinuria due to glomerular damage. Complications include edema, lipid and blood clotting abnormalities, infections, and PEM.
- Medications treat the underlying cause of proteinuria and manage complications. The diet should provide sufficient protein and energy to maintain health, but patients should avoid consuming excess protein. Other dietary adjustments can help to correct edema, lipid disorders, and nutrient deficiencies.

22.2 Acute Kidney Injury

Acute kidney injury is a syndrome characterized by the rapid deterioration of kidney function, which occurs over a period of hours or days. The loss of kidney function reduces urine output and allows nitrogenous wastes to build up in the blood. The degree of renal dysfunction varies from mild to severe. With prompt treatment, acute kidney injury is often reversible, although mortality rates are high, ranging from 60 to 70 percent in severe cases.[8] Most cases of acute kidney injury develop in the hospital, occurring in about 25 percent of patients undergoing intensive care.[9]

Causes of Acute Kidney Injury

Many disorders can lead to acute kidney injury, and it often develops as a consequence of critical illness, sepsis, or major surgery. To aid in diagnosis and treatment, its causes are classified as prerenal, intrarenal, or postrenal (see Table 22-2). *Prerenal* factors are conditions that cause a severe reduction in blood flow to the kidneys, such as heart failure, shock, or substantial blood loss. Factors that damage kidney tissue, such as infections, toxicants, drugs, or direct trauma, are classified as *intrarenal* causes of acute kidney injury. *Postrenal* factors are those that prevent urine excretion due to urinary tract obstructions.

Consequences of Acute Kidney Injury

A decline in renal function alters the composition of blood and urine. The kidneys become unable to regulate the levels of electrolytes, acid, and nitrogenous wastes in the blood. Urine may be diminished in quantity (**oliguria**) or absent (**anuria**), leading to fluid retention. Acute kidney injury is often identified when the reduced urinary output is coupled with a progressive rise in serum creatinine levels. Other laboratory findings may include abnormal levels of serum electrolytes, elevated blood urea nitrogen (BUN), and various

acute kidney injury: the rapid decline of kidney function over a period of hours or days; potentially a cause of acute renal failure.

oliguria (OL-lih-GOO-ree-ah): an abnormally low amount of urine, often less than 400 mL/day.

anuria (ah-NOO-ree-ah): the absence of urine; clinically identified as a urine output that is less than about 50 to 75 mL/day.

TABLE 22-2	Causes of Acute Kidney Injury	
PRERENAL FACTORS (60 TO 70% OF CASES)	**INTRARENAL FACTORS (25 TO 40% OF CASES)**	**POSTRENAL FACTORS (5 TO 10% OF CASES)**
• **Low blood volume or pressure:** hemorrhage, burns, sepsis or shock, severe diarrhea, advanced cirrhosis, diuretics, antihypertensive medications • **Renal artery disorders:** blood clots or emboli, stenosis, aneurysm, trauma • **Heart disorders:** heart failure, arrhythmias	• **Renal ischemia:** sepsis or shock, hemorrhage, blood clots, trauma • **Renal injury:** nephrotoxic drugs, infections, *Escherichia coli* food poisoning, environmental contaminants • **Obstructions (within kidney):** inflammation, tumors, stones, scar tissue	• **Obstructions (ureter or bladder):** strictures, tumors, stones, trauma • **Prostate disorders:** cancer, enlarged prostate • **Renal vein thrombosis** • **Bladder disorders:** neurological conditions, bladder rupture • **Pregnancy**

changes in urine chemistry. Diagnosis is sometimes difficult, however, because the clinical effects can be subtle (see Box 22-2) and vary according to the underlying cause of disease.

Fluid and Electrolyte Imbalances About one-half to two-thirds of patients with acute kidney injury experience oliguria, producing less than about 400 milliliters of urine per day (normal urine volume is about 1000 to 1500 milliliters daily).[10] The reduced excretion of fluids and electrolytes leads to sodium retention and elevated levels of potassium, phosphate, and magnesium in the blood. Elevated potassium levels (**hyperkalemia**) are of particular concern because potassium imbalances can alter heart rhythm and result in heart failure. Elevated serum phosphate levels (**hyperphosphatemia**) promote excessive secretion of parathyroid hormone, which leads to losses of bone calcium. Due to the sodium retention and reduced urine production, edema is a common symptom of acute kidney injury and may be apparent as puffiness in the face and hands and swelling of the feet and ankles.

Uremia As a result of impaired kidney function, nitrogen-containing compounds and various other waste products may accumulate in the blood—a condition referred to as **uremia**. The clinical outcome, called the **uremic syndrome**, includes a cluster of symptoms caused by impairments in multiple body systems. Although the clinical effects vary among patients, complications may include hormonal imbalances, electrolyte and acid–base imbalances, disturbed heart and gastrointestinal (GI) functioning, neuromuscular disturbances, and depressed immunity, among other abnormalities. The uremic syndrome is described in more detail later in this chapter.

Treatment of Acute Kidney Injury

Treatment of acute kidney injury involves a combination of drug therapies, **dialysis** (see Nutrition in Practice 22), and nutrition therapy to restore fluid and electrolyte balances and minimize blood concentrations of toxic waste products. Both medical care and dietary measures are highly individualized to suit each patient's needs. Correcting the underlying illness is necessary to prevent further damage to the kidneys.

In oliguric patients (those with reduced urine production), recovery from kidney injury sometimes begins with a period of **diuresis**, in which large amounts of fluid (up to 3 liters daily) are excreted. Because tubular function is minimal at this stage, electrolytes may not be sufficiently reabsorbed; consequently, both fluid depletion and electrolyte losses become a concern. Patients with this pattern of recovery (generally those with tubular injury) require close monitoring in case they need fluid and electrolyte replacement.

Drug Treatment for Acute Kidney Injury Because kidney function is required for drug excretion, patients may need to use lower doses of their usual medications to compensate for limited urine output. Conversely, dialysis treatment may increase losses of some drugs, and doses may need to be increased. Drugs that are **nephrotoxic** (including some antibiotics and nonsteroidal anti-inflammatory drugs) must be avoided until kidney function improves.

The medications prescribed for acute kidney injury depend on the cause of illness and the complications that develop. Inflammatory conditions may require treatment with immunosuppressants. Edema is treated with diuretics; furosemide (Lasix) is the usual choice. Correction of hyperkalemia may require the use of beta-agonists, insulin, or bicarbonate to drive extracellular potassium into cells; if insulin is used, glucose is usually coadministered to prevent hypoglycemia. To reduce serum phosphate levels, phosphate binders may be provided with meals to prevent phosphorus absorption. If acidosis is present, bicarbonate may be administered orally or intravenously.

Energy and Protein Acute kidney injury is often associated with other critical illnesses, so patients may be hypermetabolic, catabolic, and at high risk of wasting. Furthermore, patients with acute kidney injury frequently develop hyperglycemia and hypertriglyceridemia because they are unable to metabolize energy nutrients efficiently. For these

hyperkalemia (HIGH-per-ka-LEE-me-ah): elevated serum potassium levels.

hyperphosphatemia (HIGH-per-fos-fa-TEE-me-ah): elevated serum phosphate levels. Note that the phosphorus in body fluids is present as phosphate; hence, the terms *serum phosphate* and *serum phosphorus* are often used interchangeably.

uremia (you-REE-me-ah): the accumulation of nitrogenous and various other waste products in the blood (literally, "urine in the blood"); may also be used to indicate the toxic state that results when wastes are retained in the blood. The related term *azotemia* refers specifically to the accumulation of nitrogenous wastes in the blood.

uremic syndrome: the cluster of disorders caused by inadequate kidney function; complications include fluid, electrolyte, and hormonal imbalances; altered heart function; neuromuscular disturbances; and other metabolic derangements.

dialysis (dye-AH-lih-sis): a treatment that removes wastes and excess fluid from the blood after the kidneys have stopped functioning.

diuresis (DYE-uh-REE-sis): increased urine production.

nephrotoxic: toxic to the kidneys.

reasons, patients must ingest sufficient protein and energy to preserve muscle mass but should not be overfed. Protein recommendations are influenced by kidney function, the degree of catabolism, and the use of dialysis (dialysis removes nitrogenous wastes).

Although guidelines vary, patients are usually provided with 20 to 30 kcalories per kilogram of body weight per day, while body weight, nitrogen balance, blood glucose levels, and blood triglycerides are monitored to ensure that the energy intake is appropriate.[11] For noncatabolic patients who do not require dialysis, protein intakes should be limited to 0.8 to 1.0 gram per kilogram of body weight per day.[12] Higher intakes (1.0 to 1.7 grams per kilogram daily) may be recommended if kidney function improves, the patient is catabolic, or the treatment includes dialysis. Patients who require higher amounts of protein (such as those with burns or large wounds) require more frequent dialysis to accommodate the nitrogen load.

Fluids Health practitioners can assess fluid status by monitoring weight fluctuations, blood pressure, pulse rates, and the appearance of the skin and mucous membranes. Another method is to measure serum sodium concentrations: a low sodium level often indicates excessive fluid intake, whereas a high sodium level suggests inadequate fluid intake.

Fluid balance must be restored in patients who are either overhydrated or dehydrated. Thereafter, daily fluid needs can be estimated by measuring urine output and adding 400 to 600 milliliters to account for the water lost from skin, lungs, and perspiration.[13] An individual with fever, vomiting, or diarrhea requires additional fluid.

Electrolytes Serum electrolyte levels are monitored closely to determine appropriate electrolyte intakes. Depending on the results of laboratory tests and the clinical assessment, restrictions may be necessary for potassium, phosphorus, and sodium. Patients undergoing dialysis may be allowed more liberal intakes. As mentioned previously, oliguric patients who experience diuresis at the beginning of the recovery period may need electrolyte replacement to compensate for urinary losses.

Enteral and Parenteral Nutrition Many patients need nutrition support to obtain adequate energy and nutrients. Enteral support (tube feeding) is preferred over parenteral nutrition because it is less likely to cause infection and sepsis. Although most patients can tolerate standard enteral formulas, some enteral formulas designed for patients with acute kidney injury are more kcalorically dense and have either higher or lower protein and electrolyte concentrations than standard formulas.[14] Total parenteral nutrition is necessary only if patients are severely malnourished or cannot consume food or tolerate tube feedings for an extended period.

The Case Study in Box 22-3 checks your understanding of acute kidney injury.

Box 22-3	Case Study: Woman with Acute Kidney Injury

Catherine Garber is a 42-year-old office manager admitted to the hospital's intensive care unit. She was first seen in the emergency department with severe edema, headache, nausea and vomiting, and a rapid heart rate. She reported an inability to pass more than minimal amounts of urine in the past two days. Her son, who drove her to the emergency department, reported that she had missed work for several days and seemed confused and unusually tired. Laboratory tests revealed elevated serum creatinine, BUN, and potassium levels. After learning from her medical history that Mrs. Garber had begun taking penicillin in the previous week, the physician diagnosed acute kidney injury, probably caused by a reaction to the medication. Mrs. Garber is 5 feet 3 inches tall and weighs 125 pounds.

1. Describe the probable reason for Mrs. Garber's inability to produce urine. Is her reaction to penicillin considered a prerenal, intrarenal, or postrenal cause of kidney injury? Give examples of other medical problems that can cause acute kidney injury.

2. What medications may the physician prescribe to treat Mrs. Garber's edema and hyperkalemia? What recommendation is likely regarding her continued use of penicillin?

3. What concerns should be kept in mind when determining Mrs. Garber's energy, protein, fluid, and electrolyte needs during acute kidney injury? How would dialysis treatment alter recommendations?

4. After treatment begins, Mrs. Garber suddenly begins producing copious amounts of urine. How may this development alter dietary treatment?

22.3 Chronic Kidney Disease

Unlike acute kidney injury, in which kidney function declines suddenly and rapidly, **chronic kidney disease** is characterized by gradual, irreversible loss of kidney function that results from long-term disease or injury. Because the kidneys have a large functional reserve—they are able to increase their workload to meet demands—chronic kidney disease typically progresses over many years without causing symptoms. Patients are often diagnosed late in the course of illness, after most kidney function has been lost.

The most common causes of chronic kidney disease are diabetes mellitus and hypertension, which are estimated to cause 45 and 27 percent of cases, respectively.[15] Other conditions that lead to chronic kidney disease include inflammatory, immunological, and hereditary diseases that directly involve the kidneys. Chronic kidney disease affects approximately 13 percent of the U.S. population.[16]

Consequences of Chronic Kidney Disease

In the early stages of chronic kidney disease, the functional nephrons compensate for those that are lost or damaged: they enlarge and filter blood more rapidly so that they are able to handle the extra workload. As more nephrons deteriorate, however, there is additional work for the remaining nephrons. The overburdened nephrons continue to degenerate until eventually the kidneys are unable to function adequately, resulting in kidney failure. Once the extent of kidney damage necessitates active treatment—either dialysis or a kidney transplant—the condition is classified as **end-stage renal disease**. Without intervention at this stage, an individual cannot survive. The clinical effects of chronic kidney disease are often nonspecific (see Table 22-3 and Box 22-4), which may delay diagnosis of the condition.

Chronic kidney disease is evaluated based on the **glomerular filtration rate (GFR)**, the rate at which the kidneys form filtrate, and the degree of albuminuria, the amount of albumin lost in urine daily.[17] GFR is considered the best index of overall kidney function, whereas albuminuria reflects the extent of kidney damage and correlates well with disease progression and health risks. Table 22-4 shows how chronic kidney disease is classified according to estimated GFR. Other laboratory measures that help to assess kidney function include tests of urine quality, serum electrolyte and BUN levels, and the ratio of albumin to creatinine in a urine sample.[18]

Altered Electrolytes and Hormones As the GFR falls, the increased activity of the remaining nephrons is often sufficient to maintain electrolyte excretion; thus, fluid and electrolyte imbalances may not develop until the fourth or fifth stage of chronic kidney disease. A number of hormonal adaptations also help to regulate electrolyte levels, but these changes may cause complications of their own. The increased secretion of **aldosterone** helps to prevent increases in serum potassium but contributes to fluid overload and the development of hypertension (in patients who were not

TABLE 22-3 Clinical Effects of Chronic Kidney Disease

EARLY STAGES

- Anorexia
- Exercise intolerance
- Fatigue
- Headache
- Hypercoagulation
- Hypertension
- Proteinuria, hematuria (blood in urine)

ADVANCED STAGES

- Anemia, bleeding tendency
- Cardiovascular disease
- Confusion, mental impairments
- Electrolyte imbalances
- Fluid retention, edema
- Hormonal abnormalities
- Itching
- Metabolic acidosis
- Muscle wasting
- Nausea and vomiting
- Peripheral neuropathy
- Protein-energy malnutrition
- Reduced immunity
- Renal osteodystrophy

chronic kidney disease: a condition characterized by the gradual, irreversible loss of kidney function resulting from long-term disease or injury; also called *chronic renal failure*.

end-stage renal disease: an advanced stage of chronic kidney disease in which dialysis or a kidney transplant is necessary to sustain life.

TABLE 22-4 Evaluation of Chronic Kidney Disease[a]

STAGE OF DISEASE	DESCRIPTION	GFR[B] (mL/min per 1.73 m²)
1	Kidney damage with normal or increased GFR	≥90
2	Mildly decreased GFR	60–89
3a	Mildly to moderately decreased GFR	45–59
3b	Moderately to severely decreased GFR	30–44
4	Severely decreased GFR	15–29
5	Kidney failure	<15 (or undergoing dialysis)

[a]A complete assessment of chronic kidney disease takes into account the likelihood of health risk, as indicated by the degree of albuminuria and other markers of kidney damage.

[b]Glomerular filtration rate, or GFR, is usually estimated using the Modification of Diet in Renal Disease study equation, which is based on serum creatinine levels, age, gender, body size, and ethnicity. Normal GFR averages 125 mL/min in young adults and declines with age.

Sources: L. A. Inker and coauthors, KDOQI U.S. commentary on the 2012 KDIGO clinical practice guideline for the evaluation and management of CKD, *American Journal of Kidney Diseases* 63 (2014): 713–735; P.E. Stevens and A. Levin, Evaluation and management of chronic kidney disease: Synopsis of the kidney disease: improving global outcomes 2012 clinical practice guideline, *Annals of Internal Medicine* 158 (2013): 825–830.

previously hypertensive). Increased secretion of **parathyroid hormone** helps to prevent elevations in serum phosphate but contributes to bone loss and the development of **renal osteodystrophy**, a bone disorder common in renal patients. Electrolyte imbalances are likely when the GFR is very low (below 5 milliliters per minute), when hormonal adaptations are inadequate, or when intakes of water or electrolytes are either very restricted or excessive.

Because the kidneys are responsible for maintaining acid–base balance, acidosis often develops in chronic kidney disease. Although usually mild, the acidosis exacerbates renal bone disease because compounds in bone (for example, protein and phosphates) are released to buffer the acid in blood.

Uremic Syndrome Uremia may develop during the final stages of chronic kidney disease, when the GFR falls below about 15 milliliters per minute.[19] As mentioned previously, the many complications that result from uremia are collectively known as the *uremic syndrome*. Clinical effects may include the following:

- *Hormonal imbalances.* Diseased kidneys are unable to produce erythropoietin, causing anemia. Reduced production of active vitamin D contributes to bone disease. Altered levels or activities of various other hormones may upset growth, reproductive function (menstruation, sperm production), and blood glucose regulation.
- *Altered heart function/increased heart disease risk.* Fluid and electrolyte imbalances result in hypertension, arrhythmias, and eventual heart muscle enlargement. Excessive parathyroid hormone secretion leads to calcification of arteries and heart tissue. Patients with uremia are at increased risk of stroke, heart attack, and heart failure.
- *Neuromuscular disturbances.* Initial symptoms may be mild, and include malaise, irritability, and altered thought processes. Later effects include muscle cramping, restless leg syndrome, sensory deficits, tremor, and seizures.
- *Other effects.* Defects in platelet function and clotting factors prolong bleeding time and contribute to bruising, GI bleeding, and anemia. Skin changes include increased pigmentation and severe pruritus (itchiness). Many patients have suppressed immune responses and are at high risk of developing infections.

glomerular filtration rate (GFR): the rate at which filtrate is formed within the kidneys, normally about 125 mL/min in healthy young adults.

aldosterone: a steroid hormone secreted by the adrenal cortex that promotes sodium (and therefore water) retention and potassium excretion.

parathyroid hormone: a protein hormone secreted by the parathyroid glands that helps to regulate serum concentrations of calcium and phosphate.

renal osteodystrophy: a bone disorder that develops in patients with chronic kidney disease as a result of increased secretion of parathyroid hormone, reduced serum calcium, acidosis, and impaired vitamin D activation in the kidneys.

Malnutrition The metabolic derangements that occur in chronic kidney disease contribute to **protein-energy wasting**, a syndrome characterized by losses of muscle mass and energy reserves. The wasting occurs, in part, because the uremia-induced changes that accompany chronic kidney disease (such as chronic inflammation, metabolic acidosis, and hormonal disorders) cause the breakdown of body proteins and negative nitrogen balance.[20] In addition, patients with chronic kidney disease often eat poorly because of anorexia, dietary restrictions, depression, and the dietary challenges of other diseases. Nutrient losses contribute to malnutrition and may be a consequence of dialysis, frequent blood draws, or bleeding abnormalities. A screening method sometimes used for assessing malnutrition risk is the *Subjective Global Assessment*, described in Chapter 13 (Table 13-2 on p. 383).

Treatment of Chronic Kidney Disease

The goals of treatment for patients with chronic kidney disease are to slow disease progression and prevent or alleviate complications. Dietary measures help to prevent malnutrition and wasting. Once kidney disease reaches the final stages, dialysis or a kidney transplant is necessary to sustain life.

Drug Treatment Medications help to control some of the complications associated with chronic kidney disease. Treatment of hypertension is critical for preventing disease progression and reducing cardiovascular disease risk; thus, antihypertensive drugs are usually prescribed (see Chapter 21). Some antihypertensive drugs (such as ACE inhibitors) can reduce proteinuria, helping to prevent additional kidney damage. Anemia is usually treated by injection or intravenous administration of erythropoietin (epoetin). Other drug treatments may include phosphate binders (taken with food) to reduce serum phosphate levels, sodium bicarbonate to reverse acidosis, and cholesterol-lowering medications.

Dialysis Dialysis replaces kidney function by removing excess fluid and wastes from the blood. In **hemodialysis**, the blood is circulated through a **dialyzer** (artificial kidney), where it is bathed by a **dialysate**, a solution that selectively removes fluid and wastes. In **peritoneal dialysis**, the dialysate is infused into a person's peritoneal cavity, and the blood is filtered by the peritoneum (the membrane surrounding the abdominal cavity). After several hours, the dialysate is drained, removing unneeded fluid and wastes. Nutrition in Practice 22 provides additional information about dialysis.

Nutrition Therapy for Chronic Kidney Disease The patient's diet strongly influences disease progression, the development of complications, and serum levels of nitrogenous wastes and electrolytes. Because the dietary measures for chronic kidney disease are complex and nutrient needs change frequently during the course of illness, a dietitian who specializes in renal disease is best suited to provide nutrition therapy. Table 22-5 summarizes the general dietary guidelines for patients in different stages of illness. As patients' needs vary considerably, actual recommendations should be based on the results of a careful and complete nutrition assessment.

Energy Because malnutrition is a common complication of chronic kidney disease, patients are advised to consume enough energy to maintain a healthy body weight. Individuals at risk of protein-energy wasting should consume foods with **high energy density**; some malnourished patients may require oral supplements or tube feedings to maintain an appropriate weight. Wasting is more prevalent during maintenance dialysis than in earlier stages of illness.[21] Note that obesity has been associated with disease progression, and therefore some obese patients may benefit from weight loss.[22]

Most dialysates used in peritoneal dialysis contain glucose in order to draw fluid from the blood to the peritoneal cavity by osmosis; on average, about 64 percent of this glucose is absorbed.[23] The kcalories from glucose (as many as 600 kcalories daily) must

protein-energy wasting: a syndrome characterized by losses of muscle mass and energy reserves that result from the complications of kidney disease.

hemodialysis (HE-moe-dye-AL-ih-sis): a treatment that removes fluids and wastes from the blood by passing the blood through a dialyzer.

dialyzer (DYE-ah-LYE-zer): a machine used in hemodialysis to filter the blood; also called an *artificial kidney*.

dialysate (dye-AL-ih-sate): the solution used in dialysis to draw fluids and wastes from the blood.

peritoneal (PEH-rih-toe-NEE-al) **dialysis:** a treatment that removes fluids and wastes from the blood by using the body's peritoneal membrane as a filter.

high energy density: a high number of kcalories per unit weight of food; foods of high energy density are generally high in fat and low in water content.

TABLE 22-5 Dietary Guidelines for Chronic Kidney Disease[a]

NUTRIENT	PREDIALYSIS (STAGES 4–5)	HEMODIALYSIS	PERITONEAL DIALYSIS
Energy (kcal/kg of body weight)	35 for <60 years old 30–35 for ≥60 years old (or as necessary to maintain a healthy weight)	35 for <60 years old 30–35 for ≥60 years old (or as necessary to maintain a healthy weight)	35 for <60 years old 30–35 for ≥60 years old (or as necessary to maintain a healthy weight) Note: The energy intake includes kcalories absorbed from the dialysate.
Protein (g/kg of body weight)	0.6–0.75 (≥50% high-quality proteins)	1.2 (≥50% high-quality proteins)	1.2–1.3 (≥50% high-quality proteins)
Fat	As necessary to maintain a healthy lipid profile	As necessary to maintain a healthy lipid profile	As necessary to maintain a healthy lipid profile
Fluid (mL/day)	Unrestricted if urine output is normal	Urine output plus 500–1000 mL	2000–3000; unrestricted in some cases
Sodium (mg/day)	<2400; additional restriction (<2000) often advised to improve hypertension[b]	<2000	<2000
Potassium (mg/day)	<2400; adjust according to serum potassium levels	<2400; adjust according to serum potassium levels	3000–4000; adjust according to serum potassium levels
Phosphorus (mg/day)	800–1000 if serum phosphate or parathyroid hormone is elevated	800–1000 if serum phosphate or parathyroid hormone is elevated	800–1000 if serum phosphate or parathyroid hormone is elevated
Calcium (mg/day)	1000–1200; should not exceed 2000 from diet and medications	1000–1200; should not exceed 2000 from diet and medications	1000–1200; should not exceed 2000 from diet and medications

[a]The values in this table apply to adults; guidelines for children can be found at www.kidney.org/professionals/guidelines/guidelines_commentaries/nutrition-ckd.

[b]Sodium restriction may help to control hypertension and slow the progression of kidney disease.

Sources: T. A. Ikizler, Nutrition and kidney disease, in S. J. Gilbert and D. E. Weiner, eds., *National Kidney Foundation's Primer on Kidney Diseases* (Philadelphia: Elsevier, 2018), p. 484–492; Academy of Nutrition and Dietetics, *Nutrition Care Manual* (Chicago: Academy of Nutrition and Dietetics, 2018); National Kidney Foundation, *KDOQI clinical practice guidelines for nutrition in chronic renal failure*, kidneyfoundation.cachefly.net/professionals/KDOQI/guidelines_nutrition/doqi_nut.html.

be included in estimates of energy intake. Weight gain is sometimes a problem when peritoneal dialysis continues for a long period.

Protein A moderate protein restriction may be prescribed to slow disease progression and reduce nitrogenous wastes. Furthermore, low-protein diets supply less phosphorus than high-protein diets, reducing the risk of hyperphosphatemia. Because renal patients often develop protein-energy wasting, however, their diet must provide enough protein to meet needs and prevent wasting. During the later stages of kidney disease, the recommended protein intake is 0.6 to 0.75 grams per kilogram of body weight per day, slightly below the protein RDA for adults (0.8 grams per kilogram).[24] To ensure appropriate intakes of the essential amino acids, at least 50 percent of the protein consumed should come from high-quality protein sources (see Photo 22-1). Plant sources of protein should be included in the diet as they place less demand on the kidneys than animal proteins and are also low in phosphorus.[25] Low-protein breads, pastas, and other grain-based products are commercially available to help renal patients improve energy intakes without increasing protein consumption.

To reduce the high risk of wasting and difficulties with compliance that are associated with low-protein diets, some dietitians may suggest that patients consume higher amounts of protein to preserve health. Once dialysis has begun, protein restrictions can be relaxed because dialysis removes nitrogenous wastes and results in some amino acid losses as well.

Lipids To control elevated blood lipids and reduce heart disease risk, patients with chronic kidney disease are generally advised to limit their intakes of saturated and *trans*

Photo 22-1 Diet and Kidney Disease

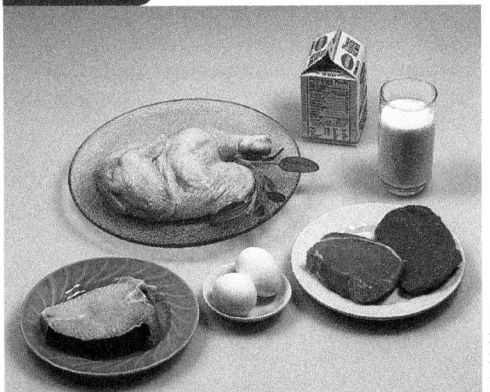

To ensure adequate intake of the essential amino acids, people with chronic kidney disease should consume high-quality protein sources such as eggs, milk products, meat, poultry, fish, and soybeans.

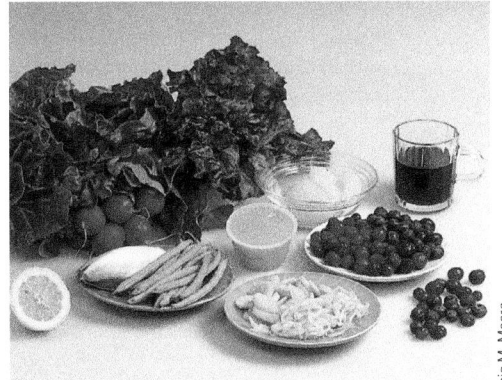

People with chronic kidney disease can consume most fruits and vegetables in limited amounts.

fats, refined sugars, and alcohol. Although renal patients are often encouraged to consume high-fat foods to improve their energy intakes, the foods they select should provide mostly unsaturated fats.

Sodium and Fluids As kidney disease progresses, patients excrete less urine and become unable to handle normal amounts of sodium and fluids. Recommendations depend on the total urine output, changes in body weight and blood pressure, and serum sodium levels. A rise in body weight and blood pressure suggests that the person is retaining sodium and fluid; conversely, declines in these measurements indicate fluid loss. Most people with kidney disease tend to retain sodium and may benefit from mild restriction; less often, a patient may have a salt-wasting condition that requires additional dietary sodium.

Fluids are not restricted until urine output decreases. For a person who is neither dehydrated nor overhydrated, the daily fluid intake should match the daily urine output. Once a person is on dialysis, sodium and fluid intakes should be controlled so that only about 2 pounds of water weight are gained daily—this excess fluid is then removed during the next dialysis treatment. Patients on fluid-restricted diets should be advised that foods such as flavored gelatin, soup, fruit ices, and frozen fruit juice bars contribute to the fluid allowance.

Potassium Most patients can handle typical intakes of potassium during stages 1 through 4 of illness. Restrictions are generally advised for patients who develop hyperkalemia, have diabetic nephropathy (which increases risk of hyperkalemia), or reach a later stage of illness. Conversely, potassium supplementation may be necessary for persons using potassium-wasting diuretics.

Dialysis patients must control potassium intakes to prevent hyperkalemia or, more rarely, **hypokalemia**. Restriction is necessary for individuals treated with hemodialysis, whereas those undergoing peritoneal dialysis can consume potassium more freely. Recommended intakes are based on serum potassium levels, renal function, medications, and the dialysis procedure used.

All fresh foods provide potassium, but some fruits and vegetables contain such high amounts that some patients must limit intakes. Table 22-6 shows the potassium content of some common fruits and vegetables. Foods in other food groups may be high in potassium as well; examples include dried beans, fish, milk and milk products, molasses, nuts and nut butters, and wheat bran. Note that salt substitutes and other

hypokalemia (HIGH-po-ka-LEE-me-ah): low serum potassium levels.

TABLE 22-6   Potassium Guide—Fruits and Vegetables

This table lists common fruits and vegetables according to their potassium content. One serving is equivalent to ½ cup raw fruit or cooked vegetable unless otherwise noted. Keep in mind that the portion size may determine how a food is categorized. Check a food composition table for additional information about the potassium content of foods.

HIGH POTASSIUM (>250 mg PER SERVING)	MEDIUM POTASSIUM (150–250 mg PER SERVING)	LOW POTASSIUM (<150 mg PER SERVING)
• Avocado	• Apple (1 medium)	• Blueberries
• Banana	• Apricots (2 whole)	• Cabbage
• Beets	• Asparagus	• Carrots (1 medium)
• Chard	• Broccoli	• Cauliflower
• Dates (3 whole)	• Cantaloupe	• Cucumbers
• Nectarine (1 small)	• Celery	• Eggplant
• Orange (1 medium)	• Corn	• Grapes
• Parsnips	• Grapefruit (½ fruit)	• Green beans
• Potatoes	• Honeydew melon	• Green pepper
• Pumpkin	• Kale	• Lettuce (4 leaves, raw)
• Raisins	• Peach (1 small)	• Onions (1 small)
• Spinach	• Pear (1 medium)	• Plum (1 small)
• Sweet potatoes	• Peas	• Strawberries
• Tomato	• Zucchini	• Watermelon

TABLE 22-7 Foods High in Phosphorus[a]

- Barley
- Bran (oat, wheat)
- Buckwheat groats
- Bulgur
- Canned iced tea
- Canned lemonade
- Coconut
- Cola beverages
- Cornmeal
- Couscous
- Dried peas and beans
- Fish
- Milk products
- Nuts and seeds
- Organ meats
- Peanut butter
- Processed foods[b]
- Soybeans, tofu

[a]For a complete list, visit the USDA's Nutrient Database at ndb.nal.usda.gov/ndb/. Click on "Nutrient Search." Then select phosphorus as the "First Nutrient," use the "Sort by" feature to select "Nutrient Content," and then click "Go."

[b]Many processed foods contain phosphate additives, which contribute significantly to phosphorus intakes.

hypercalcemia (HIGH-per-kal-SEE-me-ah): elevated serum calcium levels.

low-sodium products often contain potassium chloride, which people on a potassium-restricted diet should avoid.

Phosphorus, Calcium, and Vitamin D To minimize the risk of bone disease, serum phosphate and calcium levels are monitored in renal patients, and laboratory values help to guide recommendations. Elevated serum phosphate levels indicate the need for dietary phosphorus restriction and, if necessary, the use of phosphate binders (taken with meals). Many phosphate binders are calcium salts, and patients using these binders may be at risk of developing **hypercalcemia** in response to simultaneous calcium and vitamin D supplementation. Vitamin D supplementation is recommended only for patients with suspected deficiency;[26] note that the prevalence of vitamin D deficiency in patients with chronic kidney disease may be as high as 70 to 80 percent.[27]

High-protein foods are also high in phosphorus, so the protein-restricted diets consumed by predialysis patients curb phosphorus intakes as well. After dialysis treatments begin and protein intakes are liberalized, phosphate binders become essential for phosphorus control. Because foods that are rich in calcium (such as milk and milk products) are usually high in phosphorus and are therefore restricted, patients may rely on calcium supplements (or calcium-based phosphate binders) to meet their calcium needs. Table 22-7 lists examples of foods that are high in phosphorus.

Vitamins and Minerals The restrictive renal diet interferes with vitamin and mineral intakes, increasing the risk of deficiencies. In addition, patients treated with dialysis lose water-soluble vitamins and some trace minerals into the dialysate. Thus, multivitamin/mineral supplements are typically recommended for all patients. Supplements prescribed for dialysis patients typically supply generous amounts of folic acid and vitamin B_6—about 1 milligram and 10 milligrams per day, respectively—along with recommended amounts of the other water-soluble vitamins.[28] Supplemental vitamin C should be limited to 100 milligrams per day because excessive intakes can contribute to kidney stone formation in those at risk (see p. 644). Vitamin A supplements are not recommended because vitamin A levels tend to rise as kidney function worsens.

Iron deficiency is common in hemodialysis patients and may be due to inadequate dietary intakes, impaired iron absorption, and blood losses associated with the dialysis treatment. Intravenous administration of iron is more effective than oral iron supplementation for improving iron status in these patients.[29]

Enteral and Parenteral Nutrition Nutrition support is sometimes necessary for renal patients who cannot consume adequate amounts of food. The enteral formulas suitable for patients with chronic kidney disease are more kcalorically dense and have lower protein and electrolyte concentrations than standard formulas. **Intradialytic parenteral nutrition** is an option for supplying supplemental nutrients to dialysis patients; this technique combines parenteral infusions with hemodialysis treatments. An advantage of this approach is that the volume of parenteral solution infused can be simultaneously removed (recall that fluid intake is controlled in dialysis patients). However, clinical studies have not shown intradialytic parenteral nutrition to be more successful than oral supplementation for improving the nutrition status of malnourished dialysis patients.[30] Currently, the technique is used mainly in malnourished patients who have not responded well to oral supplements.

Dietary Compliance Adhering to a renal diet is probably the most challenging aspect of treatment for patients with chronic kidney disease. Depending on the stage of illness and the patient's laboratory values, the renal diet may limit protein, fluids, sodium, potassium, and phosphorus, thereby affecting food selections from all major food groups. In addition, adjustments in nutrient intake are required as the disease progresses. If the kidney disease was caused by diabetes, patients must also continue the dietary changes necessary for controlling blood glucose levels. Because renal diets have so many restrictions, patient compliance is often a problem. Table 22-8 shows an example of a one-day menu that includes some typical restrictions, and Box 22-5 provides suggestions to help patients comply with renal diets. The Case Study in Box 22-6 allows you to apply your knowledge about chronic kidney disease and hemodialysis.

TABLE 22-8 Chronic Kidney Disease—One-Day Menu

The menu below provides 2028 kcalories, 46 g protein, 784 mg phosphorus, 2190 mg potassium, and 1510 mg sodium.[a] The energy and protein content would be appropriate for a 135-pound predialysis patient. Note that the menu includes a number of refined and low-fiber foods due to the need to limit phosphorus and potassium.

BREAKFAST
- Corn flakes with milk (1 cup cereal, ½ cup whole milk)
- Apricot nectar (1 cup)
- Caffé latte (brewed coffee, 2 tsp sugar, ½ cup cream substitute)

LUNCH
- Turkey sandwich (2 slices white bread, 1½ oz dark meat, 5 slices cucumber, 1 tbs mayonnaise)
- Grape juice (1 cup)
- Orange sherbet (½ cup)

DINNER
- Spaghetti with tomato sauce (1 cup cooked spaghetti, ½ cup bottled tomato sauce, ½ tbs grated cheese)
- Green beans with olive oil (1 cup cooked green beans, 1 tbs olive oil)
- Biscuit with margarine (2½-inch biscuit, ½ tbs margarine)
- Baked apple with nondairy sour cream (1 large apple, ¼ cup nondairy sour cream)

[a]Energy and nutrient values were obtained from the USDA National Nutrient Database for Standard Reference at ndb.nal.usda.gov/ndb.

intradialytic parenteral nutrition: the infusion of nutrients during hemodialysis, often providing amino acids, dextrose, lipids, and some trace minerals.

Box 22-5

HOW TO Help Patients Comply with a Renal Diet

Patients with renal disease and their caregivers face considerable challenges as they learn to manage a renal diet. The following suggestions may help:

1. To keep track of fluid intake:
   - Fill a container with an amount of water equal to your total fluid allowance. Each time you consume a liquid food or beverage, discard an equivalent amount of water from the container. The amount remaining in the container will show you how much fluid you have left for the day.
   - Be sure to save enough fluid to take medications.

2. To help control thirst:
   - Chew gum or suck hard candy.
   - Suck on frozen grapes.
   - Freeze allowed beverages to a semisolid state so that they take longer to consume. Or, fill an ice-cube tray with your favorite fruit-flavored beverage and suck on flavored ice cubes during the day.
   - Add lemon juice or crumpled mint leaves to water to make it more refreshing.
   - Gargle with refrigerated mouthwash.

3. To increase the energy content of meals:
   - Add extra margarine or a flavored oil to rice, noodles, bread, crackers, and cooked vegetables. Add extra salad dressing or mayonnaise to salad.

   - Add a nondairy whipped topping to desserts.
   - Include fried foods in your diet.

4. To include more of your favorite vegetables in meals:
   - Consult your nurse or dietitian to learn whether you can safely use the process of leaching to remove some of the potassium from vegetables.
   - To leach potassium from vegetables: Cut the vegetables into $\frac{1}{8}$-inch slices and rinse. Soak the vegetables in a large amount of warm water for two hours—about 10 parts of water to 1 part of vegetables. Rinse vegetables well. Boil vegetables using 5 parts of water to 1 part of vegetables.

5. To prevent the diet from becoming monotonous:
   - Experiment with new combinations of allowed foods.
   - Substitute nondairy products for milk products. Nondairy products, which are lower in protein, phosphorus, and potassium, can substitute for milk and add energy to the diet.
   - Add flavor to foods by seasoning with garlic, onion, chili powder, curry powder, oregano, mint, basil, parsley, pepper, or lemon juice.
   - Consult a nurse or dietitian when you want to eat restricted foods. Many restricted foods can be used occasionally and in small amounts if the menu is carefully adjusted.

Box 22-6

Case Study: Man with Chronic Kidney Disease

Thomas Stone is a 55-year-old banker who developed chronic kidney disease as a result of hypertension. His condition was discovered several years ago, when routine laboratory tests revealed elevated serum creatinine levels and persistent albuminuria. Since then, he has been taking antihypertensive medications and restricting dietary sodium, but he reported difficulty following the low-protein diet that was also prescribed. Mr. Stone recently visited his doctor with complaints of low urine output and reduced sensation in his hands and feet. He also reported feeling drowsy at work and mentioned that he was bruising more than usual. The examination revealed a 9-pound weight gain since his last visit and swelling in his ankles and feet. Tests revealed that his GFR had fallen to 10 milliliters per minute. Mr. Stone is 5 feet 8 inches tall and normally weighs 160 pounds.

1. Explain how chronic kidney disease progresses. What happens to GFR, serum creatinine levels, and albuminuria as renal function declines?

2. Describe the clinical effects you would expect during the final stage of disease, when kidney failure develops. Explain the significance of each of Mr. Stone's physical complaints.

3. Explain why a low-sodium, low-protein diet was prescribed for Mr. Stone at a former visit. What energy and protein intakes were probably recommended at that time?

4. The physician determines that Mr. Stone's kidney disease has reached the final stage and prescribes hemodialysis. How will dialysis alter Mr. Stone's diet? Calculate his new protein recommendation, and compare it to the amount of protein recommended before dialysis. What other changes in nutrient intake may be necessary?

Kidney Transplants

A preferred alternative to dialysis in patients with end-stage renal disease is kidney transplantation. A successful kidney transplant restores kidney function, allows a more liberal diet, and frees the patient from routine dialysis. Given the choice, many patients would prefer transplants, but the demand for suitable kidneys far exceeds the supply. Less than 20 percent of patients with end-stage renal disease receive a kidney transplant.[31]

Immunosuppressive Drug Therapy To prevent tissue rejection following transplant surgery, patients require high doses of immunosuppressive drugs such as corticosteroids, cyclosporine, tacrolimus, and mycophenolic acid. These drugs have multiple effects that can alter nutrition status, including vomiting, diarrhea, glucose intolerance, altered blood lipids, electrolyte imbalances, weight gain, and increased infection risk (see Box 22-7).[32] Because immunosuppressive drug therapy increases the risk of foodborne infection, food safety guidelines should be provided to patients and caregivers. Box 22-8 summarizes the nutrition-related effects of immunosuppressants and other drugs mentioned in this chapter.

Nutrition Therapy after Kidney Transplant After patients recover from transplant surgery, most nutrients can be consumed at levels recommended for the general population. Patients should attempt to maintain a healthy body weight and consume a diet that reduces their risk for cardiovascular diseases.

For most transplant patients, the side effects of drugs are the primary reason that dietary adjustments may be required. Although sodium, potassium, phosphorus, and fluid intakes are usually liberalized following a successful transplant, serum electrolyte levels must be monitored because some drug therapies can cause electrolyte imbalances or fluid retention. If corticosteroids are used as immunosuppressants, calcium supplementation is recommended because the medication increases urinary calcium losses. If drug treatment leads to hyperglycemia, patients should limit intakes of refined carbohydrates and concentrated sweets; for some individuals, oral medications or insulin therapy may be necessary. Patients should continue to follow food safety guidelines to avoid foodborne illness.

Box 22-8 Diet-Drug Interactions

Check this table for notable nutrition-related effects of the medications discussed in this chapter.

Immunosuppressants (cyclosporine, tacrolimus)	**Gastrointestinal effects:** Nausea, vomiting, abdominal discomfort, diarrhea, constipation, anorexia
	Dietary interactions: Limit alcohol intake due to the potential for toxic effects; the bioavailability of tacrolimus is reduced when the drug is taken with food; grapefruit juice can raise serum concentrations of these drugs to toxic levels
	Metabolic effects: Electrolyte imbalances, hyperglycemia, hyperlipidemias, anemia, hypertension
Immunosuppressants (corticosteroids)	**Metabolic effects:** Fluid retention, hyperglycemia, hypocalcemia, hypokalemia, hypophosphatemia, increased appetite, protein catabolism, hypertension
Phosphate binders (calcium-based)	**Gastrointestinal effect:** Constipation
	Metabolic effects: Electrolyte imbalances
Potassium-exchange resins (sodium polystyrene sulfonate)	**Gastrointestinal effects:** Anorexia, constipation
	Dietary interactions: Calcium and magnesium supplements must be taken separately
	Metabolic effects: Fluid and sodium retention, hypokalemia, hypocalcemia, hypomagnesemia
Potassium citrate	**Gastrointestinal effects:** Nausea, vomiting, abdominal pain, diarrhea
	Metabolic effect: Hyperkalemia

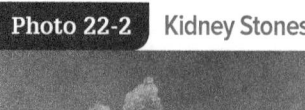

Photo 22-2 Kidney Stones

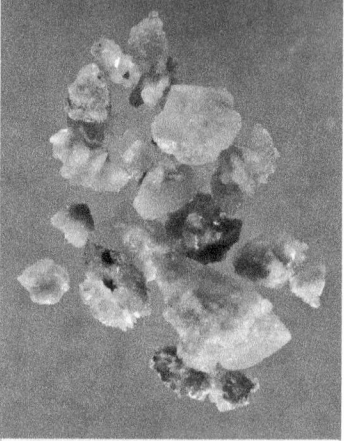

Nathan Griffith/Corbis

The most common type of kidney stone is composed of calcium oxalate crystals, as shown here. Kidney stones may be as small as a bread crumb or as large as a golf ball.

kidney stones: crystalline masses that form in the urinary tract; also called *renal calculi* or *nephrolithiasis*.

hypercalciuria (HIGH-per-kal-see-YOO-ree-ah): elevated urinary calcium levels.

hyperoxaluria (HIGH-per-ox-ah-LOO-ree-ah): elevated urinary oxalate levels.

hypocitraturia: low urinary citrate levels. Citrate is formed in the body during energy metabolism and is also a component of fruit (especially citrus fruit) and some other foods.

22.4 Kidney Stones

Approximately 11 percent of men and 7 percent of women in the United States develop one or more **kidney stones** during their lifetimes.[33] A kidney stone is a crystalline mass that forms within the urinary tract. Although stones are often asymptomatic, their passage can cause severe pain or block the urinary tract. Stones tend to recur but can be prevented with dietary measures and medical treatment.

Formation of Kidney Stones

Kidney stones develop when stone constituents become concentrated in urine, allowing crystals to form and grow. Most kidney stones are made up primarily of calcium oxalate (see Photo 22-2). Less commonly, stones are composed of calcium phosphate, uric acid, the amino acid cystine, or magnesium ammonium phosphate (the latter are known as *struvite* stones). Factors that predispose an individual to stone formation include the following:

- *Dehydration* or *low urine volume*, which promotes the crystallization of minerals and other compounds in urine.
- *Changes in urine acidity*, which affect the dissolution of urinary constituents. Some stones form more readily in acidic urine, whereas others tend to form in alkaline urine.
- *Metabolic abnormalities*, which influence the concentrations of substances that either promote or inhibit crystal growth.
- *Obstruction*, which prevents the flow of urine and encourages salt precipitation.

Calcium Oxalate Stones The most common abnormality in people with calcium oxalate stones is **hypercalciuria** (elevated urinary calcium levels). Hypercalciuria can result from excessive calcium absorption, impaired calcium reabsorption in kidney tubules, or elevated serum levels of parathyroid hormone or vitamin D.

Elevated urinary oxalate levels, or **hyperoxaluria**, also promote the formation of calcium oxalate crystals. Oxalate is a normal product of metabolism that readily binds to calcium. Hyperoxaluria reflects an increase in the body's synthesis of oxalate or increased absorption from dietary sources. Fat malabsorption can increase oxalate absorption: the malabsorbed fatty acids bind to minerals (such as calcium and magnesium) that would otherwise bind to oxalates and inhibit their absorption (see Chapter 18).

Low urinary citrate levels (**hypocitraturia**) increase the risk of forming calcium stones because the citrates in urine inhibit calcium's tendency to crystallize with oxalates and other compounds. Urinary citrate levels are influenced by genetic factors, urine acidity, some medications, and dietary factors.

Uric Acid Stones Uric acid stones develop when the urine is abnormally acidic, contains excessive uric acid, or both. These stones are frequently associated with **gout**, a metabolic disorder characterized by elevated uric acid levels in the blood and urine. A diet rich in **purines** also contributes to high uric acid levels; purines are abundant in animal proteins (meat, poultry, seafood) and degrade to uric acid in the body. In addition, a high intake of animal protein increases urine acidity, which promotes the crystallization of uric acid.

Cystine and Struvite Stones Cystine stones can form in people with the inherited disorder **cystinuria**, in which the renal tubules are unable to reabsorb the amino acid cystine. The abnormality results in high concentrations of cystine in the urine, leading to subsequent crystallization and stone formation. **Struvite** stones, composed primarily of magnesium ammonium phosphate, form in alkaline urine; the urinary pH is sometimes elevated due to the bacterial degradation of urea to ammonia. Struvite stones can accompany chronic urinary infections or disorders that interfere with urinary flow.

Consequences of Kidney Stones

In most cases, kidney stones do not pose serious medical problems. Small stones can readily pass through the ureters and out of the body with minimal treatment.

Renal Colic A stone passing through the ureter may produce severe, stabbing pain, called **renal colic** (see Box 22-9). The pain can be severe enough to cause nausea and vomiting and sometimes requires medication. Blood may appear in the urine (**hematuria**) as a result of damage to the kidney or ureter lining.

Urinary Tract Complications Depending on the location of the stone, symptoms may include urination urgency, frequent urination, or inability to urinate. Stones that are unable to pass through the ureter can cause a urinary tract obstruction and possibly lead to infection or acute kidney injury.

Prevention and Treatment of Kidney Stones

Solutes are less likely to crystallize and form stones in dilute urine. Therefore, people who form kidney stones are advised to drink 12 or more cups of fluid daily to maintain a urine volume of at least 2 liters per day (see Photo 22-3).[34] Additional fluid may be needed in hot weather or if an individual is extremely active.

Calcium Oxalate Stones Most dietary strategies and drug treatments for calcium oxalate stones aim to reduce urinary calcium and oxalate levels. Dietary measures may include adjustments in calcium, oxalate, protein, and sodium intakes.[35] Patients should consume adequate calcium from food sources (about 800 to 1200 milligrams per day) because dietary calcium combines with oxalate in the intestines, reducing oxalate absorption and helping to control hyperoxaluria.* Conversely, low-calcium diets promote oxalate absorption and higher urinary oxalate levels. Some individuals with hyperoxaluria may benefit from dietary oxalate restriction (see Table 22-9). High intakes of protein (especially from meat, fish, poultry, or eggs) and sodium increase urinary calcium excretion, so a moderate protein consumption (0.8 to 1.0 gram per kilogram of body weight per day) and a controlled sodium intake (no more than about 2000 to 3000 milligrams daily) are also advised. Patients with hypocitraturia may be advised to reduce intakes of animal proteins and increase intakes of citrus fruits and other

---

*Note that calcium supplements can elevate urinary calcium levels, so they are not as helpful as dietary sources of calcium.

Photo 22-3 Diet and Kidney Stones

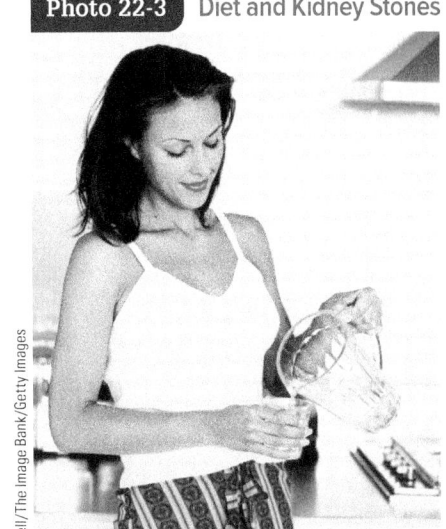

James Darell/The Image Bank/Getty Images

Drinking plenty of fluids throughout the day is the most important measure for preventing kidney stones. Acceptable fluid sources include water, tea, coffee, wine, and beer, but sugar-sweetened soft drinks should be limited because they may increase the risk of stone formation.

BOX 22-9 *Nursing Diagnosis*

Nursing diagnoses for patients with kidney stones may include *acute pain*, *impaired urinary elimination*, and *risk for infection*.

gout (GOWT): a metabolic disorder characterized by elevated uric acid levels in the blood and urine and the deposition of uric acid in and around the joints, causing acute joint inflammation.

purines (PYOO-reens): products of nucleotide metabolism that degrade to uric acid.

cystinuria (SIS-tin-NOO-ree-ah): a genetic disorder characterized by the elevated urinary excretion of several amino acids, including cystine.

struvite (STROO-vite): crystals of magnesium ammonium phosphate.

renal colic: the intense pain that occurs when a kidney stone passes through the ureter; the pain typically begins in the back and intensifies as the stone travels toward the bladder.

hematuria (HE-mah-TOO-ree-ah): blood in the urine.

TABLE 22-9	Foods High in Oxalates
Vegetables	Bamboo shoots, beets, carrots, celery, chard, collard greens, dried beans, okra, parsnips, potatoes, rutabagas, spinach, sweet potatoes, tomato sauce, turnips, yams
Fruit	Avocados, dates, grapefruit, kiwis, oranges (including orange peel), pineapple, raspberries, rhubarb, tangerines
Other	Buckwheat, chocolate, cocoa powder, cornmeal, grits, millet, miso, nuts and nut butters (including peanut butter), pumpkin seeds, rice, sesame seeds (including tahini), soybean products, sunflower seeds, tea, wheat bran, whole-wheat flour

Note: The oxalate content of many foods has not been analyzed, and few studies have been conducted to determine which foods raise urinary oxalate levels.

fruits and vegetables. Vitamin C supplements should be avoided because vitamin C degrades to oxalate.[36] Medications used to prevent calcium oxalate stones include thiazide diuretics, which reduce urinary calcium excretion; potassium citrate (a base), which inhibits crystal formation; and allopurinol (Zyloprim), which reduces uric acid production in the body and may have other effects.

Uric Acid Stones Although diets restricted in purines may help to control urinary uric acid levels, the effects on stone formation are unclear. Moreover, because all animal proteins contain purines, long-term restriction can be difficult to achieve. Drug treatments for uric acid stones include allopurinol to reduce uric acid levels and potassium citrate to reduce urine acidity.

Cystine and Struvite Stones High fluid intakes may prevent the formation of cystine stones in some patients, whereas other individuals require drug therapy to reduce cystine production in the body. Medications frequently prescribed include penicillamine (Cuprimine) and tiopronin (Thiola), which increase the solubility of cystine, and potassium citrate, which reduces urine acidity. For preventing struvite stones, preventing or promptly treating urinary tract infections is an important strategy.

Medical Treatment for Kidney Stones Medical treatment may be necessary for a kidney stone that is too large to pass, blocks urine flow, or causes severe pain or bleeding. Medications that relax the ureter and increase urine volume may be given to facilitate stone passage; examples include alpha-receptor blockers and calcium channel blockers. Some kidney stones can be fragmented into pieces that are small enough to pass in the urine; the most common method is *extracorporeal shock wave lithotripsy*, a procedure that uses high-amplitude sound waves to degrade the stone. Surgical methods that involve physical removal of kidney stones have a higher success rate but are also more invasive.

Review Notes

- Kidney stones form when stone constituents crystallize in urine. Complications include renal colic, difficulty with urination, and obstruction.
- Kidney stones may be prevented by maintaining a urine volume of at least 2 liters daily. Dietary measures include adjustments in intakes of calcium, oxalates, protein, sodium, and purines.
- Symptomatic kidney stones may be treated with medications that facilitate stone passage or surgeries that fragment or remove stones.

Nutrition Assessment Checklist for People with Kidney Diseases

MEDICAL HISTORY

Check the medical record to determine:

- ○ Degree of kidney function
- ○ Cause of the nephrotic syndrome or kidney disease
- ○ Type of dialysis, if appropriate
- ○ Whether the patient has received a kidney transplant
- ○ Type of kidney stone

Review the medical record for complications that may alter nutritional needs:

- ○ Anemia
- ○ Diabetes mellitus
- ○ Edema or oliguria
- ○ Hyperlipidemia
- ○ Hypertension
- ○ Metabolic stress or infection
- ○ Protein-energy malnutrition

MEDICATIONS

Assess risks for medication-related malnutrition related to:

- ○ Long-term use of medications
- ○ Multiple medication use, especially if medications affect nutrition status

In all patients with kidney diseases, note:

- ○ Whether medications or supplements contain electrolytes that must be controlled
- ○ Use of drugs or herbs that may be toxic to the kidneys

DIETARY INTAKE

In patients with the nephrotic syndrome, kidney disease, or a kidney transplant, assess intakes of:

- ○ Protein and energy
- ○ Fluid
- ○ Vitamins, especially vitamin D
- ○ Minerals, especially calcium, phosphorus, iron, and electrolytes

In patients with kidney stones or a history of kidney stones:

- ○ Stress the need to drink plenty of fluids throughout the day.

- ○ Assess intake of calcium, oxalates, sodium, protein, purines, or vitamin C, as appropriate for the type of stone.

ANTHROPOMETRIC DATA

Take accurate baseline height and weight measurements. Keep in mind that:

- ○ Fluid retention due to the nephrotic syndrome or kidney failure can mask malnutrition.
- ○ In dialysis patients, the weight measured immediately after the dialysis treatment (called the dry weight) most accurately reflects the person's true weight. Rapid weight gain between dialysis treatments reflects fluid retention and requires a review of the patient's fluid intake.

LABORATORY TESTS

Note that serum protein levels are often low in patients with the nephrotic syndrome or advanced kidney disease. Review the following laboratory test results to assess the degree of kidney function and response to treatments:

- ○ Albuminuria
- ○ Creatinine
- ○ Glomerular filtration rate (GFR)
- ○ Serum electrolytes

Check laboratory test results for complications associated with kidney disease, including:

- ○ Anemia
- ○ Hyperglycemia
- ○ Hyperlipidemia
- ○ Hyperparathyroidism (related to bone disease)

PHYSICAL SIGNS

In patients with the nephrotic syndrome or kidney disease, look for physical signs of:

- ○ Bone disease
- ○ Dehydration or fluid retention
- ○ Hyperkalemia
- ○ Iron deficiency
- ○ Uremia

Self Check

1. Which of the following is *not* a function of the kidneys?
   a. Activation of vitamin K
   b. Maintenance of acid–base balance
   c. Elimination of metabolic waste products
   d. Maintenance of fluid and electrolyte balances

2. The nephrotic syndrome frequently results in:
   a. the uremic syndrome.
   b. oliguria.
   c. edema.
   d. renal colic.

3. Dietary recommendations for patients with the nephrotic syndrome include:
   a. a high protein intake.
   b. sodium restriction.
   c. calcium and potassium restrictions.
   d. fluid restriction.

4. What is a common treatment for hyperkalemia?
   a. Eliminating potassium from the diet
   b. Using potassium-wasting diuretics to increase potassium losses
   c. Increasing fluid intake to maintain a high urine volume
   d. Using potassium-exchange resins, which bind potassium in the GI tract

5. If a patient with acute kidney injury should require a high protein intake, which additional treatment may be necessary?
   a. Frequent dialysis
   b. Use of diuretics
   c. Enteral nutrition support
   d. Fluid restriction

6. The most common cause of chronic kidney disease is:
   a. diabetes mellitus.
   b. hypertension.
   c. autoimmune disease.
   d. exposure to toxins.

7. A person with chronic kidney disease who has been following a renal diet for several years begins hemodialysis treatment. An appropriate dietary adjustment would be to:
   a. reduce protein intake.
   b. consume protein more liberally.
   c. increase intakes of sodium and water.
   d. consume potassium and phosphorus more liberally.

8. Which of the following nutrients may be unintentionally restricted when a patient restricts phosphorus intake?
   a. Water
   b. Calcium
   c. Potassium
   d. Sodium

9. Most kidney stones are made primarily from:
   a. struvite.
   b. uric acid.
   c. calcium oxalate.
   d. cystine.

10. Treatment for all kidney stones includes:
    a. dietary oxalate restriction.
    b. dietary protein restriction.
    c. vitamin C supplementation.
    d. a fluid intake that produces at least 2 liters of urine daily.

Answers: 1. a, 2. c, 3. b, 4. d, 5. a, 6. a, 7. b, 8. b, 9. c, 10. d

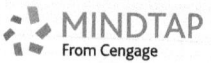 **MINDTAP** From Cengage   For more chapter resources visit **www.cengage.com** to access MindTap, a complete digital course.

Clinical Applications

1. A person with chronic kidney disease may need multiple medications to control disease progression and treat symptoms and complications. For people with diabetes and hyperlipidemias who develop chronic kidney disease, medications might include insulin, oral hypoglycemic drugs, antihypertensives, diuretics, lipid-lowering medications, and phosphate binders. Review the nutrition-related side effects of these medications. Describe the ways in which these medications may make it harder for people to maintain nutrition status.

2. Identify the recommended energy, protein, and sodium intakes for a 65-year-old hemodialysis patient who weighs 60 kilograms (use the guidelines shown in Table 22-5). Then, consider the type of diet that would be appropriate for this patient by following these steps:
   - Create a one-day menu that provides appropriate amounts of energy, protein, and sodium for this patient (use the energy and nutrient values in a food composition table).
   - Assuming that the patient's laboratory test results suggest that potassium and phosphorus restrictions are necessary, would the day's intake of these nutrients be within the ranges suggested in Table 22-5? If not, adjust the food list to better match the guidelines.
   - If this patient were to begin peritoneal dialysis, which nutrient recommendations would change? Explain why the diet would be easier to follow than the diet required during hemodialysis.

Notes

1. G. B. Appel and J. Radhakrishnan, Glomerular disorders and nephrotic syndromes, in L. Goldman and A. I. Schafer, eds., *Goldman-Cecil Medicine* (Philadelphia: Saunders, 2016), pp. 783–793.
2. Appel and Radhakrishnan, 2016.
3. S. Ananthakrishnan and G. A. Kaysen, Proteinuria and nephrotic syndrome, in R. W. Schrier, ed., *Renal and Electrolyte Disorders* (Philadelphia: Wolters Kluwer, 2018), pp. 503–541.
4. Ananthakrishnan and Kaysen, 2018; Academy of Nutrition and Dietetics, *Nutrition Care Manual* (Chicago: Academy of Nutrition and Dietetics, 2018).
5. Ananthakrishnan and Kaysen, 2018.
6. H. Trachtman, J. Hogan, and J. Radhadrishnan, Minimal change nephrotic syndrome, in S. J. Gilbert and D. E. Weiner, eds., *National Kidney Foundation's Primer on Kidney Diseases* (Philadelphia: Elsevier, 2018), pp. 175–180; Academy of Nutrition and Dietetics, 2018.
7. Academy of Nutrition and Dietetics, 2018.
8. T. S. McNees, Renal failure, in G. A. Cresci, ed., *Nutrition for the Critically Ill Patient* (Boca Raton, FL: CRC Press, 2015), pp. 483–496.
9. C. L. Edelstein, Acute kidney injury: Pathogenesis, diagnosis, and management, in R. W. Schrier, ed., *Renal and Electrolyte Disorders* (Philadelphia: Wolters Kluwer, 2018), pp. 325–400.
10. Edelstein, 2018; E. Macedo and R. L. Mehta, Clinical approach to the diagnosis of acute kidney injury, in S. J. Gilbert and D. E. Weiner, eds., *National Kidney Foundation's Primer on Kidney Diseases* (Philadelphia: Elsevier, 2018), pp. 300–310.
11. M. T. James and N. Pannu, Management of acute kidney injury, in S. J. Gilbert and D. E. Weiner, eds., *National Kidney Foundation's Primer on Kidney Diseases* (Philadelphia: Elsevier, 2018), pp. 326–332; M. S. McCarthy and S. C. Phipps, Special nutrition challenges: Current approach to acute kidney injury, *Nutrition in Clinical Practice* 29 (2014): 56–62.
12. James and Pannu, 2018.
13. Edelstein, 2018.
14. McNees, 2015; McCarthy and Phipps, 2014.
15. W. L. Whittier and E. Lewis, Development and progression of chronic kidney disease, in S. J. Gilbert and D. E. Weiner, eds., *National Kidney Foundation's Primer on Kidney Diseases* (Philadelphia: Elsevier, 2018), pp. 466–475.
16. M. Chonchol and L. Chan, Chronic kidney disease: Manifestations and pathogenesis, in R. W. Schrier, ed., *Renal and Electrolyte Disorders* (Philadelphia: Wolters Kluwer, 2018), pp. 401–436.
17. L. A. Inker and coauthors, KDOQI U.S. commentary on the 2012 KDIGO clinical practice guideline for the evaluation and management of CKD, *American Journal of Kidney Diseases* 63 (2014): doi: 10.1053/j.ajkd.2014.01.416; P.E. Stevens and A. Levin, Evaluation and management of chronic kidney disease: Synopsis of the kidney disease: improving global outcomes 2012 clinical practice guideline, *Annals of Internal Medicine* 158 (2013): 825–830.
18. W. E. Mitch, Chronic kidney disease, in L. Goldman and A. I. Schafer, eds., *Goldman-Cecil Medicine* (Philadelphia: Saunders, 2016), pp. 833–841.
19. J. A. Kraut, Chronic renal failure, in E. T. Bope and R. D. Kellerman, eds., *Conn's Current Therapy 2012* (Philadelphia: Saunders, 2012), pp. 883–888.
20. K. Nitta and K. Tsuchiya, Recent advances in the pathophysiology and management of protein-energy wasting in chronic kidney disease, *Renal Replacement Therapy* 2 (2016): doi.org/10.1186/s41100-016-0015-5.
21. J. D. Kopple, Nutrition, diet, and the kidney, in A. C. Ross and coeditors, *Modern Nutrition in Health and Disease* (Baltimore: Lippincott Williams & Wilkins, 2014), pp. 1330–1371; T. A. Ikizler, Optimal nutrition in hemodialysis patients, *Advances in Chronic Kidney Disease* 20 (2013): 181–189.
22. R. Filipowicz and S. Beddhu, Optimal nutrition for predialysis chronic kidney disease, *Advances in Chronic Kidney Disease* 20 (2013): 175–180.
23. X. Zuo and coauthors, Glucose absorption in nephropathy patients receiving continuous ambulatory peritoneal dialysis, *Asia Pacific Journal of Clinical Nutrition* 24 (2015): 394–402.
24. T. A. Ikizler, Nutrition and kidney disease, in S. J. Gilbert and D. E. Weiner, eds., *National Kidney Foundation's Primer on Kidney Diseases* (Philadelphia: Elsevier, 2018), pp. 484–492.
25. A. L. Steiber, Chronic kidney disease: Considerations for nutrition interventions, *Journal of Parenteral and Enteral Nutrition* 38 (2014): 418–426; Filipowicz and Beddhu, 2013.
26. Inker and coauthors, 2014.
27. S. U. Nigwekar, H. Tamez, and R. I. Thadhani, Vitamin D and chronic kidney disease–mineral bone disease (CKD–MBD), *BoneKEy Reports* 3 (2014): doi: 10.1038/bonekey.2013.232.
28. Kopple, 2014.
29. J. B. Wish, Anemia and other hematologic complications of chronic kidney disease, in S. J. Gilbert and D. E. Weiner, eds., *National Kidney Foundation's Primer on Kidney Diseases* (Philadelphia: Elsevier, 2018), pp. 515–525.
30. Ikizler, 2013.
31. G. Knoll and T. Fairhead, Selection of prospective kidney transplant recipients and donors, in S. J. Gilbert and D. E. Weiner, eds., *National Kidney Foundation's Primer on Kidney Diseases* (Philadelphia: Elsevier, 2018), pp. 565–576.
32. S. Chandran and F. G. Vincenti, Immunosuppression in transplantation, in S. J. Gilbert and D. E. Weiner, eds., *National Kidney Foundation's Primer on Kidney Diseases* (Philadelphia: Elsevier, 2018), pp. 589–600.
33. J. B. Ziemba and B. R. Matlaga, Epidemiology and economics of nephrolithiasis, *Investigative and Clinical Urology* 58 (2017): 299–306.
34. M. Prochaska and G. C. Curhan, Nephrolithiasis, in S. J. Gilbert and D. E. Weiner, eds., *National Kidney Foundation's Primer on Kidney Diseases* (Philadelphia: Elsevier, 2018), pp. 420–426; D. A. Bushinsky, Nephrolithiasis, in L. Goldman and A. I. Schafer, eds., *Goldman-Cecil Medicine* (Philadelphia: Saunders, 2016), pp. 811–816.
35. Prochaska and Curhan, 2018; Bushinsky, 2016.
36. Prochaska and Curhan, 2018.

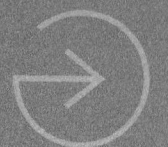
Although there is no perfect substitute for one's own kidneys, dialysis offers a life-sustaining treatment option for people with chronic kidney disease who develop renal failure. Dialysis can serve as a long-term treatment or as a temporary measure to sustain life until a suitable kidney donor can be found. Dialysis can also restore fluid and electrolyte balances in patients with acute kidney injury. Clinicians who routinely work with renal patients should understand how dialysis procedures work. This Nutrition in Practice describes the process of dialysis and outlines the various types of procedures that are available. The glossary in Box NP22-1 defines the relevant terms.

How does dialysis work?

Dialysis removes excess fluids and wastes from the blood by employing the processes of **diffusion**, **osmosis**, and **ultrafiltration** (see Figure NP22-1). The dialysate, a solution similar in composition to normal blood plasma, is carried through a compartment beside a **semipermeable membrane**; the person's blood flows in the opposite direction along the other side of the membrane. The semipermeable membrane acts like a filter: small molecules such as urea and glucose can pass through microscopic pores in the membrane, whereas large molecules are unable to cross.

In *hemodialysis*, the tiny tubes that carry blood through the dialyzer are made of materials that serve as semipermeable membranes. In *peritoneal dialysis*, the body's peritoneal membrane, rich with blood vessels, is used to filter the blood.

How are solutes separated from the blood in dialysis?

The chemical composition of the dialysate affects the movement of solutes across the semipermeable membrane. When the concentration of a substance is lower in the dialysate than in the blood, the substance—provided it can cross the membrane—will diffuse out of the blood. For example, the goal is to remove as much as possible of the waste product urea from the blood, so the dialysate contains no urea. For many other solutes, the dialysate is adjusted so that only excesses will be removed. Potassium can be removed from the blood, for example, by providing a dialysate that has a lower concentration of potassium than is found in the person's blood. The dialysate must contain some potassium, however; otherwise, the blood potassium level would fall too low.

The dialysate can also be used to add needed components back into the blood. For a person with acidosis, for example, bases such as bicarbonate are added to the

Box NP22-1 Glossary

continuous ambulatory peritoneal dialysis (CAPD): the most common method of peritoneal dialysis; involves frequent exchanges of dialysate, which remains in the peritoneal cavity throughout the day.

continuous renal replacement therapy (CRRT): a slow, continuous method of removing solutes and/or fluids from the blood by gently pumping the blood across a filtration membrane over a prolonged time period.

diffusion: movement of solutes from an area of high concentration to one of low concentration.

hemofiltration: removal of fluid and solutes from the blood by pumping the blood across a membrane; no osmotic gradients are created during the process.

oncotic pressure: the pressure exerted by fluid on one side of a membrane as a result of osmosis.

osmosis: movement of water across a membrane toward the side where solutes are more concentrated.

peritonitis: inflammation of the peritoneal membrane.

pressure gradient: the change in pressure over a given distance. In dialysis, a pressure gradient is created between the blood and the dialysate.

semipermeable membrane: a membrane that allows some, but not all, particles to pass through.

ultrafiltration: removal of fluids and solutes from the blood by using pressure to transfer the blood across a semipermeable membrane.

urea kinetic modeling: a method of determining the adequacy of dialysis treatment by calculating the urea clearance from blood.

FIGURE NP22-1 Diffusion, Osmosis, and Ultrafiltration

Diffusion

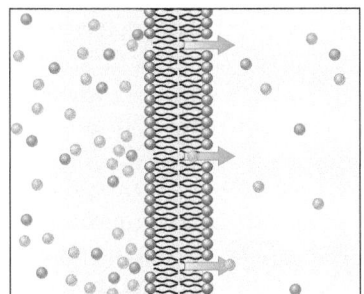

Small molecules (electrolytes and waste products) move from an area of high concentration to an area of low concentration by diffusion.

Osmosis

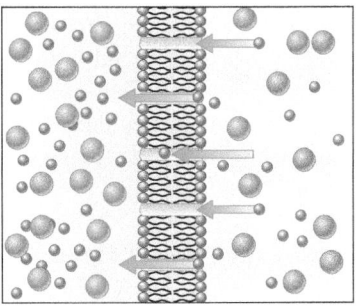

Water moves from an area of high water concentration to an area of low water concentration. In other words, water moves toward the side where solutes are more concentrated.

Ultrafiltration

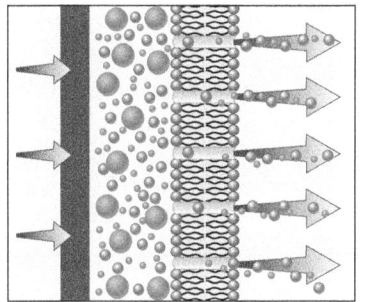

Pressure squeezes water and small molecules through the pores of a semipermeable membrane during ultrafiltration.

---

dialysate; the bases then move by diffusion into the blood to alleviate the acidosis.

How is fluid removed from the blood?

Because albumin and other plasma proteins are so adept at retaining fluids in blood, osmosis alone is not an efficient process for removing fluid. In hemodialysis, a **pressure gradient** is created between the blood and the dialysate. Most modern dialyzers produce *positive* pressure in the blood compartment and *negative* pressure in the dialysate compartment, establishing a pressure gradient that "pushes" water (and accompanying solutes) through the pores of the membrane. This process, called ultrafiltration, relies on pumps to establish an appropriate flow rate between the blood and the dialysate.

How often do patients require hemodialysis, and how long do treatments last?

Most patients undergo hemodialysis three times weekly and the treatments last three to four hours (see Photo NP22-1). Other options include short daily dialysis, performed five to six times per week for about two hours per session, and nocturnal hemodialysis, in which dialysis is done three to seven nights per week while the patient is sleeping. Although some studies have reported improved outcomes in patients who undergo more frequent dialysis, these approaches have not been widely adopted.[1] Note that most patients must visit dialysis centers to obtain treatment, as few patients have access to a dialysis machine at home.

Photo NP22-1 Hemodialysis

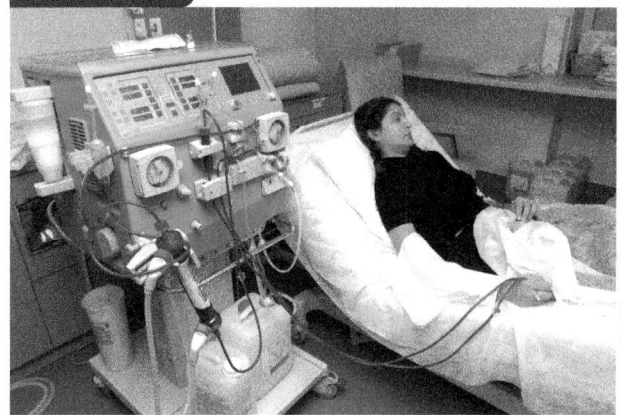

During hemodialysis, blood passes through a dialyzer where wastes are extracted, and the cleansed blood is returned to the body.

How does the health practitioner know if the dialysis treatment has been effective?

A number of methods have been devised for gauging the adequacy of dialysis treatment. The most common method is **urea kinetic modeling**, a technique that evaluates the amount of urea cleared from the blood. The formula used most often is Kt/V, where K is the amount of urea cleared, t is the time spent on dialysis, and V is the blood volume. The value obtained indicates whether the patient has undergone sufficient dialysis; the minimum goal is a *Kt/V* result of approximately 1.2. Because technical data (such as dialyzer clearance data, blood flow rate, and dialysate flow rate) need to be incorporated into the calculation, the computation is usually done by computer analysis. Current treatment guidelines recommend that hemodialysis adequacy be evaluated at least monthly, or more often if problems develop or patients are noncompliant.[2]

Are any complications associated with hemodialysis?

Yes. Although lifesaving, hemodialysis is associated with a substantial number of complications.[3] Problems at the vascular access site include infections and blood clotting. Hypotension can develop while blood is circulated through the dialyzer. Muscle cramping often occurs during the procedure, especially in the hands, legs, and feet. Blood losses can worsen anemia, which is already severe in two-thirds of patients beginning hemodialysis treatment.[4] Patients may also experience headaches, weakness, nausea, vomiting, restlessness, and agitation. Many patients are extremely fatigued after a hemodialysis treatment, and some may require rest or sleep.

How does peritoneal dialysis work?

In peritoneal dialysis, the peritoneal membrane surrounding the abdominal organs serves as a semipermeable membrane. The dialysate is infused into a catheter that empties into the peritoneal space—the space within the abdomen near the intestines (see Figure NP22-2). In the most common procedure, **continuous ambulatory peritoneal dialysis (CAPD)**, the dialysate remains in the peritoneal cavity for four to six hours, after which it is drained and replaced with fresh dialysate (about 2 to 3 liters in adults). Generally, the dialysate solution is exchanged four times daily and requires only about 30 minutes to drain and replace.

Because a pressure gradient cannot be created in the peritoneal cavity as it can in a dialyzer, the glucose concentration in the dialysate must be high enough to create sufficient **oncotic pressure** to draw fluid from the blood. As indicated in Chapter 22, a substantial amount of glucose can be absorbed into the patient's blood and may contribute to weight gain over time. The high glucose load may also cause hyperglycemia and hypertriglyceridemia in some patients.

What are the advantages and disadvantages of peritoneal dialysis?

Peritoneal dialysis offers a number of advantages over hemodialysis: vascular access is not required, dietary restrictions are fewer, and the procedure can be scheduled when convenient. The most common complication is infection, which often involves the catheter site or the peritoneal membrane (**peritonitis**).[5] Other problems that may arise include blood clotting in the catheter, catheter

---

FIGURE NP22-2   Peritoneal Dialysis

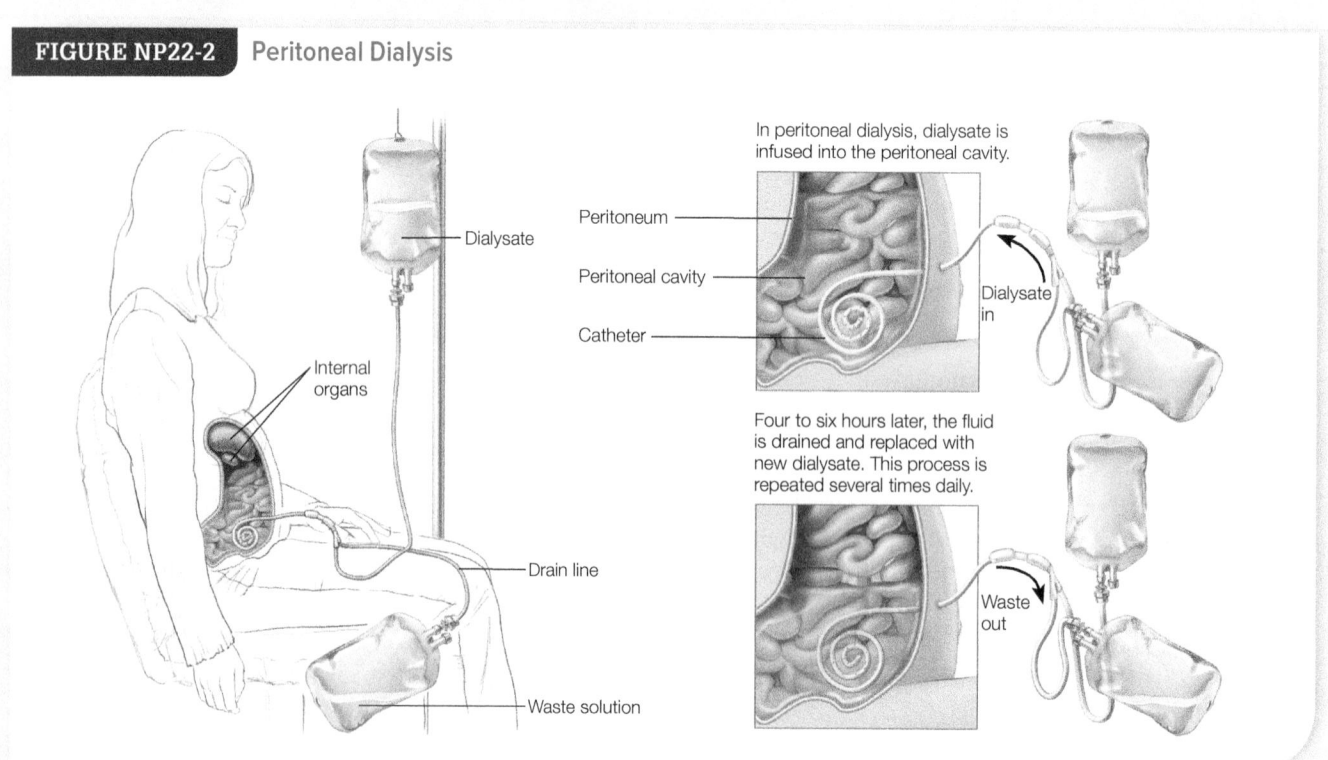

Dialysate

Internal organs

Drain line

Waste solution

In peritoneal dialysis, dialysate is infused into the peritoneal cavity.

Peritoneum

Peritoneal cavity

Catheter

Dialysate in

Four to six hours later, the fluid is drained and replaced with new dialysate. This process is repeated several times daily.

Waste out

displacement, leakage of the dialysate, and abdominal hernia due to the dialysate volume.

What are the features of continuous renal replacement therapy?

In most people with acute kidney injury, **continuous renal replacement therapy (CRRT)** removes fluids and wastes. CRRT uses the process of **hemofiltration**, in which blood is gently pumped across a filtration membrane over a prolonged time period. (This process differs from dialysis treatments that rely on the diffusion of wastes across a membrane into the dialysate.) Either a pump or the patient's own blood pressure moves the blood across the membrane. The procedure can be used to remove fluids, solutes, or both. Some patients require fluid replacement during the procedure to maintain adequate blood volume, so hydration status must be closely monitored.

The use of CRRT is advantageous in acute care situations because it corrects imbalances without causing sudden shifts in blood volume, which are poorly tolerated in acute care patients. In addition, replacement fluids can include parenteral feedings without upsetting fluid balance. Complications include clotting problems, damage to arteries, and inadequate blood flow rates in hypotensive patients.

Dialysis and CRRT help to remove the fluid and wastes that are normally removed by healthy kidneys. Although these procedures cannot restore the kidneys' hormonal functions, they provide a lifesaving means of alleviating symptoms of uremia, hypertension, and edema.

Notes

1. A. X. Garg and coauthors, Patients receiving frequent hemodialysis have better health-related quality of life compared to patients receiving conventional hemodialysis, *Kidney International* 91 (2017): 746–754; M. Misra, Hemodialysis and hemofiltration, in S. J. Gilbert and D. E. Weiner, eds., *National Kidney Foundation's Primer on Kidney Diseases* (Philadelphia: Elsevier, 2018), pp. 528–538.
2. National Kidney Foundation, KDOQI clinical practice guideline for hemodialysis adequacy: 2015 update. *American Journal of Kidney Diseases* 66 (2015): 884–930.
3. N. Tolkoff-Rubin, Treatment of irreversible renal failure, in L. Goldman and A. I. Schafer, eds., *Goldman's Cecil Medicine* (Philadelphia: Saunders, 2012), pp. 818–826.
4. Tolkoff-Rubin, 2012.
5. A. Vardhan and A. J. Hutchison, Peritoneal dialysis, in S. J. Gilbert and D. E. Weiner, eds., *National Kidney Foundation's Primer on Kidney Diseases* (Philadelphia: Elsevier, 2018), pp. 539–552.

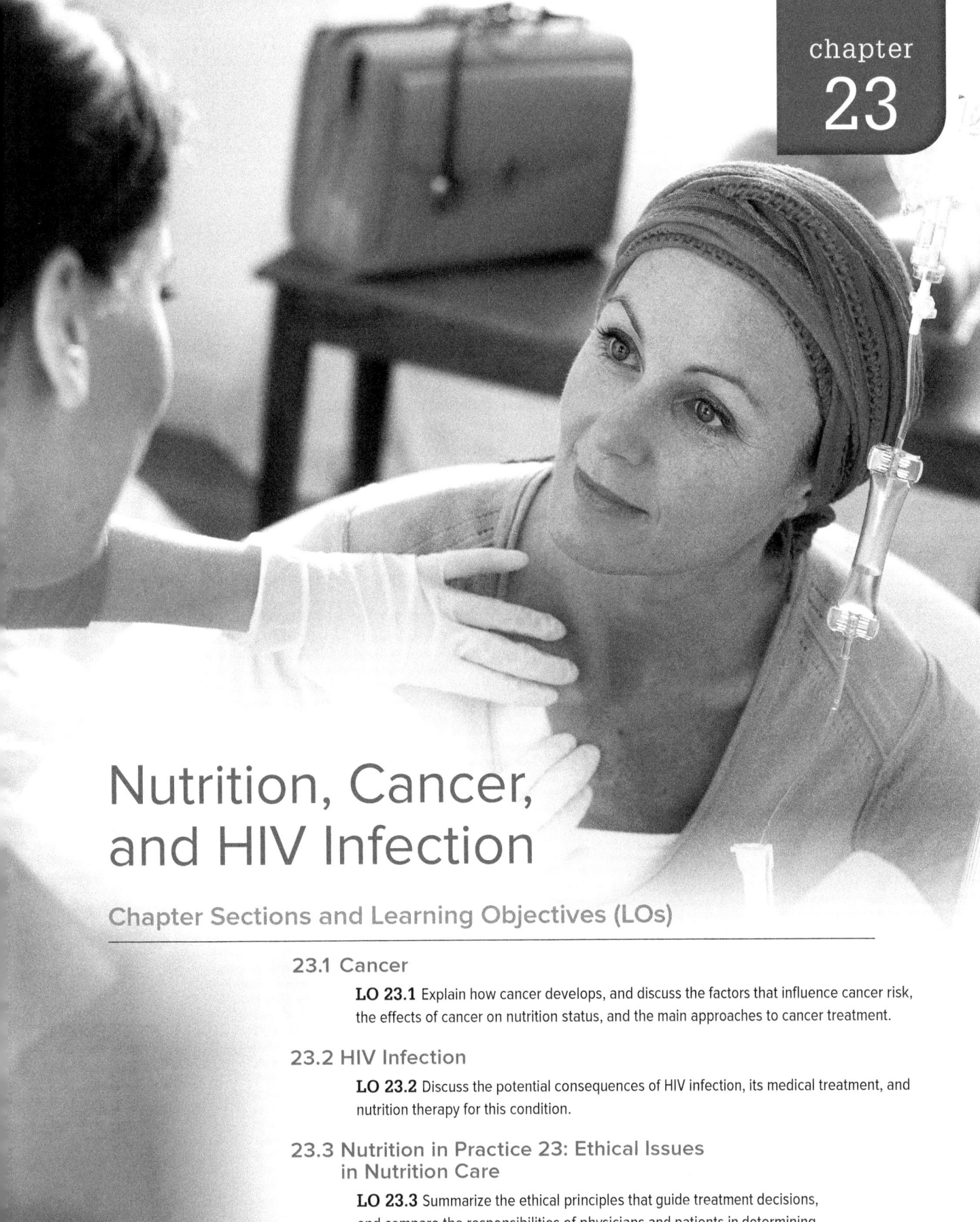

23

Nutrition, Cancer, and HIV Infection

Chapter Sections and Learning Objectives (LOs)

23.1 Cancer

LO 23.1 Explain how cancer develops, and discuss the factors that influence cancer risk, the effects of cancer on nutrition status, and the main approaches to cancer treatment.

23.2 HIV Infection

LO 23.2 Discuss the potential consequences of HIV infection, its medical treatment, and nutrition therapy for this condition.

23.3 Nutrition in Practice 23: Ethical Issues in Nutrition Care

LO 23.3 Summarize the ethical principles that guide treatment decisions, and compare the responsibilities of physicians and patients in determining the appropriate care during medical emergencies.

BURGER/PHANIE/AGE Fotostock

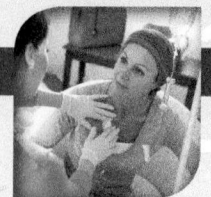

standpoint **cancers** and **human immunodeficiency virus (HIV)** infections have some similarities. Both disorders have debilitating effects that influence nutritional needs, and both can lead to severe wasting in advanced cases. These illnesses require nutrition therapy that is highly individualized based on the symptoms manifested and the tissues or organs involved.

cancers: diseases characterized by the uncontrolled growth of a group of abnormal cells, which can destroy adjacent tissues and spread to other areas of the body via the lymph or blood.

23.1 Cancer

Cancer, the growth of **malignant** tissue, is the second most common cause of death in the United States, ranking just below cardiovascular disease. Cancer is not a single disorder, however; there are many different kinds of malignant growths (see Box 23-1). The various types of cancer have different characteristics, occur in different locations in the body, take different courses, and require different treatments. Whereas an isolated, nonspreading type of skin cancer may be removed in a physician's office with no effect on nutrition status, advanced cancers—especially those of the gastrointestinal (GI) tract and pancreas—can seriously impair nutrition status. In the United States, the most common cancers are breast cancer (in women), prostate cancer (in men), lung cancer, and colorectal cancers.[1]

How Cancer Develops

The development of cancer, called **carcinogenesis**, often proceeds slowly and continues for several decades. A cancer usually arises from genetic mutations that alter gene expression in a single cell.[2] These alterations may promote cellular growth, interfere with growth restraint, or prevent cellular death. The affected cell thereby loses its built-in capacity for halting cell division and produces daughter cells with the same genetic defects. As the abnormal mass of cells, called a **tumor** (or *neoplasm*), grows, a network of blood vessels forms to supply the tumor with the nutrients it needs to support its growth. The tumor can disrupt the functioning of the normal tissue around it, and some tumor cells may **metastasize**, spreading to other regions in the body. In leukemia (cancer affecting the white blood cells), the abnormal cells do not form a tumor; they accumulate in the blood and other tissues. Figure 23-1 illustrates the steps in cancer development.

FIGURE 23-1   Cancer Development

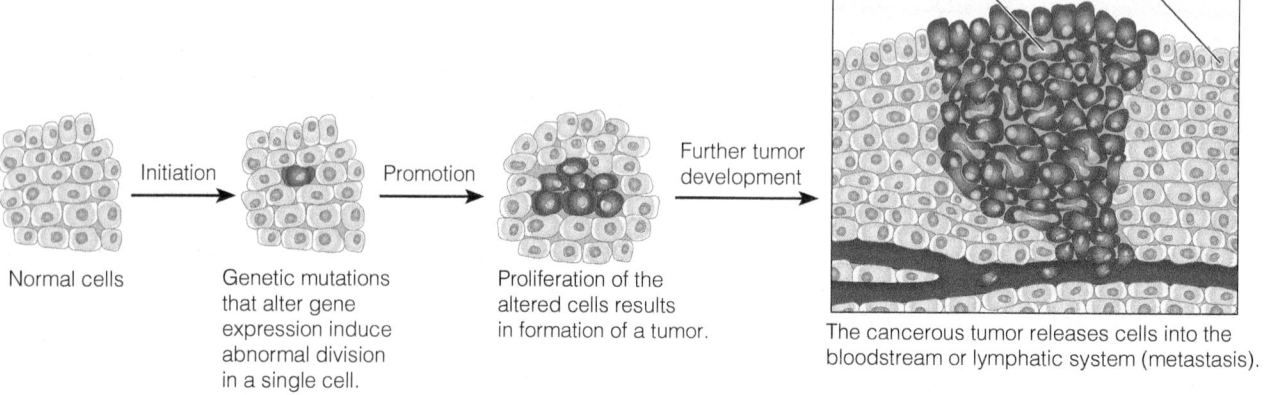

Normal cells

Initiation

Genetic mutations that alter gene expression induce abnormal division in a single cell.

Promotion

Proliferation of the altered cells results in formation of a tumor.

Further tumor development

Malignant cells   Normal cells

The cancerous tumor releases cells into the bloodstream or lymphatic system (metastasis).

TABLE 23-1 Environmental Factors That Increase Cancer Risk

ENVIRONMENTAL FACTORS	CANCER SITES
Aflatoxins (toxins in moldy peanuts or grains)	Liver
Arsenic	Skin, lung, kidney, bladder
Asbestos[a]	Larynx, lung, mesothelium (lining of lungs), ovary, pharynx, stomach, colon, rectum
Chromium (hexavalent) compounds	Nasal cavity, lung
Estrogen-progesterone menopausal therapy	Breast, cervix, liver
Infection with *Helicobacter pylori*	Stomach, lymphoid tissues
Infection with hepatitis B or hepatitis C viruses	Liver
Infection with human papillomavirus (HPV)	Cervix, vulva, vagina, penis, anus, oral cavity, tonsil, oropharynx
Ionizing radiation (X-rays, radon, radioactive isotopes, and other sources)	White blood cells (leukemia), thyroid, nasal cavity, lung, salivary glands, stomach, colon, rectum, skin, bladder, breast, bone, liver, gallbladder, kidney, brain
Tobacco[b]	Lip, oral cavity, pharynx, larynx, lung, esophagus, stomach, colon, rectum, liver, pancreas, kidney, ureter, bladder, cervix, ovary, white blood cells
Ultraviolet radiation (sun exposure)	Skin, eye, lip

[a]Risk is greatly increased in cigarette smokers.
[b]A combined exposure to tobacco and alcohol multiplies the risks of developing cancers of the oral cavity, pharynx, larynx, and esophagus.

Sources: M. J. Thun and A. Jemel, Epidemiology of cancer, in L. Goldman and A. I. Schafer, eds., *Goldman's Cecil Medicine* (Philadelphia: Saunders, 2012), pp. 1177–1182; V. J. Cogliano and coauthors, Preventable exposures associated with human cancers, *Journal of the National Cancer Institute* 103 (2011): 1827–1839.

The reasons why cancers develop are numerous and varied. Vulnerability to cancer is sometimes inherited, as when a person is born with a genetic defect that alters DNA structure, function, or repair. Some metabolic processes may initiate carcinogenesis, as when phagocytes (immune cells) produce oxidants that cause DNA damage, or when chronic inflammation increases the rate of cell division and the risk of a damaging mutation. More often, cancers are caused by interactions between a person's genes and the environment. Exposure to cancer-causing substances, or **carcinogens**, may induce genetic mutations that lead to cancer; other substances may stimulate division or proliferation of the altered cells. Table 23-1 provides examples of environmental factors that increase cancer risk.

Nutrition and Cancer Risk

Like other environmental factors, diet and lifestyle strongly influence cancer risk. Various food components can alter processes of DNA repair, gene expression, or cell differentiation in ways that affect cancer development.[3] Moreover, certain food compounds can directly damage DNA, alter carcinogen metabolism by liver enzymes, or inhibit the formation of carcinogens in the body. Energy balance and growth rate can both influence cancer risk due to their effects on cell division rates (and therefore, mutation risk) and hormones that regulate cell growth. Table 23-2 lists examples of nutrition-related factors that may increase or decrease the risk of developing cancer.

Nutrition and Increased Cancer Risk As shown in Table 23-2, obesity is a risk factor for a number of different cancers, including some relatively common cancers such as colon cancer and postmenopausal breast cancer. Obesity increases cancer risk, in part, by altering the levels of hormones that influence cell growth, such as insulin, the sex hormones, and several kinds of growth factors.[4] For example, in the case of breast cancer in postmenopausal women, the hormone estrogen is likely involved: obese women have higher estrogen levels than lean women do because adipose tissue is the

human immunodeficiency virus (HIV): the virus that causes acquired immunodeficiency syndrome (AIDS). HIV destroys immune cells and progressively impedes the body's ability to fight infections and certain cancers.

malignant (ma-LIG-nent)**:** describes a cancerous cell or tumor, which can injure healthy tissue and spread cancer to other regions of the body.

carcinogenesis (CAR-sin-oh-JEN-eh-sis)**:** the process of cancer development.

tumor: an abnormal tissue mass that has no physiological function; also called a *neoplasm* (NEE-oh-plazm). Tumors may be malignant (cancerous) or benign (noncancerous).

metastasize (meh-TAS-tah-size)**:** to spread from one part of the body to another; refers to cancer cells.

carcinogens (CAR-sin-oh-jenz or car-SIN-oh-jenz)**:** substances that can cause cancer (the adjective is *carcinogenic*).

TABLE 23-2 Nutrition-Related Factors That Influence Cancer Risk

NUTRITION-RELATED FACTORS[a]	CANCER SITES
FACTORS THAT MAY INCREASE CANCER RISK	
Obesity	Esophagus, stomach, colon, rectum, pancreas, liver, gallbladder, kidney, breast (postmenopausal), ovary, endometrium, prostate
Red meat, processed meats	Colon, rectum
Salted and salt-preserved foods	Stomach
Beta-carotene supplements	Lung[b]
High-calcium diets (over 1500 mg daily)	Prostate
Alcohol[c]	Mouth, pharynx, larynx, esophagus, stomach, colon, rectum, liver, breast
Low level of physical activity[d]	Colon, breast (postmenopausal), endometrium
FACTORS THAT MAY DECREASE CANCER RISK	
Fruits and nonstarchy vegetables	Lung, mouth, pharynx, larynx
Carotenoid-containing foods	Lung, mouth, pharynx, larynx, esophagus
Tomato products	Prostate
Allium vegetables (onion, garlic)	Stomach, colon, rectum
Vitamin C–containing foods	Esophagus
Folate-containing foods	Pancreas, colon, rectum
Fiber-containing foods	Colon, rectum
Milk products and calcium supplements	Colon, rectum
High level of physical activity[d]	Colon, breast (postmenopausal), endometrium

[a]For the dietary substances on this list, altered cancer risk is associated with high intakes of the substances listed.
[b]Cancer risk is increased in tobacco smokers and may not apply to other groups.
[c]A combined exposure to alcohol and tobacco multiplies the risks of developing cancers of the oral cavity, pharynx, larynx, and esophagus.
[d]Physical activity may influence cancer risk by altering body fatness, intestinal transit time, insulin sensitivity, hormone levels, enzyme activities, and immune responses.

Sources: World Cancer Research Fund International, *Cancer Prevention and Survival* (London: World Cancer Research Fund International, 2017); World Cancer Research Fund/American Institute for Cancer Research, *Food, Nutrition, Physical Activity, and the Prevention of Cancer: A Global Perspective* (Washington, D.C.: American Institute for Cancer Research, 2007).

BOX 23-2

To minimize carcinogen formation during cooking:

- Marinate meat before cooking.
- Use lower-heat options such as roasting, stewing, or microwaving.
- Choose lean meat for grilling, and take care not to blacken surfaces.
- To reduce smoke formation, prevent fat from dripping onto the heat source.

primary source of estrogen after menopause. The increase in circulating estrogen may create an environment that encourages carcinogenesis in breast tissue.[5]

About 1 in 30 cancer deaths can be attributed to alcohol consumption, which correlates strongly with cancers of the head and neck, liver, stomach, colon, rectum, and breast.[6] For head and neck cancers, the risk is multiplied when alcohol drinkers also smoke tobacco. Alcohol's link to cancer risk illustrates why the potential benefits of moderate alcohol consumption on cardiovascular disease risk must be weighed against the potential dangers.

Food preparation methods can influence the production of carcinogens (see Box 23-2). Cooking meat, poultry, and fish at high temperatures (by frying or broiling, for example) may cause carcinogens to form in these foods.[7] Carcinogens also accompany the smoke that adheres to foods during grilling and are present in the charred surfaces of grilled meat and fish. However, the cancer risk from eating such foods is unclear because the biological effects of these carcinogens are modulated by other dietary components, including compounds in vegetables and other plant foods. Consumption of meat carcinogens has been linked to cancers of the colon, rectum, pancreas, and kidney.[8]

Nutrition and Decreased Cancer Risk Consuming fruits and vegetables may reduce the risks of some cancers (see Table 23-2 and Photo 23-1).[9] Possible benefit has been attributed, in part, to nutrients and phytochemicals with antioxidant activity, as these substances may prevent or reduce the oxidative reactions in cells that cause DNA damage. In addition, phytochemicals may inhibit carcinogen production in the body, enhance immune responses that protect against cancer development, or promote enzyme reactions that inactivate carcinogens. The B vitamin folate (provided by certain fruits and vegetables) functions in DNA synthesis and repair; thus, inadequate folate intakes may allow DNA damage to accumulate. Fruits and vegetables also contribute dietary fiber, which may help to protect against colon and rectal cancers by diluting potential carcinogens in fecal matter and accelerating their removal from the GI tract. Table 23-3 summarizes the dietary and lifestyle practices that may help to reduce the risk of developing cancer.

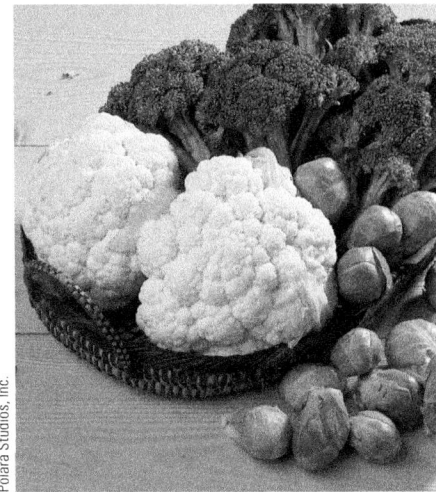

Photo 23-1 Cruciferous Vegetables and Cancer Risk

Cruciferous vegetables—such as cauliflower, broccoli, and brussels sprouts—may inhibit several types of cancer, including cancers of the prostate, bladder, and lung.

TABLE 23-3 Guidelines for Reducing Cancer Risk

Achieve and maintain a healthy body weight throughout life.
- Be as lean as possible within the normal range of body weight for your height.
- Avoid weight gain and increases in waist circumference throughout adulthood.

Be physically active as part of everyday life.
- For adults: engage in moderate physical activity (equivalent to brisk walking) for at least 30 minutes each day; increase duration or intensity of activity as fitness improves.
- For children and adolescents: engage in moderate-to-vigorous activity for at least 60 minutes each day.
- Limit sedentary habits such as watching television.

Choose a healthy diet that emphasizes plant sources.
- Limit consumption of energy-dense foods (>225 kcal per 100 g food) and sugary drinks that contribute to weight gain.
- Consume relatively unprocessed grains and/or legumes with every meal. Choose whole-grain products instead of processed (refined) grains.
- Consume at least 2½ cups of nonstarchy vegetables and fruit every day.

Limit consumption of foods that may increase cancer risk.
- Limit consumption of red meat (beef, pork, and lamb) to 18 ounces per week.
- Limit consumption of processed meats (those preserved by smoking, curing, or salting).
- Avoid salt-preserved, salted, and salty foods.
- Avoid moldy grains and legumes.

Limit consumption of alcoholic beverages.
- For women: consume no more than one drink daily.
- For men: consume no more than two drinks daily.

Aim to meet nutritional needs through the diet.
- Obtain necessary nutrients from the diet. Dietary supplements are not recommended for cancer prevention, and they may have unexpected adverse effects.

Avoid using tobacco in any form.

Sources: L. H. Kushi and coauthors, American Cancer Society guidelines on nutrition and physical activity for cancer prevention: Reducing the risk of cancer with healthy food choices and physical activity, *CA: A Cancer Journal for Clinicians* 62 (2012): 30–67; World Cancer Research Fund/American Institute for Cancer Research, *Food, Nutrition, Physical Activity, and the Prevention of Cancer: A Global Perspective* (Washington, D.C.: American Institute for Cancer Research, 2007).

Consequences of Cancer

Once cancer develops, its consequences depend on the location of the cancer, its severity, and the treatment. The complications that develop are often due to the tumor's impingement on surrounding tissues. Nonspecific effects of cancer include **anorexia**, fatigue, unexplained weight loss, fever, night sweats, skin lesions, and hyperpigmented (darkened) skin.[10] During the early stages, many cancers produce no symptoms, and the person may be unaware of the threat to health.

Anorexia and Reduced Food Intake Anorexia is a major contributor to the weight loss often associated with cancer (see Box 23-3). Some factors that contribute to anorexia or otherwise reduce food intake include the following:

- *Mental stress.* A cancer diagnosis can cause distress, anxiety, and depression, all of which may reduce appetite. Facing and undergoing cancer treatments induces additional psychological stress.
- *Chronic nausea and early satiety.* People with cancer frequently experience nausea and a premature feeling of fullness after eating small amounts of food.
- *Fatigue.* People with cancer may tire easily and lack the energy to prepare and eat meals. If substantial weight loss occurs, these tasks become even more difficult.
- *Pain.* People in pain may have little interest in eating, particularly if eating makes the pain worse.
- *Gastrointestinal obstructions.* A tumor may partially or completely obstruct a portion of the GI tract, causing complications such as nausea and vomiting, early satiety, delayed gastric emptying, and bacterial overgrowth. Some patients with obstructions are unable to tolerate oral diets.
- *Effects of cancer therapies.* Chemotherapy and radiation treatments for cancer frequently have side effects that make food consumption difficult, such as nausea, vomiting, dry mouth, altered taste perceptions, **oral mucositis** (inflamed oral mucosa), esophagitis, dysphagia, abdominal pain, and diarrhea.

Metabolic Changes The metabolic changes that arise in cancer contribute to weight loss and nutrient depletion.[11] **Cytokines**, released by both tumor cells and immune cells, induce an inflammatory and catabolic state. Cancer patients exhibit an increased rate of **protein turnover**, but reduced muscle protein synthesis. Muscle contributes amino acids for gluconeogenesis (glucose production), further depleting the body's supply of protein. Triglyceride breakdown increases, elevating serum lipids. Many patients develop insulin resistance. These metabolic abnormalities help to explain why people with cancer fail to regain lean tissue or maintain healthy body weights even when they are consuming adequate energy and nutrients.

Cancer Cachexia The combined effects of a poor appetite, accelerated and abnormal metabolism, and the diversion of nutrients to support tumor growth result in a lower supply of energy and nutrients at a time when demands are high. **Cancer cachexia**—characterized by anorexia, weight loss, muscle wasting, anemia, and fatigue—develops in 50 to 80 percent of cancer patients and is responsible for as many as 20 percent of cancer deaths (see Box 23-4).[12] Cachexia may be indicated by an involuntary weight loss of more than 5 percent of body weight over the preceding 6 months;[13] care must be taken not to overlook unintentional weight loss in patients who are overweight or obese. Unlike in starvation, nutrition intervention alone is unable to reverse cachexia.[14]

Treatments for Cancer

The primary medical treatments for cancer—surgery, chemotherapy, radiation therapy, or any combination of the three—aim to remove cancer cells, prevent further tumor growth, and alleviate symptoms.[15] The likelihood of effective treatment is highest with early detection and intervention. Because treatment decisions are difficult and cancer therapies have considerable side effects, patients rely on health care providers to help them make informed decisions.

Surgery Surgery is performed to remove tumors, determine the extent of cancer, and protect nearby tissues. Often, surgery must be followed by other cancer treatments to prevent the growth of new tumors. The acute metabolic stress caused by surgery raises protein and energy needs and can exacerbate wasting. Surgery also contributes to pain, fatigue, and anorexia, all of which can reduce food intake at a time when nutritional needs are substantial. Blood loss contributes to nutrient losses and further exacerbates malnutrition. Some surgeries can have long-term effects on nutrition status (see Table 23-4).

Chemotherapy **Chemotherapy** relies on the use of drugs to treat cancer, and is used to inhibit tumor growth, shrink tumors before surgery, and prevent or suppress metastasis. Some cancer drugs (such as **methotrexate**) interfere with the process of cell division; others sterilize cells that are in a resting phase and are not actively dividing. Unfortunately, most of these drugs have toxic effects on normal cells as well and are especially damaging to rapidly dividing cells, such as those of the GI tract, skin, and bone marrow. The bone marrow damage can impair the production of red blood cells (causing anemia) and white blood cells (causing **neutropenia**). Some of the newer drugs target properties specific to cancer cells and are better tolerated by the body's tissues. Table 23-5 describes some nutrition-related side effects that may result from chemotherapy.

TABLE 23-4 Nutrition-Related Side Effects of Cancer Surgeries

HEAD AND NECK SURGERIES
- Aspiration
- Dry or sore mouth
- Reduced chewing or swallowing ability
- Reduced sense of taste or smell

ESOPHAGEAL RESECTION
- Acid reflux
- Altered gastric motility
- Reduced swallowing ability

GASTRIC RESECTION
- Dumping syndrome
- Early satiety
- Inadequate gastric acid secretion
- Malabsorption of iron, folate, and vitamin B_{12}

INTESTINAL RESECTION
- Bile insufficiency
- Diarrhea
- Fluid and electrolyte imbalances
- General malabsorption

PANCREATIC RESECTION
- Diabetes mellitus
- General malabsorption

TABLE 23-5 Nutrition-Related Side Effects of Chemotherapy and Radiation Therapy

	REDUCED NUTRIENT INTAKE	INCREASED NUTRIENT LOSSES	ALTERED METABOLISM
Chemotherapy	Abdominal pain Anorexia Nausea and vomiting Oral mucositis Reduced taste sensation	Diarrhea Gastrointestinal inflammation Malabsorption Vomiting	Anemia, neutropenia Fluid and electrolyte imbalances as a consequence of vomiting, diarrhea, or malabsorption Hyperglycemia Interference with vitamins or body compounds Negative nitrogen and micronutrient balances Secondary effects of malnutrition, infection, or inflammation
Radiation therapy	Anorexia Damage to teeth, jaws, or salivary glands Dysphagia Esophagitis Nausea and vomiting Oral mucositis Reduced salivary secretions Reduced taste sensation	Blood loss from intestine and bladder Diarrhea Fistulas Intestinal obstructions Malabsorption Radiation enteritis Vomiting	Fluid and electrolyte imbalances as a consequence of vomiting, diarrhea, or malabsorption Secondary effects of malnutrition, infection, or inflammation

chemotherapy: the use of drugs to arrest or destroy cancer cells; these drugs are called *antineoplastic agents*.

methotrexate: an anticancer drug that inhibits cell division. Methotrexate closely resembles the B vitamin folate, which is needed for DNA synthesis; the drug works by blocking activity of the enzyme that converts folate to its active form (see Figure 14-3, p. 418).

neutropenia: a low white blood cell (neutrophil) count, which increases susceptibility to infection.

Radiation Therapy **Radiation therapy** treats cancer by bombarding cancer cells with X-rays, gamma rays, or various atomic particles. These treatments generate reactive forms of oxygen, such as superoxide and hydroxyl radicals, which can damage cellular DNA and cause cell death. Newer techniques can focus the radiation directly at tumors and minimize damage to nearby tissues. An advantage of radiation therapy over surgery is that it can shrink tumors while preserving organ structure and function. Compared with chemotherapy, radiation therapy is better able to target specific regions of the body, rather than involving all body cells. Nonetheless, radiation therapy can damage healthy tissues and sometimes has long-term detrimental effects on nutrition status (see Table 23-5). Radiation to the head and neck can damage the salivary glands and taste buds, causing inflammation, dry mouth, and a reduced sense of taste; in severe cases, the damage may be permanent. Radiation treatment in the lower abdomen can cause **radiation enteritis**, an inflammatory condition of the small intestine that causes nausea, vomiting, and diarrhea; the condition may persist for months or years and lead to chronic malabsorption in some individuals.

Hematopoietic Stem Cell Transplantation **Hematopoietic stem cell transplantation** replaces the blood-forming stem cells that have been destroyed by high-dose chemotherapy or radiation therapy. These procedures may be used to treat leukemias, lymphomas, and multiple myeloma.[16] If possible, stem cells are collected from the patient's bone marrow or circulating blood before chemotherapy or radiation treatment begins so that a separate donor is not required. If another person's cells are used, the patient must take immunosuppressive drugs to prevent **graft-versus-host disease**, in which the donor's immune cells attack the recipient's tissues, and **graft rejection**, in which the recipient's immune system rejects the donor cells. Graft-versus-host disease often damages tissues of the GI tract, leading to severe intestinal inflammation, profuse diarrhea, and bleeding.

The treatments required for stem cell transplantation can have a substantial impact on food intake and nutrition status (see Box 23-5). The high-dose chemotherapy or radiation therapy preceding the transplant and the immunosuppressive drugs often required afterward can impair immune function substantially and increase the risk of infection and foodborne illness. Other common complications include anorexia, nausea, vomiting, dry mouth, oral mucositis, altered taste sensations, diarrhea, and malabsorption. Patients are often unable to consume adequate food during or after the procedures and usually require nutrition support.

Immunotherapy Newer therapies for cancer include the use of biological molecules that stimulate immune responses against cancer cells. These substances include antibodies, cytokines, and other proteins that strengthen the body's immune defenses, enable the destruction of cancer cells, or interfere with cancer development in some way. Although side effects vary, the drugs used in immunotherapy treatments may cause a variety of symptoms—such as fever, nausea, vomiting, GI symptoms, headache, and fatigue—that reduce a person's ability or desire to consume adequate amounts of food.

Medications to Combat Anorexia and Wasting Medications prescribed to stimulate the appetite and promote weight gain include megestrol acetate (Megace), a synthetic compound similar in structure to the hormone progesterone, and dronabinol (Marinol), which resembles the psychoactive ingredient in marijuana and stimulates the appetite at doses that have minimal mental effects. Antiemetic drugs, which control nausea and vomiting, are typically coadministered with chemotherapeutic drugs to improve appetite and food intake. Under investigation are medications that promote muscle protein synthesis, induce the secretion of growth hormone or growth factors, or reduce catabolism.[17]

Alternative Therapies Many patients turn to **complementary and alternative medicine (CAM)** to assist them in their fight against cancer. Patients may use CAM because they

radiation therapy: the use of X-rays, gamma rays, or atomic particles to destroy cancer cells.

radiation enteritis: inflammation of intestinal tissue caused by radiation therapy.

hematopoietic stem cell transplantation: transplantation of the stem cells that produce red blood cells and white blood cells; the stem cells are obtained from bone marrow (*bone marrow transplantation*) or circulating blood.

haima = blood
poiesis = to make

graft-versus-host disease: a condition in which the immune cells in transplanted tissue (the graft) attack recipient (host) cells, leading to widespread tissue damage.

graft rejection: destruction of donor tissue by the recipient's immune system, which recognizes the donor cells as foreign.

complementary and alternative medicine (CAM): health care practices that have not been proved to be effective and consequently are not included as part of conventional treatment (see Nutrition in Practice 14).

wish to have more control over their treatment or because they are concerned about the effectiveness of conventional approaches. Although few abandon conventional medicine, an estimated 40 to 83 percent of cancer patients combine one or more CAM approaches with standard treatment.[18] Many patients do not discuss their use of CAM with physicians.

Multivitamin and herbal supplements are among the most frequently used CAM therapies. Although many supplements can be used without risk, some may have adverse effects or interfere with conventional treatments. Use of the herb St. John's wort, for example, can reduce the effectiveness of some anticancer drugs.[19] As another example, some studies suggest that antioxidant supplements can interfere with chemotherapy and radiation treatments.[20] Most current research suggests that dietary supplements (including multivitamins and antioxidant supplements) are unable to improve outcomes or survival after a cancer diagnosis and may actually increase mortality rates.[21]

Nutrition Therapy for Cancer

The goals of nutrition therapy for cancer patients are to maintain a healthy weight, preserve muscle tissue, prevent or correct nutrient deficiencies, and provide a diet that patients can tolerate and enjoy despite the complications of illness.[22] Appropriate nutrition care helps patients preserve their strength and improves recovery after stressful cancer treatments. Moreover, malnourished cancer patients develop more complications and have shorter survival times than patients who maintain good nutrition status.

Because there are many forms of cancer and a variety of potential treatments, nutritional needs among cancer patients vary considerably. Furthermore, a person's needs may change at different stages of illness. Patients should be screened for malnutrition when cancer is diagnosed and reassessed during the treatment and recovery periods.

Protein and Energy For patients at risk of weight loss and wasting, the focus of nutrition care is to ensure appropriate intakes of protein and energy. Protein requirements are often between 1.0 and 1.5 grams per kilogram of body weight per day, but may be higher if protein depletion is severe or if patients are older or chronically ill.[23] Patients should consume adequate energy to prevent weight loss; those who cannot eat enough food may be able to meet their needs by supplementing the diet with nutrient-dense oral supplements.[24] Box 23-6 provides suggestions that can help to increase the energy and protein content of meals.

Although weight loss is a problem for many cancer patients, breast cancer patients often gain weight.[25] The weight gain occurs during the first five years after breast cancer diagnosis and is associated with an increase in total body fat. By discussing weight maintenance soon after diagnosis and encouraging physical activity, health practitioners can help patients avoid unnecessary weight gain.

Managing Symptoms and Complications A thorough nutrition assessment often uncovers specific problems or symptoms that interfere with food consumption. Table 23-6 lists dietary considerations related to cancers affecting different sites in the body. Box 23-7 on pp. 663–664 describes dietary strategies that may alleviate symptoms and improve food intake. Patients' responses to these strategies can vary considerably, and in some cases, a number of adjustments may be necessary.

Food Safety Concerns To minimize the risk of foodborne illness and other infectious complications, patients with suppressed immunity or neutropenia (due to hematopoietic stem cell transplants or use of immunosuppressive drugs) are advised to carefully follow safe food-handling practices. Typical recommendations are to consume only well-cooked meat and eggs, pasteurized milk products, and well-washed fruits and vegetables. Foods to avoid include unpasteurized juices and milk products and unwashed raw fruits and vegetables. Nutrition in Practice 2 describes additional strategies that can help to prevent foodborne illness.

Box 23-6

HOW TO Increase Kcalories and Protein in Meals

To increase the energy content of a meal, try these suggestions:

- *Meat.* Choose high-fat meat instead of lean meat. Sauté or pan-fry meat instead of baking or roasting it, and use sauces or gravies liberally. Sprinkle bacon bits or sausage pieces on vegetable dishes.
- *Cheese.* Include cheese slices or cream cheese in sandwiches made with luncheon meat. Spread cream cheese on raw vegetables, toast, and crackers or mix into dishes that contain chopped fruit.
- *Half-and-half and cream.* Replace milk or water with half-and-half or cream in breakfast cereal, soup, mashed potatoes, sauces, hot chocolate, and desserts. Add sour cream or cream sauce to soup, vegetable dishes, and potato dishes. Add whipped cream to fruit salad and desserts.
- *Breads and cereals.* Choose high-fat grain products such as granola, pancakes, waffles, French toast, and biscuits. Prepare hot cereal with whole milk or cream, or added fat.
- *Fruit.* Mash avocados to make guacamole, or use mashed avocado as a sandwich spread. Add chopped dried fruit to salads and baked goods. Snack on dried fruit between meals.
- *Nuts.* Add chopped nuts to stir-fried vegetables, pasta dishes, fruit salad, and green salad. Use nut meats in baked products. Spread nut butters on bread or crackers.
- *Butter or margarine.* Melt on pasta, potatoes, rice, and cooked vegetables. Add to hot cereal, soup, and casseroles. Spread liberally on bread, crackers, and rolls.
- *Mayonnaise or salad dressing.* Add to pasta, tuna, and potato salads. Use as a dressing for raw or cooked vegetables.

- *Beverages.* Replace water and non-kcaloric beverages with sweetened drinks, fruit juice, and milkshakes. Drink whole milk instead of low-fat or nonfat milk. Add strawberry or chocolate syrup to plain milk to boost kcalories.

These suggestions can help to add protein to a meal:

- *Meat.* Add small chunks of meat to soup, potato salad, egg dishes, bean dishes, and casseroles. Add chunks of chicken or turkey to green salad. Add minced meat to pasta sauce and vegetable dishes.
- *Eggs.* Add raw eggs when preparing casseroles, meatballs, and hamburgers. Add chopped hard-cooked eggs to green salad, vegetable dishes, sandwich fillings, and pasta and potato salads.
- *Cheese.* Melt on scrambled eggs, vegetable dishes, potatoes, hamburgers, meat loaf, and casseroles. Add cottage cheese to egg dishes, pasta recipes, and salad dressing. Grate hard cheese and sprinkle on soup, salad, and cooked vegetables. Avoid using reduced-fat cheese.
- *Milk.* Use in place of water when preparing cereal or soup. Use cream sauce (which is made with milk) to flavor vegetable and pasta dishes.
- *Powdered milk (use full-fat milk powder if available).* Add to recipes that include milk. Dissolve extra milk powder into milk-containing beverages. Stir into hot cereal, potato dishes, casseroles, and sauces. Add to scrambled eggs, hamburgers, and meat loaf.
- *Protein supplements.* Snack on protein bars between meals. Add protein powder to beverages and shakes. Drink meal replacement formulas, such as Ensure or Boost, instead of juice or soda.

TABLE 23-6 Dietary Considerations for Specific Cancers

CANCER SITES	COMMON COMPLICATIONS[a]	POSSIBLE DIETARY MEASURES
Brain and nervous system	Chewing or swallowing difficulty, headache, altered taste or smell sensation, difficulty feeding oneself	Mechanically altered diet, use of adaptive feeding devices (see Nutrition in Practice 21)
Head and neck[b]	Chewing or swallowing difficulty, aspiration, dry mouth, altered taste or smell sensation, inflamed mucosa	Tube feeding, mechanically altered diet
Esophagus	Swallowing difficulty, aspiration, obstruction, acid reflux, inflamed mucosa	Tube feeding, mechanically altered diet
Stomach	Anorexia, early satiety, reduced secretion of gastric acid and intrinsic factor, delayed stomach emptying, dumping syndrome, malabsorption, nutrient deficiencies	Tube feeding (for obstruction or unmanageable dumping syndrome); postgastrectomy diet; small, frequent meals; limited sugar intake; modified fiber intake (see Chapter 17); nutrient supplementation
Intestine	Inflamed mucosa, bacterial overgrowth, obstruction, lactose intolerance, general malabsorption, bile insufficiency, nutrient deficiencies, short bowel syndrome (if resected), altered bowel function, fluid and electrolyte imbalances	Tube feeding or total parenteral nutrition for obstruction, enteritis, or short bowel syndrome; fat- and lactose-restricted diet (see Chapter 18); nutrient supplementation
Pancreas	Reduced secretion of digestive enzymes, bile insufficiency, general malabsorption, nutrient deficiencies, hyperglycemia	Enzyme replacement (see Chapter 18); small, frequent meals; fat-restricted diet; carbohydrate-controlled diet (see Chapter 20); nutrient supplementation

[a]Actual complications depend on the exact location of the cancer and the specific treatment methods used.
[b]Includes cancers of the salivary glands, oral and nasal cavities, pharynx, and larynx.

Box 23-7 *HOW TO* **Help Patients Handle Food-Related Problems**

In people with cancer or HIV infection, various complications can interfere with food intake. Health care providers can try to identify a patient's specific problems and offer appropriate solutions. Not every suggestion will work for each person, so encourage patients to experiment and find strategies that work best.

I just don't have an appetite.

- Eat small meals and snacks at regular times each day.
- Eat the largest meal at the time of day when you feel the best.
- Include nutrient-dense foods in meals, and consume them before other foods.
- Indulge in favorite foods throughout the day. Serve foods attractively.
- Avoid drinking large amounts of liquid before or with meals.
- Eat in a pleasant and relaxed environment. Eat with family and friends when possible.
- Listen to your favorite music or enjoy a TV or radio program while you eat.
- Ask your doctor about appetite-enhancing medications.

I am too tired to fix meals and eat.

- Let family members and friends prepare food for you.
- Obtain foods that are easy to prepare and easy to eat, such as sandwiches, ready-to-eat soups and entrees, ready-made foods from the deli counter, frozen dinners, instant breakfast drinks, and energy bars.
- Find time to rest before you attempt to prepare a large meal.
- Prepare soups, stews, and casserole dishes in sufficient quantity to provide enough for several meals, so that you will have enough to eat at times when you are too tired to cook.

Foods just don't taste right.

- Brush your teeth or use mouthwash before you eat.
- Consume foods chilled or at room temperature. Use plastic, rather than metal, eating utensils.
- Choose eggs, fish, poultry, and milk products instead of meat dishes.
- Experiment with sauces, seasonings, herbs, spices, and sweeteners to improve food taste and flavor.
- Save your favorite foods for times when you are not feeling nauseated.

I am nauseated a lot of the time, and sometimes I need to vomit.

- Consume liquid throughout the day to replace fluids.
- If you become nauseated from chemotherapy treatments, avoid eating for at least two hours before treatments.
- Consume your largest meal at a time when you are least likely to feel nauseated.
- Try consuming smaller meals, and eat slowly. Experiment with foods to see if some foods cause nausea more than others.

- Avoid foods and meals that have strong odors or are fatty, greasy, or gas forming.

I have problems chewing and swallowing food.

- Experiment with food consistencies to find the ones you can manage best. Thin liquids, dry foods, and sticky foods (such as peanut butter) are often difficult to swallow.
- Add sauces and gravies to dry foods.
- Drink fluids during meals to ease chewing and swallowing.
- Try using a straw to drink liquids. Experiment with beverage thickeners if you cannot tolerate thin beverages.
- Tilt your head forward and backward to see if you can swallow more easily when your head is positioned differently.

I have sores in my mouth, and they hurt when I eat.

- Try eating chilled or frozen foods; they are often soothing.
- Try soft foods such as ice cream, milkshakes, bananas, applesauce, mashed potatoes, cottage cheese, and macaroni and cheese. Mix dry foods with sauces or gravies.
- Cut foods into smaller pieces, so they are less likely to irritate the mouth.
- Avoid foods that irritate mouth sores, such as citrus fruits and juices, tomatoes and tomato-based products, spicy foods, foods that are very salty, foods with seeds (such as poppy seeds and sesame seeds) that can scrape the sores, and coarse foods such as raw vegetables, crackers, corn chips, and toast.
- Ask your doctor about using a local anesthetic solution such as lidocaine before eating to reduce the pain.
- Use a straw for drinking liquids, in order to bypass the sores.

My mouth is really dry.

- Rinse your mouth with warm salt water or mouthwash frequently. Avoid using mouthwash that contains alcohol.
- Drink small amounts of liquid frequently between meals.
- Ask your doctor or pharmacist about medications or saliva substitutes that can help a dry mouth condition.
- Use sour candy or chewing gum to stimulate the flow of saliva.
- Sip fluids frequently while eating. Add broth, sauces, gravies, mayonnaise, butter, or margarine to dry foods.
- Make sure you brush your teeth and floss regularly to prevent tooth decay and oral infections.

I am having trouble with constipation.

- Drink plenty of fluids. Try warm fluids, especially in the morning.
- Eat whole-grain breads and cereals, nuts, fresh fruits and vegetables, prunes, and prune juice. Avoid refined carbohydrate foods such as white bread, white rice, and enriched pasta.
- Engage in physical activity regularly.
- Try an over-the-counter bulk-forming agent, such as methylcellulose (Citrucel), psyllium (Metamucil or Fiberall), or polycarbophil (Fiber-Lax).

(Continued)

Box 23-7

HOW TO Help Patients Handle Food-Related Problems (continued)

I am having trouble with diarrhea.

- To avoid dehydration, drink plenty of fluids throughout the day. Diluted fruit juices, sports drinks, and salty broths and soups are good choices. Avoid caffeine- and alcohol-containing beverages. For severe diarrhea, try oral rehydration formulas that are commercially prepared.

- Avoid foods and beverages that increase gas, such as legumes, onions, vegetables of the cabbage family, foods that contain sorbitol or mannitol, and carbonated beverages.

- Try using lactase enzyme replacements when you use milk products in case you are experiencing lactose intolerance. Yogurt and aged cheeses may be easier to tolerate than milk and fresh cheeses.

- Avoid fatty foods if you are fat intolerant. Try reducing your intake of whole-grain breads and cereals if they worsen the diarrhea.

- Eat small, frequent meals instead of large ones. Try consuming cool or lukewarm foods instead of very cold or hot foods.

- Ask your doctor about using a bulk-forming agent or antidiarrheal medication.

In addition to instructing immunosuppressed patients about food safety, many institutions prescribe *low-microbial diets* (also called *neutropenic diets*) with more stringent recommendations for avoiding microbial contamination.[26] For example, the diet may omit fresh fruits and vegetables or include only foods that have been sterilized by cooking or canning. Note that low-microbial diets have not been standardized, and recommendations differ somewhat among institutions.[27] In addition, the benefits of using low-microbial diets have not been established, and some researchers have suggested that the diets may lead to food avoidance and malnutrition.[28]

Enteral and Parenteral Nutrition Support Tube feedings or parenteral nutrition may be necessary for patients who develop complications that interfere with food intake or have long-term or permanent GI impairment.[29] For example, many patients who undergo radiation therapy for head and neck cancers develop dysphagia or oral mucositis and may benefit from tube feeding. Parenteral nutrition is reserved for patients who have inadequate GI function, such as those with severe radiation enteritis. Whenever possible, enteral nutrition is strongly preferred over parenteral nutrition, to preserve GI function and avoid infection.

The Case Study in Box 23-8 allows you to apply information about nutrition and cancer to a clinical situation.

Box 23-8

Case Study: Woman with Cancer

Joan Monroy is a 58-year-old public relations consultant who was recently diagnosed with colon cancer after a routine colonoscopy, a procedure in which the colon is examined using a flexible tube attached to an optical device. Mrs. Monroy is scheduled to have surgery to remove the segment of colon that contains the tumor and to determine if the cancer has spread to the surrounding lymph nodes and, possibly, other organs. The nurse completing the nutrition assessment finds that Mrs. Monroy is 5 feet 5 inches tall and weighs 178 pounds. Mrs. Monroy usually spends most of the day sitting and has little time to engage in recreational exercise. Her diet typically includes red meat at both lunch and dinner, and she consumes one or two glasses of wine with both meals. She eats two or three servings of fruits and vegetables each day, although she does not like green leafy vegetables very much. She rarely drinks milk or consumes milk products.

1. Review Table 23-2 on p. 656, and describe the factors in Mrs. Monroy's diet and lifestyle that may have contributed to the development of colon cancer.

2. What symptoms and complications may arise after colon surgery and impair nutrition status? If the cancer team decides that Mrs. Monroy needs follow-up chemotherapy, how might the chemotherapy affect her nutrition status?

3. If Mrs. Monroy is unresponsive to treatment and her cancer progresses, she may develop cancer cachexia. Describe this syndrome, its causes, and its consequences.

4. Provide suggestions that may help Mrs. Monroy handle the following problems should they develop: poor appetite, fatigue, taste alterations, nausea and vomiting, chewing and swallowing difficulties, mouth sores, dry mouth, diarrhea, constipation, and weight loss.

Review Notes

- Cancer arises from altered expression of the genes that control cell division. Some dietary substances promote carcinogenesis, whereas others may help to prevent cancer.
- Cancer's effects on nutrition status depend on the type of cancer a person has, its severity, and the methods used to treat the cancer. Cancer cachexia is a frequent complication of cancer and may be a consequence of anorexia, altered metabolism, and responses to cancer treatment.
- Medical treatments for most cancers include surgery, chemotherapy, radiation therapy, and/or immunotherapy. Nutrition therapy aims to minimize weight loss and wasting, correct deficiencies, and manage complications that impair food intake.

23.2 HIV Infection

Possibly the most infamous infectious disease today is **acquired immunodeficiency syndrome (AIDS)**. AIDS develops from infection with human immunodeficiency virus (HIV), which attacks the immune system and disables a person's defenses against other diseases, including infections and certain cancers. Then these diseases—which would produce mild, if any, illness in people with healthy immune systems—destroy health and life. In the 30-plus years since AIDS has been identified, it has caused about 35 million deaths worldwide.[30]

Although the global incidence of HIV infection has been declining in recent years, its prevalence continues to be high in sub-Saharan Africa (see Table 23-7). Fortunately, remarkable progress has been made in understanding and treating HIV infection. Access to antiretroviral drugs continues to increase throughout the world, reducing AIDS-related deaths and the risk of HIV transmission.

Prevention of HIV Infection

As there is still no cure for AIDS, the best course is prevention. HIV is most often sexually transmitted and can be spread by direct contact with contaminated body fluids, such as blood, semen, vaginal secretions, and breast milk. Because many people remain symptom-free during the early stages of infection, they may not realize that they can

TABLE 23-7	The HIV and AIDS Epidemic at a Glance, 2016		
STAGE OF EPIDEMIC	**WORLD**	**SUB-SAHARAN AFRICA[a]**	**UNITED STATES**
Individuals living with HIV infection or AIDS	36,700,000	25,500,000[a]	1,123,000
Individuals newly infected with HIV	1,800,000	1,160,000	39,800
AIDS-related deaths	1,000,000	730,000	12,500

[a]Although nearly 70 percent of the world's HIV/AIDS cases are in sub-Saharan Africa, the region accounts for only 13 percent of the world's population.

Sources: Joint United Nations Programme on HIV/AIDS (UNAIDS), *Fact Sheet—World AIDS Day 2017: Global HIV Statistics,* available at www.unaids.org/sites/default/files/media_asset/UNAIDS_FactSheet_en.pdf; Centers for Disease Control and Prevention, *HIV in the United States: At a Glance,* available at www.cdc.gov/hiv/statistics/overview/ataglance.html.

acquired immunodeficiency syndrome (AIDS): the late stage of illness caused by infection with the human immunodeficiency virus (HIV); characterized by severe damage to immune function.

TABLE 23-8   Risk Factors for HIV Infection

- History of receiving blood transfusions or blood components before 1985
- Infant born to mother with HIV infection
- Intravenous drug use in which syringes are shared among users
- Sexual contact with intravenous drug users, prostitutes, or individuals with a history of HIV or other sexually transmitted diseases
- Sexual contact with multiple partners
- Unsafe sexual practices

BOX 23-9 *Nursing Diagnosis*

Nursing diagnoses appropriate for those with HIV infection may include *ineffective protection, risk for infection, impaired oral mucous membrane integrity, risk for impaired skin integrity, chronic pain, diarrhea, fatigue, imbalanced nutrition: less than body requirements, hopelessness,* and *death anxiety.*

helper T cells: lymphocytes that have a specific protein called CD4 on their surfaces and therefore are also known as *CD4+ T cells*; these are the cells most affected in HIV infection.

opportunistic infections: infections caused by microorganisms that normally do not cause disease in healthy people but are damaging to persons with compromised immune function.

AIDS-defining illnesses: diseases and complications associated with the later stages of an HIV infection, including recurrent bacterial pneumonia, opportunistic infections, certain cancers, and wasting of muscle tissue.

candidiasis: a fungal infection on the mucous membranes of the oral cavity and elsewhere; usually caused by *Candida albicans.*

herpes simplex virus: a common virus that can cause blisterlike lesions on the lips and in the mouth.

pass the infection to others. To reduce the spread of HIV infection, individuals at risk (see Table 23-8) are encouraged to undergo testing.* A blood test can usually detect HIV antibodies within several months after exposure and, often, after just two or three weeks. An estimated 15 percent of persons in the United States who have HIV infection are unaware that they are infected.[31]

Consequences of HIV Infection

HIV infection destroys immune cells that have a protein called CD4 on their surfaces.[32] The cells most affected are the **helper T cells**, also called *CD4+ T cells* because the presence of CD4 is a primary characteristic. HIV is able to enter helper T cells and induce them to produce additional copies of the virus, thus perpetuating and exacerbating the infection. Other cells that have the CD4 protein (and can be infected by HIV) include tissue macrophages and certain cells of the central nervous system. Early symptoms of HIV infection are nonspecific and may include fever, sore throat, malaise, swollen lymph nodes, skin rashes, muscle and joint pain, and diarrhea. After these symptoms subside, many people remain symptom-free for 5 to 10 years or even longer. If the HIV infection is not treated, however, the depletion of T cells eventually increases the person's susceptibility to **opportunistic infections**— that is, infections caused by microorganisms that normally do not cause disease in healthy individuals.

The term *AIDS* applies to the advanced stages of HIV infection, in which the inability to fight illness allows a number of serious diseases and complications to develop; such **AIDS-defining illnesses** include severe infections, certain cancers, and wasting of muscle tissue (see Box 23-9). Without treatment, AIDS develops in most HIV-infected persons within 7 to 10 years (in some individuals, the disease progresses more quickly).[33] Health practitioners evaluate disease progression by measuring the concentrations of helper T cells and circulating virus (called the *viral load*) and by monitoring clinical symptoms. Although drug therapies dramatically slow the progression of HIV infection, the drugs' side effects may make it difficult for patients to adhere to treatments, as discussed in several of the following sections.

Weight Loss and Wasting Even with effective treatment of HIV infection, weight loss and wasting remain common problems among HIV-infected patients. The wasting has been linked with accelerated disease progression, reduced strength, and fatigue. In the later stages of AIDS, the wasting is severe and increases the risk of death. Much as in cancer, the wasting associated with HIV infection has many causes: anorexia and inadequate food intake, nutrient malabsorption, altered metabolism, and diet-drug interactions. The *AIDS-wasting syndrome* is diagnosed when a patient has an involuntary weight loss greater than 10 percent of initial body weight plus either chronic diarrhea or chronic weakness and fever for more than 30 days.[34]

Reduced Food Intake As mentioned, inadequate food intake is a key factor in the development of wasting. Poor food intake may result from various factors, including the following:

- *Oral infections.* The oral infections associated with HIV infection may cause discomfort and interfere with food consumption. Common infections include **candidiasis** and **herpes simplex virus** infection. Oral candidiasis (commonly called *thrush;* see Photo 23-2) can cause mouth pain, dysphagia (difficulty swallowing), and altered taste sensation; an oral infection with herpes simplex virus may cause painful lesions around the lips and in the mouth.

---

*Some high-risk individuals may be prescribed an antiretroviral drug combination (named *Truvada*) to reduce their risk of contracting HIV infection; however, the drug must be taken daily and can cause multiple adverse effects.

- *Cancer.* As described earlier in this chapter, cancer leads to anorexia for numerous reasons. In addition, **Kaposi's sarcoma**, a type of cancer frequently associated with HIV infection, can cause lesions in the mouth and throat that make eating painful.
- *Medications.* The medications given to treat HIV infection, other coexisting infections, and cancer often cause anorexia, nausea and vomiting, altered taste sensation, food aversions, and diarrhea.
- *Respiratory disorders.* Respiratory infections, including pneumonia and tuberculosis, are common in people with HIV infection. Symptoms may include chest pain, shortness of breath, and cough, which interfere with eating and contribute to anorexia.
- *Emotional distress, pain, and fatigue.* The physical and social problems that accompany chronic illness may cause fear, anxiety, and depression, which contribute to anorexia. Pain and fatigue, which may be associated with some disease complications, can lead to anorexia and difficulty with eating.

GI Complications GI complications in HIV-infected patients may result from opportunistic infections, medications, or the HIV infection itself.[35] In addition to the oral infections described previously, infections may develop in the esophagus, stomach, and intestines. The medications that treat some of these infections may promote bacterial overgrowth. In addition, many patients develop nausea, vomiting, and diarrhea from the medications used to suppress HIV. As a result of these multiple problems, HIV-infected patients using standard treatments face an extremely high risk of malnutrition due to the combination of GI discomfort, bacterial overgrowth, malabsorption, and nutrient losses from vomiting, steatorrhea, and diarrhea.

Patients in the advanced stages of HIV infection may develop pathological changes in the small intestine, referred to as *AIDS enteropathy* (also called *HIV enteropathy*).[36] The condition is characterized by villus atrophy and blunting, intestinal cell losses, and inflammation. The result is a substantial reduction in the intestinal absorptive area, causing malabsorption, diarrhea, and weight loss.

Lipodystrophy Many patients who use drug therapies to suppress HIV infection develop abnormalities in body fat and fat metabolism known as **lipodystrophy**.[37] Patients may lose fat from the face and extremities, accumulate abdominal fat, or both. Also observed are breast enlargement (in both men and women), fat accumulation at the base of the neck (sometimes called a **buffalo hump**; see Photo 23-3), and benign growths composed of fat tissue (called **lipomas**). These changes in body composition are often disfiguring and may cause physical discomfort; moreover, patients often develop hypertriglyceridemia, elevated low-density lipoprotein (LDL) cholesterol levels, insulin resistance, and hyperinsulinemia. Some of the drugs (especially newer drugs) used to treat HIV infection have fewer adverse effects on lipid metabolism, and a change in medications can sometimes improve the condition.[38]

Neurological Complications Neurological complications may be a consequence of HIV infection, immunosuppression (which causes cancers and infections that target brain tissue), or the medications used to treat HIV infection.[39] Clinical features include mild to severe dementia, muscle weakness and gait disturbances, and pain, numbness, and tingling in the legs and feet. Neurological impairments are usually more pronounced in the advanced stages of AIDS.

Other Complications Patients with HIV infection can develop anemia due to nutrient malabsorption, blood loss, disturbed bone marrow function, medication side effects, or the chronic illness itself. HIV infection may also lead to skin disorders (rashes, infections, cancers), kidney diseases (nephrotic syndrome, chronic kidney disease), eye disorders (retinal infection or detachment), and coronary heart disease.

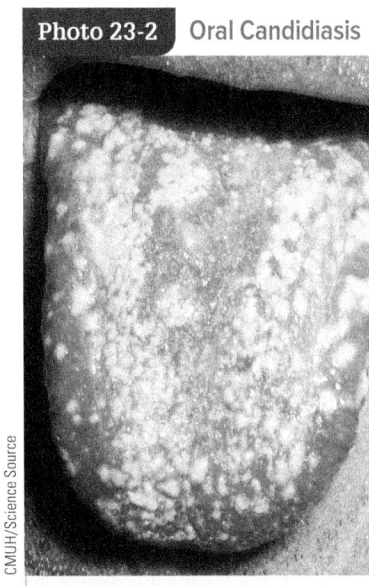

Photo 23-2 Oral Candidiasis

Oral candidiasis (also known as *thrush*) is characterized by a milky white coating or individual white patches on the tongue and other oral tissues.

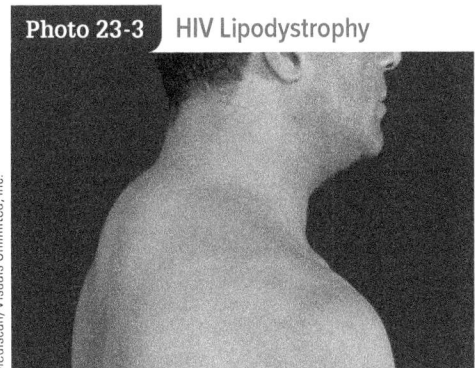

Photo 23-3 HIV Lipodystrophy

HIV-associated lipodystrophy is sometimes evident by the accumulation of fatty tissue at the base of the neck, referred to as *buffalo hump.*

Kaposi's (kah-POH-seez) **sarcoma:** a common cancer in HIV-infected persons that is characterized by lesions in the skin, lungs, and GI tract.

lipodystrophy (LIP-oh-DIS-tro-fee): abnormalities in body fat and fat metabolism that may result from drug treatments for HIV infection. The accumulation of abdominal fat is sometimes called *protease paunch.*

buffalo hump: the accumulation of fatty tissue at the base of the neck.

lipomas (lih-POE-muz): benign tumors composed of fatty tissue.

TABLE 23-9 Antiretroviral Drugs for Treatment of HIV Infection

CATEGORY	EXAMPLES	MODE OF ACTION
CCR5 antagonists	Maraviroc	CCR5 antagonists prevent HIV from entering cells by blocking a membrane receptor on the host cell.
Fusion inhibitors	Enfuvirtide	Fusion inhibitors prevent HIV from entering cells by binding a viral protein needed for its entry.
Integrase inhibitors	Raltegravir, elvitegravir, dolutegravir	Integrase inhibitors impair the function of HIV's integrase enzyme, which incorporates viral DNA into the host cell's genome.
Non-nucleoside reverse transcriptase inhibitors (NNRTIs)	Efavirenz, etravirine, nevirapine	NNRTIs bind active sites on HIV's reverse transcriptase enzyme, blocking the ability of HIV to produce DNA copies of its genetic material.
Nucleoside reverse transcriptase inhibitors (NRTIs)	Abacavir, lamivudine, zidovudine	As analogs of the nucleosides needed for DNA synthesis, NRTIs impair the ability of HIV's reverse transcriptase enzyme to produce usable copies of DNA.
Protease inhibitors (PIs)	Ritonavir, saquinavir, tipranavir	PIs inhibit HIV's protease enzyme, which cleaves HIV's gene products into usable structural proteins.

Sources: S. Safrin, Antiviral agents, in B. G. Katzung, ed., *Basic and Clinical Pharmacology* (New York: McGraw-Hill, 2018), pp. 863–894; R. M. Gulick, Antiretroviral therapy of human immunodeficiency virus and acquired immunodeficiency syndrome, in L. Goldman and A. I. Schafer, eds., *Goldman-Cecil Medicine* (Philadelphia: Saunders, 2016), pp. 2287–2292.

Treatments for HIV Infection

Although there is no cure for HIV infection, treatments can help to slow its progression, reduce complications, and alleviate pain. The standard drug treatment for suppressing HIV infection is usually a combination of three antiretroviral drugs, which should be initiated immediately after an individual is diagnosed.[40] Table 23-9 lists the major drug categories included in antiretroviral therapy and describes the drugs' modes of action. These antiretroviral agents have multiple adverse effects that make their long-term use difficult to tolerate. In addition to the GI effects discussed previously, side effects may include skin rashes, headache, anemia, tingling and numbness, hepatitis, pancreatitis, and kidney stones. Thus, although antiretroviral therapy has improved the life span and quality of life for many patients, the drug regimens are difficult to adhere to and cause complications that require continual management.

In addition to antiretroviral drugs, adjunct drug therapies may be necessary to prevent or treat infections, treat HIV-associated cancers, or manage other complications that arise over the course of illness. Medications are often prescribed to treat vomiting, anorexia, diarrhea, pain, blood lipid abnormalities, or glucose intolerance. Box 23-10 summarizes the nutrition-related effects of some of the antiretroviral agents and other drugs mentioned in this chapter.

Control of Anorexia and Wasting Anabolic hormones, appetite stimulants, and regular physical activity have been successful in reversing unintentional weight loss and increasing muscle mass in HIV-infected patients. Testosterone and human growth hormone have demonstrated positive effects on muscle tissue, especially in combination with resistance training.[41] A regular program of resistance exercise (see Photo 23-4) improves muscle mass and strength and corrects some of the metabolic abnormalities (altered blood lipids and insulin resistance) that are common in HIV-infected patients. The medications megestrol acetate and dronabinol (described on p. 660) are sometimes prescribed to stimulate appetite and improve weight gain, although much of the weight increase is attributable to a gain of fat rather than lean tissue.

Control of Lipodystrophy Treatment strategies for lipodystrophy are under investigation. Both aerobic activity and resistance training may help to reduce abdominal fat,

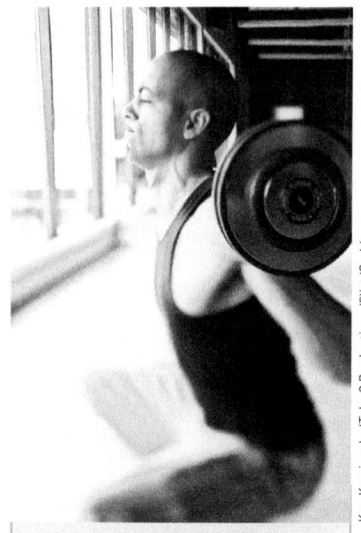

Photo 23-4 Resistance Training

Ken Kaminesky/Take 2 Productions/Flirt/Corbis

Resistance exercises force muscles to contract, improving muscle mass and strength; examples include weight-lifting, use of weight machines or stretchable bands, push-ups, chin-ups, arm raises, and leg lifts.

Box 23-10 Diet-Drug Interactions

Check this table for notable nutrition-related effects of the medications discussed in this chapter.

Appetite stimulants (megestrol acetate, dronabinol)	**Gastrointestinal effects:** Nausea, vomiting, diarrhea
	Dietary interaction: Dronabinol potentiates the effects of alcohol
	Metabolic effect: Hyperglycemia (megestrol acetate)
Abacavir	**Gastrointestinal effects:** Nausea, vomiting, anorexia, abdominal pain, diarrhea
	Dietary interaction: Avoid using alcohol while taking the drug
	Metabolic effects: Liver toxicity, pancreatitis, acidosis
Methotrexate	**Gastrointestinal effects:** Nausea, vomiting, gingivitis, diarrhea
	Dietary interaction: Reduces folate absorption
	Metabolic effects: Liver toxicity, increased serum uric acid levels, anemia
Ritonavir	**Gastrointestinal effects:** Nausea, vomiting, altered taste sensation, anorexia, diarrhea
	Dietary interaction: Must be taken with food; avoid using alcohol while taking the drug
	Metabolic effects: Hyperglycemia, liver toxicity, jaundice, hyperlipidemias (especially hypertriglyceridemia)
Zidovudine	**Gastrointestinal effects:** Nausea, vomiting, anorexia
	Dietary interactions: Do not take with a high-fat meal, which may decrease drug absorption
	Metabolic effects: Insulin resistance, diabetes, anemia, hyperlipidemias

Note: Most antiretroviral drugs used to treat HIV infection have gastrointestinal and metabolic side effects; only a few are listed here as examples.

although some patients opt for cosmetic surgery. As mentioned previously, an alternative antiretroviral drug regimen may improve the condition. Medications may be prescribed to treat abnormal blood lipids and insulin resistance.

Alternative Therapies Like cancer patients, people with HIV infection and AIDS are frequently tempted to try unconventional methods of treatment. Although many alternative therapies are harmless, some have side effects that may worsen complications or interfere with treatment. For example, herbal preparations that contain St. John's wort or garlic may reduce the effectiveness of some antiretroviral drugs.[42] Zinc megadoses may increase the progression of HIV infection.[43] Monitoring patients' use of dietary supplements is essential to reduce the likelihood of adverse effects or diet-drug interactions.

Nutrition Therapy for HIV Infection

HIV-infected individuals must learn how to maintain a healthy body weight, preserve muscle mass, prevent malnutrition, and cope with nutrition-related side effects of medications. Therefore, nutrition assessment and counseling should begin soon after a patient is diagnosed with HIV infection. The initial assessment should include an evaluation of body weight and body composition. Follow-up measurements may indicate the need to adjust dietary measures and drug therapies.

Weight Management Since the development of successful drug therapies for HIV infection, overweight and obesity have become more prevalent than wasting among

HIV-infected individuals in the United States.[44] Because excessive body weight can increase the risk of cardiovascular disease and diabetes, moderate weight loss may be recommended for patients with HIV infection who are overweight or obese.

Individuals who experience weight loss and wasting may benefit from a high-kcalorie, high-protein diet. If food consumption is difficult, small, frequent meals may be better tolerated than several large ones. The addition of nutrient-dense snacks, protein or energy bars, and oral supplements can improve intakes. Liquid formulas may be useful for the person who is too tired to eat or prepare meals. Review Box 23-6 on p. 662 for additional suggestions for adding energy and protein to the diet.

Metabolic Complications As mentioned, individuals who use antiretroviral drugs frequently develop insulin resistance and elevated triglyceride and LDL cholesterol levels. Treating these problems often requires both medications and dietary adjustments. Patients are generally advised to achieve or maintain a desirable weight, replace saturated fats with unsaturated fats, increase fiber intake, and limit intakes of *trans* fats and added sugars.[45] Fish oil supplementation has been shown to be effective for reducing blood triglyceride levels in patients with HIV infection.[46] Regular physical activity can improve both insulin resistance and blood lipid levels. If problems persist, alternative antiretroviral medications may be prescribed in an attempt to improve the metabolic abnormalities.

Vitamins and Minerals Micronutrient recommendations for patients with HIV infection are similar to those for the general population. Because nutrient deficiencies may result from reduced food intake, malabsorption, diet-drug interactions, and nutrient losses, multivitamin/mineral supplements are often recommended.[47] Patients should avoid taking high-dose supplements, however, due to the potential for adverse effects.

Symptom Management The discomfort associated with antiretroviral therapy, opportunistic GI infections, and symptoms of malabsorption can make food consumption difficult, and problems such as vomiting and diarrhea contribute to fluid and electrolyte losses. Box 23-7 on pp. 663–664 describes measures for improving food and fluid intakes in individuals with these problems.

Food Safety Concerns The depressed immunity of people with HIV infections places them at extremely high risk of developing foodborne infections. Health practitioners should caution patients about their high susceptibility to foodborne illness and provide detailed instructions about the safe handling and preparation of foods (see Nutrition in Practice 2). Water can also be a source of foodborne illness and is a common cause of **cryptosporidiosis** in HIV-infected individuals. In places where water quality is questionable, patients should consult their local health departments to determine whether the tap water is safe to drink. If not, or to take additional safety measures, water used for drinking and making ice cubes should be boiled for one minute.

Enteral and Parenteral Nutrition Support In later stages of illness, people with HIV infections may be unable to consume enough food and may need aggressive nutrition support. Tube feedings are preferred whenever the GI tract is functional; they can be provided at night as a supplement to the usual diet. Parenteral nutrition is reserved for patients who are unable to tolerate enteral nutrition, such as those with GI obstructions that prevent food intake. For individuals with severe malabsorption, orally administered hydrolyzed formulas containing medium-chain triglycerides are well tolerated and may be as effective as parenteral nutrition for reversing weight loss and wasting.[48] For either type of nutrition support, careful measures are necessary to avoid bacterial contamination of nutrient formulas and feeding equipment.

The Case Study in Box 23-11 provides an opportunity to review the nutritional concerns of a person with HIV infection.

cryptosporidiosis (KRIP-toe-spor-ih-dee-OH-sis): a foodborne illness caused by the parasite *Cryptosporidium parvum*.

Box 23-11 **Case Study: Man with HIV Infection**

Three years ago, **Alan Stratton, a 37-year-old financial planner,** sought medical help when he began feeling run-down and developed a painful white fungal infection over his mouth and tongue. The presence of thrush, recent weight loss, and anemia alerted Mr. Stratton's physician to the possibility of an HIV infection. When Mr. Stratton tested positive for HIV, he and his family and friends were devastated by the news, but those close to him have remained supportive. During the three years since Mr. Stratton began antiretroviral drug therapy, he has maintained his weight but has also developed lipodystrophy and hypertriglyceridemia. Mr. Stratton is 6 feet tall and currently weighs 185 pounds. He is occasionally anorexic and sometimes develops diarrhea.

1. Describe lipodystrophy, and discuss its typical pattern in people who have an HIV infection. What adjustments in treatment and lifestyle may be helpful for Mr. Stratton?

2. Describe an appropriate diet for Mr. Stratton. What strategies may improve his problems with anorexia and diarrhea? Suggest reasons why anorexia and diarrhea may develop in people with HIV infections.

3. Explain why an HIV infection can lead to wasting as the disease progresses to the later stages. What recommendations may be helpful for maintaining weight and health if wasting becomes a problem?

Review Notes

- By attacking immune cells, HIV causes progressive damage to immune function and may eventually lead to AIDS. Improved antiretroviral drug therapies have dramatically slowed the progression of HIV infection; the drug treatment should be started soon after diagnosis.

- HIV infection may lead to reduced food intake, GI complications, weight loss and wasting, and other problems; patients who use certain antiretroviral drugs may develop lipodystrophy.

- Patients with HIV infection who are overweight or obese may benefit from moderate weight loss; those who have experienced weight loss and wasting may need to consume a high-kcalorie, high-protein diet. To improve body weight and increase muscle mass, patients can use medications that improve muscle mass or appetite and participate in a resistance exercise program.

- People with HIV infection must pay strict attention to food safety guidelines to prevent foodborne illnesses.

Nutrition Assessment Checklist for People with Cancer or HIV Infections

MEDICAL HISTORY

Check the medical record to determine:

- ○ Type and stage of cancer
- ○ Stage of HIV infection

Review the medical record for complications that may alter nutrition therapy, including:

- ○ Altered organ function
- ○ Altered taste perception
- ○ Anorexia
- ○ Dry mouth and oral infections
- ○ GI symptoms and infections
- ○ Hyperlipidemias
- ○ Insulin resistance
- ○ Malnutrition and wasting

MEDICATIONS

For patients with cancer or HIV infections:

- ○ Check medications to identify potential diet-drug interactions.
- ○ Recommend the use of antinauseants, if needed.
- ○ Ask about the use of dietary supplements, including herbal products.

For cancer patients who require chemotherapy:

- ○ Recommend strategies to prevent food aversions.
- ○ Offer suggestions for managing drug-related complications.

For HIV-infected patients using antiretroviral drug therapy:

- ○ Remind patients that some drugs are better absorbed with foods and that others must be taken on an empty stomach.

- Help patients work out a medication schedule that suits their lifestyle and is timed appropriately with regard to food intake.
- Offer suggestions for managing drug-related complications.

DIETARY INTAKE

For patients with poor food intakes and weight loss:

- Determine the reasons for reduced food intake.
- Offer appropriate suggestions to improve food intake.
- Provide interventions before weight loss progresses further.

For patients with HIV infections who experience weight gain, elevated triglyceride or LDL cholesterol levels, or hyperglycemia:

- Assess intakes of energy, total fat, saturated fat, cholesterol, fiber, and sugars.
- For patients with hyperlipidemias, recommend a diet low in saturated fat, *trans* fat, and sugars.
- For patients with hyperglycemia, recommend a consistent carbohydrate intake at meals and snacks that emphasizes complex carbohydrates and limits concentrated sweets.
- Recommend regular physical activity for weight control and for improving blood lipid levels and insulin resistance.

ANTHROPOMETRIC DATA

Take baseline height and weight measurements, monitor weight regularly, and suggest dietary adjustments for weight maintenance, if necessary. Remember that body composition may change without affecting body weight. Perform baseline and periodic body composition measurements in HIV-infected patients who are using antiretroviral drug therapy.

LABORATORY TESTS

Note that albumin and other serum proteins may be reduced in patients with cancer or HIV infections, especially in those experiencing wasting. Check laboratory tests for indications of:

- Anemia
- Dehydration
- Elevated LDL cholesterol levels
- Elevated triglyceride levels
- Hyperglycemia

For patients with HIV infections, evaluate disease progression by checking:

- Helper T cell counts
- Viral load

PHYSICAL SIGNS

Look for physical signs of:

- Dehydration (especially in patients with fever, vomiting, or diarrhea)
- Kaposi's sarcoma
- Oral infections
- Protein-energy malnutrition and wasting

Self Check

1. Which of these dietary substances may help to protect against cancer?
   a. Alcoholic beverages
   b. Well-cooked meat, poultry, and fish
   c. Animal fats
   d. Compounds in fruits and vegetables

2. The metabolic changes that often accompany cancer include all of the following *except*:
   a. increased triglyceride breakdown.
   b. increased protein turnover.
   c. increased muscle protein synthesis.
   d. insulin resistance.

3. An advantage of radiation therapy over chemotherapy is that:
   a. radiation is not damaging to rapidly dividing cells.
   b. side effects of radiation therapy do not include malnutrition.
   c. radiation can be directed toward the regions affected by cancer.
   d. the radiation used is too weak to damage GI tissues.

4. Although many cancer patients lose weight, which type of cancer is often associated with weight gain?
   a. Kidney cancer
   b. Breast cancer
   c. Colon cancer
   d. Lung cancer

5. Which food below should be avoided by a patient taking immunosuppressive medications?
   a. Baked potato
   b. Canned tuna fish
   c. Banana
   d. Unpasteurized milk

6. HIV can enter and destroy:
   a. epithelial cells.
   b. helper T cells.
   c. liver cells.
   d. intestinal cells.

7. In patients who develop lipodystrophy, which abnormality is unlikely?
   a. Increased abdominal fat
   b. Increased fat in the arms and legs
   c. Fat accumulation at the base of the neck
   d. Hypertriglyceridemia

8. In people with HIV infection, mouth sores may be caused by all of the following, *except*:
   a. cryptosporidiosis.
   b. Kaposi's sarcoma.
   c. herpes simplex virus.
   d. candidiasis.

9. Megestrol acetate and dronabinol are:
   a. medications used to promote weight gain.
   b. protease inhibitors that fight HIV infection.
   c. medications that treat common opportunistic infections.
   d. anabolic hormones that promote the gain of muscle tissue.

10. To prevent cryptosporidiosis, a person with HIV infection may need to:
    a. wash hands carefully before meals.
    b. avoid consuming undercooked meat, poultry, and eggs.
    c. consume a high-kcalorie, high-protein diet.
    d. boil drinking water for one minute.

Answers: 1. d, 2. c, 3. c, 4. b, 5. d, 6. b, 7. b, 8. a, 9. a, 10. d

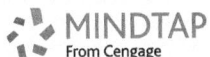 **MINDTAP** From Cengage · For more chapter resources visit **www.cengage.com** to access MindTap, a complete digital course.

Clinical Applications

1. Consider the nutrition problems that may develop in a 36-year-old woman with a malignant brain tumor that affects her ability to move the right side of her body (including the tongue) and to speak coherently. She is taking a pain medication that makes her nauseated and sleepy. Her expected survival time is only about six months.
   - If she is right-handed, how might her impairment interfere with eating? What suggestions do you have for overcoming this problem?
   - How might her nutrition status be affected by her inability to communicate effectively? What suggestions may help?
   - In what ways might the pain medication she is taking affect her nutrition status?

2. Various types of chronic conditions can lead to weight loss and wasting. For some of these conditions, such as Crohn's disease and celiac disease (Chapter 18), diet is a cornerstone of treatment. For others, such as cancer and HIV infection, nutrition plays a supportive role. What determines whether nutrition plays a primary role or a supportive role in the treatment of disease?

Notes

1. V. Kumar, A. K. Abbas, and J. C. Aster, Neoplasia, in V. Kumar and coeditors, *Robbins Basic Pathology* (Philadelphia: Elsevier, 2018), pp. 189–242.
2. Kumar, Abbas, and Aster, Neoplasia, 2018.
3. J. L. Freudenheim and E. Gower, Interaction of genetic factors with nutrition in cancer, in A. M. Coulston and coeditors, eds., *Nutrition in the Prevention and Treatment of Disease* (London: Academic Press/Elsevier, 2017), pp. 733–747.
4. K. Robien, C. L. Rock, and W. Demark-Wahnefried, Nutrition and cancers of the breast, endometrium, and ovary, in A. M. Coulston and coeditors, eds., *Nutrition in the Prevention and Treatment of Disease* (London: Academic Press/Elsevier, 2017), pp. 749–764.
5. S. D. Hursting and coauthors, Obesity, energy balance, and cancer: New opportunities for prevention, *Cancer Prevention Research* 5 (2012): 1260–1272.
6. D. E. Nelson and coauthors, Alcohol-attributable cancer deaths and years of potential life lost in the United States, *American Journal of Public Health* 103 (2013): 641–648.
7. M. Cascella and coauthors, Dissecting the mechanisms and molecules underlying the potential carcinogenicity of red and processed meat in colorectal cancer (CRC): An overview on the current state of knowledge, *Infectious Agents and Cancer* 13 (2018): doi: 10.1186/s13027-018-0174-9.
8. Z. Abid, A. J. Cross, and R. Sinha, Meat, dairy, and cancer, *American Journal of Clinical Nutrition* 100 (2014): 386S–393S.
9. W. C. Willett and coauthors, Diet, obesity, and physical activity, in B. W. Stewart and C. B. Wild, eds., *World Cancer Report* 2014 (Lyon, France: International Agency for Research on Cancer; 2014), pp. 171–184.
10. J. H. Doroshow, Approach to the patient with cancer, in L. Goldman and A. I. Schafer, eds., *Goldman-Cecil Medicine* (Philadelphia: Saunders, 2016), pp. 1206–1222.
11. V. C. Vaughan, P. Martin, and P. A. Lewandowski, Cancer cachexia: Impact, mechanisms and emerging treatments, *Journal of Cachexia, Sarcopenia, and Muscle* 4 (2013): 95–109; K. C. Fearon, The 2011 ESPEN Arvid Wretlind lecture: Cancer cachexia: The potential impact of translational research on patient-focused outcomes, *Clinical Nutrition* 31 (2012): 577–582.
12. A. M. Ryan and coauthors, Cancer-associated malnutrition, cachexia and sarcopenia: The skeleton in the hospital closet 40 years later, *Proceedings of the Nutrition Society* 75 (2016): 199–211.
13. Ryan and coauthors, 2016.
14. J. Arends and coauthors, ESPEN guidelines on nutrition in cancer patients, *Clinical Nutrition* 36 (2017): 11–48.
15. Doroshow, 2016.
16. A. Keating and M. R. Bishop, Hematopoietic stem cell transplantation, in L. Goldman and A. I. Schafer, eds., *Goldman-Cecil Medicine* (Philadelphia: Saunders, 2016), pp. 1198–1204.
17. R. Dev and coauthors, The evolving approach to management of cancer cachexia, *Oncology (Williston Park)* 31 (2017): 23–32; T. Aoyagi and

coauthors, Cancer cachexia, mechanism and treatment, *World Journal of Gastrointestinal Oncology* 7 (2015): 17–29.

18. K. Arthur and coauthors, Practices, attitudes, and beliefs associated with complementary and alternative medicine (CAM) use among cancer patients, *Integrative Cancer Therapies* 11 (2012): 232–242.

19. S. Chrubasik-Hausmann, J. Vlachojannis, and A. J. McLachlan, Understanding drug interactions with St John's wort (*Hypericum perforatum* L.): Impact of hyperforin content, *Journal of Pharmacy and Pharmacology* 70 (2018): doi: 10.1111/jphp.12858; S. Soleymani and coauthors, Clinical risks of St John's Wort (*Hypericum perforatum*) co-administration, *Expert Opinion on Drug Metabolism & Toxicology* 13 (2017): 1047–1062.

20. A. Agins, *ADA Quick Guide to Drug-Supplement Interactions* (Chicago: American Dietetic Association, 2011), pp. 19–20; M. L. Heaney and coauthors, Vitamin C antagonizes the cytotoxic effects of antineoplastic drugs, Cancer Research 68 (2008): 8031–8038; B. D. Lawenda and coauthors, Should supplemental antioxidant administration be avoided during chemotherapy and radiation therapy? *Journal of the National Cancer Institute* 100 (2008): 773–783.

21. N. S. Chandel and D. A. Tuveson, The promise and perils of antioxidants for cancer patients, *New England Journal of Medicine* 371 (2014): 177–178; C. L. Rock and coauthors, Nutrition and physical activity guidelines for cancer survivors, *CA: A Cancer Journal for Clinicians* 62 (2012): 242–274.

22. Rock and coauthors, 2012.

23. Arends and coauthors, 2017.

24. Academy of Nutrition and Dietetics, *Nutrition Care Manual* (Chicago: Academy of Nutrition and Dietetics, 2018).

25. A. L. Gross and coauthors, Weight change in breast cancer survivors compared to cancer-free women: A prospective study in women at familial risk of breast cancer, *Cancer Epidemiology, Biomarkers and Prevention* 24 (2015): 1262–1269; Rock and coauthors, 2012.

26. S. Trifilio and coauthors, Questioning the role of a neutropenic diet following hematopoetic stem cell transplantation, *Biology of Blood and Marrow Transplantation* 18 (2012): 1385–1390.

27. N. Fox and A. G. Freifeld, The neutropenic diet reviewed: Moving toward a safe food handling approach, *Oncology* 26 (2012): 572–575; S. J. Jubelirer, The benefit of the neutropenic diet: Fact or fiction? *Oncologist* 16 (2011): 704–707.

28. Arends and coauthors, 2017; E. C. van Dalen and coauthors, Low bacterial diet versus control diet to prevent infection in cancer patients treated with chemotherapy causing episodes of neutropenia, *Cochrane Database of Systematic Reviews* 9 (2012): doi: 10.1002/14651858.CD006247.pub2; Trifilio and coauthors, 2012.

29. Arends and coauthors, 2017.

30. Joint United Nations Programme on HIV/AIDS (UNAIDS), *Fact Sheet–World AIDS Day 2017: Global HIV Statistics*, available at www.unaids.org/sites/default/files/media_asset/UNAIDS_FactSheet_en.pdf.

31. A. F. Dailey and coauthors, Vital signs: Human immunodeficiency virus testing and diagnosis delays—United States, *Morbidity and Mortality Weekly Report* 66 (2017): 1300–1306.

32. F. Maldarelli, Biology of human immunodeficiency viruses, in L. Goldman and A. I. Schafer, eds., *Goldman-Cecil Medicine* (Philadelphia: Saunders, 2016), pp. 2280–2285.

33. V. Kumar, A. K. Abbas, and J. C. Aster, Diseases of the immune system, in V. Kumar and coeditors, *Robbins Basic Pathology* (Philadelphia: Elsevier, 2018), pp. 121–188.

34. V. Fuchs-Tarlovsky and E. Isenring, Nutrition therapy in patients with cancer and immunodeficiency, in G. A. Cresci, ed., *Nutrition for the Critically Ill Patient* (Boca Raton, FL: CRC Press, 2015), pp. 589–603.

35. T. A. Knox and C. Wanke, Gastrointestinal manifestations of HIV and AIDS, in L. Goldman and A. I. Schafer, eds., *Goldman-Cecil Medicine* (Philadelphia: Saunders, 2016), pp. 2302–2305.

36. E. Sakai and coauthors, Investigation of small bowel abnormalities in HIVinfected patients using capsule endoscopy, *Gastroenterology Research and Practice* 2017 (2017): doi 10.1155/2017/1932647.

37. L. B. Sacilotto and coauthors, Body composition and metabolic syndrome components on lipodystrophy different subtypes associated with HIV, *Journal of Nutrition and Metabolism* 2017 (2017): doi: 10.1155/2017/8260867; J. da Cunha and coauthors, Impact of antiretroviral therapy on lipid metabolism of human immunodeficiency virus-infected patients: Old and new drugs, *World Journal of Virology* 4 (2015): 56–77.

38. R. M. Gulick, Antiretroviral therapy of human immunodeficiency virus and acquired immunodeficiency syndrome, in L. Goldman and A. I. Schafer, eds., *Goldman-Cecil Medicine* (Philadelphia: Saunders, 2016), pp. 2287–2292; da Cunha and coauthors, 2015.

39. J. R. Berger and A. Nath, Neurologic complications of human immunodeficiency virus infection, in L. Goldman and A. I. Schafer, eds., *Goldman-Cecil Medicine* (Philadelphia: Saunders, 2016), pp. 2328–2332.

40. U.S. Department of Health and Human Services, DHHS Panel on Antiretroviral Guidelines for Adult and Adolescents, *Guidelines for the Use of Antiretroviral Agents in Adults and Adolescents Living with HIV* (updated October 17, 2017), available at www.aidsinfo.nih.gov/contentfiles/lvguidelines/AdultandAdolescentGL.pdf; Gulick, 2016.

41. M. H. Katz, HIV infection and AIDS, in M. A. Papadakis and S. J. McPhee, eds., *Current Medical Diagnosis and Treatment* 2018 (New York: Lange/McGraw-Hill, 2018), pp. 1340–1377.

42. C. E. Dennehy and C. Tsourounis, Dietary supplements and herbal medications, in B. G. Katzung, ed., *Basic and Clinical Pharmacology* (New York: McGraw-Hill, 2018), pp. 1131–1145.

43. J. Doley, HIV and cancer, in A. Skipper, ed., *Dietitian's Handbook of Enteral and Parenteral Nutrition* (Sudbury, MA: Jones and Bartlett Learning, 2012), pp. 199–216.

44. A. Willig, L. Wright, and T. A. Galvin, Practice paper of the Academy of Nutrition and Dietetics: Nutrition intervention and human immunodeficiency virus infection, *Journal of the Academy of Nutrition and Dietetics* 118 (2018): 486–498.

45. Willig, Wright, and Galvin, 2018.

46. N. Amador-Licona and coauthors, Omega 3 fatty acids supplementation and oxidative stress in HIV-seropositive patients: A clinical trial, *PLoS One* 11 (2016): doi: 10.1371/journal.pone.0151637.

47. Willig, Wright, and Galvin, 2018; Fuchs-Tarlovsky and Isenring, 2015.

48. Fuchs-Tarlovsky and Isenring, 2015; Doley, 2012.

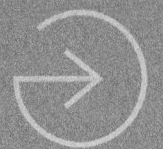

As with other medical technologies, the availability of specialized nutrition support forces health care professionals and members of our society to face difficult **ethical** decisions. When medical treatments prolong life by merely delaying death, the lifetime that remains may be of extremely low quality. This Nutrition in Practice examines the ethical dilemmas that clinicians must face when dealing with patients in critical care. Box NP23-1 defines the relevant terms.

If providing nutrition care can do little to promote recovery, is it appropriate to withhold or withdraw nutrition support?

In attempting to answer questions such as these, health professionals must consider the following ethical principles:[1]

- A patient has the right to make decisions concerning his or her own well-being (**patient autonomy**), even if refusing treatment could result in death. It is generally accepted that patients' preferences should take precedence over those of their health care providers.

- A patient should be fully informed of a treatment's benefits and risks in a fair and honest manner (**disclosure**). A patient's acceptance of a treatment that has been adequately disclosed is considered **informed consent**.

- A patient must have the mental capacity to make appropriate health care decisions (**decision-making capacity**). If a patient is mentally incapable of doing so, a person designated by the patient should serve as a **surrogate** decision maker.

- The potential benefits (**beneficence**) of any treatment should outweigh its potential harm (**maleficence**).

- Health care providers must determine whether the provision of health care to one patient would unfairly limit the care of other patients (**distributive justice**).

Box NP23-1 Glossary

advance health care directive: written or oral instructions regarding one's preferences for medical treatment to be used in the event of becoming incapacitated; also called an *advance medical directive* or a *living will*.

beneficence (be-NEF-eh-sense): actions that are taken to benefit others.

cardiopulmonary resuscitation (CPR): life-sustaining treatment that supplies oxygen and restores a person's ability to breathe and pump blood.

decision-making capacity: the ability to understand pertinent information and make appropriate decisions; known within the legal system as *decision-making competency*.

defibrillation: life-sustaining treatment in which an electronic device is used to shock the heart and reestablish a pattern of normal contractions. Defibrillation is used when the heart has arrhythmias or has experienced arrest.

dialysis: life-sustaining treatment in which a patient's blood is filtered using selective diffusion through a semipermeable membrane; substitutes for kidney function.

disclosure: the act of revealing pertinent information. For example, clinicians should accurately describe proposed tests and procedures, their benefits and risks, and alternative approaches.

distributive justice: the equitable distribution of resources.

do-not-resuscitate (DNR) order: a request by a patient or surrogate to withhold cardiopulmonary resuscitation.

durable power of attorney: a legal document (sometimes called a *health care proxy*) that gives legal authority to another (a *health care agent*) to make medical decisions in the event of incapacitation.

ethical: pertaining to accepted principles of right and wrong.

futile: describes medical care that will not improve the medical circumstances of a patient.

health care agent: a person given legal authority to make medical decisions for another in the event of incapacitation.

informed consent: a patient's or caregiver's agreement to undergo a treatment that has been adequately disclosed. Persons must be mentally competent in order to make the decision.

maleficence (mah-LEF-eh-sense): actions that are harmful to others.

mechanical ventilation: life-sustaining treatment in which a mechanical ventilator assists or replaces spontaneous breathing; substitutes for a patient's failing lungs.

patient autonomy: a principle of self-determination, such that patients (or surrogate decision makers) are free to choose the medical interventions that are acceptable to them, even if they choose to refuse interventions that may extend their lives.

persistent vegetative state: a condition resulting from brain injury in which an awake individual is unresponsive and shows no signs of higher brain function for a prolonged period; usually permanent.

surrogate: a substitute; a person who takes the place of another.

Although these principles may seem simple and obvious, it is often difficult to determine the appropriate action to take during intensive care. When clinicians and families disagree, the courts may be asked to decide.

What kinds of treatments can help to sustain a patient's life?

Nutrition support and hydration are both considered life-sustaining treatments because withholding or withdrawing either can result in death (see Photo NP23-1). Other life-sustaining treatments include **cardiopulmonary resuscitation (CPR)**, which supplies oxygen and restores a person's ability to breathe and pump blood; **defibrillation**, in which an electronic device shocks the heart and reestablishes normal contractions; **mechanical ventilation**, which substitutes for lung function; and **dialysis**, which substitutes for kidney function.

Do patients have a right to life-sustaining treatments?

Although life-sustaining treatments are readily provided to patients who have a reasonable chance of recovering from illness, it may be difficult to determine the best course of action for patients who are dying or who are unlikely to regain consciousness. Under such circumstances, the treatments may be considered **futile** because they are unable to improve the outcome of disease or increase the patient's comfort and well-being.[2] If patients or caregivers demand treatment that health practitioners have determined to be useless, a legal resolution may be required. Conversely, medical personnel may

find it objectionable to withdraw life support when they know that the inevitable consequence will be the patient's death.

How have the courts resolved conflicts involving nutrition support?

One of the landmark cases involving nutrition support concerned Nancy Cruzan, who suffered permanent and irreversible brain damage after a car crash in 1983 when she was 26 years of age.[3] After she had been in a **persistent vegetative state** for five years, her parents requested permission to discontinue tube feeding, but hospital staff refused to honor the request and the matter was taken to court. The Missouri Supreme Court determined that Nancy had never definitively stated her "right to die" wishes and that her parents were not entitled to make such a request for her. The court also stated that preserving life, no matter what its quality, should take precedence over all other considerations. Nancy's parents appealed the ruling, but in 1990, the U.S. Supreme Court upheld the Missouri Supreme Court in a 5–4 decision. Three witnesses were eventually found who could testify that Nancy would not have desired life-sustaining treatment under the circumstances, and the Court finally granted permission to remove the feeding tube. This case illustrates the importance of having an **advance health care directive** (discussed in a later section) that specifies one's preferences for medical treatment in the event of incapacitation.

In a more recent case that received widespread media attention, the spouse and parents of a patient in a persistent vegetative state fought a 10-year legal battle over her medical care. In 1990, at the age of 25, Terri Schiavo suffered a full cardiac arrest.[4] She initially fell into a coma, but her condition evolved into a persistent vegetative state that was considered irreversible. Despite the neurologists' diagnosis and a series of computed tomography (CT) and magnetic resonance imaging (MRI) scans showing extensive brain atrophy, her parents maintained that she was minimally conscious and could improve somewhat with rigorous treatment. Her husband, who was legally responsible for her care, insisted that she never would have wanted to be kept alive in a vegetative state. Like Nancy Cruzan, Terri had never expressed her wishes in an advance directive.

In 1998, Terri's husband filed a petition to have her feeding tube removed, and a Florida court approved the motion in February 2000. Although Terri's parents appealed, an appeals court affirmed the decision, and the Florida Supreme Court declined to review the case. In April 2001, Terri's physicians removed her feeding tube,

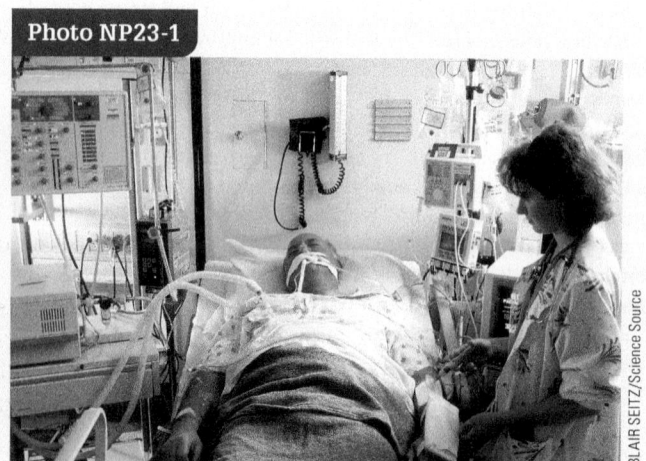

Photo NP23-1

Is it ever morally or legally appropriate to withhold or withdraw nutrition support?

BLAIR SEITZ/Science Source

but within days, a federal circuit court judge ordered it to be reinserted and reopened the case. Eventually, the various motions filed by the parents were dismissed and Terri's feeding tube was removed for the second time in October 2003. Within days, the Florida legislature passed a bill known as *Terri's Law* that gave the governor the authority to intervene, and Governor Jeb Bush ordered the feeding tube reinserted. A year later, Florida's Supreme Court declared Terri's Law to be unconstitutional. Although the governor appealed the decision, his appeal was rejected in January 2005. Terri's feeding tube was removed for the third and final time in March 2005. Despite emergency petitions by her parents and an attempt by the U.S. Congress to have her case reconsidered, the courts refused to grant a restraining order, and Terri died 13 days after her feeding tube was removed.

How can people ensure that their wishes will be considered in the event that they become incapacitated?

A person can declare preferences about medical treatments in an advance health care directive, sometimes called a *living will*. These directives include instructions about life-sustaining procedures that a person does or does not want. The documents are incorporated into the medical record and updated when appropriate; they take effect only if a physician determines that a patient lacks the ability to understand and make decisions about available treatments. If a person's preferences are unknown, decisions are based on a patient's best interests as determined by a caregiver or family member.[5]

Another important directive is a **durable power of attorney** (sometimes called a *health care proxy*), in which another person (a **health care agent**) is appointed to act as decision maker in the event of incapacitation. The agent should understand one's medical preferences and be absolutely trustworthy. Only one person can be designated, although one or two alternates may also be listed. If an agent is given comprehensive power to supervise care, he or she may make decisions about medical staff, health care facilities, and medical procedures.

Laws regarding advance directives vary from state to state. In some states, nutrition and hydration are not considered life-sustaining treatments, and a person's instructions about them may need to be indicated separately. Some states restrict the use of advance directives to terminal illness or disallow them during pregnancy. Generally, advance directives created in one state are honored in another.

How does a "do-not-resuscitate" order differ from other advance directives?

A **do-not-resuscitate (DNR) order** is frequently used to withhold CPR in the event of cardiopulmonary arrest, which occurs too suddenly for deliberate decision making. A DNR order is written in the medical record as other directives are, but it does not exclude the use of other life-prolonging measures. The DNR order is most often used in patients for whom death is expected and unavoidable, such as those with serious illnesses or advanced age. Some institutions allow a physician to write a DNR order for a patient who has a poor prognosis, but the physician must inform the patient or surrogate if this is done.

Have advance directives changed the way that medical care is provided?

Not really. Despite the availability of advance directives, less than 30 percent of people in the United States have completed one.[6] Even among severely or terminally ill patients, less than 50 percent have an advance directive.[7] In addition, many advance directives are too general or vague to guide specific treatment decisions. Furthermore, patients' preferences often change as their medical conditions evolve or they learn more about their prognosis.[8]

Physicians must often provide patient care before they have a chance to discuss treatments with patients or caregivers. For example, in emergency situations, consent is often assumed, and life-sustaining treatments are begun without the prior knowledge of patients or their decision makers.[9] In other cases, medical treatments are continued even if patients want them stopped, as when a doctor finds it difficult to withdraw a treatment (such as ventilation) that is certain to end in the patient's death.[10] Patients who are fully aware of treatment options and clearly state their preferences are more likely to be successful at obtaining the care they desire.

What resources are available to individuals who have difficulty making decisions about life-sustaining medical treatments?

Many medical institutions have ethics committees that meet regularly to update patient care policies pertaining to end-of-life treatments; these committees provide guidelines to help families and hospital staff who face difficult treatment decisions. Medical staff may also provide referrals for hospice care to dying patients who prefer comfort and palliation over invasive procedures in their final days.

Notes

1. E. J. Emanuel, Bioethics in the practice of medicine, in L. Goldman and A. I. Schafer, eds., *Goldman-Cecil Medicine* (Philadelphia: Saunders, 2016), pp. 4–9; J. M. Luce and D. B. White, A history of ethics and law in the intensive care unit, *Critical Care Clinics* 25 (2009): 221–237.

2. Emanuel, 2016; J. M. Luce, End-of-life decision making in the intensive care unit, *American Journal of Respiratory and Critical Care Medicine* 182 (2010): 6–11.

3. M. R. Andrews and J. O. Maillet, An ethics primer, in A. Skipper, ed., *Dietitian's Handbook of Enteral and Parenteral Nutrition* (Sudbury, MA: Jones and Bartlett Learning, 2012), pp. 46–56; Luce and White, 2009.

4. R. Cranford, Facts, lies, and videotapes: The permanent vegetative state and the sad case of Terri Schiavo, *Journal of Law, Medicine, and Ethics* 33 (2005): 363–372.

5. L. Snyder, American College of Physicians ethics manual: sixth edition, *Annals of Internal Medicine* 156(1 Pt 2) (2012): 73–104.

6. Emanuel, 2016.

7. Emanuel, 2016.

8. Luce and White, 2009.

9. J. Welie and H. ten Have, The ethics of forgoing life-sustaining treatment: Theoretical considerations and clinical decision making, *Multidisciplinary Respiratory Medicine* 9 (2014): doi: 10.1186/2049-6958-9-14.

10. Emanuel, 2016.

appendixes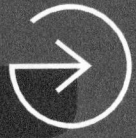

Contents

appendix A

Aids to Calculation

Many mathematical problems have been worked out in the "How To" boxes of the text. These pages provide additional help and examples.

A.1 Conversion Factors

A *conversion factor* is a numerical factor—expressed as a ratio—that can convert a quantity expressed in one unit to another unit; for example, the factor may be used to convert pounds to kilograms or feet to inches. To create a conversion factor, an equality (such as 1 *kilogram* = 2.2 *pounds*) is expressed as a fraction:

$$\frac{1 \text{ kg}}{2.2 \text{ lb}} \text{ and } \frac{2.2 \text{ lb}}{1 \text{ kg}}$$

Because a conversion factor has a value of *1* (the value in the numerator is equal to the value in the denominator), it can be used as a multiplier to change the *unit* of measure without changing the *value* of the measurement. To convert the units of a measurement, the fraction must have the desired unit in the numerator, as the unit in the denominator will cancel out the original unit.

Example 1 Convert the weight of 130 pounds to kilograms.

- Multiply 130 pounds by a conversion factor (fraction) that includes both pounds and kilograms and is arranged so that the desired unit (kilograms) is in the numerator:

$$130 \text{ lb} \times \frac{1 \text{ kg}}{2.2 \text{ lb}} = \frac{130 \text{ kg}}{2.2} = 59 \text{ kg}$$

As this example shows, the unit for *pounds* cancels out and the unit for *kilograms* remains in the solution.

Example 2 The food label on a bottle of apple juice shows the contents in both fluid ounces and liters. How many liters are contained in a bottle that holds 64 fluid ounces?

- Multiply 64 ounces by a conversion factor that includes both fluid ounces and liters, with the desired unit (liters) in the numerator:

$$64 \text{ fl oz} \times \frac{1 \text{ L}}{33.8 \text{ fl oz}} = \frac{64 \text{ L}}{33.8} = 1.89 \text{ L}$$

A.2 Percentages

A percentage expresses a fraction that has 100 in the denominator; for example, the term *50 percent* is equivalent to the fraction 50/100. Similar to other fractions, percentages are used to express a *proportion* of the *whole*; therefore, the units in the numerator and denominator must be similar. Any fraction can be expressed in hundredths and converted to a percentage by dividing the numerator by the denominator and multiplying by 100:

$$\frac{1}{4} = 0.25$$
$$0.25 \times 100 = 25\%$$

Example 3 Suppose your energy intake for the day is 2000 kcalories (kcal) and your recommended energy intake is 2400 kcalories. What percent of the recommended energy intake did you consume?

• Divide your intake by the recommended intake:

2000 kcal (your intake) ÷ 2400 kcal (recommended intake) = 0.83

• Multiply by 100 to express the decimal as a percentage:

0.83 × 100 = 83%

Example 4 A percentage can also be greater than 100. Suppose your intake of vitamin C is 120 milligrams and your RDA (male) is 90 milligrams. What percent of the RDA for vitamin C did you consume?

120 mg (your intake) ÷ 90 mg (RDA) = 1.33
1.33 × 100 = 133%

A.3 Weights and Measures

Length

1 meter (m) = 39 in
1 centimeter (cm) = 0.4 in
1 inch (in) = 2.5 cm
1 foot (ft) = 30 cm

Temperature

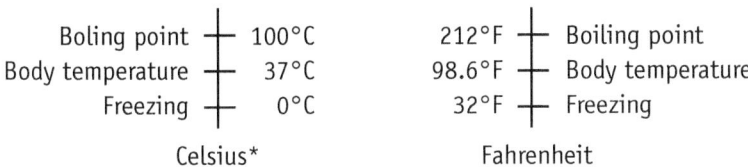

Boling point — 100°C   212°F — Boiling point
Body temperature — 37°C   98.6°F — Body temperature
Freezing — 0°C   32°F — Freezing

Celsius*   Fahrenheit

• To find degrees Fahrenheit (°F) when you know degrees Celsius (°C), multiply by 9/5 and then add 32.
• To find degrees Celsius (°C) when you know degrees Fahrenheit (°F), subtract 32 and then multiply by 5/9.

Volume

1 liter (L) = 1000 mL, 0.26 gal, 1.06 qt, 2.1 pt, or 33.8 fl oz
1 milliliter (mL) = 1/1000 L or 0.03 fl oz
1 gallon (gal) = 128 oz, 16 c, or 3.8 L
1 quart (qt) = 32 fl oz, 4 c, or 0.95 L
1 pint (pt) = 16 fl oz, 2 c, or 0.47 L
1 cup (c) = 8 fl oz, 16 tbs, about 250 mL, or 0.25 L
1 fluid ounce (fl oz) = 30 mL
1 tablespoon (tbs) = 3 tsp or 15 mL
1 teaspoon (tsp) = 5 mL

*Also known as centigrade.

Weight

1 kilogram (kg) = 1000 g or 2.2 lb

1 gram (g) = 1/1000 kg, 1000 mg, or 0.035 oz

1 milligram (mg) = 1/1000 g or 1000 μg

1 microgram (mg) = 1/1000 mg

1 pound (lb) = 16 oz, 454 g, or 0.45 kg

1 ounce (oz) = about 28 g

Energy

1 megajoule (MJ) = 240 kcal

1 kilojoule (kJ) = 0.24 kcal

1 kcalorie (kcal) = 4.2 kJ

1 g carbohydrate = 4 kcal = 17 kJ

1 g fat = 9 kcal = 37 kJ

1 g protein = 4 kcal = 17 kJ

1 g alcohol = 7 kcal = 29 kJ

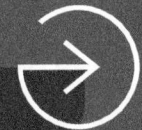

appendix B

WHO: Nutrition Recommendations

The World Health Organization (WHO) has assessed the relationships between diet and the development of chronic diseases. Its recommendations include:

- Energy intake: in balance with energy expenditure; sufficient to support growth, physical activity, and a healthy body weight (BMI between 18.5 and 24.9) and limited enough to avoid unhealthy weight gain greater than 11 pounds (5 kilograms) during adult life
- Total fat: 15 to 30 percent of total energy
- Saturated fatty acids: <10 percent of total energy
- Polyunsaturated fatty acids: 6 to 10 percent of total energy
- Omega-6 polyunsaturated fatty acids: 5 to 8 percent of total energy
- Omega-3 polyunsaturated fatty acids: 1 to 2 percent of total energy
- *Trans*-fatty acids: <1 percent of total energy
- Total carbohydrate: 55 to 75 percent of total energy
- Sugars: <10 percent of total energy, preferably <5 percent of total energy
- Protein: 10 to 15 percent of total energy
- Cholesterol: <300 mg per day
- Salt (sodium): <5 g salt per day (<2 g sodium per day), appropriately iodized
- Potassium: ≥3510 mg per day
- Fruits and vegetables: ≥400 g per day (about 1 pound)
- Total dietary fiber: >25 g per day from foods
- Physical activity: one hour of moderate-intensity activity, such as walking, on most days of the week

CONTENTS

Nutrition Recommendations from WHO

appendix C

Choose Your Foods: Food Lists for Diabetes

CONTENTS

Chapter 20 describes how a meal-planning system based on food lists can be used to control carbohydrate intakes, and this appendix provides details from the 2014 publication *Choose Your Foods: Food Lists for Diabetes*. These food lists can help people with diabetes to manage their blood glucose levels by controlling the amount and kinds of carbohydrates they consume. These lists can also be used to help in planning diets for weight management by controlling kcalorie intake.

C.1 The Food Lists

The food lists sort foods into groups by their proportions of carbohydrate, fat, and protein (Table C-1 on p. C-2). These major groups may be organized into several lists of foods (Tables C-2 through C-12 on pp. C-3–C-17). For example, the carbohydrate group includes these food lists:

- Starch
- Fruits
- Milk and Milk Substitutes (fat-free/low-fat, reduced-fat, and whole)
- Nonstarchy Vegetables
- Sweets, Desserts, and Other Carbohydrates

Then any food on a list can be substituted for any other on that same list. Note that some foods may count as choices from more than one group. For example, ½ cup black beans counts as 1 starch plus 1 lean protein choice.

C.2 Serving Sizes

The serving sizes have been carefully adjusted and defined so that a serving of any food on a given list provides roughly the same amount of carbohydrate, fat, and protein and, therefore, total energy. Any food on a list can thus be traded for any other food on the same list without significantly affecting the diet's energy–nutrient balance or total kcalories. For example, a person may select 17 small grapes or ½ large grapefruit as one fruit choice and either would provide roughly 15 grams of carbohydrate and 60 kcalories. A whole grapefruit, however, would count as 2 fruit choices.

To apply the system successfully, users must become familiar with the specified serving sizes. A convenient way to remember the serving sizes and energy values is to keep in mind a typical item from each list (review Table C-1).

C.3 The Foods on the Lists

Foods do not always appear on the food list where you might first expect to find them. They are grouped according to their energy–nutrient contents rather than by their source (such as milks), their outward appearance, or their vitamin and mineral contents. For example, cheeses are on the Protein list (not Milk and Milk Substitutes) because, like medium- and high-fat meats, cheeses contribute energy from protein and fat but provide negligible carbohydrate. For similar reasons, starchy vegetables such as corn, green peas, and potatoes are found on the Starch list with breads and cereals, not with the Nonstarchy Vegetables.

Diet planners learn to view mixtures of foods, such as casseroles and soups, as combinations of foods from different food lists. They also learn to interpret food labels with the food lists in mind.

c.4 Controlling Energy, Fat, and Sodium

The food lists help people control their energy intakes by paying close attention to serving sizes. People wanting to lose weight can limit foods from the Sweets, Desserts, and Other Carbohydrates list, and they might choose to avoid the Alcohol list altogether. The Free Foods list includes low-kcalorie choices.

The food lists alert consumers to foods that are high in fat. For example, the Starch list specifies which grain products contain extra fat (such as biscuits, taco shells, and bread stuffing by marking them with a symbol to indicate high-fat foods (the symbols are explained in the table keys). In addition, foods on the milk and protein lists are separated into categories based on their fat contents (review Table C-1). The Milk and Milk Substitutes list is subdivided for fat-free/low-fat, reduced-fat, and whole; the Protein list is subdivided for lean, medium-fat, and high-fat. The Protein list also includes plant-based protein, which tends to be rich in fiber. Notice that many of these foods bear the symbol for "good source of fiber."

People wanting to control the sodium in their diets can begin by eliminating any foods bearing the "high in sodium" symbol. In most cases, the symbol identifies foods that, in one serving, provide 480 milligrams or more of sodium. Foods on the Combination Foods or Fast Foods lists that bear the symbol provide more than 600 milligrams of sodium. Other foods may also contribute substantially to sodium intake (consult Chapter 9 for details).

TABLE C-1   The Food Lists

FOOD LISTS	TYPICAL ITEM/PORTION SIZE	CARBOHYDRATE (g)	PROTEIN (g)	FAT (g)	ENERGY^a (kcal)
CARBOHYDRATES					
Starch^b	1 slice bread	15	3	1	80
Fruits	1 small apple	15	—	—	60
Milk and milk substitutes					
Fat-free, low-fat (1%)	1 c fat-free milk	12	8	0–3	100
Reduced-fat (2%)	1 c reduced-fat milk	12	8	5	120
Whole	1 c whole milk	12	8	8	160
Nonstarchy vegetables	½ c cooked carrots	5	2	—	25
Sweets, desserts, and other carbohydrates	5 vanilla wafers	15	varies	varies	varies
PROTEINS					
Lean	1 oz chicken (no skin)	—	7	2	45
Medium-fat	1 oz ground beef	—	7	5	75
High-fat	1 oz pork sausage	—	7	8	100
Plant-based	½ c tofu	varies	7	varies	varies
FATS	1 tsp olive oil	—	—	5	45
ALCOHOL	12 fl oz beer	varies	—	—	100

^{a}The energy value for each food list represents an approximate average for the group and does not reflect the precise number of grams of carbohydrate, protein, and fat. For example, a slice of bread contains 15 grams of carbohydrate (60 kcalories), 3 grams of protein (12 kcalories), and 1 gram of fat (9 calories)—rounded to 80 kcalories for ease in calculating. A ½ cup of nonstarchy vegetables contains 5 grams of carbohydrate (20 kcalories) and 2 grams of protein (8 kcalories), which has been rounded down to 25 kcalories.
^{b}The Starch list includes cereals, grains and pasta, breads, crackers and snacks, starchy vegetables (such as corn, peas, and potatoes), and legumes (beans, peas, and lentils).

C.5 Planning a Healthy Diet

To obtain a daily variety of foods that provide healthful amounts of carbohydrate, protein, and fat, as well as vitamins, minerals, and fiber, the meal pattern for adults and teenagers should include at least:

- Three servings of nonstarchy vegetables
- Three servings of fruits
- Six servings of grains (at least three of whole grains), beans, and starchy vegetables
- Two servings of low-fat or fat-free milk or milk substitutes
- No more than 6 ounces of lower-fat protein foods
- No more than 5 to 8 servings of fat, mainly as nuts, seeds, and liquid fats (rather than solid fats)
- *Small* amounts sugar

The actual amounts are determined by age, gender, activity levels, and other factors that influence energy needs.

TABLE C-2 Starch

The Starch list includes breads, cereals, grains (including pasta and rice), starchy vegetables, crackers and snacks, and legumes (beans, peas, and lentils). 1 starch choice = 15 grams carbohydrate, 3 grams protein, 1 gram fat, and 80 kcalories.

Note: In general, one starch choice is ½ cup of cooked cereal, grain, or starchy vegetable; ⅓ cup of cooked rice or pasta; 1 ounce of bread product, such as 1 slice of bread; ¾ to 1 ounce of most snack foods.

FOOD	SERVING SIZE	FOOD	SERVING SIZE
BREAD		**BREAD—continued**	
Bagel	¼ large bagel (1 oz)	Hot dog bun or hamburger bun	½ bun (¾ oz)
! Biscuit	1 (2½ in. across)	Pancake	1 (4 in. across, ¼ in. thick)
Breads, loaf-type		Roll, plain	1 small (1 oz)
white, whole-grain, French, Italian, pumpernickel, rye, sourdough, unfrosted raisin or cinnamon	1 slice (1 oz)	! Stuffing, bread	⅓ cup
		Waffle	1 (4-in. square or 4 in. across)
		CEREALS	
✓ reduced-calorie, light	2 slices (1½ oz)	✓ Bran cereal (twigs, buds, or flakes)	½ cup
Breads, flat-type (flatbreads)		Cooked cereals (oats, oatmeal)	½ cup
chapatti	1 oz	Granola cereal	½ cup
ciabatta	1 oz	Grits, cooked	½ cup
naan	3¼-in. square (1 oz)	Muesli	¼ cup
pita (6 in. across)	½ pita	Puffed cereal	1½ cups
roti	1 oz	Shredded wheat, plain	½ cup
✓ sandwich flat buns, whole-wheat	1 bun (1½ oz)	Sugar-coated cereal	½ cup
		Unsweetened, ready-to-eat cereal	¾ cup
! taco shell	2 (each 5 in. across)	**GRAINS**[a]	
tortilla, corn	1 small (6 in. across)	Barley	⅓ cup
tortilla, flour (white or whole-wheat)	1 small (6 in. across) or ⅓ large (10 in. across)	Bran, dry	
		✓ oat	¼ cup
Cornbread	1¾-in. cube (1½ oz)	✓ wheat	½ cup
English muffin	½ muffin		

(Continued)

TABLE C-2 Starch (continued)

FOOD	SERVING SIZE
GRAINSª—continued	
✓ Bulgur	½ cup
Couscous	⅓ cup
Kasha	½ cup
Millet	⅓ cup
Pasta, white or whole-wheat	⅓ cup
Polenta	⅓ cup
Quinoa, all colors	⅓ cup
Rice, all colors and types	⅓ cup
Tabbouleh (tabouli), prepared	½ cup
Wheat germ, dry	3 Tbsp
Wild rice	½ cup
STARCHY VEGETABLESᵇ	
Breadfruit	¼ cup
Cassava or dasheen	⅓ cup
Corn	½ cup
on cob	4- to 4½-in. piece (½ large)
✓ Hominy	¾ cup
✓ Mixed vegetables with corn or peas	1 cup
Marinara, pasta, or spaghetti sauce	½ cup
✓ Parsnips	½ cup
✓ Peas, green	½ cup
Plantain	⅓ cup
Potato	
baked with skin	¼ large (3 oz)
boiled, all kinds	½ cup or ½ medium (3 oz)
! mashed, with milk and fat	½ cup
french-fried (oven-baked)ᶜ	1 cup (2 oz)
✓ Pumpkin puree, canned, no sugar added	¾ cup
✓ Squash, winter (acorn, butternut)	1 cup
✓ Succotash	½ cup
Yam or sweet potato, plain	½ cup (3½ oz)

ªServing sizes are for cooked grains, unless otherwise noted.
ᵇServing sizes are for cooked vegetables.
ᶜRestaurant-style french fries are on the Fast Foods list.
ᵈAlso found on the Protein list.

FOOD	SERVING SIZE
CRACKERS AND SNACKS	
Crackers	
animal	8
✓ crispbread	2–5 pieces (¾ oz)
graham, 2½-in. square	3
nut and rice	10
oyster	20
! round, butter-type	6
saltine-type	6
! sandwich-style, cheese or peanut butter filling	3
whole-wheat, baked	5 regular 1½-in. squares or 10 thins (¾ oz)
Granola or snack bar	1 (¾ oz)
Matzoh, all shapes and sizes	¾ oz
Melba toast	4 (2 in. by 4 in.)
Popcorn	
✓ no fat added	3 cups
!! with butter added	3 cups
Pretzels	¾ oz
Rice cakes	2 (4 in. across)
Snack chips	
baked (potato, pita)	~8 (¾ oz)
!! regular (tortilla, potato)	~13 (1 oz)
BEANS, PEAS, AND LENTILSᵈ	

The choices on this list count as 1 starch + 1 lean protein.

✓ Baked beans, canned	⅓ cup
✓ Beans (black, garbanzo, kidney, lima, navy, pinto, white), cooked or canned, drained and rinsed	½ cup
✓ Lentils (any color), cooked	½ cup
✓ Peas (black-eyed and split), cooked or canned, drained and rinsed	½ cup
ⓢ✓ Refried beans, canned	½ cup

KEY

✓ = Good source of fiber: >3 g/serving
! = Extra fat: +5 grams fat
!! = Extra fat: +10 grams fat
ⓢ = High in sodium: ≥480 mg/serving

appendix C

TABLE C-3 Fruits

FRUIT[a]

The Fruits list includes fresh, frozen, canned, and dried fruits and fruit juices.

1 fruit choice = 15 grams carbohydrate, 0 grams protein, 0 grams fat, and 60 kcalories.

Note: In general, one fruit choice is ½ cup of canned or frozen fruit or unsweetened fruit juice; 1 small fresh fruit (¾ to 1 cup); 2 tablespoons of dried fruit.

FOOD	SERVING SIZE	FOOD	SERVING SIZE
Apple, unpeeled	1 small (4 oz)	Mango	½ small (5½ oz) or ½ cup
Apples, dried	4 rings	Nectarine	1 medium (5½ oz)
Applesauce, unsweetened	½ cup	✓Orange	1 medium (6½ oz)
Apricots		Papaya	½ (8 oz) or 1 cup cubed
canned	½ cup	Peaches	
dried	8 halves	canned	½ cup
fresh	4 (5½ oz total)	fresh	1 medium (6 oz)
Banana	1 extra-small, ~4 in. long (4 oz)	Pears	
✓Blackberries	1 cup	canned	½ cup
Blueberries	¾ cup	✓fresh	½ large (4 oz)
Cantaloupe	1 cup diced	Pineapple	
Cherries		canned	½ cup
sweet, canned	½ cup	fresh	¾ cup
sweet, fresh	12 (3½ oz)	Plantain, extra-ripe (black), raw	¼ (2¼ oz)
Dates	3 small (deglet noor) or 1 large (medjool)	Plums	
		canned	½ cup
Dried fruits (blueberries, cherries, cranberries, mixed fruit, raisins)	2 Tbsp	dried (prunes)	3
		fresh	2 small (5 oz total)
Figs		Pomegranate seeds (arils)	½ cup
dried	3 small	✓Raspberries	1 cup
✓fresh	1½ large or 2 medium (3½ oz total)	✓Strawberries	1¼ cup whole
		Tangerine	1 large (6 oz)
Fruit cocktail	½ cup	Watermelon	1¼ cups diced
Grapefruit		**FRUIT JUICE**	
fresh	½ large (5½ oz)		
sections, canned	¾ cup	Apple juice/cider	½ cup
Grapes	17 small (3 oz total)	Fruit juice blends, 100% juice	⅓ cup
✓Guava	2 small (2½ oz total)	Grape juice	⅓ cup
Honeydew melon	1 cup diced	Grapefruit juice	½ cup
Kiwi	½ cup sliced	Orange juice	½ cup
Loquat	¾ cup cubed	Pineapple juice	½ cup
Mandarin oranges, canned	¾ cup	Pomegranate juice	½ cup
		Prune juice	⅓ cup

[a]The weights listed include skin, core, seeds, and rind.

KEY

✓ = Good source of fiber: >3 g/serving

TABLE C-4 Milk and Milk Substitutes

The Milk and Milk Substitutes list groups milks and yogurts based on the amount of fat they contain. Cheeses are on the Protein list because they are rich in protein and have very little carbohydrate; butter, cream, coffee creamers, and unsweetened nut milks are on the Fats list; and ice cream and frozen yogurt are on the Sweets, Desserts, and Other Carbohydrates list.

1 fat-free (skim) or low-fat (1%) milk choice = 12 grams carbohydrate, 8 grams protein, 0–3 grams fat, and 100 kcalories.

1 reduced-fat milk choice = 12 grams carbohydrate, 8 grams protein, 5 grams fat, and 120 kcalories.

1 whole-milk choice = 12 grams carbohydrate, 8 grams protein, 8 grams fat, and 160 kcalories.

1 carbohydrate choice = 15 grams carbohydrate and about 70 kcalories.

1 fat choice = 5 grams fat and 45 kcalories.

Note: In general, one milk choice is 1 cup (8 fluid ounces or ½ pint) milk or yogurt.

FOOD	SERVING SIZE	CHOICES PER SERVING
MILK AND YOGURTS		
Fat-free (skim) or low-fat (1%)		
milk, buttermilk, acidophilus milk, lactose-free milk	1 cup	1 fat-free milk
evaporated milk	½ cup	1 fat-free milk
yogurt, plain or Greek; may be sweetened with artificial sweetener	⅔ cup (6 oz)	1 fat-free milk
chocolate milk	1 cup	1 fat-free milk + 1 carbohydrate
Reduced-fat (2%)		
milk, acidophilus milk, kefir, lactose-free milk	1 cup	1 reduced-fat milk
yogurt, plain	⅔ cup (6 oz)	1 reduced-fat milk
Whole		
milk, buttermilk, goat's milk	1 cup	1 whole milk
evaporated milk	½ cup	1 whole milk
yogurt, plain	1 cup (8 oz)	1 whole milk
chocolate milk	1 cup	1 whole milk + 1 carbohydrate
OTHER MILK FOODS AND MILK SUBSTITUTES[a]		
Eggnog		
fat-free	⅓ cup	1 carbohydrate
low-fat	⅓ cup	1 carbohydrate + ½ fat
whole milk	⅓ cup	1 carbohydrate + 1 fat
Rice drink		
plain, fat-free	1 cup	1 carbohydrate
flavored, low-fat	1 cup	2 carbohydrates
Soy milk		
light or low-fat, plain	1 cup	½ carbohydrate + ½ fat
regular, plain	1 cup	½ carbohydrate + 1 fat
Yogurt with fruit, low-fat	⅔ cup (6 oz)	1 fat-free milk + 1 carbohydrate

[a]Unsweetened nut milks (such as almond and coconut milks) are on the Fats list.

appendix C

TABLE C-5   Nonstarchy Vegetables

The Nonstarchy Vegetables list includes vegetables that contain small amounts of carbohydrates and few kcalories; starchy vegetables that contain higher amounts of carbohydrate and kcalories are found on the Starch list. Salad greens (like arugula, chicory, endive, escarole, lettuce, radicchio, romaine, and watercress) are on the Free Foods list.

1 nonstarchy vegetable choice = 5 grams carbohydrate, 2 grams protein, 0 grams fat, and 25 kcalories.

Note: In general, one nonstarchy vegetable choice is ½ cup of cooked vegetables or vegetable juice or 1 cup of raw vegetables. Count 3 cups of raw vegetables or 1½ cups of cooked nonstarchy vegetables as one carbohydrate choice.

Amaranth leaves (Chinese spinach)	Hearts of palm
Artichoke	✓ Jicama
Artichoke hearts (no oil)	Kale
Asparagus	Kohlrabi
Baby corn	Leeks
Bamboo shoots	Mixed vegetables (without starchy vegetables, legumes, or pasta)
Bean sprouts (alfalfa, mung, soybean)	Mushrooms, all kinds, fresh
Beans (green, wax, Italian, yard-long)	Okra
Beets	Onions
Broccoli	Pea pods
Broccoli slaw, packaged, no dressing	Peppers (all varieties)
✓ Brussels sprouts	Radishes
Cabbage (green, red, bok choy, Chinese)	Rutabaga
✓ Carrots	🅢 Sauerkraut, drained and rinsed
Cauliflower	Spinach
Celery	Squash, summer varieties (yellow, pattypan, crookneck, zucchini)
Chayote	Sugar snap peas
Coleslaw, packaged, no dressing	Swiss chard
Cucumber	Tomato
Daikon	Tomatoes, canned
Eggplant	🅢 Tomato sauce (unsweetened)
Fennel	Tomato/vegetable juice
Gourds (bitter, bottle, luffa, bitter melon)	Turnips
Green onions or scallions	Water chestnuts
Greens (collard, dandelion, mustard, purslane, turnip)	

KEY

✓ = Good source of fiber: >3 g/serving

🅢 = High in sodium: ≥480 mg/serving

appendix C

TABLE C-6   Sweets, Desserts, and Other Carbohydrates

The Sweets, Desserts, and Other Carbohydrates list contains foods with added sugars, added fats, or both.

1 sweets, desserts and other carbohydrates choice = 15 grams carbohydrate, about 70 kcalories.

1 carbohydrate choice = 15 grams carbohydrate and about 70 kcalories.

1 fat choice = 5 grams fat and 45 kcalories.

FOOD	SERVING SIZE	CHOICES PER SERVING
BEVERAGES, SODA, AND SPORTS DRINKS		
Cranberry juice cocktail	½ cup	1 carbohydrate
Food drink or lemonade	1 cup (8 oz)	2 carbohydrates
Hot chocolate, regular	1 envelope (2 Tbsp or ¾ oz) added to 8 oz water	1 carbohydrate
Soft drink (soda), regular	1 can (12 oz)	2½ carbohydrates
Sports drink (fluid replacement type)	1 cup (8 oz)	1 carbohydrate
BROWNIES, CAKE, COOKIES, GELATIN, PIE, AND PUDDING		
Biscotti	1 oz	1 carbohydrate + 1 fat
Brownie, small, unfrosted	1¼-in. square, ⅞-in. high (~1 oz)	1 carbohydrate + 1 fat
Cake		
angel food, unfrosted	¹⁄₁₂ of cake (~2 oz)	2 carbohydrates
frosted	2-in. square (~2 oz)	2 carbohydrates + 1 fat
unfrosted	2-in. square (~1 oz)	1 carbohydrate + 1 fat
Cookies		
100-kcalorie pack	1 oz	1 carbohydrate + ½ fat
chocolate chip cookies	2, 2¼ in. across	1 carbohydrate + 2 fats
gingersnaps	3 small, 1½ in. across	1 carbohydrate
large cookie	1, 6 in. across (~3 oz)	4 carbohydrates + 3 fats
sandwich cookies with crème filling	2 small (~⅔ oz)	1 carbohydrate + 1 fat
sugar-free cookies	1 large or 3 small (¾ to 1 oz)	1 carbohydrate + 1–2 fats
vanilla wafer	5	1 carbohydrate + 1 fat
Cupcake, frosted	1 small (~1¾ oz)	2 carbohydrates + 1–1½ fats
Flan	½ cup	2½ carbohydrates + 1 fat
Fruit cobbler	½ cup (3½ oz)	3 carbohydrates + 1 fat
Gelatin, regular	½ cup	1 carbohydrate
Pie		
commercially prepared fruit, 2 crusts	⅙ of 8-in. pie	3 carbohydrates + 2 fats
pumpkin or custard	⅛ of 8-in. pie	1½ carbohydrates + 1½ fats
Pudding		
regular (made with reduced-fat milk)	½ cup	2 carbohydrates
sugar-free or sugar- and fat-free (made with fat-free milk)	½ cup	1 carbohydrate

(Continued)

appendix C

TABLE C-6 Sweets, Desserts, and Other Carbohydrates *(continued)*

FOOD	SERVING SIZE	CHOICES PER SERVING
CANDY, SPREADS, SWEETS, SWEETENERS, SYRUPS, AND TOPPINGS		
Blended sweeteners (mixtures of artificial sweeteners and sugar)	1½ Tbsp	1 carbohydrate
Candy		
chocolate, dark or milk type	1 oz	1 carbohydrate + 2 fats
chocolate "kisses"	5 pieces	1 carbohydrate + 1 fat
hard	3 pieces	1 carbohydrate
Coffee creamer, nondairy type		
powdered, flavored	4 tsp	½ carbohydrate + ½ fat
liquid, flavored	2 Tbsp	1 carbohydrate
Fruit snacks, chewy (pureed fruit concentrate)	1 roll (¾ oz)	1 carbohydrate
Fruit spreads, 100% fruit	1½ Tbsp	1 carbohydrate
Honey	1 Tbsp	1 carbohydrate
Jam or jelly, regular	1 Tbsp	1 carbohydrate
Sugar	1 Tbsp	1 carbohydrate
Syrup		
chocolate	2 Tbsp	2 carbohydrates
light (pancake-type)	2 Tbsp	1 carbohydrate
regular (pancake-type)	1 Tbsp	1 carbohydrate
CONDIMENTS AND SAUCES		
Barbecue sauce	3 Tbsp	1 carbohydrate
Cranberry sauce, jellied	¼ cup	1½ carbohydrates
Curry sauce	1 oz	1 carbohydrate + 1 fat
Gravy, canned or bottled	½ cup	½ carbohydrate + ½ fat
Hoisin sauce	1 Tbsp	½ carbohydrate
Marinade	1 Tbsp	½ carbohydrate
Plum sauce	1 Tbsp	½ carbohydrate
Salad dressing, fat-free, cream-based	3 Tbsp	1 carbohydrate
Sweet-and-sour sauce	3 Tbsp	1 carbohydrate
DOUGHNUTS, MUFFINS, PASTRIES, AND SWEET BREADS		
Banana nut bread	1-in. slice (2 oz)	2 carbohydrates + 1 fat
Doughnut		
cake, plain	1 medium (1½ oz)	1½ carbohydrates + 2 fats
hole	2 (1 oz)	1 carbohydrate + 1 fat
yeast-type, glazed	1, 3¾ in. across (2 oz)	2 carbohydrates + 2 fats
Muffin		
regular	1 (4 oz)	4 carbohydrates + 2½ fats
low-fat	1 (4 oz)	4 carbohydrates + ½ fat

(Continued)

TABLE C-6 Sweets, Desserts, and Other Carbohydrates *(continued)*

FOOD	SERVING SIZE	CHOICES PER SERVING
Scone	1 (4 oz)	4 carbohydrates + 3 fats
Sweet roll or Danish	1 (2½ oz)	2½ carbohydrates + 2 fats
FROZEN BARS, FROZEN DESSERTS, FROZEN YOGURT, AND ICE CREAM		
Frozen pops	1	½ carbohydrate
Fruit juice bars, frozen, 100% juice	1 (3 oz)	1 carbohydrate
Ice cream		
fat-free	½ cup	1½ carbohydrates
light	½ cup	1 carbohydrate + 1 fat
no-sugar-added	½ cup	1 carbohydrate + 1 fat
regular	½ cup	1 carbohydrate + 2 fats
Sherbet, sorbet	½ cup	2 carbohydrates
Yogurt, frozen		
fat-free	⅓ cup	1 carbohydrate
regular	½ cup	1 carbohydrate + 0–1 fat
Greek, lower-fat or fat-free	½ cup	1½ carbohydrates

KEY

⑤ = High in sodium: ≥480 mg/serving

TABLE C-7 Protein

The Protein list groups foods based on the amount of fat they contain.

FOOD	SERVING SIZE	FOOD	SERVING SIZE
LEAN PROTEIN		**LEAN PROTEIN—continued**	
1 lean protein choice = 0 grams carbohydrate, 7 grams protein, 2 grams fat, and 45 kcalories.		Fish	
Beef: ground (90% or higher lean/10% or lower fat); select or choice grades trimmed of fat such as roast (chuck, round, rump, sirloin), steak (cubed, flank, porterhouse, T-bone), tenderloin	1 oz	fresh or frozen, such as catfish, cod, flounder, haddock, halibut, orange roughy, tilapia, trout	1 oz
		salmon, fresh or canned	1 oz
		sardines, canned	2 small
⑤Beef jerky	½ oz	tuna, fresh or canned in water or oil and drained	1 oz
Cheeses with ≤3 g fat/oz	1 oz	⑤ smoked: herring or salmon (lox)	1 oz
Curd-style cheeses: cottage-type (all kinds); ricotta (fat-free or light)	¼ cup (2 oz)	Game: buffalo, ostrich, rabbit, venison	1 oz
Egg substitutes, plain	¼ cup	⑤ Hot dog[a] with ≤3 g fat/oz	1 (1¾ oz)
Egg whites	2	Lamb: chop, leg, or roast	1 oz
		Organ meats: heart, kidney, liver[b]	1 oz

(Continued)

TABLE C-7	Protein *(continued)*

FOOD	SERVING SIZE
Oysters, fresh or frozen	6 medium
Pork, lean	
⬛ Canadian bacon	1 oz
⬛ ham	1 oz
rib or loin chop/roast, tenderloin	1 oz
Poultry, without skin: chicken; Cornish hen; domestic duck or goose (well drained of fat); turkey; lean ground turkey or chicken	1 oz
⬛ Processed sandwich meats with ≤3 g fat/oz: chipped beef, thin-sliced deli meats, turkey ham, turkey pastrami	1 oz
⬛ Sausage with ≤3 g fat/oz	1 oz
Shellfish: clams, crab, imitation shellfish, lobster, scallops, shrimp	1 oz
Veal: cutlet (no breading), loin chop, roast	1 oz

MEDIUM-FAT PROTEIN

1 medium-fat protein choice = 0 grams carbohydrate, 7 grams protein, 5 grams fat, and 75 kcalories.

FOOD	SERVING SIZE
Beef trimmed of visible fat: ground beef (85% or lower lean/15% or higher fat), corned beef, meatloaf, prime cuts of beef (rib roast), short ribs, tongue	1 oz
Cheeses with 4–7 g fat/oz: feta, mozzarella, pasteurized processed cheese spread, reduced-fat cheeses	1 oz
Cheese, ricotta (regular or part-skim)	¼ cup (2 oz)
Egg	1
Fish: any fried	1 oz
Lamb: ground, rib roast	1 oz

ᵃMay contain carbohydrate.
ᵇMay be high in cholesterol.

FOOD	SERVING SIZE
MEDIUM-FAT PROTEIN—*continued*	
Pork: cutlet, ground, shoulder roast	1 oz
Poultry with skin: chicken, dove, pheasant, turkey, wild duck, or goose; fried chicken	1 oz
⬛ Sausage with 4–7 g fat/oz	1 oz

HIGH-FAT PROTEIN

1 high-fat protein choice = 0 grams carbohydrate, 7 grams protein, 8 grams fat, and 100 kcalories. These foods are high in saturated fat, cholesterol, and kcalories and may raise blood cholesterol levels if eaten on a regular basis. Try to eat 3 or fewer choices from this group per week.

FOOD	SERVING SIZE
Bacon, pork	2 slices (1 oz each before cooking)
⬛ Bacon, turkey	3 slices (½ oz each before cooking)
Cheese, regular: American, blue-veined, brie, cheddar, hard goat, Monterey jack, Parmesan, queso, and Swiss	1 oz
Hot dog: beef, pork, or combination	1 (10 per 1 lb-sized package)
Hot dog: turkey or chicken	1 (10 per 1 lb-sized package)
Pork: sausage, spareribs	1 oz
⬛ Processed sandwich meats with ≥8 g fat/oz: bologna, hard salami, pastrami	1 oz
⬛ Sausage with ≥8 g fat/oz: bratwurst, chorizo, Italian, knockwurst, Polish, smoked, summer	1 oz

KEY

❗ = Extra fat: +5 grams fat

⬛ = High in sodium: ≥480 mg/serving (based on the sodium content of a typical 3-oz serving of meat, unless 1 oz or 2 oz is the normal serving size)

TABLE C-7   Protein *(continued)*

Beans, peas, and lentils are also on the Starch list; nut butters in small amounts are on the Fats list. Because carbohydrate content varies among plant-based proteins, read food labels.

1 plant-based protein choice = variable grams carbohydrate, 7 grams protein, variable grams fat, and variable kcalories.

FOOD	SERVING SIZE	CHOICES PER SERVING
PLANT-BASED PROTEIN		
"Bacon" strips, soy-based	2 (½ oz)	1 lean protein
✓ Baked beans, canned	⅓ cup	1 starch + 1 lean protein
✓ Beans (black, garbanzo, kidney, lima, navy, pinto, white), cooked or canned, drained and rinsed	½ cup	1 starch + 1 lean protein
"Beef" or "sausage" crumbles, meatless	1 oz	1 lean protein
"Chicken" nuggets, soy-based	2 (1½ oz)	½ carbohydrate + 1 medium-fat protein
✓ Edamame, shelled	½ cup	½ carbohydrate + 1 lean protein
Falafel (spiced chickpea and wheat patties)	3 patties (~2 in. across)	1 carbohydrate + 1 high-fat protein
Hot dog, meatless, soy-based	1 hot dog (1½ oz)	1 lean protein
✓ Hummus	⅓ cup	1 carbohydrate + 1 medium-fat protein
✓ Lentils, any color, cooked or canned, drained and rinsed	½ cup	1 starch + 1 lean protein
Meatless burger, soy-based	3 oz	½ carbohydrate + 2 lean proteins
Meatless burger, vegetable- and starch-based	1 patty (~2½ oz)	½ carbohydrate + 1 lean protein
Meatless deli slices	1 oz	1 lean protein
Mycoprotein ("chicken" tenders or crumbles), meatless	2 oz	½ carbohydrate + 1 lean protein
Nut spreads: almond butter, cashew butter, peanut butter, soy nut butter	1 Tbsp	1 high-fat protein
✓ Peas (black-eyed and split peas), cooked or canned, drained and rinsed	½ cup	1 starch + 1 lean protein
✓ ⓢ Refried beans, canned	½ cup	1 starch + 1 lean protein
"Sausage" breakfast-type patties, meatless	1 (1½ oz)	1 medium-fat protein
Soy nuts, unsalted	¾ oz	½ carbohydrate + 1 medium-fat protein
Tempeh, plain, unflavored	¼ cup (1½ oz)	1 medium-fat protein
Tofu	½ cup (4 oz)	1 medium-fat protein
Tofu, light	½ cup (4 oz)	1 lean protein

KEY

✓ = Good source of fiber: >3 g/serving   ⓢ = High in sodium: ≥480 mg/serving

appendix C

TABLE C-8 Fats

Fats and oils have mixtures of unsaturated (polyunsaturated and monounsaturated) and saturated fats. Foods on the Fats list are grouped together based on the major type of fat they contain.

1 fat choice = 0 grams carbohydrate, 0 grams protein, 5 grams fat, and 45 kcalories.

Note: In general, one fat choice is 1 teaspoon of oil or solid fat or 1 tablespoon of salad dressing.

When used in large amounts, bacon and nut butters are counted as high-fat protein choices (see Protein list). Fat-free salad dressings are on the Sweets, Desserts, and Other Carbohydrates list. Fat-free products such as margarines, salad dressings, mayonnaise, sour cream, and cream cheese are on the Free Foods list.

FOOD	SERVING SIZE	FOOD	SERVING SIZE
UNSATURATED FATS—MONOUNSATURATED FATS		**UNSATURATED FATS—POLYUNSATURATED FATS—***continued*	
Almond milk (unsweetened)	1 cup	Mayonnaise-style salad dressing	
Avocado, medium	2 Tbsp (1 oz)	reduced-fat	1 Tbsp
Nut butters (*trans* fat-free): almond butter, cashew butter, peanut butter (smooth or crunchy)	1½ tsp	regular	2 tsp
		Nuts	
Nuts		pignolia (pine nuts)	1 Tbsp
almonds	6 nuts	walnuts, English	4 halves
Brazil	2 nuts	Oil: corn, cottonseed, flaxseed, grapeseed, safflower, soybean, sunflower	1 tsp
cashews	6 nuts		
filberts (hazelnuts)	5 nuts	Salad dressing	
macadamia	3 nuts	reduced-fat*ᵃ*	2 Tbsp
mixed (50% peanuts)	6 nuts	regular	1 Tbsp
peanuts	10 nuts	Seeds	
pecans	4 halves	flaxseed, ground	1½ Tbsp
pistachios	16 nuts	pumpkin, sesame, sunflower	1 Tbsp
Oil: canola, olive, peanut	1 tsp	Tahini or sesame paste	2 tsp
Olives		**SATURATED FATS**	
black (ripe)	8	Bacon, cooked, regular or turkey	1 slice
green, stuffed	10 large	Butter	
Spread, plant stanol ester-type		reduced-fat	1 Tbsp
light	1 Tbsp	stick	1 tsp
regular	2 tsp	whipped	2 tsp
		Butter blends made with oil	
UNSATURATED FATS—POLYUNSATURATED FATS		reduced-fat or light	1 Tbsp
Margarine		regular	1½ tsp
lower-fat spread (30–50% vegetable oil, *trans* fat-free)	1 Tbsp	Chitterlings, boiled	2 Tbsp (½ oz)
		Coconut, sweetened, shredded	2 Tbsp
stick, tub, or squeeze (*trans* fat-free)	1 tsp	Coconut milk, canned, thick	
Mayonnaise		light	⅓ cup
reduced-fat	1 Tbsp	regular	1½ Tbsp
regular	1 tsp		

(Continued)

TABLE C-8 Fats *(continued)*

FOOD	SERVING SIZE	FOOD	SERVING SIZE
SATURATED FATS—*continued*		Lard	1 tsp
Coconut milk beverage (thin), unsweetened	1 cup	Oil: coconut, palm, palm kernel	1 tsp
Cream		Salt pork	¼ oz
half-and-half	2 Tbsp	Shortening, solid	1 tsp
heavy	1 Tbsp	Sour cream	
light	1½ Tbsp	reduced-fat or light	3 Tbsp
whipped	2 Tbsp	regular	2 Tbsp
Cream cheese			
reduced-fat	1½ Tbsp (¾ oz)		
regular	1 Tbsp (½ oz)		

ᵃMay contain carbohydrate.

TABLE C-9 Free Foods

Most foods on the Free Foods list should be limited to 3 servings per day and eaten throughout the day. Eating all 3 servings at one time could raise blood glucose levels. Food and drink choices listed without a serving size can be eaten whenever you like.

1 free food choice = ≤5 grams carbohydrate and ≤20 kcalories.

FOOD	SERVING SIZE	FOOD	SERVING SIZE
LOW-CARBOHYDRATE FOODS		**REDUCED-FAT OR FAT-FREE FOODS**	
Candy, hard (regular or sugar-free)	1 piece	Cream cheese, fat-free	1 Tbsp (½ oz)
Fruits: cranberries or rhubarb, sweetened with sugar substitute	½ cup	Coffee creamers, nondairy	
Gelatin dessert, sugar-free, any flavor		liquid, flavored	1½ tsp
Gum, sugar-free		liquid, sugar-free, flavored	4 tsp
Jam or jelly, light or no-sugar-added	2 tsp	powdered, flavored	1 tsp
Salad greens (such as arugula, chicory, endive, escarole, leaf or iceberg lettuce, purslane, romaine, radicchio, spinach, watercress)		powdered, sugar-free, flavored	2 tsp
		Margarine spread	
Sugar substitutes (artificial sweeteners)		fat-free	1 Tbsp
Syrup, sugar-free	2 Tbsp	reduced-fat	1 tsp
Vegetables: any **raw** nonstarchy vegetables (such as broccoli, cabbage, carrots, cucumber, tomato)	½ cup	Mayonnaise-style salad dressing	
		fat-free	1 Tbsp
		reduced-fat	2 tsp
Vegetables: any **cooked** nonstarchy vegetables (such as carrots, cauliflower, green beans)	¼ cup	Mayonnaise-style salad dressing	
		fat-free	1 Tbsp
		reduced-fat	2 tsp

(Continued)

appendix C

TABLE C-9   Free Foods *(continued)*

FOOD	SERVING SIZE	FOOD	SERVING SIZE
REDUCED-FAT OR FAT-FREE FOODS—*continued*		**CONDIMENTS—***continued*	
Salad dressing		Sweet-and-sour sauce	2 tsp
fat-free	1 Tbsp	Taco sauce	1 Tbsp
fat-free, Italian	2 Tbsp	Vinegar	
Sour cream, fat-free or reduced-fat	1 Tbsp	Worcestershire sauce	
Whipped topping		Yogurt, any type	2 Tbsp
light or fat-free	2 Tbsp	**DRINKS/MIXES**	
regular	1 Tbsp	ⓢ Bouillon, broth, consommé	
CONDIMENTS		Bouillon or broth, low-sodium	
Barbecue sauce	2 tsp	Carbonated or mineral water	
Catsup (ketchup)	1 Tbsp	Club soda	
Chili sauce, sweet, tomato-type	2 tsp	Cocoa powder, unsweetened	1 Tbsp
Horseradish		Coffee, unsweetened or with sugar substitute	
Hot pepper sauce		Diet soft drinks, sugar-free	
Lemon juice		Drink mixes (powder or liquid drops), sugar-free	
Miso	1½ tsp	Tea, unsweetened or with sugar substitute	
Mustard		Tonic water, sugar-free	
honey	1 Tbsp	Water	
brown, Dijon, horseradish-flavored, wasabi-flavored, or yellow		Water, flavored, sugar-free	
Parmesan cheese, grated	1 Tbsp	**SEASONINGS**	
Pickle relish (dill or sweet)	1 Tbsp	Flavoring extracts (for example, vanilla, almond, or peppermint)	
Pickles		Garlic, fresh or powder	
ⓢ dill	1½ medium	Herbs, fresh or dried	
sweet, bread and butter	2 slices	Kelp	
sweet, gherkin	¾ oz	Nonstick cooking spray	
Pimento		Spices	
Salsa	¼ cup	Wine, used in cooking	
ⓢ Soy sauce, light or regular	1 Tbsp		

KEY

ⓢ = High in sodium: ≥480 mg/serving

TABLE C-10 Combination Foods

Many foods are eaten in various combinations, such as casseroles. Because "combination" foods do not fit into any one choice list, this list of choices provides some typical combination foods.

1 carbohydrate choice = 15 grams carbohydrate and about 70 kcalories.

FOOD	SERVING SIZE	CHOICES PER SERVING
ENTREES		
⑤ Casserole-type entrees (tuna noodle, lasagna, spaghetti with meatballs, chili with beans, macaroni and cheese)	1 cup (8 oz)	2 carbohydrates + 2 medium-fat proteins
⑤ Stews (beef/other meats and vegetables)	1 cup (8 oz)	1 carbohydrate + 1 medium-fat protein + 0–3 fats
FROZEN MEALS/ENTREES		
⑤✓ Burrito (beef and bean)	1 (5 oz)	3 carbohydrates + 1 lean protein + 2 fats
Dinner-type healthy meal (includes dessert and is usually <400 kcal)	~9–12 oz	2–3 carbohydrates + 1–2 lean proteins + 1 fat
"Healthy"-type entree (usually <300 kcal)	~7–10 oz	2 carbohydrates + 2 lean proteins
Pizza		
⑤ cheese/vegetarian, thin crust	¼ of a 12-in. pizza (4½–5 oz)	2 carbohydrates + 2 medium-fat proteins
⑤ meat topping, thin crust	¼ of a 12-in. pizza (5 oz)	2 carbohydrates + 2 medium-fat proteins + 1½ fats
⑤ cheese/vegetarian or meat topping, rising crust	⅙ of a 12-in. pizza (4 oz)	2½ carbohydrates + 2 medium-fat proteins
⑤ Pocket sandwich	1 sandwich (4½ oz)	3 carbohydrates + 1 lean protein + 1–2 fats
⑤ Pot pie	1 (7 oz)	3 carbohydrates + 1 medium-fat protein + 3 fats
SALADS (DELI-STYLE)		
Coleslaw	½ cup	1 carbohydrate + 1½ fats
Macaroni/pasta salad	½ cup	2 carbohydrates + 3 fats
⑤ Potato salad	½ cup	1½–2 carbohydrates + 1–2 fats
Tuna salad or chicken salad	½ cup (3½ oz)	½ carbohydrate + 2 lean proteins + 1 fat
SOUPS		
⑤✓ Bean, lentil, or split pea soup	1 cup (8 oz)	1½ carbohydrates + 1 lean protein
⑤ Chowder (made with milk)	1 cup (8 oz)	1 carbohydrate + 1 lean protein + 1½ fats
⑤ Cream soup (made with water)	1 cup (8 oz)	1 carbohydrate + 1 fat
⑤ Miso soup	1 cup (8 oz)	½ carbohydrate + 1 lean protein
⑤ Ramen noodle soup	1 cup (8 oz)	2 carbohydrates + 2 fats
Rice soup/porridge (congee)	1 cup (8 oz)	1 carbohydrate
⑤ Tomato soup (made with water), borscht	1 cup (8 oz)	1 carbohydrate
⑤ Vegetable, beef, chicken, noodle, or other broth-type soup (including "healthy"-type soups, such as those lower in sodium and/or fat)	1 cup (8 oz)	1 carbohydrate + 1 lean protein

KEY

✓ = Good source of fiber: >3 g/serving

⑤ = High in sodium: ≥600 mg/serving for main dishes/meals and ≥480 mg/serving for side dishes

appendix C

TABLE C-11 Fast Foods

The choices in the Fast Foods list are not specific fast-food meals or items, but are estimates based on popular foods. Ask the restaurant or check its website for nutrition information about your favorite fast foods. 1 carbohydrate choice = 15 grams carbohydrate and about 70 kcalories.

FOOD	SERVING SIZE	CHOICES PER SERVING
MAIN DISHES/ENTREES		
Chicken		
breast, breaded and fried[a]	1 (~7 oz)	1 carbohydrate + 6 medium-fat proteins
breast, meat only[b]	1	4 lean proteins
drumstick, breaded and fried[a]	1 (~2½ oz)	½ carbohydrate + 2 medium-fat proteins
drumstick, meat only[b]	1	1 lean protein + ½ fat
nuggets or tenders	6 (~3½ oz)	1 carbohydrate + 2 medium-fat proteins + 1 fat
thigh, breaded and fried[a]	1 (~5 oz)	1 carbohydrate + 3 medium-fat proteins + 2 fats
thigh, meat only[b]	1	2 lean proteins + ½ fat
wing, breaded and fried[a]	1 wing (~2 oz)	½ carbohydrate + 2 medium-fat proteins
wing, meat only[b]	1 wing	1 lean protein
Main dish salad (grilled chicken–type, no dressing or croutons)	1 salad (~11½ oz)	1 carbohydrate + 4 lean proteins
Pizza		
cheese, pepperoni, or sausage, regular or thick crust	⅛ of a 14-in. pizza (~4 oz)	2½ carbohydrates + 1 high-fat protein + 1 fat
cheese, pepperoni, or sausage, thin crust	⅛ of a 14-in. pizza (~2¾ oz)	1½ carbohydrates + 1 high-fat protein + 1 fat
cheese, meat, and vegetable, regular crust	⅛ of a 14-in. pizza (~5 oz)	2½ carbohydrates + 2 high-fat proteins
ASIAN		
Beef/chicken/shrimp with vegetables in sauce	1 cup (~6 oz)	1 carbohydrate + 2 lean proteins + 1 fat
Egg roll, meat	1 egg roll (~3 oz)	1½ carbohydrates + 1 lean protein + 1½ fats
Fried rice, meatless	1 cup	2½ carbohydrates + 2 fats
Fortune cookie	1	½ carbohydrate
Hot-and-sour soup	1 cup	½ carbohydrate + ½ fat
Meat with sweet sauce	1 cup (~6 oz)	3½ carbohydrates + 3 medium-fat proteins + 3 fats
Noodles and vegetables in sauce (chow mein, lo mein)	1 cup	2 carbohydrates + 2 fats
MEXICAN		
Burrito with beans and cheese	1 small (~6 oz)	3½ carbohydrates + 1 medium-fat protein + 1 fat
Nachos with cheese	1 small order (~8)	2½ carbohydrates + 1 high-fat protein + 2 fats
Quesadilla, cheese only	1 small order (~5 oz)	2½ carbohydrates + 3 high-fat proteins
Taco, crisp, with meat and cheese	1 small (~3 oz)	1 carbohydrate + 1 medium-fat protein + ½ fat
Taco salad with chicken and tortilla bowl	1 salad (1 lb including bowl)	3½ carbohydrates + 4 medium-fat proteins + 3 fats
Tostada with beans and cheese	1 small (~5 oz)	2 carbohydrates + 1 high-fat protein
SANDWICHES		
Breakfast sandwiches		

(Continued)

TABLE C-11 Fast Foods *(continued)*

FOOD	SERVING SIZE	CHOICES PER SERVING
⑤ breakfast burrito with sausage, egg, cheese	1 (~4 oz)	1½ carbohydrates + 2 high-fat proteins
⑤ egg, cheese, meat on an English muffin	1	2 carbohydrates + 3 medium-fat proteins + ½ fat
⑤ egg, cheese, meat on a biscuit	1	2 carbohydrates + 3 medium-fat proteins + 2 fats
⑤ sausage biscuit sandwich	1	2 carbohydrates + 1 high-fat protein + 4 fats
Chicken sandwiches		
⑤ grilled with bun, lettuce, tomatoes, spread	1 (~7½ oz)	3 carbohydrates + 4 lean proteins
⑤ crispy with bun, lettuce, tomatoes, spread	1 (~6 oz)	3 carbohydrates + 2 lean proteins + 3½ fats
Fish sandwich with tartar sauce and cheese	1 (5 oz)	2½ carbohydrates + 2 medium-fat proteins + 1½ fats
Hamburger		
regular with bun and condiments (catsup, mustard, onion, pickle)	1 (~3½ oz)	2 carbohydrates + 1 medium-fat protein + 1 fat
⑤ 4 oz meat with cheese, bun, and condiments (catsup, mustard, onion, pickle)	1 (~8½ oz)	3 carbohydrates + 4 medium-fat proteins + 2½ fats
Hot dog with bun, plain	1 (~3½ oz)	1½ carbohydrates + 1 high-fat protein + 2 fats
Submarine sandwich (no cheese or sauce)		
⑤ <6 g fat	1 6-in. sub	3 carbohydrates + 2 lean proteins
⑤ regular	1 6-in. sub	3 carbohydrates + 2 lean proteins + 1 fat
⑤ Wrap, grilled chicken, vegetables, cheese, and spread	1 small (~4–5 oz)	2 carbohydrates + 2 lean proteins + 1½ fats
SIDES/APPETIZERS		
⑤! French fries	1 small order (~3½ oz)	2½ carbohydrates + 2 fats
	1 medium order (~5 oz)	3½ carbohydrates + 3 fats
	1 large order (~6 oz)	4½ carbohydrates + 4 fats
⑤ Hash browns	1 cup/medium order (~5 oz)	3 carbohydrates + 6 fats
⑤ Onion rings	1 serving (8–9 rings, ~4 oz)	3½ carbohydrates + 4 fats
Salad, side (no dressing, croutons, or cheese)	1 small	1 nonstarchy vegetable
BEVERAGES AND DESSERTS		
Coffee, latte (fat-free milk)	1 small (~12 oz)	1 fat-free milk
Coffee, mocha (fat-free milk, no whipped cream)	1 small (~12 oz)	1 fat-free milk + 1 carbohydrate
Milkshake, any flavor	1 small (~12 oz)	5½ carbohydrates + 3 fats
	1 medium (~16 oz)	7 carbohydrates + 4 fats
	1 large (~22 oz)	10 carbohydrates + 5 fats
Soft-serve ice cream cone	1 small	2 carbohydrates + ½ fat

^aDefinition and weight refer to food **with** bone, skin, and breading.

^bDefinition refers to food **without** bone, skin, and breading.

KEY

✓ = Good source of fiber: >3 g/serving

! = Extra fat: +5 grams fat

⑤ = High in sodium: ≥600 mg/serving for main dishes/meals and ≥480 mg/serving for side dishes

appendix C

TABLE C-12 Alcohol

Note: For those who choose to drink alcohol, guidelines suggest limiting alcohol intake to 1 drink or less per day for women, and 2 drinks or less per day for men. To reduce the risk of low blood glucose (hypoglycemia), especially when taking insulin or a diabetes pill that increases insulin, alcohol should always be consumed with food. While alcohol, by itself, does not directly affect blood glucose, be aware of the carbohydrate (for example, in mixed drinks, beer, and wine) that may raise blood glucose.

1 alcohol equivalent = variable grams carbohydrate, 0 grams protein, 0 grams fat, and 100 kcalories.

Alcoholic Beverage[a]	Serving Size	Choices per Serving
Beer		
light (<4.5% abv)	12 fl oz	1 alcohol equivalent + ½ carbohydrate
regular (~5% abv)	12 fl oz	1 alcohol equivalent + 1 carbohydrate
dark (>5.7% abv)	12 fl oz	1 alcohol equivalent + 1–1½ carbohydrates
Distilled spirits (80 or 86 proof): vodka, rum, gin, whiskey, tequila	1½ fl oz	1 alcohol equivalent
Liqueur, coffee (53 proof)	1 fl oz	½ alcohol equivalent + 1 carbohydrate
Sake	1 fl oz	½ alcohol equivalent
Wine		
champagne/sparkling	5 fl oz	1 alcohol equivalent
dessert (sherry)	3½ fl oz	1 alcohol equivalent + 1 carbohydrate
dry, red or white (10% abv)	5 fl oz	1 alcohol equivalent

[a]"%abv" refers to the percentage of alcohol by volume.

The Food Lists are the basis of a meal planning system designed by a committee of the American Diabetes Association and the Academy of Nutrition and Dietetics. While originally designed for people with diabetes and others who must follow special diets, the Food Lists are based on principles of good nutrition that apply to everyone. (c) 2014 by the American Diabetes Association and the Academy of Nutrition and Dietetics.

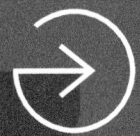
Physical Activity and Energy Requirements

Chapter 6 described how to calculate your estimated energy requirements by using an equation that accounts for your gender, age, weight, height, and physical activity level. This appendix presents tables that provide a shortcut to estimating total energy requirements, as developed by the Dietary Guidelines for Americans, and based on the equations of the Committee on Dietary Reference Intakes.

Table D-1 describes activity levels for three groups of people: sedentary, moderately active, or active. Once you have found an activity level that approximates your own, find your daily kcalorie need in Table D-2.

CONTENTS

TABLE D-1 Sedentary, Moderately Active, and Active People

Sedentary	A lifestyle that includes only the light physical activity associated with typical day-to-day life.
Moderately active	A lifestyle that includes physical activity equivalent to walking about 1.5 to 3 miles per day at 3 to 4 miles per hour in addition to the light physical activity associated with typical day-to-day life.
Active	A lifestyle that includes physical activity equivalent to walking more than 3 miles per day at 3 to 4 miles per hour in addition to the light physical activity associated with typical day-to-day life.

TABLE D-2 Estimated kCalorie Needs per Day by Age, Gender, and Physical Activity Level (Detailed)

Estimated amounts of kcalories needed to maintain kcalorie balance for various gender and age groups at three different levels of physical activity. The estimates are rounded to the nearest 200 kcalories. An individual's kcalorie needs may be higher or lower than these average estimates.[a]

	GENDER/ACTIVITY LEVEL					
AGE (YEARS)	MALE/ SEDENTARY	MALE/ MODERATELY ACTIVE	MALE/ACTIVE	FEMALE[b]/ SEDENTARY	FEMALE[b]/ MODERATELY ACTIVE	FEMALE[b]/ ACTIVE
2	1000	1000	1000	1000	1000	1000
3	1000	1200	1400	1000	1200	1400
4	1200	1400	1600	1200	1400	1400
5	1200	1400	1600	1200	1400	1600
6	1400	1600	1800	1200	1400	1600
7	1400	1600	1800	1200	1600	1800
8	1400	1600	2000	1400	1600	1800
9	1600	1800	2000	1400	1600	1800
10	1600	1800	2200	1400	1800	2000
11	1800	2000	2200	1600	1800	2000

(Continued)

appendix D

| TABLE D-2 | Estimated kCalorie Needs per Day by Age, Gender, and Physical Activity Level (Detailed) *(continued)* |

| | GENDER/ACTIVITY LEVEL | | | | | |
AGE (YEARS)	MALE/ SEDENTARY	MALE/ MODERATELY ACTIVE	MALE/ACTIVE	FEMALE[b]/ SEDENTARY	FEMALE[b]/ MODERATELY ACTIVE	FEMALE[b]/ ACTIVE
12	1800	2200	2400	1600	2000	2200
13	2000	2200	2600	1600	2000	2200
14	2000	2400	2800	1800	2000	2400
15	2200	2600	3000	1800	2000	2400
16–18	2400	2800	3200	1800	2000	2400
19–20	2600	2800	3000	2000	2200	2400
21–25	2400	2800	3000	2000	2200	2400
26–30	2400	2600	3000	1800	2000	2400
31–35	2400	2600	3000	1800	2000	2200
36–40	2400	2600	2800	1800	2000	2200
41–45	2200	2600	2800	1800	2000	2200
46–50	2200	2400	2800	1800	2000	2200
51–55	2200	2400	2800	1600	1800	2200
56–60	2200	2400	2600	1600	1800	2200
61–65	2000	2400	2600	1600	1800	2000
66–75	2000	2200	2600	1600	1800	2000
76+	2000	2200	2400	1600	1800	2000

[a]Based on Estimated Energy Requirements (EER) equations, using reference heights (average) and reference weights (healthy) for each age-gender group. For children and adolescents, reference height and weight vary. For adults the reference man is 5 feet 10 inches tall and weighs 154 pounds. The reference woman is 5 feet 4 inches tall and weighs 126 pounds. EER equations are from the Institute of Medicine. *Dietary Reference Intakes for Energy, Carbohydrate, Fiber, Fat, Fatty Acids, Cholesterol, Protein, and Amino Acids.* Washington, D.C.: The National Academies Press, 2002.

[b]Estimates for females do not include women who are pregnant or breastfeeding.

Source: U.S. Department of Health and Human Services and U.S. Department of Agriculture, *2015–2020 Dietary Guidelines for Americans*, 8th ed. (2015), health.gov/dietaryguidelines/2015/guidelines.

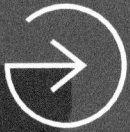
Chapter 13 describes data from nutrition assessments that allow health professionals to evaluate their patients' nutrition status and nutritional needs. This appendix provides additional information that may be useful for complete assessments.

E.1 Weight Gain during Pregnancy

Chapter 10 describes desirable weight-gain patterns during pregnancy. Figure E-1 shows prenatal weight-gain grids, which are used to plot the rate of weight gain during pregnancy.

CONTENTS

Weight Gain during Pregnancy
Growth Charts
Measures of Body Fat and Lean Tissue
Nutritional Anemias
Cautions about Nutrition Assessment

FIGURE E-1   Recommended Prenatal Weight Gain Based on Prepregnancy Weight

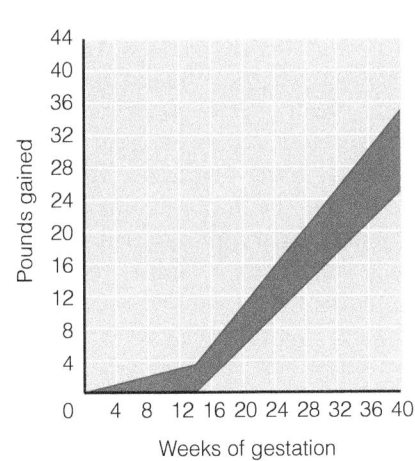

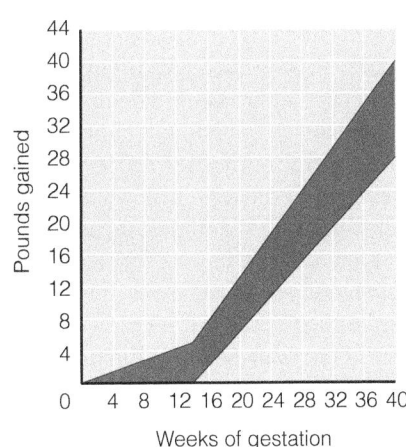

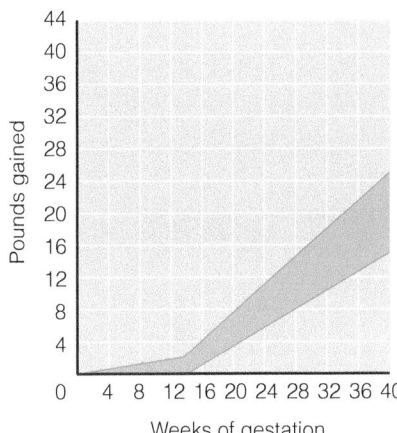

Normal-weight women should gain about 3¹/₂ pounds in the first trimester and just under 1 pound/week thereafter, achieving a total gain of 25 to 35 pounds by term.

Underweight women should gain about 5 pounds in the first trimester and just over 1 pound/week thereafter, achieving a total gain of 28 to 40 pounds by term.

Overweight women should gain about 2 pounds in the first trimester and ²/₃ pound/week thereafter, achieving a total gain of 15 to 25 pounds.

E.2 Growth Charts

Health professionals evaluate physical development by monitoring children's growth rates and comparing these rates with those on standard growth charts. Standard charts compare length or height to age, weight to age, weight to length, head circumference to age, and body mass index (BMI) to age (see Box E-1). Although individual growth patterns vary, a child's growth curve will generally stay at about the same percentile throughout childhood. In children whose growth has been impaired, nutrition rehabilitation will ideally allow height and weight to increase to higher percentiles. In overweight children, the goal is for weight to remain stable as height increases, until weight becomes appropriate for height.

BOX E-1

The *body mass index (BMI)* is a measure of body size, determined by dividing a person's weight by the square of their height:

$$BMI = \frac{Weight\ (kg)}{Height\ (m)^2}$$

appendix E

How to Determine a Child's Weight Percentile

- Select the appropriate chart based on age and sex.
- Locate the child's age along the horizontal axis on the bottom of the chart.
- Locate the child's weight in pounds or kilograms along the vertical axis.
- Mark the chart where the age and weight lines intersect, and read off the percentile.

BOX E-3

Common sites for skinfold measures:

- Triceps
- Biceps
- Subscapular (below shoulder blade)
- Suprailiac (above hip bone)
- Abdomen
- Upper thigh

To evaluate growth in infants, the assessor uses a chart such as those in Figures E-2 through E-5 (pp. E-3 to E-6). For example, the assessor follows the steps in Box E-2 to determine the weight percentile. For other measures, the assessor follows a similar procedure using the appropriate chart. (When length is measured, use the chart for birth to 36 months; when height is measured, use the chart for 2 to 20 years.) Ideally, the height, weight, and head circumference should be in roughly the same percentile.

Head circumference is generally measured in children who are under two years of age. Because the brain grows rapidly before birth and during early infancy, extreme and chronic malnutrition during these periods can impair brain development, curtailing the number of brain cells and reducing head circumference. Nonnutritional factors, such as certain disorders and genetic variation, can also influence head circumference.

E.3 Measures of Body Fat and Lean Tissue

Significant weight changes in both children and adults can reflect overnutrition or undernutrition with respect to energy and protein. To estimate the degree to which fat stores or lean tissues are affected by malnutrition, several anthropometric measurements are useful.

Skinfold Measures Skinfold measures provide a good estimate of total body fat and a fair assessment of the fat's location (see Box E-3). Most body fat lies directly beneath the skin, and the thickness of this subcutaneous fat correlates with total body fat. In some parts of the body, such as the back of the arm over the triceps muscle, this fat is loosely attached. As illustrated in Figure E-6, an assessor can measure the thickness of the fat with calipers that apply a fixed amount of pressure. If a person gains body fat, the skinfold increases proportionally; if the person loses fat, it decreases. Measurements taken from central-body sites reflect changes in fatness better than those taken from upper sites (arm and back). Because subcutaneous fat may be thicker in one area than in another, skinfold measurements are often taken at three or four different places on the body (including upper-, central-, and lower-body sites); the sum of these measures is then compared to standard values. In some situations, the triceps skinfold measurement alone may be used because it is easily accessible. Triceps skinfold measures greater than 15 millimeters in men or 25 millimeters in women suggest excessive body fat.

Waist Circumference Chapter 6 explains how fat distribution correlates with health risks and mentions that the waist circumference is a valuable indicator of abdominal fat. To measure waist circumference, the assessor places a nonstretchable tape around the person's body, crossing just above the upper hip bones and making sure that the tape remains on a level horizontal plane on all sides (see Figure E-7). The tape is tightened slightly, but without compressing the skin.

Waist-to-Hip Ratio The waist-to-hip ratio assesses abdominal obesity but offers no advantage over the waist circumference alone. To calculate the waist-to-hip ratio, divide the waist measurement by the hip measurement (in a woman with a 28-inch waist and 38-inch hips, the waist-to-hip ratio would be 28 ÷ 38 = 0.74). In general, women and men with waist-to-hip ratios above 0.8 and 0.9, respectively, are at increased risk of developing diabetes and cardiovascular diseases.

Waist-to-Height Ratio The waist-to-height ratio helps to assess the health risks associated with excessive abdominal fat. To calculate the waist-to-height ratio, divide the waist measurement by the height measurement (in a woman with a 28-inch waist who is 63 inches tall, the waist-to-height ratio would be 28 ÷ 63 = 0.44). Women and men with waist-to-height ratios above 0.5 may be at increased risk of developing diabetes and cardiovascular diseases.

FIGURE E-2 Length-for-Age and Weight-for-Age Percentiles

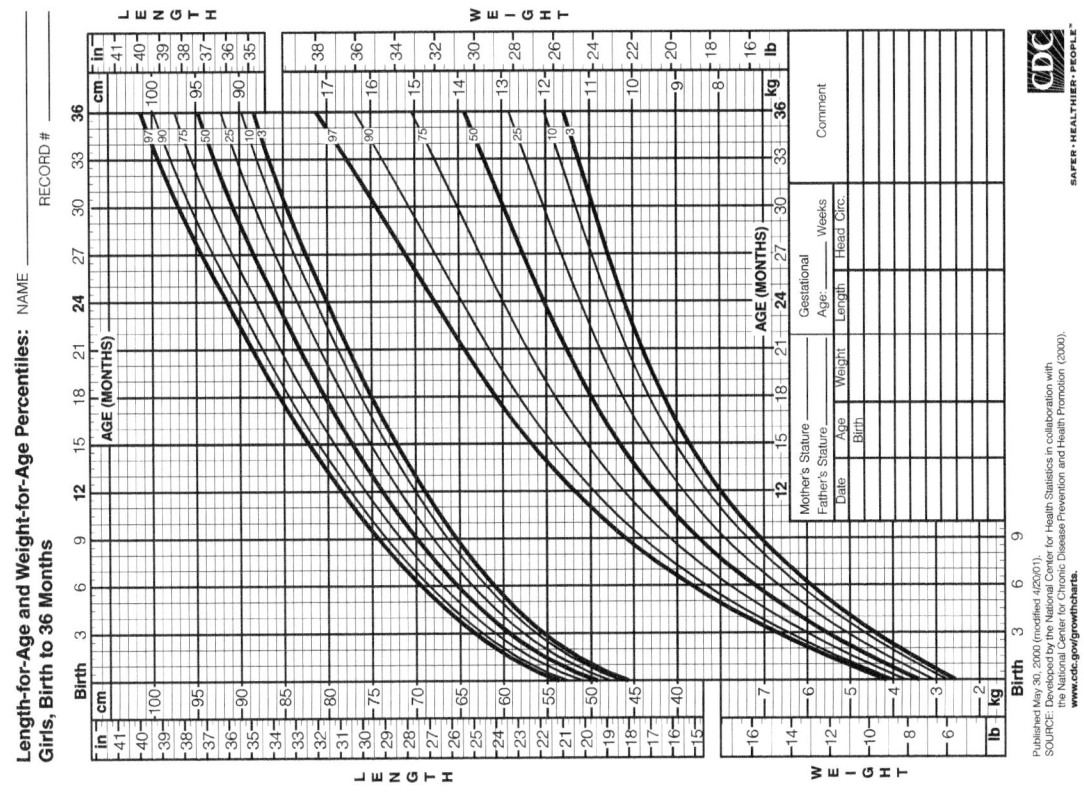

Length-for-Age and Weight-for-Age Percentiles: Girls, Birth to 36 Months

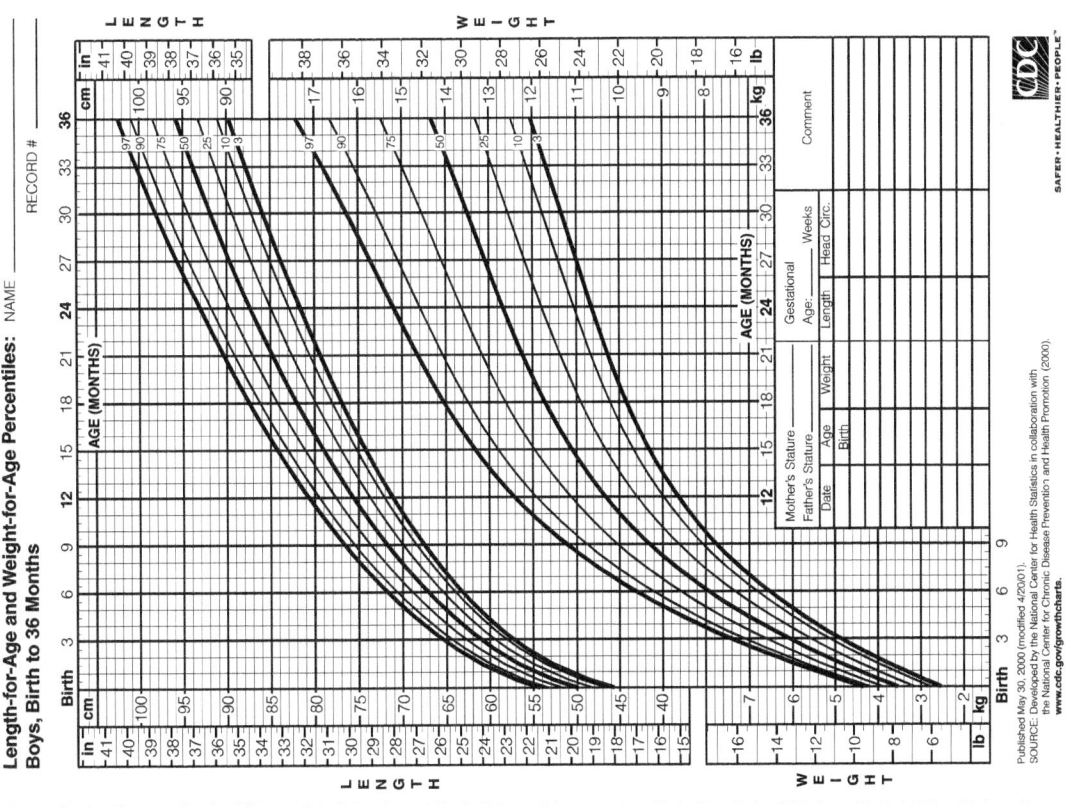

Length-for-Age and Weight-for-Age Percentiles: Boys, Birth to 36 Months

FIGURE E-3 Head Circumference-for-Age and Weight-for-Length Percentiles

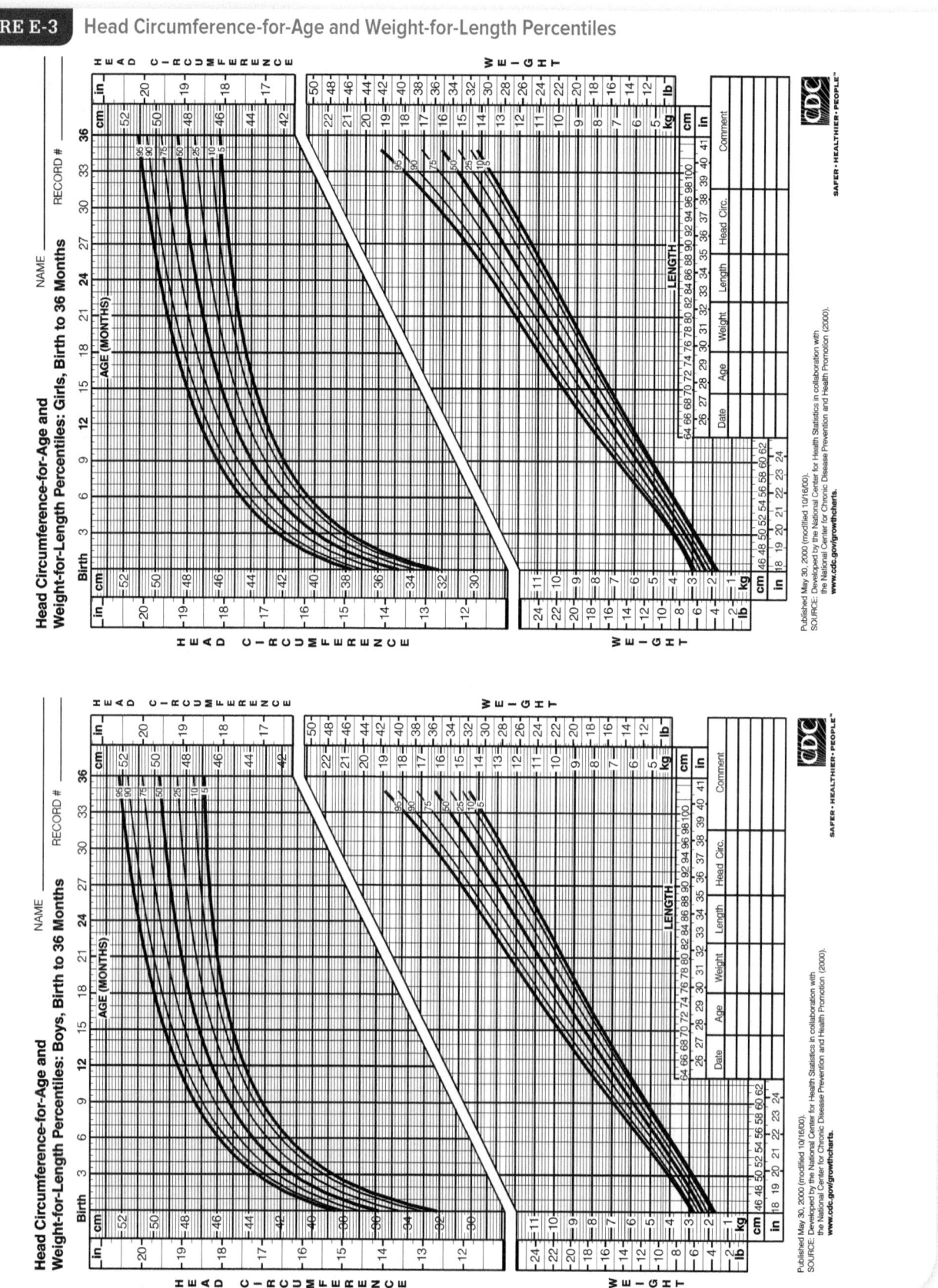

FIGURE E-4 Stature-for-Age and Weight-for-Age Percentiles

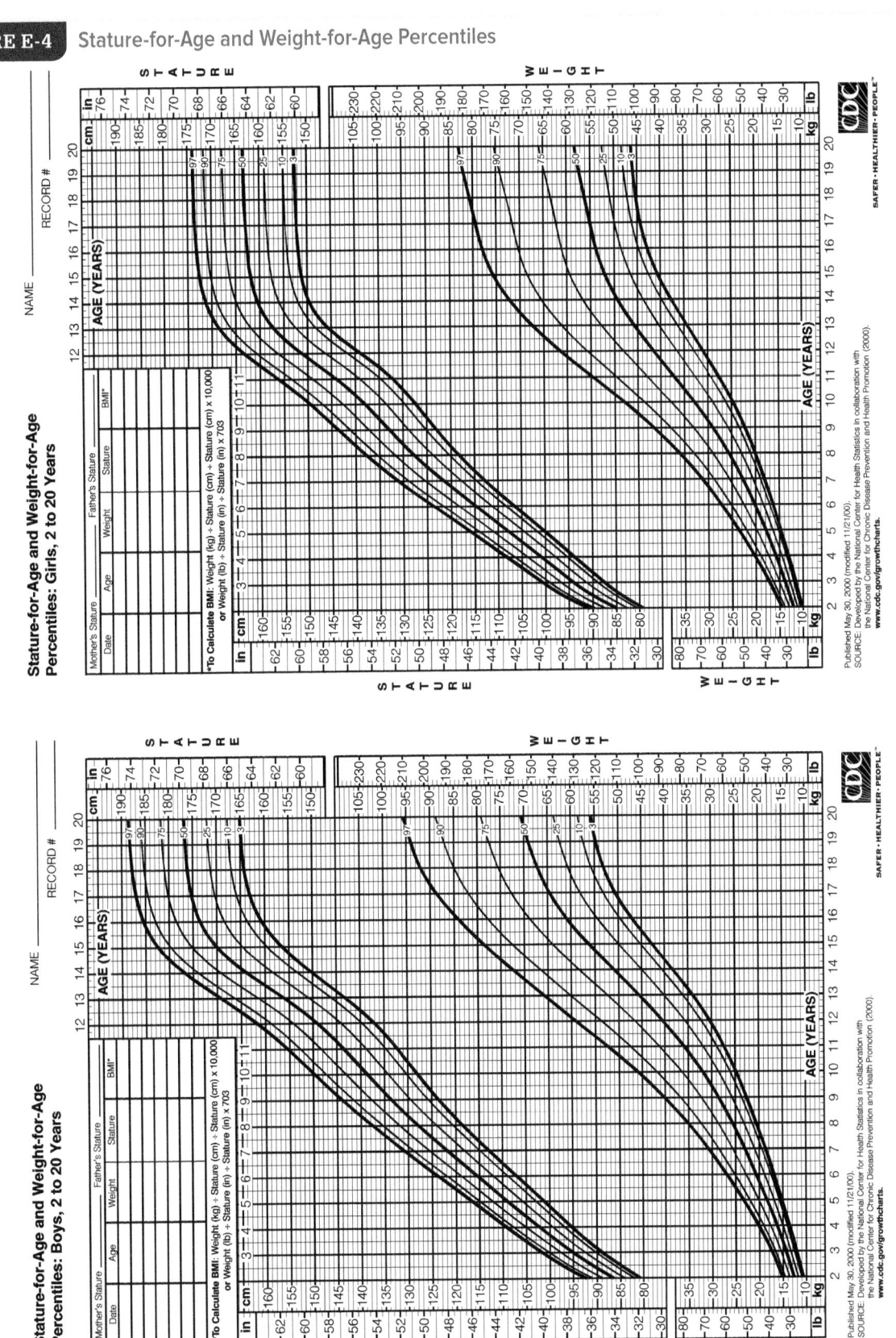

FIGURE E-5 Body Mass Index-for-Age Percentiles

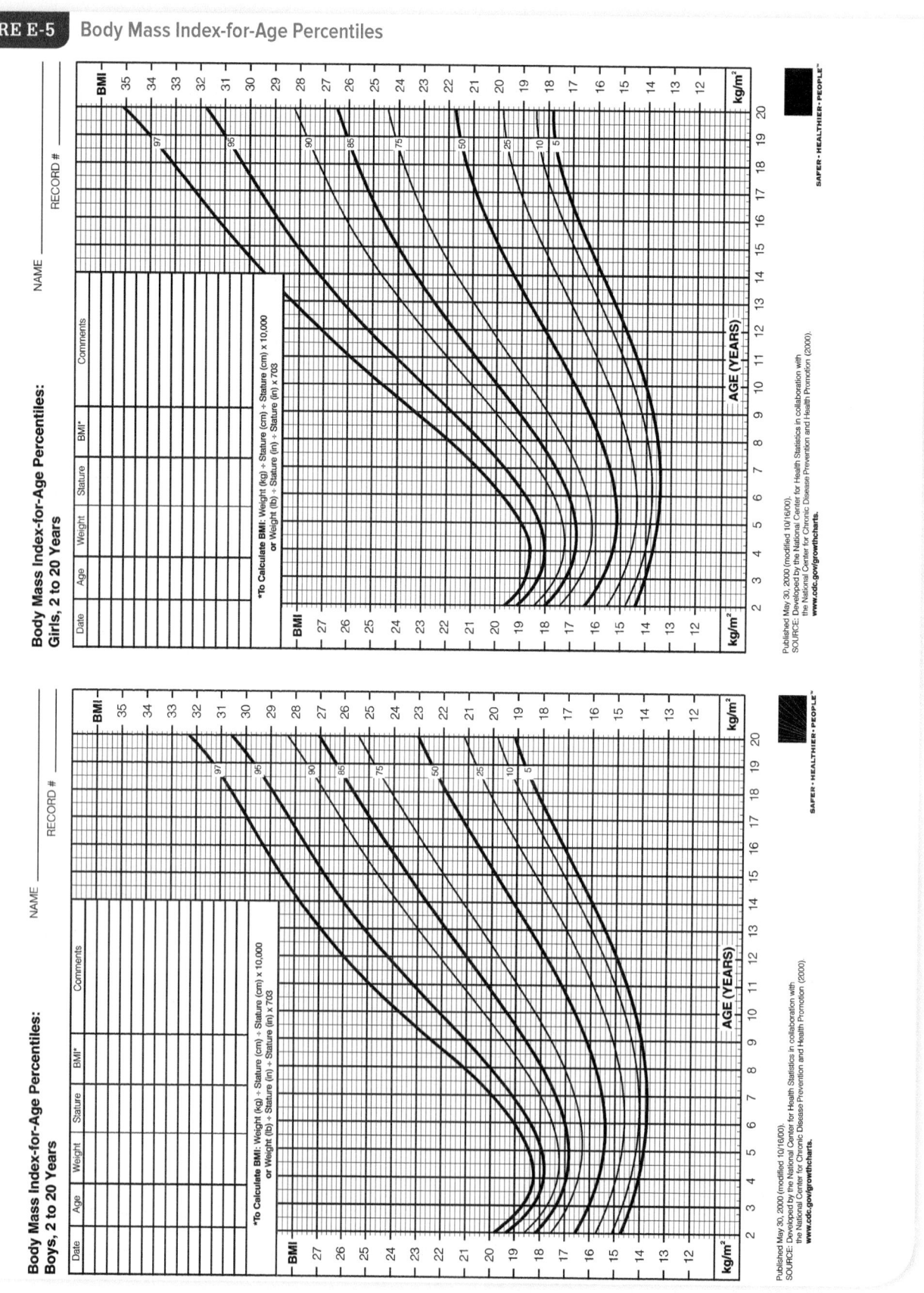

Body Mass Index-for-Age Percentiles:
Girls, 2 to 20 Years

Body Mass Index-for-Age Percentiles:
Boys, 2 to 20 Years

FIGURE E-6 How to Measure the Triceps Skinfold

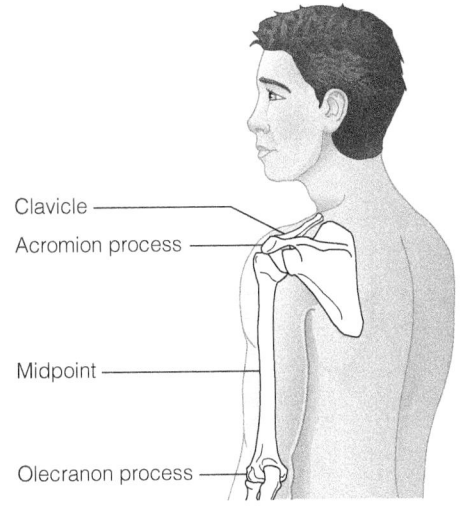
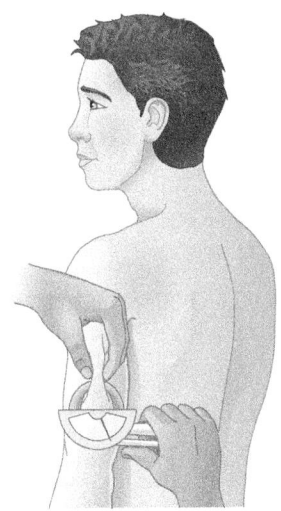

Clavicle

Acromion process

Midpoint

Olecranon process

A. Find the midpoint of the arm:
1. Ask the subject to bend his or her arm at the elbow and lay the hand across the stomach. (If he or she is right-handed, measure the left arm, and vice versa.)
2. Feel the shoulder to locate the acromion process. It helps to slide your fingers along the clavicle to find the acromion process. The olecranon process is the tip of the elbow.
3. Place a measuring tape from the acromion process to the tip of the elbow.

Divide this measurement by 2 and mark the midpoint of the arm with a pen.
B. Measure the skinfold:
1. Ask the subject to let his or her arm hang loosely to the side.
2. Grasp a fold of skin and subcutaneous fat between the thumb and forefinger slightly above the midpoint mark. Gently pull the skin away from the underlying muscle. (This step takes a lot of practice. If you want to be sure you don't have muscle as well as fat, ask the subject to

contract and relax the muscle. You should be able to feel if you are pinching muscle.)
3. Place the calipers over the skinfold at the midpoint mark, and read the measurement to the nearest 1.0 millimeter in two to three seconds. (If using plastic calipers, align pressure lines, and read the measurement to the nearest 1.0 millimeter in two to three seconds.)
4. Repeat steps 2 and 3 twice more. Add the three readings, and then divide by 3 to find the average.

Hydrodensitometry To estimate body density using hydrodensitometry, the person is weighed twice—first on land and then again when submerged in water. Underwater weighing usually generates a good estimate of body fat and is useful in research, although the technique has drawbacks: it requires bulky, expensive, and nonportable equipment. Furthermore, submerging some people in water (especially those who are very young, very old, ill, or fearful) is difficult and not well tolerated.

Bioelectrical Impedance To measure body fat using the bioelectrical impedance method, a very low-intensity electrical current is briefly sent through the body by way of electrodes placed on the wrist and ankle. Fat impedes the flow of electricity; thus, the magnitude of the current is influenced by the body-fat content. Recent food intake and hydration status can influence results. As with other anthropometric methods, bioelectrical impedance requires standardized procedures and calibrated instruments.

FIGURE E-7 How to Measure Waist Circumference

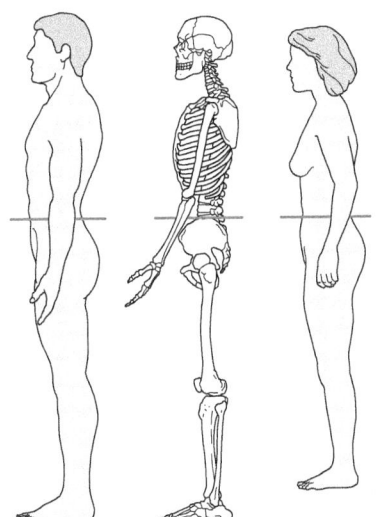

Place the measuring tape around the waist just above the bony crest of the hip. The tape runs parallel to the floor and is snug (but does not compress the skin). The measurement is taken at the end of normal expiration.

Source: National Institutes of Health Obesity Education Initiative, *Clinical Guidelines on the Identification, Evaluation, and Treatment of Overweight and Obesity in Adults* (Washington, D.C.: U.S. Department of Health and Human Services, 1998), p. 59.

appendix E

TABLE E-1	Methods of Estimating Body Fat Content

Air-displacement plethysmography (Bod Pod®): Estimates body density by measuring the body's volume (density = mass/volume); the density value allows derivation of the body's fat and lean tissue contents

Bioelectrical impedance assay: Measures the magnitude of an electrical current passed through the body; electrical conductivity is higher in lean tissues than in fat tissue

Dual energy X-ray absorptiometry: Analyzes the change in X-rays after they contact body tissues; fat and lean tissue have different effects on X-rays, allowing quantification of these tissues

Hydrodensitometry: Estimates body density by comparing the body's weight on land and in water or by measuring the body's volume (density = mass/volume); the density value allows derivation of the body's fat and lean tissue contents

Isotope dilution—deuterated water: Measures total body water content by analyzing the dilution of heavy water (water with a heavy form of hydrogen) in body tissues; allows an estimate of lean tissue (and by difference, the body fat content)

Skinfold: Estimates subcutaneous fat in several regions of the body by using calipers to measure skinfold thicknesses

Ultrasound: Estimates subcutaneous fat in several regions of the body by using ultrasound to measure skinfold thicknesses

A number of other methods are sometimes used to estimate the body's content of body fat. Table E-1 describes common techniques often used in the clinical or research setting.

E.4 Nutritional Anemias

Anemia, which can result from a wide variety of medical problems, is characterized by a significant reduction in the blood's oxygen-carrying capacity. Iron, folate, and vitamin B$_{12}$ deficiencies—caused by inadequate intake, poor absorption, or abnormal metabolism of these nutrients—are the most common causes of the nutrition-related anemias. Some nonnutritional causes of anemia include massive blood loss, infection, hereditary blood disorders such as sickle-cell anemia, and chronic liver or kidney disease. Table E-2 lists laboratory tests that are useful for diagnosing or evaluating anemia.

Assessment of Iron Status

Chapter 9 describes the progression of iron deficiency in detail, as well as the roles of some of the proteins involved in iron metabolism. This section describes the various tests that assess iron status, and Table E-3 (p. E-10) provides acceptable values. Although other tests are more specific for detecting the early stages of iron deficiency, hemoglobin levels and hematocrit values are most often used to detect iron-deficiency anemia because they are inexpensive and easily measured.

Serum Ferritin In the initial stage of iron deficiency, iron stores diminish (see Box E-4).

BOX E-4

Iron deficiency progresses as follows:

1. Iron stores diminish
2. Transport iron decreases
3. Hemoglobin production falls

Serum Ferritin In the initial stage of iron deficiency, iron stores diminish (see Box E-4). Iron is stored in the protein ferritin, which is located in the liver, spleen, and bone marrow. Serum ferritin values provide a noninvasive estimate of iron stores because the ferritin levels in blood reflect the amounts present in tissues. Serum ferritin is not a reliable indicator of iron deficiency, however, because its concentrations are increased by infection, inflammation, alcohol consumption, and liver disease.

Serum Iron and Total Iron-Binding Capacity (TIBC) Early stages of iron deficiency are characterized by reduced levels of serum iron, which represent the amount of iron bound to transferrin, the iron transport protein. Total iron-binding capacity (TIBC) is a measure of the total amount of iron that the blood can carry; thus, it is an indirect

TABLE E-2 Laboratory Tests for Anemia

TEST OR TEST RESULT	WHAT IT REFLECTS
For Anemia (general)	
Hemoglobin (Hb)	Total amount of hemoglobin in the red blood cells (RBCs)
Hematocrit (Hct)	Percentage of RBCs in the total blood volume
Red blood cell (RBC) count	Number of RBCs
Mean corpuscular volume (MCV)	RBC size; helps to determine if anemia is microcytic (iron deficiency) or macrocytic (folate or vitamin B_{12} deficiency)
Mean corpuscular hemoglobin concentration (MCHC)	Hemoglobin concentration within the average RBC; helps to determine if anemia is hypochromic (iron deficiency) or normochromic (folate or vitamin B_{12} deficiency)
Bone marrow aspiration	The manufacture of blood cells in different developmental states
For Iron-Deficiency Anemia	
↓ Serum ferritin	Early deficiency state with depleted iron stores
↓ Transferrin saturation	Progressing deficiency state with diminished transport iron
↓ Erythrocyte protoporphyrin	Later deficiency state with limited hemoglobin product
For Folate-Deficiency Anemia	
↓ Serum folate	Progressing deficiency state
↓ RBC folate	Later deficiency state
For Vitamin B_{12}–Deficiency Anemia	
↓ Serum vitamin B_{12}	Progressing deficiency state
↑ Serum methylmalonic acid	Vitamin B_{12} deficiency
Schilling test	Adequacy of vitamin B_{12} absorption

measure of the transferrin content of blood. During iron deficiency, the liver produces more transferrin in an effort to increase iron transport capacity, and therefore iron depletion is characterized by an increase in TIBC. TIBC reflects liver function as well as changes in iron metabolism.

Transferrin Saturation The percentage of transferrin that is saturated with iron is an indirect measure derived from the serum iron and total iron-binding capacity measures, as follows:

$$\% \text{ Transferrin saturation} = \frac{\text{serum iron}}{\text{total iron-binding capacity}} \times 100$$

During iron deficiency, transferrin saturation decreases. The transferrin saturation value is a useful indicator of iron status because it includes information about both the iron and transferrin content of the blood.

appendix E

TABLE E-3	Criteria for Assessing Iron Status

LABORATORY TEST	ACCEPTABLE VALUES	EFFECT OF IRON DEFICIENCY
Serum ferritin	Male: 20–250 ng/mL Female: 10–120 ng/mL	Lower than normal
Serum iron	Male: 60–175 µg/dL Female: 50–170 µg/dL	Lower than normal
Total iron-binding capacity	250–450 µg/dL	Higher than normal
Transferrin saturation	Male: 20–50% Female: 15–50%	Lower than normal
Erythrocyte protoporphyrin	<70 µg/dL red blood cells	Higher than normal
Hemoglobin (Hb), whole blood	Male: 13.5–17.5 g/dL Female: 12.0–16.0 g/dL	Lower than normal
Hematocrit (Hct)	Male: 39–49% Female: 35–45%	Lower than normal
Mean corpuscular volume (MCV)	80–100 fL	Lower than normal

Note: ng = nanogram; µg = microgram; dL = deciliter; fL = femtoliter
Source: L. Goldman and A. I. Schafer, eds., Goldman-Cecil Medicine (Philadelphia: Saunders, 2016).

Erythrocyte Protoporphyrin The iron-containing molecule in hemoglobin is heme, which is formed from iron and protoporphyrin. Protoporphyrin accumulates in the blood when iron supplies are inadequate for the formation of heme. However, levels of protoporphyrin may increase when hemoglobin synthesis is impaired for other reasons, such as lead poisoning or inflammation.

Hemoglobin When iron stores are depleted, hemoglobin production is impaired, and symptoms of anemia may eventually develop. Hemoglobin's usefulness in evaluating iron status is limited, however, because hemoglobin concentrations drop fairly late in the development of iron deficiency, and other nutrient deficiencies and medical conditions can also alter hemoglobin concentrations.

Hematocrit The hematocrit value reflects the percentage of the total blood volume occupied by red blood cells. To measure the hematocrit, a clinician spins the blood samples in a centrifuge to separate the red blood cells from the plasma. Low values indicate a reduced number or size of red blood cells. Although this test is not specific for iron status, it can help to detect the presence of iron-deficiency anemia.

Mean Corpuscular Volume (MCV) The hematocrit value divided by the red blood cell count provides a measure of the average size of a red blood cell, referred to as the mean corpuscular volume (MCV). This measure helps to classify the type of anemia that is present. In iron deficiency, the red blood cells are smaller than average (microcytic cells).

Assessment of Folate and Vitamin B_{12} Status

Folate deficiency and vitamin B_{12} deficiency present a similar clinical picture—an anemia characterized by abnormally large, misshapen, and immature red blood cells (megaloblastic cells). Distinguishing between folate and vitamin B_{12} deficiency is essential, however, because their treatments differ. Giving folate to a person with vitamin B_{12} deficiency can improve many of the test results indicative of vitamin B_{12} deficiency, but this would be a dangerous treatment because vitamin B_{12} deficiency causes nerve damage that folate cannot correct. Thus, inappropriate folate administration can mask vitamin B_{12}–deficiency anemia, and nerve damage could worsen. For this reason, it is critical to determine whether an anemia characterized by macrocytic cells results from a folate deficiency or from a vitamin B_{12} deficiency. Several of the following assessment measures can help in making this distinction.

Mean Corpuscular Volume (MCV) As previously mentioned, MCV is a measure of red blood cell size. In folate and vitamin B_{12} deficiencies, the red blood cells are larger than average, or macrocytic. Macrocytic cells are not necessarily indicative of nutrient deficiency, however, as they may also result from a high alcohol intake, liver disease, or various medications.

Serum Folate and Vitamin B_{12} Levels Analyses of serum folate and vitamin B_{12} levels are usually among the first tests conducted to determine the cause of macrocytic red blood cells. The presence of low serum levels of either nutrient is consistent with a deficiency of that nutrient, whereas adequate levels can help to rule out deficiency. Folate levels are not a specific measure of folate status, however, as they may increase after folate consumption and decrease because of alcohol consumption, pregnancy, or use of anticonvulsants. The folate level in red blood cells—called erythrocyte folate—correlates well with folate stores and can help in the diagnosis of folate deficiency, but this test is not available at all institutions. Table E-4 shows the acceptable values for tests used in assessing folate and vitamin B_{12} status.

Homocysteine and Methylmalonic Acid Levels To determine whether a nutrient deficiency is present, clinicians can measure the levels of substances that accumulate when the functions of that nutrient are impaired. For example, blood levels of the amino acid homocysteine are usually increased by both folate and vitamin B_{12} deficiency because both nutrients are needed for its metabolism. Methylmalonic acid, a breakdown product of several amino acids, requires vitamin B_{12} for its metabolism; hence, serum levels increase as a result of vitamin B_{12} deficiency. Because methylmalonic acid levels are not

TABLE E-4 Criteria for Assessing Folate and Vitamin B_{12} Status

LABORATORY TEST	ACCEPTABLE VALUES	EFFECT OF FOLATE OR VITAMIN B_{12} DEFICIENCY
Serum folate	2.6–12.2 ng/mL	Reduced in folate deficiency
Erythrocyte folate	103–411 ng/mL packed cells	Reduced in folate deficiency
Serum vitamin B_{12}	> 200 pg/mL	Reduced in vitamin B_{12} deficiency
Serum methylmalonic acid	70–270 nmol/L	Increased in vitamin B_{12} deficiency
Serum homocysteine	5–14 μmol/L	Increased in folate or vitamin B_{12} deficiency

Note: ng = nanogram; pg = picogram; nmol = nanomole; μmol = micromole

Sources: L. Goldman and A. I. Schafer, eds., *Goldman-Cecil Medicine* (Philadelphia: Saunders, 2016).

influenced by folate status, this measure is useful for distinguishing between folate and vitamin B_{12} deficiency.

Schilling Test As Chapter 8 explains, vitamin B_{12} deficiency most often results from malabsorption, not poor intake. The Schilling test can help to diagnose malabsorption of vitamin B_{12}: after the patient takes an oral dose of radioactive vitamin B_{12}, a urine test determines whether the vitamin B_{12} was absorbed. The Schilling test is rarely performed at present because it involves the administration of a radioactive reagent.

Antibodies to Intrinsic Factor The presence of serum antibodies to intrinsic factor can help to confirm a diagnosis of pernicious anemia, an autoimmune disease characterized by destruction of the cells that produce intrinsic factor (a protein required for vitamin B_{12} absorption; see Chapter 8). Serum antibodies to the parietal cells that produce and release intrinsic factor may also indicate pernicious anemia, but these antibodies may be present in various other conditions as well.

E.5 Cautions about Nutrition Assessment

The tests outlined in this appendix yield information that becomes meaningful only when they are conducted and interpreted by a skilled clinician. Potential sources of error may be introduced at any step, from the collection of samples to the analysis and reporting of data. Equipment must be regularly calibrated to ensure accuracy of measurements. In addition, the assessor must keep in mind that few tests may be specific to the nutrient of interest alone, and lab results may reflect physiological processes other than the ones being tested. Furthermore, because many tests are not sensitive enough to detect the early stages of deficiency, follow-up testing is often necessary to identify a nutrition problem.

appendix F

Enteral Formulas

The large number of enteral formulas available allows patients to meet a wide variety of medical needs. The first step in choosing a formula depends on the patient's ability to digest and absorb nutrients. Table F–1 lists examples of standard formulas for patients who have adequate gastrointestinal function, and Table F–2 provides examples of elemental formulas for patients with limited ability to digest or absorb nutrients. Each formula is listed only once, although a formula may have more than one use. A high-protein formula, for example, may also be a fiber-containing formula. Tables F–3 and F–4 list modules that can be used to prepare modular formulas or enhance enteral formulas.

The information shown in this appendix reflects the literature provided by manufacturers and does not suggest endorsement by the authors. Manufacturers frequently add new formulas, discontinue old ones, and change formula composition. Consult the manufacturers' literature and websites for updates and additional examples of enteral formulas.* The following products are listed in this appendix:

- Abbott Nutrition: Glucerna 1.0 Cal, Jevity 1.0 Cal, Jevity 1.5 Cal, Nepro with Carb Steady, Osmolite 1.0 Cal, Oxepa, Pivot 1.5 Cal, Polycose, Promote, Promote with Fiber, Pulmocare, Suplena with Carb Steady, Vital 1.0 Cal
- Nestlé Nutrition: Beneprotein, Compleat, Compleat Pediatric, Diabetisource AC, Fibersource HN, Glytrol, Impact, Impact Advanced Recovery, Impact Peptide 1.5, Isosource HN, MCT Oil, Microlipid, Novasource Renal, Nutren 1.0, Nutren 1.0 Fiber, Nutren 1.5, Nutren 2.0, Nutren Junior, Nutren Pulmonary, NutriHep, Peptamen, Peptamen Junior, Replete, Replete Fiber, Vivonex Pediatric, Vivonex T.E.N.

*Sources for the information in this appendix: Abbott Nutrition, www.abbottnutrition.com; Nestlé Nutrition, www.nestlehealthscience.us/brands.

TABLE F-1	Standard Formulas					
PRODUCT[a]	VOLUME TO MEET 100% RDI[b] (mL)	ENERGY (kcal/mL)	PROTEIN OR AMINO ACIDS (g/L)	CARBOHYDRATE (g/L)	FAT (g/L)	NOTES
General-Use Adult Formulas						
Compleat	1400	1.06	48	136	40	Blenderized formula, 8 g fiber/L
Nutren 1.0	1500	1.00	40	136	34	20% fat from MCT
Osmolite 1.0 Cal	1321	1.06	44	144	35	20% fat from MCT
Fiber-Enhanced Formulas						
Jevity 1.0 Cal	1321	1.06	44	155	35	14 g fiber/L
Nutren 1.0 Fiber	1500	1.00	40	148	34	15 g fiber/L
Promot with Fiber	1000	1.00	63	138	28	High in protein; 14 g fiber/L

(Continued)

TABLE F-1	Standard Formulas *(continued)*					
PRODUCT[a]	VOLUME TO MEET 100% RDI[b] (mL)	ENERGY (kcal/mL)	PROTEIN OR AMINO ACIDS (g/L)	CARBOHYDRATE (g/L)	FAT (g/L)	NOTES
High-kCalorie Formulas						
Jevity 1.5 Cal	1000	1.50	64	216	50	22 g fiber/L
Nutren 1.5	1000	1.50	68	176	60	20% fat from MCT
Nutren 2.0	750	2.00	84	216	92	50% fat from MCT
High-Protein Formulas						
Fibersource HN	1250	1.20	54	164	40	20% fat from MCT, 15 g fiber/L
Isosource HN	1250	1.20	54	156	40	20% fat from MCT, low fiber
Promote	1000	1.00	63	130	26	19% fat from MCT, low fiber
Specialized Formulas: Pediatric (1 to 13 Years)						
Compleat Pediatric	1–8 yr: 1000 mL; 9–13 yr: 1500 mL	1.00	38	136	38	Blenderized formula, 8 g fiber/L
Nutren Junior	1–8 yr: 1000 mL; 9–13 yr: 1500 mL	1.00	30	110	50	20% fat from MCT
Specialized Formulas: Glucose Intolerance						
Diabetisource AC	1250	1.20	60	100	59	33% kcal from carbohydrate, 15 g fiber/L
Glucerna 1.0 Cal	1420	1.00	42	96	54	34% kcal from carbohydrate, 14 g fiber/L
Glytrol	1500	1.00	45	100	48	40% kcal from carbohydrate, 15 g fiber/L
Specialized Formulas: Immune System Support						
Impact	1500	1.00	56	132	28	Enriched with arginine, nucleotides, and omega-3 fatty acids
Impact Advanced Recovery	Information unavailable	1.20	101	84	45	Same as above; very high protein (35% of kcals)
Impact Peptide 1.5	1000	1.50	94	140	64	Enriched with arginine, nucleotides, and omega-3 fatty acids

(Continued)

TABLE F-1	Standard Formulas *(continued)*

PRODUCT[a]	VOLUME TO MEET 100% RDI[b] (mL)	ENERGY (kcal/mL)	PROTEIN OR AMINO ACIDS (g/L)	CARBOHYDRATE (g/L)	FAT (g/L)	NOTES
Specialized Formulas: Chronic Kidney Disease (CKD)						
Nepro with Carb Steady	944	1.80	81	161	96	Low in potassium and phosphorus; to be used after dialysis has been instituted
Novasource Renal	1000	2.00	91	183	100	Low in electrolytes; to be used after dialysis has been instituted
Suplena with Carb Steady	1000	1.80	45	196	96	Low in protein, potassium, phosphorus, and calcium; for stage 3 and 4 CKD
Specialized Formulas: Respiratory Insufficiency						
Nutren Pulmonary	1000	1.50	68	100	95	57% kcal from fat, 40% fat from MCT
Oxepa	946	1.50	63	105	94	Enriched with omega-3 fatty acids and antioxidants; for mechanically ventilated patients
Pulmocare	947	1.50	63	106	93	55% kcal from fat, 20% fat from MCT, enriched with antioxidant nutrients
Specialized Formulas: Wound Healing						
Replete	1500	1.00	64	112	34	For patients recovering from surgery, burns, or pressure injuries
Replete Fiber	1500	1.00	64	124	34	Same as above; 15 g fiber/L

[a]All formulas listed are both gluten-free and suitable for patients with lactose intolerance.

[b]RDI = Reference Daily Intakes, which are labeling standards for vitamins, minerals, and protein. Consuming 100% of the RDI will meet the nutrient needs of most people using the product.

Note: MCT = medium-chain triglycerides

TABLE F-2   Elemental Formulas

PRODUCT[a]	VOLUME TO MEET 100% RDI[b] (mL)	ENERGY (kcal/mL)	PROTEIN OR AMINO ACIDS (g/L)	CARBOHYDRATE (g/L)	FAT (g/L)	NOTES
Specialized Elemental Formula: Hepatic Insufficiency						
NutriHep	1000	1.50	40	290	21	High in branched-chain amino acids and low in aromatic amino acids; 70% fat from MCT
Specialized Elemental Formula: Immune System Support						
Pivot 1.5 Cal	1000	1.50	94	172	51	High in protein; enriched with arginine, glutamine, omega-3 fatty acids, and antioxidants
Specialized Elemental Formulas: Malabsorption						
Peptamen	1500	1.00	40	128	39	70% fat from MCT
Vital 1.0 Cal	1422	1.00	40	130	38	Enhanced with prebiotics and antioxidants
Vivonex T.E.N.	2000	1.00	38	206	3	Powder form, 100% free amino acids, very low fat
Specialized Elemental Formulas: Pediatric (1 to 13 Years)						
Peptamen Junior	1–8 yr: 1000 mL; 9–13 yr: 1500 mL	1.00	30	136	38	60% fat from MCT
Vivonex Pediatric	1–8 yr: 1000 mL; 9–13 yr: 1500 mL	0.80	24	128	23	Powder form, 100% free amino acids

[a]All formulas listed are both gluten-free and suitable for patients with lactose intolerance.
[b]RDI = Reference Daily Intakes, which are labeling standards for vitamins, minerals, and protein. Consuming 100% of the RDI will meet the nutrient needs of most people using the product.

Note: MCT = medium-chain triglycerides

TABLE F-3   Protein and Carbohydrate Modules

PRODUCT	MAJOR INGREDIENT	ENERGY (kcal/g)	NUTRIENT CONTENT (g/100 g)
Beneprotein	Whey protein powder	3.6	86 g protein
Polycose	Hydrolyzed cornstarch (powder)	3.8	94 g carbohydrate

TABLE F-4   Fat Modules

PRODUCT	MAJOR INGREDIENT	ENERGY (kcal/mL)	FAT CONTENT (g/100 mL)
MCT Oil	Coconut and/or palm kernel oil	7.7	93
Microlipid	Safflower oil	4.5	50

Glossary

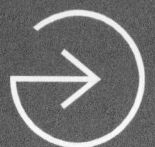

24-hour dietary recall: a record of foods consumed during the previous day or in the past 24 hours; sometimes modified to include foods consumed in a typical day.

2-in-1 solution: a parenteral solution that contains dextrose and amino acids, but excludes lipids.

abscesses (AB-sess-es)**:** accumulations of pus.

Academy of Nutrition and Dietetics: the professional organization of dietitians in the United States; formerly the Academy of Nutrition and Dietetics. The Canadian equivalent is Dietitians of Canada, which operates similarly.

Acceptable Daily Intake (ADI): the amount of a nonnutritive sweetener that individuals can safely consume each day over the course of a lifetime without adverse effect. It includes a 100-fold safety factor.

Acceptable Macronutrient Distribution Ranges (AMDR): ranges of intakes for the energy-yielding nutrients that provide adequate energy and nutrients and reduce the risk of chronic disease.

acetaldehyde (ah-set-AL-deh-hide)**:** an intermediate in alcohol metabolism that, in excess, can damage the body's tissues and interfere with cellular functions.

acetate (AH-seh-tate)**:** the product of alcohol metabolism that is used as a source of energy by many tissues in the body.

acetone breath: a distinctive fruity odor on the breath of a person with ketosis.

achalasia (ack-ah-LAY-zhah)**:** an esophageal disorder characterized by the absence of peristalsis and impaired relaxation of the lower esophageal sphincter.

achlorhydria (AY-clor-HIGH-dree-ah)**:** absence of gastric acid secretions.

acid regurgitation: the sensation of gastric contents backing up into the esophagus, possibly reaching the throat or mouth.

acid–base balance: the balance maintained between acid and base concentrations in the blood and body fluids.

acidosis: acid accumulation in body tissues; depresses the central nervous system and may lead to disorientation and, eventually, coma.

acids: compounds that release hydrogen ions in a solution.

acquired immunodeficiency syndrome (AIDS): the late stage of illness caused by infection with the human immunodeficiency virus (HIV); characterized by severe damage to immune function.

acupuncture (AK-you-PUNK-chur)**:** a therapy that involves inserting thin needles into the skin at specific anatomical points, allegedly to correct disruptions in the flow of energy within the body.

acute kidney injury: the rapid decline of kidney function over a period of hours or days; potentially a cause of acute renal failure.

acute respiratory distress syndrome (ARDS): respiratory failure triggered by severe lung injury; a medical emergency that causes dyspnea and pulmonary edema and usually requires mechanical ventilation.

acute-phase response: changes in body chemistry resulting from infection, inflammation, or injury; characterized by alterations in plasma proteins.

added sugars: sugars and other kcaloric sweeteners that are added to foods during processing or preparation or at the table. Added sugars do not include the naturally occurring sugars found in fruit and in milk products.

adequacy: the characteristic of a diet that provides all the essential nutrients, fiber, and energy necessary to maintain health and body weight.

Adequate Intakes (AI): a set of values that are used as guides for nutrient intakes when scientific evidence is insufficient to determine an RDA.

adipokines (AD-ih-poh-kynz)**:** protein hormones made and released by adipose tissue (fat) cells.

adiponectin (AH-dih-poe-NECK-tin)**:** a hormone produced by adipose cells that improves insulin sensitivity.

adipose tissue: the body's fat, which consists of masses of fat-storing cells called adipose cells.

adiposity-based chronic disease: a medical name for obesity. *Adiposity* refers to fat cells and tissues and identifies them as the source of the disease.

adolescence: the period of growth from the beginning of puberty until full maturity. Timing of adolescence varies from person to person.

advance health care directive: written or oral instructions regarding one's preferences for medical treatment to be used in the event of becoming incapacitated; also called an *advance medical directive* or a *living will*.

advanced glycation end products (AGEs): reactive compounds formed after glucose combines with protein; AGEs can damage tissues and lead to diabetic complications.

adverse reactions: unusual responses to food (including intolerances and allergies).

aerobic physical activity: activity in which the body's large muscles move in a rhythmic manner for a sustained period of time. Aerobic activity, also called *endurance activity*, improves cardiorespiratory fitness. Brisk walking, running, swimming, and bicycling are examples.

AIDS-defining illnesses: diseases and complications associated with the later stages of an HIV infection, including wasting, recurrent bacterial pneumonia, opportunistic infections, and certain cancers.

albuminuria: the presence of albumin (a blood protein) in the urine, a sign of diabetic nephropathy.

alcohol abuse: the continued use of alcohol despite the development of health, psychological, social, or legal problems; also known as *alcohol misuse* or *alcohol use disorder*.

alcoholic liver disease: liver disease that is related to excessive alcohol consumption. Disorders that may develop include fatty liver, hepatitis, and cirrhosis, which may lead to liver failure.

alcohol-related birth defects (ARBD): a condition caused by prenatal alcohol exposure that is diagnosed when there is a history of substantial, regular maternal alcohol intake or heavy episodic drinking and birth defects known to be associated with alcohol exposure.

alcohol-related neurodevelopmental disorder (ARND): a condition caused by prenatal alcohol exposure that is diagnosed when there is a confirmed history of substantial, regular maternal alcohol intake or heavy episodic drinking and behavioral, cognitive, or central nervous system abnormalities known to be associated with alcohol exposure.

aldosterone (al-DOS-ter-own): a hormone secreted by the adrenal glands that stimulates the reabsorption of sodium by the kidneys; also regulates chloride and potassium concentrations.

alkalosis: excessive base in the blood and body fluids.

alpha-lactalbumin (lact-AL-byoo-min): a major protein in human breast milk, as opposed to *casein* (CAY-seen), a major protein in cow's milk.

alveoli (al-VEE-oh-lee): air sacs in the lungs. One air sac is an *alveolus*.

Alzheimer's disease: a progressive, degenerative disease that attacks the brain and impairs thinking, behavior, and memory.

amenorrhea (ay-MEN-oh-RE-ah): the absence of or cessation of menstruation. Primary amenorrhea is menarche delayed beyond 16 years of age. Secondary amenorrhea is the absence of three to six consecutive menstrual cycles.

amino acids: building blocks of protein. Each contains an amino group, an acid group, a hydrogen atom, and a distinctive side group, all attached to a central carbon atom.

amniotic (am-nee-OTT-ic) **sac:** the "bag of waters" in the uterus in which the fetus floats.

amylase (AM-uh-lace): an enzyme that splits amylose (a form of starch).

anaphylactic (AN-ah-feh-LAC-tic) **shock:** a life-threatening whole-body allergic reaction to an offending substance.

anencephaly (AN-en-SEF-a-lee): an uncommon and always fatal type of neural tube defect; characterized by the absence of a brain.

aneurysm (AN-you-rih-zum): an abnormal enlargement or bulging of a blood vessel (usually an artery) caused by weakness in the blood vessel wall.

angina (an-JYE-nah or AN-ji-nah) **pectoris:** a condition caused by ischemia in the heart muscle that results in discomfort or dull pain in the chest region. The pain often radiates to the left shoulder, arms, neck, back, or jaw.

anorexia nervosa: an eating disorder characterized by restriction of energy intake relative to requirements, leading to a significantly low body weight, self-starvation to the extreme, and a disturbed perception of body weight and shape; seen (usually) in adolescent girls and young women.

anorexia: lack of appetite.

anthropometric (AN-throw-poe-MEH-trik): related to physical measurements of the human body, such as height, weight, body circumferences, and percentage of body fat.

antibodies: large proteins of the blood and body fluids, produced in response to invasion of the body by unfamiliar molecules (mostly proteins) called *antigens*. Antibodies inactivate the invaders and so protect the body.

anticonvulsants: drugs that treat epileptic seizures.

antidiuretic hormone (ADH): a hormone released by the pituitary gland in response to high salt concentrations in the blood. The kidneys respond by reabsorbing water. ADH elevates blood pressure and so is also called *vasopressin* (VAS-oh-PRES-in).

antiemetics: drugs that prevent vomiting.

antigens: substances that elicit the formation of antibodies or an inflammation reaction from the immune system. A bacterium,

a virus, a toxin, and a protein in food that causes allergy are all examples of antigens.

antineoplastic drugs: drugs that control or kill cancer cells.

antioxidant (anti-OX-ih-dant): a compound that protects other compounds from oxygen by itself reacting with oxygen. *Oxidation* is a potentially damaging effect of normal cell chemistry involving oxygen.

antioxidants: as a food additive, preservatives that delay or prevent rancidity of foods and other damage to food caused by oxygen.

antiretroviral drugs: drugs that treat retroviral infections, such as infection with human immunodeficiency virus (HIV).

anuria (ah-NOO-ree-ah): the absence of urine; often defined as a urine output that is less than about 50 to 75 mL/day.

anus (AY-nus): the terminal outlet of the GI tract.

appendix: a narrow blind sac extending from the beginning of the colon that stores lymph cells.

appetite: the psychological desire to eat; a learned motivation that is experienced as a pleasant sensation that accompanies the sight, smell, or thought of appealing foods.

aromatherapy: inhalation of oil extracts from plants to cure illness or enhance health.

aromatic amino acids: the amino acids phenylalanine, tyrosine, and tryptophan, which have carbon rings in their side groups.

artery: a vessel that carries blood away from the heart.

arthritis: inflammation of a joint, usually accompanied by pain, swelling, and structural changes.

artificial fats: zero-energy fat replacers that are chemically synthesized to mimic the sensory and cooking qualities of naturally occurring fats but are totally or partially resistant to digestion.

ascites (ah-SIGH-teez): an abnormal accumulation of fluid in the abdominal cavity.

ascorbic acid: one of the two active forms of vitamin C. Many people refer to vitamin C by this name.

-ase (ACE): a suffix denoting an enzyme. The root of the word often identifies the compound the enzyme works on.

aspiration: drawing in by suction or inhalation; a common complication of enteral feedings in which substances from the GI tract are drawn into the lungs. Aspiration risk is high in patients with esophageal disorders, neuromuscular diseases, and conditions that reduce consciousness or cause dementia.

aspiration pneumonia: pneumonia that results from the abnormal entry of foreign material; may be caused by either bacterial infection or irritation of the lower airways.

atherogenic: able to initiate or promote atherosclerosis.

atherosclerosis (ath-er-oh-scler-OH-sis): a type of artery disease characterized by accumulations of lipid-containing material on the inner walls of the arteries (see Chapter 21).

atrophic gastritis (a-TRO-fik gas-TRI-tis): chronic gastritis characterized by destruction of gastric mucosal tissue due to chronic inflammation; eventually the gastric epithelium may be replaced with another type of tissue.

autoimmune: refers to an immune response directed against the body's own tissues.

ayurveda: a traditional medical system from India that promotes the use of diet, herbs, meditation, massage, and yoga for preventing and treating illness.

bacterial overgrowth: excessive bacterial colonization of the stomach and small intestine; may be due to low gastric acidity, altered GI motility, mucosal damage, or contamination.

bacterial translocation: the migration of viable bacteria and/or bacterial products from the GI tract to normally sterile tissues such as the bloodstream, lymph nodes, or internal organs, potentially causing infection or tissue injury.

balance: the dietary characteristic of providing foods in proportion to one another and in proportion to the body's needs.

bariatric (BAH-ree-AH-trik) surgery: surgery that treats severe obesity.

Barrett's esophagus: a condition in which esophageal cells damaged by chronic exposure to stomach acid are replaced by cells that resemble those in the stomach or small intestine, sometimes becoming cancerous.

basal metabolic rate (BMR): the rate of energy use for metabolism under specified conditions: after a 12-hour fast and restful sleep, without any physical activity or emotional excitement, and in a comfortable setting. It is usually expressed as kcalories per kilogram of body weight per hour.

basal metabolism: the energy needed to maintain life when a person is at complete digestive, physical, and emotional rest. Basal metabolism is normally the largest part of a person's daily energy expenditure.

bases: compounds that accept hydrogen ions in a solution.

behavior-modification: the changing of behavior by the manipulation of *antecedents* (cues or environmental factors that trigger behavior), the behavior itself, and *consequences* (the penalties or rewards attached to behavior).

beneficence (be-NEF-eh-sense): the act of performing beneficial services rather than harmful ones.

beriberi: the thiamin-deficiency disease; characterized by loss of sensation in the hands and feet, muscular weakness, advancing paralysis, and abnormal heart action.

beta-carotene: a vitamin A precursor made by plants and stored in human fat tissue; an orange pigment.

BHA, BHT: preservatives commonly used to slow the development of "off" flavors, odors, and color changes caused by oxidation.

bicarbonate: an alkaline secretion of the pancreas; part of the pancreatic juice. (Bicarbonate also occurs widely in all cell fluids.)

bile: an emulsifier that prepares fats and oils for digestion; made by the liver, stored in the gallbladder, and released into the small intestine when needed.

binders: chemical compounds in foods that combine with nutrients (especially minerals) to form complexes the body cannot absorb. Examples include *phytates* and *oxalates*.

binge eating disorder: an eating disorder characterized by recurring episodes of eating a significant amount of food in a short period of time with marked feelings of lack of control.

bioactive food components: compounds in foods (either nutrients or phytochemicals) that alter physiological processes in the body.

bioavailability: the rate and extent to which a nutrient is absorbed and used.

bioelectrical or bioelectromagnetic therapies: therapies that involve the unconventional use of electric or magnetic fields to cure illness.

biofeedback training: instruction in techniques that allow individuals to gain voluntary control of certain physiological processes, such as skin temperature or brain wave activity, to help reduce stress and anxiety.

biofield therapies: healing methods based on the belief that illnesses can be cured by manipulating energy fields that purportedly surround and penetrate the body. Examples include *acupuncture, qi gong,* and *therapeutic touch.*

blastocyst (BLASS-toe-sist): the developmental stage of the zygote when it is about 5 days old and ready for implantation.

blenderized formulas: enteral formulas that are prepared by using a food blender to mix and puree whole foods.

blind loops: bypassed sections of small intestine that are cut off from the normal flow of food material, allowing bacteria to flourish; created in certain types of gastrectomy procedures.

bloating: the sensation of swelling in the abdominal area; often due the accumulation of stomach or intestinal gas or fluid.

body mass index (BMI): an index of a person's weight in relation to height; determined by dividing the weight (in kilograms) by the square of the height (in meters).

bolus (BOH-lus) feeding: feedings with delivery rates of about 250 to 500 milliliters of formula over a 5- to 15-minute period.

bolus (BOH-lus): the portion of food swallowed at one time.

Bowman's (BOE-minz) capsule: a cuplike component of the nephron that surrounds the glomerulus and collects the filtrate that is passed to the tubules.

branched-chain amino acids: the essential amino acids leucine, isoleucine, and valine, which have side groups with a branched structure.

bronchi (BRON-key), bronchioles (BRON-key-oles): the main airways of the lungs. The singular form of bronchi is *bronchus.*

brown sugar: refined white sugar with molasses added; 95 percent pure sucrose.

buffalo hump: the accumulation of fatty tissue at the base of the neck.

buffers: compounds that can reversibly combine with hydrogen ions to help keep a solution's acidity or alkalinity constant.

bulimia (byoo-LEM-ee-uh) nervosa: an eating disorder characterized by repeated episodes of binge eating combined with a fear of becoming fat, usually followed by self-induced vomiting, misuse of laxatives or diuretics, fasting, or excessive exercise.

built environment: the buildings, roads, utilities, homes, fixtures, parks, and all other manufactured entities that form the physical characteristics of a community.

calciferol (kal-SIF-er-ol): vitamin D.

calorie counts: estimates of food energy (and often, protein) consumed by patients for one or more days.

calories: a measure of *heat* energy. Food energy is measured in **kilocalories** (1000 calories equal 1 kilocalorie), abbreviated **kcalories** or kcal. One kcalorie is the amount of heat necessary to raise the temperature of 1 kilogram (kg) of water 1°C. The scientific use of the term *kcalorie* is the same as the popular use of the term *calorie.*

cancer cachexia (ka-KEK-see-ah): a wasting syndrome associated with cancer that is characterized by anorexia, muscle wasting, weight loss, and fatigue.

cancers: diseases characterized by the uncontrolled growth of a group of abnormal cells, which can destroy adjacent tissues and spread to other areas of the body via the lymph or blood.

candidiasis: a fungal infection on the mucous membranes of the oral cavity and elsewhere; usually caused by *Candida albicans.*

capillaries: small vessels that branch from an artery; connect arteries to veins. Oxygen, nutrients, and waste materials are exchanged across capillary walls.

carbohydrates: energy nutrients composed of monosaccharides.

carbohydrate-to-insulin ratio: the amount of carbohydrate that can be handled per unit of insulin; on average, every 15 grams of carbohydrate requires about 1 unit of rapid- or short-acting insulin.

carcinogenesis (CAR-sin-oh-JEN-eh-sis): the process of cancer development.

carcinogens (CAR-sin-oh-jenz or car-SIN-oh-jenz): substances that can cause cancer (the adjective is *carcinogenic*).

cardiac arrhythmias: abnormal heart rhythms.

cardiac cachexia: severe malnutrition that develops in heart failure patients; characterized by weight loss and tissue wasting.

cardiac output: the volume of blood pumped by the heart within a specified period of time.

cardiopulmonary resuscitation (CPR): life-sustaining treatment that supplies oxygen and restores a person's ability to breathe and pump blood.

cardiovascular disease (CVD): a general term for all diseases of the heart and blood vessels (see Chapter 21).

cariogenic (KAH-ree-oh-JEN-ik)**:** conducive to the development of dental caries.

cataracts: clouding of the eye lenses that impairs vision and can lead to blindness.

cathartics (ca-THART-ics)**:** strong laxatives.

catheter: a thin tube placed within a narrow lumen (such as a blood vessel) or body cavity; can be used to infuse or withdraw fluids or keep a passage open.

CDC (Centers for Disease Control and Prevention): a branch of the Department of Health and Human Services that is responsible for, among other things, identifying, monitoring, and reporting food-borne illnesses and outbreaks (www.cdc.gov).

celiac (SEE-lee-ack) **disease:** an immune disorder characterized by an abnormal immune response to wheat gluten and related proteins; also called *gluten-sensitive enteropathy* or *celiac sprue*.

central obesity: excess fat around the trunk of the body; also called *abdominal fat* or *upper-body fat*.

central veins: the large-diameter veins located close to the heart.

cerebral cortex: the outer surface of the cerebrum, which is the largest part of the brain.

Certified Diabetes Educator: a health care professional who specializes in diabetes management education; certification is obtained from the National Certification Board for Diabetes Educators.

cesarean (see-ZAIR-ee-un) **section:** surgical childbirth, in which the infant is taken through an incision in the woman's abdomen.

chemotherapy: the use of drugs to arrest or destroy cancer cells; these drugs are called *antineoplastic agents*.

chiropractic (KYE-roh-PRAK-tic)**:** a method of treatment based on the unproven theory that spinal manipulation can restore health.

- According to chiropractic theory, a *subluxation* is a misaligned vertebra or other spinal alteration that may cause illness.
- *Adjustment* is the manipulative therapy practiced by chiropractors.

choline: a nonessential nutrient that can be made in the body from an amino acid.

chromosomes: structures within the nucleus of a cell that contain the cell's DNA and associated proteins.

chronic bronchitis (bron-KYE-tis)**:** a lung disorder characterized by persistent inflammation and excessive secretions of mucus in the main airways of the lungs.

chronic diseases: diseases characterized by slow progression, long duration, and degeneration of body organs due in part to such personal lifestyle elements as poor food choices, smoking, alcohol use, and lack of physical activity.

chronic hypertension: in pregnant women, hypertension that is present and documented before pregnancy; in women whose prepregnancy blood pressure is unknown, the presence of sustained hypertension before 20 weeks of gestation.

chronic kidney disease: a condition characterized by the gradual, irreversible loss of kidney function resulting from long-term disease or injury; also called *chronic renal failure*.

chronic malnutrition: malnutrition caused by long-term food deprivation; characterized in children by short height for age (stunting).

chronic obstructive pulmonary disease (COPD): a group of lung diseases characterized by persistent obstructed airflow through the lungs and airways; includes chronic bronchitis and emphysema.

chronological age: a person's age in years from his or her date of birth.

chylomicrons (kye-lo-MY-crons)**:** the lipoproteins that transport lipids from the intestinal cells into the body. The cells of the body remove the lipids they need from the chylomicrons, leaving chylomicron remnants to be picked up by the liver cells.

chyme (KIME)**:** the semiliquid mass of partly digested food expelled by the stomach into the duodenum (the top portion of the small intestine).

cirrhosis (sih-ROE-sis)**:** an advanced stage of liver disease in which extensive scarring replaces healthy liver tissue, causing impaired liver function and liver failure.

claudication (CLAW-dih-KAY-shun)**:** pain in the legs while walking; usually due to an inadequate supply of blood to muscles.

clear liquid diet: a diet that consists of foods that are liquid at body temperature, require minimal digestion, and leave little residue (undigested material) in the colon.

clinical pathways: coordinated programs of treatment that merge the care plans of different health practitioners; also called *care pathways*, *care maps*, or *critical pathways*.

clinically severe obesity: a BMI of 40 or greater, or a BMI of 35 or greater with one or more serious conditions such as hypertension. Another term used to describe the same condition is *morbid obesity*.

closed feeding system: a formula delivery system in which the sterile formula is packaged in a container that can be attached directly to the feeding tube for administration.

coenzyme (co-EN-zime)**:** a small molecule that works with an enzyme to promote the enzyme's activity. Many coenzymes contain B vitamins as part of their structure.

cognitive behavioral therapy: psychological therapy aimed at changing undesirable behaviors by changing the underlying thought processes contributing to these behaviors. In anorexia nervosa, a goal is to replace false beliefs about body weight, eating, and self-worth with health-promoting beliefs.

cognitive skills: as taught in behavior therapy, changes to conscious thoughts with the goal of improving adherence to lifestyle modifications; examples are problem-solving skills or the correction of false-negative thoughts, termed *cognitive restructuring*.

colectomy: removal of a portion or all of the colon.

collagen: the characteristic protein of connective tissue.

collateral vessels: blood vessels that enlarge or newly form to allow an alternative pathway for diverted blood.

colostomy (co-LAH-stoe-me)**:** a surgical passage through the abdominal wall into the colon.

colostrum (co-LAHS-trum)**:** a milklike secretion from the breasts, present during the first few days after delivery before milk appears; rich in protective factors.

complement: a group of plasma proteins that assist the activities of antibodies and phagocytes.

complementary and alternative medicine (CAM): health care practices that have not been proved to be effective and consequently are not included as part of conventional treatment (see Nutrition in Practice 14).

complementary foods: nutrient- and energy-containing solid or semisolid foods (or liquids) fed to infants in addition to breast milk or infant formula.

complementary proteins: two or more proteins whose amino acid assortments complement each other in such a way that the essential amino acids missing from one are supplied by the other.

concentrated fruit juice sweetener: a concentrated sugar syrup made from dehydrated, deflavored fruit juice, commonly grape juice; used to sweeten products that can then claim to be "all fruit."

conditionally essential amino acid: an amino acid that is normally nonessential but must be supplied by the diet in special circumstances when the need for it becomes greater than the body's ability to produce it.

confectioners' sugar: finely powdered sucrose; 99.9 percent pure.

conjugated linoleic acid: a collective term for several fatty acids that have the same chemical formulas as linoleic acid but with different configurations.

continuous ambulatory peritoneal dialysis (CAPD): the most common method of peritoneal dialysis; involves frequent exchanges of dialysate, which remains in the peritoneal cavity throughout the day.

continuous feedings: feedings that are delivered slowly and at a constant rate over an 8- to 24-hour period.

continuous glucose monitoring: continuous monitoring of tissue glucose levels using a small sensor placed under the skin.

continuous parenteral nutrition: continuous administration of parenteral solutions over a 24-hour period.

continuous renal replacement therapy (CRRT): a slow, continuous method of removing solutes and/or fluids from the blood by gently pumping the blood across a filtration membrane over a prolonged time period.

corn sweeteners: corn syrup and sugar solutions derived from corn.

corn syrup: a syrup, mostly glucose, partly maltose, produced by the action of enzymes on cornstarch. It may be dried and used as *corn syrup solids*.

cornea (KOR-nee-uh): the hard, transparent membrane covering the outside of the eye.

coronary heart disease (CHD): a chronic, progressive disease characterized by obstructed blood flow in the coronary arteries; also called *coronary artery disease*.

C-reactive protein: an acute-phase protein produced in substantial amounts during acute inflammation; it binds dead or dying cells to activate certain immune responses. C-reactive protein is considered the best clinical indicator of the acute-phase response although it is elevated during many chronic illnesses.

creatinine: the waste product of creatine, a nitrogen-containing compound in muscle cells that supplies energy for muscle contraction.

cretinism (CREE-tin-ism): an iodine-deficiency disease characterized by mental and physical retardation.

critical period: a finite period during development in which certain events occur that will have irreversible effects on later developmental stages; usually a period of rapid cell division.

Crohn's disease: an inflammatory bowel disease that usually occurs in the lower portion of the small intestine and the colon; the inflammation may pervade the entire intestinal wall.

cross-contamination: the contamination of food by bacteria that occurs when the food comes into contact with surfaces previously touched by raw meat, poultry, or seafood.

cryptosporidiosis (KRIP-toe-spor-ih-dee-OH-sis): a foodborne illness caused by the parasite *Cryptosporidium parvum*.

cultural competence: an awareness and acceptance of one's own and others' cultures, combined with the skills needed to interact effectively with people of diverse cultures.

cyanosis (sigh-ah-NOH-sis): a bluish cast in the skin due to the color of deoxygenated hemoglobin. Cyanosis is most evident in individuals with lighter, thinner skin; it is mostly seen on lips, cheeks, and ears and under the nails.

cyclic feedings: continuous feedings conducted for 8 to 16 hours daily, allowing patient mobility and bowel rest during the remaining hours of the day.

cyclic parenteral nutrition: administration of parenteral solutions over an 8- to 14-hour period each day.

cystic fibrosis: a genetic disorder characterized by abnormal chloride and sodium levels in exocrine secretions; often leads to respiratory illness and pancreatic insufficiency.

cystinuria (SIS-tin-NOO-ree-ah): a genetic disorder characterized by the elevated urinary excretion of several amino acids, including cystine.

cytokines (SIGH-toe-kines): signaling proteins produced by the body's cells; the cytokines that promote inflammation and catabolism include tumor necrosis factor-α, interleukin-1, interleukin-6, and γ-interferon.

Daily Values: reference values developed by the FDA specifically for use on food labels.

dawn phenomenon: morning hyperglycemia that is caused by the early-morning release of growth hormone, which reduces insulin sensitivity.

debridement: the surgical removal of dead, damaged, or contaminated tissue resulting from burns or wounds; helps to prevent infection and hasten healing.

decision-making capacity: the ability to understand pertinent information and make appropriate decisions; known as *decision-making competency* within the legal system.

deep vein thrombosis: formation of a stationary blood clot (thrombus) in a deep vein, usually in the leg, which causes inflammation, pain, and swelling, and is potentially fatal.

defibrillation: life-sustaining treatment in which an electronic device is used to shock the heart and reestablish a pattern of normal contractions. Defibrillation is used when the heart has arrhythmias or has experienced arrest.

deficient: in regard to nutrient intake, describes the amount below which almost all healthy people can be expected, over time, to experience deficiency symptoms.

dehydration: the loss of water from the body that occurs when water output exceeds water input. The symptoms progress rapidly from thirst, to weakness, to exhaustion and delirium, and end in death if not corrected.

denaturation (dee-nay-cher-AY-shun): the change in a protein's shape brought about by heat, acid, or other agents. Past a certain point, denaturation is irreversible.

dental calculus: mineralized dental plaque, often associated with inflammation and progressive gum disease.

dental caries (KAH-reez): infectious disease of the teeth that causes the gradual decay and disintegration of tooth structures.

dental plaque (PLACK): a film of bacteria and bacterial by-products that accumulates on the tooth surface.

dermatitis herpetiformis (HER-peh-tih-FOR-mis): a gluten-sensitive disorder characterized by a severe skin rash.

dextrose, anhydrous dextrose: forms of glucose.

diabetes (DYE-ah-BEE-teez) **mellitus:** a group of metabolic disorders characterized by hyperglycemia and disordered insulin metabolism.

diabetic coma: a coma that occurs in uncontrolled diabetes; may be due to diabetic ketoacidosis, hyperosmolar hyperglycemic syndrome, or severe hypoglycemia. Diabetic coma was a frequent cause of death before insulin was routinely used to manage diabetes.

diabetic nephropathy (neh-FRAH-pah-thee): damage to the kidneys that results from long-term diabetes.

diabetic neuropathy (nur-RAH-pah-thee): nerve damage that results from long-term diabetes.

diabetic retinopathy (REH-tih-NAH-pah-thee): retinal damage that results from long-term diabetes.

dialysate (dye-AL-ih-sate): the solution used in dialysis to draw wastes and fluids from the blood.

dialysis (dye-AH-lih-sis): a treatment that removes wastes and excess fluid from the blood after the kidneys have stopped functioning.

dialyzer (DYE-ah-LYE-zer): a machine used in hemodialysis to filter the blood; also called an *artificial kidney.*

diet manual: a resource that specifies the foods or preparation methods to include in or exclude from modified diets and provides sample menus.

diet orders: specific instructions regarding dietary management; also called *diet prescriptions* or *nutrition prescriptions.*

diet progression: a change in diet as a patient's tolerances permit.

dietary antioxidants: compounds typically found in plant foods that significantly decrease the adverse effects of oxidation on living tissues. The major antioxidant vitamins are vitamin E, vitamin C, and beta-carotene.

dietary fibers: a general term denoting in plant foods the polysaccharides cellulose, hemicellulose, pectins, gums, and mucilages, as well as the nonpolysaccharide lignins, which are not digested by human digestive enzymes, although some are digested by GI tract bacteria.

dietary folate equivalents (DFE): the amount of folate available to the body from naturally occurring sources, fortified foods, and supplements, accounting for differences in bioavailability from each source.

Dietary Reference Intakes (DRI): a set of values for the dietary nutrient intakes of healthy people in the United States and Canada. These values are used for planning and assessing diets.

dietary supplements: products that are added to the diet and contain any of the following ingredients: a vitamin, a mineral, an herb or other botanical, an amino acid, a metabolite, a constituent, or an extract.

dietetic technicians: persons who have completed a minimum of an associate's degree from an accredited college or university and an approved dietetic technician program. A dietetic technician, registered (DTR) has also passed a national examination and maintains registration through continuing professional education.

dietetics: the application of nutrition principles to achieve and maintain optimal human health.

differentiation: the development of specific functions different from those of the original.

diffusion: movement of solutes from an area of high concentration to one of low concentration.

digestion: the process by which complex food particles are broken down to smaller absorbable particles.

digestive system: all the organs and glands associated with the ingestion and digestion of food.

dipeptide: two amino acids bonded together.

disaccharides (dye-SACK-uh-rides): pairs of sugar units bonded together.

disclosure: the act of revealing pertinent information. For example, clinicians should accurately describe proposed tests and procedures, their benefits and risks, and alternative approaches.

disordered eating: eating behaviors that are neither normal nor healthy, including restrained eating, fasting, binge eating, and purging.

distributive justice: the equitable distribution of resources.

diuresis (DYE-uh-REE-sis): increased urine production.

diuretics (dye-yoo-RET-ics): medications that promote the excretion of water through the kidneys.

diverticulitis (DYE-ver-tic-you-LYE-tis): inflammation or infection involving diverticula.

diverticulosis (DYE-ver-tic-you-LOH-sis): an intestinal condition characterized by the presence of small herniations (called diverticula) in the intestinal wall.

do-not-resuscitate (DNR) order: a request by a patient or surrogate to withhold cardiopulmonary resuscitation.

drink: volume of an alcoholic beverage that contains about ½ ounce of pure ethanol; equivalent to 12 oz of beer, 5 oz of wine, or 1½ oz of 80-proof distilled spirits such as gin, rum, vodka, and whiskey.

dumping syndrome: a cluster of symptoms that result from the rapid emptying of an osmotic load from the stomach into the small intestine.

duodenum (doo-oh-DEEN-um, doo-ODD-num): the top portion of the small intestine (about "12 fingers' breadth long" in ancient terminology).

durable power of attorney: a legal document (sometimes called a *health care proxy*) that gives legal authority to another (a *health care agent*) to make medical decisions in the event of incapacitation.

dyspepsia: symptoms of pain or discomfort in the upper abdominal area, often called "indigestion"; a symptom of illness rather than a disease itself.

dysphagia (dis-FAY-jah): difficulty swallowing.

dyspnea (DISP-nee-ah): shortness of breath.

eating disorder: a disturbance in eating behavior that jeopardizes a person's physical and psychological health.

eating pattern: customary intake of foods and beverages over time.

eclampsia (eh-KLAMP-see-ah): a severe complication during pregnancy in which seizures occur.

edamame: fresh green soybeans.

edema (eh-DEEM-uh): the swelling of body tissue caused by leakage of fluid from the blood vessels and accumulation of the fluid in the interstitial spaces.

eicosanoids (eye-KO-sa-noids): 20-carbon molecules derived from dietary fatty acids that help to regulate blood pressure, blood clotting, and other body functions.

electrolyte solutions: solutions that can conduct electricity.

electrolyte: a salt that dissolves in water and dissociates into charged particles called ions.

elemental formulas: enteral formulas that contain proteins and carbohydrates that are partially or fully hydrolyzed; also called *hydrolyzed, chemically defined,* or *monomeric formulas.*

embolism (EM-boh-lizm): the obstruction of a blood vessel by an embolus, causing sudden tissue death.

- *embol* = to insert, plug

embolus (EM-boh-lus): an abnormal particle, such as a blood clot or air bubble, that travels in the blood.

embryo (EM-bree-oh): the developing infant from two to eight weeks after conception.

emergency kitchens: programs that provide meals to be eaten on-site; often called soup kitchens.

emetic (em-ET-ic): an agent that causes vomiting.

emphysema (EM-fih-ZEE-mah): a progressive lung disease characterized by the breakdown of the lungs' elastic structure and destruction of the walls of the respiratory bronchioles and alveoli, reducing the surface area involved in respiration.

empty kcalories: kcalories provided by added sugars and solid fats with few or no other nutrients.

emulsifier: a substance that mixes with both fat and water and that disperses the fat in the water, forming an emulsion.

endothelial cells: cells that line the inner surfaces of blood vessels, lymphatic vessels, and body cavities.

end-stage renal disease: an advanced stage of chronic kidney disease in which dialysis or a kidney transplant is necessary to sustain life.

energy density: a measure of the energy a food provides relative to the amount of food (kcalories per gram).

energy-yielding nutrients: the nutrients that break down to yield energy the body can use. The three energy-yielding nutrients are carbohydrate, protein, and fat.

engorgement: overfilling of the breasts with milk.

enrichment: the addition to a food of nutrients to meet a specified standard. In the case of refined bread or cereal, five nutrients have been added: thiamin, riboflavin, niacin, and folate in amounts approximately equivalent to, or higher than, those originally present and iron in amounts to alleviate the prevalence of iron-deficiency anemia.

enteral (EN-ter-al) **nutrition:** the provision of nutrients using the GI tract; usually refers to the use of tube feedings.

enteric coated: refers to medications or enzyme preparations that are coated to withstand stomach acidity and dissolve only at the higher pH of the small intestine.

environmental tobacco smoke (ETS): the combination of exhaled smoke (mainstream smoke) and smoke from lighted cigarettes, pipes, or cigars (sidestream smoke) that enters the air and may be inhaled by other people.

enzymes: protein catalysts. A catalyst is a compound that facilitates chemical reactions without itself being changed in the process.

EPA, DHA: omega-3 fatty acids made from linolenic acid. The full name for EPA is *eicosapentaenoic* (EYE-cosa-PENTA-ee-NO-ick) *acid*. The full name for DHA is *docosahexaenoic* (DOE-cosa-HEXA-ee-NO-ick) *acid*.

epigenetics: processes that cause heritable changes in gene expression that are separate from the DNA nucleotide sequence.

epiglottis (epp-ih-GLOTT-iss): cartilage in the throat that guards the entrance to the trachea and prevents fluid or food from entering it when a person swallows.

epinephrine: one of the stress hormones secreted whenever emergency action is needed; prescribed therapeutically to relax the bronchioles during allergy or asthma attacks.

epithelial cells (ep-i-THEE-lee-ul): cells on the surface of the skin and mucous membranes.

epithelial tissue: tissue composing the layers of the body that serve as selective barriers between the body's interior and the environment (examples are the cornea, the skin, the respiratory lining, and the lining of the digestive tract).

erythrocyte (er-RITH-ro-cite) **hemolysis** (he-MOLL-uh-sis): rupture of the red blood cells, caused by vitamin E deficiency.

erythrocyte protoporphyrin (PRO-toh-PORE-fe-rin): a precursor to hemoglobin.

erythropoietin (eh-RITH-ro-POY-eh-tin): a hormone made by the kidneys that stimulates red blood cell production.

esophageal (eh-SOF-ah-JEE-al): involving the esophagus.

esophageal dysphagia: difficulty passing food through the esophagus; usually caused by an obstruction or a motility disorder.

esophageal (ee-SOF-a-GEE-al) **sphincter:** a sphincter muscle at the upper or lower end of the esophagus. The *lower esophageal sphincter* is also called the *cardiac sphincter*.

esophagus (ee-SOFF-ah-gus): the food pipe; the conduit from the mouth to the stomach.

essential amino acids: amino acids that the body cannot synthesize in amounts sufficient to meet physiological needs. Nine amino acids are known to be essential for human adults: histidine, isoleucine, leucine, lysine, methionine, phenylalanine, threonine, tryptophan, and valine.

essential fatty acids: fatty acids that the body requires but cannot make and so must be obtained through the diet.

essential nutrients: nutrients a person must obtain from food because the body cannot make them for itself in sufficient quantities to meet physiological needs.

Estimated Average Requirements (EAR): the average daily nutrient intake levels estimated to meet the requirements of half of the healthy individuals in a given age and gender group; used in nutrition research and policymaking and as the basis on which RDA values are set.

Estimated Energy Requirement (EER): the dietary energy intake level that is predicted to maintain energy balance in a healthy adult of a defined age, gender, weight, and physical activity level consistent with good health.

ethical: in accordance with accepted principles of right and wrong.

ethnic diets: foodways and cuisines typical of national origins, races, cultural heritages, or geographic locations.

evaporated cane juice: raw sugar from which impurities have been removed.

exclusive breastfeeding: an infant's consumption of human milk with no supplementation of any type (no water, no juice, no nonhuman milk, and no foods) except for vitamins, minerals, and medications.

exocrine: pertains to external secretions, such as those of the mucous membranes or the skin. Opposite of *endocrine*, which pertains to hormonal secretions into the blood.

expected outcomes: patient-oriented goals that are derived from nursing diagnoses.

extracellular fluid: fluid residing outside the cells; includes the fluid between the cells (*interstitial fluid*), plasma, and the water of structures such as the skin and bones. Extracellular fluid accounts for about one-third of the body's water.

faith healing: the use of prayer or belief in divine intervention to promote healing.

fasting hyperglycemia: hyperglycemia that typically develops in the early morning after an overnight fast of at least eight hours.

fat replacers: ingredients that replace some or all of the functions of fat in foods and may or may not provide energy.

fats: lipids that are solid at room temperature (70°F or 21°C).

fatty acids: organic compounds composed of a chain of carbon atoms with hydrogen atoms attached and an acid group at one end.

fatty liver: an accumulation of fat in liver tissue; also called *hepatic steatosis*.

fatty streaks: accumulation of cholesterol and other lipids along the walls of the arteries.

female athlete triad: used to refer to the syndrome characterized by low energy availability (with or without disordered eating), menstrual dysfunction (including **amenorrhea**), and low bone mineral density.

fermentation: the anaerobic (without oxygen) breakdown of carbohydrates by microorganisms that releases small organic compounds along with carbon dioxide and energy.

fertility: the capacity of a woman to produce a normal ovum periodically and of a man to produce normal sperm; the ability to reproduce.

fetal alcohol spectrum disorders (FASD): a spectrum of physical, behavioral, and cognitive disabilities caused by prenatal alcohol exposure.

fetal alcohol syndrome (FAS): the cluster of symptoms seen in an infant or child whose mother consumed excessive alcohol during her pregnancy. FAS includes, but is not limited to, brain damage, growth retardation, mental retardation, and facial abnormalities.

fetus (FEET-us): the developing infant from eight weeks after conception until its birth.

fibrinogen (fye-BRIN-oh-jen): a liver protein that promotes blood clot formation.

filtrate: the substances that pass through the glomerulus and travel through the nephron's tubules, eventually forming urine.

fistulas (FIST-you-luz): abnormal passages between organs or tissues that allow the passage of fluids or secretions.

fitness: the characteristics that enable the body to perform physical activity; more broadly, the ability to meet routine physical demands with enough reserve energy to rise to a physical challenge; the body's ability to withstand stress of all kinds.

flatulence: the condition of having excessive intestinal gas, which causes abdominal discomfort.

fluid and electrolyte balance: maintenance of the necessary amounts and types of fluid and minerals in each compartment of the body fluids.

fluorapatite (floor-APP-uh-tite)**:** the stabilized form of bone and tooth crystal, in which fluoride has replaced the hydroxy portion of hydroxyapatite.

fluorosis (floor-OH-sis)**:** mottling of the tooth enamel from ingestion of too much fluoride during tooth development.

FODMAPs: an acronym for *fermentable oligosaccharides, disaccharides, monosaccharides, and polyols,* which are incompletely digested or poorly absorbed carbohydrates that are fermented in the large intestine; a low-FODMAP diet may help to reduce flatulence, abdominal distention, and diarrhea.

follicle (FOLL-i-cul)**:** a group of cells in the skin from which a hair grows.

food allergy: an adverse reaction to food that involves an immune response; also called *food-hypersensitivity reactions.*

food aversions: strong desires to avoid particular foods.

food banks: facilities that collect and distribute food donations to authorized organizations feeding the hungry.

food cravings: deep longings for particular foods.

food deserts: urban and rural low-income areas with limited access to affordable and nutritious foods.

food frequency questionnaire: a survey of foods routinely consumed. Some questionnaires ask about the types of food eaten and yield only qualitative information; others include questions about portions consumed and yield semiquantitative data as well.

food group plan: a diet-planning tool that sorts foods into groups based on nutrient content and then specifies that people should eat certain amounts of food from each group.

food insecurity: limited or uncertain access to foods of sufficient quality or quantity to sustain a healthy and active life.

food intolerances: adverse reactions to foods or food additives that do not involve the immune system.

food pantries: community food collection programs that provide groceries to be prepared and eaten at home.

food poverty: hunger occurring when enough food exists in an area but some of the people cannot obtain it because they lack money, are being deprived for political reasons, live in a country at war, or suffer from other problems such as lack of transportation.

food record: a detailed log of food eaten during a specified time period, usually several days; also called a *food diary.* A food record may also include information about medications, disease symptoms, and physical activity.

food recovery: the collection of wholesome food for distribution to low-income people who are hungry.

food security: access to enough food to sustain a healthy and active life.

foodborne illness: illness transmitted to human beings through food and water, caused by either an infectious agent (foodborne infection) or a poisonous substance (foodborne intoxication); commonly known as **food poisoning.**

foodways: the eating habits and culinary practices of a people, region, or historical period.

fortification: the addition to a food of nutrients that were either not originally present or present in insignificant amounts. Fortification can be used to correct or prevent a widespread nutrient deficiency, to balance the total nutrient profile of a food, or to restore nutrients lost in processing. The terms *fortified* and *enriched* may be used interchangeably.

free radicals: highly reactive chemical forms that can cause destructive changes in nearby compounds, sometimes setting up a chain reaction.

French units: units of measure for a feeding tube's outer diameter; 1 French equals ⅓ millimeter.

fructosamine test: a measurement of glycated serum proteins that reflects glycemic control over the preceding two to three weeks; also known as the *glycated albumin test* or the *glycated serum protein test.*

fructose: a monosaccharide; sometimes known as *fruit sugar.*

functional foods: whole, fortified, enriched, or enhanced foods that have a potentially beneficial effect on health when consumed as part of a varied diet on a regular basis at effective levels.

futile: describes medical care that will not improve the medical circumstances of a patient.

galactose: a monosaccharide; part of the disaccharide lactose.

galactosemia (ga-LAK-toe-SEE-me-ah)**:** an inherited disorder that impairs galactose metabolism; may cause damage to the brain, liver, kidneys, and lens in untreated patients.

gallbladder: the organ that stores and concentrates bile. When it receives the signal that fat is present in the duodenum, the gallbladder contracts and squirts bile through the bile duct into the duodenum.

gangrene: death of tissue due to a deficient blood supply and/or infection.

gastrectomy (gah-STREK-ta-mie)**:** the surgical removal of part of the stomach (partial gastrectomy) or the entire stomach (total gastrectomy).

gastric banding: a surgical means of producing weight loss by restricting stomach size with a constricting band.

gastric bypass: surgery that restricts stomach size and reroutes food from the stomach to the lower part of the small intestine; creates a chronic, lifelong state of malabsorption by preventing normal digestion and absorption of nutrients.

gastric decompression: the removal of stomach contents (such as GI secretions, air, or blood) in patients with motility problems or obstructions that prevent stomach emptying; the procedure may be used to reduce discomfort, vomiting, or various complications during critical illness or after certain surgeries.

gastric glands: exocrine glands in the stomach wall that secrete gastric juice into the stomach.

gastric juice: the digestive secretion of the gastric glands containing a mixture of water, hydrochloric acid, and enzymes. The principal enzymes are pepsin (acts on proteins) and lipase (acts on emulsified fats).

gastric outlet obstruction: an obstruction that prevents the normal emptying of stomach contents into the duodenum.

gastric residual volume: the volume of formula and GI secretions remaining in the stomach after a previous feeding.

gastrin: a hormone secreted by cells in the stomach wall. Target organ: the glands of the stomach. Response: secretion of gastric acid.

gastritis: inflammation of stomach tissue. (The suffix *-itis* refers to the presence of inflammation in an organ or tissue.)

gastroesophageal reflux disease (GERD): a condition characterized by frequent reflux (backward flow) of the stomach's acidic contents into the esophagus.

gastrointestinal motility: spontaneous motion in the digestive tract accomplished by involuntary muscular contractions.

gastrointestinal (GI) tract: the digestive tract. The principal organs are the stomach and intestines.

gastroparesis (GAS-troe-pah-REE-sis): delayed stomach emptying; most often a consequence of diabetes, gastric surgery, or neurological disorders.

gatekeeper: with respect to nutrition, a key person who controls other people's access to foods and thereby exerts a profound impact on their nutrition. Examples are the spouse who buys and cooks the food, the parent who feeds the children, and the caregiver in a daycare center.

gene expression: the process by which a cell converts the genetic code into RNA and protein.

gene therapy: treatment for inherited disorders in which DNA sequences are introduced into the chromosomes of affected cells, prompting the cells to express the protein needed to correct the disease.

genes: segments of DNA that contain the information needed to make proteins.

genetic counseling: support for families at risk of genetic disorders; involves diagnosis of disease, identification of inheritance patterns within the family, and review of reproductive options.

genome (JEE-nome): the full complement of genetic material in the chromosomes of a cell.

genomics (jee-NO-miks): the study of genomes.

gestation: the period of about 40 weeks (three trimesters) from conception to birth; the term of a pregnancy.

gestational diabetes: glucose intolerance with first onset or first recognition during pregnancy.

gestational hypertension: high blood pressure that develops in the second half of pregnancy and usually resolves after childbirth.

ghrelin (GRELL-in): a hormone produced primarily by the stomach cells. It signals the hypothalamus of the brain to stimulate appetite and food intake.

GI microbiota: the collection of microbes found in the GI tract, sometimes called the *microflora* or *gut flora*. The collection of genes and genomes of the microbiota is called the *microbiome*.

gingiva (jin-JYE-va, JIN-jeh-va): the gums.

gingivitis (jin-jeh-VYE-tus): inflammation of the gums, characterized by redness, swelling, and bleeding.

glands: cells or groups of cells that secrete materials for special uses in the body. Glands may be *exocrine* (EKS-oh-crin) *glands*, secreting their materials "out" (into the digestive tract or onto the surface of the skin), or *endocrine* (EN-doe-crin) *glands*, secreting their materials "in" (into the blood).

glomerular filtration rate (GFR): the rate at which filtrate is formed within the kidneys, normally about 125 mL/min in healthy young adults.

glomerulus (gloh-MEHR-yoo-lus): a tuft of capillaries within the nephron that filters water and solutes from the blood as urine production begins (plural: *glomeruli*).

glucagon (GLOO-ka-gon): a hormone that is secreted by special cells in the pancreas in response to low blood glucose concentration and that elicits release of glucose from storage.

glucose: a monosaccharide; the sugar common to all disaccharides and polysaccharides; also called *blood sugar* or *dextrose*.

gluten-free: a food that contains less than 20 parts per million of gluten from any source: synonyms include *no gluten, free of gluten,* or *without gluten.*

glycated hemoglobin (HbA₁c): hemoglobin that has nonenzymatically attached to glucose; the level of HbA$_{1c}$ in the blood helps to diagnose diabetes and evaluate long-term glycemic control. Also called *glycosylated hemoglobin.*

glycemic (gly-SEE-mic): pertaining to blood glucose.

glycemic index: a method of classifying foods according to their potential for raising blood glucose.

glycemic response: the extent to which a food raises the blood glucose concentration and elicits an insulin response.

glycerol (GLISS-er-ol): an organic compound, three carbons long, that can form the backbone of triglycerides and phospholipids.

glycogen (GLY-co-gen): a polysaccharide composed of glucose, made and stored by liver and muscle tissues of human beings and animals as a storage form of glucose. Glycogen is not a significant food source of carbohydrate and is not counted as one of the polysaccharides in foods.

glycosuria (GLY-co-SOOR-ee-ah): the presence of glucose in the urine.

goiter (GOY-ter): an enlargement of the thyroid gland due to an iodine deficiency, malfunction of the gland, or overconsumption of a thyroid antagonist. Goiter caused by iodine deficiency is sometimes called *simple goiter.*

goitrogen (GOY-troh-jen): a substance that enlarges the thyroid gland and causes *toxic goiter*. Goitrogens occur naturally in such foods as cabbage, kale, brussels sprouts, cauliflower, broccoli, and kohlrabi.

gout (GOWT): a metabolic disorder characterized by elevated uric acid levels in the blood and urine and the deposition of uric acid in and around the joints, causing acute joint inflammation.

graft rejection: destruction of donor tissue by the recipient's immune system, which recognizes the donor cells as foreign.

graft-versus-host disease: a condition in which the immune cells in transplanted tissue (the graft) attack recipient (host) cells, leading to widespread tissue damage.

granulated sugar: white sugar.

half-life: in blood tests, refers to the length of time that a substance remains in plasma. The albumin in plasma has a half-life of 14 to 20 days, meaning that half of the amount circulating in plasma is degraded in this time period.

Hazard Analysis and Critical Control Points (HACCP) systems: management systems that address food safety by analyzing biological, chemical, and physical hazards that may arise during the preparation, storage, handling, and administration of food products; commonly referred to as *HASS-ip.*

health: a range of states with physical, mental, emotional, spiritual, and social components. At a minimum, health means freedom from physical disease, mental disturbances, emotional distress, spiritual discontent, social maladjustment, and other negative states. At a maximum, health means *wellness.*

health care agent: a person given legal authority to make medical decisions for another in the event of incapacitation.

health care communities: living environments for people with chronic conditions, functional limitations, or need for supervision or assistance; include assisted living facilities, group homes, short-term rehabilitation facilities, skilled nursing facilities, and hospice facilities.

health claims: statements that characterize the relationship between a nutrient or other substance in food and a disease or health-related condition.

Healthy People: a national public health initiative under the jurisdiction of the U.S. Department of Health and Human Services (DHHS) that identifies the most significant preventable threats to health and focuses efforts toward eliminating them.

heartburn: a burning sensation in the chest region.

heart failure: a condition characterized by the heart's inability to pump adequate blood to the body's cells, resulting in fluid accumulation in the tissues; also called *congestive heart failure.*

Helicobacter pylori (H. pylori): a species of bacterium that colonizes the GI mucosa; a primary cause of gastritis and peptic ulcer disease.

helper T cells: lymphocytes that have a specific protein called CD4 on their surfaces and therefore are also known as *CD4+ T cells*; these are the cells most affected in HIV infection.

hematocrit (hee-MAT-oh-crit)**:** measurement of the volume of the red blood cells packed by centrifuge in a given volume of blood.

hematopoietic stem cell transplantation: transplantation of the stem cells that produce red blood cells and white blood cells; the stem cells are obtained from bone marrow (*bone marrow transplantation*) or circulating blood.

hematuria (HE-mah-TOO-ree-ah)**:** blood in the urine.

hemochromatosis (heem-oh-crome-a-TOH-sis)**:** iron overload characterized by deposits of iron-containing pigment in many tissues, with tissue damage. Hemochromatosis is usually caused by a hereditary defect in iron absorption.

hemodialysis (HE-moe-dye-AL-ih-sis)**:** a treatment that removes fluids and wastes from the blood by passing the blood through a dialyzer.

hemofiltration: removal of fluid and solutes from the blood by pumping the blood across a membrane; no osmotic gradients are created during the process.

hemoglobin: the oxygen-carrying protein of the red blood cells.

hemolytic (HE-moh-LIT-ick) **anemia:** the condition of having too few red blood cells as a result of erythrocyte hemolysis.

hemophilia (HE-moh-FEEL-ee-ah)**:** an inherited bleeding disorder characterized by deficiency or malfunction of a plasma protein needed for clotting blood.

hemorrhagic (hem-oh-RAJ-ik) **disease:** the vitamin K–deficiency disease in which blood fails to clot.

hemorrhagic strokes: strokes caused by bleeding within the brain, which destroys or compresses brain tissue.

hepatic coma: loss of consciousness resulting from severe liver disease.

hepatic encephalopathy (en-sef-ah-LOP-ah-thie)**:** a neurological complication of advanced liver disease that is characterized by changes in personality, mood, behavior, mental ability, and motor functions.

hepatic portal vein: the blood vessel that conducts nutrient-rich blood from the digestive tract to the liver.

hepatic vein: the vein that collects blood from the liver capillaries and returns it to the heart.

hepatitis (hep-ah-TYE-tis)**:** inflammation of the liver.

hepatomegaly (HEP-ah-toe-MEG-ah-lee)**:** enlargement of the liver.

hepcidin (HEP-sid-in)**:** a hormone secreted by the liver in response to elevated blood iron. Hepcidin reduces iron's absorption from the intestine and its release from storage.

herpes simplex virus: a common virus that can cause blisterlike lesions on the lips and in the mouth.

hiatal hernia: a condition in which the upper portion of the stomach protrudes above the diaphragm; most cases are asymptomatic.

high energy density: a high number of kcalories per unit weight of food; foods of high energy density are generally high in fat and low in water content.

high-density lipoproteins (HDL): lipoproteins that help to remove cholesterol from the bloodstream by transporting it to the liver for reuse or disposal.

high-fructose corn syrup: a widely used commercial kcaloric sweetener made by adding enzymes to cornstarch to convert a portion of its glucose molecules into sweet-tasting fructose.

high-quality proteins: dietary proteins containing all the essential amino acids in relatively the same amounts that human beings require; may also contain nonessential amino acids.

high-risk pregnancy: a pregnancy characterized by risk factors that make it likely the birth will be surrounded by problems such as

premature delivery, difficult birth, retarded growth, birth defects, and early infant death.

histamine-2 receptor blockers: a class of drugs that suppress acid secretion by inhibiting receptors on acid-producing cells; commonly called *H2 blockers*. Examples include cimetidine (Tagamet), ranitidine (Zantac), and famotidine (Pepcid).

homeopathic (HO-mee-oh-PATH-ic) **medicine:** a practice based on the theory that "like cures like"; that is, substances believed to cause certain symptoms are prescribed at extremely low concentrations for curing diseases with similar symptoms.

homeostasis (HOME-ee-oh-STAY-sis)**:** the maintenance of constant internal conditions (such as chemistry, temperature, and blood pressure) by the body's control system.

homocysteine: an amino acid produced during the conversion of methionine to cysteine; blood homocysteine levels are influenced by intakes of folate, vitamin B_{12}, and vitamin B_6.

honey: a concentrated solution primarily composed of glucose and fructose; produced by enzymatic digestion of the sucrose in nectar by bees.

hormones: chemical messengers. Hormones are secreted by a variety of glands in the body in response to altered conditions. Each travels to one or more target tissues or organs and elicits specific responses to restore normal conditions.

human genome (GEE-nome)**:** the complete set of genetic material (DNA) in a human being.

human immunodeficiency virus (HIV): the virus that causes acquired immune deficiency syndrome (AIDS). HIV destroys immune cells and progressively impedes the body's ability to fight infections and certain cancers.

hunger: the physiological need to eat, experienced as a drive to obtain food; an unpleasant sensation that demands relief.

hydrochloric acid (HCl): an acid composed of hydrogen and chloride atoms; normally produced by the gastric glands.

hydrogenation (high-dro-gen-AY-shun)**:** a chemical process by which hydrogen atoms are added to monounsaturated or polyunsaturated fats to reduce the number of double bonds, making the fats more saturated (solid) and more resistant to oxidation (protecting against rancidity). Hydrogenation produces *trans*-fatty acids.

hyperactivity: inattentive and impulsive behavior that is more frequent and severe than is typical of others of a similar age; professionally called **attention-deficit/hyperactivity disorder (ADHD)**.

hypercalcemia (HIGH-per-kal-SEE-me-ah)**:** elevated serum calcium levels.

hypercalciuria (HIGH-per-kal-see-YOO-ree-ah)**:** elevated urinary calcium levels.

hypercapnia (high-per-CAP-nee-ah)**:** excessive carbon dioxide in the blood.

hyperglycemia: elevated blood glucose concentrations. Normal fasting plasma glucose levels are less than 100 mg/dL. Fasting plasma glucose levels between 100 and 125 mg/dL suggest prediabetes; values of 126 mg/dL and above suggest diabetes.

hyperinsulinemia: abnormally high levels of insulin in the blood.

hyperkalemia (HIGH-per-ka-LEE-me-ah)**:** elevated serum potassium levels.

hypermetabolism: a higher-than-normal metabolic rate.

hyperosmolar hyperglycemic syndrome: a condition of extreme hyperglycemia associated with dehydration, hyperosmolar blood, and altered mental status; sometimes called the *hyperosmolar hyperglycemic nonketotic state*.

hyperosmolar: having an abnormally high osmolarity; osmolarity refers to the concentration of osmotically active particles in solution. Hyperglycemia may cause some body fluids to become hyperosmolar.

hyperoxaluria (HIGH-per-ox-ah-LOO-ree-ah): elevated urinary oxalate levels.

hyperphosphatemia (HIGH-per-fos-fa-TEE-me-ah): elevated serum phosphate levels. Note that the phosphorus in body fluids is present as phosphate; hence, the terms *serum phosphate and serum phosphorus* are often used interchangeably.

hypertension: high blood pressure.

hypertonic formula: a formula with an osmolality greater than that of blood serum.

hypertriglyceridemia: elevated blood triglyceride levels.

hypnotherapy: a technique that uses hypnosis and the power of suggestion to improve health behaviors, relieve pain, and promote healing.

hypoalbuminemia: low plasma albumin concentrations. Plasma proteins such as albumin help to maintain fluid balance within the blood; thus, low levels contribute to edema.

hypocaloric feedings: a reduced-calorie regimen that includes sufficient protein and micronutrients to maintain nitrogen balance and prevent malnutrition; also called *permissive underfeeding*.

hypochlorhydria (HIGH-poe-clor-HIGH-dree-ah): abnormally low gastric acid secretions.

hypocitraturia: low urinary citrate levels. Citrate is formed in the body during energy metabolism and is also a component of fruit (especially citrus fruit) and some other foods.

hypoglycemia: abnormally low blood glucose concentrations. In diabetes, hypoglycemia is treated when plasma glucose falls below 70 mg/dL.

hypokalemia (HIGH-po-ka-LEE-me-ah): low serum potassium levels.

hyponatremia (HIGH-po-na-TREE-me-ah): abnormally low sodium levels in the blood; a possible result of fluid overload.

hypothalamus (high-poh-THAL-ah-mus): a brain center that controls activities such as maintenance of water balance, regulation of body temperature, and control of appetite.

hypoxemia (high-pock-SEE-me-ah): insufficient oxygen in the blood.

hypoxia (high-POCK-see-ah): insufficient oxygen in body tissues.

ileocecal (ill-ee-oh-SEEK-ul) **valve:** the sphincter separating the small and large intestines.

ileostomy (ill-ee-AH-stoe-me): a surgical passage through the abdominal wall into the ileum.

ileum (ILL-ee-um): the last segment of the small intestine.

imagery: the use of mental images of things or events to aid relaxation or promote self-healing.

immunity: the body's ability to defend itself against diseases.

implantation: the stage of development in which the blastocyst embeds itself in the wall of the uterus and begins to develop; occurs during the first two weeks after conception.

inborn error of metabolism: an inherited trait (one that is present at birth) that causes the absence, deficiency, or malfunction of a protein that has a critical metabolic role.

indirect calorimetry: a method of estimating resting energy expenditure by measuring a person's oxygen consumption and carbon dioxide production.

inflammation: an immunological response to cellular injury characterized by an increase in white blood cells.

inflammatory response: a group of nonspecific immune responses to infection or injury.

informed consent: a patient's or caregiver's agreement to undergo a treatment that has been adequately disclosed. Persons must be mentally competent in order to make the decision.

inherited disorders: medical conditions resulting from genetic defects.

inorganic: not containing carbon or pertaining to living organisms. The two classes of nutrients that are inorganic are minerals and water.

insoluble fibers: the tough, fibrous structures of fruits, vegetables, and grains; indigestible food components that do not dissolve in water.

insulin resistance: reduced sensitivity to insulin in muscle, adipose, and liver cells.

insulin: a pancreatic hormone that regulates glucose metabolism; its actions are countered mainly by the hormone *glucagon.*

intermittent feedings: feedings with delivery rates of about 250 to 400 milliliters of formula over 30 to 45 minutes.

intestinal adaptation: physiological changes in the small intestine that increase its absorptive capacity after resection.

intestinal juice: the secretion of the intestinal glands; contains enzymes for the digestion of carbohydrate and protein and a minor enzyme for fat digestion.

intestinal flora: the bacterial inhabitants of the GI tract.

intractable: not easily managed or controlled.

intractable vomiting: vomiting that is not easily managed or controlled.

intradialytic parenteral nutrition: the infusion of nutrients during hemodialysis, often providing amino acids, dextrose, lipids, and some trace minerals.

intrinsic factor: a substance secreted by the stomach cells that binds with vitamin B_{12} in the small intestine to aid in the absorption of vitamin B_{12}. Anemia that reflects a vitamin B_{12} deficiency caused by lack of intrinsic factor is known as *pernicious anemia.*

invert sugar: a mixture of glucose and fructose formed by the splitting of sucrose in an industrial process. Sold only in liquid form and sweeter than sucrose, invert sugar forms during certain cooking procedures and works to prevent crystallization of sucrose in soft candies and sweets.

iron deficiency: the condition of having depleted iron stores.

iron-deficiency anemia: a blood iron deficiency characterized by small, pale red blood cells; also called *microcytic hypochromic anemia.*

iron overload: toxicity from excess iron.

irritable bowel syndrome: an intestinal disorder of unknown cause that disturbs the functioning of the large intestine; symptoms include abdominal pain, flatulence, diarrhea, and constipation.

ischemia (iss-KEE-mee-a): inadequate blood supply within a tissue due to obstructed blood flow.

ischemic strokes: strokes caused by the obstruction of blood flow to brain tissue.

isotonic formula: a formula with an osmolality similar to that of blood serum (about 300 milliosmoles per kilogram).

jaundice (JAWN-dis): yellow discoloration of the skin and eyes due to an accumulation of bilirubin, a breakdown product of hemoglobin that normally exits the body via bile secretions.

jejunum (je-JOON-um): the first two-fifths of the small intestine beyond the duodenum.

Kaposi's (kah-POH-seez) **sarcoma:** a common cancer in HIV-infected persons that is characterized by lesions in the skin, lungs, and GI tract.

kcalorie (energy) control: management of food energy intake.

kcalorie counts: estimates of food energy (and often, protein) consumed by patients for one or more days.

keratin (KERR-uh-tin): a water-insoluble protein; the normal protein of hair and nails. Keratin-producing cells may replace mucus-producing cells in vitamin A deficiency.

keratomalacia (KARE-ah-toe-ma-LAY-shuh): softening of the cornea that leads to irreversible blindness; a sign of severe vitamin A deficiency.

ketoacidosis (KEY-toe-ass-ih-DOE-sis): an acidosis (lowering of blood pH) that results from the excessive production of ketone bodies.

ketone bodies: acidic, water-soluble compounds produced by the liver during the breakdown of fat when carbohydrate is not available. Small amounts of ketone bodies are normally produced during energy metabolism, but when their blood concentration rises, they spill into the urine. The combination of a high blood concentration of ketone bodies (*ketonemia*) and ketone bodies in the urine (*ketonuria*) is called *ketosis*.

ketonuria (KEY-toe-NOOR-ee-ah): the presence of ketone bodies in the urine.

ketosis (key-TOE-sis): elevated levels of ketone bodies in body tissues.

kidney stones: crystalline masses that form in the urinary tract; also called *renal calculi* or *nephrolithiasis*.

kwashiorkor: severe malnutrition characterized by failure to grow and develop, edema, changes in the pigmentation of the hair and skin, fatty liver, anemia, and apathy.

lactation: production and secretion of breast milk for the purpose of nourishing an infant.

lacto-ovo vegetarian diet: an eating pattern that includes milk, milk products, eggs, vegetables, grains, legumes, fruit, and nuts; excludes meat, poultry, and seafood.

lactose: a disaccharide composed of glucose and galactose; commonly known as *milk sugar*.

lactose intolerance: intolerance to lactose-containing foods due to the loss or reduction of intestinal lactase; symptoms may include flatulence, bloating, and diarrhea.

lacto-vegetarian diet: an eating pattern that includes milk, milk products, vegetables, grains, legumes, fruit, and nuts; excludes meat, poultry, seafood, and eggs.

laparoscopic weight-loss surgery: a weight-loss surgery procedure in which surgeons gain access to the abdomen via several small incisions. A tiny video camera is inserted through one of the incisions and surgical instruments through the others. The surgeons watch their work on a large-screen monitor.

lapses: periods of returning to old habits.

large intestine or colon: the lower portion of intestine that completes the digestive process. Its segments are the ascending colon, the transverse colon, the descending colon, and the sigmoid colon.

lecithins: one type of phospholipid.

legumes (lay-GYOOMS, LEG-yooms): plants of the bean and pea family with seeds that are rich in protein compared with other plant-derived foods.

length: the distance from the top of the head to the soles of the feet while a person is recumbent (lying down). In contrast, *height* is measured while a person is standing upright.

leptin: a hormone produced by fat cells under the direction of the (*ob*) gene. It decreases appetite and increases energy expenditure.

letdown reflex: the reflex that forces milk to the front of the breast when the infant begins to nurse.

life expectancy: the average number of years lived by people in a given society.

life span: the maximum number of years of life attainable by a member of a species.

limiting amino acid: an essential amino acid that is present in dietary protein in the shortest supply relative to the amount needed for protein synthesis in the body.

linoleic acid, linolenic acid: polyunsaturated fatty acids that are essential for human beings.

lipids: a family of compounds that includes triglycerides (fats and oils), phospholipids, and sterols. Lipids are characterized by their insolubility in water.

lipodystrophy (LIP-oh-DIS-tro-fee): abnormalities in body fat and fat metabolism that may result from drug treatments for HIV infection. The accumulation of abdominal fat is sometimes called *protease paunch*.

lipomas (lih-POE-muz): benign tumors composed of fatty tissue.

lipoprotein lipase (LPL): an enzyme mounted on the surface of fat cells (and other cells) that hydrolyzes triglycerides in the blood into fatty acids and glycerol for absorption into the cells. There they are metabolized or reassembled for storage.

lipoproteins: clusters of lipids associated with proteins that serve as transport vehicles for lipids in the lymph and blood.

listeriosis: a serious foodborne infection that can cause severe brain infection or death in a fetus or newborn; caused by the bacterium *Listeria monocytogenes*, which is found in soil and water.

liver: the organ that manufactures bile. (The liver's other functions are described in Chapter 19.)

longevity: long duration of life.

low birthweight (LBW): a birthweight less than 5½ lb (2500 g); indicates probable poor health in the newborn and poor nutrition status of the mother during pregnancy. Optimal birthweight for a full-term infant is 6.8 to 7.9 lb (about 3100 to 3600 g). Low-birthweight infants are of two different types. Some are **premature**; they are born early and are of a weight **appropriate for gestational age (AGA)**. Others have suffered growth failure in the uterus; they may or may not be born early, but they are **small for gestational age (SGA)**.

low-density lipoproteins (LDL): lipoproteins that transport cholesterol in the blood.

low-risk pregnancy: a pregnancy characterized by factors that make it likely the birth will be normal and the infant healthy.

lymph (LIMF): the body fluid found in lymphatic vessels. Lymph consists of all the constituents of blood except red blood cells.

lymphatic system: a loosely organized system of vessels and ducts that conveys the products of digestion toward the heart.

macrobiotic diet: a philosophical eating pattern based on mostly plant foods such as whole grains, legumes, and certain vegetables, with small amounts of fish, fruit, nuts, and seeds.

macrocytic anemia: large-cell anemia; also known as *megaloblastic anemia*.

macrosomia (MAK-roh-SOH-mee-ah): the condition of having an abnormally large body; in infants, refers to birth weights of 4000 grams (8 pounds, 13 ounces) and above.

macrovascular complications: disorders that affect large blood vessels, including the coronary arteries and arteries of the limbs.

macular (MACK-you-lar) **degeneration:** deterioration of the macular area of the eye that can lead to loss of central vision and eventual blindness. The **macula** is a small, oval, yellowish region in the center of the retina that provides the sharp, straight-ahead vision so critical to reading and driving.

major minerals: essential mineral nutrients required in the adult diet in amounts greater than 100 milligrams per day.

maleficence (mah-LEF-eh-sense): the act of doing evil or harm.

malignant (ma-LIG-nent): describes a cancerous cell or tumor, which can injure healthy tissue and spread cancer to other regions of the body.

malnutrition: any condition caused by deficient or excess energy or nutrient intake or by an imbalance of nutrients.

malt syrup: a sweetener made from sprouted barley.

maltose: a disaccharide composed of two glucose units; sometimes known as *malt sugar*.

maple syrup: a concentrated solution of sucrose derived from the sap of the sugar maple tree, mostly sucrose. This sugar was once common but is now usually replaced by sucrose and artificial maple flavoring.

marasmic kwashiorkor: a particularly lethal form of SAM, in which a child's dangerous loss of lean tissue (wasting) is masked by edema, making it harder to detect.

marasmus (ma-RAZZ-mus): severe malnutrition characterized by poor growth, dramatic weight loss, loss of body fat and muscle, and apathy.

massage therapy: manual manipulation of muscles to reduce tension, increase blood circulation, improve joint mobility, and promote healing of injuries.

mast cells: cells within connective tissue that produce and release histamine.

mastitis: infection of a breast.

mechanical ventilation: life-sustaining treatment in which a mechanical ventilator assists or replaces spontaneous breathing; substitutes for a patient's failing lungs.

medical nutrition therapy: nutrition care provided by a registered dietitian; includes assessing nutrition status, diagnosing nutrition problems, and providing nutrition care.

meditation: a self-directed technique of calming the mind and relaxing the body.

medium-chain triglycerides (MCT): triglycerides with fatty acids that are 6 to 12 carbons in length. MCT do not require digestion and can be absorbed in the absence of lipase or bile.

metabolic stress: a disruption in the body's chemical environment due to the effects of disease or injury. Metabolic stress is characterized by changes in metabolic rate, heart rate, blood pressure, hormonal status, and nutrient metabolism.

metabolic syndrome: a cluster of interrelated disorders, including abdominal obesity, insulin resistance, high blood pressure, and abnormal blood lipids, which together increase risk of diabetes and cardiovascular disease.

metabolites: products of metabolism; compounds produced by a biochemical pathway.

metastasize (meh-TAS-tah-size): to spread from one part of the body to another; refers to cancer cells.

methotrexate: an anticancer drug that inhibits cell division. Methotrexate closely resembles the B vitamin folate, which is needed for DNA synthesis; the drug works by blocking activity of the enzyme that converts folate to its active form.

methylation: the addition of methyl ($-CH_3$) groups.

microarray technology: research technology that monitors the expression of thousands of genes simultaneously.

microbes (MY-krobes): microscopically small organisms including bacteria, viruses, fungi, and protozoa; also called microorganisms. *mikros* 5 small

microbiota: the mix of microbial species of a community; for example, all of the bacterium, fungi, and viruses present in the human digestive tract.

microvascular complications: disorders that affect small blood vessels, including those in the retina and kidneys.

microvilli (MY-cro-VILL-ee or MY-cro-VILL-eye): tiny, hairlike projections on each cell of every villus that can trap nutrient particles and transport them into the cells. The singular form is **microvillus**.

miso: fermented soybean paste used in Japanese cooking.

minute ventilation: the volume of air a person inhales or exhales each minute.

moderate-intensity physical activity: physical activity that requires some increase in breathing and/or heart rate and expends 3.5 to 7 kcalories per minute. Walking at a speed of 3 to 4.5 miles per hour (about 15 to 20 minutes to walk one mile) is an example.

moderation: the provision of enough, but not too much, of a substance.

modified diet: a diet that contains foods altered in texture, consistency, or nutrient content or that includes or omits specific foods; may also be called a *therapeutic diet*.

modular formulas: enteral formulas prepared in the hospital from *modules* that contain single macronutrients; used for people with unique nutrient needs.

molasses: a thick, brown syrup left over from the refining of sucrose from sugarcane. The major nutrient in molasses is iron, a contaminant from the machinery used in processing it.

molybdenum (mo-LIB-duh-num): a trace element.

monoglycerides: molecules of glycerol with one fatty acid attached. A molecule of glyceride with two fatty acids attached is a *diglyceride*.

monosaccharides (mon-oh-SACK-uh-rides): single sugar units.

monounsaturated fatty acid (MUFA): a fatty acid that has one point of unsaturation; for example, the oleic acid found in olive oil.

mouth: the oral cavity containing the tongue and teeth.

mucous membrane: membrane composed of mucus-secreting cells that lines the surfaces of body tissues. (Reminder: *Mucus* is the smooth, slippery substance secreted by these cells.)

mucus (MYOO-cuss): a mucopolysaccharide (a relative of carbohydrate) secreted by cells of the stomach wall that protects the cells from exposure to digestive juices (and other destructive agents). The cellular lining of the stomach wall with its coat of mucus is known as the *mucous membrane*. (The noun is *mucus*; the adjective is *mucous*.)

multigene or polygenic: involving a number of genes, rather than a single gene.

mutation: a heritable change in the DNA sequence of a gene.

myocardial (MY-oh-CAR-dee-al) **infarction** (in-FARK-shun): death of heart muscle caused by a sudden obstruction in blood flow to the heart; also called a *heart attack*.

myoglobin: the oxygen-carrying protein of the muscle cells.

naturally occurring sugars: sugars that are not added to a food but are present as its original constituents, such as the sugars of fruit or milk.

naturopathic (NAY-chur-oh-PATH-ic) **medicine:** an approach to health care using practices alleged to enhance the body's natural healing abilities. Treatments may include a variety of alternative therapies including dietary supplements, herbal remedies, exercise, and homeopathy.

nephron (NEF-ron): the functional unit of the kidneys, consisting of a glomerulus and tubules.

nephrotic (neh-FROT-ik) **syndrome:** a syndrome caused by significant urinary protein losses (more than 3 to 3½ grams daily), as a result of severe glomerular damage.

nephrotoxic: toxic to the kidneys.

neural tube defects (NTD): malformations of the brain, spinal cord, or both that occur during embryonic development. The two main types of neural tube defects are *spina bifida* (literally, "split spine") and *anencephaly* ("no brain").

neural tube: the embryonic tissue that later forms the brain and spinal cord.

neurofibrillary tangles: snarls of the threadlike strands that extend from the nerve cells, commonly found in the brains of people with Alzheimer's dementia.

neurons: nerve cells; the structural and functional units of the nervous system. Neurons initiate and conduct nerve transmissions.

neutropenia: a low white blood cell (neutrophil) count, which increases susceptibility to infection.

niacin equivalents (NE): the amount of niacin present in food, including the niacin that can theoretically be made from tryptophan, its precursor, present in the food.

night blindness: the slow recovery of vision after exposure to flashes of bright light at night; an early symptom of vitamin A deficiency.

nitrogen balance: the amount of nitrogen consumed (N in) as compared with the amount of nitrogen excreted (N out) in a given period of time. The laboratory scientist can estimate the protein in a sample of food, body tissue, or excreta by measuring the nitrogen in it.

noncoding sequences: regions of DNA that do not code for proteins. Some noncoding sequences may have regulatory or structural properties, but most have no known function.

nonessential amino acids: amino acids that the body can synthesize.

nonnutritive sweeteners: synthetic or natural food additives that offer sweet flavor but with negligible or no calories per serving; also called *artificial sweeteners, intense sweeteners, noncaloric sweeteners,* and *very-low-calorie sweeteners.*

nonpathogenic: not capable of causing disease.

nucleotides: the subunits of DNA and RNA molecules. These compounds—cytosine (C), thymine (T), uracil (U), guanine (G), and adenine (A)—are each composed of a phosphate group, a five-carbon sugar (ribose), and a nitrogen-containing base.

nursing bottle tooth decay: extensive tooth decay due to prolonged tooth contact with formula, milk, fruit juice, or other carbohydrate-rich liquid offered to an infant in a bottle.

nursing diagnoses: clinical judgments about actual or potential health problems that provide the basis for selecting appropriate nursing interventions.

nutrient claims: statements that characterize the quantity of a nutrient in a food.

nutrient density: a measure of the nutrients a food provides relative to the energy it provides. The more nutrients and the fewer kcalories, the higher the nutrient density.

nutrient profiling: ranking foods based on their nutrient composition.

nutrients: substances obtained from food and used in the body to provide energy and structural materials and to serve as regulating agents to promote growth, maintenance, and repair. Nutrients may also reduce the risks of some diseases.

nutrition care plans: strategies for meeting an individual's nutritional needs.

nutrition: the science of foods and the nutrients and other substances they contain, and of their ingestion, digestion, absorption, transport, metabolism, interaction, storage, and excretion. A broader definition includes the study of the environment and of human behavior as it relates to these processes.

nutrition and dietetics technician, registered (NDTR): see **dietetic technicians**

nutritional genomics: the study of dietary effects on genetic expression; also known as *nutrigenomics.*

nutritionists: all registered dietitians are nutritionists, but not all nutritionists are registered dietitians. Some state licensing boards set specific qualifications for holding the title. For states that regulate this title, the definition varies from state to state. To obtain some "nutritionist" credentials requires little more than a payment.

nutrition care process: a systematic approach used by dietetics professionals to evaluate and treat nutrition-related problems.

nutrition screening: an assessment procedure that helps to identify patients who are malnourished or at risk for malnutrition.

nutrition support: see **specialized nutrition support**

nutrition support teams: health care professionals responsible for the provision of nutrients by tube feeding or intravenous infusion.

nutrition support: the delivery of nutrients using a feeding tube or intravenous infusions.

nutritive sweeteners: sweeteners that yield energy, including both the sugars and the sugar alcohols.

obese: having too much body fat with adverse health effects; BMI 30 or more.

obesogenic (oh- BES-oh-JEN-ick) **environment:** all the factors surrounding a person that promote weight gain, such as an increased food intake—especially of unhealthy choices—and decreased physical activity.

oils: lipids that are liquid at room temperature (70°F or 21°C).

olestra: a synthetic fat made from sucrose and fatty acids that provides zero kcalories per gram; also known as *sucrose polyester.*

oliguria (OL-lih-GOO-ree-ah): an abnormally low amount of urine, often less than 400 mL/day.

omega-3 fatty acids: polyunsaturated fatty acids in which the endmost double bond is three carbons back from the end of the carbon chain. Linolenic acid is an example.

omega-6 fatty acid: a polyunsaturated fatty acid with its endmost double bond six carbons back from the end of its carbon chain. Linoleic acid is an example. Chemists use the term *omega,* the last letter of the Greek alphabet, to refer to the position of the last double bond in a fatty acid.

oncotic pressure: the pressure exerted by fluid on one side of a membrane as a result of osmosis.

open feeding system: a formula delivery system that requires the transfer of the formula from its original packaging to a feeding container.

opportunistic infections: infections caused by microorganisms that normally do not cause disease in healthy people but are damaging to persons with compromised immune function.

opsin (OP-sin): the protein portion of the visual pigment molecule.

oral glucose tolerance test: a test that evaluates a person's ability to tolerate an oral glucose load.

oral mucositis: inflammation of the oral mucosa; signs may include swelling, redness, mouth sores, bleeding, or ulcerations in mucosal tissue.

oral nutrition support: nutrition care that allows a malnourished patient to meet nutritional requirements by mouth; may include oral nutritional supplements, nutrient-dense foods and snacks, or fortified foods.

organic: in chemistry, substances or molecules containing carbon–carbon bonds or carbon–hydrogen bonds. The four organic nutrients are carbohydrate, fat, protein, and vitamins.

oropharyngeal (OR-row-fah-ren-JEE-al): involving the mouth and pharynx.

oropharyngeal dysphagia: difficulty transferring food from the mouth and pharynx to the esophagus to initiate the swallowing process; usually due to a neurological, muscular, or structural disorder.

osmolality (OZ-moe-LAL-ih-tee): the concentration of osmotically active solutes in a solution, expressed as milliosmoles (mOsm) per kilogram of solvent. Osmotically active solutes affect *osmosis,* the movement of water across semipermeable membranes.

osmolarity: the concentration of osmotically active solutes in a solution, expressed as milliosmoles per liter of solution (mOsm/L). *Osmolality* (mOsm/kg) is an alternative measure used to describe a solution's osmotic properties.

osmosis: movement of water across a membrane toward the side where solutes are more concentrated.

osteoarthritis: a painful, chronic disease of the joints that occurs when the cushioning cartilage in a joint breaks down; joint structure is usually altered, with loss of function; also called *degenerative arthritis.*

osteomalacia (os-tee-oh-mal-AY-shuh): a bone disease characterized by softening of the bones. Symptoms include bending of the spine and bowing of the legs. The disease occurs most often in adults with renal failure or malabsorption disorders.

osteopathic (OS-tee-oh-PATH-ic) manipulation: a CAM technique performed by a doctor of osteopathy (D.O., or osteopath) that includes deep tissue massage and manipulation of the joints, spine, and soft tissues. A D.O. is a fully trained and licensed medical physician, although osteopathic manipulation has not been proved to be an effective treatment.

osteoporosis (os-tee-oh-pore-OH-sis): literally, porous bones; reduced density of the bones, also known as *adult bone loss*.

outbreaks: two or more cases of a similar illness resulting from the ingestion of a common food.

overnutrition: overconsumption of food energy or nutrients sufficient to cause disease or increased susceptibility to disease; a form of malnutrition.

overweight: body weight greater than the weight range that is considered healthy; BMI 25.0 to 29.9.

ovo-vegetarian diet: an eating pattern that includes eggs, vegetables, grains, legumes, fruits, and nuts; excludes meat, poultry, seafood, and milk and milk products.

ovum (OH-vum): the female reproductive cell, capable of developing into a new organism upon fertilization; commonly referred to as an egg.

oxalates: plant compounds found in green leafy vegetables and some other foods; these compounds can bind to minerals in the GI tract and form complexes that cannot be absorbed.

oxidation (OKS-ee-day-shun): the process of a substance combining with oxygen.

pancreas: a gland that secretes digestive enzymes and juices into the duodenum. (The pancreas also secretes hormones that help to maintain glucose homeostasis into the blood.)

pancreatic (pank-ree-AT-ic) juice: the exocrine secretion of the pancreas, containing enzymes for the digestion of carbohydrate, fat, and protein. Juice flows from the pancreas into the small intestine through the pancreatic duct. The pancreas also has an endocrine function, the secretion of insulin and other hormones.

paracentesis (pah-rah-sen-TEE-sis): a surgical puncture of a body cavity with an aspirator to draw out excess fluid.

parathyroid hormone: a protein hormone secreted by the parathyroid glands that helps to regulate serum concentrations of calcium and phosphate.

parenteral (par-EN-ter-al) nutrition: the provision of nutrients by vein, bypassing the intestine.

partial vegetarian diet: a term sometimes used to describe an eating pattern that includes seafood, poultry, eggs, milk and milk products, vegetables, grains, legumes, fruit, and nuts; excludes or strictly limits certain meats, such as red meat. Also called *semi-vegetarian*.

pasteurization: heat processing of food that inactivates some, but not all, microorganisms in the food; not a sterilization process. Bacteria that cause spoilage are still present.

pathogenic: capable of causing disease.

pathogens (PATH-oh-jens): microorganisms capable of producing disease.

patient autonomy: a principle of self-determination, such that patients (or surrogate decision makers) are free to choose the medical interventions that are acceptable to them, even if they choose to refuse interventions that may extend their lives.

pellagra (pell-AY-gra): the niacin-deficiency disease. Symptoms include the "4 Ds": diarrhea, dermatitis, dementia, and, ultimately, death.

pepsin: a protein-digesting enzyme (gastric protease) in the stomach. It circulates as a precursor, pepsinogen, and is converted to pepsin by the action of stomach acid.

peptic ulcer: an open sore in the GI mucosa; may develop in the esophagus, stomach, or duodenum.

pernicious anemia: vitamin B_{12} deficiency that results from lack of intrinsic factor; may be evidenced by macrocytic anemia, muscle weakness, and neurological damage.

periodontal disease: disease that involves the connective tissues that support the teeth.

periodontitis: inflammation or degeneration of the tissues that support the teeth.

periodontium: the tissues that support the teeth, including the gums, cementum (bonelike material covering the dentin layer of the tooth), periodontal ligament, and underlying bone.

peripheral artery disease: impaired blood flow in the arteries of the legs; may cause pain and weakness in the legs and feet, especially during exercise. The presence of pain or discomfort while walking is known as *intermittent claudication*.

peripheral parenteral nutrition (PPN): the infusion of nutrient solutions into peripheral veins, usually a vein in the arm or back of the hand.

peripheral vascular disease: a condition characterized by impaired blood circulation in the limbs.

peripheral veins: the small-diameter veins that carry blood from the limbs.

peristalsis (peri-STALL-sis): successive waves of involuntary muscular contractions passing along the walls of the GI tract that push the contents along.

peritoneal (PEH-rih-toe-NEE-al) dialysis: a treatment that removes fluids and wastes from the blood by using the body's peritoneal membrane as a filter.

peritonitis: inflammation of the peritoneal membrane.

pernicious (per-NISH-us) anemia: a blood disorder that reflects a vitamin B_{12} deficiency caused by lack of intrinsic factor and characterized by large, immature red blood cells and damage to the nervous system (*pernicious* means "highly injurious or destructive").

persistent vegetative state: a condition resulting from brain injury in which an awake individual is unresponsive and shows no signs of higher brain function for a prolonged period; usually permanent.

PES statement: a statement that describes a nutrition problem in a format that includes the problem (P), the etiology or cause (E), and the signs and symptoms (S).

pH: the concentration of hydrogen ions. The lower the pH, the stronger the acid. Thus, pH 2 is a strong acid; pH 6 is a weak acid; pH 7 is neutral; and a pH above 7 is alkaline.

phagocytes (FAG-oh-sites): immune cells (neutrophils and macrophages) that have the ability to engulf and destroy antigens.

pharynx (FAIR-inks): the passageway leading from the nose and mouth to the larynx and esophagus, respectively.

phenylketonuria (FEN-il-KEY-toe-NU-ree-ah) or PKU: an inherited disorder characterized by a defect in the enzyme phenylalanine hydroxylase, which normally converts the essential amino acid phenylalanine to the amino acid tyrosine. The condition is named after the phenylalanine metabolites—called *phenylketones*—that are excreted in the urine of individuals who have the disorder.

phlebitis (fleh-BYE-tiss): inflammation of a vein.

phospholipids: one of the three main classes of lipids; compounds that are similar to triglycerides but have *choline* (or another compound) and a phosphorus-containing acid in place of one of the fatty acids.

physiological age: a person's age as estimated from her or his body's health and probable life expectancy.

phytates: nonnutrient components of grains, legumes, and seeds. Phytates can bind minerals such as iron, zinc, calcium, and magnesium in insoluble complexes in the intestine, and the body excretes them unused.

phytochemicals (FIGH-toe-CHEM-ih-cals): compounds in plants that confer color, taste, and other characteristics. Some phytochemicals are bioactive food components in functional foods. Nutrition in Practice 8 provides details.

pica (PIE-ka): a craving for nonfood substances; also known as *geophagia* (jee-oh-FAY-jee-uh) when referring to clay-eating behavior.

piggyback: the administration of a second solution using a separate port in an intravenous catheter.

pigment: a molecule capable of absorbing certain wavelengths of light so that it reflects only those that we perceive as a certain color.

pituitary (pit-TOO-ih-tary) **gland:** in the brain, the "king gland" that regulates the operation of many other glands.

placenta (pla-SEN-tuh): an organ that develops inside the uterus early in pregnancy, in which maternal and fetal blood circulate in close proximity and exchange materials. The fetus receives nutrients and oxygen across the placenta; the mother's blood picks up carbon dioxide and other waste materials to be excreted via her lungs and kidneys.

plant sterols: steroid compounds produced in plants; those added to commercial food products are extracted from soybeans and pine tree oils. Plant sterols can be hydrogenated to produce *plant stanols*, which have LDL-lowering effects similar to those of plant sterols.

plaque (PLACK): an accumulation of fatty deposits, smooth muscle cells, and fibrous connective tissue that develops in the artery walls. Plaque associated with atherosclerosis is known as **atheromatous** (ATH-er-OH-ma-tus) **plaque.**

plasminogen activator inhibitor-1: a protein that promotes blood clotting by inhibiting blood clot degradation within blood vessels.

polydipsia (POL-ee-DIP-see-ah): excessive thirst.

polymorphisms: variations in DNA sequences of a particular gene. A *single-nucleotide polymorphism*, the most common type of polymorphism, involves the insertion, deletion, or substitution of a single nucleotide in the DNA strand.

polypeptide: 10 or more amino acids bonded together. An intermediate strand of between 4 and 10 amino acids is an *oligopeptide*.

polyphagia (POL-ee-FAY-jee-ah): excessive hunger or food intake.

polysaccharides: long chains of monosaccharide units arranged as starch, glycogen, or fiber.

polyunsaturated fatty acids (PUFA): fatty acids with two or more points of unsaturation. For example, linoleic acid has two such points, and linolenic acid has three. Thus, polyunsaturated *fat* is composed of triglycerides containing a high percentage of PUFA.

polyuria (POL-ee-YOOR-ree-ah): excessive urine production.

portal hypertension: elevated blood pressure in the hepatic portal vein due to obstructed blood flow through the liver and a greater inflow of portal blood.

portion sizes: the quantity of food served or eaten at one meal or snack; *not* a standard amount.

prebiotics: indigestible substances in foods that stimulate the growth of nonpathogenic bacteria within the large intestine.

precursors: compounds that can be converted into other compounds; with regard to vitamins, compounds that can be converted into active vitamins; also known as *provitamins*.

prediabetes: the state of having plasma glucose levels that are higher than normal but not high enough to be diagnosed as diabetes (100–125 mg/dL when fasting or 140–199 mg/dL when measured two hours after ingesting 75 grams of glucose); occurs in individuals who have metabolic defects that often lead to type 2 diabetes.

preeclampsia (PRE-ee-KLAMP-see-ah): a condition characterized by hypertension and protein in the urine during pregnancy.

preformed vitamin A: vitamin A in its active form.

prehypertension: blood pressure values that predict hypertension.

prenatal supplements: nutrient supplements specifically designed to provide the nutrients needed during pregnancy, particularly folate, iron, and calcium, without excesses or unneeded constituents.

pressure gradient: the change in pressure over a given distance. In dialysis, a pressure gradient is created between the blood and the dialysate.

pressure sores: regions of skin and tissue that are damaged due to prolonged pressure on the affected area by an external object, such as a bed, wheelchair, or cast; vulnerable areas of the body include buttocks, hips, and heels. Also called *decubitus* (deh-KYU-bih-tus) *ulcers*.

primary hypertension: hypertension with an unknown cause; also known as **essential hypertension.**

probiotics: live microorganisms from foods or supplements that confer a health benefit when taken in sufficient amounts.

processed foods: foods that have been intentionally changed by the addition of substances, or a method of cooking, preserving, milling, or such.

processed meat: meat that has been preserved or flavored by additives, curing, salting, or smoking. Examples include bacon, ham, hot dogs, jerky, luncheon meats, salami, and other sausages.

promoter: a region of DNA involved with gene activation.

protein digestibility: a measure of the amount of amino acids absorbed from a given protein intake.

protein isolates: proteins that have been isolated from foods.

protein turnover: the continuous breakdown and synthesis of body proteins involving the recycling of amino acids.

protein-energy malnutrition (PEM): a state of malnutrition characterized by depletion of tissue proteins and energy stores, usually accompanied by micronutrient deficiencies.

protein-energy wasting: a syndrome characterized by losses of muscle mass and energy reserves that result from the complications of kidney disease.

proteins: compounds made from strands of amino acids composed of carbon, hydrogen, oxygen, and nitrogen atoms. Some amino acids also contain sulfur atoms.

proteinuria (PRO-teen-NOO-ree-ah): the presence of protein in the urine. When only urinary albumin is measured, the term used is *albuminuria*.

proton-pump inhibitors: a class of drugs that inhibit the enzyme that pumps hydrogen ions (protons) into the stomach. Examples include omeprazole (Prilosec) and lansoprazole (Prevacid).

pruritis: itchy skin.

puberty: the period in life in which a person becomes physically capable of reproduction.

purines (PYOO-reens): products of nucleotide metabolism that degrade to uric acid.

pyloric (pie-LORE-ic) **sphincter:** the circular muscle that separates the stomach from the small intestine and regulates the flow of partially digested food into the small intestine; also called *pylorus* or *pyloric valve*.

qi gong (chee-GUNG): a traditional Chinese system that combines movement, meditation, and breathing techniques and allegedly cures illness by enhancing the flow of qi (energy) within the body.

quality of life: a person's perceived physical and mental well-being.

radiation enteritis: inflammation of intestinal tissue caused by radiation therapy.

radiation therapy: the use of X-rays, gamma rays, or atomic particles to destroy cancer cells.

rancid: the term used to describe fats when they have deteriorated, usually by oxidation. Rancid fats often have an "off" odor.

raw sugar: the first crop of crystals harvested during sugar processing. Raw sugar cannot be sold in the United States because it contains too much filth (dirt, insect fragments, and the like). Sugar sold as "raw sugar" is actually evaporated cane juice.

rebound hyperglycemia: hyperglycemia that results from the release of counterregulatory hormones following nighttime hypoglycemia; also called the *Somogyi effect*.

Recommended Dietary Allowances (RDA): a set of values reflecting the average daily amounts of nutrients considered adequate to meet the known nutrient needs of practically all healthy people in a particular life stage and gender group; a goal for dietary intake by individuals.

rectum: the muscular terminal part of the intestine, extending from the sigmoid colon to the anus.

RED-S (relative energy deficiency in sport): a syndrome of impaired physiological function including, but not limited to, metabolic rate, menstrual function, bone health, immunity, protein synthesis, and cardiovascular health caused by relative energy deficiency.

refeeding syndrome: a condition that sometimes develops when a severely malnourished person is aggressively fed; characterized by electrolyte and fluid imbalances and hyperglycemia.

refined grain: a grain or grain product from which the bran, germ, and husk have been removed, leaving only the endosperm.

reflexology: a technique that applies pressure or massage on areas of the hands or feet to allegedly cure disease or relieve pain in other areas of the body; sometimes called *zone therapy*.

reflux esophagitis: inflammation in the esophagus resulting from the reflux of acidic stomach contents.

registered dietitian (RD): an alternative term for an RDN.

registered dietitian nutritionists (RDNs): food and nutrition experts who have earned a minimum of a bachelor's degree from an accredited university or college after completing a program of coursework approved by the Academy of Nutrition and Dietetics (or Dietitians of Canada); also called registered dietitians (RDs). The dietitians must serve in an approved, supervised internship or coordinated program to practice the necessary skills, pass the registration examination, and maintain competency through continuing education. Many states require licensing for practicing dietitians. Licensed dietitians (LDs) have met all state requirements to offer nutrition advice.

regular diet: a diet that includes all foods and meets the nutrient needs of healthy people; may also be called a *standard diet, general diet, normal diet,* or *house diet.*

renal (REE-nal): pertaining to the kidneys.

renal colic: the intense pain that occurs when a kidney stone passes through the ureter; the pain typically begins in the back and intensifies as the stone travels toward the bladder.

renal osteodystrophy: a bone disorder that develops in patients with chronic kidney disease as a result of increased secretion of parathyroid hormone, reduced serum calcium, acidosis, and impaired vitamin D activation by the kidneys.

renal threshold: the blood concentration of a substance that exceeds the kidneys' capacity for reabsorption, causing the substance to be passed into the urine.

renin (REN-in): an enzyme released by the kidneys in response to low blood pressure that helps them retain water through the renin–angiotensin mechanism.

requirement: the lowest continuing intake of a nutrient that will maintain a specified criterion of adequacy.

resection: the surgical removal of part of an organ or body structure.

residue: material left in the intestine after digestion; includes mostly dietary fiber, undigested starches and proteins, GI secretions, and cellular debris.

resistance training: the use of free weights or weight machines to provide resistance for developing muscle strength, power, and endurance; also called *weight training.* A person's own body weight may also be used to provide resistance, as when a person does push-ups, pull-ups, or abdominal crunches.

resistant starches: starches that escape digestion and absorption in the small intestine of healthy people.

resistin (re-ZIST-in): a hormone produced by adipose cells that promotes insulin resistance.

respiratory failure: a potentially life-threatening condition in which inadequate respiratory function impairs gas exchange between the air and circulating blood, resulting in abnormal levels of tissue gases.

respiratory stress: a condition characterized by abnormal oxygen and carbon dioxide levels in body tissues due to abnormal gas exchange between the air and blood.

responsive feeding: an interactive feeding process in which a young child signals hunger and satiety vocally, through facial expressions, and through motor actions; the caregiver recognizes these cues and responds promptly in an emotionally supportive and developmentally appropriate manner. In this way, the child experiences a predictable response to hunger and satiety signals that supports healthy eating behaviors.

resting metabolic rate (RMR): a measure of the energy use of a person at rest in a comfortable setting—similar to the BMR but with less stringent criteria for recent food intake and physical activity. Consequently, the RMR is slightly higher than the BMR.

retina (RET-in-uh): the layer of light-sensitive nerve cells lining the back of the inside of the eye; consists of rods and cones.

retinol activity equivalents (RAE): a measure of vitamin A activity; the amount of retinol that the body will derive from a food containing preformed retinol or its precursor beta-carotene.

retinol-binding protein (RBP): the specific protein responsible for transporting retinol. Measurement of the blood concentration of RBP is a sensitive test of vitamin A status.

rheumatoid arthritis: a disease of the immune system involving painful inflammation of the joints and related structures.

rhodopsin (ro-DOP-sin): a light-sensitive pigment of the retina; contains the retinal form of vitamin A and the protein opsin.

rickets: the vitamin D–deficiency disease in children.

rooting reflex: a reflex that causes an infant to turn toward whichever cheek is touched, in search of a nipple.

saliva: the secretion of the salivary glands. The principal enzyme is salivary amylase.

salivary glands: exocrine glands that secrete saliva into the mouth.

salts: compounds composed of charged particles (ions). An example of a salt is potassium chloride (K^+C^-).

sarcopenia (SAR-koh-PEE-nee-ah): age-related loss of skeletal muscle mass, muscle strength, and muscle function.

satiation (say-she-AY-shun): the feeling of satisfaction and fullness that occurs during a meal and halts eating. Satiation determines how much food is consumed during a meal.

satiety: the feeling of fullness and satisfaction that occurs after a meal and inhibits eating until the next meal. Satiety determines how much time passes between meals.

saturated fatty acid: a fatty acid carrying the maximum possible number of hydrogen atoms (having no points of unsaturation).

screen time: sedentary time spent using an electronic device, such as a television, computer, or video-game player.

scurvy: the vitamin C–deficiency disease.

secondary hypertension: hypertension that results from a known physiological abnormality.

segmentation: periodic squeezing or partitioning of the intestine by its circular muscles that both mixes and slowly pushes the contents along.

selective menus: menus that provide choices in some or all menu categories.

self-efficacy: a person's belief in his or her ability to succeed in an undertaking.

self-monitoring of blood glucose: home monitoring of blood glucose levels using a glucose meter.

semipermeable membrane: a membrane that allows some, but not all, particles to pass through.

senile dementia: the loss of brain function beyond the normal loss of physical adeptness and memory that occurs with aging.

senile plaques: clumps of the protein fragment beta-amyloid on the nerve cells, commonly found in the brains of people with Alzheimer's dementia.

sepsis: a whole-body inflammatory response caused by infection; characterized by signs and symptoms similar to those of *systemic inflammatory response syndrome*.

set-point theory: the theory that the body tends to maintain a certain weight by means of its own internal controls.

severe acute malnutrition (SAM): malnutrition caused by recent severe food restriction; characterized in children by underweight for height (wasting).

shear stress: a stress that occurs sideways against a surface rather than perpendicular to a surface. In blood vessels, disturbed blood flow can be harmful to endothelial cells, whereas regular blood flow is protective against atherosclerosis.

short bowel syndrome: the malabsorption syndrome that follows resection of the small intestine; characterized by inadequate absorptive capacity in the remaining intestine.

shock: a severe reduction in blood flow that deprives the body's tissues of oxygen and nutrients; characterized by reduced blood pressure, raised heart and respiratory rates, and muscle weakness.

sinusoids: the small, capillary-like passages that carry blood through liver tissue.

Sjögren's (SHOW-grenz) syndrome: an autoimmune disease characterized by the destruction of secretory glands, resulting in dry mouth and dry eyes.

skinfold measure: a clinical estimate of total body fatness in which the thickness of a fold of skin on the back of the arm (over the triceps muscle), below the shoulder blade (subscapular), or in other places is measured with a caliper.

small intestine: a 10-foot length of small-diameter intestine that is the major site of digestion of food and absorption of nutrients. Its segments are the duodenum, jejunum, and ileum.

soaps: chemical compounds formed from fatty acids and positively charged minerals.

solid fats: fats that are not usually liquid at room temperature; commonly found in most foods derived from animals and vegetable oils that have been hydrogenated. Solid fats typically contain more saturated and *trans* fats than most oils.

soluble fibers: indigestible food components that readily dissolve in water and often impart gummy or gel-like characteristics to foods. An example is pectin from fruit, which is used to thicken jellies.

soy milk: a milk-like beverage made from ground soybeans. Soy milk should be fortified with vitamin A, vitamin D, riboflavin, and calcium to approach the nutritional equivalency of milk.

spasm: a sudden, forceful, and involuntary muscle contraction.

Special Supplemental Nutrition Program for Women, Infants, and Children (WIC): a high-quality, cost-effective health care and nutrition services program administered by the U.S. Department of Agriculture for low-income women, infants, and children who are nutritionally at risk. WIC provides supplemental foods, nutrition education, and referrals to health care and other social services.

specialized formulas: enteral formulas for patients with specific illnesses; also called *disease-specific formulas* or *specialty formulas*.

specialized nutrition support: the delivery of nutrients using a feeding tube or intravenous infusions, often referred to simply as *nutrition support*.

sphincter (SFINK-ter): a circular muscle surrounding, and able to close, a body opening. Sphincters are found at specific points along the GI tract and regulate the flow of food particles.

spina (SPY-nah) bifida (BIFF-ih-dah): one of the most common types of neural tube defects; characterized by the incomplete closure of the spinal cord and its bony encasement.

standard formulas: enteral formulas that contain mostly intact proteins and polysaccharides; also called *polymeric formulas*.

starch: a plant polysaccharide composed of glucose and digestible by human beings.

steatohepatitis (STEE-ah-to-HEP-ah-TYE-tis): liver inflammation that is associated with fatty liver.

steatorrhea (stee-AT-or-REE-ah): excessive fat in the stool due to fat malabsorption; characterized by stools that are loose, frothy, and foul smelling due to a high fat content.

sterile: free of microorganisms such as bacteria.

steroids (STARE-oids): medications used to reduce tissue inflammation, to suppress the immune response, or to replace certain steroid hormones in people who cannot synthesize them.

sterols: one of the main classes of lipids; includes cholesterol, vitamin D, and the sex hormones (such as testosterone).

stoma (STOE-ma): a surgically created opening in a body tissue or organ.

stomach: a muscular, elastic, saclike portion of the digestive tract that grinds and churns swallowed food, mixing it with acid and enzymes to form chyme.

stress fractures: bone damage or breaks caused by stress on bone surfaces during exercise.

stress response: the chemical and physical changes that occur within the body during stress.

stricture: abnormal narrowing of a passageway; often due to inflammation, scarring, or a congenital abnormality.

stroke: sudden death of brain cells due to impaired blood flow to the brain or rupture of an artery in the brain; also called a *cerebrovascular accident*.

structure–function claims: statements that describe how a product may affect a structure or function of the body; for example, "calcium builds strong bones." Structure–function claims do not require FDA authorization.

struvite (STROO-vite): crystals of magnesium ammonium phosphate.

stunting: low height for age, indicating restriction of potential growth in children.

subcutaneous (sub-cue-TAY-nee-us): beneath the skin.

subcutaneous fat: fat stored directly under the skin.

sucrose: a disaccharide composed of glucose and fructose; commonly known as *table sugar*, *beet sugar*, or *cane sugar*.

sugar alcohols: sugarlike compounds in the chemical family *alcohol* derived from fruits or manufactured from carbohydrates; sugar alcohols are absorbed more slowly than other sugars, are metabolized differently, and do not elevate the risk of dental caries. Examples are maltitol, mannitol, sorbitol, isomalt, lactitol, and xylitol.

sushi: vinegar-flavored rice and seafood, typically wrapped in seaweed and stuffed with colorful vegetables. Some sushi is stuffed with raw fish; other varieties contain cooked seafood.

syringes: devices used for injecting medications. A syringe consists of a hypodermic needle attached to a hollow tube with a plunger inside.

systemic (sih-STEM-ic): affecting the entire body.

systemic inflammatory response syndrome (SIRS): a whole-body inflammatory response caused by severe illness or trauma; characterized by raised heart and respiratory rates, abnormal white blood cell counts, and fever.

tannins: compounds in tea (especially black tea) and coffee that bind iron.

teratogenic (ter-AT-oh-jen-ik): causing abnormal fetal development and birth defects.

therapeutic touch: a technique of passing hands over a patient to purportedly identify energy imbalances and transfer healing power from therapist to patient; also called *laying on of hands*.

thermic effect of food: an estimation of the energy required to process food (digest, absorb, transport, metabolize, and store ingested nutrients).

thrombosis (throm-BOH-sis): the formation or presence of a blood clot in blood vessels. A *coronary thrombosis* occurs in a coronary artery, and a *cerebral thrombosis* occurs in an artery that supplies blood to the brain.

thrombus: a blood clot formed within a blood vessel that remains attached to its place of origin.

tocopherol (tuh-KOFF-er-ol): a general term for several chemically related compounds, one of which has vitamin E activity.

Tolerable Upper Intake Levels (UL): a set of values reflecting the highest average daily nutrient intake levels that are likely to pose no risk of toxicity to almost all healthy individuals in a particular life stage and gender group. As intake increases above the UL, the potential risk of adverse health effects increases.

tolerance level: the maximum amount of residue permitted in a food when a pesticide is used according to the label directions.

total nutrient admixture (TNA): a parenteral solution that contains dextrose, amino acids, and lipids; also called a **3-in-1 solution** or an **all-in-one solution**.

total parenteral nutrition (TPN): the infusion of nutrient solutions into a central vein.

trace minerals: essential mineral nutrients required in the adult diet in amounts less than 100 milligrams per day.

traditional Chinese medicine (TCM): an approach to health care based on the concept that illness can be cured by enhancing the flow of qi (energy) within a person's body. Treatments may include herbal therapies, physical exercises, meditation, acupuncture, and remedial massage.

transcription factors: proteins that bind DNA at specific sequences to regulate gene expression.

***trans*-fatty acids:** fatty acids in which the hydrogen atoms next to the double bond are on opposite sides of the carbon chain.

transferrin (trans-FERR-in): the body's iron-carrying protein.

transient ischemic attacks (TIAs): brief ischemic strokes that cause short-term neurological symptoms.

transjugular intrahepatic portosystemic shunt: a passage within the liver that connects a portion of the portal vein to the hepatic vein using a stent; access to the liver is gained via the jugular vein in the neck.

traveler's diarrhea: nausea, vomiting, and diarrhea caused by consuming food or water contaminated by any of several organisms, most commonly *E. coli*, *Shigella*, *Campylobacter jejuni*, and *Salmonella*.

triglycerides (try-GLISS-er-rides): one of the main classes of lipids: the chief form of fat in foods and the major storage form of fat in the body; composed of glycerol with three fatty acids attached.

trimester: a period representing one-third of the term of gestation. A trimester is about 13 to 14 weeks.

tripeptide: three amino acids bonded together.

tube feedings: liquid formulas delivered through a tube placed in the stomach or intestine.

tubules: tubelike structures of the nephron that process filtrate during urine production. The tubules are surrounded by capillaries that reabsorb substances retained by tubule cells.

tumor: an abnormal tissue mass that has no physiological function; also called a *neoplasm* (NEE-oh-plazm). Tumors may be malignant (cancerous) or benign (noncancerous).

turbinado (ter-bih-NOD-oh) **sugar:** raw sugar from which the filth has been washed; legal to sell in the United States.

type 1 diabetes: diabetes that is characterized by absolute insulin deficiency, usually resulting from the autoimmune destruction of pancreatic beta cells.

type 2 diabetes: diabetes that is characterized by insulin resistance coupled with insufficient insulin secretion.

ulcerative colitis (ko-LY-tis): an inflammatory bowel disease that involves the rectum and colon; the inflammation affects the mucosa and submucosa of the intestinal wall.

ultrafiltration: removal of fluids and solutes from the blood by using pressure to transfer the blood across a semipermeable membrane.

umbilical (um-BIL-ih-cul) **cord:** the ropelike structure through which the fetus's veins and arteries reach the placenta; the route of nourishment and oxygen into the fetus and the route of waste disposal from the fetus.

undernutrition: underconsumption of food energy or nutrients severe enough to cause disease or increased susceptibility to disease; a form of malnutrition.

underweight: body weight lower than the weight range that is considered healthy; BMI below 18.5.

unsaturated fatty acid: a fatty acid with one or more points of unsaturation where hydrogen atoms are missing (includes monounsaturated and polyunsaturated fatty acids).

urea (yoo-REE-uh): the principal nitrogen-excretion product of protein metabolism; generated mostly by removal of amine groups from unneeded amino acids or from the sacrifice of amino acids to meet a need for energy.

urea kinetic modeling: a method of determining the adequacy of dialysis treatment by calculating the urea clearance from blood.

uremia (you-REE-me-ah): the accumulation of nitrogenous and various other waste products in the blood (literally, "urine in the blood"); may also be used to indicate the toxic state that results when wastes are retained in the blood. The related term *azotemia* refers specifically to the accumulation of nitrogenous wastes in the blood.

uremic syndrome: the cluster of disorders caused by inadequate kidney function; complications include fluid, electrolyte, and hormonal imbalances; altered heart function; neuromuscular disturbances; and other metabolic derangements.

USDA Food Patterns: the USDA's food group plan for ensuring dietary adequacy that assigns foods to five major food groups.

uterus (YOO-ter-us): the womb, the muscular organ within which the infant develops before birth.

varices (VAH-rih-seez): abnormally dilated blood vessels (singular: *varix*).

variety: consumption of a wide selection of foods within and among the major food groups (the opposite of monotony).

vegan diet: an eating pattern that includes only plant-based foods: vegetables, grains, legumes, fruit, seeds, and nuts; excludes all animal-derived foods; also called *strict vegetarian, pure vegetarian,* or *total vegetarian*.

vegetarian diet: a general term used to describe an eating pattern that includes plant-based foods and eliminates some or all animal-derived foods.

vein: a vessel that carries blood back to the heart.

very-low-density lipoproteins (VLDL): lipoproteins that transport triglycerides from the liver to other tissues; in clinical practice, VLDL are commonly referred to as *blood triglycerides*.

vigorous-intensity physical activity: physical activity that requires a large increase in breathing and/or heart rate and expends more than 7 kcalories per minute. Walking at a very brisk pace (>4.5 miles per hour) or running at a pace of at least 5 miles per hour are examples.

villi (VILL-ee or VILL-eye): fingerlike projections from the folds of the small intestine. The singular form is **villus**.

visceral fat: fat stored within the abdominal cavity in association with the internal abdominal organs, as opposed to fat stored directly under the skin (subcutaneous fat); also called *intra-abdominal fat*.

viscous: having a gel-like consistency.

vitamin A: a fat-soluble vitamin with three chemical forms: *retinol* (the alcohol form), *retinal* (the aldehyde form), and *retinoic acid* (the acid form).

vitamin D_2: vitamin D derived from plants in the diet; also called *ergocalciferol* (ER-go-kal-SIF-er-ol).

vitamin D_3: vitamin D derived from animals in the diet or made in the skin from 7-dehydrocholesterol, a precursor of cholesterol, with the help of sunlight; also called *cholecalciferol* (KO-lee-kal-SIF-er-ol).

vitamins: essential, non-kcaloric, organic nutrients needed in tiny amounts in the diet.

voluntary activities: the component of a person's daily energy expenditure that involves conscious and deliberate muscular work—walking, lifting, climbing, and other physical activities. Voluntary activities normally require less energy in a day than basal metabolism does.

warfarin: an anticoagulant that works by interfering with vitamin K's blood-clotting function; patients using warfarin need to maintain a consistent vitamin K intake from day to day.

waist circumference: a measurement used to assess a person's abdominal fat.

warfarin: an anticoagulant that works by interfering with vitamin K's blood-clotting function; patients using warfarin need to maintain a consistent vitamin K intake from day to day.

wasting: in malnutrition, thinness for height, indicating recent rapid weight loss, often from severe, acute malnutrition.

water balance: the balance between water intake and water excretion that keeps the body's water content constant.

water intoxication: the rare condition in which body water contents are too high. The symptoms may include confusion, convulsion, coma, and even death in extreme cases.

wean: to gradually replace breast milk with infant formula or other foods.

weight cycling: repeated rounds of weight loss and subsequent regain, with reduced ability to lose weight with each attempt; also called *yo-yo dieting*.

wellness: maximum well-being; the top range of health states; the goal of the person who strives toward realizing his or her full potential physically, mentally, emotionally, spiritually, and socially.

Wernicke-Korsakoff syndrome: severe thiamin deficiency in people who abuse alcohol; symptoms include disorientation, loss of short-term memory, jerky eye movements, and staggering gait.

wheat gluten (GLU-ten): a family of water-insoluble proteins in wheat; includes the gliadin (GLY-ah-din) fractions that are toxic to persons with celiac disease.

white sugar: granulated sucrose or "table sugar," produced by dissolving, concentrating, and recrystallizing raw sugar; 99.9 percent pure.

whole foods: fresh foods such as vegetables, grains, legumes, meats, and milk that are unprocessed or minimally processed.

whole grains: grains or foods made from them that contain all the essential parts and naturally occurring nutrients of the entire grain seed (except the inedible husk).

xerophthalmia (zer-off-THAL-mee-uh): progressive blindness caused by inadequate mucus production due to severe vitamin A deficiency.

xerosis (zee-ROW-sis): abnormal drying of the skin and mucous membranes; a sign of vitamin A deficiency.

xerostomia (ZEE-roh-STOE-me-ah): dry mouth caused by reduced salivary flow.

zygote (ZY-goat): the product of the union of ovum and sperm; a fertilized ovum.

Index

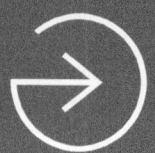

Note: Page numbers in bold indicate where a term is defined; those with f, t, or b indicate figures, tables, and boxes, respectively.

Alpha-lactalbumin, **307**
Alpha-tocopherol, **211**
Altered stomach acidity, 416
Alternative feeding routes, 413
Alternative sweeteners, 73–77
    on food labels, 79f
    nonnutritive sweeteners, 79–81
    sugar alcohols, **78–79**
Alveoli, **477–478**
Alzheimer's disease, **357–359**, 358t
Amenorrhea, **167**
American Academy of Pediatrics
    (AAP), 291, 300, 307
American College of Cardiology
    (ACC), 599
American College of Sports Medicine
    (ACSM), 17
American Heart Association (AHA),
    104, 599
American Heart Association Dietary
    Guidelines and Strategies for
    Children, 348t
Amino acids, **126**, 126f, 218, 450
    composition, 137
    supplements, 135–136, 136t
    vitamin C in amino acid
        metabolism, 222
Amniotic sac, **273**
Amylase, **45**
Anaphylactic shock, **323**
Anemia, 254, 321, 503, 635
    laboratory tests for, E-9
    normal and anemic blood cells, 254f
Anencephaly, **278**
Aneurysm, **596**, 597
Angina pectoris, **596**, 597
Angiotensin-converting enzyme
    (ACE), 627
Anhydrous dextrose, **77**
Animal protein, 249
Anorexia, **380**, **658**
    control, 668
Anorexia nervosa, 161, **166**, 167
    bulimia nervosa *vs.*, 169–170
    risk for, 168
Antacids, 495
Anthropometric data, **389**, 389–391
    anthropometric assessment in
        infants and children, 391
    body weight, 389, 390t, 392b
    circumferences of waist and
        limbs, 391
    head circumference, 390–391, 391t
    height (or length), 389, 390t
    rate of involuntary weight loss
        associated with nutritional risk,
        391t
Antibodies, **131**, 309t
    to intrinsic factor, E-12
Anticonvulsants, **418**
Antidiabetic drugs, 583, 583t
Antidiuretic hormone (ADH), **239**

Antiemetic drugs, 660
Antiemetics, **416**
Antigens, **131**, **322**
Antihypertensive drugs, 635
"Anti-infective" vitamin, 204
Antineoplastic drugs, **416**
Antioxidants, **99**, **204**, **229**
    beta-carotene's role as, 204
    nutrient, 258
    supplements, 268, 604–605
    vitamin C as, 222
    vitamin E as, 211
Antiretroviral drugs, **416**
Antiulcer drugs, **416**
Anuria, **630**
Anus, **40**, **42**
Appendix, **40**, 42
Appetite, **177–178**
    control, 185
Aromatic amino acids, **551**
Artery, **50**
Arthritis, **356**
Artificial fats, **113**
Ascites, **550**, **614**
Ascorbic acid, **222**
-ase, 45
Aspartame, 81
Aspartate aminotransferase (AST), 546
Aspiration, **437**
    pneumonia, **437**
Associations, 3
Asthma, 163
Atazanavir, 418
Atherogenic lipoproteins, **598**
Atheromatous plaque, **345**
Atherosclerosis, **102**, 230, **346**, 512,
    596, 597–598
    causes, 597–598
    consequences, 597
Athletes, eating disorders in, 168
Atrophic gastritis, **221**, **362**, **498**
Attention-deficit/hyperactivity
    disorder (ADHD), **324**
Attitude, behavior and, 186–188
Autoimmune, **567**
Autonomic neuropathy, 572
Availability, 4–5

B

Bacterial overgrowth, **503**, **521**, 521
Bacterial translocation, **521**, **544**
Balance, **13**
Bariatric surgery, **500**, 503–505
    altering dietary habits to achieving
        and maintaining weight loss, 505
    bariatric surgical procedures,
        503–504
    nutrition care after bariatric surgery,
        504–505
    postsurgical concerns, 505
Barrett's esophagus, **495**
Basal insulin, 580

Basal metabolic rate (BMR), **152**,
    153t, 185. *See also* Resting
    metabolic rate (RMR)
Basal metabolism, **152**
Bases, **131**
Behavior
    changes in overweight children, 329
    hunger and, 320
    iron deficiency and, 320
    modification, **186**, 187b
Behavior and attitude, 186–188
    aware of behaviors, 186–187
    cognitive skills, 188
    personal attitude, 188
    small changes, 187
Beneficence, **675**
Beriberi, **215**
Beta-carotene, **203–207**
    conversion and toxicity, 206, 206f
    in foods, 207
    role as antioxidant, 204
Beverages, 338
Bicarbonate, **45**, **46**
Bifidus factors, 309t
Bile, **45**, **46**
Bile acid
    binders, 416
    sequestrants, 605
Binders, **248**
Binge eating, 170
    disorder, **166**
Bioactive food components, **2**, **229**
Bioavailability, **201**
Biochemical analysis, 392–394
    albumin, 392–394
    CRP, 394
    routine laboratory tests with
        nutritional implications,
        393t–394t
    serum proteins, 392
    transferrin, 394
    transthyretin and retinol-binding
        protein, 394
Bioelectrical impedance, E-7
Bioelectrical therapies, **429**
Bioelectromagnetic therapies, **429**
Biofeedback training, **426**
Biofield therapies, **429**
Biologically based therapies, 426
Biotin, 215
    deficiency, 218
Blastocyst, **274**
Blenderized formulas, **439**
Blenderized liquid diet, 410
Blind loops, **521**
Bloating, **496**
    and stomach gas, 497
Blood
    fluid removed from, 649
    glucose regulation, 72–73
    lipid, 627
    lipid profile. *See* Lipoprotein profile

Colectomy, **530**
Colestid, 605
Collagen, **222**
Collagen formation, vitamin C's role in, 222
Collateral vessels, **550**
Colon, diverticular disease of, 535–536
Colostomy, **536–538**
    diarrhea, 538
    nutrition care for patients with ostomies, 536–537
    obstructions, 537
    reducing gas and odors, 537
Colostrum, **307–308**
Combat anorexia and wasting, medications to, 660
Combination foods, C-16
Competitive foods, 335
Complement, **470, 473**
Complementary and alternative medicine (CAM), 424t, 424–430, 660–661
    alleged effects of "energy" therapies, 429–430
    alternative medical systems, 425–426
    biologically based therapies, 426
    cleansing practices, 428–429
    health care professionals, 430
    herbal products, 427t, 427–428
    herbal remedies, 426–427
    knowledge of, by health professionals, 424
    mind-body practices, 426
    physical manipulation, 429
    practices, 424
    in United States, 424
Complementary foods, **311**
Complementary proteins, 137, 138f, **138**
Computed tomography (CT), 676
Concentrated fruit juice sweetener, **77**
Conditionally essential amino acid, **127**
Confectioners' sugar, **77**
Conjugated linoleic acid, **100**
Constipation, 286, 514–516
    causes, 514
    laxatives, 515–516
    medical interventions, 516
    treatment, 514–515
Continuous ambulatory peritoneal dialysis (CAPD), 650
Continuous feedings, **443**, 444
Continuous glucose monitoring, **574**
Continuous parenteral nutrition, **454**
Continuous renal replacement therapy (CRRT), **651**
Contraindications to breastfeeding, 294–296
    alcohol, 295
    maternal illness, 295–296
    medications and illicit drugs, 295
    tobacco and caffeine, 295

Controlling potassium distribution, 244
Convenience, 4–5
Conversion factors, A-2
Copper, 260
    copper recommendations and food sources, 260
    deficiency, 260
    toxicity, 260
Cornea, **203**
Corn sweeteners, **77**
Coronary artery disease. *See* Coronary heart disease (CHD)
Coronary heart disease (CHD), 345, 346, **596**, 599–607
    drug therapies for CHD prevention, 605
    evaluating risk for, 599–600
    heart-healthy diet, 604t
    laboratory measures, 599t
    lifestyle changes for hypertriglyceridemia, 605
    lifestyle management to reducing CHD risk, 600–603, 601t
    symptoms, 599
    treatment of heart attack, 607
    vitamin supplementation and CHD risk, 603–605
Corticosteroids, 420, 641
Coumadin, 419
Cow's milk, transition to, 311
Cranberries, 231
Creatinine, **626**
Crestor, 605
Cretinism, **260**
Critical periods, **275–276**
Crohn's disease, **528–531**
    comparison with ulcerative colitis, 529t
    complications, 529–530
    management of symptoms and complications, 531t
    nutrition therapy for, 530
Crying, 306
Cryptosporidiosis, **670**
Cultural competence, 2
Cuprimine, 644
Cyanosis, **481**
Cyclic feedings, **444**
Cyclic parenteral nutrition, **454**
Cyclosporine, 641
Cystic fibrosis, **464**, **524**, 524–525
    consequences, 524–525
    nutrition therapy for, 525
Cystine stones, 643, 644
Cystinuria, **643**
Cytokines, **470, 472, 591, 592, 658**

D

Daily meals
    calcium to, 249b
    iron to, 257b

Daily Values, **26**, 27t
Dancers, eating disorders in, 168
Daraprim, 416
DASH Eating Plan, 603, 612, 612t
Dawn phenomenon, **583**
Debridement, **474**
Decision-making capacity, **675**
Deep vein thrombosis, **627**
Defibrillation, **676**
Deficiency diseases, 355
Degenerative arthritis, 356
Dehydration, **238**, 239t, 362, 396, 642
Dehydroepiandrosterone (DHEA), 428
Denaturation, **131**
Dental calculus, **510**
Dental caries, **74**, **509**
    nutrient deficiencies affecting development, 510t
    sugar and, 75–76
Dental diseases
    adverse effects on health effects on teeth, 512
    chronic diseases influencing person's risk, 511
    dental plaque contributing to, 510
Dental plaque, **509**
    contributing to dental diseases, 510
Depression, 365
Dermatitis herpetiformis condition, **527**
Desserts, C-8–C-10
Developmental origins of health and disease, 346
Dextrose, **77**
    monohydrate, 452
Diabetes. *See* Diabetes mellitus
Diabetes mellitus, **72**, 82, 163, 283, 511, 512, **566**, 598
    antidiabetic drugs, 583, 583t
    chronic complications, 571–572
    diagnosis, 567
    diet-drug interactions, 584b
    effects of insulin insufficiency, 570f
    insulin therapy, 580–583
    nutrition therapy, 575–580
    physical activity and diabetes management, 584–585
    in pregnancy, 586–587
    sick-day management, 585
    symptoms, 566–567, 567t
    treatment, 573–585
    types, 567–569
Diabetic coma, **566**, 571
Diabetic ketoacidosis in type 1 diabetes, 570
Diabetic nephropathy, **566, 572**
Diabetic neuropathy, **566, 572**
Diabetic retinopathy, **566, 572**
Dialysate, **635**, 648–650
Dialysis, **631**, 635, 648–651, **676**
    advantages and disadvantages of peritoneal dialysis, 650–651

Faith healing, **426**
Fashion criterion, 157
Fast foods, C-17–C-18
    meals, 207
Fasting, 149–151, 150f
    energy deficit, 149
    glucose needed for brain, 150
    glycogen, 150
    hazards of fasting, 151
    hyperglycemia, **583**
    intermittent fasting, 151
    protein breakdown and ketosis, 150
    slowed metabolism, 151
Fat cell, 96f
    development, 176, 176f
    enlargement, 148f
Fatigue, 658, 667
Fat malabsorption, 502–503, 519–521,
        552
    consequences, 519–520
    fat-restricted diet, 520t, 521f
    nutrition therapy for, 520–521
Fat-restricted diets, 411, 522b
Fats, 6, 117–122, 276–278, 361–362,
        555, C-13–C-14. *See also* Lipids
    in children, 317
    comparison of dietary fats, 112f
    controlling, C-2
    digestion and absorption, 103t
    distinguishing good from bad,
        117–118, 121
    excess, 148
    on food labels, 113–114
    in foods, 107–109, 108t
    health effects and recommended
        intakes, 102–107
    and heart health, 103–106
    heart health and, 110–111b
    and kcalories, 110–112, 111f
    messages about, changes in, 117
    modules, F-5
    recommendations, 106–107
    recommended intakes of, 117
    replacers, **113**
    solid, 110–114
    soluble vitamins, 201–202, 202t
    unsaturated, choosing, 110–114
    USDA food patterns, 122t
Fat-soluble vitamins, 202–214, 214t.
        See also Water-soluble vitamins
    vitamin A and beta-carotene,
        203–207
    vitamin D, 207–211
    vitamin E, 211–212
    vitamin K, 212–214
Fatty acids, **98**–100, 99f
    chain length and saturation, 98
    in children, 317
    essential, 100
    hard and soft fat, 98
    hydrogenation, **99**
    linoleic acid, 100

stability, 99
    trans-fatty acids, 99–100, 100f
    unsaturated, **98**, 99f
Fatty foods, 348
Fatty liver, **546**–547
Fatty streaks, **346**
Feasting, 148, 149f
    excess carbohydrate, 148
    excess fat, 148
    excess protein, 149
Feeding America, 376
Feeding disabilities, 620–623
    ability to eat affected by, 620
    adaptive feeding devices, 621,
        622f
    conditions leading to, 620t
    energy needs altered by, 620
    family life affected by, 623
    health professionals who evaluate
        and treat, 620–621
    interventions, 621t
    physical symptoms of disease
        leading to, 620
Feeding picky eaters, tips for, 332t
Feeding route selection, 434f
Female athlete triad, 166, **167**
Fermentable oligosaccharides,
        disaccharides, monosaccharides,
        and polyols (FODMAPs), **516**
Fermentation, **71**
Fertility, **272**
Fetal alcohol spectrum disorders
        (FASD), **290**
Fetal alcohol syndrome (FAS),
        290, 290f
Fetal chromosomes, 288
Fetal programming, 346
Fetus, **275**, 275f
Fiber, 361
    in carbohydrate-rich foods, 276
    in children, 317
    content, 439
    restriction, 411
    supplements, 515
Fibrates, 605
Fibrinogen, **591**, **593**
Fight-or-flight hormones, 471
Filtrate, **626**
Fish, 602
    oil supplements, 605
Fistulas, **435**, **529**
Fitness, **17**
Fitness guidelines, 16–17. *See also*
        Physical activity
Flatulence, **516**
Flavonoids, **229**, **230**
Flaxseed, **229**, **231**
Fluid and electrolyte balance, 130–131,
        240–241
Fluid retention, **131**, 627
Fluid(s), 452
    in acute kidney injury, 632

in chronic kidney disease, 637
    and electrolyte imbalances, 631
    removed from blood, 649
    retention, 395
Fluorapatite, **261**
Fluoride, 261, 308t
Fluorosis, **261**
Folate, 219–220, 220f, 362, 418f
    alcohol, and drugs, 219
    in foods, 219–220
    status assessment, E-10–E-12
    and vitamin B$_{12}$, 278–279
Folic acid, 219, 278
Follicle, **205**
Food-drug interactions. *See* Diet-drug
        interactions
Food allergy, 313–314, **322**, 322–324
    adverse reactions, 323–324
    allergy detection, 322
    anaphylactic shock, 323
    food dislikes, 324
    food labeling, 323
    immediate and delayed reactions,
        322–323
Food and Drug Administration (FDA),
        25, 35, 57, 79, 210, 230, 310
    FDA-approved drugs for weight
        loss, 181t
Food and nutrition history, 386
Food assistance programs, 281–282,
        320, 376
    for older adults, 365–366t
Foodborne illness, **57**–65, 289
    avoiding, 366
    cause of, 59
    distinguished from food
        intoxications, 57–59
    microbes, 58t
    preventing, 60, 60f, 61–62t
Food group plan, **18**. *See also* USDA
        Food Patterns
Food labels, 24–30, 28–29t, 323. *See
        also* Nutrition Facts panel
    carbohydrates, 86–87
    claims on labels, 27–30
    fats on, 113–114
    ingredient list, 24
    protein on, 138
    sugar alternatives on, 79f
Food(s)
    additives, 324
    allergens, 323f
    aversions, **285**
    banks, **376**
    beta-carotene in, 207
    calcium in, 248
    choices, 2–6
    combining, 49
    composition, 152, 201
    cravings, **285**
    deserts, **178**, **374**

Glycated hemoglobin levels (HbA_{1c} levels), **567**
Glycemic control, **573**
Glycemic index (GI), **82**, 90, **576**
  blood glucose response to high-GI and low-GI foods, 90f
  factors influencing, 92
  high-GI foods, avoiding, 93
  low-GI diet and chronic disease risk, 92–93
  measuring, 90–92
  recommendations, 93
  of selected foods, 91t
Glycemic load (GL), 90
Glycemic response, **82**
Glycogen, **69**, 70f, 150
Glycomacropeptide, 466
Glycosuria, **566**, **567**
Goiter, **259**
Goitrogen, **259**
Gout, **223**, **643**
Graft rejection, **660**
Graft-*vs.*-host disease, **660**
Grains, 84–86
  fats in, 109
Granulated sugar, **77**
Grapefruit juice-drug interactions, 419t
Green vegetables, 217
Growth, 155
  charts, E-1–E-2
  factors, 309t
  nutrients to support, 304–305
  in overweight children, 327

H

Habit, 2
Halal, 3
Half-life, **394**
Hard fat, 98
Harmful bacteria, 310
Hazard Analysis and Critical Control Points (HACCP), **57**, **59**, **414**, **442**
Hazards of fasting, 151
Health, **2**, 5–6
  criterion, 157
  dietary guidelines, fitness guidelines, and food guides, 13–24
  ethnic food choices, 4t
  food choices, 2–6
  food labels, 24–30
  GI tract, 53–54
  health line, 3f
  national nutrition surveys, 11–12
  nutrient recommendations, 8–10
  nutrients, 6–7
  protein and, 132–136
  vitamin D's potential roles in, 208
Health care
  agent, 677
  communities, **361**

professionals, 36–37, 382
  proxy, 677
Health claims, **29**, 30f
  carbohydrates, 86–87
Healthful eating plan, 182–184
  lower energy density, 184
  nutritional adequacy, 183
  realistic energy intake, 182–183
  small portions, 183–184
  sugar and alcohol, 184
Health risks, 161–163
  of overweight and obesity, 162–163
  risk from obesity, 163
  of underweight, 161
Healthy body weight, 156, 157t
  BMI, 157–159
  criterion of fashion, 157
  criterion of health, 157
Healthy dietary pattern, 600
Healthy diet, planning, C-3–C-19
Healthy foods, 178–179
Healthy obese, 162
Healthy people, **11**, 12t
Healthy support tissues, 273–274
Heart attack, treatment of, 607
Heartburn, 286, **495**
Heart disease, 81–82, 134–135, **273**, 401, 512. *See also* Cardiovascular diseases (CVD); Coronary heart disease (CHD)
  sugar and, 75
Heart failure, **614**–615
  consequences, 614
  medical management, 615
Heart health, fats and, 103–106, 110–111b. *See also* Cholesterol
Helicobacter pylori, **498**
Helper T cells, **666**
Hematocrit, **254**, E-10
Hematopoietic stem cell transplantation, **660**
Hematuria, **643**
Hemicellulose, 71
Hemochromatosis, **255**
Hemodialysis, **635**, 648, 649
  complications associating with, 650
  patients requiring, 649
Hemofiltration process, **651**
Hemoglobin, **251**, **254**, E-10
  structure, 127f
Hemolytic anemia, **211**
Hemophilia, **464**
Hemorrhagic disease, **212**
Hemorrhagic strokes, **607**–608
Hepatic coma, **551**
Hepatic encephalopathy, **551**, 551t
Hepatic portal vein, **50**, **549**
Hepatic vein, **50**
Hepatitis, 547–548
  nutrition therapy for, 548
  symptoms and signs, 548

treatment, 548
  viral, 547–548
Hepatitis A virus (HAV), 547
Hepatitis B virus (HBV), 547
Hepatitis C virus (HCV), 547–548
Hepatomegaly, **546**
Hepcidin, **253**, **470**, **473**
Herb-drug interaction, 428t
Herbal remedies, 426
Herbal supplements, 288
Herpes simplex virus infection, **666**
Hiatal hernia, **494**
High blood pressure. *See* Hypertension
High-density lipoproteins (HDL), **51**, **598**
High-dose chemotherapy, 660
High energy density, **635**
High-fructose corn syrup (HFCS), **68**, **77**
High-kcalorie diet, 412, 412t
High-protein diets, 412, 412t, 628
High-protein foods, 638
High-protein supplements, 278
High-quality proteins, **137**
High-risk pregnancy, **275**, 276t
Histamine-2 receptor blockers (H2 blockers), **495**
HIV enteropathy. *See* Acquired immunodeficiency syndrome (AIDS)—enteropathy
Home enteral nutrition, 457–458
Home nutrition support, 457–458
Homeopathy, **425**–426
Homeostasis, **53**
Home parenteral nutrition, 458
Homocysteine, **598**, 604
Honey, **77**
Honeymoon period, 582
Hormonal imbalances, 634
Hormone(s), **53**, 131–132, 428
  altered, 633–634
  hepcidin, 280
Human genome, **130**, 399f
Human Genome Project, 400
Human immunodeficiency virus (HIV), 295, 655
  alternative therapies, 669
  antiretroviral drugs for treatment of, 668
  complications, 667
  consequences, 666–667
  control of anorexia and wasting, 668
  control of lipodystrophy, 668–669
  enteral and parenteral nutrition support, 670
  food safety concerns, 670
  GI complications, 667
  HIV/AIDS, 511, 665t
  infection, 665–673
  lipodystrophy, 667
  man with, 671
  metabolic complications, 670
  neurological complications, 667
  nutrition therapy for, 669–671

Wean, **309**
Weight
    maintenance, 188
    and measures, A-3–A-4
    reduction, 603
    weight-bearing physical activity, 247
Weight, body. *See* Body weight
Weight cycling, **166**
Weight gain
    energy-dense foods, 189
    extra snacks, 190
    insulin therapy and, 582
    juice and milk, 190
    large portions, 190
    meals daily, 190
    physical activity to build muscles,
        189
    pregnancy, 282t, 282–283, 283f
    during pregnancy, E-1
    strategies for, 189–190, 190t
Weight loss, 293, 666
    behavior and attitude, 186–188
    healthful eating plan, 182–185
    physical activity, 185–188
    after pregnancy, 283

scams, 197t
strategies, 182–189, 189t
weight maintenance, 188
Weight management, 79, 83, 173–190,
    669–670
    aggressive treatments of obesity,
        180–181
    causes of obesity, 174–179
    inappropriate obesity treatments,
        179–180
    obesity treatment, 179
    strategies for weight gain,
        189–190
    strategies for weight loss, 182–189
Wellness, 2
Wernicke-Korsakoff syndrome,
    216
What We Eat in America, 11
Wheat gluten, **526**
White sugar, **77**
Whole foods, **5**
Whole grains, **70**
WIC program, 320
Woman in first pregnancy, 294b

World Health Organization (WHO),
    205, 295–296, 300
    nutrition recommendations, B-1

X

Xerophthalmia, **205**
Xerosis, **205**
Xerostomia (dry mouth), **490**

Y

Yohimbe, 427
Young children, 288–289

Z

Zinc, 256–258, 258f, 280, 307,
    363
    deficiency, 257
    foods to providing, and 313
    recommendations and food sources,
        258
    toxicity, 258
Zygote, **274**
Zyloprim, 644

Daily Values for Food Labels

The Daily Values are standard values developed by the Food and Drug Administration (FDA) for use on food labels. The values are based on 2000 kcalories a day for adults and children over 4 years old.

Nutrient	Amount
Biotin	30 µg
Choline	550 mg
Folate	400 µg DFE
Niacin	16 mg NE
Pantothenic acid	5 mg
Riboflavin	1.3 mg
Thiamin	1.2 mg
Vitamin A	900 µg RAE
Vitamin B$_6$	1.7 mg
Vitamin B$_{12}$	2.4 µg
Vitamin C	90 mg
Vitamin D	20 µg
Vitamin E (α-tocopherol)	15 mg
Vitamin K	120 µg
Calcium	1300 mg
Chloride	2300 mg
Chromium	35 µg
Copper	0.9 mg
Iodine	150 µg
Iron	18 mg
Magnesium	420 mg
Manganese	2.3 mg
Molybdenum	45 µg
Phosphorus	1250 mg
Potassium	4700 mg
Selenium	55 µg
Sodium	2300 mg
Zinc	11 mg

Food Component	Amount	Calculation Factors
Fat	65 g	30% of kcalories
Saturated fat	20 g	10% of kcalories
Cholesterol	300 mg	Same regardless of kcalories
Carbohydrate (total)	300 g	60% of kcalories
Fiber	28 g	14 g per 1000 kcalories
Protein	50 g	10% of kcalories

GLOSSARY
OF NUTRIENT MEASURES

kcal: kcalories; a unit by which energy is measured (Chapter 1 provides more details).

g: grams; a unit of weight equivalent to about 0.03 ounces.

mg: milligrams; one-thousandth of a gram.

µg: micrograms; one-millionth of a gram.

IU: international units; an old measure of vitamin activity determined by biological methods (as opposed to new measures that are determined by direct chemical analyses). Many fortified foods and supplements use IU on their labels.

- For vitamin A, 1 IU = 0.3 µg retinol, 3.6 µg β-carotene, or 7.2 µg other vitamin A carotenoids.
- For vitamin D, 1 IU = 0.02 µg cholecalciferol.
- For vitamin E, 1 IU = 0.67 natural α-tocopherol (other conversion factors are used for different forms of vitamin E).

mg NE: milligrams niacin equivalents; a measure of niacin activity (Chapter 8 provides more details).

- 1 NE = 1 mg niacin
  = 60 mg tryptophan (an amino acid).

µg DFE: micrograms dietary folate equivalents; a measure of folate activity (Chapter 8 provides more details).

- 1 µg DFE = 1 µg food folate.
  = 0.6 µg fortified food or supplement folate.
  = 0.5 µg supplement folate taken on an empty stomach.

µg RAE: micrograms retinol activity equivalents; a measure of vitamin A activity (Chapter 8 provides more details).

- 1 µg RAE = 1 µg retinol.
  = 12 µg β-carotene.
  = 24 µg other vitamin A carotenoids.

mmol: millimoles; one-thousanth of a mole, the molecular weight of a substance. To convert mmol to mg, multiply by the atomic weight of the substance.

- For sodium, mmol × 23 = mg Na.
- For chloride, mmol × 35.5 = mg Cl.
- For sodium chloride, mmol × 58.5 = mg NaCl.

Body Mass Index (BMI)

Find your height along the left-hand column and look across the row until you find the number that is closest to your weight. The number at the top of that column identifies your BMI. Chapter 6 describes how BMI correlates with disease risks and defines obesity. The area shaded in blue represents healthy weight ranges.

Height	Under-weight (<18.5)	Healthy Weight (18.5–24.9)						Overweight (25–29.9)					Obese (≥30)										
	18	19	20	21	22	23	24	25	26	27	28	29	30	31	32	33	34	35	36	37	38	39	40
Body Weight (pounds)																							
4'10"	86	91	96	100	105	110	115	119	124	129	134	138	143	148	153	158	162	167	172	177	181	186	191
4'11"	89	94	99	104	109	114	119	124	128	133	138	143	148	153	158	163	168	173	178	183	188	193	198
5'0"	92	97	102	107	112	118	123	128	133	138	143	148	153	158	163	168	174	179	184	189	194	199	204
5'1"	95	100	106	111	116	122	127	132	137	143	148	153	158	164	169	174	180	185	190	195	201	206	211
5'2"	98	104	109	115	120	126	131	136	142	147	153	158	164	169	175	180	186	191	196	202	207	213	218
5'3"	102	107	113	118	124	130	135	141	146	152	158	163	169	175	180	186	191	197	203	208	214	220	225
5'4"	105	110	116	122	128	134	140	145	151	157	163	169	174	180	186	192	197	204	209	215	221	227	232
5'5"	108	114	120	126	132	138	144	150	156	162	168	174	180	186	192	198	204	210	216	222	228	234	240
5'6"	112	118	124	130	136	142	148	155	161	167	173	179	186	192	198	204	210	216	223	229	235	241	247
5'7"	115	121	127	134	140	146	153	159	166	172	178	185	191	198	204	211	217	223	230	236	242	249	255
5'8"	118	125	131	138	144	151	158	164	171	177	184	190	197	203	210	216	223	230	236	243	249	256	262
5'9"	122	128	135	142	149	155	162	169	176	182	189	196	203	209	216	223	230	236	243	250	257	263	270
5'10"	126	132	139	146	153	160	167	174	181	188	195	202	209	216	222	229	236	243	250	257	264	271	278
5'11"	129	136	143	150	157	165	172	179	186	193	200	208	215	222	229	236	243	250	257	265	272	279	286
6'0"	132	140	147	154	162	169	177	184	191	199	206	213	221	228	235	242	250	258	265	272	279	287	294
6'1"	136	144	151	159	166	174	182	189	197	204	212	219	227	235	242	250	257	265	272	280	288	295	302
6'2"	141	148	155	163	171	179	186	194	202	210	218	225	233	241	249	256	264	272	280	287	295	303	311
6'3"	144	152	160	168	176	184	192	200	208	216	224	232	240	248	256	264	272	279	287	295	303	311	319
6'4"	148	156	164	172	180	189	197	205	213	221	230	238	246	254	263	271	279	287	295	304	312	320	328
6'5"	151	160	168	176	185	193	202	210	218	227	235	244	252	261	269	277	286	294	303	311	319	328	336
6'6"	155	164	172	181	190	198	207	216	224	233	241	250	259	267	276	284	293	302	310	319	328	336	345